Rehabilitation for the Postsurgical Orthopedic Patient

Rehabilitation for the Postsurgical Orthopedic Patient

SECOND EDITION

Edited by

Lisa Maxey, PT
Private Practice
Calabasas, California

Jim Magnusson, PT, ATC
Co-Owner
Performance Therapy Center, Inc.
Oxnard and Camarillo, California
Team Physical Therapist
Oxnard College
Team Physical Therapist
Pacifica High School Football
Sports Medicine Consultant
The Tennis Channel

MOSBY

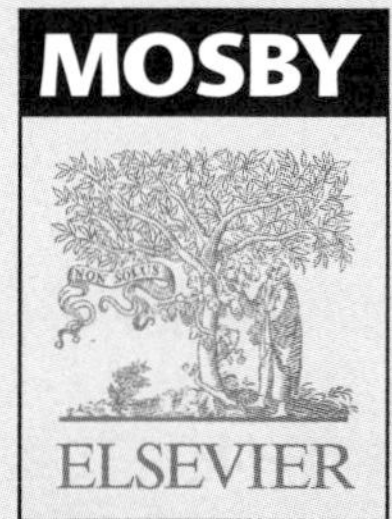

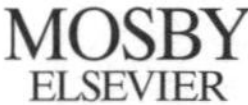

11830 Westline Industrial Drive
St. Louis, Missouri 63146

REHABILITATION FOR THE POSTSURGICAL ORTHOPEDIC PATIENT, ED 2 ISBN-13: 978-0-323-03474-6
ISBN-10: 0-323-03474-8

Notice

Neither the Publisher nor the Editors assume any responsibility for any loss or injury and/or damage to persons or property arising out of or related to any use of the material contained in this book. It is the responsibility of the treating practitioner, relying on independent expertise and knowledge of the patient, to determine the best treatment and method of application for the patient.

The Publisher

Previous edition copyrighted 2001

ISBN-13: 978-0-323-03474-6
ISBN-10: 0-323-03474-8

Publishing Director: Linda Duncan
Senior Editor: Kathy Falk
Senior Developmental Editor: Christie Hart
Publishing Services Manager: Julie Eddy
Project Manager: Andrea Campbell
Design Direction: Louis Forgione

Printed in the United States of America

Last digit is the print number: 9 8 7 6 5 4 3 2 1

Contributors

Mayra Saborio Amiran, PT
Physical Therapist
Thousand Oaks, California

James R. Andrews, MD
Clinical Professor of Surgery
UAB School of Medicine, Division of Orthopaedic Surgery
Birmingham, Alabama;
Clinical Professor of Orthopaedics & Sports Medicine
University of Virginia Medical School
Charlottesville, Virginia;
Clinical Professor
Department of Orthopaedic Surgery
University of Kentucky Medical Center
Lexington, Kentucky;
Senior Orthopaedic Consultant
Washington Redskins Professional Football Team
Washington, DC;
Medical Director
Tampa Bay Devil Rays Professional Baseball Team
Tampa Bay, Florida;
Co-Medical Director
Intercollegiate Sports at Auburn University
Auburn, Alabama;
Orthopaedic Surgeon
Alabama Sports Medicine & Orthopaedic Center
Birmingham, Alabama

Mark T. Bastan, DPT, CSCS
Coordinator of Clinical Research and Development
Elite Physical Therapy
Warwick, Rhode Island

Clive E. Brewster, MS, PT
Administrator
Department of Orthopedic/Sports Medicine
Kerlan-Jobe Orthopaedic Clinic
Los Angeles, California

Andrew A. Brooks, MD, FACS
Attending Orthopedic Surgeon
Southern California Orthopedic Institute
Van Nuys, California;
Attending Orthopedic Surgeon
Encino Hospital
Encino, California;
Attending Orthopedic Surgeon
Motion Picture and Television Hospital
Woodland Hills, California;
Attending Orthopedic Surgeon
Specialty Surgical Center
Encino, California and Beverly Hills, California

Nora P. Cacanindin, PT
Director/Owner
PROActive Therapy
San Francisco, California

James H. Calandruccio, MD
Assistant Professor
University of Tennessee–Campbell Clinic
Department of Orthopaedic Surgery
Campbell Clinic, Inc.
Germantown, Tennessee

Douglas N. Calhoun, MD
Orthopedic Surgeon
Hand Surgery
Knoxville Orthopedic Clinic
Knoxville, Tennessee

Robert I. Cantu, MMSc, PT, MTC
Sr. Group Director
Physiotherapy Associates
Atlanta, Georgia;
Assistant Professor
Department of Physical Therapy
University of St. Augustine for Health Sciences
St. Augustine, Florida;
Adjunct Instructor
Department of Occupational Therapy
University of Indianapolis
Indianapolis, Indiana

Christina M. Clark, OTR, CHT
Van Nuys, California

Deborah Mandis Cozen, RPT
Physical Therapist
Pasadena, California

Curtis A. Crimmins, MD
Board Certified Hand Surgeon
Hand Surgery, Ltd.
Milwaukee, Wisconsin

Rick B. Delamarter, MD
Director
The Spine Institute
St. John's Medical Center
Santa Monica, California

Robert Donatelli, PhD, PTOCS
National Director of Sports Specific
Rehabilitation and Performance Enhancement
Physiotherapy Associates
Las Vegas, Nevada

Daniel A. Farwell, PT, DPT
Adjunct Professor of Clinical Physical Therapy
Department of Biokinesiology and Physical Therapy
University of Southern California
Los Angeles, California;
Owner/Director
Private Practice
Body RX Physical Therapy
Glendale, California

Richard D. Ferkel, MD
Associate Clinical Professor
Department of Orthopedic Surgery
UCLA
Los Angeles, California;
Attending Surgeon & Sports Medicine Fellowship Director
Southern California Orthopedic Institute
Van Nuys, California

Freddie H. Fu, MD
David Silver Professor and Chairman
Department of Orthopaedic Surgery
University of Pittsburgh School of Medicine;
UPMC Hospitals
Department of Orthopaedic Surgery
Pittsburgh, Pennsylvania

Mark Ghilarducci, MD
Department of Orthopedic Surgery
St. Johns Regional Medical Center;
Department of Sports Medicine
Ventura Orthopedic Medical Group
Oxnard, California

Terry Gillette, PT
Gillette and Associates Physical Therapy
Woodland Hills, California

David Girard, PT/CHT
Pacific Coast Healthcare
Saugus, California

Eric Giza, MD
Central Maine Orthopedics Group
Auburn, Maine

Patricia A. Gray, MS, PT
Physical Therapist
San Francisco, California

Jane Gruber, PT, DPT, MS, OCS
Director of Rehabilitation Services
Newton Wellesley Hospital
Newton, Massachusetts

Carlos A. Guanche, MD
Attending Physician
Southern California Orthopedic Institute
Van Nuys, California

Will Hall, PT, DPT, OCS
Group Director
Physiotherapy Associates
Cumming, Georgia

Jason T. Huffman, MD
Comprehensive Spine Care
Sonoma, California

Wendy J. Hurd, PT
University of Delaware
Newark, Delaware

Frank W. Jobe, MD
Associate
Kerlan-Jobe Orthopaedic Clinic;
Clinical Professor
Department of Orthopaedics
University of Southern California–Keck School of Medicine
Los Angeles, California;
Medical Director
Biomechanics Laboratory
Centinela Freeman Hospital
Inglewood, California;
Orthopaedic Consultant
Los Angeles Dodgers
Los Angeles, California;
PGA Tour
Senior PGA Tour

Kelly Akin Kaye, PT, CHT
Staff Therapist
Department of Physical Therapy
Campbell Clinic Orthopedics
Germantown, Tennessee

Linda J. Klein, OTR, CHT
Lead Therapist
Hand Therapy Department
Hand Surgery, Ltd.
Milwaukee, Wisconsin

Kristen Griffith Lowrance, OTR/L, CHT
Clinic Manager
Therapy Services
Campbell Clinic
Germantown, Tennessee

Bert R. Mandelbaum, MD
Assistant Professor
Division of Orthopedic Surgery
Department of Surgery
University of California, Los Angeles
Los Angeles, California;
Chief Surgeon
Medical Plaza Orthopedic Surgery Center
Santa Monica, California;
Chief of Orthopedics
Department of Orthopedic Surgery
St. John's Hospital and Health Center
Santa Monica, California

Benjamin Maser, MD
Attending Plastic Surgeon
Plastic Surgery
Palo Alto Medical Foundation
Palo Alto, California

Joel M. Matta, MD
Associate Professor of Clinical Orthopaedics
University of Southern California School of Medicine
John C. Wilson Jr. Chair of Orthopaedic Surgery
Good Samaritan Hospital
Santa Monica, California

Erica V. Pablo, PT, DPT
Physical Therapist
Knight Physical Therapy
Garden Drive, California;
Physical Therapy Consultant
Chapman University Women's Basketball
Orange, California

David Pakozdi, PT, OCS
Director
Kinetic Orthopaedic Physical Therapy
Santa Monica, California

Mark R. Phillips, MD
Clinical Assistant Professor
Department of Orthopedic Surgery
University of Illinois College of Medicine at Peoria;
Department of Orthopedic Surgery
Methodist Medical Center;
Department of Orthopedic Surgery
Proctor Hospital
Peoria, Illinois

Haideh V. Plock, MSPT, OCS, ATC, FAAOMPT
Director
Emerald Bay Physical Therapy
Physical Rehabilitation Network
South Lake Tahoe, California

Luga Podesta, MD
Physiatrist
Kerlan-Jobe Orthopaedic Clinic
Los Angeles, California;
Physiatrist
Ventura Orthopedics
Thousand Oaks, California

Ben B. Pradhan, MD
Spine Surgeon
Director of Clinical Research
Los Angeles, California;
The Spine Institute
Santa Monica, California

Edward Pratt, MD
Memphis Spine Center
Germantown, Tennessee

Christine M. Prelaz, PT, MS, OCS, CSCS
Staff Physical Therapist
Sports Physical Therapy
University of Kentucky
Lexington, Kentucky

Brian E. Prell, MSPT, RRT
Clinical Director
Physiotherapy Associates
Athens, Georgia

Michael M. Reinold, PT, DPT, ATC, CSCS
Adjunct Faculty
Department of Physical Therapy
Northeastern University;
Assistant Athletic Trainer
Boston Red Sox Baseball Club
Boston, Massachusetts

Michael D. Ries, MD
Professor
Department of Orthopaedic Surgery
University of California, San Francisco;
Chief of Arthroplasty
Department of Orthopaedic Surgery
University of California, San Francisco
San Francisco, California

Diane R. Schwab, MS, RPT
Owner
Champion Rehabilitation
San Diego, California

Jessie Scott, PT, MBA
California Pacific Medical Center
San Francisco, California

Chris A. Sebelski, PT, DPT, OCS, CSCS
Assistant Professor of Clinical Physical Therapy
Department of Biokinesiology and Physical Therapy
University of Southern California
Los Angeles, California

Paul Slosar, MD
Spine Care Medical Group
Daly City, California

Jason A. Steffe, DPT, OCS, MTC
Group Director
Physiotherapy Associates
Atlanta, Georgia

Derrick G. Sueki, PT, DPT, GCPT
Adjunct Orthopedic Faculty
Department of Physical Therapy
Mount St. Mary's College;
Clinical Assistant Professor
Department of Biokinesiology and Physical Therapy
University of Southern California
Los Angeles, California;
Owner/Clinical Director
Knight Physical Therapy
Garden Grove, California;
Physical Therapy Consultant
Chapman University Women's Basketball
Orange, California;
Physical Therapist
Association of Volleyball Professionals

Steven R. Tippett, PT, PhD, SCS, ATC
Associate Professor and Associate Chair
Department of Physical Therapy and Health Science
Bradley University
Peoria, Illinois

Timothy F. Tyler, MS, PT, ATC
Clinical Research Associate
Nicholas Institute of Sports and Athletic Trauma
Lenox Hill Hospital
New York, New York;
Director
Pro Sports Physical Therapy Westchester
Scarsdale, New York

Kurt R. Weiss, MD
Resident Surgeon
Department of Orthopaedic Surgery
University of Pittsburgh Medical Center
Pittsburgh, Pennsylvania

Arthur White, MD
Founder
Spine Care Medical Group
Daly City, California

Kevin E. Wilk, PT, OPT
Adjunct Assistant Professor
Physical Therapy Department
Marquette University
Milwaukee, Wisconsin;
Clinical Director
Champion Sports Medicine;
Vice President of Education
Benchmark Medical Inc.
Birmingham, Alabama

Julie Wong, PT, CLT
Owner
ProActive Therapy
San Francisco, California

James E. Zachazewski, PT, DPT, ACT, SCS
Adjunct Clinical Assistant Professor
Department of Physical Therapy
Massachusetts General Hospital Institute of Health Professions;
Clinical Director
Massachusetts General Hospital Sports Medicine
Department of Physical Therapy
Massachusetts General Hospital
Boston, Massachusetts

Craig Zeman, MD
Department of Orthopedics
St. Johns Hospital
Oxnard, California

Boris A. Zelle, MD
Department of Orthopaedic Surgery
University of Pittsburgh School of Medicine
Pittsburgh, Pennsylvania

DEDICATION

In thanksgiving for all His blessings.
Lisa Maxey

To my two children, Nicholas and Michelle.
Jim Magnusson

Foreword

One of the editors of this book, Lisa Maxey, whom I have known for over ten years, has asked me to contribute a foreword to this revised edition of *Rehabilitation for the Postsurgical Orthopedic Patient*, to which I have contributed a chapter on Anterior Capsular Reconstruction. I have been a physical therapist for almost thirty years, specializing in orthopedics and sports medicine, and I have had the privilege to work with some of whom I consider to be the greatest orthopedic surgeons in the country, if not the world (at Kerlan-Jobe Orthopedic Clinic and elsewhere). In addition, I have had the honor to be mentored by some of the best therapists of my time. And, in my later years, I have found that I am working with some of the greatest upcoming talents in contemporary physical therapy. Needless to say, I believe most strongly that physical therapy has a bright future from what I have been able to witness from the work of student and "fledgling" physical therapists. I wholeheartedly believe that the whole field of physical therapy will continue to grow, and offer more and better solutions to the problems of rehabilitation of those who continue to present us with orthopedic and sports medicine-related injuries.

While working alongside some of the greatest surgeons in the world, I have had the opportunity to observe how they have introduced innovative surgical techniques, which have prolonged the careers of professional athletes, in addition to helping the general public (whom we may sometimes refer to as the "industrial athlete"). This has given many individuals a new lease on life as they work toward achieving complete recovery. As these surgeons developed innovative techniques, I too have been called upon to develop new rehabilitative protocols to support these surgical interventions.

This textbook gives you valuable insights into the important part physical therapy plays in the process of rehabilitation. Though I have written many protocols, I urge you to keep in mind that protocols should serve solely as reference points rather than step-by-step "recipes" to be slavishly followed. Remember that every patient is different, every patient has a different pain tolerance, every patient has a different tissue type and every patient has a different perception of what he/she expects to get out of the rehabilitation process. Something as simple as the questions you ask the patient and your interpretation of the answers can go a long way to giving you a sense of the patient's physical and mental state. The answer to the first or second question you may ask the patient regarding their injury may not be a true indicator as to how the patient is actually doing. We must be able to isolate the questions and thereby force the patient to reveal the true nature of their progress, as specifically related to their injury.

As physical therapists, we have the great opportunity to learn and evaluate patients' injuries from the outside, while the physician may have the opportunity to look at x-rays, MRIs, scans, and, eventually, to use a surgical procedure to determine what is wrong with the patient. We as physical therapists must depend on our evaluation skills. I cannot emphasize too strongly how important your evaluation skills should be. The better your evaluation skills, combined with your understanding of the options of a rehabilitation program, the more successful your patients' outcomes will be. Of course, there are many parts to an evaluation, with palpation and the understanding of body mechanics, and a thorough knowledge of anatomy, kinesiology, and physiology, all specific to the patient's skill level, which can be of great assistance to your final outcome. Now that the interaction between the physician and the physical therapist has become more dynamic, these evaluation skills are of the utmost importance.

What's more, it has to be kept in mind that physical therapy is a communication profession. You must learn to communicate at one level with your patients and at another level with the physicians. However, sometimes you may find that those levels may be harder to distinguish. Mind you, we are not saying that physicians do not understand the physical therapy process. What I am trying to say is that it is incumbent on physical therapists to keep the physician abreast of the patients' progress or lack thereof. We are also called upon to communicate with case managers, employers, and network providers. With the Internet and growing importance of the computer, the new generation of physical therapists must be extremely communication savvy.

All in all, a complete rehab no longer consists of merely getting the patient to the point of having good levels of strength, range of motion, flexibility, and endurance. Everything now is measured in terms of function. Therefore, regardless of whether he/she is an athlete, your success is grounded in how well patients can return as closely as possible to their pre-injury level of activity. In terms of sporting activity, it is important that we become familiar with the demands of the sport and the mechanics of the specific position that the athlete plays. In the everyday/industrial athlete, we have familiarized ourselves with the mechanics of standing, walking, lying, sitting, rising up, lifting, carrying, etc. Likewise, for the athlete's rehabilitation to be successful, we must have some understanding/knowledge of the mechanics specific to a range of sports.

In conclusion, I love being a physical therapist, and I continue to be fascinated by the entire process and how complicated, yet simple, it can be. I feel as though my own journey only began with my education, and I think you will find that learning is a lifelong process in your never-ending quest for astuteness in the physical therapy profession.

Clive E. Brewster, MS, PT

Preface

We initially set out on this project to help bring knowledge that was lacking to the medical field regarding postoperative rehabilitation for the orthopedic patient population. We knew it was a project that would only grow in the coming years as further evidence would necessitate revisions. Our purpose remains the same with this second edition and, with the addition of new chapters and updates of existing chapters, we are confident that this book provides the clinician with the most comprehensive evidence-based view of post-operative orthopedic rehabilitation.

We are very excited about the CD accompanying this book. It provides the clinician with a review of soft tissue and contains video on selected orthopedic surgeries as well as downloadable and adaptable Home Maintenance Program handouts.

This second edition begins with an overview regarding the principles of soft tissue healing and treatment presented by experts in their field. Clinicians must remember the biology of the healing process and the many factors that influence it. Some of the concepts touched on are controversial and experimental (e.g., gene therapy), but the material is presented to provide a glimpse of what potentials the future may have in store. It also encourages the clinician to visualize the healing process from the cellular level.

The practice of physical therapy continues to undergo transformations. Over the past 60 years it has evolved into a science that is continually being scrutinized by third-party payers challenging us to prove that what we do is effective and efficient. We are at a crucial point in our profession in which we need to justify how many treatments are necessary to manage a condition or ICD-9 code; at times this practice ignores the person we are treating. This book is *not* a "cookbook" for success but rather a compass from which the clinician can find guidance. This text is our effort to provide a resource that the clinician can reference as a guideline in the rehabilitation of the postsurgical patient.

We feel this is second edition continues to be an invaluable resource in that we have brought together more than 40 authors from around the country. Many of the authors are widely published and some are just plain good clinicians who are willing to share their experiential philosophy. We wanted the clinicians to be able to visualize the common surgical approaches to each case (through the physicians' portion) and then follow the therapist(s) guidelines to establish an efficient treatment plan. The prototype of this text had not been explored, to our knowledge, in this much depth (and with this many contributors). Especially with Appendix A—*Transitioning the Throwing Athlete Back to the Field*, and the additions of Appendix B—*Transitioning the Jumping Athlete Back to the Court* and Appendix C—*New Approaches in Total Hip Replacement: The Anterior Approach for Minimally Invasive Total Hip Arthroplasty.*

We expect that, with progression and enhancement of surgical techniques, rehabilitation will continue to evolve as well. Our hope is that this second edition of our book will continue to enhance our profession through the exchange of information, and that subsequent editions will continue to respond to the changing needs of the postoperative patient.

How to Use this Book

This second edition has evolved and expanded as has our knowledge base over the last 7 years. We have added 7 new chapters (*Pathogenesis of Soft Tissue and Bone Repair, SLAP Repair, Total Shoulder Replacement, Tendon Repair in the Hand, Cervical Spine Fusion, Transitioning the Jumping Athlete Back to the Court*, and *New Approach to Total Hip Arthroplasty*). We have also made the table guidelines and Home Maintenance Programs easier to follow. We believe that these additions to the book make it an invaluable tool for every clinician treating postoperative orthopedic patients.

The book gives the physical therapist a clear understanding of the surgical procedures required for various injuries so that a rehabilitation program can be fashioned appropriately. Each chapter presents the indications and considerations for surgery; a detailed look at the surgical procedure, including the surgeon's perspective regarding rehabilitation concerns; and therapy guidelines to use in designing the rehabilitation program. Areas that might prove troublesome are noted, with appropriate ways to address problems.

The indications and considerations for surgery and the surgery itself are described by an outstanding surgeon specializing in each area. All of the information presented should be valuable in understanding the mechanics of the injury and the repair process.

The therapy guidelines section is divided into three parts:

- Evaluation
- Phases of rehabilitation
- Suggested home maintenance

Every rehabilitation program begins with a thorough evaluation at the initial physical therapy visit. This provides pertinent information for formulating the treatment program. As the patient progresses through the program, assessment continues. Activities that are too stressful for healing tissues at one point are delayed and then reassessed when the tissue is ready for the stress. Treatment measures are outlined in tabular format for easy reference.

The phases each patient faces in rehabilitation are clearly indicated both as a way to break the program into manageable segments and to provide reassurance to the patient that rehabilitation will proceed in an orderly fashion. The time span covered by each phase and the goals of the rehabilitation process during that phase are noted. The exercises are carefully explained and photographs are provided for assistance.

Home maintenance for the postsurgical patient is an essential component of the rehabilitation program. Even when the therapist is able to follow the patient routinely in the clinic, the patient is still on his or her own for most of the day. The patient must understand the importance of compliance with the home program to maximize postoperative results. In the successful home maintenance program, the patient is the primary force in rehabilitation, with the therapist acting as an informed and effective communicator, an efficient coordinator, and a motivator. When the therapist successfully fulfills these obligations and the patient is motivated and compliant, the home maintenance program can be especially rewarding.

When the patient is not motivated or not compliant or possesses less-than-adequate pain tolerance, a no-nonsense and forthright dialogue with the surgeon, referring physician, rehabilitation nurse, or any other professional involved is essential. Timely, accurate, and straightforward documentation also is significant in the case of the "problem" patient. Emphasizing active patient involvement in an exercise program at home is even more imperative in light of the prescriptive nature of current managed care dictums.

The keys to an effective home maintenance program are structure, individuality, prioritization, and conciseness. The term *structure* refers to exercises that are well defined in terms of sets, repetitions, frequency, resistance, and technique. The patient must know what to do and how to do it. Home programs with photographs or video demonstrations are helpful in assisting the patient to visualize what is intended. Some computer-generated home exercise programs also offer adequate visual descriptions of the desired exercises. Stick figures and drawings that the physical therapist makes are often unclear and confusing to the patient.

Individuality, in the clearest sense, involves prescribing exercises that address the specific needs of a patient at a specific point in time. It includes being flexible enough to allow the patient to work the home program into the daily schedule as opposed to following only an "ideal" treatment schedule. Other components inherent in the concept of individuality include assistance available to the patient at home, financial implications, geographical concerns that influence follow-up, and the patient's cognitive abilities.

Prioritization and *conciseness* involve maximizing the use of the patient's time to perform the exercises at home. If the patient is being seen in the clinic, home exercises should stress activities not routinely performed in the clinic. If the patient is constrained for time, the therapist can identify the most beneficial exercises and prescribe them. It is best not to prescribe too many exercises to be done at home. Ideally, the patient should have to concentrate on no more than five or six at a time. To help keep the number of exercises manageable, the therapist should discontinue less taxing exercises as new exercises are added to the program.

Lisa Maxey
Jim Magnusson

Acknowledgments

I would like to give my sincere appreciation to all the contributors for their commitment to their work and for sharing their time and knowledge with us for the benefit of patients. Special thanks to Clive Brewster for his insights into book writing. Finally, thanks to my colleagues—I've been fortunate to have worked with good people.

> *"A smile must always be on our lips for any child to whom we offer help, for any to whom we give companionship or medicine. It would be very wrong to offer only our cures; we must offer to all our hearts."*
> —Mother Teresa of Calcutta

Lisa Maxey

I would like to acknowledge my wife, Tracy, who continues to amaze me with her patience and understanding. My parents, Nancy and Chuck, who gave me the foundations of respect, honesty, and love. My brothers, Bill and Bob, who remind me of the value of faith, being humble, challenging ourselves, and never giving up on your dreams, and my favorite—James 3:13.

My grandfather, Dr. James Logie, who helped me understand the dedication of those who aspire to become the best in their profession. I studied some of his own hand drawings of the human anatomy when he was in school and have seen how, through his dedication to serving his patients, his life has been blessed. He has taught me the importance of patience and showed me the art of fly fishing.

In the course of a lifetime, we meet people who have made impressions on us. Good or bad, they change us and shape our vision of who we want to become. In my experience (25 years) working in the field of physical therapy, I also have worked with individuals who, not only through clinical work but also through life experience, have taught me the value of compassion, dedication, empathy, and respect. Although a number of physical therapists have individually helped, the ones I've singled out also have positively influenced countless other therapists: Dee Lilly, Rick Katz, Gary Souza, and Charles Magistro.

I continue to thank God (and Dee) for helping me to find that special person in my wife, partner in life, and peer—Tracy Magnusson, PT.

Jim Magnusson

Contents

PART 1

INTRODUCTION

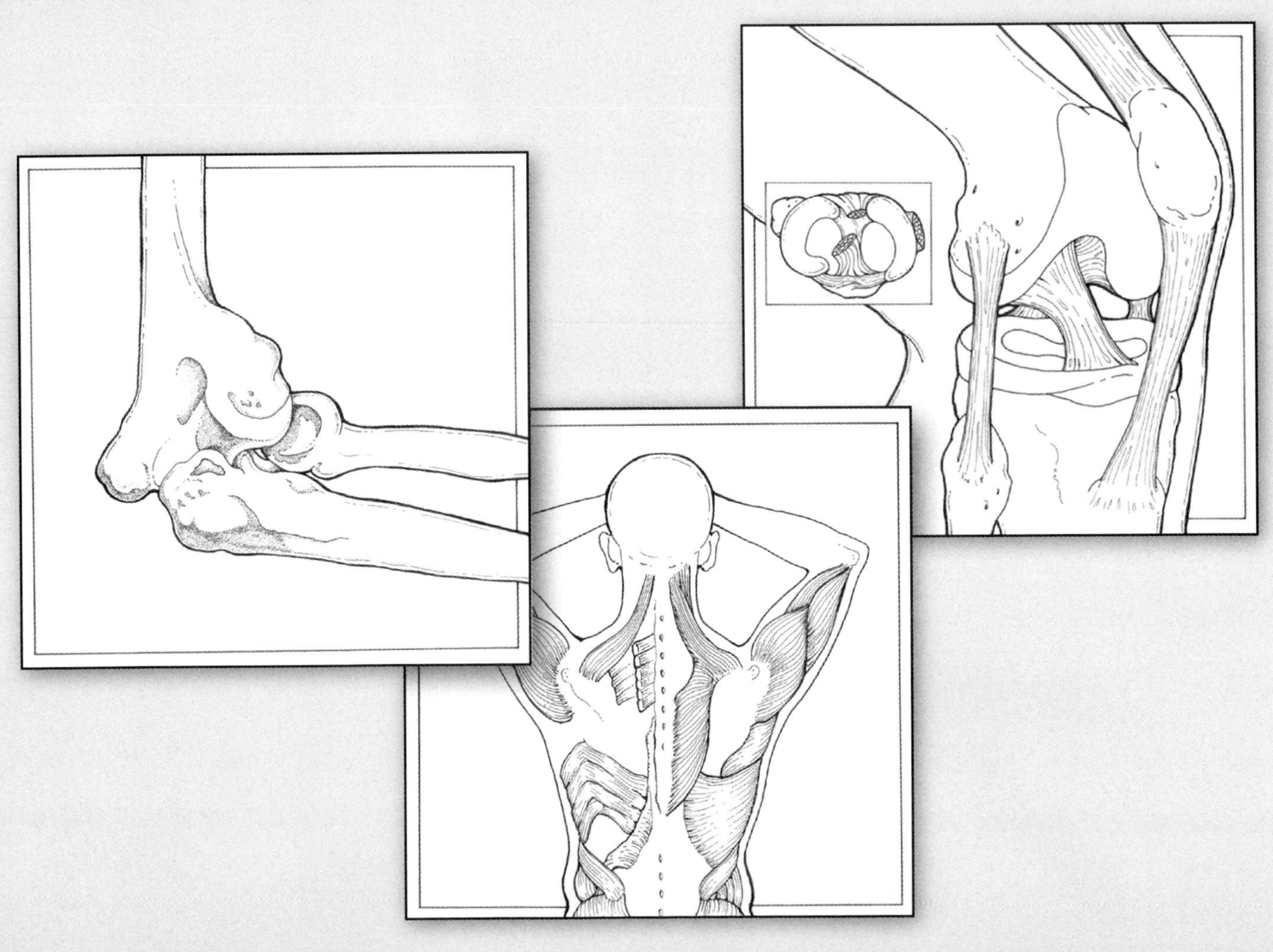

CHAPTER 1

Pathogenesis of Soft Tissue and Bone Repair

Boris A. Zelle
Kurt R. Weiss
Freddie H. Fu

INTRODUCTION

Musculoskeletal injuries usually result from supraphysiologic stresses that overwhelm the intrinsic stability of the musculoskeletal apparatus. The consequence is injury to the bone, tendon, muscle, ligaments, or a combination of these structures. The physiologic healing response varies among these tissues and is influenced by various intrinsic and extrinsic factors. Among these are the degree and anatomic location of the injury, the patient's preinjury condition, and the mode of treatment rendered. The aim of this chapter is to review the concept of soft tissue and bone healing and to describe the factors that can positively and negatively influence the healing response.

The healing process of soft tissue is dependent on forces that acted on it in creating the wound or trauma. As an introduction, the authors will focus on the incision (epithelial tissue) and progress into the other more complex soft tissue healing timeframes. Two factors to consider regarding the rate of healing of soft tissue deal with the forces causing the injury (i.e., high energy and velocity) and the magnitude of the injury (i.e., type of tissue involved, direction of force in relation to the tissue stress alignment).

For the purposes of discussing epithelial tissue, the incision is considered to be the "controlled trauma."

Incision and wound healing begins immediately after surgery and progresses through four distinct phases: (1) coagulation phase (Fig. 1-1), (2) inflammatory phase, (3) granulation phase (Fig. 1-2), and (4) scar formation and maturation phase. Table 1-1 gives an approximate time frame for each of these phases with hallmarks of what each phase accomplishes.

Wound healing requires a clean environment, good circulation, good approximation of wound edges, and a balance of the cellular mechanisms that ensure a proper immune response in the wound environment (chemotaxis). With a proper environment, scarring will be minimal. However, it must be kept in mind that there will be scar formation and that many internal factors (e.g., age, metabolic and circulatory disorders, physiology of the environment, mechanism of the injury) and external factors (e.g., nutrition, hydration, smoking, wound exposure and cleaning) will influence the amount of scarring that occurs.

LIGAMENT INJURIES AND HEALING

Ligament Anatomy and Function

Ligaments are anatomic structures of dense, fibrous connective tissue. They can be divided into two major subgroups: (1) those connecting the elements of the bony skeleton (skeletal subgroup) and (2) those connecting other organs, such as suspensory ligaments in the abdomen (visceral subgroup). The several hundred skeletal ligaments in the human body are the focus of this chapter. The nomenclature of the ligaments usually goes by their anatomic location and their bony attachments (i.e., medial collateral, posterior talofibular), as well as their shape and function (i.e., triangular, cruciate, deltoid ligament).

The macroscopic and microscopic structures of ligaments are similar to tendons. They contain rows of fibroblasts within parallel bundles of collagen fibers. Approximately two thirds of the wet weight of ligament is water, whereas collagen fibers account for approximately 70% of the dry weight. More than 90% of the collagen in ligaments is type I collagen. Trace amounts of other collagens exist, such as type III, V, X, XII, and XIV.[32] The primary structure of the type I collagen consists of a polypeptide chain with high concentrations of glycine, proline, and hydroxyproline. Almost two thirds of the primary structure of type I collagen consists of these three amino acids. Intermolecular forces cause three polypeptide chains to combine into a triple helical collagen molecule.

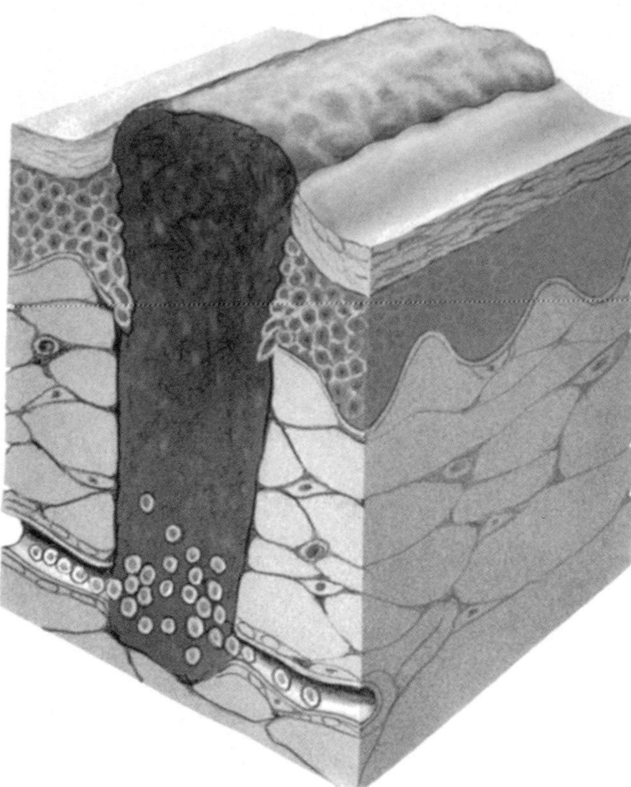

Fig. 1-1 Coagulation phase of wound healing; wound gap is filled with blood clot.
(From Browner BD et al: *Skeletal trauma—basic science, management, and reconstruction*, ed 3, Philadelphia, 2003, Elsevier, p 76.)

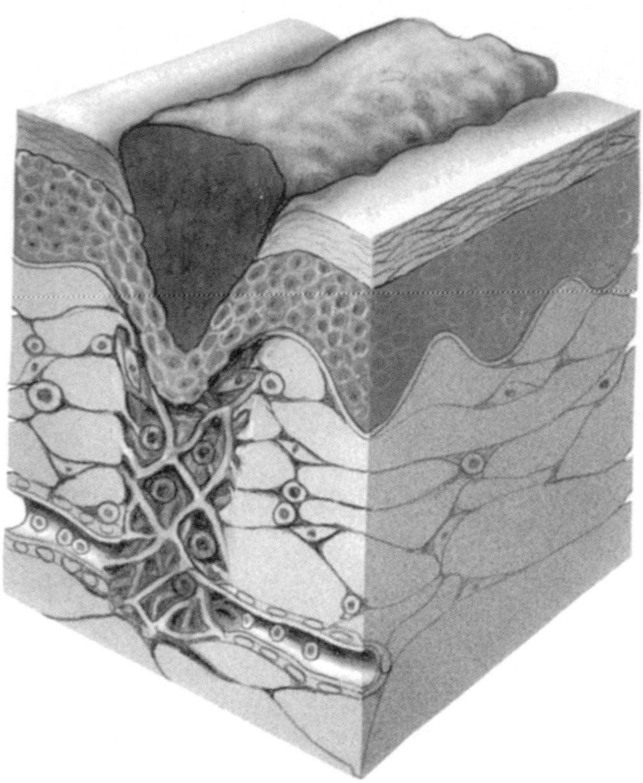

Fig. 1-2 Granulation Phase of wound healing, fibroplasias, angiogenesis, epithelialization, and wound contraction.
(From Browner BD et al: *Skeletal trauma—basic science, management, and reconstruction*, ed 3, Philadelphia, 2003, Elsevier, p 78.)

Table 1-1 Epithelial Tissue Healing

Coagulation Phase (see Fig. 1-1)	Vasoconstriction, platelet aggregation, clot formation	Begins immediately and lasts minutes
Inflammatory Phase	Vasodilation, polymorphonuclear (PMN) leukocytes, phagocytes	At the edges of wounds, epidermis immediately begins thickening; within the first 48 hours entire wound is epithelialized; lasts hours
Granulation Phase	Fibroplasia, epithelialization, wound contraction	Fibroblasts appear by day 2-3 and are dominant cell by day 10
Scar Formation/ Maturation Phase (see Fig.1-2)	Collagen synthesis; rarely regain full elasticity and strength	Lasts weeks to months and even up to 1 year

(Adapted from Browner BD et al: *Skeletal trauma—basic science, management, and reconstruction*, ed 3, Philadelphia, 2003, Elsevier.)

This configuration imparts great tensile strength properties, much like a braided rope (Fig. 1-3). Within the ligament, the collagen fibrils are usually organized in a longitudinal pattern and are held in place by the extracellular matrix (see Fig. 1-1).[13] Collagen fibers in the extracellular matrix are surrounded by water-soluble molecules such as proteoglycans, glycosaminoglycans, and structural glycoproteins. Although these molecules represent only approximately 1% of the dry weight of ligaments, they are important for proper ligament formation and organization of the ligament meshwork. Their hydrophilic properties are crucial for the viscoelastic capacity of ligament tissue and ensure adequate tissue lubrication and proper gliding of the fibers. Moreover, it has been shown that proteoglycans couple adjacent collagen fibrils together and thus help to guarantee the overall mechanical integrity of the ligaments.[45]

Ligament Injury

Clinically, ligamentous injuries are classified into three grades.[39] Grade I injuries include mild sprains. The

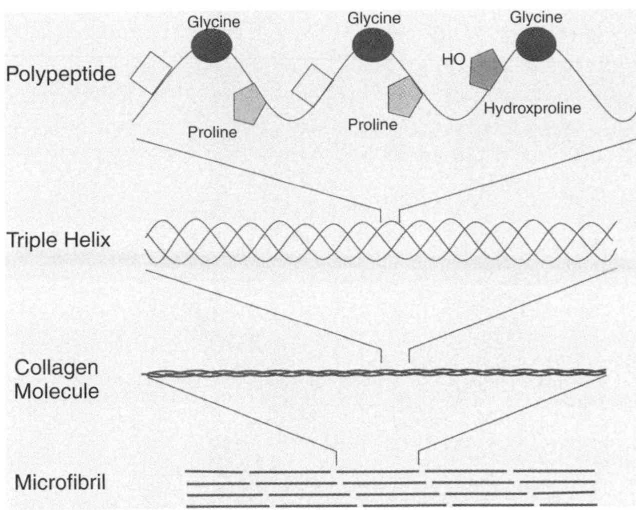

Fig. 1-3 Schematic drawing of the collagen structure. A linear polypeptide with a high perecentage of proline, glycine, and hydroxyproline is folded into an α-helix. Three polypeptide chains form a triple helix. The collagen molecules are packed to form the microfibrils.
(Adapted from Gamble JC, Edward C, Max S: Enzymatic adaptation of ligaments during immobilization, *Am J Sports Med* 12:221-228, 1984.)

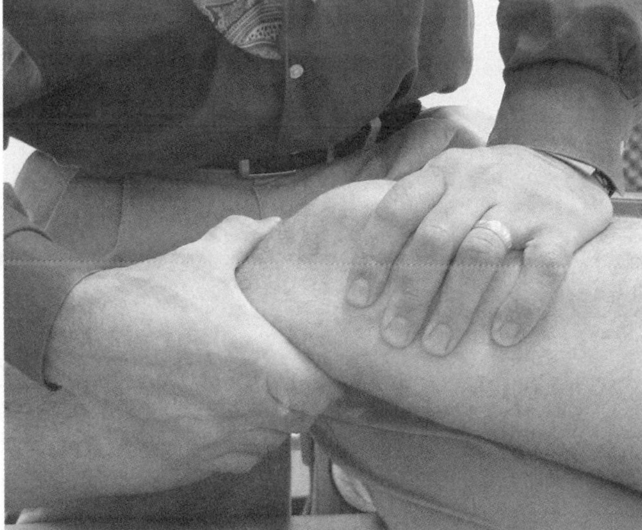

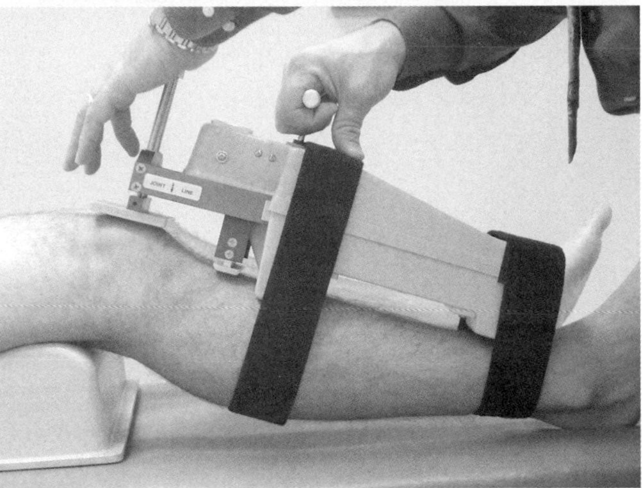

Fig. 1-4 Clinical examination of the anteroposterior knee stability using the Lachman test (**A**) and the KT-1000 (**B**).

ligament midsubstance is intact although edema, swelling, and punctate ligament bleeding may be present. In grade II injuries individual fibrils are torn, whereas the overall continuity of the ligament is maintained. Significant edema and bleeding is usually noted, and ligament stability is reduced. Grade III injuries are characterized by complete disruption of the ligament substance. Most ligamentous injuries can be diagnosed clinically by joint stability tests. Common examples include the clinical tests for diagnosing anterior cruciate ligament (ACL) injuries including the pivot-shift test, Lachman test, anterior drawer sign, and the KT-1000 (MedMetric Inc., San Diego, CA) (Fig. 1-4, *A* and *B*). Magnetic resonance imaging (MRI) represents the most commonly performed imaging study for diagnosing ligamentous injuries (Fig. 1-5, A and B).

The medial collateral ligament of the knee (MCL) has been studied most extensively after injury, and it has provided most of our knowledge on the healing process of ligaments. The healing phases of ligaments are traditionally divided by their morphologic appearance into an inflammatory phase (first days postinjury), a proliferative phase (1 to 6 weeks postinjury), and a remodeling phase (beginning at 7 weeks postinjury) (Table 1-2).[25] It is important to appreciate that these three phases represent a continuum of the healing process rather than discrete temporal divisions. The predominant cell types in the inflammatory phase are inflammatory cells and erythrocytes. As the ligament ruptures, its torn ends retract and have a ragged, mop end appearance. The gap between these torn ends is filled with hematoma from ruptured capillaries. Histologically, the inflammatory reaction is characterized by increased vasodilation, capillary permeability, and migration of leucocytes. During the inflammatory phase, increases in water and glycosaminoglycan contents of the injured tissue have been described. During the proliferative phase, a highly cellular scar develops, with fibroblasts as the dominating cell type. New collagen fibrils can be identified as early as 4 days after the injury. After approximately 2 weeks, the newly formed collagen fibrils bridge the gap between the torn ligament ends. However, the water content of the scar remains elevated, the collagen density remains low, and the collagen fibrils still appear less organized than in normal ligament tissue. During the remodeling phase, cellularity and vascularity decrease while collagen density increases. Moreover, the collagen arrangement becomes more organized along the axis of the ligament.

Long-term investigations in MCL healing studies in rabbits demonstrated the remodeling phase is a long ongoing process.[11] At 10 months after ligament midsubstance injuries, the scar could be identified macroscopically and

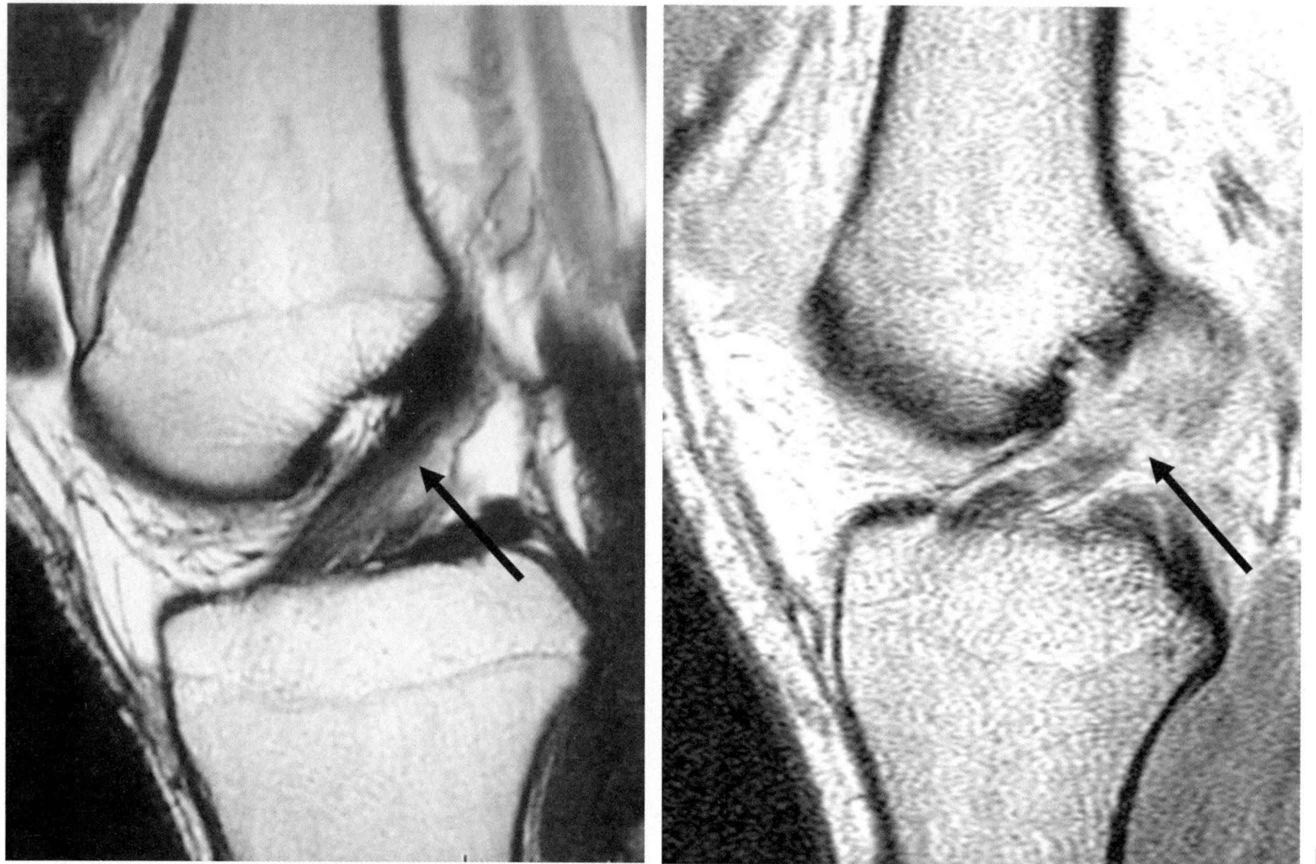

Fig. 1-5 Magnetic resonance imaging (MRI) evaluation of the knee joint. **A**, An intact anterior cruciate ligament (ACL) (*arrow*) in the sagittal cuts. **B**, The ACL fibers are torn (*arrow*).

Table 1-2 Ligament Healing

Inflammatory Phase	Vasodilation, fibrin clot formation, increased capillary permeability, and migration of leucocytes	Begins immediately and lasts minutes to hours
Proliferative Phase	Fibroblasts the dominate cell type, collagen fibrils (as early as 4 days postinjury)	1-6 weeks postinjury
Remodeling Phase	Collagen synthesis and increased density; rarely regain full elasticity and strength	7 weeks up to 1 year

a significantly increased cross-sectional area of the scar was noticed at 10 months postinjury. This scar tissue demonstrated an increased cellularity and highly organized scar tissue was not achieved, even at 10 months postinjury. Although the water content returned to normal values, the glycosaminoglycan content of the scar tissue remained elevated at 10 months. In contrast, the collagen concentration of the scar remained decreased at 10 months postinjury. Although a gradual increase was noted after 3 weeks, the collagen content plateaued at 70% of uninjured ligament tissues. In addition, the collagen types in the ligament scar varied from the normal tissues, with type III collagen being increased in the scar tissue.[11] This increase in type III collagen imparts biomechanical inferiority to the healed tendon, which seldom achieved preinjury strength.

The MCL is an extra-articular ligament with the potential to heal spontaneously. In some other ligamentous injuries, such as ACL injuries, spontaneous healing does usually not occur; various explanations have been suggested for this phenomenon. It must be assumed that the high stress carried by the ACL prevents the ruptured ligament ends from having sufficient contact. In addition, the ACL is not embedded in a strong soft tissue envelope. Moreover, the ACL is an intra-articular structure; when it ruptures, the blood is diluted by the synovial fluid, preventing hematoma formation and hence initiation of the healing mechanism. Finally, it has been suggested that the synovial fluid is a hostile environment for soft tissue healing. Thus in ACL-deficient knees, the levels of pro-inflammatory cytokines are elevated, leading to a potentially unfavorable intra-articular microenvironment.[4]

Effect of Mobilization and Immobilization on Ligament Healing

An important aspect for the rehabilitation of patients with ligament injuries represents the timing of postinjury mobilization. Although aggressive mobilization obviously results in disruption of the scar tissue, prolonged immobilization may decrease the morphologic and biomechanical properties of the newly formed scar. Thus the following question arises: What degree of immobilization is appropriate for healing ligaments?

The role of mobilization versus immobilization on ligament healing has been investigated in numerous animal studies.[18,44,54] In an MCL healing study in rats, Vailas et al[54] compared the healing properties of the transected MCL across the following four groups: (1) surgical repair with 2 weeks of immobilization and 6 weeks of normal cage activity, (2) surgical repair with 2 weeks of immobilization and 6 weeks of treadmill exercise, (3) surgical repair with 8 weeks of immobilization, and (4) no surgical repair and no exercise. All animals were sacrificed at 8 weeks. These authors reported that the wet ligament weight, dry ligament weight, total collagen content of the ligament, and the ultimate load at failure of the ligament substance was lowest in the completely immobilized group (3) and highest in the exercised group (2).[54] In an MCL transection model in the rabbit, Gomez et al[18] investigated the effect of continuous tension, as achieved by the implantation of a steel pin applying continuous stress on the healing MCL. At 12 weeks after MCL transection, the additional implantation of a tension pin resulted in a significantly decreased varus and valgus laxity, decreased cellularity of the scar tissue, and a more longitudinal alignment of the collagen fibers. Thus these authors concluded that the application of controlled stress helped to augment the biochemical, morphological, and biomechanical properties of the healing MCL.[18] In a more recent study, Provenzano et al[44] investigated the effect of hind limb immobilization on the healing response of transected MCLs in a rat model. These authors reported significantly superior biomechanical ligament properties in the mobilized group. Microscopic analysis revealed abnormal scar formation and cell distribution in the immobilized group, as suggested by disoriented fiber bundles and discontinuities in the extracellular ligament matrix. Therefore these authors independently suggested that stress deprivation in healing ligaments results in malalignment of the collagen fibrils and subsequently in unfavorable tensile ligament properties.[44]

These experimental data clearly emphasize the importance of stress and motion for the functional recovery of healing ligaments. However, the ideal amount of mobilization and immobilization during ligament healing is difficult to determine by animal studies, because animal studies are limited by the differing physiology and joint kinematics of animals. In addition, the amount of mobilization is difficult to control, and an exact titration of the stress cannot be performed with current in vivo models. Therefore future clinical trials are necessary to determine the optimal amount of applied stress for the various ligament injuries.

TENDON INJURIES AND HEALING

Tendon Anatomy and Function

Tendons are bands of dense, fibrous connective tissue interposed between muscles and bones. They transmit the forces created in the muscles to the bone, making joint motion possible. Some tendons may also connect two muscle bellies (e.g., digastrics, omohyoid). The gross tendon structure varies considerably from tendon to tendon, ranging from cylindrical rounded cords to flattened bands, called *aponeuroses*. The cross-sectional area of the more rounded tendons usually correlates with the isometric strength of the muscle from which they arise.[6] The bony insertion site of the tendon is often accompanied by a small synovial bursa (e.g., subacromial bursa, pes anserinus, retrocalcaneal bursa). The tendon bursae are usually located in those anatomic sites where a bony prominence might otherwise compress and wear the gliding tendon.

Microscopically, tendon and ligament are similar. The tendon tissue is a complex composite consisting of parallel collagen fibrils embedded in a matrix; cells are relatively rare, and fibroblasts represent the predominant cell type within the tendon; the fibroblasts are arranged in parallel rows between the collagen fibrils (Fig. 1-6, A and B). The biochemical composition of ligaments and tendons are similar. Water is the major constituent of the wet tendon weight, whereas type I collagen accounts for approximately 70% to 80% and elastin for approximately 1% to 2% of the dry tendon substance. As in ligaments, other collagen types exist only in small amounts. The proteoglycans and glycosaminoglycans in the extracellular matrix play an important role for the viscoelastic properties and the tensile strength of the tendon. Their hydrophilic capacity provides the tendon with lubrication and facilitates gliding of the fibrils during tensile stress.

According to their envelope, tendons can be divided into tendons within a synovial sheath (i.e., sheathed tendons) and paratenon-covered tendons. In particular, tendons in the hand and foot are often enclosed in a synovial tendon sheath. The tendon sheath directs the path of the tendon and produces a synovial fluid, which allows tendon gliding and contributes to the tendon nutrition. True tendon sheaths are only found in areas with an increased friction or sharp bending of the tendons (i.e., flexor tendons of the hand). A simple membranous thickening of the surrounding soft tissue called the *paratenon* usually surrounds tendons without a true synovial

A

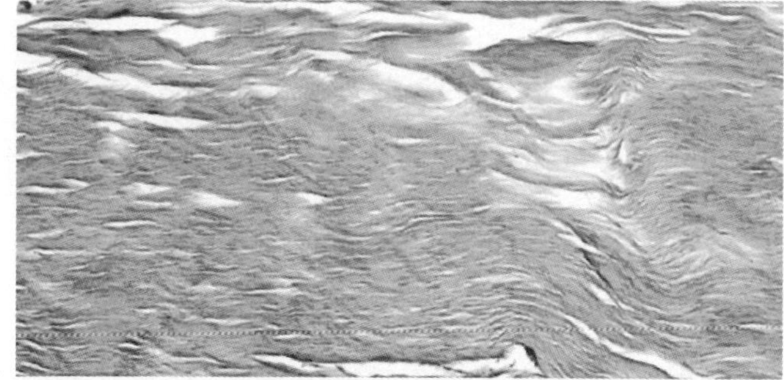

B

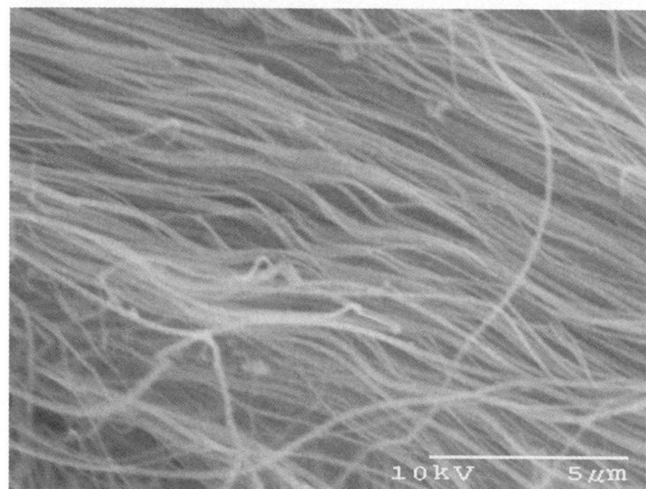

Fig. 1-6 Microscopic longitudinal sections of the patellar tendon. **A**, The hematoxylin-and-eosin (H&E) staining demonstrates the parallel arrangement of the collagen fibers and the fibroblasts under the light microscope. **B**, Electron microscopy demonstrates the wavy pattern of the fibers (i.e., "crimp").
(From Fu FH, Zelle BA: Ligaments and tendons: basic science and implications for rehabilitation. Mary Ann Wilmarth, editor: *Clinical applications for orthopaedic basic science: independent study course,* La Crosse, WI, 2004, American Physical Therapy Association, Inc, pp 1-25.)

tendon sheath, such as the Achilles tendon. The paratenon is composed of loose fibrillar tissue. It also functions as an elastic sleeve and permits free movement of the tendon against the surrounding tissue, although not as efficient as a true tendon sheath.

Like ligaments, tendons have a poor blood supply. The vascular supply of tendons was identified by injection studies, which demonstrated that the blood vessels form a network within and around the tendon.[28] Arteries supplying the tendon might come from the attached muscle, the bony insertion site, and the paratenon and tendon sheath along the length of the tendon. However, there seems to be a difference between the nutrition of the sheathed tendons and the paratenon-covered tendons. The paratenon-covered tendons receive the majority of their blood supply from vessels in the paratenon. In sheathed tendons, the synovial sheath minimizes the vascular supply to the tendon substance, and avascular regions have been identified within the midsubstance of these tendons.[19,28,33,57] Hence the diffusion of nutrients through the synovial fluid of sheathed tendons is critical for their homeostasis. Indeed, in sheathed tendons this process may be even more important than vascular perfusion. For example, the digital flexor tendons receive up to 90% of their nutrition by diffusion.[36,37] For this reason, sheathed tendons have also been referred to as *avascular tendons*, whereas the paratenon-covered tendons have been referred to as *vascular tendons*.

Tendon Injury

Tendon injuries may occur as a result of direct or indirect trauma (Fig. 1-7, A and B). Direct trauma includes contusions and lacerations, such as lacerations of the flexor tendons of the hand. Indirect tendon injuries are usually a consequence of tensile overload. Because most tendons can withstand higher tensile forces than their associated muscles or osseous insertion sites, avulsion fractures and ruptures at the myotendinous junctions are more likely than midsubstance ruptures. Midsubstance ruptures of the tendon after indirect trauma are usually associated with pre-existing tendon degeneration. This has been supported by histologic investigations of ruptured Achilles tendons, which demonstrated increased tenocyte necrosis, loss of fiber structure, increased vascularity, decreased collagen content, and increased glycosaminoglycan content in the substance of previously-ruptured tendons.[5,34,52]

Tendon Healing

The repair process in paratenon-covered tendons is also initiated by the influx of extrinsic inflammatory cells. As in ligaments, the healing of the ruptured tendon proceeds through an inflammatory phase, a proliferative phase, and a remodeling phase.[17,35,38,48] During the inflammatory phase the healing is initiated by formation of a blood clot bridging the gap between the ruptured ends. During the first few days after the injury, the proliferative phase begins; disorganized fibroblasts are the dominating cell types, and collagen synthesis can be detected. During the remodeling phase the collagen fibers orient themselves along the axis of the tendon. The remodeling phase continues for many months. It is characterized by increased organization of the collagen fibers, an increase in the number of intermolecular bonds between the collagen fibers, subsequent reduction of the scar tissue, and increase of tensile strength (Table 1-3).

Although it seems well accepted that the healing response in paratenon-covered tendons is initiated by immigration of extrinsic inflammatory cells, the initiation of the healing response of sheathed tendons remains controversial. Both an intrinsic mechanism and an extrinsic mechanism have been proposed. The extrinsic concept suggests that, similar to paratenon-covered tendons, the healing of sheathed tendons occurs by

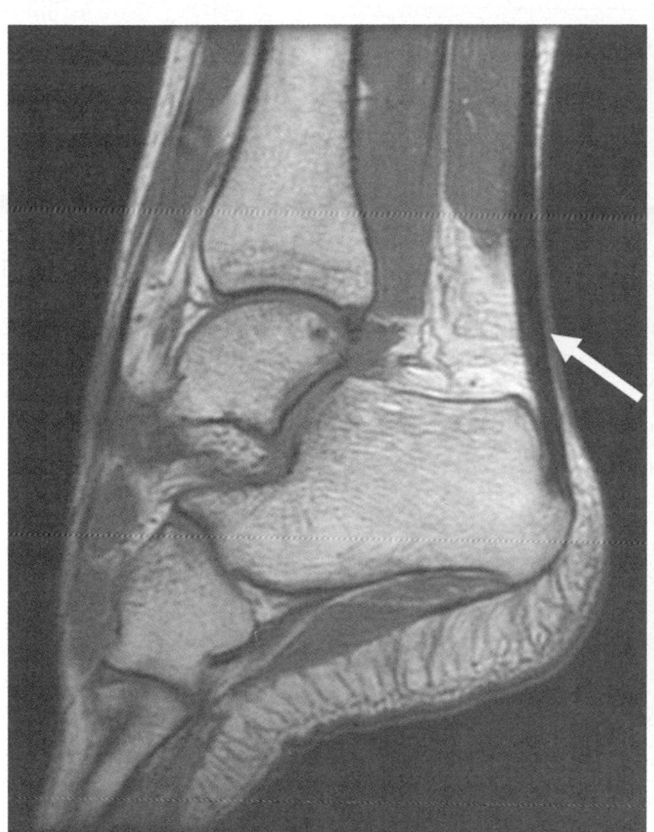

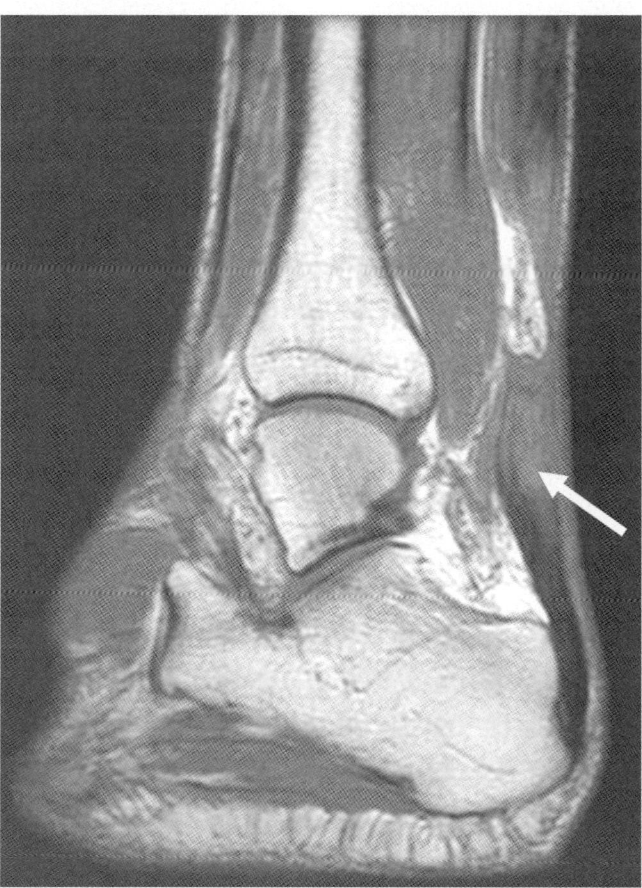

Fig. 1-7 Magnetic resonance imaging (MRI) evaluation of the Achilles tendon. The T1-weighted sagittal cuts show normal continuity of the Achilles tendon (**A**) (*arrow*) and a ruptured Achilles tendon (**B**) (*arrow*).

Table 1-3 Tendon Healing

Inflammatory Phase	Vasodilation, hematoma formation to bridge the defect (or gap), increased capillary permeability, and migration of leucocytes; influx of extrinsic/intrinsic inflammatory cells	Begins immediately and lasts minutes to hours
Proliferative Phase	Fibroblasts the dominate cell type, collagen synthesis	1-6 weeks postinjury
Remodeling Phase	Collagen synthesis and increased density	Can last for several months

granulation from the tendon sheath and the surrounding tissue, although the tenocytes themselves play no important role in this repair. According to the intrinsic theory, cells from within the tendon proliferate at the wound site, leading to collagen and extracellular matrix production.[35,38] With regard to the initiation of the healing response, it appears probable that both intrinsic and extrinsic healing exist.

Effect of Mobilization and Immobilization on Tendon Healing

The ideal mobilization regimen for the various tendon injuries is beyond the scope of this discussion. Clearly, overaggressive early mobilization may result in rerupture of the tendon.

However, sufficient scientific evidence shows that motion and stress increase collagen production, accelerate remodeling, and improve the biomechanical properties of healing tendons.[10,29,40] However, the optimal level of stress and motion of the healing tendon must be established based on clinical evidence.

SKELETAL MUSCLE INJURIES AND HEALING

Anatomy and Function of Skeletal Muscle

Skeletal muscle represents the largest tissue mass in the body and accounts for up to 45% of the total body weight.[15] Skeletal muscle originates from bone and inserts into bone via tendon. The primary function of skeletal muscle is to provide mobility to the bony skeleton. This is accomplished by muscle contraction (i.e., shortening) and force transmission through the muscle-tendon-bone complex.

The basic structural element of the skeletal muscle is the muscle fiber (diameter 10 to 100 μm, length up to 10 cm). The muscle fiber is a syncytium of many cells fused together with multiple nuclei. The muscle fibers consist of contractile elements, the myofibrils (diameter 0.5 to 1 μm), which give skeletal muscle tissue a striated appearance by light microscopy. The myofibrils consist of myofilaments (actin and myosin filaments).

Individual muscle fibers are organized into muscle by surrounding connective tissues (i.e., endomysium, perimysium, epimysium) that provide integrated motion among the muscle fibers. The endomysium surrounds the individual muscle fibers. Groups of muscle fibers are arranged together to fascicles surrounded by the perimysium. The fascicles are grouped together by the epimysium to form the whole muscle belly.

Skeletal muscle contraction is accomplished by sliding of its filaments.[22,23] The basic contractile unit is the sarcomere. The active contractile units within the sarcomere are the actin and the myosin filaments. These myofilaments are arranged in a parallel fashion in which the larger myosin filaments interdigitate between the small actin filaments. The actin filaments actively slide along the surface of the myosin filaments through cross-bridges originating from the myosin. The coordinated sliding of actin and myosin filaments throughout the muscle translates into contraction of the entire unit, which generates force and motion.

Muscle Injuries and Healing

Skeletal muscle injuries constitute the majority of sports-related injuries.[7,14] Skeletal muscle injuries can be classified as indirect and direct injuries. Indirect injuries result from an overload that overwhelms the muscle's ability to respond normally, such as muscle strains and delayed-onset muscle soreness. Direct injuries are usually a result of external forces, such as muscle contusions and muscle lacerations. Most injuries are diagnosed clinically. MRI has been found to be highly sensitive to muscle edema and hemorrhage and is the primary imaging modality for determining the type of injury and the degree of muscle involvement (Fig. 1-8).[49,51] Muscle injuries have a limited healing capacity, and the repair process in larger insults usually results in the formation of scar tissue.[30] Severe muscle injuries may result in the inability to train or compete for several weeks, and they have a high tendency to recur.[43,55]

Similar to ligaments and tendons, injured skeletal muscle undergoes phases of disruption and degeneration, inflammation, proliferation, and fibrosis (Table 1-4). After the trauma to the muscle, the disrupted muscle ends retract and the gap is filled by a local hematoma. Disruption of the muscle fibers leads to increased extracellular calcium levels, activation of the complement cascade, and myofiber necrosis. Inflammation is an early response to muscle tissue injury. Neutrophils rapidly invade the injury site and release inflammatory cytokines followed by an increase in macrophages that phagocytose cell debris. Certain subpopulations of macrophages also play a role in muscle regeneration.[53] Structural damage of the muscle fibers usually heals with formation of scar tissue (Fig. 1-9, A-D).[49]

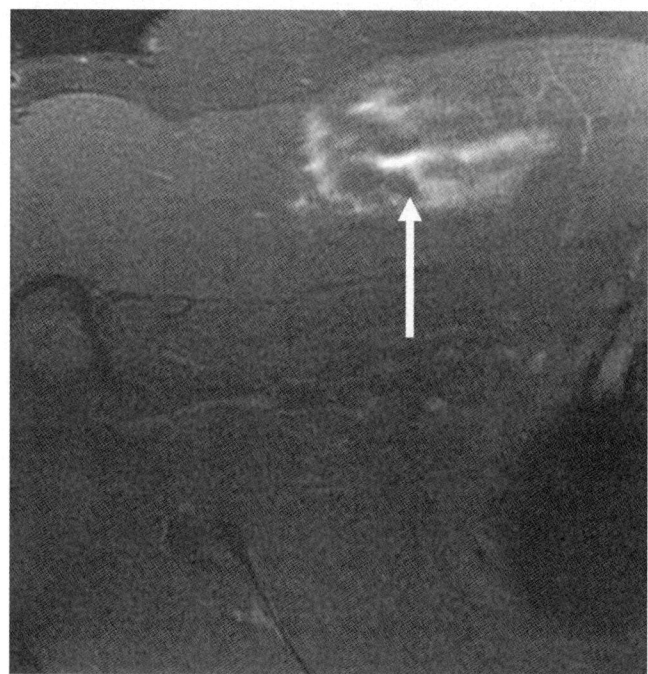

Fig. 1-8 Magnetic resonance imaging (MRI) evaluation of a partial tear of the pectoralis muscle. The T2-weighted axial cuts depict the edema formation (*arrow*) within the pectoralis muscle.

Table 1-4 Muscle Healing (Involving Disruption of Muscle Cell Structure)

Phase	Events	Timing
Inflammatory Phase (Disruption and degeneration)	Vasodilation, hematoma formation, increased capillary permeability, increased extracellular calcium, and migration of leucocytes	Begins immediately and lasts minutes to hours
Proliferative Phase	Neutrophil and macrophage migration	1-6 weeks postinjury
Remodeling/Fibrosis Phase	Collagen synthesis and increased density; scar formation	Can last for several months

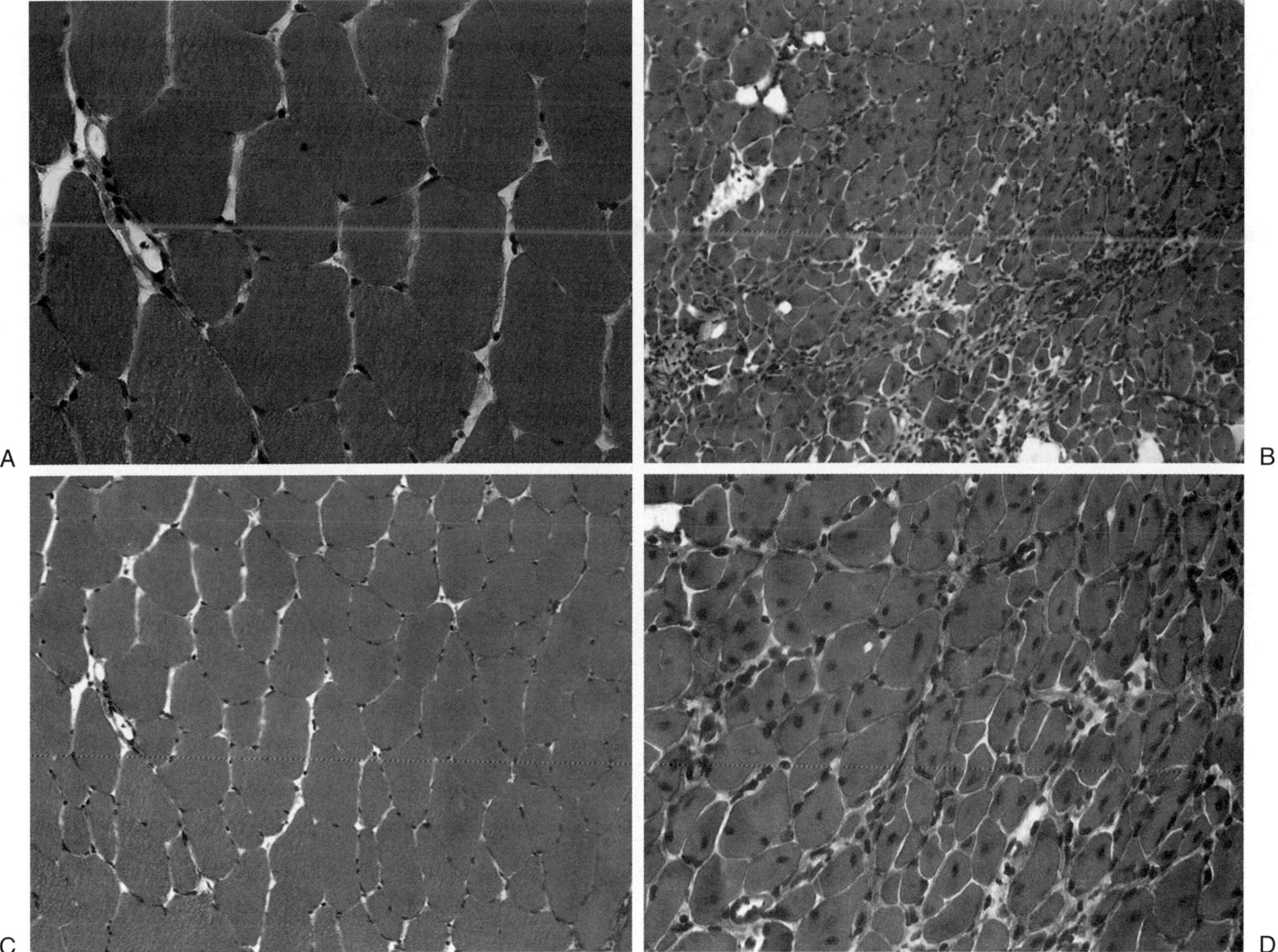

Fig. 1-9 Histologic pictures of muscle tissue from mice. **A** and **B** show normal muscle tissue. **C** and **D** show evidence of fibrosis and regenerating myofibers in the trichrome stain at 2 weeks after experimental muscle laceration.

The most common muscle injuries include delayed-onset muscle soreness (DOMS), muscular contusion, muscular strain, and muscular laceration. Among these types of injuries, the mechanism of injury, pathologic changes, treatment, and outcome vary greatly. Therefore these issues will be discussed in detail for each of these muscle injuries.

Delayed Onset Muscle Soreness

DOMS is a consequence of extensive exercise and usually occurs approximately 12 to 48 hours after exercise. The symptoms of DOMS occur when the amount of stress applied to the muscle exceeds its ability to elongate without disrupting the structural integrity. The symptoms of DOMS are particularly intense after eccentric muscle contraction exercises, whereas repetitive submaximal muscle contractions cause less severe symptoms.[12,15,50] DOMS is characterized by alterations of the structural integrity, an inflammatory response, and the loss of functional capacity.[2,31] The inflammatory component is most likely a response to the damage of the structural muscle integrity and usually lasts for 2 to 3 days.[42] To reduce the inflammatory response, the treatment during the first 2 to 3 days consists of rest, ice, compression, and elevation. Stretching exercises are recommended thereafter to allow superior scar tissue remodeling and fiber alignment of the repair tissue. However, most competitive athletes resume their normal activities quickly after DOMS onset. Permanent impairment after DOMS does not occur.[12]

Muscular Contusion

Muscular contusions are caused by direct blunt trauma to the muscle resulting in damage and partial disruption of the muscle fibers. Frequently, muscle contusions are associated with capillary rupture and local hematoma formation. This is associated with an inflammatory reaction, including increased neutrophil and phagocytic activity, release of inflammatory cytokines, prostaglandin production, and local edema. Clinical signs and symptoms may include ecchymosis, superficial and deep soft tissue swelling, pain, local tenderness, and decreased or abnormal range of motion (ROM). Jackson and Feagin[26] classified the muscular contusions into three degrees, according to the clinical symptoms. A mild contusion is characterized by localized tenderness, near normal ROM, and near normal gait pattern. A moderate contusion usually includes a swollen tender muscle mass, decrease of ROM by 50%, and antalgic gait. A severe contusion is characterized by marked tenderness and swelling, decrease of ROM by 75%, and severe limp.[26]

The initial treatment consists of rest, ice, compression, and elevation to avoid further hemorrhage. This is followed by active and passive ROM exercises and eventually heat, whirlpool, and ultrasound. Functional rehabilitation includes strengthening exercises. Muscular contusions heal by formation of dense connective scar tissue with variable amounts of muscle regeneration. Early stretching exercises of the injured muscle play an important role in the functional scar tissue remodeling process and normal alignment of the newly formed collagen fibers. In contrast, it seems that prolonged immobilization is associated with inferior recovery of muscle function.[26]

Muscular Strain

Muscular strains are tears in the muscle, which may occur as a result of excessive stress (i.e., acute strain) or constant overuse (i.e., chronic strain).[50] In particular, muscles that cross two joints, such as the hamstring muscles and the gastrocnemius, seem to be particularly susceptible to muscular strains.[42] Chronic muscle strains usually occur as a result of repetitive overuse causing fatigue of the muscle. Acute strains, on the other hand, are the result of an excessive force applied to the muscle. The injury usually occurs at the weakest part of the muscle, the myotendinous junction.[15] Histologically, muscle strains are characterized by hemorrhage and an inflammatory response. However, the extent of muscle strain may vary. Mild strains occur when no appreciable structural damage exists to the muscle tissue and pathologic changes are confined to an inflammatory response with swelling and edema, causing discomfort with exercise. With moderate damage, an appreciable muscular defect occurs and the inflammatory response, edema, and discomfort are increased as compared with mild strains. Severe strains are characterized by complete rupture of the muscle belly or the myotendinous junction.

The treatment of muscular strains is completely dependent on the grade of the injury. Although mild strains are usually treated symptomatically with rest, ice, compression, and elevation, severe strains may often require surgical reconstruction. Muscular strains usually heal with the formation of fibrous scar tissue that may be appreciated by MRI.[49]

Muscular Laceration

Muscle lacerations may be caused by penetrating trauma to the muscle and the surrounding soft tissue. Recovery of the muscle function depends on the orientation of the laceration. Lacerations perpendicular to the muscle fibers may create a denervated segment, which is associated with a poor recovery.[3,16] Suture repair of these lesions usually results in scar formation across the laceration. Thus muscle regeneration does not occur across the laceration site, and the functional continuity is usually not restored after muscle laceration.[3,16] In addition, the distal segment is often denervated, and even surgical repair of the muscle belly may not restore the innervation of this part of the muscle. Therefore the functional recovery after muscle laceration is usually limited.

Myositis Ossificans

The term *myositis ossifcans* is used to describe ectopic calcifications within a muscle. Myositis ossificans represents a common complication after muscle injuries. Although common locations of myositis ossificans are the anterior thigh and the upper arm, it may occur in any muscle of the body. The clinical symptoms suggesting myositis ossificans include localized tenderness, swelling, and lack of stretch. Calcifications can usually be detected on plain radiographs (Fig. 1-10, A and B). MRI studies may provide additional information with regard to location within the muscle and extent of the lesion. In addition, nuclear bone scans may play a role in the early detection of the lesion and may help judging the activity of the process. The pathogenesis of myositis ossificans is not completely understood. It has been suggested that myositis ossificans commonly occurs adjacent to the bone shaft, and it appears logical to assume that bone-forming cells from the periosteum migrate into the muscle tissue and form calcifications within the injured muscle or the muscle hematoma.[1,27,56] In some cases, however, the ectopic calcifications occur within the muscle and are not in the close proximity of the bone. For these lesions, the pathogenesis remains unclear. Possible theories include that after the muscle injury the circulation in the traumatized area decreases, which eventually leads to ossification.[20] Other authors theorize that after the muscle injury, rapidly proliferating nondifferentiated connective tissue forms calcifications within the muscle.[24]

In the early stages of myositis ossificans, RICE (rest, ice, compression, elevation) represents the preferred treatment.[1,56] A major issue in orthopaedics is ectopic calcifi-

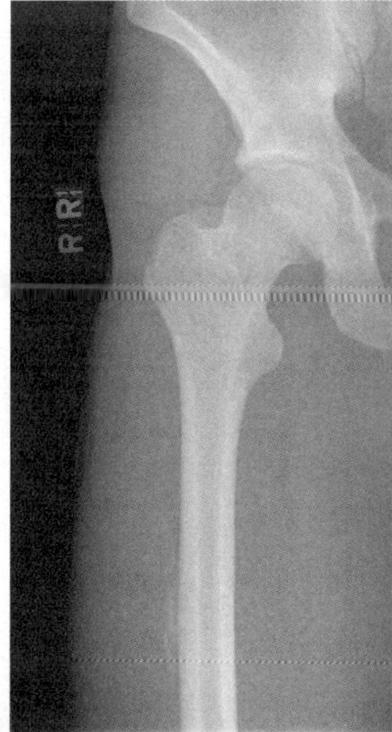

A

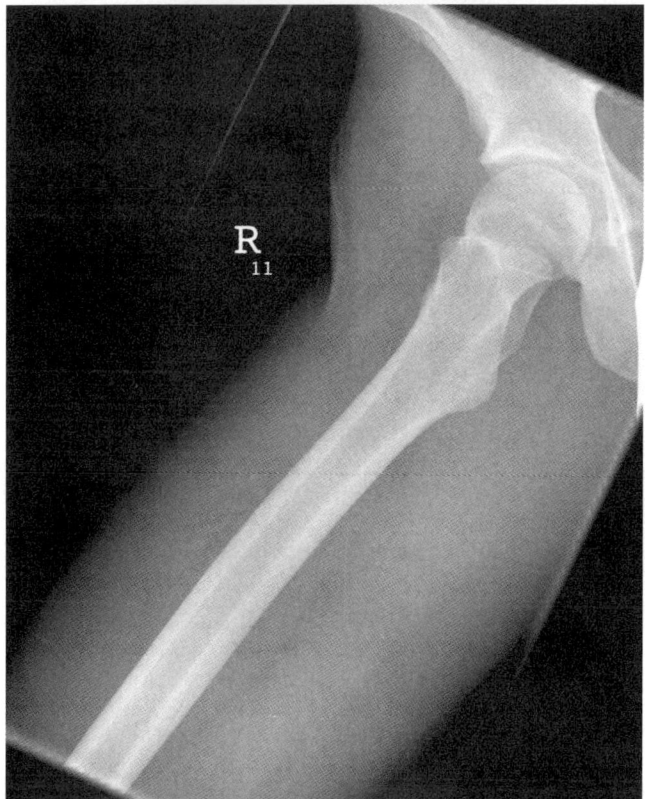

B

Fig. 1-10 Radiographs of the right femur with anteroposterior (A) and lateral view (B) demonstrate an ectopic bone formation lateral to the femur in the middle third of the bone.

cation in the soft tissues surrounding the hip joint after total hip replacement or treatment of acetabular fractures. A meta-analysis of the literature demonstrated that treatment with moderate to high doses of nonsteroidal anti-inflammatory drugs (NSAIDs), such as indomethacin, at the time of surgery decreases the risk of ectopic bone formation.[41] The method by which NSAIDs prevent ectopic bone formation has not been completely understood, but early inhibition of prostaglandin-dependent osteogenic cells appears to be a likely mechanism.[27] Early surgery is contraindicated in myositis ossificans because reossification is likely. Surgical exploration and excision of heterotopic bone formations is only indicated in symptomatic patients and when bone scans and consecutive radiographs suggest low activity and mature bone formation.[27]

BONE INJURY AND HEALING

Bone Morphology

Bone is a composite of material consisting of minerals, proteins, water, cells, and other macromolecules (i.e., lipids, sugar). The composition of the bone tissue varies and depends on age, diet, and general health status. In general, minerals account for 60% to 70% of the bone tissue, water accounts for 5% to 10% of the bone tissue, and the organic bone matrix makes up the remainder. The mineral component is mainly composed of tricalcium phosphate ($Ca_{10}[PO_4]_6[OH]_2$), an analogue of calcium hydroxyapatite. Approximately 90% of the organic bone matrix is type I collagen; the remainder consists of minor collagen types, noncollagenous proteins, and other macromolecules.

The major cell types of bone tissue are osteoblasts, osteocytes, and osteoclasts. The osteoblasts and osteocytes represent the bone-forming cells. Although osteoblasts line the surface of the bone, the osteocytes are encased by mineralized bone matrix. Both cell types are derived from the same osteoprogenitor cell line. A layer of unmineralized bone matrix (i.e., osteoid), which lies between the osteoblast and the mineralized bone matrix, usually surrounds osteoblasts. Once an osteoblast becomes surrounded by mineralized bone matrix, it is referred to as an *osteocyte.* Osteocytes are characterized by a higher nucleus-to-cytoplasm ratio and contain fewer cell organelles than osteoblasts. Osteoclasts are the major resorptive cells of bone and are characterized by their large size and multiple nuclei. Osteoclasts derive from pluripotent cells of the bone marrow, which are hematopoietic precursors that also give rise to monocytes and macrophages. Osteoclasts are characterized by their ability to resorb bone. They lie in regions of bone resorption in pits called *Howship's lacunae.*

Bone Injuries and Healing

A bone fracture is a complete or partial break in the continuity of the bone. Fractures usually occur as a result of trauma and may arise from low energy forces that are cyclically repeated over a long time period (i.e., stress fractures) or from forces having sufficient magnitude to cause structural failure after a single impact. Most

Table 1-5 Bone Healing for a Stable Fracture

Inflammatory Phase	Hemorrhage, necrotic cells; hematoma and fibrin clot formed to bridge the gap	Begins immediately
Soft Callus Phase	Fibrous and cartilaginous tissue formed between the fracture ends, increase in vascularity and ingrowth of capillaries into the fracture callus; increase in cellular proliferation, osteoclasts remove dead bone fragments	1-6 weeks postinjury
Hard Callus Phase	Woven bone develops when the callus converts from fibrocartilaginous; osteoclasts continue removing dead bone; osteoblast activity abundant	4-6 weeks postinjury
Remodeling Phase	Woven bone slowly changes to lamellar bone; medullary canal is then reconstituted; fracture diameter decreases to the original width	6 weeks and up to several months or years (depends on a number of anatomic and physiologic factors)

fractures can be identified on plain radiographs. In some cases, computed tomography (CT) scans or MRI may provide additional information on the fracture pattern. Fracture repair is unique in that healing occurs without scar formation, and only mature bone remains in the fracture site at the end of the repair process. This repair process consists of four stages including inflammation, soft callus, hard callus, and remodeling (Table 1-5).

The inflammation period begins immediately after the fracture is sustained and is characterized by the presence of hemorrhage, necrotic cells, hematoma and fibrin clot. The predominant cell types are platelets, polymorphonuclear neutrophils, monocytes, and macrophages. Shortly thereafter, fibroblasts and osteoprogenitor cells appear and blood vessels start growing into the defect. This neoangiogenesis is initiated and maintained by a tissue oxygen gradient in the tissue and is enhanced by angiogenic factors that are released by macrophages.

The stage of soft callus is characterized by fibrous or cartilaginous tissue within the fracture gap and a great increase in vascularity (Fig. 1-11, A and B). The bony ends are no longer freely moveable. Clinically, subsiding pain and swelling characterize this stage.

During the stage of hard callus, the fibrous callus is replaced by immature woven bone. (Fig. 1-12, A and B). The transition of soft callus to hard callus is somewhat arbitrary, and overlap exists between these two stages because different regions may progress at different rates. During the remodeling process, the woven bone slowly converts to lamellar bone and the trabecular structure responds to the loading conditions according to Wolff's law.[46] The remodeling process may continue for years after the fracture.

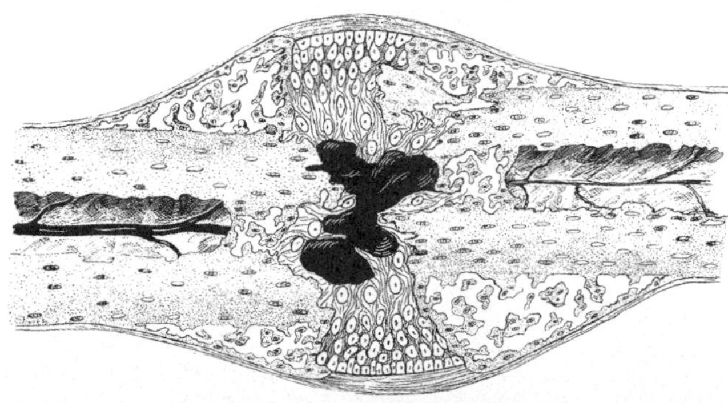

A

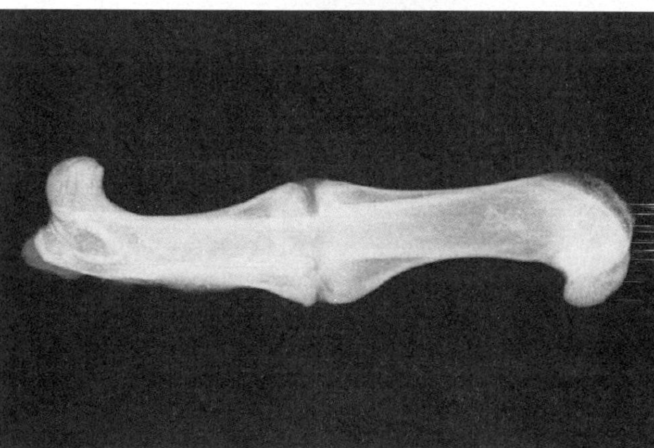

B

Fig. 1-11 In the second stage of structural fracture healing (i.e., soft callus), subperiosteal bone and medullary callus have formed in the adjacent region, but the central region has filled with cartilage and fibrous tissue, and the peripheral region covers them with dense fibrous tissue forming a new periosteum (**A**), which is not evident radiographically (**B**).
(From Browner BD et al: *Skeletal trauma—basic science, management, and reconstruction*, ed 3, Philadelphia, 2003, Elsevier, p 164.)

The vast majority of fractures (90% to 95%) are treated successfully.[8] However, a variety of local and systemic factors may affect fracture healing. Local factors that may impede fracture healing include extensive injury to the surrounding soft tissue envelope, decreased local blood supply, inadequate reduction, inadequate mobilization, local infection, or malignant tissue at the fracture site. Systemic factors may include endocrinologic factors (e.g., diabetes mellitus, menopause), general bone loss (e.g., osteopenia, osteoporosis), and patient nutrition (e.g., smoking, insufficient vitamin or calcium uptake). In many fractures that do not heal, multiple risk factors may exist. Impaired bone healing may present as delayed osseous union or osseous nonunion. Delayed union is usually defined as the failure of the fractured bone to heal within

A

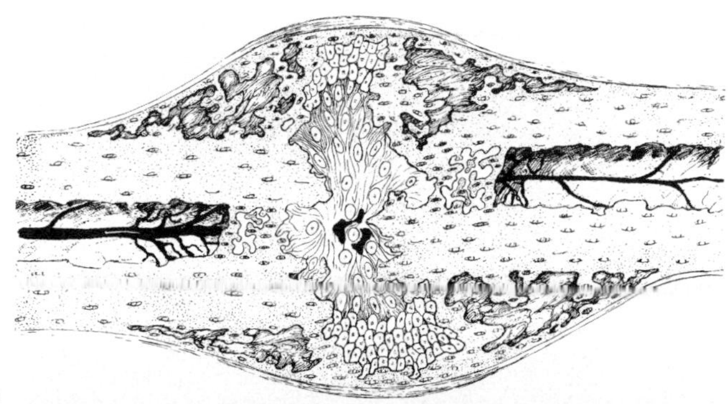

B

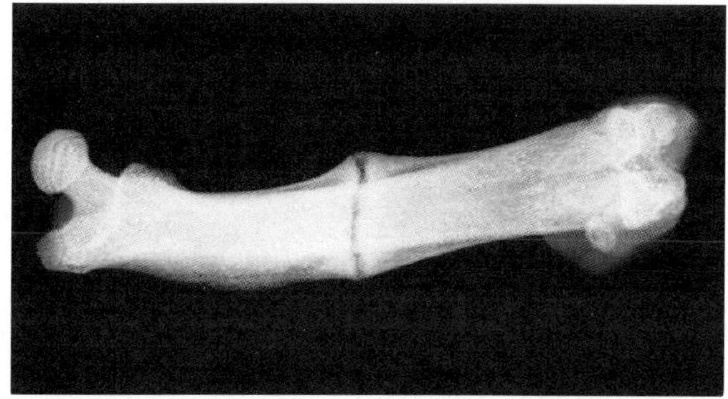

Fig. 1-12 The third stage of structural fracture healing (i.e., hard callus). **A**, Bone begins to form in the peripheral callus region supplied by vascular invasion from the surrounding soft tissues. **B**, This early bone formation may be very thin and not radiographically dense, and the central region is still the bulk of the bridging tissues.
(From Browner BD et al: *Skeletal trauma—basic science, management, and reconstruction*, ed 3, Philadelphia, 2003, Elsevier, p 165.)

the expected time course, while maintaining the potential to heal. Nonunion is defined as a state in which all healing processes have ceased before fracture healing has occurred. **Nonunions can be classified as hypertrophic/vascular and atrophic/avascular. Nonunions lack the potential to heal and require further interventions. Hypertrophic nonunions demonstrate excessive vascularity and callus formation. They are typically the result of biomechanical instability and have a good biologic healing potential. Treatment of hypertrophic nonunions requires biomechanical stabilization of the fracture site. Atrophic nonunions have a limited healing potential, decreased vascularity, and show decreased callus formation. Treatment of atrophic nonunions is challenging, and the treatment may include débridement, stabilization, and utilization of osteoconductive and osteoinductive agents.**

BIOLOGIC TREATMENT APPROACHES

The successful treatment of musculoskeletal injuries remains challenging. Both ligaments and tendons have a poor vascular supply and a low cell turnover. Recent experimental investigations have attempted to establish novel biologic treatment methods, such as growth factor stimulation. Although most of these novel techniques have not been established in the clinical practice, we provide a brief review of the current research and discuss future perspectives in this area.

Growth Factors and Gene Therapy

Growth factors are proteins that can be synthesized by both the resident cells (e.g., fibroblasts) and by immigrating cells (e.g., macrophages, platelets). Growth factors have the ability to stimulate cell proliferation, cell migration, and cell differentiation. Several authors have investigated the role of growth factors in stimulating the musculoskeletal healing response. Stimulating effects of various growth factors have been demonstrated in a variety of tissues (Table 1-6).[21]

The use of most of these growth factors is limited by their short biologic half-lives, requiring repeated applications.[9,47] To overcome this problem, gene transfer techniques have been tested in experimental studies. Gene therapy is based on the modification of cellular genetic information (Fig. 1-13). Thus the genes encoding for growth factors are transferred into local cells at the injury site to modify their genetic codes so that growth factors are continuously produced. This continuous excretion of growth factors will result in an uninterrupted stimulation of the injured musculoskeletal tissue. To achieve gene expression, the DNA encoding for the growth factors must be transferred into the nucleus of the host cells. After gene transfer, the treated cells plentifully express the intended factor (Fig. 1-14). Usually, viral vectors are used for the gene transfer, with adenoviruses and retroviruses representing the most commonly used vectors. Two strategies are used for the transfection of the host cells: (1) the in vivo approach and (2) the ex vivo approach.[9,47] The in vivo approach includes the injection of a virus (usually an adenovirus) encoding the growth factor gene at the injury site. The ex vivo approach includes harvesting cells from the host, genetic modification in vitro (usually by a retrovirus), and reinjection of the modified cells to the injury site. Although the in vivo approach appears to be technically simpler, the ex vivo approach appears to be safer because the transfection of the cells occurs under controlled conditions in vitro.

Although experimental data have demonstrated the great potential of gene therapy techniques, gene therapy has not been established as a standard treatment in patients with musculoskeletal injuries. The major concern surrounding gene therapy is the safety of this technique. Potential risk factors include uncontrolled overstimulation and overgrowth of the repair tissue, mutation of the viral vectors, development of malignancies, and immunologic reactions. Future research is required to investigate and optimize the safety of gene therapy to translate this treatment approach into clinical practice.

Table 1-6 Effects of Growth Factors on Musculoskeletal Tissues

	Muscle	Cartilage	Meniscus	Ligament/Tendon	Bone
GF-1	+	+	+	+	+
(a,b) FGF	+	+	+	+	+
NGF	+				
PDGF (AA,AB,BB)	+		+	+	+
EGF		+	+	+	
TGF-α			+		
TGF-β		+	+	+	+
BMP-2		+	+		+
BMP-4					+
BMP-7					+
VEGF					+

BMP-2, Bone morphogenetic protein-2; *BMP-4*, bone morphogenetic protein-4; *BMP-7*, bone morphogenetic protein-7; *EGF*, endothelial growth factor; *FGF*, fibroblast growth factor; *IGF-1*, insulin-like growth factor-1; *NGF*, nerve growth factor; *PDGF*, platelet-derived growth factor; *TGF-α*, transforming growth factor-alpha; *TGF-β*, transforming growth factor-beta; *VEGF*, vascular endothelial growth factor.

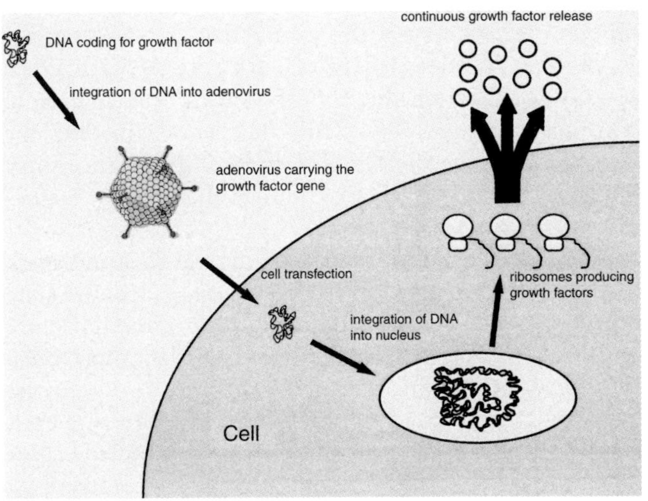

Fig. 1-13 Gene expression pathway. The DNA encoding for a growth factor is inserted into a viral vector. The viral vector is transfecting the cell, and the growth factor gene is inserted into the cell nucleus. The growth factor is then produced by the transfected cells and released into the extracellular space. (Adapted from Lattermann C, Fu FH: Gene therapy in orthopaedics. In Huard J, Fu FH, editors: *Gene therapy and tissue engineering in orthopaedics and sports medicine,* New York, NY, 2000, Birkhauser Boston, c/o Springer Verlag.)

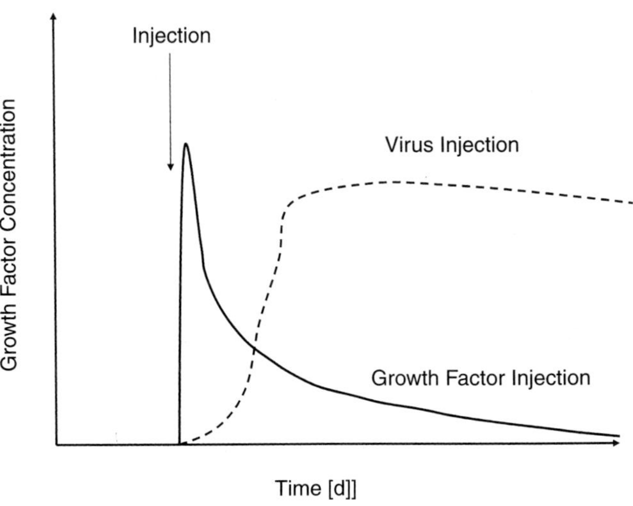

Fig. 1-14 Growth factor concentration after injection of the pure protein versus gene therapy. After injection of the pure growth factor, the concentration reaches a maximum and returns instantly to the baseline level. Gene therapy results in a continuous growth factor concentration in the target tissue over a longer time period. (Reprinted from Fu FH, Zelle BA: Ligaments and tendons: basic science and implications for rehabilitation. Mary Ann Wilmarth, editor: *Clinical applications for orthopaedic basic science: independent study course,* La Crosse, WI, 2004, American Physical Therapy Association, Inc, pp 1-25.)

References

1. Arrington ED, Miller MD: Skeletal muscle injuries, *Orthop Clin North Am* 26:411-422, 1995.
2. Barash IA et al: Desmin cytoskeletal modifications after a bout of eccentric exercise in the rat, *Am J Physiol Regul Integr Comp Physiol* 283:958-963, 2002.
3. Botte MJ et al: Repair of severe muscle belly lacerations using tendon grafts, *J Hand Surg* 12A:406-412, 1987.
4. Cameron M et al: The natural history of the anterior cruciate ligament-deficient knee. Changes in synovial fluid cytokine and keratan sulfate concentrations, *Am J Sports Med* 25:751-754, 1997.
5. Cetti R, Junge J, Vyberg M: Spontaneous rupture of the Achilles tendon is preceded by widespread and bilateral tendon damage and ipsilateral inflammation: a histopathologic study of 60 patients, *Acta Orthop Scand* 74:78-84, 2003.
6. Cook CS, McDonagh MJN: Measurement of muscle and tendon stiffness in man, *Eur J Appl Physiol Occup Physiol* 72:380-382, 1996.
7. Croisier JL et al: Hamstring muscle strain recurrence and strength performance disorders, *Am J Sports Med* 30:199-203, 2002.

8. Einhorn TA: Enhancement of fracture healing, *J Bone Joint Surg Am* 77:940-956, 1995.
9. Evans C, Robbins PD: Possible orthopaedic applications of gene therapy, *J Bone Joint Surg Am* 77:1103-1114, 1995.
10. Feehan LM, Beauchene JG: Early tensile properties of healing chicken flexor tendons: early controlled passive motion versus postoperative mobilization, *J Hand Surg [Am]* 15:63-68, 1990.
11. Frank CB et al: Medial collateral ligament healing: a multidisciplinary assessment in rabbits, *Am J Sports Med* 11:379-389, 1983.
12. Friden J, Sjostrom M, Ekblom B: Myofibrillar damage following intense eccentric exercise in man, *Int J Sports Med* 4:170-176, 1983.
13. Fu FH, Zelle BA: Ligaments and tendons: basic science and implications for rehabilitation. In Mary Ann Wilmarth, editor: *Clinical applications for orthopaedic basic science: independent study course,* La Crosse, WI, 2004, American Physical Therapy Association, Inc, pp 1-25.
14. Garrett WE Jr: Muscle strain injuries, *Am J Sports Med* 24(suppl 6):S2-S8, 1996.
15. Garrett WE, Best TM: Anatomy, physiology, and mechanics of the skeletal muscle. In Simon SR, editor: *Orthopaedic basic science,* Rosemont, IL, 1994, American Academy of Orthopaedic Surgeons.
16. Garrett WE et al: Recovery of skeletal muscle after laceration and repair, *J Hand Surg* 9A:683-692, 1984.
17. Gelberman RH et al: Flexor tendon repair in vitro: a comparative histologic study of the rabbit, chicken, dog, and monkey, *J Orthop Res* 2:39-48, 1984.
18. Gomez MA et al: The effects of increased tension on healing medial collateral ligaments, *Am J Sports Med* 19:347-354, 1991.
19. Hergenroeder PT, Gelberman RH, Akeson WH: The vascularity of the flexor pollicis longus tendon, *Clin Orthop* 162:298-303, 1982.
20. Hierton C: Regional blood flow in experimental myositis ossificans, *Acta Orthop Scand* 54:58-63, 1983.
21. Huard J: Gene therapy and tissue engineering for sports medicine, *J Gene Med* 5:93-108, 2003.
22. Huxley HE: The mechanism of muscular contraction, *Science* 164:1356-1366, 1969.
23. Huxley AF, Simmons RM: Proposed mechanism of force generation in striated muscle, *Nature* 233:533-538, 1971.
24. Illes T et al: Characterization of bone forming cells in post traumatic myositis ossificans by lectins, *Pathol Res Pract* 188:172-176, 1992.
25. Jack EA: Experimental rupture of the medial collateral ligament, *J Bone Joint Surg Br* 32:396-402, 1950.
26. Jackson DW, Feagin JA: Quadriceps contusions in young athletes, *J Bone Joint Surg Am* 55:95-105, 1973.
27. King JB: Post-traumatic ectopic calcification in the muscles of athletes: a review, *Br J Sports Med* 32:287-290, 1998.
28. Kolts I, Tillmann B, Lullmann-Rauch R: The structure and vascularization of the biceps brachii long head tendon, *Ann Anat* 176;75-80, 1994.
29. Kubota H et al: Effect of motion and tension on injured flexor tendons in chickens, *J Hand Surg [Am]* 21:456-463, 1996.
30. Lehto M, Jarvinen M, Nelimarkka O: Scar formation after skeletal muscle injury. A histological and autoradiographical study in rats, *Arch Orthop Trauma Surg* 104:366-370, 1986.
31. Lieber RL, Shah S, Friden J: Cytoskeletal disruption after eccentric contraction-induced muscle injury, *Clin Orthop* 403:S90-S99, 2002.
32. Liu SH et al: Collagen in tendon, ligament, and bone healing, *Clin Orthop* 318:265-278, 1995.
33. Lundborg G, Myrhage R, Rydevik B: The vascularization of human flexor tendons with the digital synovial sheath region: structural and functional aspects, *J Hand Surg [Am]* 2:417-427, 1977.
34. Maffulli N, Barrass V, Ewen SW: Light microscopic histology of Achilles tendon ruptures: a comparison with unruptured tendons, *Am J Sports Med* 28:857-863, 2000.
35. Manske PR et al: Intrinsic flexor-tendon repair: a morphological study in vitro, *J Bone Joint Surg Am* 66:385-396, 1984.
36. Manske PR, Lesker PA: Comparative nutrient pathways to the flexor profundus tendons in zone II of various experimental animals, *J Surg Res* 34:83-93, 1983.
37. Manske PR, Lesker PA: Nutrient pathways to extensor tendons within the extensor retinacular compartments, *Clin Orthop* 181:234-237, 1983.
38. Manske PR, Lesker PA: Histologic evidence of intrinsic flexor tendon repair in various experimental animals: an in vitro study, *Clin Orthop* 182:297-304, 1984.
39. Marshall JL, Rubin RM: Knee ligament injuries: a diagnostic and therapeutic approach, *Orthop Clin North Am* 8:641-668, 1977.
40. Mass DP et al: Effects of constant mechanical tension on the healing of rabbit flexor tendons, *Clin Orthop* 296:301-306, 1993.
41. Neal BC et al: A systematic overview of 13 randomized trials of non-steroidal anti-inflammatory drugs for prevention of heterotopic bone formation after major hip surgery, *Acta Orthop Scand* 71:122-128, 2000.
42. Nikolaou PK et al: Biomechanical and histological evaluation of muscle after controlled strain injury, *Am J Sports Med* 15:9-13, 1987.
43. Orchard J, Best TM: The management of muscle strain injuries: an early return versus the risk of recurrence, *Clin J Sport Med* 12:3-5, 2002.
44. Provenzano PP et al: Hindlimb unloading alters ligament healing, *J Appl Physiol* 94:314-324, 2002.
45. Raspanti M, Congiu T, Guizzardi S: Structural aspects of the extracellular matrix of tendon: an atomic force and scanning electron microscopy study, *Arch Histol Cytol* 65:37-43, 2002.
46. Regling G, editor: *Wolff's law and connective tissue regulation: modern interdisciplinary comments on Wolff's law of connective tissue regulation and rational understanding of common clinical problems*, Berlin, NY, 1992, W de Gruyter.
47. Robbins PD, Ghivizzani S: Viral vectors for gene therapy, *Pharmacol Ther* 80:35-47, 1998.
48. Russell JE, Manske PR: Collagen synthesis during primate flexor tendon repair in vitro, *J Orthop Res* 8:13-20, 1990.
49. Speer KP, Lohnes J, Garrett WE Jr: Radiographic imaging of muscle strain injury, *Am J Sports Med* 21:89-95, 1993.

50. Stauber WT: Eccentric action of muscles physiology, injury, and adaptation, *Exerc Sport Sci Rev* 17:157-185, 1989.
51. Steinbach LS, Fleckenstein JL, Mink JH: Magnetic resonance imaging of muscle injuries, *Orthopedics* 17:991-999, 1994.
52. Tallon C, Maffulli N, Ewen SWB: Ruptured Achilles tendons are significantly more degenerated than tendinopathic tendons, *Med Sci Sports Exerc* 33:1983-1990, 2001.
53. Tidball JG: Inflammatory cell response to acute muscle injury, *Med Sci Sports Exerc* 27:1022-1032, 1995.
54. Vailas AC et al: Physical activity and its influence on the repair process of medial collateral ligaments, *Connect Tissue Res* 9:25-31, 1981.
55. Verrall GM et al: Clinical risk factors for hamstring muscle strain injury: a prospective study with correlation of injury by magnetic resonance imaging, *Br J Sports Med* 35:435-439, 2001.
56. Young JL, Laskowski ER, Rock MG: Thigh injuries in athletes, *Mayo Clin Proc* 68:1099-1106, 1993.
57. Zbrodowski A, Gajisin S, Grodecki J: Vascularization of the tendons of the extensor pollicis longus, extensor carpi radialis longus and extensor carpi radialis brevis muscles, *J Anat* 135:235-244, 1982.

CHAPTER 2

Soft Tissue Healing Considerations after Surgery

Robert I. Cantu
Jason A. Steffe

Physical therapists work daily on connective tissues that are dynamic and have the capacity for change. Changes in these tissues are driven by a number of factors, including trauma, surgery, immobilization, posture, and repeated stresses. The physical therapist must have a good working knowledge of the normal histology and biomechanics of connective tissue and understand the way connective tissue responds to immobilization, trauma, and remobilization. Both experienced and novice physical therapists can benefit from a good "mental picture" of connective tissues in operation.

SURGERY DEFINED

Because this text primarily considers postsurgical rehabilitation, an operational definition of *surgery* is in order. For the purpose of considering injury and repair of soft tissues, surgery may be defined as *controlled trauma produced by a trained professional to correct uncontrolled trauma.* The reason for this unusual definition is that connective tissues respond in characteristic ways to immobilization and trauma. Because surgery is itself a form of trauma that is usually followed by some form of immobilization, the physical therapist must understand the way tissues respond to both immobilization and trauma.

This chapter begins by dealing with the basic histology and biomechanics of connective tissue. It then presents the histopathology and pathomechanics of connective tissues (i.e., the way connective tissues respond to immobilization, trauma, and remobilization). Finally it addresses some basic principles of soft tissue mobilization based on the connective tissue response to immobilization, trauma, and remobilization.

HISTOLOGY AND BIOMECHANICS OF CONNECTIVE TISSUE

The connective tissue system in the human body is quite extensive. Connective tissue makes up 16% of the body's weight and holds 25% of the body's water.[9] The "soft" connective tissues form ligaments, tendons, periosteum, joint capsules, aponeuroses, nerve and muscle sheaths, blood vessel walls, and the bed and framework of the internal organs. If the bony structures were removed, then a semblance of structure would remain from the connective tissues.

A majority of the tissues affected by mobilization are connective tissues. During joint mobilization, for example, the tissues being mobilized are the joint capsule and the surrounding ligaments and connective tissues. The facet joint space is merely a "space built for motion." Arthrokinematic rules are followed, but the tissue being mobilized is classified as connective tissue. Therefore, background knowledge of the histology and histopathology of connective tissues is essential for the practicing physical therapist.

Normal Histology and Biomechanics of Connective Tissue Cells

Connective tissue has two components: (1) the cells and (2) the extracellular matrix. The cell of primary importance is the fibroblast. The fibroblast synthesizes all the inert components of connective tissue, including collagen, elastin, reticulin, and ground substance.

Extracellular Matrix

The extracellular matrix of connective tissue includes connective tissue fibers and ground substance. The

Table 2-1 Classification of Connective Tissue

Tissue Type	Specific Structures	Characteristics of the Tissue
Dense regular	Ligaments, tendons	Dense, parallel arrangement of collagen fibers; proportionally less ground substance
Dense irregular	Aponeurosis, periosteum, joint capsules, dermis of skin, areas of high mechanical stress	Dense, multidirectional arrangement of collagen fibers; able to resist multidirectional stress
Loose irregular	Superficial fascial sheaths, muscle and nerve sheaths, support sheaths of internal organs	Sparse, multidirectional arrangement of collagen fibers; greater amounts of elastin present

(From Cantu R, Grodin A: *Myofascial manipulation: theory and clinical application*, Gaithersburg, MD, 1992, Aspen.)

connective tissue fibers include collagen (the most tensile), elastin, and reticulin (the most extensible). Collagen, elastin, and reticulin provide the tensile support that connective tissue offers. Extensibility or the lack of it is driven by the relative density and percentage of the connective tissue fibers. Tissues with less collagen density and a greater proportion of elastin fibers are more pliable than tissues with a greater density and proportion of collagen fibers.

The ground substance of connective tissue plays a very different role in the connective tissue response to immobility, trauma, and remobilization. The ground substance is the viscous, gel-like substance in which the cells and connective tissue fibers lie. It acts as a lubricant for collagen fibers in conditions of normal mobility and maintains a crucial distance between collagen fibers. The ground substance also is a medium for the diffusion of nutrients and waste products and acts as a mechanical barrier for invading microorganisms. It has a much shorter half-life than collagen and, as will be discussed, is much more quickly affected by immobilization than collagen.[16]

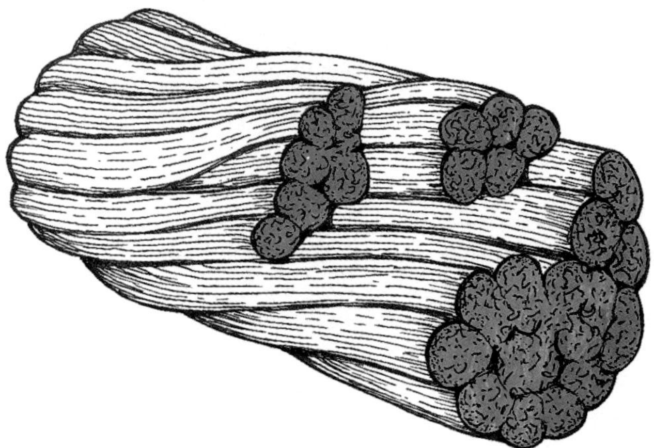

Fig. 2-1 Dense regular connective tissue. The parallel compact arrangement of the collagen fibers should be noted.
(Modified from Williams P, Warwick R, editors: *Gray's anatomy,* ed 35, Philadelphia, 1973, WB Saunders.)

Three Types of Connective Tissue

Connective tissue is classified according to fiber density and orientation. The three types of connective tissue found in the human body are (1) dense regular, (2) dense irregular, and (3) loose irregular (Table 2-1).[7,24]

Dense regular connective tissue includes ligaments and tendons (Fig. 2-1).[25] The fiber orientation is unidirectional for the purpose of attenuating unidirectional forces. The high density of collagen fibers accounts for the high degree of tensile strength and lack of extensibility in these tissues. Relatively low vascularity and water content account for the slow diffusion of nutrients and resulting slower healing times. Dense regular connective tissue is the most tensile and least extensible of the connective tissue types.

Dense irregular connective tissue includes joint capsules, periosteum, and aponeuroses. The primary difference between dense regular and dense irregular connective tissue is that dense irregular connective tissue has a multidimensional fiber orientation (Fig. 2-2). This multidimensional orientation allows the tissue to attenuate forces in numerous directions. The density of collagen fibers is high, producing a high degree of tensile strength and a low degree of extensibility. Dense irregular connective tissue also has low vascularity and water content, resulting in slow diffusion of nutrients and slower healing times.

Loose irregular connective tissue includes, but is not limited to, the superficial fascial sheath of the body directly under the skin, the muscle and nerve sheaths, and the bed and framework of the internal organs. Similarly to dense irregular connective tissue, loose irregular connective tissue has a multidimensional tissue orientation. However, the density of collagen fibers is much less than that of dense irregular connective tissue. The relative vascularity and water content of loose irregular connective tissue is much greater than dense regular and dense irregular connective tissue. Therefore it is much more pliable and extensible and exhibits faster healing times after trauma. Loose irregular connective tissue also is the easiest to mobilize.

Normal Biomechanics of Connective Tissue

Connective tissues have unique deformation characteristics that enable them to be effective shock attenuators. This is

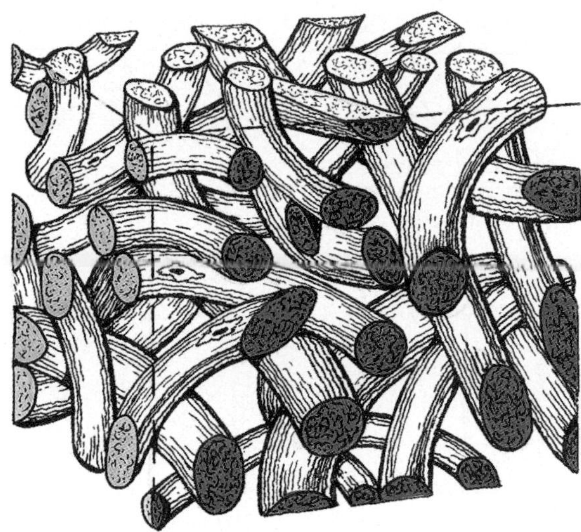

Fig. 2-2 Dense irregular connective tissue with multidimensional compact arrangement of collagen fibers.
(Modified from Williams P, Warwick R, editors: *Gray's anatomy,* ed 35, Philadelphia, 1973, WB Saunders.)

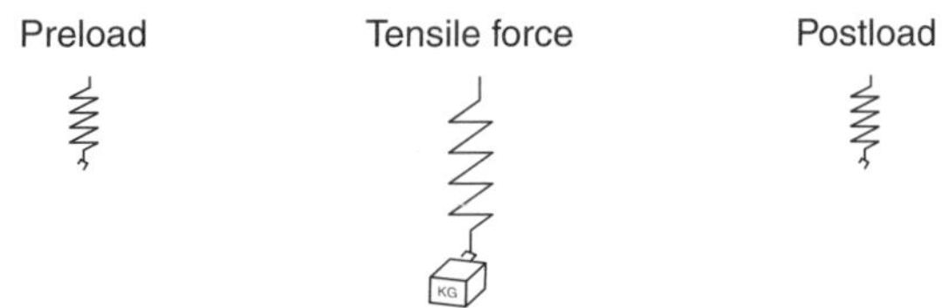

Fig. 2-3 The elastic component of connective tissue.
(From Grodin A, Cantu R: *Myofascial manipulation: theory and clinical management,* Centerpoint, NY, 1989, Forum Medical Publishers.)

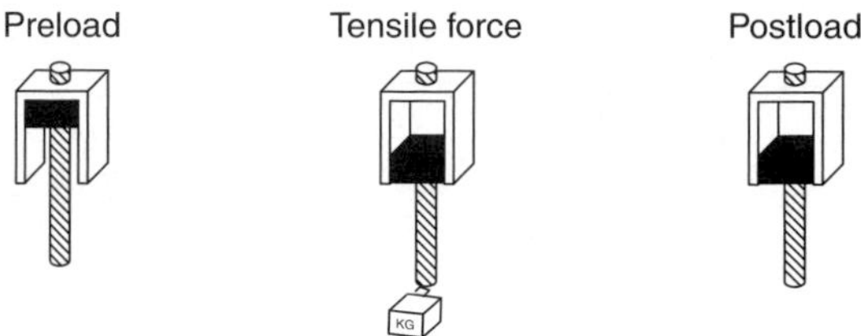

Fig. 2-4 The viscous, or plastic, component of connective tissue.
(From Grodin A, Cantu R: *Myofascial manipulation: theory and clinical management,* Centerpoint, NY, 1989, Forum Medical Publishers.)

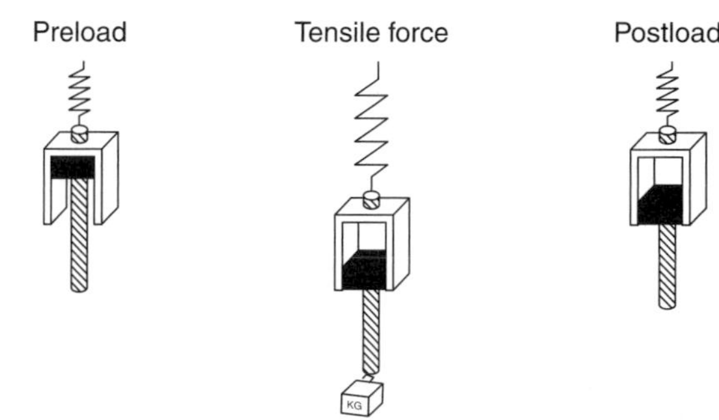

Fig. 2-5 The viscoelastic nature of connective tissue.
(From Grodin A, Cantu R: *Myofascial manipulation: theory and clinical management,* Centerpoint, NY, 1989, Forum Medical Publishers.)

termed the *viscoelastic nature of connective tissue.*[26] This viscoelasticity is the very characteristic that makes connective tissue able to change based on the stresses applied to it. The ability of connective tissue to thicken or become more extensible based on outside stresses is the basic premise to be understood by the manual therapist seeking to increase mobility.

In the viscoelastic model, two components combine to give connective tissues its dynamic deformation attributes. The first is the *elastic* component, which represents a temporary change in the length of connective tissue subjected to stress (Fig. 2-3). A spring, which elongates when loaded and returns to its original position when unloaded, illustrates this. This elastic component is the "slack" in connective tissue.

The *viscous,* or plastic, component of the model represents the permanent change in connective tissue subjected to outside forces. A hydraulic cylinder and piston illustrates this (Fig. 2-4). When a force is placed on the piston, the piston slowly moves out of the cylinder. When the force is removed, the piston does not recoil but remains at the new length, indicating permanent change. These permanent changes result from the breaking of intermolecular and intramolecular bonds between collagen molecules, fibers, and cross-links.

The viscoelastic model combines the elastic and plastic components just described (Fig. 2-5). When subjected to a mild force in the midrange of the tissue, the tissue elongates in the elastic component and then returns to its original length. If, however, the stress pushes the tissue to the end range, then the elastic component is depleted and plastic deformation occurs. When the stress is released, some permanent deformation has occurred. It should be noted that not all the elongation (only a portion) is permanently retained.

Clinically, this phenomenon occurs frequently. For example, a client with a frozen shoulder that has only 90 degrees of elevation is mobilized to reach a range of motion (ROM) of 110 degrees by the end of the treatment session. When the client returns in a few days, the ROM of that shoulder is less than 110 degrees but more than 90 degrees. Some degree of elongation is lost and some is retained.

This viscoelastic phenomenon can be further illustrated by the use of stress-strain curves. By definition, stress is the force applied per unit area, and strain is the percent change in length. When connective tissue is initially stressed or loaded, very little force is required to elongate the tissue. However, as more stress is applied and the slack or spring is taken up, more force is required and less change

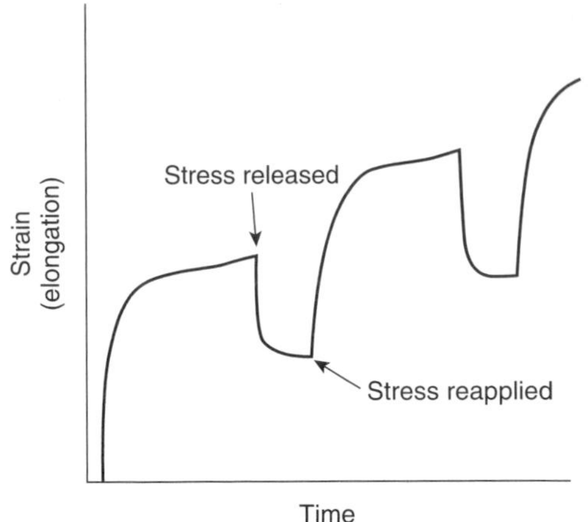

Fig. 2-6 Stress-strain curves indicating the progressive elongation of connective tissue with repeated stresses.
(From Grodin A, Cantu R: *Myofascial manipulation: theory and clinical management,* Centerpoint, NY, 1989, Forum Medical Publishers.)

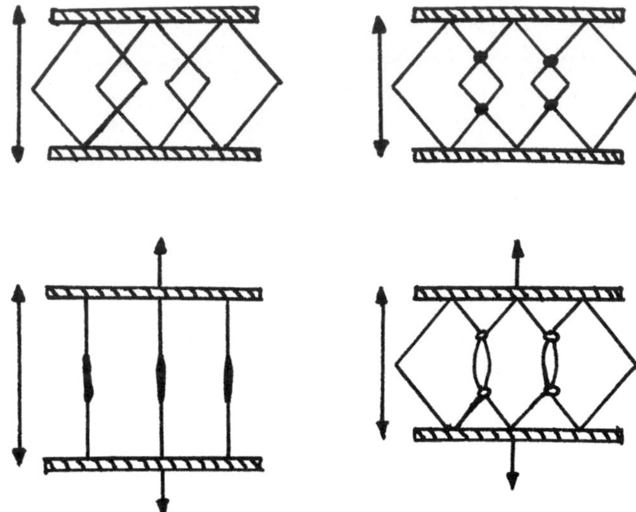

Fig. 2-7 The basket weave configuration of connective tissue. With immobilization, the distance between fibers is diminished, forming cross-link adhesions.
(From Cantu R, Grodin A: *Myofascial manipulation: theory and clinical application,* Gaithersburg, MD, 1992, Aspen Publishers.)

occurs in the tissue (Fig. 2-6). When the tissue is subjected to repeated stresses, the curve shows that after each stress the tissue elongates and then only partially returns to its original length. Some length is gained each time the tissue is taken into the plastic range. This phenomenon is seen clinically in repeated sessions of therapy. ROM is gained during a session, with some of the gain being lost between sessions.

EFFECTS OF IMMOBILIZATION, REMOBILIZATION, AND TRAUMA ON CONNECTIVE TISSUE

Immobilization

Immobilization and trauma significantly change the histology and normal mechanics of connective tissue. A majority of the hallmark studies in the area of immobilization follow the same basic experimental mode.[1-5,26] Laboratory animals are fixated internally for varying periods. The fixation is removed and the animals are then sacrificed. Histochemical and biomechanical analyses are performed to determine changes in the tissues. In some studies the fixation is removed and the animals are allowed to move the fixated joint for a period before the analysis is performed. This is done to determine the reversibility of the effects of immobilization.[11]

Macroscopically, fibrofatty infiltrate is evident in the recesses of the immobilized tissues. With prolonged immobilization the infiltrates develop a more fibrotic appearance, creating adhesions in the recesses. These fibrotic changes occur in the absence of trauma. Histologic and histochemical analyses show significant changes primarily in the ground substance, with no significant loss of collagen. The changes in the ground substance consist of substantial losses of glycosaminoglycans and water. Because a primary function of ground substance is binding water to assist in hydration, the loss of ground substance results in a related loss of water.

Another purpose of ground substance is to lubricate adjacent collagen fibers and maintain a crucial interfiber distance. If collagen fibers approximate too closely, then the fibers will adhere to one another. These cross-links create a series of microscopic adhesions that limit the pliability and extensibility of the tissues (Fig. 2-7). **In addition, collagen that has been immobilized for extended periods of time demonstrates less tissue strength and quicker failure during stress-strain studies and load-to-failure studies.**[13,14,17,19,21,23,27-29]

Furthermore, because movement affects the orientation of newly synthesized collagen, the collagen in the immobilized joints studied was laid down in a more haphazard, "haystack" arrangement. This orientation restricts tissue mobility further by adhering to existing collagen fibers (Fig. 2-8).

Biomechanical analysis reveals that as much as ten times more torque is necessary to mobilize fixated joints than normal joints. After repeated mobilizations, these joints gradually return to normal. The authors of these studies implicate both fibrofatty microadhesions and increased microscopic cross-linking of collagen fibers in the decreased extensibility of connective tissues.

Remobilization

Available research seems to suggest that mobility and remobilization prevent the haystack development of collagen fibers within ligaments and tendons, as well as

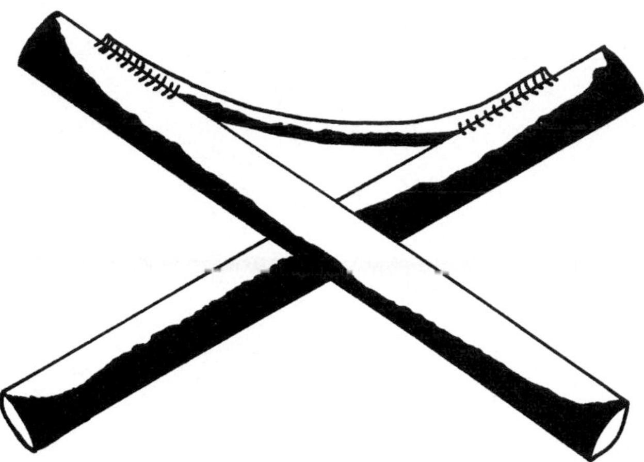

Fig. 2-8 The random haystack arrangement of immobilized scar tissue creating additional adhesions.
(From Cantu R, Grodin A: *Myofascial manipulation: theory and clinical application,* Gaithersburg, MD, 1992, Aspen Publishers.)

stimulate the production of ground substance. When connective tissue is stressed with movement, the tissue rehydrates, collagen cross-links are diminished, and new collagen is laid down in a more orderly fashion.

The collagen tends to be laid down in the direction of the forces applied and in an appropriate length. In addition, early mobilization leads to enhanced ligament and tendon strength, resistance to tensile forces, greater joint stability, and improved resistance of the ligament to avulsion.[13-16,18-20,22,27-29]

Additionally, macroadhesions formed during the immobilization period partially elongate and partially rupture during the remobilization process, increasing the overall mobility of the tissue. Both passive mobilization and active ROM produce similar results.

Trauma

These studies have limited application because they involve the immobilization of normal, healthy joints. To complete this discussion, we must superimpose the effects of trauma and scar tissue on immobilization.

Scar

Scar tissue mechanics differ somewhat from normal connective tissue mechanics. Normal connective tissue is mature and stable, with limited pliability. Immature scar tissue is much more dynamic and pliable. Scar tissue formation occurs in four distinct phases. Each of these phases shows characteristic differences during phases of immobilization and mobilization.[9,10]

The first phase of scar tissue formation is the inflammatory phase. This phase occurs immediately after trauma. Blood clotting begins almost instantly and is followed by migration of macrophages and histiocytes to start débriding the area. This phase usually lasts 24 to 48 hours, and immobilization is usually important because of the potential for further damage with movement. Some exceptions to routine immobilization exist. For example, in an anterior cruciate ligament (ACL) reconstruction in which the graft is safely fixated and damage from gentle movement is unlikely, there may be a great advantage in moving the tissue as early as the first day after surgery. Research indicates that early mobilization leads to more rapid ligament regeneration and ultimate load to failure strength in surgically repaired ACLs.[21]

The second phase of scar tissue formation is the granulation phase. This phase is characterized by an uncharacteristic increase in the relative vascularity of the tissue. Increased vascularity is essential to ensure proper nutrition to meet the metabolic needs of the repairing tissue. The granulation phase varies greatly depending on the type of tissue and the extent of the damage. Generally speaking, the entire process of scar tissue formation is lengthened if the damaged tissue is less vascular in its nontraumatized state. For example, tendons and ligaments require more time for scar tissue formation than muscle or epithelial tissue. Movement is helpful in this phase, although the scar tissue can be easily damaged. The physician and therapist need to work closely to determine the extent of movement relative to the risk.

The third phase of scar tissue formation is the fibroplastic stage. In this stage the number of fibroblasts increases, as does the rate of production of collagen fibers and ground substance. Collagen is laid down at an accelerated rate and binds to itself with weak hydrostatic bonds, making tissue elongation much easier. This stage presents an excellent window of opportunity for the reshaping and molding of scar tissue without great risk of tissue reinjury. This stage lasts 3 to 8 weeks depending on the histologic makeup and relative vascularity of the damaged tissue. Scar tissue at this phase is less likely to be injured but is still easily remodeled with stresses applied (Fig. 2-9).

The final phase of scar tissue formation is the maturation phase. Collagen matures, solidifies, and shrinks during this phase. Maximal stress can be placed on the tissue without risk of tissue failure. Because collagen synthesis is still accelerated, significant remodeling can take place when appropriate mobilizations are performed. Conversely, if they are left unchecked, then the collagen fibers can cross-link and the tissue can shrink significantly. At the end of the maturation phase, tissue remodeling becomes significantly more difficult because the tissue reverts to a more mature, inactive, and nonpliable status.

Surgical Perspective

Surgery has been defined in this chapter as controlled trauma produced by a trained professional to correct uncontrolled trauma. Postsurgical cases are subject to the effects of immobilization, trauma, and scar formation. However, they have the advantage of resulting from

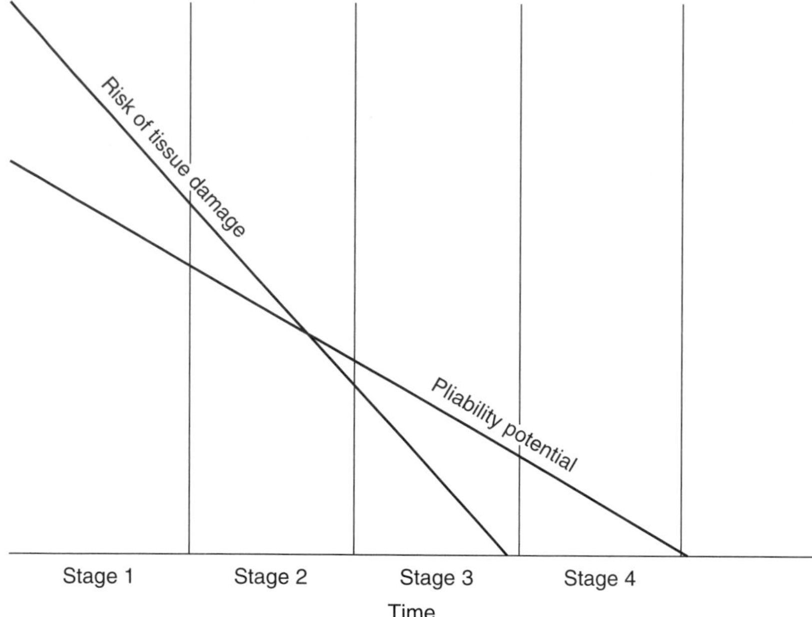

Fig. 2-9 Relationship of tissue pliability to relative risk of injury.

controlled trauma. The scar tissue formed by surgery is usually more manageable than scar tissue formed by uncontrolled trauma or overuse.

When dealing with scar tissue after surgery, the physical therapist should remember the following guidelines:

- Assess the approximate stage of development of the scar tissue. Although the timelines vary, vascular tissue matures faster than nonvascular tissue.
- Whenever possible, movement is helpful in controlling the direction and length of the scar tissue. **Communicate with the referring physician regarding the amount of movement that is appropriate.** In a study performed by Flowers and Pheasant,[12] casted joints regained mobility much faster than fixated joints. This is probably because a cast does not provide the same immobilization as rigid fixation. The small amounts of movement allowed in casted joints may be enough to prevent some of the changes caused by rigid fixation.
- Recognize the window of opportunity to stress scar tissue, and keep in mind the associated risk of tissue injury or microtrauma (see Fig. 2-9). Although the potential to change scar tissue may be greater in earlier stages, the risk of damage is higher. The third stage appears to be the stage at which the reward of mobility work exceeds the risk. **The therapist should proceed with caution in the second stage of scar tissue formation, recognizing that some risk may be necessary if optimal results are to be obtained.**

GOALS OF MOBILITY WORK

- In 1945, John Mennell[20] said, "There are only two possible effects of any movement or massage: they are reflex and mechanical." The following summary emphasizes the goals of the mechanical changes of mobility work:

- Mobility work allows for the hydration and rehydration of connective tissues.
- Mobility work causes the breaking and subsequent prevention of cross-links in collagen fibers.
- Mobility work allows for the breaking and prevention of macroadhesions.
- Mobility work allows for the plastic deformation and permanent elongation of connective tissues.
- Mobility work allows for the laying down of collagen fibers and scar tissue in the appropriate length and direction of the stresses applied.
- Mobility work allows for the molding and remolding of collagen fibers during the fibroplastic and maturation stages of scar tissue formation.
- Mobility work prevents scar tissue shrinkage.
- Mobility work allows for the more generalized effects of increased blood flow, increased venous and lymphatic return, and increased cellular metabolism.

PRINCIPLES FOR MOBILIZATION OF CONNECTIVE TISSUES

This section attempts to integrate the principles of basic scientific research and years of clinical experience into a series of techniques useful for the physical therapist in treating immobilized tissue.

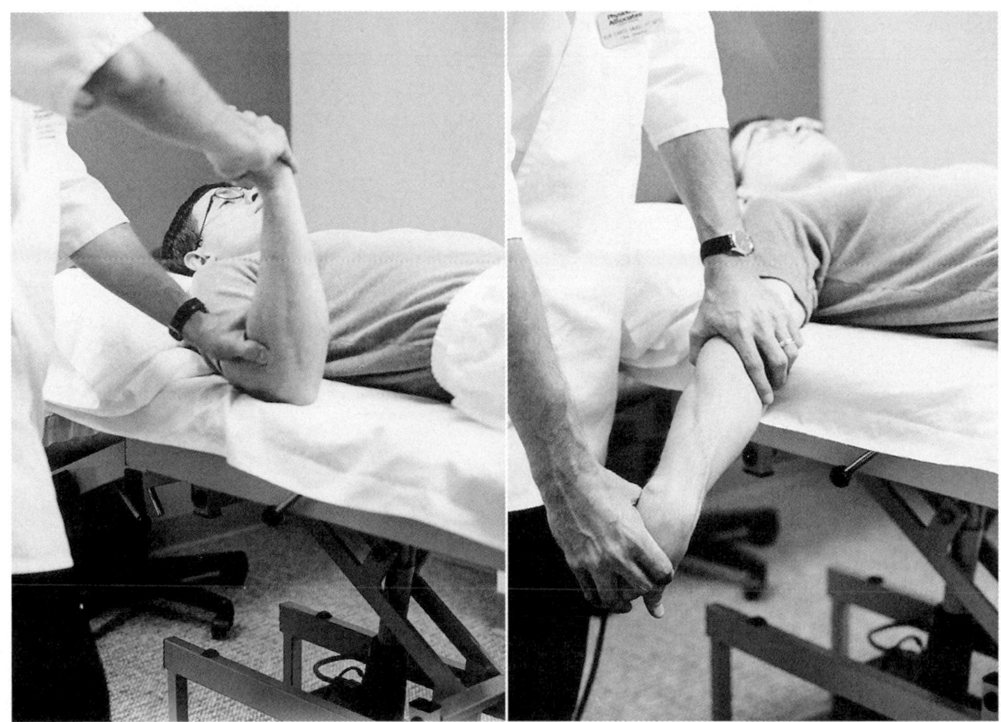

Fig. 2-10 The principle of short and long. Soft tissue immobilization is performed in a shortened range, then immediately elongated.

Three-Dimensionality of Connective Tissue

Connective tissue is three-dimensional. Especially after trauma and immobilization, the scar tissue can follow lines of development not consistent with the kinesiology or arthrokinematics of the area. Therefore the ability to feel the location and direction of the restriction becomes important in the mobilization of scar tissue.

Creep

Creep is another term for the plastic deformation of connective tissue. Active scar tissue is more "creepy" than normal connective tissue (i.e., it is more easily elongated by external forces). Creep occurs when all the "slack" has been let out of the tissue. It is best accomplished with low-load, prolonged stretching but also can be accomplished with other manual techniques. Dynamic splinting is another technique used to elongate connective tissue. The tissue should be elongated along the lines of normal movement; however, at times the restrictive lesion may not follow the line of movement. The therapist must identify the direction of the restriction and mobilize directly into the restriction. This may be a transverse or horizontal plane. Mobilizing the scar in the direction of the restriction usually results in more movement along conventional planes.

Principle of Short and Long

The principle of short and long is the idea that tissues mobilized in a shortened range often become more extensible when they are immediately elongated (Fig. 2-10). For example, in a lateral epicondylitis, cross-friction massage may be performed over the lateral epicondyle with the elbow passively flexed and the wrist passively extended. Immediately after the cross-friction in the shortened range, the tissue is stretched into the plastic range. In the shortened range, deeper tissues can be accessed. When tissue is taut, only the more superficial layers can be accessed. When the tissue has some slack, the deeper tissues can be accessed and prepared for stretching.

The principle of short and long has neuromuscular implications as well. If a muscle is guarded, then shortening the muscle by mobilizing it has an inhibitory effect that makes immediate elongation easier.

TECHNIQUES FOR MOBILIZATION OF CONNECTIVE TISSUES

The following techniques and associated photographs illustrate some simple manual techniques effective in mobilizing soft tissues.

Muscle Splay

Muscle splay is a term that implies a widening or separation of longitudinal fibers of muscle or connective tissues that have adhered to one another (Fig. 2-11). These adhesions limit the ability of the tissue to be lengthened passively or shortened actively. When muscle bundles or connective tissue bundles stick together, the muscle fibers become

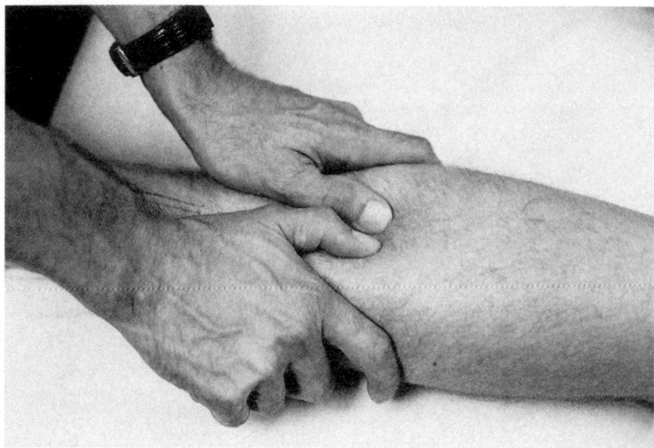

Fig. 2-11 The splaying, or longitudinal separation, of fascial planes.

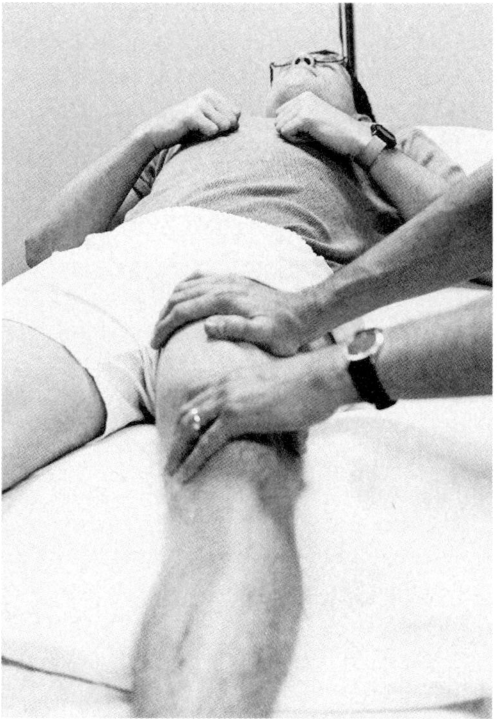

Fig. 2-12 The bending of the fascial sheath surrounding the muscles.

less efficient in their contractions. For example, muscle splay in the wrist flexors often produces a slightly greater grip strength immediately after soft tissue work. This is not greater strength, but greater muscle efficiency produced by increased soft tissue pliability. The muscle can contract more efficiently within its connective tissue compartments.

Transverse Muscle Bending

Transverse muscle bending takes the contractile unit and mobilizes it perpendicular to the fibers (Fig. 2-12). This

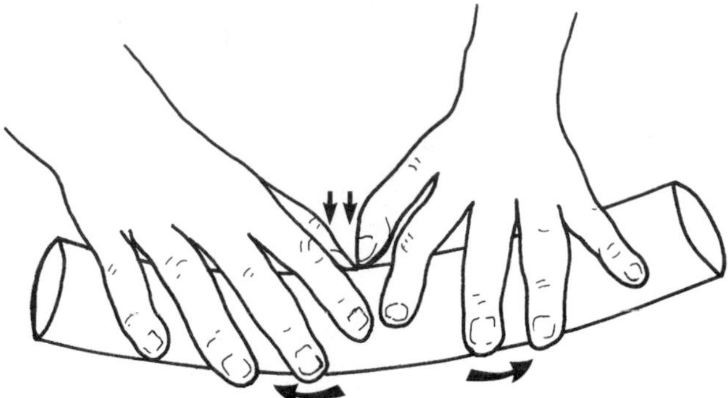

Fig. 2-13 Transverse movement of fascial planes.

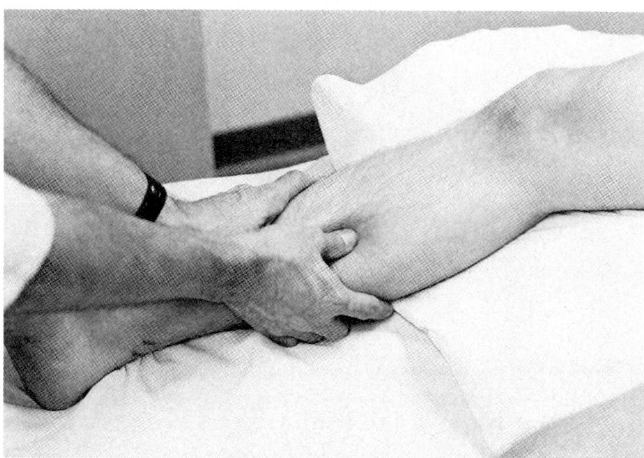

Fig. 2-14 Longitudinal stroke clearing fascia away from a bony surface.

perpendicular bending mobilizes connective tissues in a way similar to the bending of a garden hose (Fig. 2-13). The connective tissue sheath surrounding a muscle may be likened to the hose itself, with the muscle being analogous to the water inside it. If the connective tissue sheath is stiff and rigid, then the muscle inside has difficulty contracting. The unforgiving sheath does not allow the muscle to expand transversely, creating a lack of efficiency and a low-grade "compartment syndrome." By mobilizing these muscle sheaths, overall mobility is enhanced along planes of normal movement.

Bony Clearing

Bony clearing is similar to muscle splay, except the mobilization is applied longitudinally along the soft tissues that border or attach to a bony surface (Fig. 2-14). A good example of this is longitudinal stroking of the anterior lateral border of the tibia in conditions such as shin splints. The connective tissues along the border of the tibia thicken and become adhered, and the therapist attempts to mobilize the tissues in this plane.

Cross-Friction

Cross-friction massage, which was developed and advocated by the late James Cyriax, is excellent for mobilizing scar tissue and nonvascular connective tissues. It is an aggressive form of soft tissue mobilization designed to break scar tissue adhesions and temporarily increase the blood flow to nonvascular areas. Ligaments and tendons struggling to heal completely are excellent candidates for cross-friction massage. This technique can be used on scar tissue as well, and it should be performed in many different angles to access fibers in all directions.

IMPORTANT MUSCLES BY REGION

Individual muscles can be grouped together according to their response to dysfunction. Typically, *postural* muscles (which can also be thought of as prime movers of the limbs and joints) respond to injury, abnormal stress, and surgery by tightening or becoming facilitated. *Phasic* muscles (which may also be thought of as stabilizers of joints) tend to respond to injury, abnormal stress, and surgery by weakening or becoming inhibited.[6]

Each joint complex in the body has groups of muscles that are dedicated to functioning as stabilizers and muscles that function as prime movers. For example, it is well known that the vastus medialis oblique (VMO) at the knee functions to stabilize the patella during knee flexion and extension. It is also well known that the VMO responds to dysfunction by weakening, becoming inhibited, and displaying atrophy. Conversely, the hamstring muscle group functions as a prime mover of the knee during locomotion, and it responds to dysfunction by tightening.[6]

During postsurgical rehabilitation, the therapist should expect to provide manual treatment for the postural muscles that act on the involved joint and strengthen (when healing constraints permit) the phasic muscles that have invariably weakened. A prime example is the shoulder after rotator cuff surgery. Initially, during the acute and protective phases of rehab, the therapist should treat latissimus dorsi, levator scapulae, trapezius, subscapularis, teres major, and pectoralis minor (all prime movers or postural muscles that act on the shoulder complex). After the patient enters into the active phase of rehab, efforts should be shifted to strengthening of the rotator cuff, lower traps, rhomboids, and serratus anterior (all phasic muscles that stabilize the shoulder complex).[6]

Tables 2-2 to 2-4 illustrate and summarize the groupings of postural and phasic muscles by region, and agonist-antagonist relationships.

SUMMARY

This chapter outlines the basic principles and guidelines for soft tissue management after surgery and discusses the stages of scar tissue formation.

The time frames for these stages are variable based on the vascularity of the tissues and the surgical procedure performed. They are delineated in more detail in the following chapters.

The physical therapist must understand connective tissue responses to immobilization, trauma, remobilization, and scar remodeling to treat injured tissues effectively. Awareness of these principles along with good physician-client communication ensures consistently effective management of postsurgical rehabilitation.

Table 2-2 Classification of Postural and Phasic Muscles of the Shoulder

Postural	Phasic
Upper traps	Lower traps/middle lower rhomboids
Levator scapulae	Latissimus dorsi
Pectoralis major	Middle traps
Pectoralis minor	Rhomboids
Subscapularis	Teres minor, infraspinatus, supraspinatus
Teres major	

(From Cantu R, Grodin A: *Myofascial manipulation: theory and clinical application*, Gaithersburg, MD, 1992, Aspen.)

Table 2-3 Classification of Postural and Phasic Muscles of the Hip

Postural	Phasic
Iliopsoas	Gluteus maximus
Tensor fasciae latae	Gluteus medius/minimus
Hip adductors	Hip external rotators
Hip internal rotators	

(From Cantu R, Grodin A: *Myofascial manipulation: theory and clinical application*, Gaithersburg, MD, 1992, Aspen.)

Table 2-4 Classification of Postural and Phasic Muscles of the Knee

Postural	Phasic
Hamstrings	Quadriceps (vastus medialis oblique [VMO])
Gastrocnemius	Dorsiflexors

(From Cantu R, Grodin A: *Myofascial manipulation: theory and clinical application*, Gaithersburg, MD, 1992, Aspen.)

References

1. Akeson WH, Amiel D: The connective tissue response to immobility: a study of the chondroitin 4 and 6 sulfate and dermatan sulfate changes in periarticular connective tissue of control and immobilized knees of dogs, *Clin Orthop* 51:190, 1967.
2. Akeson WH, Amiel D: Immobility effects of synovial joints: the pathomechanics of joint contracture, *Biorheology* 17:95, 1980.
3. Akeson WH et al: The connective tissue response to immobility: an accelerated aging response, *Exp Gerontol* 3:289, 1968.
4. Akeson WH et al: The connective tissue response to immobilization: biochemical changes in periarticular connective tissue of the rabbit knee, *Clin Orthop* 93:356, 1973.
5. Akeson WH et al: Collagen cross-linking alterations in the joint contractures: changes in the reducible cross-links in periarticular connective tissue after 9 weeks of immobilization, *Connect Tissue Res* 5:15, 1977.
6. Cantu R, Grodin A: *Myofascial manipulation: theory and clinical application*, Gaithersburg, MD, 1992, Aspen.
7. Copenhaver WM, Bunge RP, Bunge MB: *Bailey's textbook of histology,* Baltimore, MD, 1971, Williams & Wilkins.
8. Cummings GA: *Soft tissue contractures: clinical management continuing education seminar,* course notes, Atlanta, GA, March 1989, Georgia State University.
9. Cummings GS, Crutchfield CA, Barnes MR: *Orthopedic physical therapy series: soft tissue changes in contractures,* Atlanta, 1983, Stokesville Publishing.
10. Dicke E, Schliack H, Wolff A: *A manual of reflexive therapy of the connective tissue,* Scarsdale, NY, 1978, Sidney S. Simon.
11. Evans E et al: Experimental immobilization and mobilization of rat knee joints, *J Bone Joint Surg* 42A:737, 1960.
12. Flowers KR, Pheasant SD: The use of torque angle curves in the assessment of digital stiffness, *J Hand Therapy,* p. 69, Jan-March 1988.
13. Gelberman RH et al: Effects of early intermittent passive mobilization on healing canine flexor tendons, *J Hand Surg [Am]* 7(2):170-175, 1982.
14. Goldstein WM, Barmada R: Early mobilization of rabbit medial ligament and collateral ligament repairs: biomechanics and histological study, *Arch Phys Med Rehab* 65(5):239-242, 1984.
15. Gomez, MA et al: The effects of increased tension on healing medial collateral ligaments, *Acta Orthop Scand* 54(6):917-23. 1983.
16. Ham AW, Cormack DH: *Histology,* Philadelphia, 1979, JB Lippincott.
17. Hart DP, Dahners LE: Healing of the medial collateral ligament in rats. The effects of repair, motion, and secondary stabilizing ligaments, *J Bone Joint Surg Am* 69(8):1194-1199, 1987.
18. Inoue M et al: Effects of surgical treatment and immobilization on the healing of the medial collateral ligament: a long-term multidisciplinary study, *Connect Tissue Res* 25(1):13-26, 1990.
19. Lechner CT, Dahners LE: Healing of the medial collateral ligament in unstable rat knees, *Am J Sports Med* 19(5):508-512, 1991.
20. Mennell JB: *Physical treatment by movement, manipulation and massage,* ed 5, London, 1945, Churchill Livingstone.
21. Muneta T et al: Effects of postoperative immobilization on the reconstructed anterior cruciate ligament. An experimental study in rabbits, *Am J Sports Med* 21(2):305-313, 1993.
22. Piper TL, Whiteside LA: Early mobilization after knee ligament repair in dogs: an experimental study, *Clin Orthop Relat Res* Jul-Aug (150): 277-282, 1980.
23. Thornton GM, Shrive NG, Frank CB: Healing ligaments have decreased cyclic modulus compared to normal ligaments and immobilization further compromises healing ligament response to cyclic loading, *J Orthop Res* 21(4):716-722, 2003.
24. Sapega AA et al: Biophysical factors in range-of-motion exercise, *Phys Sportsmed* 9:57, 1981.
25. Warwick R, Williams PL: *Gray's anatomy,* ed 35, Philadelphia, 1973, WB Saunders.
26. Woo S et al: Connective tissue response to immobility, *Arthritis Rheum* 18:257, 1975.
27. Woo S et al: The biomechanical and morphological changes in the medial collateral ligament of the rabbit after immobilization and remobilization, *J Bone Joint Surg Am* 69(8):1200-1211, 1987.
28. Woo SL et al: New experimental procedures to evaluate the biomechanical properties of healing canine medial collateral ligaments, *J Orthop Res* 5(3):425-432. 1987.
29. Woo SL et al: Treatment of the medial collateral ligament injury. II: Structure and function of canine knees in response to differing treatment regimens, *Am J Sports Med* 15(1):22-29, 1987.

PART 2

UPPER EXTREMITY

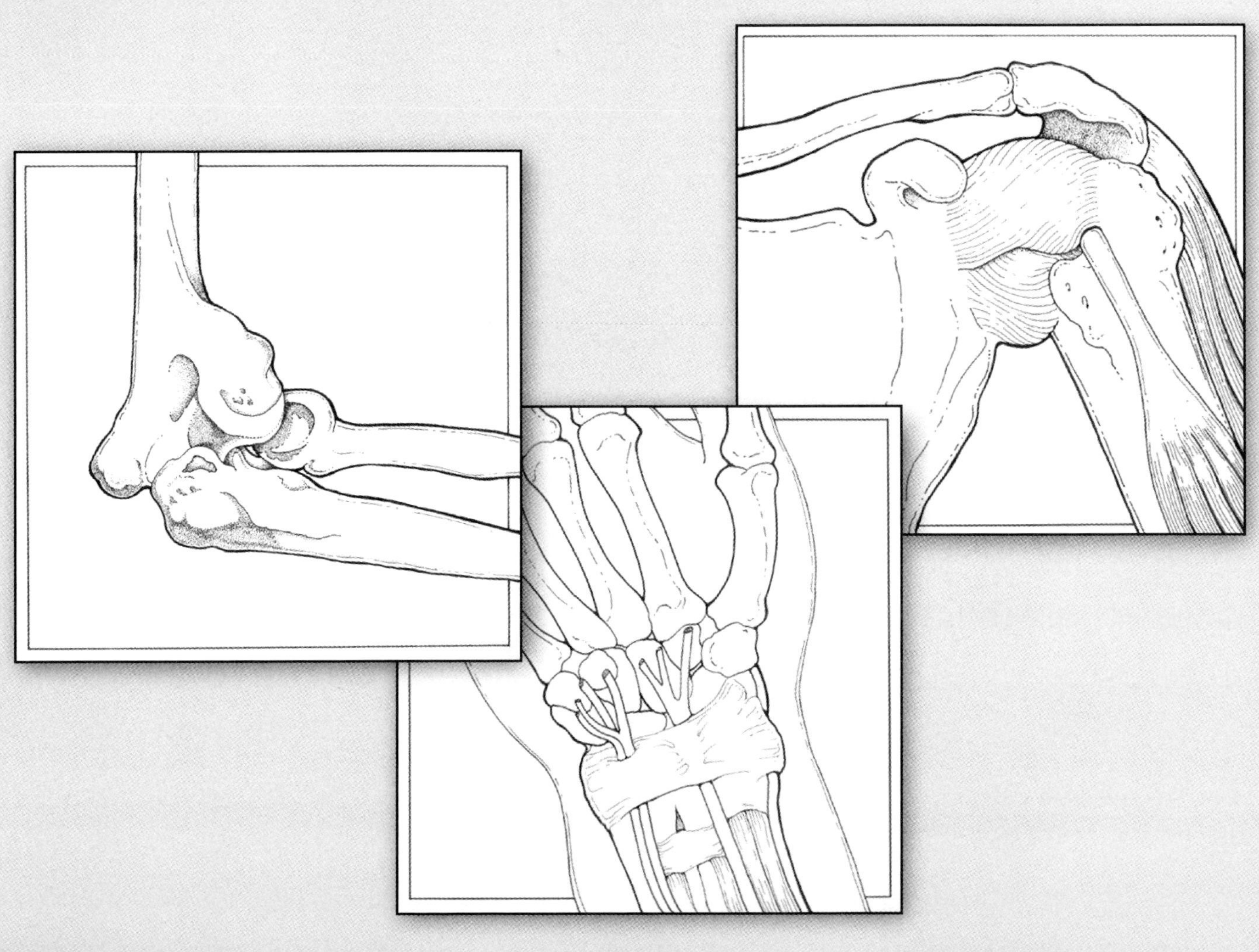

CHAPTER 3

Acromioplasty

Mark R. Phillips
Steven R. Tippett

Before the broad topic of acromioplasty is addressed, the topic of subacromial impingement syndrome must be explored. In 1972, Neer[47] described subacromial impingement as a distinct clinical entity in his landmark article. He correlated the anatomy of the subacromial space with the bony and soft tissue relationships and described the impingement zone. Neer[48] also described a continuum of three clinical and pathologic stages. This study provides a basis for understanding the impingement syndrome, which ranges from reversible inflammation to full-thickness rotator cuff tearing. The relationships among the anterior third of the acromion, coracoacromial ligament, and acromioclavicular (AC) joint and the underlying subacromial soft tissues, including the rotator cuff, remain the basis for most of the subsequent surgery-related impingement studies. Many other researchers have contributed to current knowledge of the subacromial shoulder impingement syndrome. The works of Meyer,[45] Codman,[15] Armstrong,[4] Diamond,[17] and McLaughlin and Asherman[44] provide a historical perspective.

SURGICAL INDICATIONS AND CONSIDERATIONS

Anatomic Etiologic Factors

Any abnormality that disrupts the intricate relationship within the subacromial space may lead to impingement. Both intrinsic (intratendinous) and extrinsic (extratendinous) factors have been implicated as etiologies of the impingement process. The role of muscle weakness within the rotator cuff has been described as leading to tension overload, humeral head elevation, and changes in the supraspinatus tendon, which is used most often in high-demand, repetitive overhead activities.[50,51] Authors[3,32,67] also have described inflammation and thickening of the bursal contents and their relationship to the impingement syndrome. Jobe[31] and Jobe, Kvitne, and Giangarra[32] studied the role of microtrauma and overuse in intrinsic tendonitis and glenohumeral instability and their implications for overhead-throwing athletes. Intrinsic degenerative tenopathy also has been discussed as an intrinsic cause of subacromial impingement symptoms.[54]

Extrinsic or extratendinous etiologic factors form the second broad category of causes of impingement syndrome. Rare secondary extrinsic factors (e.g., neurologic pathology secondary to cervical radiculopathy, supraspinatus nerve entrapment) are not discussed here, but the primary extrinsic factors and their anatomic relationships are of primary surgical concern. The unique anatomy of the shoulder joint sandwiches the soft tissue structures of the subacromial space (i.e., rotator cuff tendons, coracoacromial ligament, long head of biceps, bursa) between the overlying anterior acromion, AC joint, and coracoid process and the underlying greater tuberosity of the humeral head and the superior glenoid rim. Toivonen, Tuite, and Orwin[65] have supported Bigliani, Morrison, and April's description[8] of three primary acromial types and their correlation to impingement and full-thickness rotator cuff tears. AC degenerative joint disease also can be an extrinsic primary cause of impingement disease.[47,48] Many authors support Neer's original position on the contribution of AC degenerative joint disease to the impingement process.[35,70] The os acromiale, the unfused distal acromial epiphysis, also has been discussed as a separate entity and a potential etiologic factor related to impingement.[7] Glenohumeral instability is a secondary extrinsic cause or contribution to impingement. Its relationship to the impingement syndrome is poorly understood, but it helps explain the failure of acromioplasty in the subset of young, competitive, overhead-throwing athletes with a clinical impingement syndrome.[22,24,32]

Diagnosis and Evaluation of the Impingement Syndrome

History and physical examinations are crucial in diagnosing subacromial impingement syndrome. Findings may be subtle, and symptoms may overlap in the various differential diagnoses; therefore appreciating the impingement syndrome symptom complex may be difficult. The classic history has an insidious onset and a chronic component that develops over months, usually in a patient over 40 years old. The patient frequently describes repetitive activity during recreation, recreational sports, competitive athletics, and work. Pain is the most common symptom, especially pain with specific high-demand or repetitive away-from-the-chest and overhead shoulder activities. Night pain is seen later in impingement syndrome, after the inflammatory response has heightened. Weakness and stiffness may occur secondary to pain inhibition. If true weakness persists after the pain is eliminated, then the differential diagnoses of rotator cuff tearing or neurologic cervical entrapment type of pathologies must be addressed. If stiffness persists, then frozen shoulder–related conditions (e.g., adhesive capsulitis, inflammatory arthritis, degenerative joint disease) must be ruled out.[49] Younger athletic and throwing patients need continual assessment for glenohumeral instability.

The physical examination of a patient with impingement syndrome focuses on the shoulder and neck regions. Physical examination of the neck helps rule out cervical radiculopathy, degenerative joint disease, and other disorders of the neck contributing to referred pain complexes in the shoulder area. The shoulder evaluation includes a general inspection for muscle asymmetry or atrophy, with emphasis on the supraspinatus region. Range of motion (ROM) and muscle strength testing and generalized glenohumeral stability testing are emphasized during the evaluation. The Neer impingement sign[48] and Hawkins-Kennedy sign[27] are gold standard tests to help diagnose impingement. The impingement test, which includes subacromial injection of a Xylocaine type of compound and repeated impingement sign maneuvers, is most helpful in ascertaining the presence of an impingement syndrome. The AC joint also is addressed during the shoulder evaluation. The clinician should note AC joint pain with direct palpation and pain on horizontal adduction of the shoulder. Selective AC joint injection also may be helpful. Long head biceps tendon pathology, including ruptures, is rare but may occur in this subset of patients. Physical examination will define the tendon's contribution to the symptom complex. Instability testing, especially in the younger athletic patient, also should be performed. The clinician should assess for classic apprehension signs and perform the Jobe relocation test, recording any positive findings.

Radiographic Evaluation

Standard radiographic evaluation is carried out with special attention to anteroposterior (AP), 30-degree caudal tilt AP, and outlet views of the shoulder.[25,55] These plain studies are helpful in demonstrating acromial anatomy types, hypertrophic coracoacromial ligament spurring, AC joint osteoarthrosis, and calcific tendonitis. These views, in combination with an axillary view, can uncover os acromiale lesions. Magnetic resonance imaging (MRI) also is helpful in revealing relationships in impingement syndrome, especially if rotator cuff tear and other internal derangement pathologies (e.g., glenolabral or biceps tendon pathologies) are suspected.[6]

SURGICAL PROCEDURE

Subacromial impingement syndrome that has not responded to rehabilitation techniques and nonoperative means may require surgery. If proven trials of rehabilitation, activity modification, use of nonsteroidal anti-inflammatory agents (NSAIDs), and judicious use of subacromial cortisone injections are unsuccessful, then acromioplasty and subacromial decompression (SAD) should be considered.

Historically, open acromioplasties produced excellent results and still have a significant role in surgical treatment.[7,47,60] Ellman[20] is credited with the first significant arthroscopic SAD techniques and studies, and many surgeons and investigators have developed techniques and arthroscopic SAD advancements for the surgical treatment of subacromial impingement syndrome.[1,21,33,37,57,61] Indications for surgery to correct subacromial impingement syndrome include persistent pain and dysfunction that have failed to respond to nonsurgical treatment, including physician- or therapist-directed physical therapy, trials of NSAIDs, subacromial cortisone or lidocaine injections, and activity modification.

The most controversial surgical indication topic concerns the amount of time that should elapse before nonoperative management is considered a failure.[7] Most surgeons and investigators recommend a trial period of approximately 6 months. However, this depends on the individual patient and pathologic condition and should be tailored to the circumstances. For example, a 42-year-old patient with a history of several months of progressive symptoms has an occupation or recreational activity that requires high-demand, repetitive overhead movement. In the absence of instability, with a hooked acromion (type III) and MRI-documented, partial-thickness tearing, this patient need not endure the 6-month trial period to meet surgical indications for the treatment of his condition. On the other hand, a noncompliant patient in a worker's compensation–related situation who has a flat acromion and equivocal, inconsistent clinical findings may never meet the surgical indications.

Procedure

Both open acromioplasty and the arthroscopic SAD procedure are discussed in the following sections. Open acromioplasty techniques have been well documented, their outcomes have been well researched, and their results have been rated as very good to excellent in numerous studies.[1,5,21,47,60] Because of these factors and the high technical demands of arthroscopic decompression, surgeons should never completely abandon this proven technique for the surgical management of persistent shoulder impingement. Surgeons also may resort to these open techniques in the event of arthroscopic procedure failure or intraoperative difficulties. Depending on surgical experience and expertise, an open procedure may be used in deference to an arthroscopic SAD procedure.

Arthroscopic SAD for the surgical treatment of impingement syndrome has a number of advantages. First, the arthroscopic technique allows evaluation of the glenohumeral joint for associated labral, rotator cuff, and biceps pathology, as well as assessment of the AC joint and surgical treatment of any condition contributing to impingement. Second, this technique produces less postoperative morbidity and is relatively noninvasive, minimizing deltoid muscle fiber detachment. However, arthroscopic SAD is a technically demanding procedure with a learning curve that can be higher than for other orthopedic procedures.

Many different arthroscopic techniques have been described, but the authors of this chapter recommend the modified technique initially described by Caspari.[13] The patient is usually anesthetized with both a general and a scalene block regional anesthetic. In most community settings this combination has been highly successful in allowing patients to have this procedure done on an outpatient basis. A scalene regional block and home patient-controlled analgesia (PCA) provide acceptable pain control and ensure a comfortable postoperative course.

After the patient has reached the appropriate depth of anesthesia, the shoulder is evaluated in relationship to the contralateral side in both a supine and a semisitting beach chair position. Any concern regarding stability testing can be further assessed at this time, taking advantage of the complete anesthesia. Then, using the standard beach chair positioning, the surgeon begins the arthroscopic procedure. An inflow pressure pump (Davol) is used to maintain appropriate tissue space distention. Epinephrine is added to the irrigation solution to a concentration of 1 mg/L, thus enhancing hemostasis.

Specific portal placement is important to eliminate technical difficulties. Carefully addressing the palpable bony topography of the shoulder and marking the acromion, clavicle, AC joint, and coracoid process greatly facilitate portal placement (Fig. 3-1). First, the sulcus is palpated directly posterior to the AC joint. From this universal landmark, appropriate orientation can be obtained and consistent reproducible posterior, anterior, and lateral portal placement achieved.

Using the standard posterior portal, the surgeon inserts the arthroscope into the glenohumeral joint. In a routine and sequential fashion, the glenohumeral joint is evaluated with attention directed to the biceps tendon and the labral and rotator cuff anatomy. Any incidental pathology can be addressed arthroscopically at this point. Subacromial space arthroscopy can now be performed.

For subacromial procedures, a long diagnostic double-cannula arthroscope is recommended. The cannula with blunt trocar is placed from the posterior portal superior to the cuff, exiting the anterior portal.

Using this cannula as a switch stick equivalent, the surgeon places a cannula with a plastic diaphragm over the arthroscopic instrument and returns it to the subacromial space. Gently retracting the arthroscopic cannula and inserting the arthroscope allows the inflow and arthroscopic cannulas to be close together. Adequate distention and maintenance of inflow and outflow are crucial for visualization and indirect hemostasis. This technique has been successful in achieving these goals. At this point the lateral portal is fashioned, generally on the lateral aspect of the acromion just posterior and inferior to a line drawn by extending the topographic anatomy of the anterior AC complex (see Fig. 3-1). A spinal needle may assist in the accurate placement of this portal, which is crucial to instrument placement and subsequent visualization.

Starting from the posterior portal and using an aggressive synovial resector with the inflow in the anterior portal, the surgeon uses the lateral portal to perform a bursectomy and débride the soft tissues of the subacromial space. This is done in a sequential manner, working from the lateral bursal area to the anterior and medial AC regions. Spinal needles can be placed in the anterolateral and AC joint region to facilitate visualization and reveal spatial relationships. After the subacromial bursectomy and denudement of the undersurface of the acromion, the superior rotator cuff can be visualized along with the AC joint and anterior acromial anatomy is more easily defined. The surgeon must take care not to violate the coracoacromial ligament during this initial bursectomy procedure.

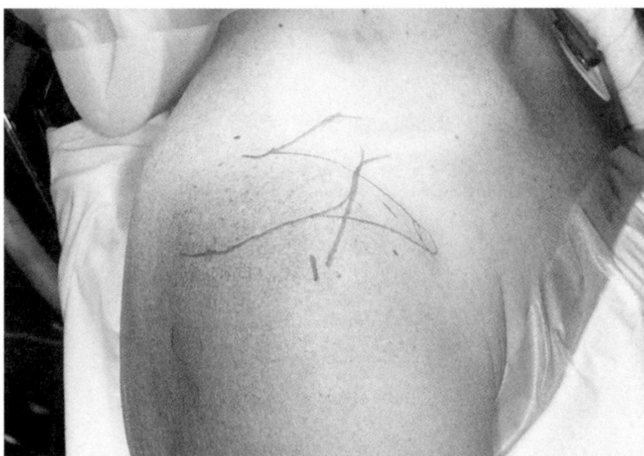

Fig. 3-1 The lateral portal is fashioned on the lateral aspect of the acromion just posterior and inferior to a line drawn by extending the topographic anatomy of the anterior acromioclavicular (AC) complex.

At this point the surgeon inserts the arthroscope in the lateral portal for visualization. Using the posterior portal and following the posterior slope of the normal acromion, the surgeon performs sequential acromioplasty with an acromionizer instrument. In the technique described by Caspari,[13] the shank of the acromionizer is directed flat against the posterior acromial slope and acromioplasty is completed from the posterior to the anterior aspect. This accomplishes two goals. First, it provides a reliable and reproducible template to convert any abnormal hooked, sloped, or curved acromion to the therapeutic goal of a flat, type I configuration. Second, it allows for the removal of the coracoacromial ligament from its bony attachment with minimal chance for coracoacromial artery bleeding, thereby maximizing arthroscopic visualization and minimizing technical difficulties. At this point any further modification or "fine tuning" may be done through both the lateral and the anterior portals. Any residual coraco-acromial ligament is removed from its acromial insertion while its bursal extension is excised.

The AC joint also may be assessed at this stage, and minimal inferior osteophytes may be excised. Depending on the results of the preoperative evaluation, distal clavicle procedures can be performed at this point either through directed arthroscopic techniques or, as the authors of this chapter prefer, through a small incision located over the AC joint region. If AC joint symptoms are present with horizontal adduction and direct palpation, if radiographs confirm the pathology, or if both occur, then the surgeon should proceed with a distal clavicle excision. A T-type capsular incision is located over the AC joint region, with the anterior and posterior capsular leaves elevated subperiosteally from the distal clavicle. Using small Homan retractors, the surgeon can excise the distal clavicle (usually 1.5 to 2 cm) with an oscillating saw. The distal clavicle can then be easily palpated and rasped smooth. With a simple digital confirmation, the undersurface of the acromion also can be checked and any residual osteophytes rasped through this minimal-incision technique.

The soft tissue is then closed in anatomic fashion with essentially no deltoid detachment. A routine subcuticular skin closure is used. The patient is placed in a post-operative pouch sling, and cryotherapy is frequently suggested. The patient is discharged to continue treatment as an outpatient; if insurance or health demands require it, overnight observation is used. Physical therapy may begin immediately on the first postoperative day and should follow the standard program discussed in this chapter.

Outcomes

The surgical outcomes for arthroscopic SAD, partial acromioplasties, and distal clavicle excisions[8,37,57] have been most favorable. Many studies have compared open and closed techniques and obtained similar overall findings.[5,7,23] SAD procedures have three general goals:

1. To return the patient to a premorbid ROM and strength perimeters
2. To eliminate pain
3. To eliminate the anatomic mechanical component of the impingement syndrome

Challenges and Precautions

The most common causes of surgical failures are associated with incomplete bone resection and not addressing AC joint arthropathy. By carefully considering surgical techniques and including (if necessary) distal clavicle excision or combined open techniques, these common pitfalls can be eliminated. Another common reason for failure of arthroscopic SAD surgery is inappropriate diagnosis or patient selection. Again, with careful assessment, especially regarding instability, underlying lesions, and differential diagnoses, these failures can be dramatically lessened.

Rehabilitation Concerns: The Surgeon's Perspective

Therapists spend more time with postoperative patients than most surgeons do, and their input and direction are important in achieving a successful outcome. Their understanding of the procedure, postoperative pain, patient apprehension, and general medical concerns is vital. Physical therapy–directed early diagnosis of any wound problems (evidenced by erythema) or superficial infection can eliminate potential major complications. Postoperative inflammation also can be assessed with careful observation. Stiffness in frozen shoulder syndrome, although rare, can develop postoperatively and is addressed optimally with early diagnosis and progressive physical therapy.

THERAPY GUIDELINES FOR REHABILITATION

The goal of the therapeutic exercise program after a SAD procedure is to augment the surgical decompression by increasing the subacromial space. Additional clearance for subacromial structures can be gained by strengthening the scapular upward rotators and humeral head depressors. Exercises to enhance the surgical decompression are straightforward.

The challenge for the physical therapist is to implement the appropriate therapeutic exercise regimen without overloading healing tissue.

The postoperative rehabilitation program can be divided into three phases:

Box 3-1 Components of the Physical Therapy Evaluation

Background information
- Status of capsule
- Status of rotator cuff
- Status of articular cartilage
- Previous procedures
- Associated medical problems that can influence rehabilitation (e.g., cardiovascular concerns, diabetes mellitus)
- Work-related injury
- Insurance status
- Motivation
- Comprehension

Subjective information
- Previous level of function
- Present level of function
- Patient's goals and expectations
- Intensity of pain
- Location of pain
- Frequency of pain
- Presence of night pain
- Assistance at home
- Access to rehabilitation facilities
- Medication (dose, effect, tolerance, compliance)

Objective information
- Observation:
  Muscle wasting
  Resting posture
  Use of sling
  Wound status
  Swelling
  Color
- Range of motion (ROM) (active/passive):
  Upper thoracic spine
  Scapulothoracic joint
  Sternoclavicular joint
  Acromioclavicular (AC) joint
  Scapulothoracic rhythm
- Strength

(Note: Strength testing should be delayed until safe and appropriate. Bicep testing could be performed earlier than the deltoid strength test. Care must be taken so that the recovering tissues are not compromised and irritated.)
  - Rotator cuff
  - Scapular upward rotators
  - Scapular retractors
  - Scapular protractors
  - Deltoid
  - Biceps

1. Phase one emphasizes *a return of ROM.*
2. Phase two stresses *regaining muscle strength.*
3. Phase three stresses *endurance and functional progression.*

These three phases are not distinct entities and they do overlap. Together they serve as a template on which the physical therapist can build a management protocol for the post-SAD patient. An absence of pain is the primary guideline for progressing to more strenuous activities.[12] The phases are simply guidelines and should be adapted to each patient. Patients with significant rotator cuff involvement, articular cartilage defects, significant preoperative motion or strength loss, perioperative or intraoperative complications, and glenohumeral instability require special consideration and may not progress as rapidly as indicated in the standard rehabilitation program, which assumes that no glenohumeral instability exists and that the rotator cuff tendons are intact.

Signs that therapeutic activities are too aggressive include the following:

- Increased levels of referred pain to the area of insertion of the deltoid
- Night pain
- Pain that lasts more than 2 hours after exercising[52]
- Pain that alters the performance of an activity or exercise[52]

Evaluation

Every rehabilitation program begins with a thorough evaluation at the initial physical therapy visit. This evaluation provides pertinent information for formulating a treatment program. As the patient progresses through the program, assessment is ongoing. Activities that are too stressful for healing tissue at one point are reassessed when the tissue is ready for the stress. Measures to be included in the physical therapy evaluation are provided in Box 3-1.

Phase I

TIME: First 2-3 weeks after surgery
GOALS: Emphasis on measures to control normal postoperative inflammation and pain, protect healing soft tissues, and minimize the effects of immobilization and activity restriction (Table 3-1)

Control of inflammation and pain

The surgeon may have prescribed NSAIDs to control normal postoperative inflammation and pain. These can be an adjunct to the other means the physical therapist uses to decrease inflammation (i.e., gentle therapeutic exercise, cryotherapy).

Table 3-1 Acromioplasty

Rehabilitation Phase	Criteria to Progress to this Phase	Anticipated Impairments and Functional Limitations	Intervention	Goal	Rationale
Phase Ia Postoperative 1-2 days	◆ Postoperative	◆ Pain ◆ Edema ◆ Dependent upper extremity (usually in a sling or airplane splint depending on degree of repair)	◆ Cryotherapy 20-30 minutes ◆ Monitoring of incision site ◆ Grip strength exercises (with arm elevated if swollen)	◆ Decrease pain ◆ Prevent infection ◆ Minimize wrist and hand weakness from disuse	◆ Self-manage pain and manage edema ◆ Prevent complications during healing ◆ Minimize disuse atrophy and promote circulation
Phase Ib Postoperative 3-10 days	◆ No wound drainage or presence of infection	◆ As in phase Ia	◆ Continue intervention as in Phase Ia with addition of the following: ◆ PROM of shoulder as indicated ◆ Isometrics—Submaximal to maximal internal and external rotation in sling or supported out of sling in neutral resting position ◆ AROM—Scapular retraction/protraction (position as with isometrics) ◆ Joint mobilization to the SC and AC joints as indicated	◆ Improve PROM avoiding aggravating surgical site ◆ Produce fair to good muscular contraction of rotators ◆ Restore/maintain scapula mobility ◆ Reduce pain/ joint stiffness	◆ Increase PROM preparing to advance AROM exercises ◆ Minimize reflex inhibition of rotator cuff ◆ Minimize disuse atrophy of scapula stabilizers ◆ Use low-grade (resistance free) mobilizations to decrease muscle guarding and progress grades as tolerated to restore arthrokinematics
Phase Ic Postoperative 11-14 days	◆ Comfortable out of sling ◆ No signs of infection or night pain	◆ Intermittent pain ◆ Limited upper extremity use with reaching/lifting activities ◆ Limited ROM ◆ Limited strength	Continue as in Phases Ia & Ib: ◆ AROM—External rotation (at 60- degrees to 90-degrees abduction) Supine flexion ◆ AROM—Supine scapular protraction (elbow extended) "punches" side-lying (midrange) external rotation with support (i.e., towel) in axilla Prone scapular retraction ◆ Pool therapy (with appropriate waterproof dressing if incision site not fully closed) ◆ Cardiovascular exercise (bike, walking program) ◆ Depending on job activities, return to limited work duties	◆ Flexion PROM to 150 degrees ◆ External/internal rotation PROM to functional levels (or full ROM) ◆ Scapulothoracic PROM to full mobility ◆ Supine AROM flexion to 120 degrees ◆ Symmetric AC/SC mobility ◆ Increase AROM tolerance in water to 100-degree flexion ◆ Minimize cardiovascular deconditioning ◆ Improve general muscular strength and endurance	◆ Increase capsular extensibility with flexion/elevation and rotation exercises ◆ Make rotator cuff ready for supine elevation ◆ Initiate strengthening of scapula stabilizers (proximal stability) ◆ Support axilla to allow for vascular supply to cuff during exercises ◆ Encourage AC/SC accessory motions required for full shoulder mobility ◆ Note that buoyant effects of water allow an environment where the water assists with flexion ◆ Prescribe lower-extremity conditioning exercises to promote healing and improve cardiovascular fitness ◆ Provide ergonomic education early to prevent future complications

PROM, Passive range of motion; *AROM,* active range of motion; *ROM,* range of motion; *SC,* sternoclavicular; *AC,* acromioclavicular.

The therapist should determine whether a scalene block was performed in addition to the general anesthetic. If a block was performed, then the onset of immediate postoperative pain may be delayed; the patient should be monitored for signs of delayed motor return and prolonged or abnormal hypesthesia. If narcotics are used past the first few postoperative days, then the therapist must undertake the therapeutic exercise program cautiously.

Cryotherapy can be used to help manage postoperative pain. Crushed ice conforms nicely to the shoulder, but commercially available cryotherapy and compression units (PolarCare, Cryocuff), although tedious to use, can be less messy. Sterile postoperative liners allow the source of the cold to be placed under the initial bulky dressing. The physical therapist should be aware of reimbursement practices for these units and use them accordingly.

Protection of Healing Soft Tissues

Decreased use of the upper extremity is required to protect healing soft tissues after SAD. Depending on the surgeon's protocol and operative findings, a sling may be prescribed. The sling helps decrease the forces on the supraspinatus tendon by centralizing the head of the humerus in the glenoid fossa in a dependent position. Use of the sling is encouraged for the first 2 to 3 days after surgery in most cases, with the patient's level of discomfort dictating the degree of sling use.

Although the sling is used to minimize pain, it can add to the patient's discomfort. A "critical zone" of hypovascularity in the supraspinatus tendon initially described by Rathbun and McNab[58] may contribute to shoulder pain in a resting-dependent position. Some authors debate the existence of this critical zone, but recent work by Lohr and Ulthoff[40] corroborates Rathbun and McNab's initial findings. This critical zone corresponds to the anastomoses between osseous vessels and vessels within the supraspinatus tendon. Vessels in this critical zone fill poorly when the arm is at the side,[48] but this wringing out of the supraspinatus tendon is not observed when the arm is abducted.[14] If the patient experiences increased shoulder discomfort after prolonged periods with the arm at the side, then he or she should place a small bolster (2 to 3 inches in diameter) in the axilla (resting the arm in a supported, slightly abducted position) to help decrease the pain.

Immobilization and Restricted Activities

Although the sling protects the healing tissue around the glenohumeral joint, motion should be encouraged at proximal and distal joints. Scapular protraction, retraction, and elevation can be performed in the sling. The patient should remove the arm from the sling at least three to four times daily to perform supported elbow, wrist, and hand ROM exercises.

The patient should always perform warm-up activities. This enhances the rate of muscular relaxation, increases the mechanical efficiency of muscle by decreasing viscous resistance, allows for greater hemoglobin and myoglobin dissociation in the time spent working, decreases resistance in the vascular bed, increases nerve conduction velocity, decreases the risk for electrocardiographic abnormalities, and increases metabolism.[71]

The physical therapist should educate the patient and help him or her to understand that discomfort experienced with passive stretching into external rotation comes from the capsule and occurs because the supraspinatus muscle is slack. Patients with sedentary occupations who do not have lifting duties typically can return to work during phase one. Those returning to work should perform scapular, elbow, wrist, and hand exercises during working hours.

> **Q** Carl arrives for therapy 5 weeks after a shoulder acromioplasty. He is having difficulty performing shoulder flexion and scaption exercises correctly. He occasionally demonstrates a mild shoulder hike with arm elevation exercises above 70 degrees of elevation. How can the therapist sequence his exercises to maximize his ability to elevate his arm above shoulder height?

Phase II

TIME: From 3 to at least 6 weeks after surgery
GOALS: Emphasis on muscle strengthening, with continued work on rotator cuff musculature and scapula stabilizer strengthening (Table 3-2)

Many of the exercises used to strengthen the rotator cuff and scapular stabilizers have been assessed by electromyography (EMG).[11] EMG (both superficial and fine wire) has been used to document electrical activity in the rotator cuff and intrascapular musculature during the performance of various therapeutic exercises. Strengthening of the rotator cuff muscles can be selectively progressed from supine active exercises to upright resistive exercises.[43] Muscles of the rotator cuff (especially the supraspinatus) have relatively small cross-sectional areas and short lever arms. When working with them, the therapist should apply minimal resistance, starting at 8 oz, then increase to 1 lb, and then advance in ½ or 1 lb increments as tolerated. Weights seldom have to exceed 3 to 5 lb for the supraspinatus. The infraspinatus and subscapularis can be stressed to a greater degree, and weights can be progressed from 5 to 8 lb. The therapist should emphasize scapular stabilizer efforts for proximal stability before addressing distal mobility.

Townsend, Jobe, and Pink[66] assessed the EMG output of three slips of deltoid, pectoralis major, latissimus dorsi, and the four rotator cuff muscles during 17 exercises. Findings from this study indicate that the majority of the muscles studied are most effectively recruited with the following:

Table 3-2 Acromioplasty

Rehabilitation Phase	Criteria to Progress to this Phase	Anticipated Impairments and Functional Limitations	Intervention	Goal	Rationale
Phase IIa Postoperative 3-6 weeks	◆ AROM to 120-degrees flexion ◆ AROM improving trend ◆ Gait with normal arm swing ◆ Strength of rotators to $\frac{4}{5}$ (MMT—$\frac{5}{5}$ normal) ◆ Self-manage pain	◆ Limited reach and lifting abilities, especially above shoulder height ◆ Limited strength and endurance of arm above shoulder height ◆ Limited AROM	Continue exercises from previous phases as indicated: ◆ PREs—Elastic tubing exercises for internal rotation and scapular retraction; at 3 weeks add external rotation and scapular protraction ◆ Isotonics—Side-lying external rotation (with axilla support) with $\frac{1}{2}$ to 1 lb ◆ Standing scaption with shoulder externally rotated ◆ Standing shoulder flexion with $\frac{1}{2}$ to 1 lb ◆ Elbow and wrist PREs with appropriate weight ◆ Assess lateral scapular slide	◆ PROM full in all ranges ◆ Symmetric AROM flexion ◆ Symmetric accessory motions of glenohumeral and SC/AC joints ◆ AROM flexion in standing to shoulder height without substitution from scapulothoracic region ◆ Symmetric strength scapula stabilizers and shoulder rotators	◆ Restore previous functional use and ROM of upper extremity ◆ Begin strengthening; internal rotators (subscapularis) usually not affected by surgery ◆ Initiate scapular retraction as long lever arm forces are minimal (versus protraction) ◆ Progress exercise to include external rotators and scapula protraction as tolerance to exercises improves ◆ Recognize that supraspinatus is secondary mover for straight plane external rotation ◆ Strengthen upper-quarter musculature ◆ Accompany gravity-resisted shoulder flexion and abduction by substitution with scapular elevation
Phase IIb Postoperative 6-8 weeks	◆ Gravity-resisted flexion and abduction without scapulothoracic substitution ◆ Symmetric strength of external rotators	◆ Unable to work overhead for prolonged periods of time ◆ Unable to participate in overhead-throwing athletics	◆ Continue with exercises from previous phases as indicated; maintain rotator cuff strength ◆ AROM PREs—Standing scaption with shoulder internal rotation (empty can); perform below 70-degrees scaption ◆ Prone or bent over horizontal abduction with shoulder at 100-degrees abduction ◆ Begin exercises unresisted, then add weight, beginning with $\frac{1}{2}$ lb ◆ Progress weight as indicated ◆ Initiate throwing program when able as outlined in Appendix A ◆ Begin gentle plyometrics	◆ Symmetric strength of supraspinatus and deltoid ◆ Restoration of normal arm strength ratios (involved/uninvolved) ◆ Return to previous levels of activities/sport as indicated by strength and tolerance ◆ Prevention of poor mechanics with throwing ◆ Preparation of upper extremity for advanced activities	◆ Continue to restore ROM and strength of upper-quarter musculature ◆ Strengthen supraspinatus as a prime mover ◆ Advance strength demand on the scapula stabilizers ◆ Progress resistance on a conservative basis ◆ Progress activity on a sequential basis

AROM, Active range of motion; *PREs,* progressive resistance exercises; *PROM,* passive range of motion; *ROM,* range of motion; *MMT,* manual muscle test ; *SC,* sternoclavicular; *AC,* acromioclavicular.

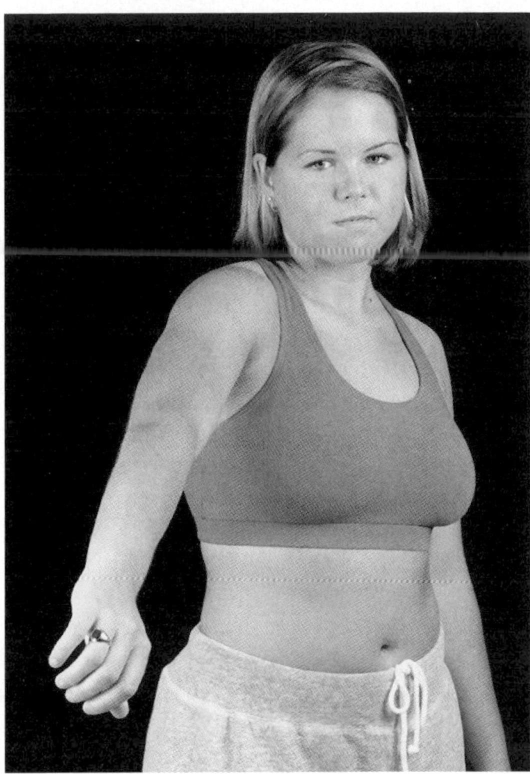

Fig. 3-2 Scaption with internal rotation should be performed below 90 degrees to prevent impinging subacromial structures.

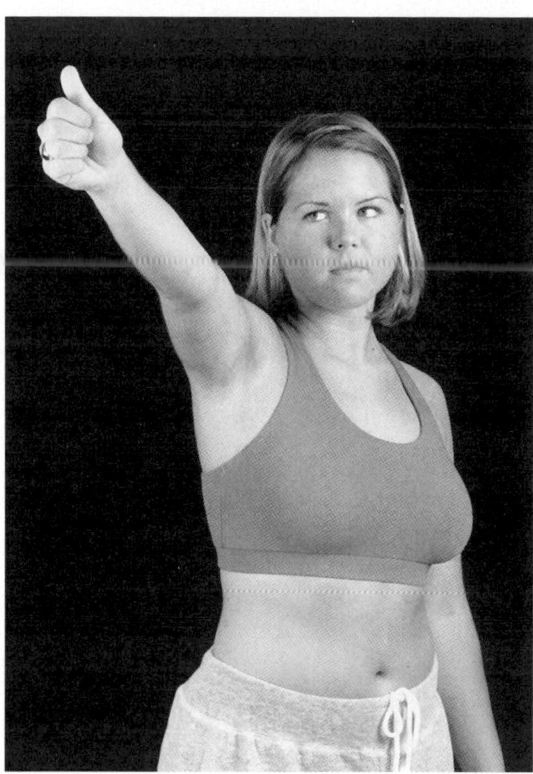

Fig. 3-3 Scaption with external rotation can safely be performed through full available range of motion (ROM).

- Scaption (with internal shoulder rotation)
- Flexion
- Horizontal abduction with external rotation
- Press-ups

Because the supraspinatus is the most frequently involved cuff muscle necessitating a subacromial decompression, diligent efforts to return supraspinatus strength are vital. The most effective exercise position to maximally recruit the supraspinatus has been evaluated in numerous studies with varying results. Elevation in the plane of the scapula (i.e., scaption) with the shoulder internally rotated is referred to as the *empty-can position* (Fig. 3-2). **To decrease the likelihood of compressing the supraspinatus between the greater tuberosity of the humerus and the subacromial structures, care should be taken never to perform the empty-can exercise past 60 to 70 degrees of elevation.** Scaption can also be performed with the humerus externally rotated (Fig. 3-3). Another position that is very effective in recruiting the supraspinatus is prone horizontal abduction of the shoulder with the shoulder abducted to 100 degrees (Fig. 3-4). Box 3-2 summarizes research findings relative to the most effective exercise position to recruit the supraspinatus.[9,30,34,42,59,62,74]

Although isolation of specific muscles is vital to ensure a comprehensive strengthening program, work with muscles contracting in synchrony about a joint also is an important consideration. Wilk[72] and Toivonen, Tuite, Orwin[65] note that in overhead activities the subscapularis is counterbalanced by the infraspinatus and teres minor in the transverse plane, whereas the deltoid is opposed by the infraspinatus and teres minor in the coronal plane. Because overhead movements are incorporated in the rehabilitation program, the physical therapist also should address the force couple of the upper and lower trapezius for scapular upward rotation.

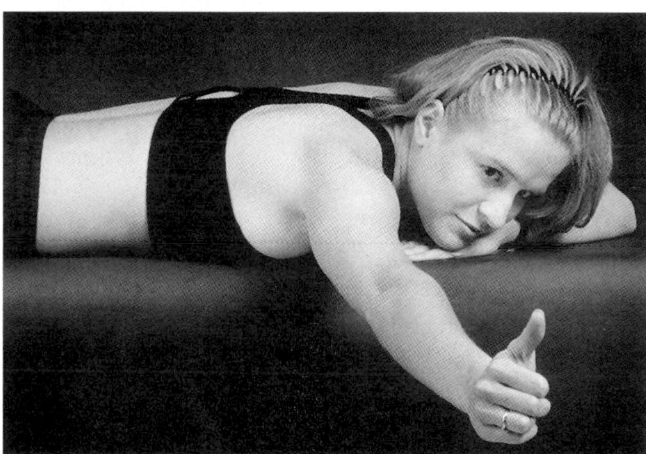

Fig. 3-4 Prone horizontal abduction with the humerus abducted to 100 degrees. The physical therapist should take care with patients with concomitant anterior glenohumeral instability.

Box 3-2 Supraspinatus Strengthening Exercises*

Jobe	EC
Blackburn	HA (100° abduction) > EC
Townsend	MP > EC
Worrell	HA (100° abduction) > EC
Malanga	EC = FC
Kelly	EC = FC
Takeda	EC = FC > HA
Reinold	HA (100° abduction) > ER

**EC,* Empty can; *FC,* full can; *HA,* horizontal abduction; *MP,* military press.

When strengthening the shoulder internal rotators, do not work with the patient in a side-lying position. Lying on the involved shoulder often increases shoulder pain; therefore internal rotation should be performed in the standing or prone position. When working on strengthening the supraspinatus and standing flexion and abduction in the same exercise session, perform the gravity-resisted elevation exercises before the strengthening ones. This sequence allows a nonfatigued supraspinatus to contribute effectively to achieve an adequate force couple.

A If the patient is going to be strengthening the supraspinatus and performing shoulder elevation exercises (i.e., shoulder flexion, abduction, or scaption exercises), he should perform the gravity-resisted elevation exercises first. The supraspinatus works more efficiently, without fatigue, to achieve an adequate force couple, thereby helping Carl to execute the elevation exercises correctly.

Q Drew is a 55-year-old plumber. He has a history of shoulder pain over the past 2 years and has a slouched posture. He had an acromioplasty performed 8 weeks ago. He still has minimal deficits with AROM for reaching overhead objects and cannot reach into his back pocket. On evaluation, Drew demonstrates near full PROM for shoulder flexion. PROM for IR and a combined movement of IR with shoulder extension is limited. What are some essential points to address and treatment techniques to use during Drew's treatment?

Exercise combinations can be used effectively to strengthen the muscles of the shoulder girdle. Wolf[73] describes a "four square" combination of tubing-resisted flexion, extension, external rotation, and IR followed by stretching of the external rotators and abductors. A combination of "around the world" exercises of flexion, abduction, and horizontal abduction followed by rotator cuff stretching also can be used during phase two. The physical therapist should use care when performing flexibility exercises of the rotator cuff because horizontal adduction can reproduce or cause impingement symptoms.

Strong scapular stabilizers are required to provide a stable base for the glenohumeral joint, elevate the acromion, and provide for retraction and protraction around the thoracic wall.[36] Moseley et al[46] studied eight scapular muscles via indwelling EMG and identified a core group of four strengthening exercises that include scaption with external rotation (i.e., full can), rowing, press-ups, and push-ups with a plus. Ludewig et al[41] found a push-up with a plus to be effective in recruiting the serratus anterior with less activity of the trapezius musculature. Lear and Gross[39] noted increased serratus anterior activity during a push-up with a plus with the feet elevated. Decker et al[16] noted push-ups with a plus (both traditional and on the knees), punching, scaption, and a dynamic hug all resulted in serratus anterior activity greater than 20% maximal voluntary contraction. Ekstrom, Donatelli, and Soderberg[19] found a seated shoulder diagonal movement of forward flexion, horizontal adduction, and external rotation to be most effective in recruiting the serratus anterior when compared with nine other open-chain exercises.

In addition to careful observation of scapulohumeral rhythm during overhead motions, scapular stabilizer efficiency can be assessed with the lateral scapular slide test. This test, which was initially described by Kibler,[36] involves observing and measuring scapular motion during abduction of the shoulder. The steps of the modified lateral scapular slide test are described in Box 3-3. The lateral scapular slide is a valid tool to assess scapular motion.[63] Kibler[36] described side-to-side differences of 1 cm as an indicator of scapulohumeral dysfunction. Other authors assessing the reliability of the lateral scapular slide, however, note that a 1 cm difference cannot be used as an indicator of dysfunction and that 1 cm can fall within intertester variability.[53]

Box 3-3 Modified Kibler's Lateral Scapular Slide Test*

1. Patient stands with the arms resting against the sides.
2. Therapist palpates the spinous process immediately between the inferior angles of the scapula (usually T-7).
3. Therapist measures and records the distance from the spinous process to each scapular inferior angle.
4. Patient abducts the arms to 90 degrees.
5. Patient internally rotates the shoulders so that the thumbs point to the floor.
6. Therapist measures and records the distance from the spinous processes to each scapular inferior angle.

*Normal test is symmetry between right and left sides.

A After correction of Drew's posture he was able to reach higher above his head. His slouched posture had previously restricted full active shoulder flexion. The shoulder capsule needs to be assessed immediately for restrictions. Emphasizing capsular mobilization of a restricted capsule allows for better joint arthrokinematics and increased ROM. The anterior, posterior, and inferior capsule were all restricted. General mobilizations were performed for all areas of the capsule, and specific mobilizations were performed for the anterior capsule. Drew then performed ROM and stretching to the shoulder, including stretches with the hand behind the back. A considerable increase in PROM and AROM for the hand behind the back was noted after this treatment.

Q Kelly had an acromioplasty on her right shoulder 6 weeks ago. She complains of a pinching pain when reaching above her head, through the last 20 degrees of shoulder flexion and abduction. She also has a pinching pain when actively reaching across her body in horizontal adduction. With PROM for horizontal adduction, shoulder flexion, and abduction, she has pain near the end of the ranges. What type of treatment may be helpful during her next session?

Continue ROM efforts during phase two, especially if limited capsular extensibility detrimentally affects physiologic motion. In addition to aggressive stretching exercises and mobilization of the glenohumeral joint, self-mobilizations also may be of benefit.[28] Patients with glenohumeral laxity also require special consideration as ROM and strengthening exercises progress. For patients with anterior instability, exercises should not stress extremes of horizontal abduction and external rotation. Posterior glenohumeral instability requires care with horizontal adduction and IR. Strengthening programs for patients with glenohumeral instability are best performed in the plane of the scapula.

A Kelly was treated with joint mobilizations to the glenohumeral joint as usual to increase shoulder flexion and shoulder abduction. AC mobilizations have been performed in the past, with the arm in anatomic position while the patient was supine. However, today AC mobilizations were performed with the shoulder in horizontal adduction and again with the shoulder in flexion above 140 degrees. An assistant was required to hold the extremity of the patient in place while the therapist performed the mobilizations. AROM for shoulder flexion, abduction, and horizontal adduction increased by 10 degrees of pain free motion. In addition, the complaints of pain intensity were less when experienced. After one more visit of the same treatment the patient exhibited full ROM.

Phase III

TIME: Weeks 9-12

GOALS: Emphasis on enhancing kinesthesia and joint position sense, building endurance, strengthening the scapular stabilizer, and performing work-specific and sport-specific tasks (Table 3-3)

After the patient has progressed through the first two phases, the obvious deficits resulting from surgery (i.e., pain, limited motion, decreased strength) have essentially been eliminated. Deficits in endurance and proprioception are not as readily apparent. Violation of the capsule, decreased use of the shoulder, and abnormal or restricted movement of the shoulder may decrease endurance and proprioception. One study[10] has demonstrated decreased proprioception in lax shoulders, with patients able to sense external rotation movements with greater ease than IR, especially at end range. Exercises to improve both passive detection of shoulder movement and active joint repositioning may help enhance kinesthesia and joint position sense, respectively. Voight et al[69] noted decreased glenohumeral joint proprioception with muscle fatigue of the rotator cuff.

Decreasing the weight used with strengthening exercises and increasing the repetitions address endurance training.

Table 3-3 Acromioplasty

Rehabilitation Phase	Criteria to Progress to this Phase	Anticipated Impairments and Functional Limitations	Intervention	Goal	Rationale
Phase III Postoperative 9-12 weeks	◆ Symmetric ROM and strength of upper quarter	◆ Decreased work- or sport-specific endurance	◆ Formal return to throwing and overhead activities	◆ Unrestricted Overhead work and sporting activity	◆ Create a specific training principle to return patient to desired activity

ROM, Range of motion.

Scapular stabilizer strengthening has been performed in sets of 30 repetitions to this point, and repetitions can be increased as required. Work- and sport-specific tasks should be used as guidelines to the number of prescribed repetitions. The supraspinatus tendon is the one most frequently involved in the injury, so it should be strengthened last.

The physical therapist also can address proprioception by having the patient perform functional tasks and emphasizing the timing of muscle contraction and movement without substitution. When rehabilitating overhead-throwing athletes, Pappas, Zawacki, and McCarthy[56] suggest timing muscle recruitment to correlate with the throwing sequence of active abduction, horizontal extension, and external rotation. Appropriate timing of muscle contraction also can be addressed using proprioceptive neuromuscular facilitation techniques.[38]

A functional progression program can be used to enhance the return of proprioception and endurance. Functional progression involves a series of sport- or work-specific basic movement patterns graduated according to the difficulty of the skill and the patient's tolerance. Providing a comprehensive functional progression program for every job or sport that a patient is involved in is impossible. Programs to return the patient to throwing, swimming, and tennis activities can be found in other sources.[2,64] Plyometric activities help restore endurance, proprioception, and muscle power.[26,68]

Q Cynthia had an acromioplasty on her right shoulder 5 days ago. She complains of moderate to severe pain intermittently throughout the day. She also has difficulty sleeping secondary to shoulder pain. She is a mother of young children. Patient uses arm for light activities of daily living (ADLs) when possible. ROM is limited in all directions. Strength is not tested secondary to healing tissues and pain levels. How did the therapist advise her and treat her for pain management?

SUGGESTED HOME MAINTENANCE FOR THE POSTSURGICAL PATIENT

The home maintenance box on page 44 outlines the shoulder rehabilitation the patient is to follow. The physical therapist can use it in customizing a patient-specific program.

Unlike more complex arthroscopic procedures or sophisticated open operative procedures, the need for structured clinic-based rehabilitation of the SAD patient should be the exception rather than the rule. Most of the rehabilitation for the patient after an uneventful SAD procedure can take place through a comprehensive home exercise program. Special cases may warrant a more formal and structured treatment program after the SAD procedure to detect problems. These special situations typically involve patients with the following conditions:

- Inadequate preoperative ROM
- Full-thickness rotator cuff pathology
- Biceps tendon or labral pathology
- Articular cartilage involvement
- Secondary "impingement"
- Tendency for excessive scarring
- History of regional complex pain syndrome or reflex sympathetic dystrophy (RSD)

A The therapist encouraged her to use a sling for a couple of days to prevent overuse of the healing extremity. She was told to use the sling when she was up and about for protection and for rest. Children as well as others would be less likely to bump or grab her arm. She was also encouraged to use cryotherapy intermittently throughout the day. The therapist advised her to try sleeping in a recliner chair or a semireclined position with her shoulder supported in a loose packed position. Treatment consisted of assessing the cervical area. Gentle mobilizations were done in the cervical area along with massage to the cervical and scapular musculature to decrease muscle guarding and spasms. Patient's pain level decreased slightly after the treatment. Pain began subsiding over the next couple days.

TROUBLESHOOTING

1. Scapulothoracic concerns. If the patient cannot perform gravity-resisted flexion or abduction without substituting with scapular elevation, then keep all efforts within the substitution-free ROM. Monitor scapular dynamic stability with the lateral scapular slide test. Because breakdown of the normal scapulothoracic muscle is more obvious with slow, controlled arm lowering, pay special attention to the eccentric component of gravity-resisted flexion and abduction.
2. Appropriate exercise dose. Dye[18] has described the *envelope of function,* which is defined as the range of load that can be applied across a joint in a given period without overloading it. The challenge is to stress the healing tissue to maximize functional collagen cross-linking without exceeding the envelope of function. As functional levels are increased, alter the therapeutic exercise dose. In cases of significant scapulothoracic dysfunction (long thoracic nerve neuropathy), scapulothoracic taping or figure-eight strapping may be used for additional stability.[29]

3. Monitoring for complications. Postoperative complications after SAD are rare, but the therapist must guard against RSD. Pain disproportionate to the patient's condition should be construed as RSD until proven otherwise. Institute aggressive ROM and pain control efforts daily. Prolonged (i.e., more than 3 weeks after surgery) loss of accessory joint motions may predispose the patient to adhesive capsulitis. Give treatments three times a week for mobilization and aggressive ROM.
4. Loading contractile tissue. Progressively load contractile tissue. Stress healing tissue initially as a secondary mover (receiving assistance from other muscles) before using the tissue in its role as a prime mover.
5. Prevention. As the old adage goes, an ounce of prevention is worth a pound of cure. Preventing early primary impingement symptoms from becoming chronic may eliminate the need for surgery. Nirschl[50] notes the following factors as keys in preventing chronic impingement syndrome: relief of inflammation, strengthening (especially the external rotators, abductors, and scapular stabilizers), flexibility (especially shoulder internal rotators and adductors), general fitness, education, and proper equipment.

SUMMARY

This chapter discusses the surgical procedure of SAD along with principles that govern postoperative rehabilitation. A surgeon with sound diagnostic, management, and surgical skills, along with a physical therapist with the expertise to advance the patient through the postoperative phase, typically produces a favorable result. Of even greater importance is the rapport established between surgeon and therapist and the relationship between the health care providers and the patient.

SUGGESTED HOME MAINTENANCE FOR THE POSTSURGICAL PATIENT

Week 1

GOAL FOR THE WEEK: Control pain and swelling and begin regaining range of motion (ROM) for joints.

Days 0-2: Perform grip strength exercises. Elevate your arm if it is swollen.

Days 3-7:

1. Do pendulum exercises for 2 minutes, 3 to 4 times each day.
2. Go through the active ROM for your elbow, wrist, and hand. Do three sets of 15 repetitions in all directions, 3 to 4 times each day.
3. Do internal and external rotation isometrics for 10 seconds each, with 10 repetitions 10 times each day.
4. Apply ice after you exercise.

Week 2

GOAL FOR THE WEEK: Prevent disuse atrophy.

Days 8-10: Continue your program from days 3 to 7 and add these exercises:

1. Active assisted supine flexion to tolerance. Do three sets of 15 repetitions, twice a day.
2. Supine scapular protraction at 90 degrees of flexion. Do three sets of 30 repetitions, twice a day.
3. Side-lying unresisted outward rotation to parallel with the floor. Do three sets of 15 repetitions twice a day.

Days 11-14: Discontinue the exercises you did on days 3 to 7 and only do the ones listed for days 8 to 10. Continue to apply ice after you exercise.

Week 3 (Only One Visit Required)

GOAL FOR THE WEEK: Prevent adhesive capsulitis and minimize disuse atrophy.

1. If passive ROM is not within normal limits and symmetrical, then institute organized outpatient treatment for mobilization. Schedule three times per week.
2. Begin tubing- or Theraband-resisted IR. Do three sets of 15 repetitions each twice a day.
3. Begin tubing- or Theraband-resisted scapular retraction exercises. Do three sets of 30 repetitions each twice a day.
4. Begin side-lying external rotation (support under arms) using 8 oz to 1 lb weights. Do three sets of 15 repetitions each twice a day.
5. Begin progressive resistance exercises (PREs) for elbow flexion and extension.
6. Assess lateral scapular slide.

Weeks 3-6 (Only One or Two Visits Required Over 3-Week Period)

GOAL FOR THE PERIOD: Supply added resistance for greater demand on scapular stabilizers.

1. Add tubing- or Theraband-resisted external rotation. Do three sets of 15 repetitions twice each day.
2. Do full ROM unresisted exercises for standing forward flexion and abduction. Begin PREs using 8 oz or 1 lb weights.
3. Continue IR as previously, but decrease to daily; then every other day.
4. Add gravity-resisted scaption with the shoulder externally rotated and unresisted. Do three sets of 15 repetitions twice each day.
5. Add tubing- or Theraband-resisted scapular protraction exercises. Do three sets of 30 repetitions twice each day.
6. Continue scapular retraction exercises as previously described.
7. Expand cardiovascular activities to include upper extremity use (e.g., using stair-climbing machine, rowing machine, upper body ergometer [UBE]).

Weeks 7-8

GOALS FOR THE PERIOD: Return to normal work or sports (with restricted activities as needed) and normal dominant-to-nondominant muscle strength ratios.

1. Add scaption with the shoulder internally rotated (use an empty can) at no greater than 70 degrees of abduction. Begin with unresisted exercises; then add weight beginning with 8 oz and progressing in 8 oz to 1 lb increments. Do three sets of 15 repetitions twice each day.
2. Add prone and bent over horizontal abduction with the shoulder at 100 degrees of abduction. Begin unresisted exercises in the middle range. Do three sets of 15 repetitions twice each day.
3. Begin return to throwing program (Appendix A).
4. Begin gentle plyometrics.

Weeks 9-12 (Only One or Two Visits Required Over 4 Weeks)

GOALS FOR THE PERIOD: Obtain ROM and muscle strength sufficient to reintroduce more aggressive occupational or sports demands.

1. Make formal return to throwing and overhead activities.

References

1. Altchek DW et al: Arthroscopic acromioplasty: technique and results, *J Bone Joint Surg Am* 72-A:1198, 1990.
2. Andrews JR, Whiteside JA, Wilk KE: Rehabilitation of throwing and racquet sport injuries. In Buschbachler RM, Braddom RL, editors: *Sports medicine and rehabilitation: a sport-specific approach*, Philadelphia, 1994, Hanley & Belfus.
3. Ark JW et al: Arthroscopic treatment of calcific tendinitis of the shoulder, *Arthroscopy* 8:183, 1992.
4. Armstrong JR: Excision of the acromion in treatment of the supraspinatus syndrome, report of ninety-five excisions, *J Bone Joint Surg Am* 31-B(3):436, 1949.
5. Basamania CJ, Wirth MA, Rockwood CA Jr: Treatment of rotator cuff tendonopathy by open techniques, *Sports Med Arthroscopy Rev* 3:68.
6. Beltran J: The use of magnetic resonance imaging about the shoulder, *J Shoulder Elbow Surg* 1:321, 1992.
7. Bigliani LU, Levine WN: Current concepts review. Subacromial impingement syndrome, *J Bone Joint Surg Am* 79-A(12):8154, 1997.
8. Bigliani LU, Morrison DS, April EW: The morphology of the acromion and its relationship to rotator cuff tears, *Orthop Trans* 10:228, 1986.
9. Blackburn TA et al: EMG analysis of posterior rotator cuff exercises, *J Athl Train* 25(1):40, 1980.
10. Blasier RB, Carpenter JE, Huston LJ: Shoulder proprioception: effect of joint laxity, joint position, and direction of motion, *Orthop Rev* 23(1):45, 1994.
11. Bradley JP, Tibone JE: Electromyographic analysis of muscle action about the shoulder, *Clin Sports Med* 15(4):789, 1991.
12. Buuck DA, Davidson MR: Rehabilitation of the athlete after shoulder arthroscopy, *Clin Sports Med* 15(4):655, 1996.
13. Caspari R: A technique for arthroscopic S.A.D., *Arthroscopy* 8(1):23, 1992.
14. Chansky HA, Ianotti JP: The vascularity of the rotator cuff, *Clin Sports Med* 10(4):807, 1991.
15. Codman EA: Rupture of the supraspinatus tendon and other lesions in or about the subacromial bursa. In Codman EA, editor: *The shoulder,* Boston, 1934, Thomas Todd.
16. Decker MJ et al: Serratus anterior muscle activity during selected rehabilitation exercises, *Am J Sports Med* 27(6):784, 1999.
17. Diamond B: *The obstructing acromion: underlying diseases, clinical development and surgery,* Springfield, IL, 1964, Charles C. Thomas.
18. Dye SF: The knee as a biologic transmission with an envelope of function: a theory, *Clin Orthop* 323:10, 1996.
19. Ekstrom RA, Donatelli RA, Soderberg GL: Surface electromyographic analysis of exercises for the trapezius and serratus anterior muscles, *J Orthop Sports Phys Ther* 33(5):247, 2003.
20. Ellman H: Arthroscopic subacromial decompression: analysis of one-to three-year results, *Arthroscopy* 3:173, 1987.
21. Esch JC et al: Arthroscopic subacromial decompression: results according to the degree of rotator cuff tear, *Arthroscopy* 4:241, 1988.
22. Fu FH, Harner CD, Klein AH: Shoulder impingement syndrome. A critical review, *Clin Orthop* 269:162, 1991.
23. Gartsman GM et al: Arthroscopic subacromial decompression. An anatomical study, *Am J Sports Med* 16:48, 1988.
24. Glousman RE: Instability versus impingement syndrome in the throwing athlete, *Orthop Clin North Am* 24:89, 1993.
25. Gold RH, Seeger LL, Yao L: Imaging shoulder impingement, *Skeletal Radiol* 22:555, 1993.
26. Goldstein TS: *Functional rehabilitation in orthopaedics,* Gaithersburg, MD, 1995, Aspen.
27. Hawkins RJ, Kennedy JC: Impingement syndrome in athletes, *Am J Sports Med* 8:151,1980.
28. Hertling D, Kessler RM: The shoulder and shoulder girdle. In Hertling D, Kessler RM, editors: *Management of common musculoskeletal disorders: physical therapy principles and methods,* ed 3, Philadelphia, 1996, Lippincott.
29. Host HH: Scapular taping in the treatment of anterior shoulder impingement, *Phys Ther* 75(9):803, 1995.
30. Jobe FW, Moynes DR: Delineation of diagnostic criteria and a rehabilitation program for rotator cuff injuries, *Am J Sports Med* 10:336, 1982.
31. Jobe FW: Impingement problems in the athlete. In Nicholas JA, Hershmann EB, editors: *The upper extremity in sports medicine,* St Louis, 1990, Mosby.
32. Jobe FW, Kvitne RS, Giangarra CE: Shoulder pain in the overhand or throwing athlete. The relationship of anterior instability and rotator cuff impingement, *Orthop Rev* 18:963, 1989.
33. Johnson LL: *Diagnostic and surgical arthroscopy of the shoulder,* St Louis, 1993, Mosby.
34. Kelly BT, Kadrmas WR, Speer KP: The manual muscle examination for rotator cuff strength: an electromyographic investigation, *Am J Sports Med* 24:581, 1996.
35. Kessel L, Watson M: The painful arc syndrome. Clinical classification as a guide to management, *J Bone Joint Surg Am* 59-B(2):166, 1977.
36. Kibler WB: The role of the scapula in the overhead throwing motion, *Contemp Orthop* 22(5):525, 1991.
37. Kuhn JE, Hawkins RJ: Arthroscopically assisted techniques in diagnosis and treatment of rotator cuff tendonopathy, *Sports Med Arthroscopy Rev* 3:60, 1995.
38. Lephart SM, Kocher MS: The role of exercise in the prevention of shoulder disorders. In Matsen FA, Fu FH, Hawkins RJ, editors: *The shoulder: a balance of mobility and stability,* Rosemont, IL, 1992, American Academy of Orthopaedic Surgeons.
39. Lear LJ, Gross MT: An electromographical study of the scapular stabilizing synergists during a push-up progression, *J Orthop Sports Phys Ther* 28(3):146, 1998.
40. Lohr JF, Ultoff HK: The microvascular pattern of the supraspinatus tendon, *Clin Orthop* 254:35, 1990.
41. Ludewig PM et al: Relative balance of serratus anterior and upper trapezius muscle activity during push-up exercises, *Am J Sports Med* 32(2):484, 2004.
42. Malanga GA et al: EMG analysis of shoulder positioning in testing and strengthening of the supraspinatus, *Med Sci Sports Exerc* 28:661, 1996.
43. McCann PD, Wooten ME, Kadaba MP: A kinematic and electromyographic study of shoulder rehabilitation exercises, *Clin Orthop* 288:179, 1993.

44. McLaughlin HL, Asherman EG: Lesions of the musculotendinous cuff of the shoulder. IV. Some observations based upon the results of surgical repair, *J Bone Joint Surg Am* 33-A:76, 1951.
45. Meyer AW: The minute anatomy of attrition lesions, *J Bone Joint Surg Am* 13:341, 1931.
46. Moseley JB et al: EMG analysis of the scapular muscles during a shoulder rehabilitation program, *Am J Sports Med* 20(2):128, 1992.
47. Neer CS II: Anterior acromioplasty for the chronic impingement syndrome in the shoulder. A preliminary report, *J Bone Joint Surg Am* 54-A:41, 1972.
48. Neer CS II: Impingement lesions, *Clin Orthop* 173:70, 1983.
49. Nevaiser RJ, Nevaiser TJ: Observations on impingement, *Clin Orthop* 254:60, 1990.
50. Nirschl RP: Rotator cuff tendinitis: basic concepts of patho-etiology. In The American Academy of Orthopedic Surgeons, editors: *Instructional course lectures,* vol 38, Park Ridge, IL, 1989, The American Academy of Orthopedic Surgeons.
51. Nirschl RP: Rotator cuff tendinitis: basic concepts of patho-etiology. In Nicholas JA, Hershman EB, editors: *The upper extremity in sports medicine,* St Louis, 1990, Mosby.
52. O'Connor FG, Sobel JR, Nirschl RP: Five-step treatment for overuse injuries, *Phys Sportsmed* 20(10)128, 1992.
53. Odom CJ, Hurd CE, Denegar CR: Intratester and intertester reliability of the lateral scapular slide test and its ability to predict shoulder pathology, J *Athl Train* 30(2):S-9, 1995.
54. Ogata S, Uhthoff HK: Acromial enthesopathy and rotator cuff tear. A radiologic and histologic postmortem investigation of the coracoacromial arch, *Clin Orthop* 254:39, 1990.
55. Ono K, Yamamuro T, Rockwood CA: Use of a thirty-degree caudal tilt radiograph in the shoulder impingement syndrome, *J Shoulder Elbow Surg* 1:246, 1992.
56. Pappas AM, Zawacki RM, McCarthy CF: Rehabilitation of the pitching shoulder, *Am J Sports Med* 13(4)223, 1985.
57. Paulos LE, Franklin JC: Arthroscopic S.A.D. Development and application: a 5 year experience, *Am J Sports Med* 18:235, 1990.
58. Rathbun JB, McNab I: The microvascular pattern of the rotator cuff, *J Bone Joint Surg Am* 52B:540, 1970.
59. Reinold MM et al: Electromyographic analysis of the rotator cuff and deltoid musculature during common shoulder external rotation exercises, *J Orthop Sports Phys Ther* 34(7): 385, 2004.
60. Rockwood CA Jr, Lyons FR: Shoulder impingement syndrome: diagnosis, radiographic evaluation, and treatment with a modified Neer acromioplasty, *J Bone Joint Surg Am* 75-A:409, 1993.
61. Snyder SJ: A complete system for arthroscopy and bursoscopy of the shoulder, *Surg Rounds Orthop* p 57, July 1989.
62. Takeda Y et al: The most effective exercise for strengthening the supraspinatus muscle: evaluation by magnetic resonance imaging, *Am J Sports Med* 30(3)374, 2002.
63. Tippett SR, Kleiner DM: Objectivity and validity of the lateral scapular slide test, *Athletic Training* 31(2):S-40, 1996.
64. Tippett SR, Voight ML: *Functional progressions for sport rehabilitation,* Champaign, IL, 1995, Human Kinetics.
65. Toivonen DA, Tuite MJ, Orwin JF: Acromial structure and tears of the rotator cuff, *J Shoulder Elbow Surg* 4:376, 1995.
66. Townsend H, Jobe FW, Pink M: Electromyographic analysis of the glenohumeral muscles during a baseball rehabilitation program, *Am J Sports Med* 19(3):264, 1991.
67. Uhthoff HK et al: The role of the coracoacromial ligament in the impingement syndrome. A clinical, radiological and histological study, *Int Orthop* 12:97, 1988.
68. Voight ML, Draovitch P, Tippett SR: Plyometrics. In Albert M, editor: *Eccentric muscle training in sports and orthopaedics,* ed 2, New York, 1995, Churchill Livingstone.
69. Voight ML et al: The effects of muscle fatigue and the relationship of arm dominance to shoulder proprioception, *J Orthop Sports Phys Ther* 23(6):348, 1996.
70. Watson M: The refractory painful arc syndrome, *J Bone Joint Surg* 60-B(4):544, 1978.
71. Wenger HA, McFayeden R: Physiological principles of conditioning. In Zachazewski JE, Magee DJ, Quillen WS, editors: *Athletic injuries and rehabilitation,* Philadelphia, 1996, WB Saunders.
72. Wilk KE: The shoulder. In Malone TR, McPoil T, Nitz AJ, editors: *Orthopaedic and sports physical therapy,* ed 3, St Louis, 1997, Mosby.
73. Wolf WB: Shoulder tendinoses, *Clin Sports Med* 11(4):871, 1992.
74. Worrell TW, Corey BJ, York SL: An analysis of supraspinatus EMG activity and shoulder isometric force development, *Med Sci Sports Exerc* 24(7):744, 1992.

CHAPTER 4

Anterior Capsular Reconstruction

Frank W. Jobe
Diane R. Schwab
Clive E. Brewster

Although it often goes undiagnosed, shoulder instability is the cause of shoulder pain in many patients.[1,2] The frequency of instability causing shoulder pain increases with the activity level of the patient and decreases somewhat with age. It is more likely in younger, more active patients—especially if they engage in overhead activities during vocational or recreational pursuits.[3] Understanding of the kinetics and root causes of shoulder pain is increasing; both factors must be addressed to redress the problem.

SURGICAL INDICATIONS AND CONSIDERATIONS

Shoulder instability is not an isolated diagnosis, but rather one point on a continuum of pathology. It is often associated with impingement of either the "inside" or "outside" type and can be found in patients of all ages and activity levels. Group I patients are generally older; shoulder instability is seldom found in younger patients. A subset of this group also experiences impingement of the undersurface of the rotator cuff (Fig. 4-1).

Group II patients are usually younger than group I patients. They have instability and impingement, but their impingement is secondary to repetitive trauma. These patients are often engaged in overhead athletic sports. On clinical evaluation, both relocation and impingement signs are usually positive. Under anesthesia, the pass-through sign is seen and excessive anterior translation of the humeral head is often evident. Both the anterior inferior capsule and the posterior superior labrum show signs of repetitive trauma; a bare spot also may be seen on the posterior aspect of the humeral head. Other common findings are a tear on the undersurface of the supraspinatus or infraspinatus and laxity in the glenohumeral (GH) ligaments, especially in external rotation.

Young patients with generalized ligamentous laxity fall into group III. They too have a positive relocation test and internal impingement. Finally, group IV patients suffer from instability (usually subluxation, rarely dislocation) resulting from a traumatic episode. These patients show no evidence of impingement. They can have a positive relocation sign but seldom a positive apprehension sign. Under arthroscopic examination a Bankart lesion, and occasionally cartilaginous erosion of the posterior humeral head, may be noted.

Younger, more active patients with shoulder pain and signs of impingement can fall into any of the four groups. Their activity demands test the limits of strength and endurance of their shoulders. If either is insufficient, then brief episodes of anterior instability follow. Associated tightness of the posterior capsule can contribute another force vector driving the humeral head forward. The humeral head, now riding anterior and superior, causes posterior impingement and labral pathology. If left unchecked, then the impingement can lead to a frank tear of the supraspinatus portion of the rotator cuff.

Some patients have signs of impingement or a diagnosis of rotator cuff tendonitis, bursitis, bicipital tendonitis, or arthritis and have been referred by an occupational medicine clinic or a gatekeeper in a managed-care office. These patients have persistent pain and limitation of activity despite a course of care that may have included nonsteroidal anti-inflammatory drugs (NSAIDs), other modalities (e.g., heat, ice, ultrasound, electrical stimulation), mobilization, exercise, and rest. They may have some temporary symptom relief but no lasting change in underlying difficulties. Some of these patients have subacromial decompression. Even after surgery they may report either no improvement or that the condition is worse than before the surgery.

All shoulder pain is not caused by anterior instability. Sometimes, the presence of a superior labral anteroposterior (SLAP) lesion complicates the clinical picture. Investigative arthroscopy may be necessary to determine the correct diagnosis if a conservative care program is not successful. Sometimes patients report relief of symptoms

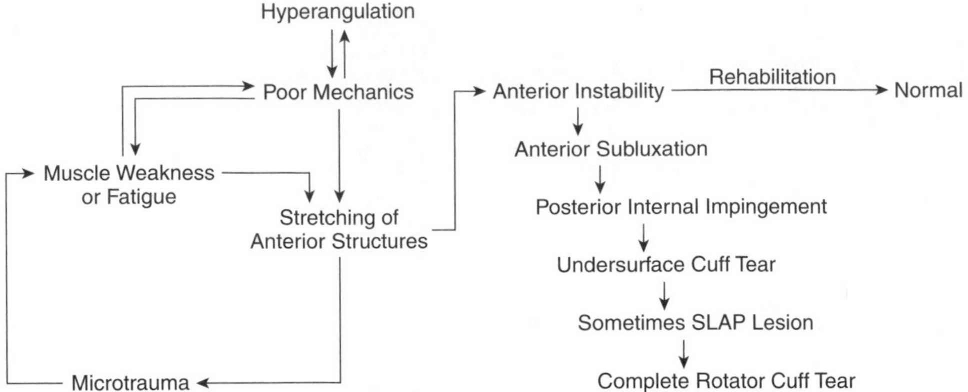

Fig. 4-1 Instability continuum.

after rehabilitation. Because they have a normal shoulder under examination, they may return to normal activities too early and consequently report recurring pain and difficulty. In these instances the therapist should determine whether faulty mechanics in their activities of choice is the culprit. It does not matter how well the patient's shoulder is rehabilitated if the offending stimulus is repeated.

However, when the diagnosis of anterior shoulder instability is the correct one and is made early during the pathologic course, as many as 95% of patients can return to their previous level of competition.[3] The later the diagnosis is made during the pathologic course, the lower the percentage of successful return with only conservative treatment. For any of these patients to return to their previous activities, the appropriate exercise program must be prescribed, supervised, and performed. While following this program the authors of this chapter have not needed to use mobilizations, massage, or modalities other than ice. The core group of exercises protects the anterior shoulder, strengthens the rotator cuff, and emphasizes the scapular muscles. Details of these exercises follow. Performing them only once or twice a week is futile. Performing them incorrectly is not beneficial and may even be harmful. Persistence and attention to detail are both essential to a successful outcome—the elimination of pain and a return to full activity without surgical intervention.

During this era of cost containment and rationed services, some may feel that this emphasis on supervision and performance detail is an unnecessary expenditure of medical dollars. However, by providing effective rehabilitation, the physical therapist can relieve pain and restore function, saving medical dollars in the long run. If the therapist and patient are willing to accept lesser goals, then less attention to rehabilitative detail will have to suffice.

When dysfunction persists despite the best efforts of orthopedist, therapist, and patient, an anterior capsulolabral reconstruction (ACLR) is the procedure most likely to eliminate pain while permitting the range of motion (ROM) and strength needed for premorbid performance.[4,5]

Traditionally, surgeons and therapists believed that any procedure that restabilized the shoulder (i.e., kept it from slipping out the front) would improve the patient's condition. Rehabilitation was prolonged and arduous after some of the more common procedures (e.g., Bankart repair, modified Bristow repair). Patients were managed with extended immobilization for weeks or months depending on the surgeon and the procedure. Full motion was seldom regained after surgery. Stability was re-established but at the expense of flexibility; patients were never able to perform at the preoperative level again.

SURGICAL PROCEDURE

Open Procedure

In the ACLR, an axillary incision is made 2 to 3 cm distal and lateral to the coracoid process and extending distally into the anterior axillary crease. The skin is undermined to provide access to the deltoid groove and allow visualization of the deltopectoral groove. This interval is then developed with blunt and sharp dissection. The clavipectoral fascia is incised along the lateral margin of the conjoined tendon from the inferior margin of the humeral head to the coracoid process. The surgeon dissects laterally to the fleshy portion of the coracobrachialis muscle, rather than medially at the lateral border of the tendinous short head of the biceps. The conjoined tendon is dissected bluntly and retraced medially.

External rotation of the arm brings the subscapularis into view. It is split longitudinally between the upper two thirds and lower third. After identifying the interval between the subscapularis and the capsule, the surgeon extends capsular exposure medially and laterally. The retractor should be placed under direct vision to avoid injury to neurovascular structures. The capsule is incised longitudinally, and tag sutures are placed at the capsule margin just lateral to the labrum. The capsulotomy may be completed carefully down to the level of the glenoid labrum.

The glenoid labrum should be palpated carefully to assess for the presence of a Bankart lesion. The capsule must be palpated for integrity, volume, and ability to buttress the anterior inferior joint margin. The degree of capsular shift must be tailored to the degree of laxity. If a Bankart lesion is present, then it is repaired by suture fixation to the prepared anterior scapular neck with Mitek bone anchors.

If the capsule is lax or incompetent, it is overlapped to obliterate the redundancy. The surgeon incises it down to the labrum and medial glenoid neck for subperiosteal elevation. The inferior leaf of the capsule contains most of the inferior GH ligament and is used to reconstruct it by advancing the tissue along the anterior glenoid rim and shifting it proximally. The superior portion of the capsule is brought over the inferior portion and labrum, resting along the anterior scapular neck. The reconstruction is fixed using No. 2 nonabsorbable sutures from the Mitek bone anchors. The inferior leaf is secured superiorly (Fig. 4-2), and the superior leaf is secured inferiorly (Fig. 4-3) using a vest-over-pants technique with non-absorbable sutures. If the labrum is intact, then it does not require removal and repair. The surgeon can simply split the capsule and overlap it, thereby reducing the volume of the joint.

The anterior glenoid labrum may be absent or defective. In this case or in the presence of a Bankart lesion, the capsule must be affixed to the prepared anterior scapular neck. Usually, both a capsular shift and a reattachment must be performed.

After the capsule is closed, the surgeon takes the arm through a ROM to note areas of tension on the repair. Immediately after surgery, the patient may begin active motion within this zone. The surgeon must communicate with the therapist for each patient to ensure that this safe zone is observed. Usually, avoiding abduction above 90 degrees in the scapular plane and external rotation beyond 45 degrees to 90 degrees is indicated. The palmaris longus may be used as a further capsular reinforcement in patients with hyperelasticity.

After determining safe postoperative motion, the surgeon reapproximates the subscapularis. All retractors are removed after a thorough irrigation of the operative field. Neither the deltoid nor the pectoralis muscles normally require surgical repair, and the skin is closed subcuticularly, with the addition of adhesive strips (Steri-Strips). The arm is splinted in abduction and external rotation. The splint may be removed for bathing and postoperative ROM assessment. If the patient has generalized ligamentous laxity, then no splint is necessary (motion will be easy to reacquire).

Arthroscopic Surgical Procedure

As minimally invasive surgical skills have improved, arthroscopic ACLR has gained recognition as a viable treatment method for anterior shoulder instability. Collective experience over the past two decades has refined knowledge of patient selection, operative technique, and postoperative rehabilitation to improve the outcome so that, for the general patient population, recent reports of arthroscopic stabilization have shown success rates comparable to those of open techniques.

For the throwing athlete, whose shoulder is subjected to tremendous torque, motion, and stress, the open ACLR currently is still our gold standard of treatment for anterior

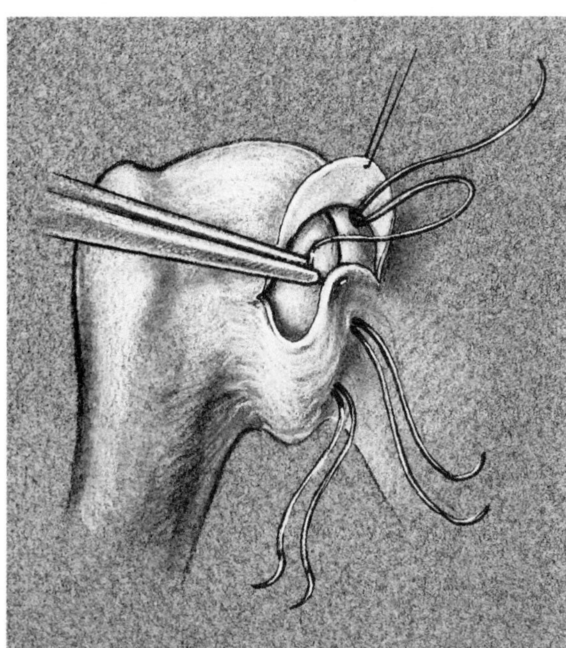

Fig. 4-2 The inferior lead is secured superiorly.

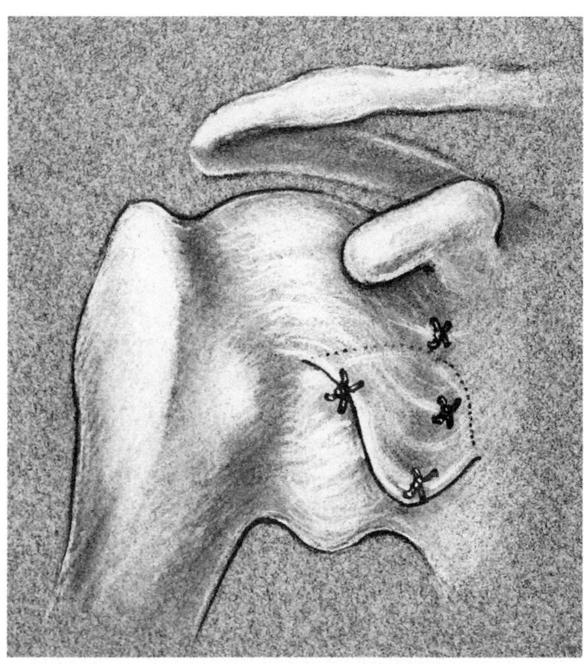

Fig. 4-3 The superior lead is secured inferiorly.

shoulder instability. It remains difficult to achieve the exacting degree of anterior tightness and rotation by operating through the arthroscope. It also remains to be seen whether GH stability can be achieved in a pitcher's shoulder with proximal tissue imbrication through a row of sutures and anchors along the anterior-inferior glenoid rim, without incision, flap creation, and a true shift of the capsulolabral structures. Although some surgeons treat these patients with the arthroscope, the authors still prefer to treat this one subset of patients with the open version of the procedure. In the hands of an experienced surgeon, other patients can be corrected adequately with the arthroscopic variation. In the future, as experience develops, the arthroscopic technique may demonstrate effectiveness similar to the open technique for the throwing athlete patient subset.

The rehabilitation program for a shoulder after arthroscopic stabilization is similar to the program after open techniques. Without the larger incision and soft tissue dissection of the open approach, the arthroscopic technique results in less initial postoperative pain. This decrease in morbidity, while desirable, may put the arthroscopically stabilized shoulder at a disadvantage: The patient feels better and may proceed too quickly through increase in activities and ROM. Premature return to high-level throwing activity will stretch the reconstructed soft tissue and render the stabilization ineffective.

A comparison examination under anesthesia of the shoulders with the patient in supine position is performed to assess the ROM and the degree and direction of instability. The patient is then placed in lateral decubitus or beach chair position according to the surgeon's preference, and a standard diagnostic arthroscopy of the GH joint is performed. The shoulder is placed through a functional ROM with the arthroscope in place, paying close attention to the shoulder positions specific to the patient's sport, to evaluate for the presence of intra-articular pathologies. If no contraindication to arthroscopic procedure is detected (e.g., glenoid bone stock insufficiency, engaging Hill-Sachs lesion), then arthroscopic stabilization can proceed; otherwise the surgeon should be prepared to reposition the patient and perform an open capsulolabral reconstruction. The capsulolabral soft tissues are elevated from the anterior-inferior glenoid edge with arthroscopic instruments through the anterior portal. This important step frees the soft tissue for sufficient mobilization and shift. Suture anchors are placed along the anterior-inferior margin of the glenoid, and then starting with the most inferior anchor, one limb of each suture is passed through capsulolabral structures. The location of the suture passage depends on the desired amount of tightening; the more inferior the suture limb is passed, the more the tissue will be shifted superiorly and the more the shoulder tightened. A knot is tied before the suture for the next anchor is passed through the soft tissue, to allow assessment of the amount of superior shift with each suture and each knot. In addition to tightening the shoulder anteriorly, the tissue imbricated with each suture passage and arthroscopic knot also creates a soft tissue "bumper" at the edge of the glenoid. Similar to a wedge, the bumper works in concert with the superiorly shifted capsulolabral structures to physically block the humeral head from sliding forward. The stability of the shoulder is again examined through a ROM to judge if the degree of tightening is appropriate. As described elsewhere, it is normal for the elite throwing athlete to have increased external rotation in the dominant shoulder; this difference has to be recognized and respected during the stabilization procedure, or the lack of external rotation after surgery will become problematic on the pitching mechanics. The portals are closed with sutures, and the shoulder is placed in an immobilizer.

Arthroscopic reconstruction provides important advantages over the open method:

1. Decreased soft tissue dissection and the potential for reduced pain in the immediate postoperative period
2. Ability to visually evaluate the entire GH and subacromial spaces to diagnose and possibly treat concomitant pathologies
3. Potentially shorter operative time

Important contraindications include:

1. Significant loss of bone in the anterior-inferior glenoid or "inverted pear" glenoid contour
2. Large and engaging Hill-Sachs lesion
3. Poor GH ligament tissue integrity

In these patients, open stabilization with possible glenoid bone stock augmentation remains the treatment of choice. Participation in contact sports was noted in earlier reports as a contraindication to arthroscopic stabilization, although recent results have shown that high success rates can still be achieved in these patients.

Overall, if the arthroscopic repair is elected, then the timing of the rehabilitation program does not change. In one sense, patients who have this less-invasive procedure may have an additional problem: Because their shoulder morbidity is so much less, they feel better faster—almost too fast! Ironically, an arthroscopic repair is almost a disservice; patients feel so much better so quickly that they do too much too soon.

Sometimes, if the patient is a thrower and is feeling great by 7 months postoperatively, then he or she will have talked a trainer into allowing the patient to pitch. This is too early because the repair will stretch and lose its effectiveness.

THERAPY GUIDELINES FOR REHABILITATION

Because no muscles are cut in this reconstruction procedure, rehabilitation proceeds briskly with two familiar general goals:

Table 4-1 Anterior Capsular Reconstruction

Rehabilitation Phase	Criteria to Progress to this Phase	Anticipated Impairments and Functional Limitations	Intervention	Goal	Rationale
Phase 1 Postoperative 1 day-2 weeks	◆ Postoperative	◆ Postoperative pain ◆ Postoperative edema ◆ Dependent UE in a sling or airplane splint ◆ Limited ROM ◆ Limited strength ◆ Limited reach, lift, and carry with UE	◆ Cryotherapy ◆ Electrical stimulation ◆ Isometrics Shoulder—All movements in a neutral position ◆ Assisted AROM—Shoulder—Flexion, internal rotation, external rotation, and abduction avoiding stress on the anterior capsule ◆ Wand exercises—Begin shoulder flexion after sling/ splint is removed ◆ AROM—Shoulder—Flexion, internal rotation, external rotation, and abduction, avoiding stress on the anterior capsule ◆ AROM elbow—Flexion, extension, pronation, supination ◆ AROM wrist—Flexion, extension	◆ Control pain ◆ Manage edema ◆ Produce good-quality contraction of shoulder muscles ◆ Produce 135 degrees of flexion in the scapular plane and 35 degrees of external rotation ◆ Allow ADLs below shoulder height with minimal difficulty, assisting with involved UE	

UE, Upper extremity; *ROM,* range of motion; *AROM,* active range of motion.

1. Strengthen dynamic GH and scapulothoracic stabilizers
2. Restore structural flexibility

The program primarily consists of active range of motion (AROM) exercises and resistive exercises. The therapist must monitor these exercises and enforce the correct execution for good progress to occur. This program includes concurrent exercises for all parts of the trinity of normalcy: ROM, strength, and endurance. The key to success is to work on all three portions without waiting for completion of any one part. The therapist should not wait for full ROM before strengthening or be overly aggressive in pushing for all movement early. Furthermore, the therapist should not wait for full strength before beginning endurance work, particularly in patients with hyperelasticity. The best plan is an integrated one. Programs to restore strength, motion, and endurance should overlap one another, rather than run in sequential phases.

Phase I

TIME: 1 day to 2 weeks after surgery (Table 4-1)

Shoulder

- The patient may be in an airplane type of abduction splint for 1 or 2 weeks. The physician may place patients with greater than normal tissue laxity in a sling instead. **These patients will have no difficulty regaining their motion but need to tighten up before moving.**
- AROM 1 day after surgery should consist of removing the arm from the sling or splint and flexing and abducting in the scapular plane. Use active assisted motion as needed.
- Strengthening begins when the splint is removed. Use active isometric contractions for internal rotation, external rotation, flexion, extension, and abduction (Fig. 4-4).
- After the splint or sling is removed, begin wand exercises for elevation. Make sure that the motion includes both flexion and abduction with external rotation. Do not stress the anterior capsule.

It is important to obtain necessary motion by 2 months after surgery.

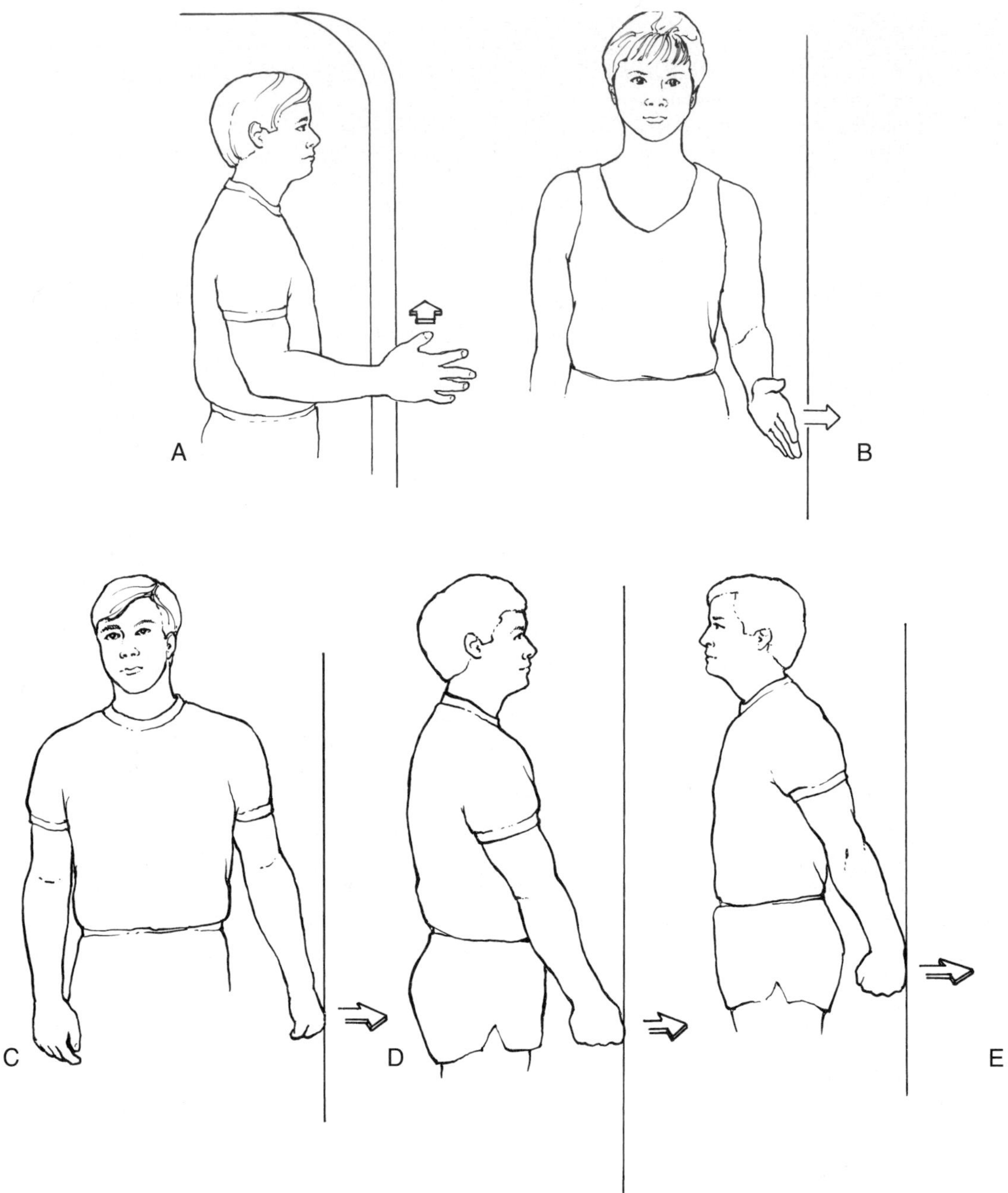

Fig. 4-4 **A,** Isometric shoulder internal rotation. **B,** Isometric shoulder external rotation. **C,** Isometric shoulder abduction. **D,** Isometric shoulder flexion. **E,** Isometric shoulder extension. (From Jobe FW: *Operative techniques in upper extremity sports injuries*, St Louis, 1996, Mosby.)

Avoid stressing the anterior joint capsule during the first postoperative month, then work gradually but insistently to get full range. After 2 months, it can be difficult to acquire additional motion. However, full ROM is different for different patients. Improved function is the goal of the therapist. Function is different for a shipyard worker than for a baseball pitcher. The function of the opposite side may not be a reasonable yardstick either, depending on the patient's requirements.

Elbow, Wrist, Hand

- Active elbow flexion and extension may begin on postoperative day 1.
- Active forearm supination and pronation may begin on postoperative day 1.
- Active wrist flexion and extension may begin on postoperative day 1.
- Patient should immediately begin squeezing a ball or plastic egg-shaped hand exerciser.
- Use cryotherapy for pain control.

Table 4-2 Anterior Capsular Reconstruction

Rehabilitation Phase	Criteria to Progress to this Phase	Anticipated Impairments and Functional Limitations	Intervention	Goal	Rationale
Phase II Postoperative 3 weeks-3 months	◆ No signs of infection ◆ No increase in pain ◆ Pain controlled with medication or modalities ◆ No loss of ROM	◆ Out of sling or splint as appropriate ◆ Limited ROM ◆ Limited strength ◆ Limited tolerance of UE for reach, lift, and carry activities	Continue exercises as in Phase I: ◆ Resisted internal and external rotation using elastic bands ◆ AROM—Shoulder—At 4 weeks add horizontal abduction; at 5 weeks add supine horizontal adduction in scapular plane; at 6 weeks add supraspinatus exercise using an empty can ◆ Add exercises from Tables 3-1 and 3-2 inclusive of isotonics and elastic tubing	By 2 months the following should occur: ◆ Shoulder AROM full ◆ Strength 60%-70% ◆ No pain during all ADLs ◆ Lift 5 lb ◆ Return to sedentary work By 3 months the following should occur: ◆ Shoulder strength 80% ◆ Carry 5 lb	◆ Progress rapidly after getting full ROM while avoiding stress on the anterior capsule ◆ Strengthen scapula stabilizers and rotator cuff muscles ◆ Increase tolerance of anterior shoulder muscles to movement ◆ Avoid impingement while exercising rotator cuff ◆ Strengthen entire UE and improve cardiovascular fitness in an effort to return patient to previous level of function

ROM, Range of motion; *UE*, upper extremity; *ADLs*, activities of daily living.

> **Q** John is a 35-year-old surfer. He had several episodes of shoulder dislocation while paddling his surfboard. He also complained of anterior shoulder pain. Conservative treatment failed, so he underwent an anterior capsular reconstruction 11 weeks ago. Passive range of motion (PROM) and AROM are good. John's main complaint is continuing anterior shoulder pain. The pain can be elicited by palpation over the biceps tendon and transverse humeral ligament. This symptom has delayed progress with strengthening. How was the patient treated?

Phase II

TIME: 3 weeks to 3 months after surgery (Table 4-2)

Shoulder

◆ Resistive exercises may begin during week 3 after surgery. Emphasize the internal and external rotators of the rotator cuff. Use elastic band resistance and position the arm at the side. An axillary roll may be used to increase the emphasis on the teres minor. Eliminate the axillary roll to increase the emphasis on the infraspinatus muscle.

◆ Extension is best done prone on a table or standing and leaning forward from the waist. The elbow should be in full extension, and the extensor motion should end at the plane of the trunk (Fig. 4-5).

◆ Horizontal abduction begins in week 4, using the same starting position as for extension. Again, keep the elbow straight and make certain that motion does not continue beyond the plane of the trunk. Watch carefully to ensure that scapular adduction and trunk rotation are not substituted for true horizontal abduction.

◆ An axillary roll may be used to emphasize the teres minor muscle. By eliminating the axillary roll, emphasis should be placed on the infraspinatus muscle.

◆ Horizontal adduction begins in week 4 or 5, supine, in the scapular plane. To get the arm in this position, use a towel or pillow under the humerus, ensuring that the start and finish positions are in front of the plane of the trunk (Fig. 4-6).

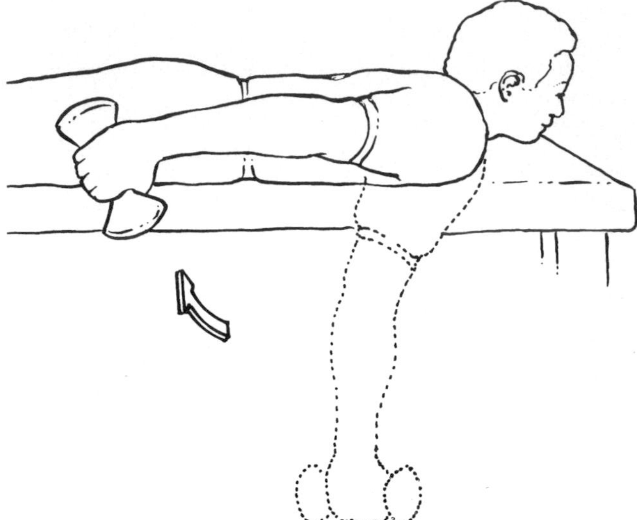

Fig. 4-5 Prone shoulder extension.
(From Jobe FW: *Operative techniques in upper extremity sports injuries*, St Louis, 1996, Mosby.)

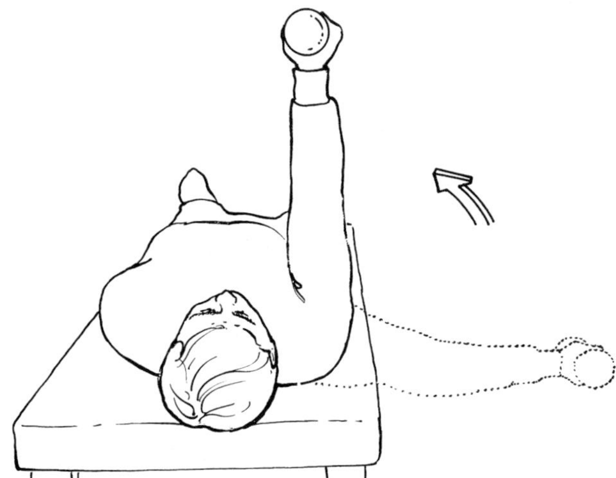

Fig. 4-6 Horizontal adduction.
(From Jobe FW: *Operative techniques in upper extremity sports injuries*, St Louis, 1996, Mosby.)

- Increase the difficulty of the rotation exercises; progress the external rotation to side lying, using hand weights (Fig. 4-7). Put a bolster under the lateral chest wall for internal rotation.
- Supraspinatus exercises are done standing, within a pain-free range only. Start using only the weight of the arm as resistance, and add hand weights only when both the form is perfect and the pain has disappeared.

Shoulder, Elbow, Wrist, Hand

- Add an upper body ergometer (UBE) work for endurance training. Begin with low resistance for early sessions. Start with an easy 5-minute program such as the following:

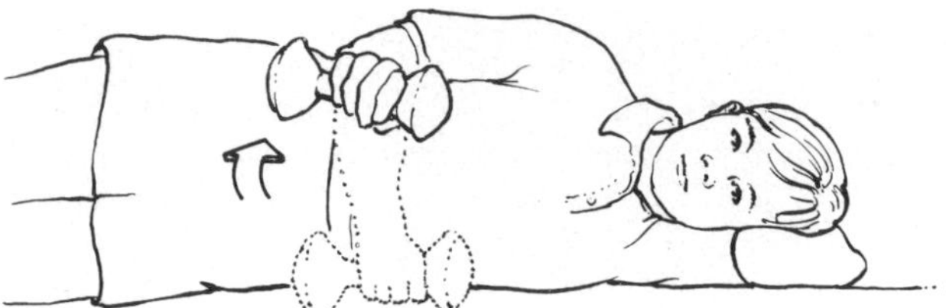

Fig. 4-7 Side-lying external rotation.
(From Jobe FW: *Operative techniques in upper extremity sports injuries*, St Louis, 1996, Mosby.)

  - 1-minute forward
  - 1-minute rest
  - 1-minute backward
  - 1-minute rest
  - 1-minute forward

A John was treated for biceps tendonitis, or inflammatory symptoms occurring in the area of the proximal biceps tendon and transverse humeral ligament. Despite the structural corrections, these tissues may remain irritable. Because the posterior capsule also was slightly restricted, posterior capsular mobilizations were performed to allow the humeral head to articulate with the glenoid at its normal contact point, eliminating this as a source of continuing aggravation for these anterior structures.

Q Peter is a 20-year-old pitcher for a baseball team. He had right-shoulder laxity and a painful shoulder secondary to impingement problems. He underwent capsular reconstruction on his right shoulder 10 weeks ago. His shoulder flexion and abduction with PROM is still limited by 15 degrees for flexion and 20 degrees for abduction. PROM for internal rotation also is limited by 20 degrees. At this time, should decreased ROM be a concern? If yes, what techniques were used to improve ROM?

Phase III

TIME: 3 to 4 months after surgery (Table 4-3)

Shoulder

- Add eccentric rotator cuff exercises.
- Add serratus anterior work, beginning with wall push-ups and then move on to regular push-ups with a stop at a modified, hands-and-knees push-up (Fig. 4-8). The most important part of the push-up is at the end when the patient emphasizes scapular protraction.
- Isokinetic training begins when the patient can lift at least 5 lb in side-lying external rotation and 10 to 15 lb in side-lying internal rotation without pain.

Table 4-3 Anterior Capsular Reconstruction

Rehabilitation Phase	Criteria to Progress to this Phase	Anticipated Impairments and Functional Limitations	Intervention	Goal	Rationale
Phase III Postoperative 3-4 months	◆ Pain self-managed and primarily associated with increased activity ◆ No loss of ROM ◆ No loss of strength	◆ Limited strength and endurance of UE ◆ Unable to perform sustained or repetitive reaching and overhead activities ◆ Limited tolerance to carrying objects	Continue strengthening and ROM exercises as noted in phases I and II: ◆ PREs—Eccentric rotator cuff exercises; wall push-up plus progressing to horizontal push-up plus (emphasizing scapular protraction at end of push-up) ◆ Isokinetics for internal and external rotation at 200 degree/sec ◆ Sport-specific drills when strength is 80% (see Appendix A) Note: Despite how good a patient feels, allowing the patient to return to pitching at 7 months is too early and will compromise the repair.	◆ 80% overhead lifting strength compared with uninvolved extremity ◆ 80% carrying strength below shoulder height	◆ Work on endurance of scapula and shoulder muscles before achieving full strength ◆ Increase static and dynamic control of rotator cuff for return to previous activities ◆ Strengthen and improve endurance of shoulder muscles using high-speed resistance training ◆ Return to sport or activity safely and without injury

ROM, Range of motion; *UE*, upper extremity; *PREs*, progressive resistance exercises.

- **Sport-specific drills do not begin until the involved side has 70% to 80% of the strength of the uninvolved side.** The authors of this chapter use an isokinetic machine for strength testing at 120 degrees/second for internal rotation and 240 degrees/second for external rotation. Keep in mind that a pitcher's dominant arm is always stronger than his or her nondominant arm. ROM in the dominant arms exceeds that in the non-dominant.
- If the patient has pain, reduce some or all of the following: number of throws, speed of the throw, distances thrown, or number of days spent throwing. **Keep the speed below three quarters of maximum until 7 months after surgery. Full speed is reasonable after 1 year.**
- Occasionally after beginning to throw, the patient will experience pain posteriorly. Check the teres minor for inflammation and the posterior capsule for tightness. Refer to the chapter on transitional throwing programs. Modified throwing programs for pitchers, throwing programs for position players, an exercise program for tennis players, and a rehabilitation program for golfers are detailed in Boxes 4-1 through 4-4. An additional throwing program is detailed in Appendix A.
- Normal ROM is relative. Again, function is the goal, and function is different for a shipyard worker than for a baseball pitcher.

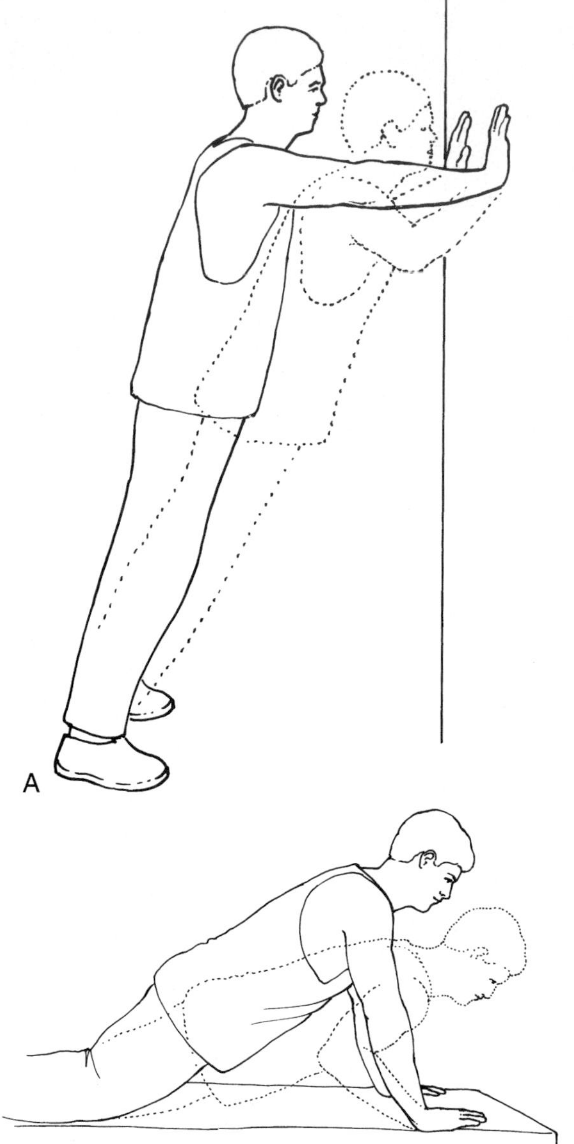

Fig. 4-8 **A**, Wall push-ups. **B**, Modified hands-and-knees push-ups. (From Jobe FW: *Operative techniques in upper extremity sports injuries*, St Louis, 1996, Mosby.)

> **A** On further investigation a tight posterior capsule was noted. The therapist used posterior capsular mobilizations in the next treatment to increase shoulder flexion and internal rotation. The patient gained 10 to 15 degrees more for flexion and internal rotation and 5 to 10 degrees more for abduction. After mobilization and PROM were performed, the patient executed AROM exercises for shoulder flexion, abduction, and internal rotation.

SUGGESTED HOME MAINTENANCE FOR THE POSTSURGICAL PATIENT

Because the correct execution of the exercises is vital, the authors of this chapter do not give a home exercise program. Instead, the authors prefer to monitor the exercises in the clinic. When a patient graduates to a transitioning sports program, home exercises may be given.

TROUBLESHOOTING

Misapprehending Quality of Patient's Tissues

Patients with "normal" or tight connective tissue must work early and diligently to reacquire motion, while avoiding stress on the anterior joint capsule during the first postoperative month. The therapist should not push patients with hyperelasticity. They will reacquire motion quickly and should be allowed to heal before attempting extremes of motion.

Anterior Shoulder Pain

Despite surgery, some patients still have anterior shoulder pain on palpation of the proximal biceps tendon or transverse humeral ligament. This may be considered "leftover inflammation." The structural problem may have been rectified surgically, but the residual inflammation does not disappear overnight. The therapist and patient should use modalities to reduce discomfort. In addition, the physical therapist should ensure that the posterior cuff and capsule are stretched so that the humeral head can articulate with the glenoid at its normal contact point, eliminating this as a source of continuing irritation for these anterior structures.

Posterior Shoulder Pain

In addition to anterior shoulder pain, many patients also note pain in the posterior shoulder, especially with activity that requires elevation above 120 degrees and motion that requires horizontal abduction posterior to the frontal plane. Another potentially difficult motion is hyperextension posterior to the plane of the body. The therapist may note pain on palpation of the posterior cuff insertion, the posterior capsule, or the proximal third of the axillary border of the scapula, and he or she should ensure that the patient has adequate excursion of the posterior capsule. Occasionally patients develop a tendonitis of the rotator cuff external rotators, specifically the teres minor. This tendonitis may be treated symptomatically with modalities, stretching (if necessary), and progressive strengthening.

Box 4-1 Rehabilitation Throwing Program for Pitchers*

Step 1: Toss the ball (no windup) against a wall on alternate days. Start with 25 to 30 throws, build up to 70 throws, and gradually increase the throwing distance.

Number of Throws	Distance (ft)
20	20 (warm-up)
25-40	30-40
10	20 (cool down)

Step 2: Toss the ball (playing catch with easy windup) on alternate days.

Number of Throws	Distance (ft)
10	20 (warm-up)
10	30-40
30-40	50
10	20-30 (cool down)

Step 3: Continue increasing the throwing distance while still tossing the ball with an easy windup.

Number of Throws	Distance (ft)
10	20 (warm-up)
10	30-40
30-40	50-60
10	30 (cool down)

Step 4: Increase throwing distance to a maximum of 60 feet. Continue tossing the ball with an occasional throw at no more than one-half speed.

Number of Throws	Distance (ft)
10	30 (warm-up)
10	40-45
30-40	60-70
10	30 (cool down)

Step 5: During this step, gradually increase the distance to 150 feet maximum.

Phase 5-1

Number of Throws	Distance (ft)
10	40 (warm-up)
10	50-60
15-20	70-80
10	50-60
10	40 (cool down)

Phase 5-2

Number of Throws	Distance (ft)
10	40 (warm-up)
10	50-60
20-30	80-90
20	50-60
10	40 (cool down)

Phase 5-3

Number of Throws	Distance (ft)
10	40 (warm-up)
10	60
15-20	100-110
20	60
10	40 (cool down)

Phase 5-4

Number of Throws	Distance (ft)
10	40 (warm-up)
10	60
15-20	120-150
20	60
10	40 (cool down)

Step 6: Progress to throwing off the mound at one-half to three-fourths speed. Try to use proper body mechanics, especially when throwing off the mound:

- Stay on top of the ball.
- Keep the elbow up.
- Throw over the top.
- Follow through with the arm and trunk.
- Use the legs to push.

Phase 6-1

Number of Throws	Distance (ft)
10	60 (warm-up)
10	120-150 (lobbing)
30	45 (off the mound)
10	60 (off the mound)
10	40 (cool down)

Phase 6-2

Number of Throws	Distance (ft)
10	50 (warm-up)
10	120-150 (lobbing)
20	45 (off the mound)
20	60 (off the mound)
10	40 (cool down)

Phase 6-3

Number of Throws	Distance (ft)
10	50 (warm-up)
10	60
10	120-150 (lobbing)
10	45 (off the mound)
30	60 (off the mound)
10	40 (cool down)

Phase 6-4

Number of Throws	Distance (ft)
10	50 (warm-up)
10	120-150 (lobbing)
10	45 (off the mound)
40-50	60 (off the mound)
10	40 (cool down)

At this time, if the pitcher has successfully completed phase 6-4 without pain or discomfort and is throwing approximately three-fourths speed, then the pitching coach and trainer may allow the pitcher to proceed to step 7: up-down bullpens. Up-down bullpens is used to simulate a game. The pitcher rests between a series of pitches to reproduce the rest period between innings.

Step 7: Up-down bullpens: (one-half to three-fourths speed)

Continued

Box 4-1 Rehabilitation Throwing Program for Pitchers*—cont'd

Day 1

Number of Throws	Distance (ft)
10 warm-up throws	120-150 (lobbing)
10 warm-up throws	60 (off the mound)
40 pitches	60 (off the mound)
Rest 10 minutes	
20 pitches	60 (off the mound)

Day 2

Off

Day 3

Number of Throws	Distance (ft)
10 warm-up throws	120-150 (lobbing)
10 warm-up throws	60 (off the mound)
30 pitches	60 (off the mound)
Rest 10 minutes	
10 warm-up throws	60 (off the mound)
20 pitches	60 (off the mound)
Rest 10 minutes	
10 warm-up throws	60 (off the mound)
20 pitches	60 (off the mound)

Day 4

Off

Day 5

Number of Throws	Distance (ft)
10 warm-up throws	120-150 (lobbing)
10 warm-up throws	60 (off the mound)
30 pitches	60 (off the mound)
Rest 8 minutes	
20 pitches	60 (off the mound)
Rest 8 minutes	
20 pitches	60 (off the mound)
Rest 8 minutes	
20 pitches	60 (off the mound)

At this point the pitcher is ready to begin a normal routine, from throwing batting practice to pitching in the bullpen. This program can and should be adjusted as needed by the trainer or physical therapist. Each step may take more or less time than listed, and the trainer, physical therapist, and physician should monitor the program. The pitcher should remember that it is necessary to work hard but not overdo it.

*Patients start at the step that is appropriate for them. Postsurgical patients begin at step 1. Patients progress depending on the maintenance of their pain-free status and their strength and endurance.

(From Jobe FW: *Operative techniques in upper extremity sports injuries*, St Louis, 1996, Mosby.)

Box 4-2 Rehabilitation Program for Catchers, Infielders, and Outfielders

- Note: Perform each step three times.
- All throws should have an arc or "hump."
- The maximum distance thrown by infielders and catchers is 120 feet.
- The maximum distance thrown by outfielders is 200 feet.

Step 1: Toss the ball with no windup. Stand with your feet shoulder-width apart and face the player to whom you are throwing. Concentrate on rotating and staying on top of the ball.

Number of Throws	Distance (ft)
5	20 (warm-up)
10	30
5	20 (cool down)

Step 2: Stand sideways to the person to whom you are throwing. Feet are shoulder-width apart. Close up and pivot onto your back foot as you throw.

Number of Throws	Distance (ft)
5	30 (warm-up)
5	40
10	50
5	30 (cool down)

Step 3: Repeat the position in step 2. Step toward the target with your front leg and follow through with your back leg.

Number of Throws	Distance (ft)
5	50 (warm-up)
5	60
10	70
5	50 (cool down)

Step 4: Assume the pitcher's stance. Lift and stride with your lead leg. Follow through with your back leg.

Number of Throws	Distance (ft)
5	60 (warm-up)
5	70
10	80
5	60 (cool down)

Step 5: Outfielders: Lead with your glove-side foot forward. Take one step, crow hop, and throw the ball.

Infielders: Lead with your glove-side foot forward. Take a shuffle step and throw the ball. Throw the last five throws in a straight line.

Number of Throws	Distance (ft)
5	70 (warm-up)
5	90
10	100
5	80 (cool down)

Step 6: Use the throwing technique used in step 5. Assume your playing position. Infielders and catchers, do

Box 4-2 Rehabilitation Program for Catchers, Infielders, and Outfielders—cont'd

not throw farther than 120 feet. Outfielders, do not throw farther than 150 feet (mid-outfield).

Number of Throws	Infielders' and Catchers' Distance (ft)	Outfielders' Distance (ft)
5	80 (warm-up)	80 (warm-up)
5	80-90	90-100
5	90-100	110-125
5	110-120	130-150
5	80 (cool down)	80 (cool down)

Step 7: Infielders, catchers, and outfielders all may assume their playing positions.

Number of Throws	Infielders' and Catchers' Distance (ft)	Outfielders' Distance (ft)
5	80 (warm-up)	80-90 (warm-up)
5	80-90	110-130
5	90-100	150-175
5	110-120	180-200
5	80 (cool down)	90 (cool down)

Step 8: Repeat step 7. Use a fungo bat to hit to the infielders and outfielders while in their normal playing positions.

(From Jobe FW: *Operative techniques in upper extremity sports injuries*, St Louis, 1996, Mosby.)

Box 4-3 Rehabilitation Program for Tennis Players

The following tennis protocol is designed to be performed every other day. Each session should begin with the warm-up exercises as outlined following. Continue with your strengthening, flexibility, and conditioning exercises on the days you are not following the tennis protocol.

Warm-up

Lower extremity:

- Jog four laps around the tennis court.
- Stretches:
  - Gastrocnemius
  - Achilles tendon
  - Hamstring
  - Quadriceps

Upper extremity:

- Shoulder stretches:
  - Posterior cuff
  - Inferior capsule
  - Rhomboid
- Forearm/wrist stretches
  - Wrist flexors
  - Wrist extensors

Trunk:

- Side bends
- Extension
- Rotation

Forehand ground strokes:

- Hit toward the fence on the opposite side of the court.
- Do not worry about getting the ball in the court.

During all of the strokes listed previously, remember these key steps:

- Bend your knees.
- Turn your body.
- Step toward the ball.
- Hit the ball when it is out in front of you.

Avoid hitting with an open stance, because this places undue stress on your shoulder. This is especially more stressful during the forehand stroke if you have had anterior instability or impingement problems. This is also true during the backhand if you have had problems of posterior instability.

On the very first day of these sport-specific drills, start with bouncing the ball and hitting it. Try to bounce the ball yourself and hit it at waist level. This will allow for consistency in the following:

- How the ball comes to you
- Approximating your timing between hits
- Hitting toward a target to ensure follow-through and full extension
- Using the proper mechanics, thereby placing less stress on the anterior shoulder

Week 1

Day 1:
25 forehand strokes
25 backhand strokes

Day 2:
If no problems occur after the first-day workout, increase the number of forehand and backhand strokes.
50 forehand strokes
50 backhand strokes

Day 3:
50 forehand strokes (waist level)
50 backhand strokes (waist level)
25 high forehand strokes
25 high backhand strokes

Week 2

Progress to having the ball tossed to you in a timely manner, giving you enough time to recover from your deliberate follow-through (i.e., wait until the ball bounces on the other side of the court before tossing another ball). Always aim the ball at a target or at a spot on the court.

If you are working on basic ground strokes, have someone bounce the ball to you consistently at waist height.

Continued

Box 4-3 Rehabilitation Program for Tennis Players—cont'd

If you are working on high forehands, have the ball bounced to you at shoulder height or higher.

Day 1:
25 high forehand strokes
50 waist-height forehand strokes
50 waist-height backhand strokes
25 high backhand strokes

Day 2:
25 high forehand strokes
50 waist-height forehand strokes
50 waist-height backhand strokes
25 high backhand strokes

Day 3:
Alternate hitting the ball cross court and down the line, using waist-high and high forehand and backhand strokes.
25 high forehand strokes
50 waist-height forehand strokes
50 waist-height backhand strokes
25 high backhand strokes

Week 3

Continue the three-times-per-week schedule. Add regular and high forehand and backhand volleys. At this point you may begin having someone hit tennis balls to you from a basket of balls. This will allow you to get the feel of the ball as it comes off another tennis racket. Your partner should wait until the ball that you hit has bounced on the other side of the court before hitting another ball to you. This will give you time to emphasize your follow-through and not hurry to return for the next shot. As always, emphasis is placed on proper body mechanics.

Day 1:
25 high forehand strokes
50 waist-height forehand strokes
50 waist-height backhand strokes
25 high backhand strokes
25 low backhand and forehand volleys
25 high backhand and forehand volleys

Day 2:
Same as day 1, week 3

Day 3:
Same as day 2, week 3, with emphasis on direction (i.e., down the line and crosscourt). Remember, good body mechanics is still a must:

- Keep knees bent.
- Hit the ball on the rise.
- Hit the ball in front of you.
- Turn your body.
- Do not hit the ball with an open stance.
- Stay on the balls of your feet.

Week 4

Day 1:
Continue having your partner hit tennis balls to you from out of a basket. Alternate hitting forehand and backhand strokes with lateral movement along the baseline. Again, emphasis is on good mechanics as described previously.

Alternate hitting the ball down the line and crosscourt. This drill should be done with a full basket of tennis balls (100 to 150 tennis balls).

Follow this drill with high and low volleys using half a basket of tennis balls (50 to 75 balls). This drill also is performed with lateral movement and returning to the middle of the court after the ball is hit.

Your partner should continue allowing enough time for you to return to the middle of the court before hitting the next ball. This is to avoid your rushing the stroke and using faulty mechanics.

Day 2:
Same drill as day 1, week 4

Day 3:
Same drills as day 2, week 4

Week 5

Day 1:
Find a partner able to hit consistent ground strokes (able to hit the ball to the same area consistently [e.g., to your forehand with the ball bouncing about waist height]).

Begin hitting ground strokes with this partner alternating hitting the ball to your backhand and to your forehand. Rally for about 15 minutes, then add volleys with your partner hitting to you from the baseline. Alternate between backhand and forehand volleys and high and low volleys. Continue volleying another 15 minutes. You will have rallied for a total of 30 to 40 minutes.

At the end of the session, practice a few serves while standing along the baseline. First, warm up by shadowing for 1 to 3 minutes. Hold the tennis racquet loosely and swing across your body in a figure eight. Do not swing the racquet hard. When you are ready to practice your serves using a ball, be sure to keep your toss out in front of you, get your racquet up and behind you, bend your knees, and hit up on the ball. Forget about how much power you are generating, and forget about hitting the ball between the service lines. Try hitting the ball as if you are hitting it toward the back fence.

Hit approximately 10 serves from each side of the court. Remember, this is the first time you are serving, so do not try to hit at 100% of your effort.

Day 2:
Same as day 1, week 5, but now increase the number of times you practice your serve. After working on your ground strokes and volleys, return to the baseline and work on your second serve: Hit up on the ball, bend your knees, follow through, and keep the toss in front of you. This time hit 20 balls from each side of the court (i.e., 20 into the deuce court and 20 into the ad court).

Day 3:
Same as day 2, week 5, with ground strokes, volleys, and serves. Do not add to the serves. Concentrate on the following:

Box 4-3 Rehabilitation Program for Tennis Players—cont'd

- Bending your knees
- Preparing the racket
- Using footwork
- Hitting the ball out in front of you
- Keeping your eyes on the ball
- Following through
- Getting in position for the next shot
- Keeping the toss in front of you during the serve

The workout should be the same as day 2, but if you emphasize the proper mechanics listed previously, then you should feel as though you had a harder workout than in day 2.

Week 6

Day 1:
After the usual warm-up program, start with specific ground stroke drills, with you hitting the ball down the line and your partner on the other side hitting the ball crosscourt. This will force you to move quickly on the court. Emphasize good mechanics as mentioned previously.

Perform this drill for 10 to 15 minutes before reversing the direction of your strokes. Now have your partner hit down the line while you hit crosscourt.

Proceed to the next drill with your partner hitting the ball to you. Return balls using a forehand, then a backhand, then a put-away volley. Repeat this sequence for 10 to 15 minutes. End this session by serving 50 balls to the ad court and 50 balls to the deuce court.

Day 2:
Day 2 should be the same as day 1, week 6, plus returning serves from each side of the court (deuce and ad court). End with practicing serves, 50 to each court.

Day 3:
Perform the following sequence: warm-up; crosscourt and down-the-line drills; backhand, forehand, and volley drills; return of serves; and practice serves.

Week 7

Day 1:
Perform the warm-up program. Perform drills as before and practice return of serves. Before practicing serving, work on hitting 10 to 15 overhead shots. Continue emphasizing good mechanics. Add the approach shot to your drills.

Day 2:
Same as day 1, week 7, except double the number of overhead shots (25 to 30 overheads).

Day 3:
Perform warm-up exercises and crosscourt drills. Add the overhead shot to the backhand, forehand, and volley drill, making it the backhand, forehand, volley, and overhead drill.

If you are a serious tennis player, you will want to work on other strokes or other parts of your game. Feel free to gradually add them to your practice and workout sessions. Just as in other strokes, the proper mechanics should be applied to drop volley, slice, heavy topspin, drop shots, and lobs (offensive and defensive).

Week 8

Day 1:
Warm up and play a simulated one-set match. Be sure to take rest periods after every third game. Remember, you will have to concentrate harder on using good mechanics.

Day 2:
Perform another simulated game but with a two-set match.

Day 3:
Perform another simulated game, this time a best-of-three match.

If all goes well, you may make plans to return to your regular workout and game schedule. You also may practice or play if your condition allows it.

(From Jobe FW: *Operative techniques in upper extremity sports injuries*, St Louis, 1996, Mosby.)

Box 4-4 Rehabilitation Program for Golfers

This sport-specific protocol is designed to be performed every other day. Each session should begin with the warm-up exercises outlined here. Continue the strengthening, flexibility, and conditioning exercises on the days you are not playing or practicing golf. Advance one stage every 2 to 4 weeks, depending on the severity of the shoulder problem, as each stage becomes pain free in execution.

Warm-up

Lower extremities: Jog or walk briskly around the practice green area three or four times; stretch the hamstrings, quadriceps, and Achilles tendon.

Upper extremities: Stretch the shoulder (i.e., posterior cuff, inferior cuff, rhomboid) and wrist flexors and extensors.

Trunk: Do side bends, extension, and rotation stretching exercises.

Stage 1		
Putt	50	3 times/week
Medium long	0	0 times/week
Long	0	0 times/week
Stage 2		
Putt	50	3 times/week
Medium long	20	2 times/week
Long	0	0 times/week
Stage 3		
Putt	50	3 times/week
Medium long	40	3 times/week
Long	0	0 times/week

Continued

Box 4-4 Rehabilitation Program for Golfers—cont'd

Not more than one-third best distance

Stage 4

Putt	50	3 times/week
Medium long	50	3 times/week
Long	10	2 times/week

Up to one-half best distance

Stage 5

Putt	50	3 times/week
Medium long	50	3 times/week
Long	10	3 times/week

Stage 6

Putt	50	3 times/week
Medium long	50	3 times/week
Long	20	3 times/week

Play a round of golf in lieu of one practice session per week.

(From Jobe FW: *Operative techniques in upper extremity sports injuries*, St Louis, 1996, Mosby.)

Insufficient Range of Motion

If too much time elapses after surgery before the patient regains normal motion, adhesive capsulitis may develop. The best defense for this problem is a good offense: The physical therapist should know the patient's tissue type and encourage motion early. As noted earlier, normal ROM differs for different patients. A baseball pitcher may require 130 degrees of external rotation for function. Most other patients have more modest requirements. **An athlete does need this external rotation, but too much external rotation can lead to instability.** A very narrow margin exists between being able to perform and having a problem. Precisely correct mechanics is crucial to prevention of recurrence.

Strength and Endurance

Often rehabilitation programs concentrate on increasing strength. However, for most patients, including overhead throwers, endurance is probably much more important to overall function than strength. Endurance training is equally important for patients who are hurt on the job. With inadequate endurance, the patient substitutes muscles and alters mechanics for a given task or sport to continue functioning. Such substitutions and alterations are often the forerunners of tissue breakdown. The therapist should strengthen specific muscle groups and prescribe the appropriate exercises (e.g., separate programs for rotator cuff, scapular rotators, shoulder flexors, and abductors) while paying special attention to the rotator cuff and the upward rotators of the scapula. These upward rotators are essential if the patient is to avoid impingement. The rhomboids and the serratus anterior should be strengthened (in addition to the more obvious rotator cuff program). To get the inferior portion of the serratus anterior, use a military press with the arms at no more than 150 degrees of elevation to avoid any possibility of impingement.

Stretching

Patients with anterior instability can have a tight posterior capsule. Despite surgical correction, the posterior tightness may remain and, if left untreated, lead to a recurrence of the original complaint. Sometimes, especially for older patients, the pectoralis minor is tight. The therapist should be suspicious if the patient has rounded shoulders and a protracted scapula. The goal should be to stretch the pectoralis minor and the posterior capsule as shown in Fig. 4-9. **The therapist must not stretch the anterior shoulder structures of any throwing athlete unless he or she is certain that tightness exists.** By and large, all these patients can demonstrate anterior laxity in the dominant shoulder. Stretching the pectoralis minor can forestall or alleviate symptoms of impingement symptoms. When the scapula does not rotate freely, tendons of the cuff will be compressed during elevation.

Mechanics

Even though the patient may have good ROM, strength, and endurance, important work remains to be done. Poor mechanics may be one of the reasons the patient was injured in the first place. Understanding the mechanics of the sport the patient is resuming is essential. For throwers, the physical therapist must ensure that the front foot is pointing toward the plate, the stride is not too long, the balance is correct, and the front foot does not hit the ground before the arm is ready to begin acceleration. An awareness of the mechanics of tennis, volleyball, swimming, and golf also is important. Without incorporating a review of mechanics and a "tune up" when necessary, it is likely that the player will return to old habits formed before the shoulder injury, despite conservative care and operative reconstruction (open or arthroscopic).

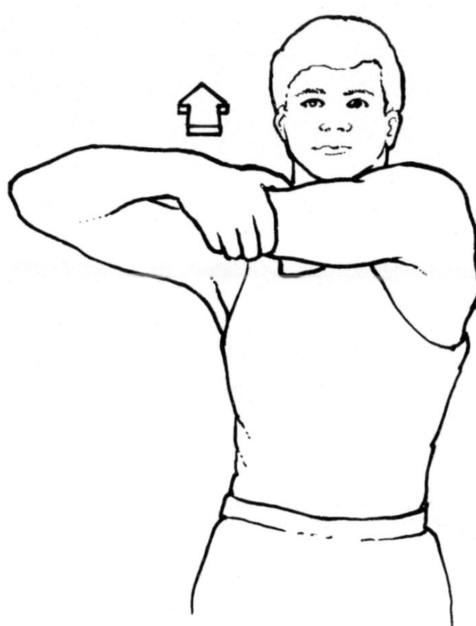

Fig. 4-9 Posterior cuff stretch.
(From Jobe FW: *Operative techniques in upper extremity sports injuries*, St Louis, 1996, Mosby.)

References

1. Garth WP, Allman FL, Armstrong WS: Occult anterior subluxation of the shoulder in noncontact sports, *Am J Sports Med* 15:579, 1987.
2. Jobe FW, Moynes DR: Delineation of diagnostic criteria and a rehabilitation program for rotator cuff injuries, *Am J Sports Med* 10:336, 1982.
3. Jobe FW, Glousman RE: *Anterior instability in the throwing athlete.* Instructional course lecture presented at the American Orthopaedic Society for Sports Medicine, Palm Desert, CA, June 1988.
4. Jobe FW, Glousman RE: Anterior capsulolabral reconstruction. In Paulous LE, Tibone JE, editors: *Operative technique in shoulder surgery,* Gaithersburg, MD, 1992, Aspen.

CHAPTER 5

Rotator Cuff Repair and Rehabilitation

Mark Ghilarducci
Lisa Maxey

SURGICAL INDICATIONS AND CONSIDERATIONS

Cause

Rotator cuff disorders are generally thought to have a multifactorial cause, including trauma, glenohumeral (GH) instability, scapulothoracic dysfunction, congenital abnormalities, and degenerative changes of the rotator cuff. Intrinsic tendon degeneration and extrinsic mechanical factors have been described extensively and are felt to be the primary contributors of rotator cuff pathology. In 1931, Codman and Akerson[20] suggested that degenerative changes in the rotator cuff lead to tears. Microvascular studies of the vascular pattern of the rotator cuff have demonstrated a hypovascular zone in the supraspinatus adjacent to the supraspinatus insertion into the humerus.[58,67,70] Relative ischemia in this hypovascular zone is felt to lead to decreased tendon cellularity and the eventual disruption of the rotator cuff attachment to bone with aging.

Compression of the rotator cuff between the acromion and the humeral head may subject the cuff to wear as the supraspinatus passes under the coracoacromial arch. Neer[61,62] postulated that 95% of rotator cuff tears are caused by impingement of the rotator cuff under the acromion. Neer[61] classified three stages of impingement as a continuum that eventually led to cuff tears. Stage I was characterized by subacromial edema and hemorrhage of the rotator cuff and usually occurs in patients younger than 25 years old. Stage II includes fibrosis and tendinosis of the rotator cuff and occurs more commonly in patients 25 to 40 years old. Stage III is a continued progression characterized by partial or complete tendon tears and bone changes. Typically, this involves patients older than 40 years old.[61] Bigliani, Morrison, and April[10] described three types of acromion shapes: (1) Type I is flat, (2) Type II is curved, and (3) Type III is hooked. An increased incidence of rotator cuff tears is associated with a curved (Type II) or a hooked (Type III) acromion. Other sources of impingement postulated include acromioclavicular (AC) osteophytes, the coracoid process, and the posterosuperior aspect of the glenoid.[35]

A rotator cuff tear may occur spontaneously after a sudden movement or a traumatic event.[23] Ruptures of the rotator cuff have been estimated to occur in up to 80% of persons older than 60 years of age with GH dislocations.[65] Cuff tears usually occur late in the shoulder deterioration process (after secondary impingements) and in older adults.

In athletes who participate in repetitive overhead activities (e.g., throwers, swimmers, tennis players), small rotator cuff tears may appear late in the deterioration process from secondary impingement. Secondary impingement is caused by instability of the GH joint or by functional scapulothoracic instability.[14] The primary underlying GH instability may progress along a continuum from anterior subluxation to impingement to rotator cuff tearing. Treatment must be directed to the primary instability problem.[49]

The throwing athlete also may have secondary impingement caused by functional scapular instability. Fatigue of the scapular stabilizers from repetitive throwing leads to abnormal positioning of the scapula. As a result, humeral and scapular elevation lose synchronization and the acromion is not elevated enough to allow free rotator cuff movement.[14] The rotator cuff abuts the acromion, causing microtrauma and impingement. A tear may gradually or spontaneously occur.

In summary, rotator cuff disease has a multifactorial cause. Vascular factors, impingement, degenerative processes, and developmental factors all contribute to the overall evolution and progression of rotator cuff disorders (Box 5-1).

Clinical Evaluation

History

The majority of patients with rotator cuff dysfunction have pain. They may complain of fatigue, functional catching, stiffness, weakness, and symptoms of instability.

Box 5-1 Rotator Cuff Deterioration Process

In older persons or laborers
Osteophyte develops
↓
Decreased subacromial space (more accentuated with a slouched posture)
↓
Continuous microtrauma from impingement leads to degenerative cuff changes
↓
Gradual partial tear or complete tear develops

In athletes secondary to glenohumeral (GH) instability
Overused biceps tendon and rotator cuff become weak and fatigued
↓
Passive restraints are overloaded
↓
Cuff laxity
↓
Anterosuperior GH instability
↓
Humeral head migrates superiorly and impinges the rotator cuff
↓
Continuous microtrauma from recurrent impingement leads to degenerative cuff changes
↓
Gradual or sudden rotator cuff tear occurs

Secondary to functional scapular instability
Weak scapulothoracic muscles
↓
Abnormal scapular positioning
↓
Humeral head elevation is not synchronized with scapular elevation and upward rotation (disrupted scapulohumeral rhythm)
↓
Acromion requires more elevation to allow unrestricted movement of the rotator cuff
↓
Rotator cuff impinged under the coracoacromial arch
↓
Continuous microtrauma from a recurrent impingement leads to degenerative cuff changes
↓
Gradual partial tear or a complete tear develops

An acute or macrotraumatic presentation is important to distinguish from an overuse or microtrauma presentation.

Pain is typically localized in the upper arm in the region of the deltoid tuberosity and anterior lateral acromion. Pain is usually worse at night. Overhead activities often induce the patient's symptoms. Typical findings are loss of endurance during activities, catching, crepitus, weakness, and stiffness.

Physical Examination

A thorough examination of the shoulder should include evaluation of the cervical spine and an upper-extremity neurologic examination. The opposite shoulder must also be examined for comparison. Inspection, palpation for tenderness, and range of motion (ROM) should be completed. Palpation should include the AC joint, sternoclavicular (SC) joint, subacromial space, biceps tendon, and trapezius muscle. Impingement signs as described by Hawkins, Misamore, and Hobeika[38] (i.e., forward flexion to 90 degrees and internal rotation) and by Neer and Welch[63] (forward elevation and internal rotation) are performed for eliciting pain. If these tests produce pain, then they are considered positive signs of impingement and suggest rotator cuff dysfunction. The rotator cuff muscle is tested for strength. Subscapularis muscle strength tests include the lift-off test and the belly-press test. The lift-off test places the arm behind the back and up the spine. The patient is then asked to lift the hand off the back against restriction. The belly-press test places the arms onto the elbows bent to 90 degrees, and the elbows are then lifted anteriorly against restriction. Examination for instability is performed. Apprehension sign, a positive-relocation test, or inferior sulcus sign are all indicative of instability. Stability testing should be performed in different positions (i.e., seated, supine) to eliminate instability as the cause of secondary impingement. Evidence of rotator cuff pathology includes painful impingement signs or weakness and a painful arc of motion.[61]

Diagnostic Testing

Diagnostic testing includes radiographs, arthrogram or magnetic resonance imaging (MRI), and injections. An impingement test (subacromial space injection with 10 ml of 1% Lidocaine) is invaluable. Physical examination several minutes after the injection, including ROM, impingement signs, strength, and instability should be completed. Resolution of symptoms without instability indicates primary rotator cuff pathology or impingement. Relief of pain with evidence of instability indicates possible primary instability with secondary rotator cuff changes because of altered shoulder mechanics.

Arthrography had been the gold standard for identification of rotator cuff tears. Although reliable for the diagnosis of complete rotator cuff tears, it is less reliable for the evaluation of partial-thickness rotator cuff tears. MRI has evolved to provide an excellent noninvasive tool in the diagnosis of rotator cuff pathology and the shoulder labrum. MRI provides information not available by other diagnostic testing, including muscle atrophy, amount of rotator cuff retraction in full-thickness tears, bursal swelling, the status of the AC joint, and the shoulder articular cartilage. The combination of intra-articular contrast (gadolinium) and MRI (magnetic resonance arthrography) has been developed to better delineate abnormalities of the rotator cuff and labrum including partial surface rotator cuff tears.[64,69]

Treatment

Symptoms of rotator cuff dysfunction are usually treated initially in a nonoperative fashion (tendonitis, partial or full-thickness rotator cuff tears). Nonsteroidal anti-inflammatory drugs (NSAIDs), heat, ice, relative rest, cortisone injection, and rehabilitation programs are used in the treatment. The initial goal of treatment is restoration of normal ROM. This is followed by a rotator cuff strengthening program. Stretch cords for resistance are initiated and are followed by free weights as tolerated. To avoid aggravation of the rotator cuff, initially, all strength training should be below shoulder level.

Nonoperative treatment programs usually continue for 4 to 6 months. Success varies from 50% to 90%.[19,34,71-73] Approximately 50% of patients with complete symptomatic rotator cuff tears have satisfactory results with nonoperative measures, but these results may deteriorate with time.[41] This wide range of outcomes is likely the result of lack of uniformity in classification, indications, and treatment. Some individuals have rotator cuff tears with no pain and normal function, whereas others may have debilitating pain. This demonstrates a need for better understanding of the factors that lead to symptoms.

Indications for Surgery

Indications for rotator cuff surgery include failure of 4 to 6 months of conservative care or an acute full-thickness tear in an active patient younger than 50 years. Failure of treatment can be determined before an entire rehabilitation course is completed. Indication for earlier surgical treatment can include return to full strength with persistent symptoms, failure to tolerate therapy because of pain, or plateau of initial improvement with persistent symptoms. Early surgical intervention is also indicated for patients sustaining acute trauma with full-thickness tears associated with significant rotator cuff weakness and posterior cuff involvement, particularly in young patients with higher functional demands. In addition, patients with acute tears or extension of chronic cuff tears may benefit from early surgery.[40]

In general, the duration of nonoperative treatment must be individualized based on pathology involved, the patient's response to treatment, and individual functional demands and expectations.

Surgical Goals

The primary goal of rotator cuff surgery is decreased pain, including rest pain, night pain and pain with activities of daily living (ADLs). Arrest of the progression of rotator cuff pathology and improved shoulder function are additional surgical goals.

SURGICAL PROCEDURES

Tendonitis and Partial Rotator Cuff Tear

Surgical management for impingement and partial-thickness rotator cuff tears generally involve open anterior acromioplasty as described by Neer[61] or arthroscopic subacromial decompression (SAD) with release or partial release of the coracoacromial ligament. Partial rotator cuff tears greater than 50% of the width of the tendon generally are treated with takedown and repair of the rotator cuff either mini-open or arthroscopic repair.[85] Repair improves results compared with débridement alone in this patient group.

Full-Thickness Tears

The mainstay of treatment for full-thickness tears is surgical repair. The type, pattern, and size of the tear, as well as the surgeon's preference, dictate whether the repair is a full-arthroscopic, mini-open, or completely open procedure.

Small- or moderate-sized (3 cm or less) partial- or full-thickness supraspinatus or infraspinatus tears may be repaired fully with arthroscopic or mini-open technique. Large width (3 to 5 cm) tears may also be repaired mini-open or arthroscopic if the cuff is mobile enough to allow anatomic repair.

Large, immobile cuff tears involving the subscapularis or teres minor, as well as tears of the musculotendinosis junction may require an open approach. Massive chronic atrophic cuff tears should be considered for arthroscopic débridement for pain control.

SURGICAL TECHNIQUE

All operative procedures discussed in recent literature for primary repair of rotator cuff tears include use of an anterioinferior acromioplasty to decompress the subacromial space. The author presently performs GH arthroscopy and subacromial bursoscopy on all patients undergoing surgery for cuff pathology.

Shoulder arthroscopy and decompression is performed as previously described. After acromioplasty, the bursal surface of the rotator cuff is evaluated. With shoulder rotation, the cuff can be completely visualized. Mobile tears maybe treated with mini-open technique or with arthroscopic repair.

Arthroscopic Rotator Cuff Repair

Arthroscopic repair involves the same general steps as mini-open or open rotator cuff repair. Multiple arthroscopic portals are made. Posterior, anterior, and lateral portals are made for all athroscopic repairs. Additional portals are made depending on the rotator cuff tear configuration and include posterior lateral, anterior lateral, and lateral acromial portals. These allow access to various rotator cuff configurations and for suture anchor placement.

GH joint arthroscopy is followed by subacromial bursoscopy. The subacromial bursa is excised, and the anterior acromion is flattened with a burr. If symptomatic, then the AC joint is excised arthroscopically. The greater tuberosity of the humerus is lightly decorticated with a burr. The rotator cuff is visualized and is repaired to bone with suture anchors.

Mini-Open Rotator Cuff Repair

In the mini-open procedure, the lateral subacromial portal incision is extended either longitudinally or transversely to expose the deltoid fascia. The deltoid fascia is then split in line with its fibers directly over the tear. The anterior deltoid insertion of the anterior acromion is preserved. The deltoid fibers should not be split more than 4 cm lateral to the lateral acromion to avoid axillary nerve injury (Fig. 5-1). Rotation of the arm provides access to the tear. Digital palpation can be used to assess the adequacy of the acromioplasty. A bony trough is prepared in the greater tuberosity of the humerus. The rotator cuff may then be repaired through a bony bridge or with suture anchors. The permanent sutures are tied, pulling the rotator cuff down into its trough on the humerus.

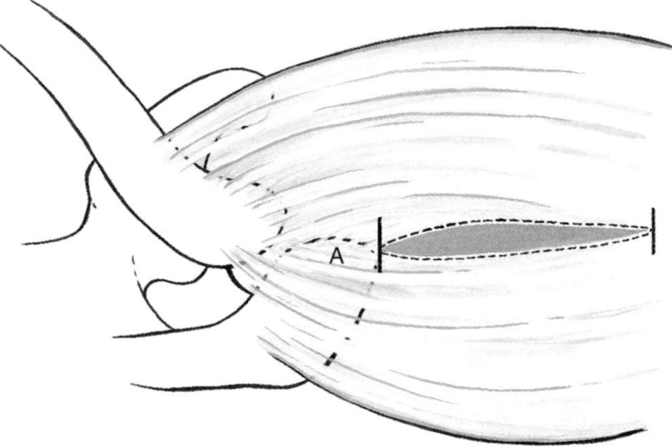

Fig. 5-1 Line of incision for partially open repair. The deltoid split begins at the lateral edge of the acromion (A) and should not extend more than 4 cm lateral to the acromion to avoid injury to the axillary nerve.

Open Rotator Cuff Repair

Tears that are fixed, retracted, but reparable, may be repaired open using principles developed by Neer.[61,62] An oblique incision in Lagers line from the anterior edge of the acromion to a point about 2 cm lateral to the coracoid process is made. The anterior deltoid is released from the anterior aspect of the acromion and splitting the deltoid no more than 4 cm lateral to the acromion (Fig. 5-2). The deltoid origin over the acromion is elevated subperiosteally. The coracoacromial ligament is released.

The anterior acromion is osteotomized. The acromion anterior to the anterior aspect of the clavicle is removed, and the undersurface of the acromion is flattened from anterior to posterior. The AC joint may be removed if arthritic and symptomatic. The distal clavicle is excised parallel to the AC joint so that no contact occurs with adduction of the arm.

The cuff tear is visualized and mobilized. A bony trough 0.5 cm in width parallel to the junction of the humeral articular cartilage and greater tuberosity of the humerus is made. The rotator cuff tear is repaired to bone with suture anchors or through a bony bridge in the

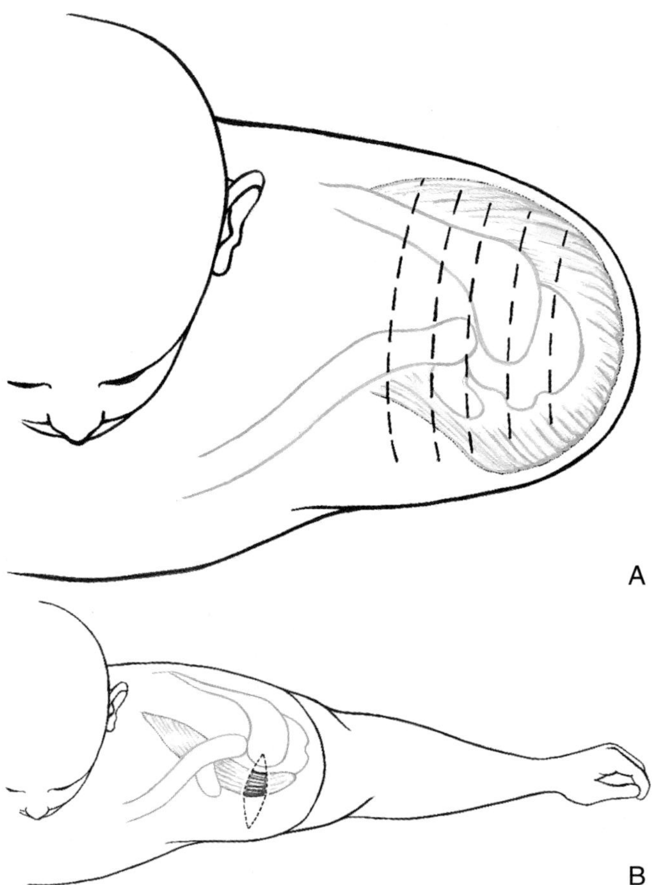

Fig. 5-2 Incision placed in Langer's lines produces the best cosmesis.

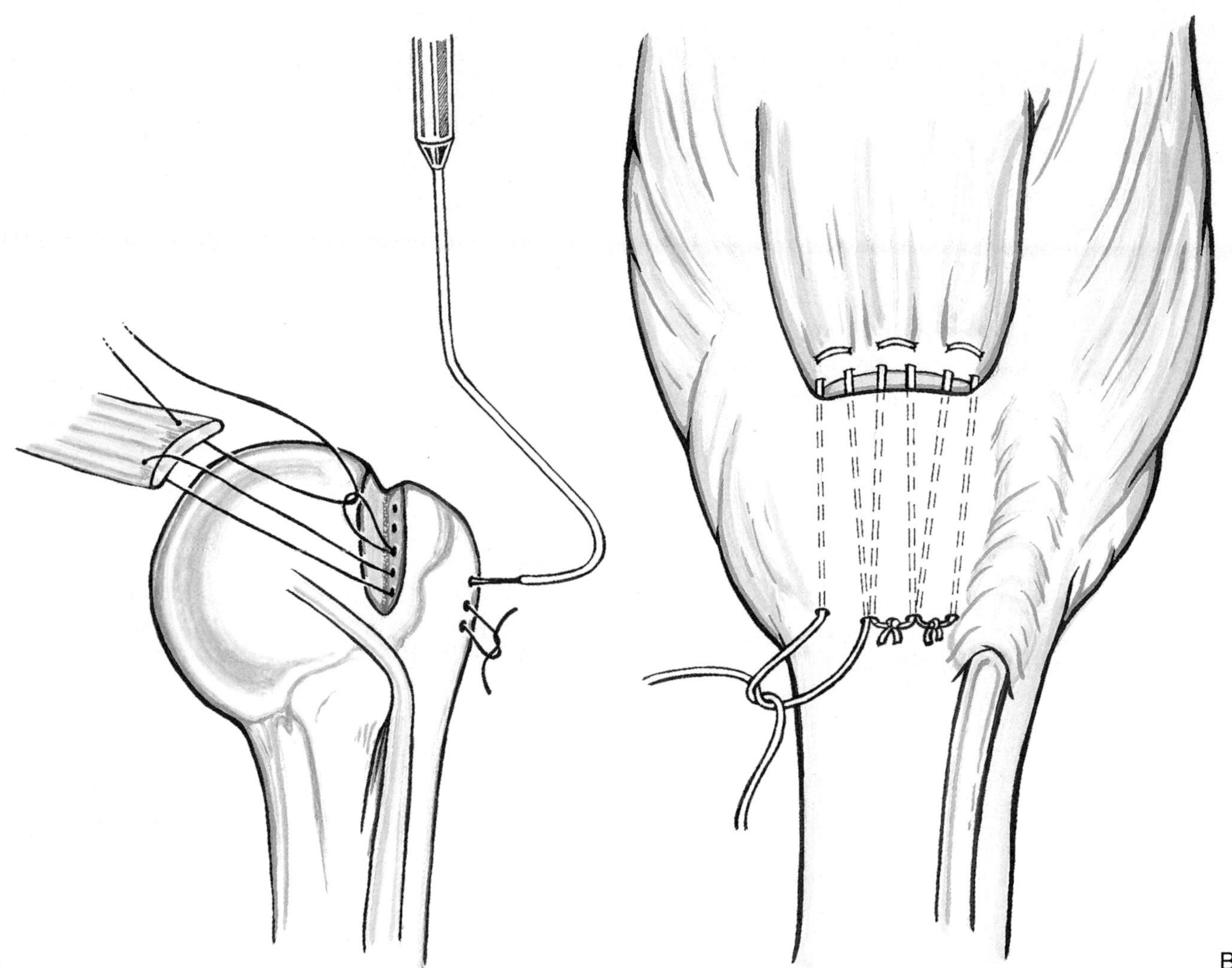

Fig. 5-3 Transosseous repair of rotator cuff tendon. A trough is created in the proximal humerus just lateral to the articular surface. Sutures are tied over the bone bridge in the greater tuberosity.

greater tuberosity using permanent sutures (Fig. 5-3). The goal is to repair the cuff with minimal tension with the arm at the side.

Watertight repairs are not necessary for good functional outcome. Excellent and good results have been shown in patients with residual cuff holes.[18,53] The anterior deltoid is repaired back to the acromion by preserved periosteum or through drill holes with permanent sutures. Routine skin closure is performed.

Postoperative management of cuff repairs must be individualized to incorporate tear size, tissue quality, difficulty of repair, and patient goals. Passive motion is initiated immediately. In general, supine active-assisted motion is started on the first postoperative day. Waist-level use of the hand can usually be started after surgery. Active ROM and isotonic strengthening are started 6 to 8 weeks after surgery. Progress of strengthening is individualized with full rehabilitation taking from 6 to 12 months. Function can continue to improve for 1 year after surgery.

MANAGEMENT OF MASSIVE TENDON DEFECTS

The management of massive irreparable tendon defects remains controversial. Options include SAD and débridement of nonviable cuff tissue without attempt at repair, use of autogenous or allograft tendon grafts, and use of active tendon transfers. Operations that require tendon transfer to nonanatomic sites to cover rotator cuff defects are likely to alter mechanics of the shoulder unfavorably.[15] Débridement may be pursued (either open or arthroscopic).

RESULTS OF TREATMENT OF FULL-THICKNESS ROTATOR CUFF TEARS

Satisfactory results after rotator cuff repair for pain relief occur 85% to 95% of the time [21,37,38,61] and appear to correlate with the adequacy of the acromioplasty and SAD. Functional outcomes correlate with integrity of the cuff repair, preoperative size of the cuff tear, and quality of the tendon issue. Poor outcomes are also associated with deltoid detachment or deneravation.[10]

Arthroscopic-assisted mini-open rotator cuff repair provides favorable clinical results. Results comparable with open cuff repair have been reported for small- and moderate-sized rotator cuff repair (less than 3 cm.).[6,51,53] These studies have shown the most important factor affecting outcome was cuff tear size. Tears of small or moderate size had better results. Belvin et al,[11] in a retrospective study, have shown 83% good or excellent results regardless of cuff size. Most studies have shown more rapid return to full activities with mini-open repair.

Fully arthroscopic repair studies have shown outcomes approaching the results of open rotator cuff repair or mini-open rotator cuff repair.[16,45,60,74,83]

A surgical technique that initially includes arthroscopy has the advantage of providing identification and treatment of intra-articular pathology (articular cartilage, labrum, biceps tendon). Additional advantages of arthroscopic rotator cuff repair include decreased soft tissue dissection, improved cosmesis, preservation of the deltoid attachment, decreased postoperative pain, and earlier return to ROM.

Unfortunately, rehabilitation cannot be accelerated for arthroscopic or mini-open cuff repairs because the limiting factor, tendon-to-bone healing, is not changed by the surgical technique.

No ideal surgical technique exists. Each surgeon must individualize treatment based on the type of lesion present, as well as the expertise of the physician. As the frequency of shoulder arthroscopy increases, surgical experience improves, and technical advances continue, a transition from open to mini-open to fully arthroscopic cuff repairs will proceed with arthroscopic repairs continuing to increase in frequency.

THERAPY GUIDELINES FOR REHABILITATION

The general guidelines that follow are for the rehabilitation of a type 2 rotator cuff tear (a medium-to-large rotator cuff tear that is larger than 1 cm and smaller than 5 cm). The protocol is designed for active patients (i.e., recreational athletes, laborers). An older, more sedentary individual progresses through the stages more slowly and is not an appropriate candidate for more aggressive exercises. The size of the tear and the tissue status will affect the rehabilitation process. An older patient with poor tissue status and a massive tear will be lacking in strength and endurance. These guidelines are designed to help guide therapists and provide treatment ideas. The scope of this chapter does not include instructions on treatment methods or applications. All modalities, mobilizations, and exercises suggested in this chapter are recommended only for therapists who have been trained in the methods and can appropriately apply them. The therapist must choose the treatment ideas that are beneficial for each patient within the restrictions outlined by the operative surgeon.

Q Jim is a 38-year-old weekend athlete who sustained a large rotator cuff tear after falling onto an outstretched arm during a flag football game. At 3 weeks after rotator cuff repair surgery, he complains of moderate shoulder pain that radiates through the upper-trapezius area and into the superior medial scapular area. Jim also complains of neck stiffness that has worsened over the past few days. He remains guarded through most of his range when performing PROM. During today's session, what areas should the therapist address to improve the quality of movement and increase the ROM?

Phase I

TIME: 1 to 4 weeks after surgery

GOALS: Comfort, increasing ROM as tolerated, decreased pain and inflammation, minimal cervical spine stiffness, protection of the surgical site, maintenance of full elbow and wrist ROM, and initiate voluntary muscle firing (Table 5-1)

Refer to Box 5-2 for a shoulder evaluation following a rotator cuff repair. The therapist must place the protection of the patient and the surgical repair while obtaining an evaluation; therefore, some tests will need to be deferred until later in the treatment process.

To reduce pain and swelling, use ice packs. Electrical stimulation may also be used for pain reduction. Instruct the patient in posturing for comfort. Encourage the patient to experiment with different positions. Usually a loose packed GH position (shoulder in some flexion, abduction, and internal rotation) with the arm supported by pillows while supine or sitting is the most comfortable. If the patient cannot sleep much initially after surgery in the supine position, then suggest sleeping semireclined in a recliner chair with the upper extremity supported in the loose packed position.

Gentle mobilizations using grades I and II help reduce pain, muscle guarding, and spasms. These mobilizations also help maintain nutrient exchange and therefore prevent

Box 5-2 Components of the Physical Therapy Evaluation

Background information
- Status of the capsule
- Status of rotator cuff
- Status of articular cartilage
- Previous procedures
- Associated medical problems that can influence rehabilitation (e.g., cardiovascular concerns, diabetes mellitus)
- Work-related injury
- Insurance status
- Comprehension

Subjective information
- Previous level of function
- Present level of function
- Patient's goals and expectations
- Intensity of pain
- Location of pain
- Frequency of pain
- Irritability of symptoms
- Presence of night pain
- Amount of hours able to sleep at night
- Assistance at home
- Access to rehabilitative facilities
- Medication (i.e., dose, effect, tolerance, compliance)

Objective information

Observations
- Muscle wasting
- Muscle spasms
- Resting posture
- Use of sling
- Wound status
- Swelling
- Color

Passive range of motion (PROM) of shoulder
- Shoulder flexion within the limits of tolerance
- Shoulder abduction within the limits of tolerance
- Shoulder external rotation
- Scapulothoracic joint

Palpation
- Biceps tendon (when tenderness and swelling near the surgical site has decreased)
- Trapezius muscle
- Cervical musculature
- Upper-thoracic spine
- Sternoclavicular (SC) joint
- Acromioclavicular (AC) joint (2 weeks s/p surgery)

Modified cervical spine evaluation

Delay active range of motion (AROM) testing of the shoulder until 7-8 weeks postsurgery

Delay strength testing until tissues have appropriately healed and testing can be done without irritating the shoulder

the painful and degenerating effects immobilization produces (i.e., a swollen and painful joint with a limited ROM).[36] Passive range of motion (PROM) and pendulum exercises are essential for increasing shoulder ROM. The passive exercises also provide nourishment to the articular cartilage and assist in collagen tissue synthesis and organization.[2,26,30] The organization of collagen may then follow stress patterns, and adverse collagen tissue formation may be minimized. PROM exercises are done in guarded and protected planes, with the patient and therapist taking care not to overstretch healing tissues. **Therefore horizontal adduction, extension, and internal rotation are not performed initially.**

> **A** The cervical spine needs to be assessed to determine whether it may be contributing to some of the patient's complaints, particularly the neck stiffness and the superior medial scapular pain. If cervical spine joint stiffness or soft tissue tightness is noted, then appropriate joint or soft tissue mobilizations may decrease these symptoms. As pain decreases, muscle guarding will lessen, allowing the shoulder to move more freely.

Perform PROM exercises for shoulder flexion and abduction (initiate these movements in the functional planes before progressing to straight planes of movement). Perform external rotation (ER) at zero degrees initially, then perform it in a functional plane, as treatments continue progress toward 45 degrees of abduction and finally 90 degrees of abduction. Move into the range so that a mild stretch is held for a second or two, and then repeat it approximately 10 times for several sets. A general guideline to use in judging the force or stretch is slight discomfort with a slight increase in motion after several repetitions. Remain sensitive and aware of the feedback the patient's body is exhibiting during ROM or mobilization techniques. The patient's response will dictate the amount of force applied or the plane of movement chosen. If muscle guarding continues to increase after several repetitions, the force being applied should be reduced or the plane of movement chosen needs to be slightly altered (or both need to be done) to avoid pinching sensations or increase of pain. The therapist usually can find a groove (i.e., line of movement that can be progressed more easily) or line of motion with less muscle guarding. Therefore constantly assess treatment application while treating the patient with manual PROM. Vary the treatment application as the patient's feedback dictates (i.e., exact plane of move-

Table 5-1 Rotator Cuff Repair

Rehabilitation Phase	Criteria to Progress to this Phase	Anticipated Impairments and Functional Limitations	Intervention	Goal	Rationale
Phase 1 Postoperative 1-4 weeks	◆ Postoperative	◆ Limited ROM ◆ Limited Strength ◆ Pain ◆ Initially restricted to PROM of the shoulder ◆ Dependent upper extremity immobilized in sling or airplane splint	◆ Cryotherapy ◆ Electrical stimulation ◆ PROM—Pendulum exercises, shoulder flexion, external rotation, and abduction in protected planes ◆ Isometrics (at 3 weeks) submaximal (without increasing pain); shoulder flexion and internal rotation; elbow flexion and extension; at 4 weeks initiate shoulder abduction and external rotation ◆ AROM—Elbow flexion, extension; cervical spine all ranges ◆ PREs—Hand gripping, exercises with putty ◆ Joint mobilization resistance free to the shoulder	◆ Decrease pain ◆ Manage edema ◆ Improve PROM and tolerance to movement ◆ Increase quality of muscle recruitment ◆ Maintain and improve ROM of joints proximal and distal to surgical site ◆ Maintain and improve distal muscle strength ◆ Control pain	◆ Pain control ◆ Edema management ◆ Prevention of joint stiffness ◆ Promotion of healthy articular surface and collagen synthesis and organization ◆ Prevention of further atrophy of upper-extremity musculature ◆ Eliminate neuromuscular inhibition ◆ Prevention of associated weakness, stiffness, and dysfunction of neighboring joints ◆ Gaiting of pain and preparation for stretches into resistance

ROM, Range of motion; *PROM*, passive range of motion; *AROM*, active range of motion; *PREs*, progressive resistance exercises.

ment, force and repetitions). An increase in ROM will often accompany a decrease in pain if executed with a sensitive hand. However general treatment soreness may be expected. Treatment soreness is usually more pronounced when progressing the patient from PROM to active range of motion (AROM) and then again when progressing to resisted ROM exercises.

During shoulder flexion, lead with the thumb up or palm up to clear the greater tuberosity from under the coracoacromial arch. Performing PROM in the scapular plane is beneficial because of decreased tension on the capsuloligament-tendon complex.[44] "In some cases, such as after RCR [rotator cuff repair] under tension, rotation exercises should be initiated at 45 degrees of abduction to minimize tension across the repair."[44]

Submaximal isometrics can be initiated in the later part of this phase to eliminate neuromuscular inhibition, reinitiate muscle firing, and retard muscle atrophy. Restoring voluntary control of the rotator cuff is imperative for proper function. At 3 weeks after the operation, the patient can begin submaximal and subpainful isometric exercises. Do not allow patients to perform isometrics at near maximal effort until the repair site has had sufficient time for healing.

Table 5-2 Rotator Cuff Repair

Rehabilitation Phase	Criteria to Progress to this Phase	Anticipated Impairments and Functional Limitations	Intervention	Goal	Rationale
Phase II Postoperative 5-8 weeks	◆ Incision area well healed ◆ Decreased pain to minimum levels ◆ Improved ROM ◆ Improved sleep patterns	◆ Limited tolerance to ROM ◆ Limited strength ◆ Relatively dependent upper extremity	◆ Continue phase I exercises ◆ Initiate A/AROM (supine) at 6 weeks progressing toward AROM ◆ Initiate A/AROM at 6 weeks for upper-extremity (PNF) D1 and D2 patterns using elbow and wrist movements in supine and progress to AROM ◆ A/AROM for shoulder flexion, external rotation, abduction, and scaption ◆ Soft tissue mobilization as needed after incision has healed ◆ Cardiovascular conditioning (e.g., bicycling, walking program)	◆ PROM shoulder flexion/ abduction 150-180 degrees, external rotation 70 degrees, internal rotation 55 degrees ◆ A/AROM reach above head height ◆ Prevent increase of pain ◆ Improve scar mobility; decrease pain ◆ Improve fitness level	◆ Continuing phase I exercises to minimize stiffness of adjacent joints ◆ Mimicking and strengthening of functional movements ◆ Improvement of ROM and strength ◆ Improvement of tolerance to movement and preparation for AROM ◆ Performance of exercises to ease subacromial pressures ◆ Normalization of skin mobility and desensitization of scar ◆ Provision of a good healing environment and normalization of arm swing with gait

ROM, Range of motion; *A/AROM,* active/assisted range of motion; *AROM,* active range of motion; *PNF,* proprioceptive neuromuscular facilitation; *PROM,* passive range of motion.

Q Brent is a 27-year-old who had a rotator cuff repair for a large tear. He has progressed nicely with PROM. At 9 weeks after surgery, Brent can elevate his arm above his head with little effort. However, he demonstrates a mild shoulder hike with elevation above 70 degrees. How much weight should Brent begin lifting when performing elevation exercises to 90 degrees?

Phase II

TIME: 5 to 8 weeks after surgery
GOALS: Protection of surgical site, improvement of ROM, increase in strength, decrease in pain and inflammation, maintenance of elbow and wrist ROM, and minimizing of cervical stiffness (Table 5-2)

During the second phase the therapist should avoid overstretching muscles into positions that could compromise the repaired tissues (e.g., horizontal adduction, internal rotation beyond 70 degrees, shoulder extension).

Strength should begin to improve, with the patient progressing from PROM to active/assisted range of motion (A/AROM) to AROM movements against gravity. A/AROM can begin at 6 weeks, and AROM can be initiated as able after 7 to 8 weeks. The therapist can incorporate active assistive proprioceptive neuromuscular facilitation (PNF) D1 and D2 patterns to mimic functional movements and strengthen the areas in functional planes.[66] In the D1 pattern the shoulder moves into flexion-abduction-external rotation. With the D2 pattern the shoulder moves into extension-adduction-internal rotation.[47,78] Initiate these exercises in the supine position with the assistance of the therapist. Then progress to

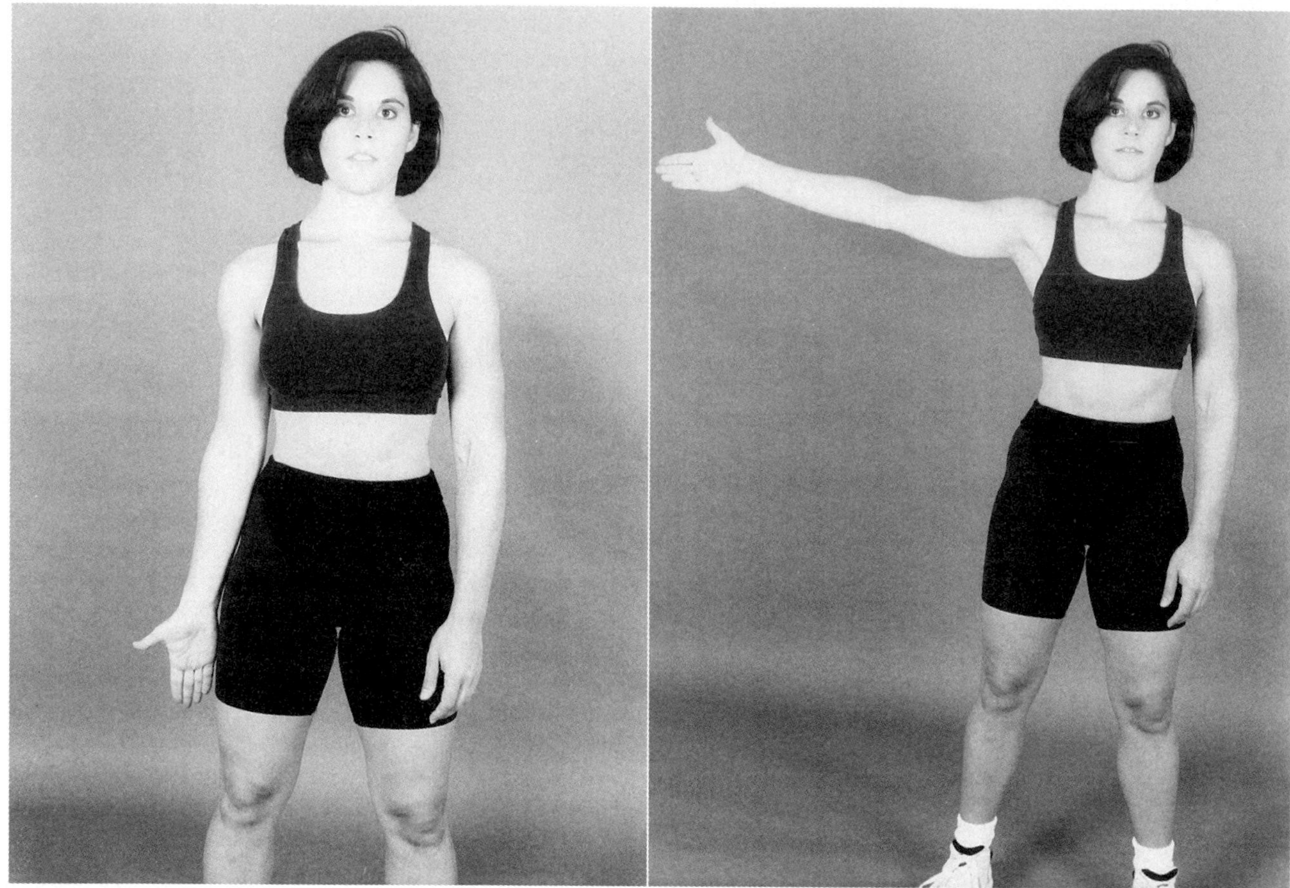

Fig. 5-4 Isotonic scaption exercises. These are elevation exercises done in the scapular plane. The patient holds the arm with the thumb up and the elbow straight and lifts the arm at a 45-degree angle to shoulder level. Patient progresses to full elevation and then gradually adds weight.

independent performance of the PNF patterns in supine advancing to a standing position when able. Eventually, active shoulder flexion, external rotation, and scaption exercises (Fig. 5-4) are performed after 7 weeks. Active shoulder flexion and scaption are usually initiated between zero and 70 degrees and progress according to the patient's ability to execute these exercises correctly. Incorrect performance of shoulder elevation exercises can lead to impingement problems.

Patients usually exhibit protective muscle guarding from the necessary insult of the surgery and the preceding shoulder pathology. Muscle guarding is present in the cervical region and the shoulder musculature. Therefore patients perform cervical AROM exercises and stretches. Appropriate cervical spine mobilization techniques may be valuable for decreasing cervical joint stiffness and muscle guarding, allowing more unrestricted movement of the shoulder complex.

Precautions at this stage include no heavy resisted exercises for 8 weeks. However, ROM exercises within pain tolerance can be performed after 7 weeks. Marked increases in swelling, pain, or wound drainage (or the presence of red, streaking marks) must be reported immediately, and exercises should be discontinued.

A Brent should not lift any weights above 70 degrees during shoulder elevation until he can execute the exercise correctly. He should practice maintaining voluntary humeral head depression with active elevation in front of a mirror. He should only do resisted exercises through the range he can correctly perform. Brent also can continue to perform appropriate resisted strengthening exercises for the serratus anterior muscle and the rotator cuff muscles. When he can elevate the arm correctly above 70 degrees, he can begin adding weight for resisted elevation above 70 degrees.

Phase III

TIME: 8 to 12 weeks after surgery
GOALS: Expansion of ROM, avoidance of impingement problems, gaining of full ROM, increase strength, alleviation of pain, increased function, and decreased soft tissue restrictions and scarring (Table 5-3)

Table 5-3 Rotator Cuff Repair

Rehabilitation Phase	Criteria to Progress to this Phase	Anticipated Impairments and Functional Limitations	Intervention	Goal	Rationale
Phase III Postoperative 8-12 weeks	◆ Steady improvement in ROM and strength (tolerance to movement) ◆ Pain controlled with therapy and medication ◆ Strength > $\frac{3}{5}$ generally	◆ Limited AROM ◆ Limited tolerance to use of upper extremity ◆ Limited reaching ◆ Limited lifting	◆ Continue exercises from phases I and II as indicated. ◆ AROM—Wand exercises (i.e., flexion, extension, abduction) progress to independent use of wand ◆ AROM progressing to PREs ◆ Begin shoulder ER with light weights and progress to using Theraband ◆ PREs (elastic tubing) for shoulder ER and IR with axillary roll ◆ Progressing to PREs (elastic tubing) for shoulder flexion and extension when able ◆ Isotonics—Shoulder flexion and abduction, modified military press ◆ Scapular exercises—Reverse rows; horizontal abduction (see Fig. 5-8); prone at 90-degree abduction, then ER without weight ◆ Scaption performed initially without weight ◆ Prone shoulder extension ◆ Standing push-ups against the wall ◆ Initiate low-level Body Blade exercises, then progress as appropriate ◆ Manual resistance added to PNF patterns	◆ Increase exercises that patient can perform at home ◆ Full PROM ◆ Strength of shoulder generally >55% ◆ Minimal pain associated with overhead activity ◆ Able to perform self-care activities using involved upper extremity	◆ Promotion of self-management ◆ Transition to AROM program with emphasis as appropriate on PROM ◆ Strengthening of shoulder and upper-quarter musculature with a variety of resistance devices and positions ◆ Scapular exercises to promote proximal stability for distal mobility ◆ Progression from AROM to PREs as tolerance to activity improves ◆ Performance of cuff -stabilization exercises with pain-free ranges

ROM, Range of motion; A/AROM, active/assisted range of motion; *AROM,* active range of motion; *PREs,* progressive resistance exercises; *PROM,* passive range of motion; *ER,* external rotation; *IR,* internal rotation.

Q Barbara is a 68-year-old woman who had a massive rotator cuff repair 12 weeks ago. Her favorite hobby is making jewelry. To work with the jewelry she needed to make a sawing motion with her affected (right dominant) upper extremity. At this point the patient had $-\frac{3}{5}$ strength for flexion and abduction. She exhibited $+\frac{3}{5}$ for ER and IR. Patient did not have the strength to make this sawing motion against much resistance throughout the range. She was weak, and her endurance was low. Tissue status was fair. How should the therapist exercise this patient?

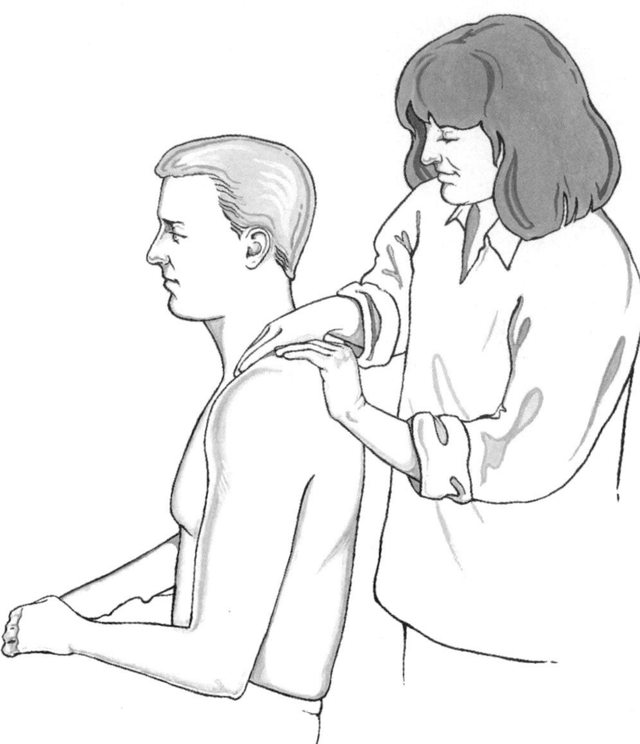

Fig. 5-5 Acromioclavicular (AC) mobilization through posteroanterior (PA) movement. The therapist stabilizes the midclavicle while applying a PA pressure through the spine of the scapula.

To advance to this phase the patient should have minimal pain, near full ROM, and greater than three-fifths strength generally throughout the shoulder movements. Often when progressing a patient to a new level of exercises (i.e., going from A/AROM to AROM), treatment soreness, muscle soreness, or both will be more pronounced initially. The patient will usually adapt to the new demands of the program within the first week.

During the period from 9 to 12 weeks after surgery, the patient's ROM should progress to full ROM. The repaired tissues are now strong enough to tolerate stretching within the patient's tolerance level. Passive stretching of the internal and external rotators is important. Tightness in these areas could promote abnormal shoulder mechanics, particularly in the throwing athlete. Tight external rotators lead to anterior translation and superior migration of the humeral head, which can produce impingement problems.[13]

AC joint pain is common in many patients who have undergone rotator cuff repair. The symptoms may result from a previous trauma, be caused by primary generalized osteoarthritis (OA), or follow abnormalities in the GH joint such as degeneration and rupture of the rotator cuff.[20] When the AC joint is hypomobile and symptomatic, mobilization can help alleviate a portion of the symptoms and allow greater mobility (Fig. 5-5).

After the incision is healed and closed, the therapist can apply soft tissue mobilization over the incision areas and instruct the patient in massaging the scarred area. Early movement minimizes tightness from scarring. Normal skin mobility allows normal movement to occur.[24]

Resistance exercises are initiated. Patients should demonstrate correct active movements before resistance is added in a particular range. The patient must perform the resisted exercises correctly or the movement needs to be altered (i.e., resisted shoulder abduction zero to 60° instead of 0 to 160°) so that the patient can successfully perform the exercise. Isotonic exercises are important for strengthening and promoting dynamic shoulder stabilization. The humeral head stabilizers are emphasized during this phase. The supraspinatus, infraspinatus, teres minor, and subscapularis muscles pull the humeral head securely into the glenoid and control humeral rotation so that the humeral head stays in good alignment with the glenoid.[2] In addition, it should be noted that the primary depressors of the humeral head during shoulder elevation are the infraspinatus, teres minor, and subscapularis muscles. Because the infraspinatus is involved in two critical force couples about the GH joint, the quality of shoulder motion is directly related to its function.[44]

When resisted exercises are initiated, begin ER with hand held weights with the patient in a side-lying position on the unaffected side. The elbow is maintained in 90 degrees of flexion, and the patient starts with the shoulder in internal rotation (IR), then moves into ER (Fig. 5-6, A and B). Eventually the patient can be progressed to concentric-eccentric movements using Theraband for ER and IR. An axillary roll can be placed under the shoulder to avoid a fully adducted position, which can cause a vascular stress on the supraspinatus and biceps tendon.[67,70] Resisted elbow flexion exercises can be done with exercise tubing for the biceps. The long head of the biceps brachialis has been revealed as a strong humeral head depressor and acts to steer.[44] Baylis and Wolf[7] described a "four square" combination of tubing-resisted exercises for shoulder flexion, shoulder extension, internal rotation, and external rotation, followed by stretching of the external rotators and abductors.

Remember that proximal stability is essential for controlling distal mobility.[47] Moseley et al[59] reported that four exercises appeared to significantly enhance recruitment of the scapular muscles. These exercises included shoulder elevation in the scapular plane, upright rowing, a press-up, and a push-up with a "plus."[44] Shoulder flexion and abduction exercises in the scapular plane (instead of the straight planes) are more functional and less problematic to the rotator cuff. Prone rowing can also be done (Fig. 5-7). Rowing is excellent for all portions of the trapezius, levator scapula, and rhomboids. These muscles help maintain the scapula in good alignment during shoulder movements. The higher- and the lower-trapezius musculature stabilizes the scapula for overhead activities. In addition, prone

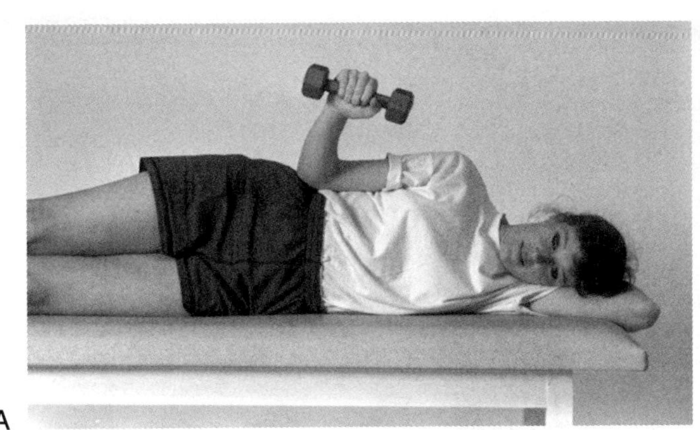

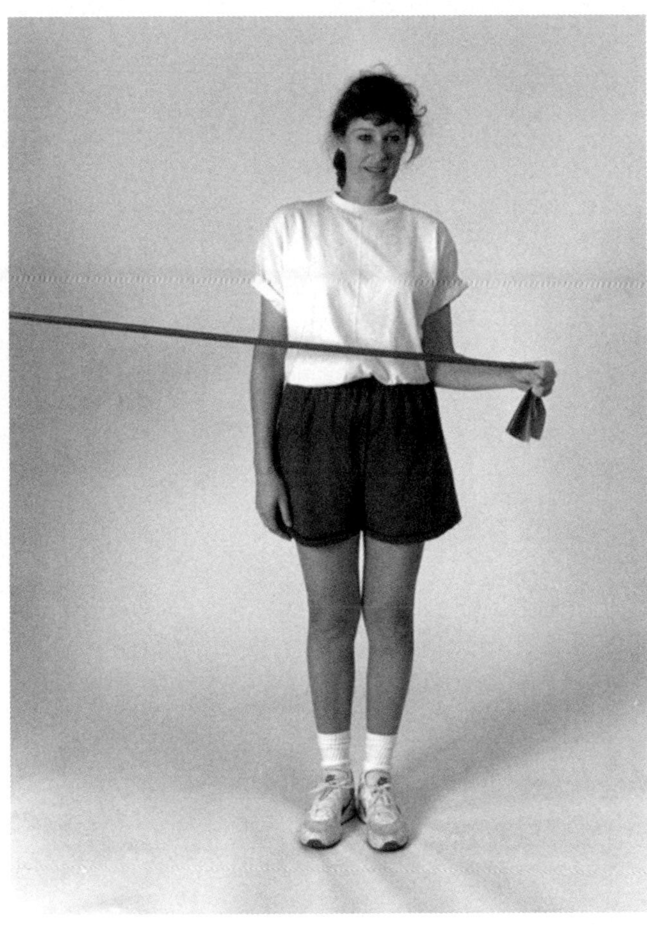

Fig. 5-6 A, Patient lies on the unaffected side, in the side-lying position. Patient maintains a 90-degree bend in the elbow while holding a hand held weight and moving the arm into external rotation. B, Again, the patient maintains the elbow in 90 degrees of flexion while externally rotating the shoulder against resistance of the band.

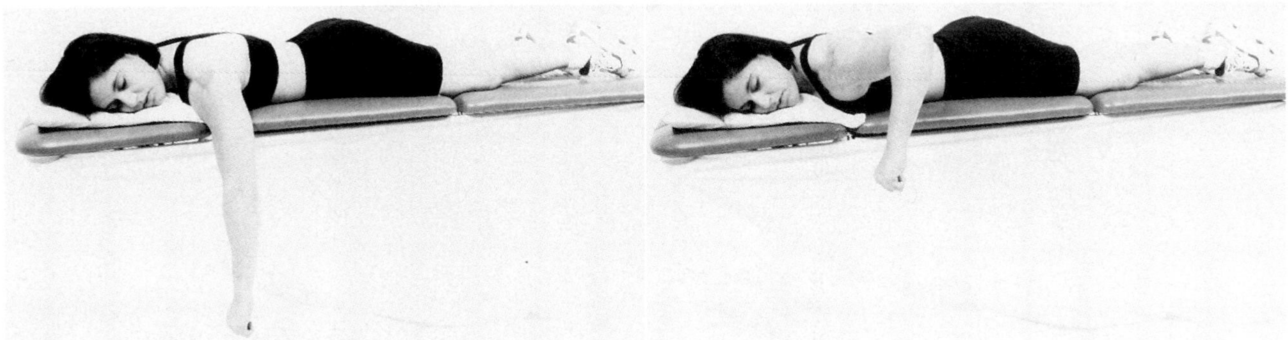

Fig. 5-7 Prone rowing. Patient hangs arm over edge of table, pulls hand upward while bending the elbow and tightening the scapular muscles, and slowly releases.

horizontal abduction can be incorporated to strengthen rhomboids major and minor and the middle trapezius (Fig. 5-8).[59] Progressive push-up exercises will strengthen the serratus anterior and the pectoralis minor muscles. A seated push-up with a plus was found to be effective in recruiting the serratus anterior with less activity of the trapezius musculature[59] (Fig. 5-9). Push-ups are initiated into the wall at this stage; later they can be progressed to table height, then performed on the floor "ladies' style," and finally some patients are progressed to a complete push-up. Press-ups are done with active patients. They can be initiated with support from the lower extremities and eventually progressed to only balance assisted by the lower extremities. These exercises help strengthen the serratus anterior muscle, which encourages humeral head depression with shoulder elevation. Older more sedentary

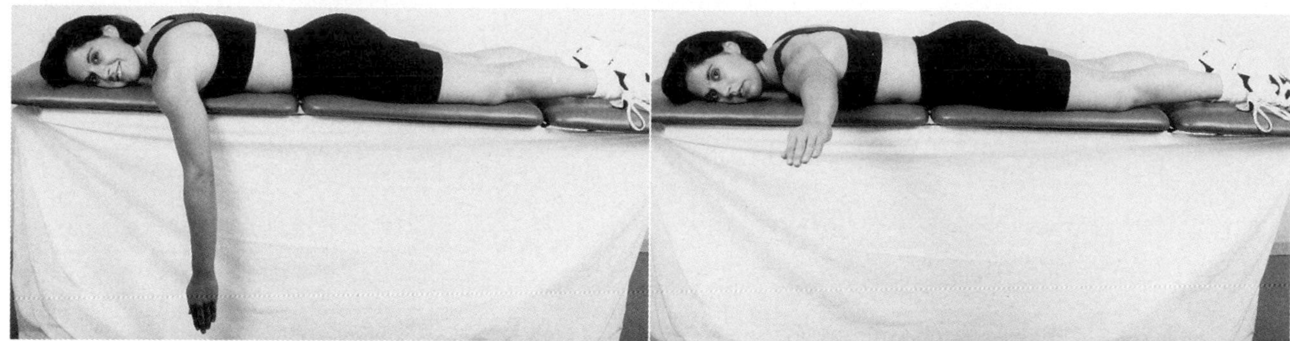

Fig. 5-8 Horizontal abduction in neutral, prone position with external rotation of the humeral head. Patient lies prone with elbow extended and arm hanging down. Therapist instructs patient to abduct the arm horizontally. Patient can start without weights, then gradually add resistance.

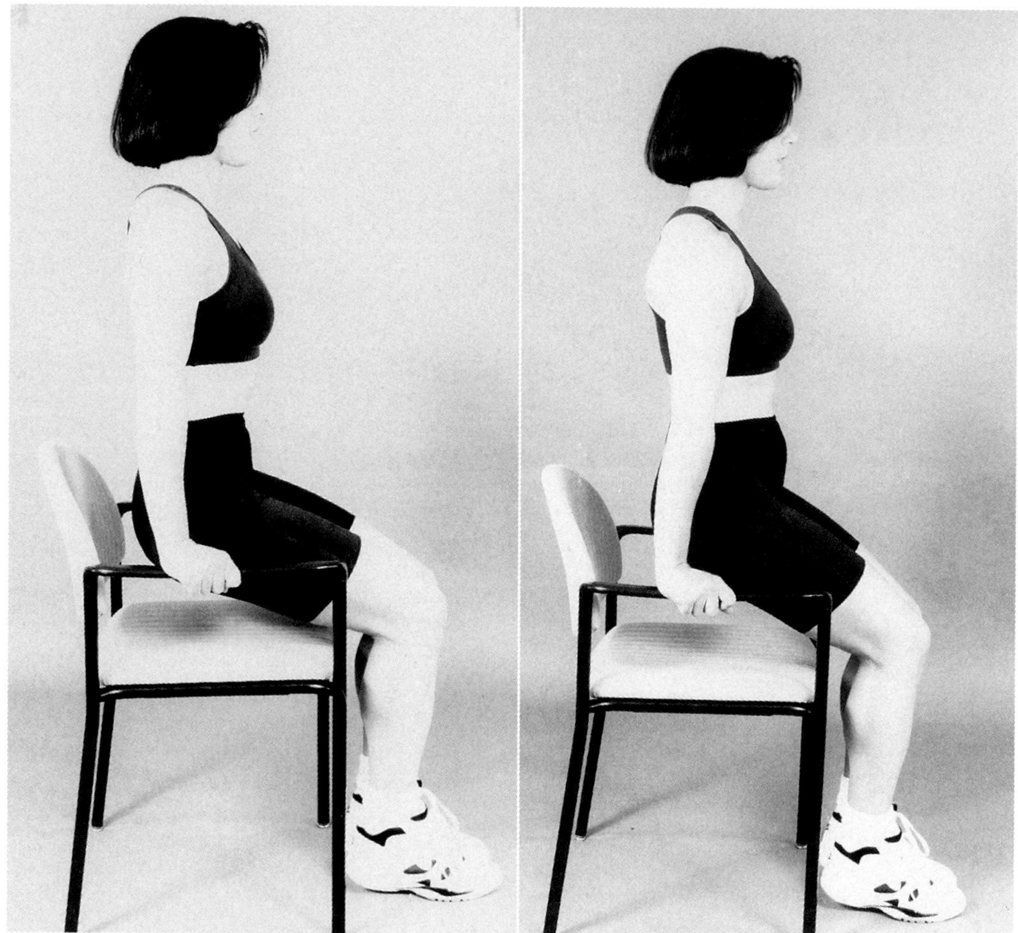

Fig. 5-9 Seated push-ups with a plus. Patient depresses the shoulders while maintaining straight elbows, thereby lifting the torso. Patient then slowly lowers torso, attempting to avoid excessive superior translation of the humeral head.

patients can strengthen their serratus anterior muscle using a Swiss ball (Fig. 5-10).

Resisted exercises also are performed in PNF patterns to strengthen the muscles in functional patterns. A frequently used pattern is the D2 pattern using both concentric and eccentric contractions. This is particularly effective in throwers. Manual resistance is again incorporated for rhythmic stabilization exercises and slow reversal hold techniques.[47,78] During rhythmic stabilization the most commonly used angles are 30, 60, 90, and 140 of shoulder elevation.[44] This movement will stimulate muscle contractions around the GH joint, promoting the joint force couples to work more efficiently and encourage better dynamic stabilization of the humeral head.[44] Good

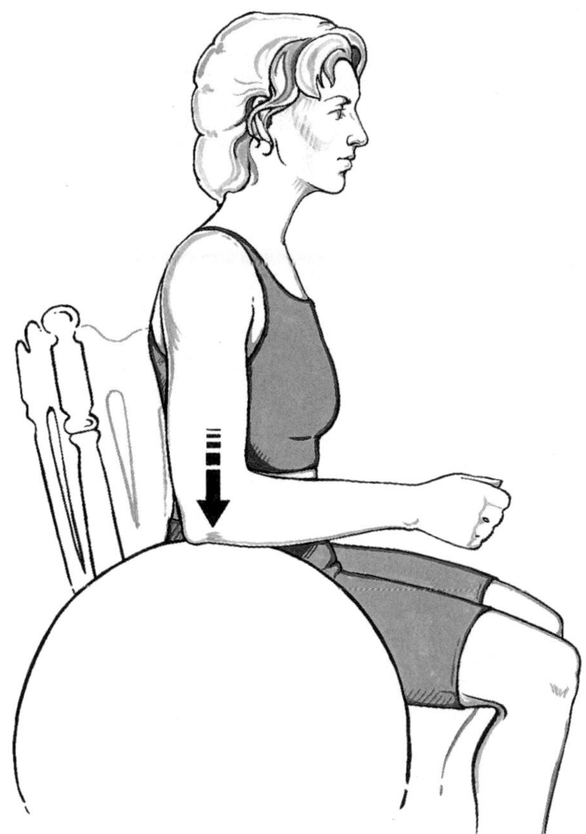

Fig. 5-10 Shoulder girdle depressions using a Swiss ball. Patient sits next to Swiss ball and places elbow on the ball. Patient maintains a 90-degree bend in the elbow while depressing the scapula to push the elbow down into the ball. This exercise is good for those who cannot or should not perform seated push-ups with a plus (e.g., older patients).

angles to work on with rhythmic stabilization are areas of increased weakness; therefore one can specifically strengthen at the weakest point, allowing improvement for the entire movement.

In the author's experience, the Body Blade has been helpful for active patients. Exercises with the Body Blade are initiated with the shoulder and upper arm against the trunk. Eventually patients progress to operating the Body Blade with the arm extended away from the body and elevated. In even more advanced stages, patterns of motion can be followed while maintaining the oscillations of the blade and proper body mechanics. These exercises enhance contractions around a joint, increase strength, increase proprioception, as well as improve coordination and increase endurance.

Often times, older patients with fair tissue status and massive tears have difficulty progressing to active shoulder flexion against gravity. Eccentric shoulder flexion exercises without weights help provide these patients with a transition to active shoulder flexion. Help patients lift their arms in the scapular plane above their heads; then instruct them to lower their arms without allowing them to fall. These patients also need to emphasize strengthening of their humeral head depressors. Finally, have them exercise in front of a mirror so that they can readily correct the tendency to shoulder hike.

Strengthening of the trunk and legs is important for athletes. Numerous studies indicate that the trunk and legs are responsible for more than 50% of the kinetic energy expended during throwing (refer to Appendix A).

Endurance training also begins during this phase. Patients begin on the upper body ergometer (UBE) with short-duration and low-intensity bouts, and then they advance to longer durations and higher-intensity bouts. Modalities are minimally used during this stage. Pain is generally minimal but will increase with moderate to dramatic changes in activity levels.

Precautions are necessary when initiating isotonic shoulder elevation exercises. Patients must be able to elevate their arms correctly without substitution patterns. Perform the exercises within a range over which the patient has control, and perform them correctly. All exercises should be performed with little or no joint pain. Complaints of muscle discomfort are acceptable and even desirable.[75] **However, if the patient complains of sharp pain through particular ranges, then the therapist needs to modify the exercises to avoid a painful arc.**

A Patient had full PROM throughout the affected shoulder. The therapist mostly performed manual assisted and resisted exercises with this patient to maximize strengthening at her weakest points in the range. The therapist performed PNF patterns for the upper extremity and the scapular muscles. Manual resisted exercises for serratus anterior strengthening and rotation strengthening. Resisted shoulder depression exercises were also done. In addition, rhythmic stabilization was used. Shoulder eccentric lowering was done for shoulder flexion strengthening because she could not perform AROM shoulder flexion against gravity (AROM shoulder flexion to 30 degrees before initiating a shoulder hike). Manual exercises with light resistance were done (and progressed) to mimic the sawing motion used with making jewelry. Surprisingly, patient did return to making jewelry after 5 to 6 weeks of exercising in physical therapy, along with home exercises. This patient was motivated and compliant.

Q Christine is a young mother who had a rotator cuff repair 6 months ago. She is returning to therapy because of stiffness issues in her shoulder. Her main complaints are reaching behind to grasp objects. Particularly difficult to reach toward the back seat of the car, which she needs to do frequently. She

Continued

Table 5-4 Rotator Cuff Repair

Rehabilitation Phase	Criteria to Progress to this Phase	Anticipated Impairments and Functional Limitations	Intervention	Goal	Rationale
Phase IV Postoperative 13-16 weeks	◆ Full ROM or near full ROM ◆ Pain controlled and self-managed ◆ No loss of strength with addition of phase III exercises ◆ No increase in night pain	◆ Limited tolerance to overhead activities ◆ Pain with activities involving prolonged use of upper extremity ◆ Limited strength of rotator cuff	◆ Exercises for phase III continued and progressed as appropriate ◆ Stretches—Corner wall stretch if necessary (see Fig. 5-11); posterior capsule stretch if restricted (see Fig. 5-12); hand behind back (see Fig. 5-13) ◆ PREs progressed—Prone horizontal abduction at 90 degrees and ER of the shoulder; closed-chain exercises; wall push-ups plus progressing to table push-ups, then floor push-ups if able; seated push-ups plus for active patients (see Fig. 5-9); shoulder girdle depressions using a Swiss ball for sedentary patients (see Fig. 5-10) ◆ May initiate plyometrics if appropriate at end of phase ◆ Progress with Body Blade exercises ◆ Trunk- and leg-strengthening exercises for return to previous level of functioning ◆ Stretching/mobilization to cervical and thoracic spine as needed	◆ Self-management of home exercises ◆ Full AROM ◆ Strength > 70% (dependent on extent of tear) ◆ Self-management of pain associated with overhead activity ◆ Reach in front and to side for light-weight objects ◆ Carry light weight for short periods (e.g., grocery bags)	◆ Preparation of patient for discharge and continued self-management ◆ Improvement of capsular mobility ◆ Restore end-range joint arthrokinematics ◆ Strengthening of upper quarter, especially scapula stabilizers in a stable but challenging environment ◆ Cocontraction exercises to enhance dynamic joint stability ◆ Preparation of patient for activity-specific demands ◆ Maintenance and improvement of cardiovascular fitness incorporating upper extremities ◆ Restore end-range joint arthrokinematics

ROM, Range of motion; *AROM,* active range of motion; *PREs,* progressive resistance exercises.

also would like to clasp her bra from the back. Upon evaluation she exhibited minimal restrictions for shoulder flexion and shoulder abduction near the end of the ranges. Shoulder internal rotation and extension were also limited, but the combined movement of IR and extension with hand-behind-the-back movements was the most restricted. Patient's thumb actively reached to T11 behind the back. What types of mobilization techniques would be particularly helpful?

Phase IV

TIME: 13 to 16 weeks after surgery

GOALS: Maintenance of full ROM, increased strength and endurance, improved function (Table 5-4)

The patient should have full ROM by 13 to 16 weeks. If this is not the case, then progressing with ROM needs to be the primary focus during treatments until this has been achieved. The therapist can emphasize more aggressive mobilization using grades +3 and +4 on the GH capsule

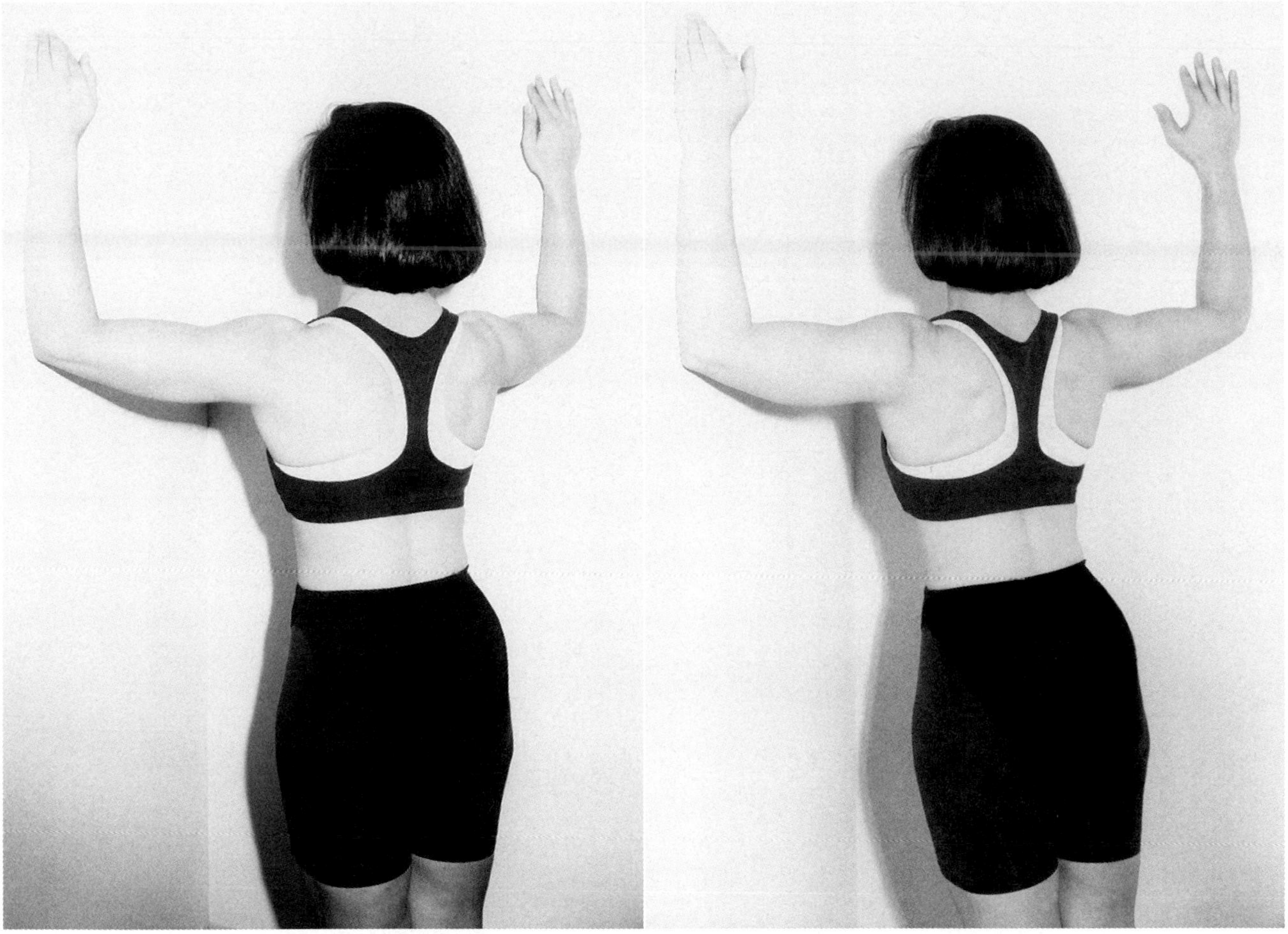

Fig. 5-11 Corner wall stretch. Patient stands facing a corner approximately one stride length away. The patient then places the forearms on the wall, keeping the elbows at shoulder height. The therapist instructs the patient to lean into the corner until he or she feels a stretch on the anterior portion of the shoulders.

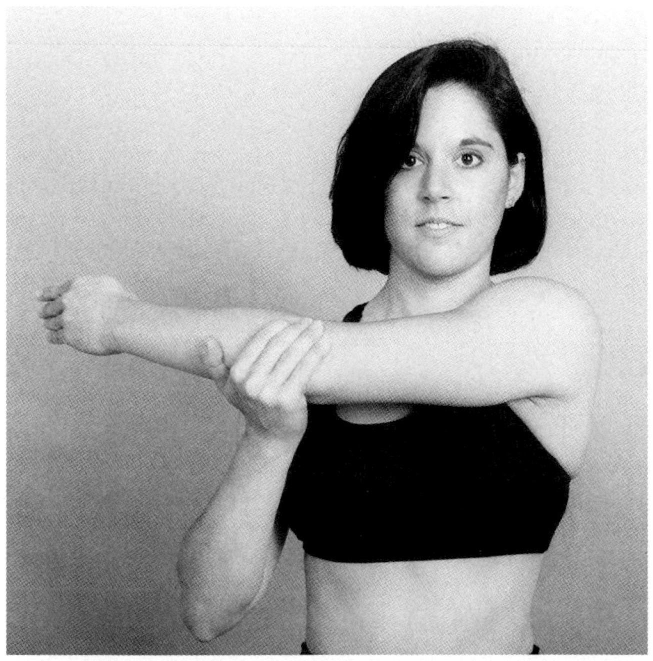

Fig. 5-12 Posterior capsular stretch. Patient horizontally adducts arm across body and then uses the other hand to pull the affected arm into further horizontal adduction.

to stretch the specific areas of capsular restrictions, thereby normalizing arthrokinematics at the GH joint. These mobilizations also can be performed near the physiologic end ROM, and they can be performed near end of ranges in conjunction with combined movements (refer to the last question-and-answer scenario for an application example). Adequate capsule laxity is necessary to allow normal rolling and gliding between the bony surfaces of a joint.[88] Patients should continue the necessary stretches to gain and maintain ROM in restricted areas (Figs. 5-11 through 5-13 illustrate some of the suggested stretches). **It should be noted that with throwing athletes the anterior capsule does not need to be stretched as much. Patients with anterior instability issues should not exercise near extreme ranges of abduction and external rotation. Those with posterior GH instabilities should avoid extreme ranges of horizontal adduction and internal rotation.**

If the patient cannot elevate the arm without shoulder hiking (i.e., scapulothorasic substitution), then continue with the humeral head-stabilizing exercises and exercise the humeral head depressors. Remember the primary function of the rotator cuff is to provide good humeral

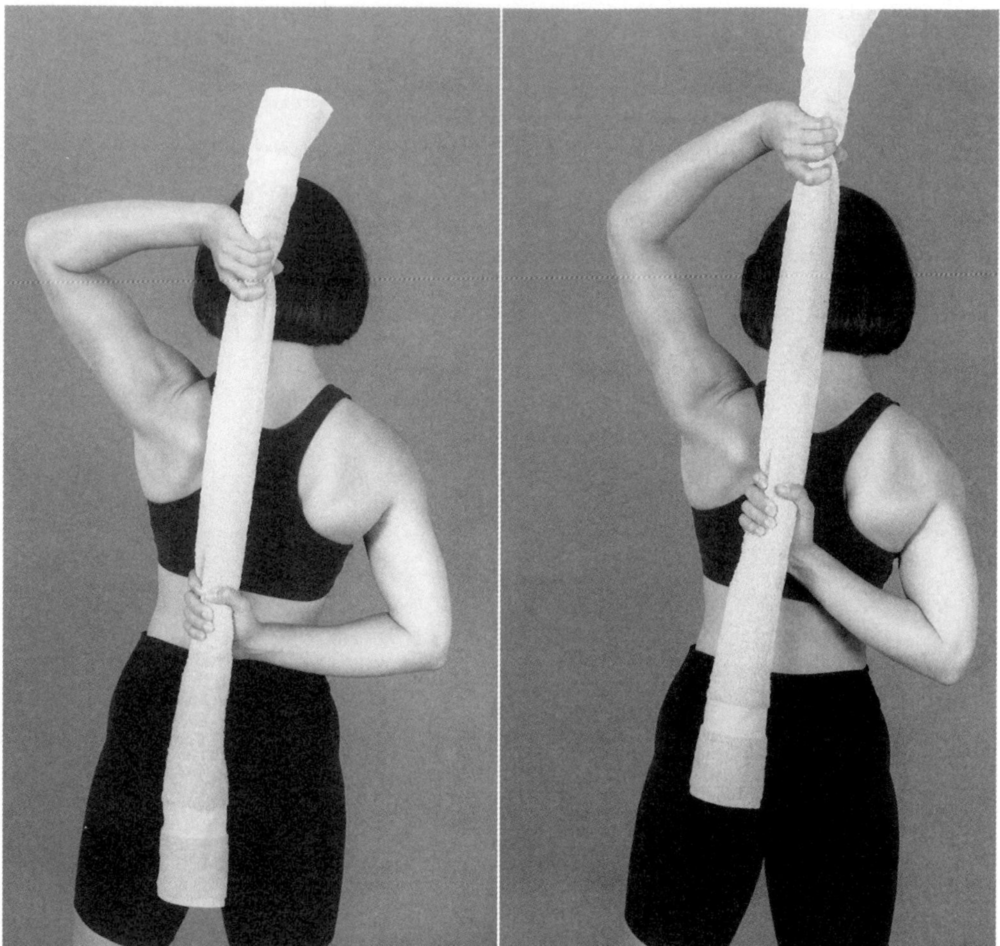

Fig. 5-13 Hand-behind-back stretch. Patient stands with towel in both hands and places the involved arm behind the buttock or low back. Patient places the uninvolved arm behind the head and slowly pulls with the superior hand up the back until he or she feels a stretch.

head alignment with the glenoid fossa; this must be mastered before any complex movements are initiated. The efficiency of the GH force couples is vital for success. The primary couples of the GH joint are the subscapularis counterbalanced by the infraspinatus and teres minor and the anterior deltoid and supraspinatus counterbalanced by the infraspinatus and teres minor.

Strengthening exercises are progressed with PREs. The supraspinatus and infraspinatus muscles (also known as *decelerators*) produce slow, controlled movements. These muscles are subjected to larger stresses and also are injured more frequently in overhead sporting activities.[4] Through the use of electromyographic (EMG) studies, Blackburn found that the best isolation for the infraspinatus and teres minor muscles occurs during prone exercises incorporating horizontal abduction and external rotation. An optimal exercise for GH congruity and stability is prone external resistance with the shoulder at 90-degrees abduction and the elbow flexed to 90 degrees. These exercises should be performed at a functional speed starting without weight then adding resistance.[25] Most older patients with massive repairs would have difficulty doing this exercise with resistance.

Continue with push-ups while leaning into a wall and progress to ladies' style if able. More active patients or athletes can progress to the standard push-ups on the floor, as previously mentioned. Closed-chain exercises help promote cocontractions and enhance dynamic joint stability.[46]

Therapists must also consider the neuromuscular system that provides joint stability through proprioceptive awareness, because proprioceptive training of the shoulder can lead to improved neuromuscular control, which can improve the overall dynamic stability of the GH joint.[87] Appropriate shoulder exercises using the Body Blade provide proprioceptive training, dynamic-stabilization training, and endurance training. Eventually (during the later stages of rehabilitation) the patient can be progressed using the Body Blade through a vast range of shoulder movements, allowing athletes and workers to train and exercise in specific patterns or postures that mimic a pattern of movement or a position used during a sport or work activity.

Table 5-5 Rotator Cuff Repair

Rehabilitation Phase	Criteria to Progress to this Phase	Anticipated Impairments and Functional Limitations	Intervention	Goal	Rationale
Phase V Postoperative 17-26 weeks	◆ Progression through phase IV without loss of strength or increase in pain ◆ Potential to return to high-level functional use of the upper extremity (i.e., competitive athletics)	◆ Limited strength and endurance of rotator cuff muscles ◆ Continued manageable pain with overhead activities	◆ Continuation of phase IV exercises as indicated ◆ Joint mobilization as appropriate ◆ PREs progressed ◆ Initiate strengthening in sport-specific activity ◆ Initiate isokinetic exercises ◆ Plyometrics ◆ Theraband for ER with the shoulder abducted at 90 degrees and elbow at 90 degrees ◆ Initiate throwing program when appropriate (see Appendix A)	◆ Pain-free with overhead activity ◆ Able to perform ADLs without increased pain ◆ Return to previous level of functioning ◆ Increase strength, endurance, and neuromuscular control	◆ Strengthening of rotator cuff in specific ranges (overhead and reaching to the side) ◆ Provision of optimal ROM for the client to perform the associated activity ◆ Provision of a vehicle for the client to return at or close to the previous level of functioning

PREs, Progressive resistance exercises; *ADLs,* activities of daily living; *ER,* external rotation.

A Mobilizations were performed in various areas of the capsule to improve all functional ranges. Mobilizations were also done near end ranges with combined movements using grades 3 and +4 to improve her hand-behind-the-back motions. The patient used her unaffected upper extremity to hold her other hand behind her back while the therapist applied a posterior-anterior force to the superior humerus. This was done to stretch the anterior capsule of the GH joint near its end range of combined movement. This was followed by the, hand-behind-the-back stretch, using a towel as shown in Fig. 5-13. The patient's range improved dramatically after two treatments with the execution of home exercises that reinforced the hand-behind-the-back movements, as well as other limited movements.

Phase V

TIME: 17 to 21 weeks after surgery

GOALS: Maintenance of full ROM, increased strength and endurance, improvement of neuromuscular control, return to functional activities, initiation of sport-specific activities (Table 5-5)

The therapist can continue the stretching program and instruct the patient in self-mobilization techniques if indicated. The patient can maintain a shoulder-strengthening program and continue PREs with increasing hand weights up to 6 to 10 lb for athletes or 1 to 5 lb for more sedentary people. Isokinetic exercises may be initiated with athletes when they are able to lift 5 to 10 lb in external rotation and 15 to 20 lb in internal rotation without pain or significant edema.[12] The patient should begin strength and endurance training at 200 degrees/second.[12] Athletes and other appropriate patients can begin plyometric exercises, which involve a stretch-shortening cycle of the muscle. Plyometrics can be performed two times a week. All sporting movements involve this explosive stretch-shortening cycle (e.g., jumping, throwing, running, swimming).[88] These exercises are excellent progressive steps between traditional strengthening exercises and training activities before initiating throwing drills.[87]

Resisted exercises using tubing with concentric-eccentric contractions, isokinetics, and scapulothorasic strengthening can be done. Progressive plyometric exercises are done with appropriate patients who exhibit correct execution of the exercises. Recreational and competitive athletes perform exercises at higher speeds, using more eccentric muscle contractions and higher-level progressions. Athletes or workers required to do continuous overhead activities can perform exercises with T-band for ER, starting with an axillary pillow between the trunk and arm, then to the scapular plane position, and then to the 90/90 position if able. D2 diagonal patterns can be executed with tubing, and latissimus strengthening and scapular retraction exercises can be performed using Theraband. Athletes and higher-level patients can perform these exercises at faster and higher speed while maintaining control over the movement. They can also perform at a slower and more deliberate pace. Initiate sport-specific drills for athletes along with an interval sports program (refer to Appendix A). Throwing techniques need to be evaluated. **If the patient is using bad body mechanics, using improper techniques while throwing, or both, then tissues may be overstressed, eventually causing rotator cuff problems once again.** Older, sedentary patients should work on specific ADLs. As appropriate, patients may progress to more difficult tasks.

Phase VI

TIME: 22 and more weeks after surgery
GOAL: Return to normal activities, maintenance of full ROM, continued strengthening and endurance, gradual return to full activities. Athletes can return to their sports usually between 6 and 12 months

During weeks 22 to 26 patients maintain a stretching and strengthening program. Athletes continue on strengthening and on a sports interval program. Others gradually progress to recreational activities. Older individuals continue to progress with PREs and work on more advanced ADLs. The ability to return to more high-level activities ranges from 26 weeks to more than 1 year after surgery. After 26 weeks, patients continue with their stretching and strengthening program as long as they anticipate using the shoulder aggressively in ADLs or sports.

SUGGESTED HOME MAINTENANCE FOR THE POSTSURGICAL PATIENT

The home maintenance box on page 88 outlines ideas for rehabilitation the patient can follow after rotator cuff repair. The physical therapist can use it in customizing a patient-specific program. Patients require a program that suits their needs and abilities. Some exercises may be appropriate for certain patients but not for others. Some patients progress slower than others. The therapist must take into account the patient's age, the condition of the repaired tissues, the size of the tear, the cause of the tear, the rate of healing, and the patient's abilities and previous level of function.

TROUBLESHOOTING

Considering influential factors outside the GH joint during treatment will aid the therapist in helping the patient progress more efficiently. General suggestions are given; however, it is beyond the scope of this book to instruct therapists in the use and application of techniques. The following areas are addressed:

- Cervical spine
- Thoracic spine
- Adverse neural tension (ANT)
- AC joint
- Sternoclavicular (SC) joint
- Scapulothoracic joint

Cervical Spine

Evaluation of the cervical spine may prove vital in addressing cervical issues that may be inhibiting progress. Although the cervical spine is not the primary cause of shoulder dysfunction when dealing with rotator cuff repairs, it may be a contributory factor. Often cervical spine disorders occur in conjunction with a traumatic shoulder injury (e.g., falling onto the upper extremity may cause injury to the shoulder and the cervical spine). Furthermore, prolonged muscle guarding secondary to the shoulder injury or pathology affects the cervical area. Muscles in spasm originating or inserting along the cervical spine can lead to cervical symptoms. Thus a patient may have a combination of cervical and shoulder signs and symptoms. Treatment to the appropriate cervical joints can alleviate a portion of the symptoms and signs, thereby decreasing the complaints of pain and potentially allowing more GH movement and function. Clinicians may notice that after treating cervical spine dysfunctions, treatment of the shoulder is more effective.

Common patterns in cervical pathology are addressed to assist clinicians with differentiating shoulder and cervical symptoms, because they frequently occur together. Spinal disorders may cause referred pain (Fig. 5-14). Joint movement disorders may cause joint pain and be associated with an altered range of cervical spine joint movement or shoulder movement. Therefore the cervical spine should be assessed for additional joint disorders that may be causing local pain or pain that is referred into the shoulder and arm region.[22] (Suggested reading for treatment of the cervical spine are *Practical Orthopedic Medicine* by Corrigan and Maitland[22] and *Vertebral Manipulation* by Maitland.[56])

Thoracic Spine

Thoracic mobility affects shoulder mobility. During unilateral shoulder flexion, contralateral side flexion of the spine occurs; bilateral shoulder flexion produces spinal extension.[43] Therefore decreased thoracic extensibility or increased thoracic kyphosis can inhibit shoulder ROM.[5]

Postural education is important, especially with patients who can voluntarily correct and maintain good posture. Maintaining an erect posture while performing upper-extremity activities allows greater ROM at the shoulders. Better posture decreases the amount of impingement, which a patient can see in the following maneuver:

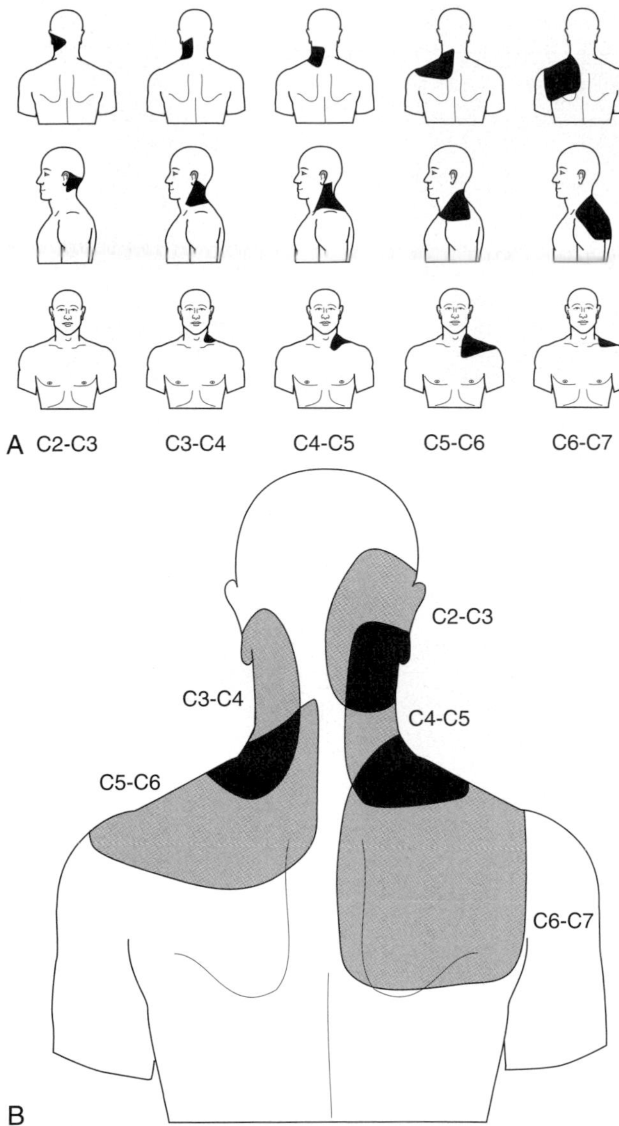

Fig. 5-14 **A,** Patterns of pain evoked by stimulating the zygapophyseal joints at segments C2-C3 to C6-C7. **B,** A composite map depicting the characteristic distribution of pain from zygapophyseal joints at segments C2-C3 to C6-C7.
(From Dwyer A, Aprill C, Bogduk N: Cervical zygapophyseal joint pain patterns. I. A study in normal volunteers, *Spine* 15(6):453, 1990.)

1. Have the patient flex the shoulder through its available ROM while in a seated slouched position.
2. Ask the patient to flex the shoulder while seated with good posture.

The patient will be able to lift the arm higher when maintaining a more upright posture. A slouched position causes depressed forward-displaced shoulders and GH internal rotation. The potential for shoulder impingement increases with this type of posture.[5]

Evaluation and treatment of the thoracic spine may prove helpful for patients having difficulty progressing in ROM in the latter stages. Addressing issues of hypomobility and decreased ROM of the thoracic spine and treating them appropriately allows for better progress. Mobilization of a hypomobile thoracic spine and ROM exercises to increase thoracic extension (e.g., supine on a Swiss ball) can be beneficial. A foam roll also may be used when appropriate to increase thoracic spinal extension and mobility (Fig. 5-15). (*Vertebral Manipulation*[56] offers instruction on evaluation and treatment of the thoracic spine.) With regard to positioning, the therapist also must consider protection of the shoulder and the surgery site.

Adverse Neural Tension

The nervous system can be directly mobilized through tension tests and their derivatives.[17] Adhesions in neural tissue can limit shoulder movement and may influence the patient's progress. However, the therapist must be aware of any precautions or contraindications. A good evaluation is necessary for addressing ANT issues. Neural tissue mobilization can be effective when used with appropriate patients to help relieve some of the symptoms and potentially improve ROM and strength. These issues may be better addressed during the latter phases of rehabilitation when the patient is well healed and shoulder ROM is only minimally limited or not restricted. Clinicians trained in neural tissue mobilization should only perform treatment to the nervous system. Avoid placing a stretch on the nerves. **The objective is to move the nerves, mobilizing them without stretching them. Increase in symptoms, like pain, numbness, tingling, and paresthesias down the arm may indicate the nerves are being stretched.**

Acromioclavicular Joint

OA in the AC joint is not uncommon.[27] It may result from previous trauma or be part of a primary generalized OA, impingement, or capsulitis. OA in the AC joint also may follow other abnormalities in the GH joint (e.g., degeneration and rupture of the rotator cuff) that allow the head of the humerus to sublux upward.[22] In the experience of the authors of this chapter, many patients with repaired and unrepaired rotator cuff tears have some symptoms arising from the AC joint.

Because the movement of all of the joints affects the shoulder complex, it is essential to evaluate and treat the entire shoulder complex to improve upper-extremity function.[52] Box 5-3 shows all the joint movements that occur within the shoulder complex. Restrictions in one area will affect other areas of the shoulder complex.

Complaints of AC joint pain are usually localized over the joint. An active movement that may best implicate this joint as a source of pain is horizontal adduction of the arm across the chest. The therapist may determine whether the AC joint is hypomobile or hypermobile by passive accessory movement tests of the joint.[81] If the AC joint is stiff and tender, then its mobilization often relieves a portion of the symptoms and promotes better shoulder ROM.

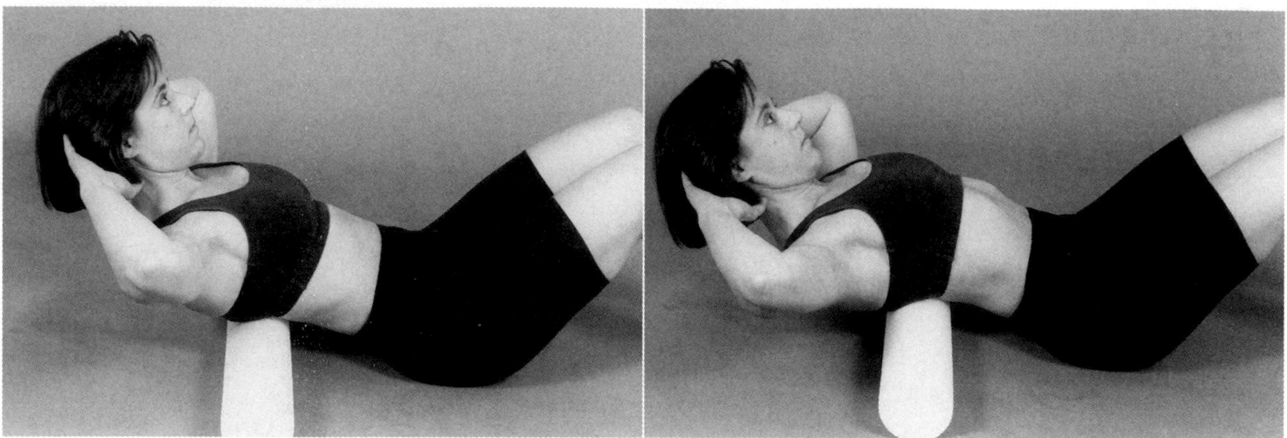

Fig. 5-15 Thoracic extension on foam roll or using tennis balls. Patient lies supine with both knees bent and places roll or balls at the middle thoracic spine levels. Patient then places hands under head and slowly leans back (taking care not to arch over the roll or balls) until a stretch is felt.

Box 5-3 Shoulder Complex—Range and Axis of Motion*

Joint Motion	Range (degrees)	Axis of Motion
Sternoclavicular (SC) rotation (counterclockwise)	0-50	Longitudinal axis of clavicle
Elevation	0-30	Oblique through
Depression	0-5	costoclavicular ligament
Protraction	0-15	Vertical through
Retraction	0-15	costoclavicular ligament
Glenohumeral (GH) flexion	0-180	Coronal through
Hyperflexion	0-55	GH joint
Abduction	0-180	Sagittal through
Horizontal adduction	0-145	GH joint Vertical through GH joint
Internal rotation	0-90	Vertical axis through
External rotation	0-90	shaft of humerus
Acromioclavicular (AC) winging of scapula	0-50	Vertical axis through AC joint
Abduction of scapula	0-30	Anteroposterior axis
Inferior angle of scapula tilts away	0-30	Coronal axis from chest wall
Scapulothoracic		
Upward rotation	0-60	From 0-30° near vertebral border on spine of scapula; from 30-60° near acromial end of spine of scapula
Elevation	Translatory	No axis
Depression	Translatory	No axis
Protraction	Translatory	No axis
Retraction	Translatory	No axis

*Data for this box was compiled from references 1, 2, 4, 9, 14, 18, 21. When conflicting information occurred, the most frequently cited numbers were used.

Accessory movements can be applied to the clavicle or acromion. When applied to the clavicle, they affect only the AC joint; however, when applied to the acromion, they affect both the AC and GH joint.[64] Accessory AC joint movements should be used within the limits of pain. To increase motion at the AC joint, the therapist can use an anterior glide to the acromion through the posterior spine of the scapula while stabilizing the midclavicle. This allows mobilization of the AC joint without direct manual pressure over the joint or inflamed tissues. As the available shoulder ROM progresses, this same technique can be applied with the shoulder in some degree of available flexion or in horizontal adduction (see Fig. 5-5).

Corrigan and Maitland[22] describe a similar technique for the AC joint. In this method an anterior-posterior movement is produced by applying pressure over the anterior surface of the outer third of the clavicle with counter pressure along the spine of the scapula.

Sternoclavicular Joint

Degenerative changes are not found as commonly in the SC joint as in the AC joint but may occur as the result of trauma or overuse of the shoulder.[28] Movements such as shoulder abduction or flexion may increase pain originating from this joint because of rotation of the inner end of the clavicle. SC joint pain is usually localized to the SC area, but it may radiate to other areas. Signs that implicate the SC joint as a contributing factor include reproduction of pain with horizontal flexion and passive accessory movements of the SC joint. The capsule and surrounding ligaments are likely to be thickened and tender.[81]

Treatment of the SC area includes rest, modalities, and mobilization, depending on the condition of the joint.[22] A hypomobile SC joint may be correctly mobilized in several ways depending on its restrictions. To increase shoulder elevation, a caudal glide to the proximal clavicle can be used.[22,57]

Scapulothoracic Joint

Scapular muscles have been included in the rotator cuff repair protocol. However, some patients require more intense conditioning of these muscles. The scapula moves with concentric-eccentric motions. Patients with poor eccentric control of the scapular stabilizers demonstrate scapula winging on the return from full shoulder flexion. These same patients may have full ROM and normal movement during flexion. If muscle weakness is apparent, then ensuring normal muscle strength around the scapulothoracic and GH joints is the goal. If the scapular muscles are weak and overstretched, then scapular motion during arm elevation may result in excessive lateral gliding of the scapula.

The therapist can use various PNF techniques such as scapular slow reversal holds, rhythmic stabilization, and timing for emphasis to intensify the dynamic control and kinesthesia of the scapulothoracic joint. Other recommended exercises are scapular protraction, retraction, elevation, and depression against manual resistance.[86]

Exercises that enhance dynamic control of the scapulothoracic musculature are encouraged.[86] These should be directed to the scapular rotator muscles (i.e., the serratus anterior, rhomboid, trapezius, levator scapula) to position the glenoid and coracoid appropriately for the humerus. Exercises that mimic the rowing motion and shoulder horizontal abduction are both excellent for all portions of the trapezius and for the levator scapulae and rhomboid muscles. Flexion and scaption (i.e., scapular plane elevation) exercises are valuable for most of the scapular muscles (see Fig. 5-4). In addition, shoulder shrugs and press-ups with a plus are essential exercises for the levator scapula, upper trapezius, serratus anterior, and pectoralis minor muscles. Also refer to the "Prone Program Plus" on page 103 for more exercise ideas.

SUMMARY

The general guidelines described in this chapter help guide therapists and provide treatment ideas. Rotator cuff repairs vary in size from small to massive. The condition of the torn tissue and the joints (i.e., AC, GH) varies. Along with these differences, therapists must consider the patient's unique history, profile, and abilities. They must consider each case and choose the treatment ideas that will work best, constantly assessing the patient's responses. Therapists must always address the individual when deciding on a treatment plan.

SUGGESTED HOME MAINTENANCE FOR THE POSTSURGICAL PATIENT

Older, more sedentary patients will progress more slowly than younger, more active patients. Some of the exercises suggested may be inappropriate for the older patient. The therapist can alter the home exercise prescription according to the individual's abilities, status, and needs.

Weeks 1-4

GOALS FOR THE PERIOD: Achieve control of pain and inflammation; increase ROM as tolerated, and promote firing of muscles.

1. Do active cervical spine rotations.
2. Do upper-trapezius (UT) stretches.
3. Do pendulum exercises.
4. Begin submaximal isometrics at 3 weeks for shoulder flexion and internal rotation.
5. Begin submaximal isometrics at 4 weeks for shoulder abduction and external rotation.
6. Begin wand exercises or pulley exercises (for passive range of motion [PROM]) when able to do so.
7. Apply a cold or ice pack intermittently throughout the day for pain control and inflammation.
8. Instruct the patient in the use of pillows to maintain the shoulder in a more loose packed position when supine, sitting, semireclined, or side-lying.

Weeks 5-8

GOALS FOR THE PERIOD: Continue to increase ROM, decrease pain and inflammation, and increase muscle activity.

1. Use cold or ice packs as needed.
2. Continue with previous exercises.
3. Initiate wand exercises for A/AROM at 6 weeks, then progress to active range of motion (AROM) in supine when able to do so (with the authorization of the surgeon).
4. Add active shoulder flexion in supine position when cleared by the surgeon (usually 6-8 weeks postsurgery).
5. Massage the scar area when the incision has appropriately healed.

Weeks 8-12

GOALS FOR THE PERIOD: Increase range of motion (ROM) to full, and continue to increase strength. Use upper extremity for light activities of daily living (ADLs).

1. Continue with wand exercises for ROM.
2. Continue with active cervical ROM and UT stretches as needed.
3. Instruct the patient in self-mobilization of the T/S using tennis balls or foam roll if needed (may not be appropriate for older or kyphotic patients).
4. Perform active shoulder flexion and abduction in the functional plane while facing a mirror; be sure to maintain voluntary humeral head depression (keeping the shoulder from hiking).
5. Initiate isotonic exercises within a controlled ROM (without substitution patterns) for the following:
   a. Deltoid
   b. Supraspinatus
   c. Elbow flexors
   d. Scapular muscles
   e. Scaption exercises
6. Use tubing or Theraband for external and internal rotation while working with an axillary roll.
7. Do standing reverse rows using tubing or Theraband.
8. Perform prone horizontal abduction in neutral position with external rotation of the humeral head without weight initially, then progress to light weights if able to do so.
9. Do push-ups with a plus while standing and using a wall.
10. If necessary, add shoulder depression exercises using a Swiss Ball for resistance (see Fig. 5-10).

Weeks 13-16

GOALS FOR THE PERIOD: Increase ROM, strength, and endurance, and begin transitioning into higher activity levels.

1. Continue with the wand exercises.
2. Continue with active ROM of the cervical spine, UT stretches, and T/S mobilizations into higher activity levels.
3. Perform a corner wall stretch for pectoralis muscles and the anterior capsule if needed.
4. Use a horizontal adduction stretch for the posterior capsule.
5. Place a hand behind the back and stretch, using a towel for assistance.
6. Continue and progress with isotonic exercises for endurance and strength training.
7. Continue and progress resistance with tubing and Theraband exercises.
8. Consider seated push-ups with a plus if a more active patient (see Fig. 5-11).
9. Perform prone horizontal abduction exercises with a dumbbell.

Weeks 17-21

1. Continue with previous stretches as needed.
2. Continue with progressive resistance exercises (PREs) (i.e., isotonics).
3. Continue to progress with tubing and Theraband exercises for reverse rows.
4. Complete proprioceptive neuromuscular facilitation (PNF) patterns using a Theraband for resistance.
5. Begin an interval sports program for athletes (see Appendix A).

Weeks 22-26

1. Continue stretches.
2. Continue PREs.
3. Progress with interval sports program.

References

1. Abrams JS: Special shoulder problems in the throwing athlete: pathology, diagnosis and nonoperative management, *Clin Sports Med* 10:839, 1991.
2. Akeson WH, Woo SLY, Amiel D: The connective tissue response to immobility: biomechanical changes in periarticular connective tissue of the immobilized rabbit knee, *Clin Orthop* 93:356, 1973.
3. Anderson L et al: The effects of a Theraband exercise program on shoulder internal rotation strength, *Phys Ther* (suppl) 72(6):540, 1992.
4. Andrews JR, Kupferman SP, Dillman CJ: Labral tears in throwing and racquet sports, *Clin Sports Med* 10(4):901, 1991.
5. Ayoub E: Posture and the upper quarter. In Donatelli R, editor: *Physical therapy of the shoulder,* New York, 1987, Churchill Livingstone.
6. Baker CL, Liu SH: Comparison of open and arthroscopically assisted rotator cuff repairs, *Am J Sports Med* 23:99, 1995.
7. Baylis RW, Wolf EM: *Arthroscopic rotator cuff repair: clinical and arthroscopic second-look assessment.* Paper presented at annual meeting of the Arthroscopy Association of North America, San Francisco, May 1995.
8. Bigliani LU, Morrison DS, April EW: The morphology of the acromion and its relationship to rotator cuff tears, *Orthop Trans* 10:216, 1986.
9. Bigliani LU et al: Operative management of failed rotator cuff repairs, *Orthop Trans* 12:674, 1988.
10. Bigliani LU et al: Operative treatment of failed repairs of the rotator cuff, *Am J Bone Joint Surg* 74A:1505, 1992.
11. Blevins FT et al: Arthroscopic assisted rotator cuff repair: results using a mini-open deltoid splitting approach, *Arthroscopy* 12:50, 1996.
12. Brewster C, Moynes-Schwab D: Rehabilitation of the shoulder following rotator cuff injury or surgery, *J Orthop Sports Phys Ther* 18(2):422, 1993.
13. Bross R et al: Optimal number of exercise bouts per week for isokinetic eccentric training of the rotator cuff musculature, *Wisc Phys Ther Assoc Newsletter* 21(5):18, 1991 (abstract).
14. Brotzman BS: *Clinical orthopaedic rehabilitation,* St Louis, 1996, Mosby.
15. Burkhart S: Reconciling the paradox of rotator cuff repair versus debridement: a unified biomechanical rationale for treatment of rotator cuff tears, *Arthroscopy* 10(1):4, 1994.
16. Burkhart SS, Danaaceau SM, Pearce CE Jr: Arthroscopic rotator cuff repair: analysis of results by tear size and by repair technique margin convergence versus direct tendon to bone repair, *Arthroscopy* 17: 905, 2001.
17. Butler DS: *Mobilization of the nervous system,* New York, 1991, Churchill Livingstone.
18. Calvert PT, Packer NP, Staker DJ: Arthrography of the shoulder after operative repair of the torn rotator cuff, *Br J Bone Joint Surg* 68:147, 1986.
19. Caspari RB, Thal R: A technique for arthroscopic subacromial decompression, *Arthroscopy* 8:23, 1992.
20. Codman EA, Akerson IB: The pathology associated with rupture of the supraspinatus tendon, *Am Surg* 93:348, 1931.
21. Cofield R et al: Surgical repair of chronic rotator cuff tears, *Am J Bone Joint Surg* 83A:71, 2005.
22. Corrigan B, Maitland GD: *Practical orthopaedic medicine,* London, 1987, Butterworth.
23. Craven WM: Traumatic avulsion tears of the rotator cuff. In Andrews JR, Wilk KE, editors: *The athlete's shoulder,* New York, 1994, Churchill Livingstone.
24. Cyriax J: *Textbook of orthopaedic medicine: diagnosis of soft tissue lesions,* vol 1, Baltimore, 1975, Williams and Wilkins.
25. Davies GJ, Dickoff-Hoffman S: Neuromuscular testing and rehabilitation of the shoulder complex, *J Orthop Sports Phys Ther* 18(2):449, 1993.
26. Dehne E, Tory R: Treatment of joint injuries by immediate mobilization, based upon the spinal adaptation concept, *Clin Orthop* 77(218): 1971.
27. De Palma AF: *Degenerative changes in the sternoclavicular and acromioclavicular joints in various decades,* Springfield, IL, 1957, Thomas.
28. De Palma AF, Callery G, Bennett CA: Variational anatomy and degenerative lesions of the shoulder bone, *J Am Acad Orthop Surg* 16:255, 1949.
29. De Palma AF, Cooke AJ, Prabhakar M: The role of the subscapularis in recurrent anterior dislocations of the shoulder, *Clin Orthop* 54:35, 1967.
30. Eriksson E: Rehabilitation of muscle function after sport injury: a major problem in sports medicine, *Int J Sports Med* 2(1): 1981.
31. Eriksson E, Haggmark T: Comparison of isometric muscle training and electric stimulation supplementing isometric muscle training in the recovery after major knee ligament surgery, *Am J Sports Med* 7:169, 1979.
32. Elvey R: *Treatment of conditions accompanied by signs of abnormal brachial plexus tension.* Proceedings of the Manipulative Therapists Association of Australia, Neck and Shoulder Symposium, Queensland, Australia, 1983.
33. Esch JC et al: Arthroscopic subacromial decompression: results according to degree of rotator cuff tear, *Arthroscopy* 4:241, 1988.
34. Gartsman GM: Arthroscopic acromioplasty for lesions of the rotator cuff, *Am J Bone Joint Surg* 72:169, 1990.
35. Gerber C, Terrier F, Fane R: The role of the coracoid process in the chronic impingement syndrome, *Am J Bone Joint Surg* 67B:703, 1985.
36. Grieve G: Manual mobilizing techniques in degenerative arthrosis of the hip, Bulletin of the Orthopaedic Section, *J Am Phys Ther Assoc* 2(1):7, 1977.
37. Harryman DT II et al: Repairs of the rotator cuff: correlation of functional results with integrity of the cuff, *Am J Bone Joint Surg* 73:982, 1991.
38. Hawkins RJ, Misamore GW, Hobeika PE: Surgery for full-thickness rotator cuff tears, *Am J Bone Joint Surg* 67A:139, 1985.
39. Iannotti JP: Full thickness rotator cuff tears: factors affecting surgical outcome, *J Am Acad Orthop Surg* 2:87, 1994.
40. Iannotti JP et al: Prospective evaluation of rotator cuff repair, *J Shoulder Elbow Surg* 2:69, 1993.
41. Itoi E, Tabata S: Conservative treatment of rotator cuff tear, *Clin Orthop* 275:165, 1992.

42. Jenp NY et al: Activation of the rotator cuff in generating isometric shoulder rotation torque, *Am J Sports Med* 24(4):477, 1996.
43. Kapangi IA: *Physiology of joints,* vol 1, New York, 1970, Churchill Livingstone.
44. Kelly M, Clark W: *Orthopedic therapy of the shoulder,* Philadelphia, 1995, Lippincott.
45. Kim S et al: Arthroscopic versus mini-open salvage repair of rotator cuff tear, *Arthroscopy* 19(7):746, 2003.
46. Kisner C, Colby LA: *Therapeutic exercise foundations and techniques,* Philadelphia, 1985, FA Davis Company.
47. Knott M, Voss D: *Proprioceptive neuromuscular facilitation,* New York: Hoeber Medical Division, Harper and Row, 1968, p 84.
48. Kopp S et al: Degenerative disease of the temporal mandibular, metatarso-phalangeal and sternoclavicular joints: an autopsy study, *Acta Odontol Scand* 23:34, 1976.
49. Kvitne RS, Jobe FW: The diagnosis and treatment of anterior instability in the throwing athlete, *Clin Orthop* 291:107, 1993.
50. Lazarus MD et al: Comparison of open and arthroscopic subacromial decompression, *J Shoulder Elbow Surg* 3:1, 1994.
51. Levy HJ, Uribe JW, Delaney LG: Arthroscopically assisted rotator cuff repair. Preliminary results, *Arthroscopy* 6:55, 1990.
52. Lucas DB: Biomechanics of the shoulder joint, *Arch Surg* 107:425, 1973.
53. Lui SH: Arthroscopically-assisted rotator cuff repair, *Br J Bone Joint Surg* 76:592, 1994.
54. Lui SH, Baker CL: Arthroscopically-assisted rotator cuff repair: correlation of functional results with integrity of the cuff, *Arthroscopy* 10:54, 1991.
55. MacConaill MA, Basmajian JV: Muscles and movements: a basis for human kinesiology, Baltimore, 1969, Williams and Wilkins.
56. Maitland GD: *Vertebral manipulations,* ed 5, Newton, MA, 1986, Butterworth.
57. Maitland GD: *Peripheral joint manipulation,* ed 3, Newton, MA, 1991, Butterworth.
58. Moseley HF, Goldie I: The arterial pattern of the rotator cuff of the shoulder, *Br J Bone Joint Surg* 45:780, 1963.
59. Moseley VB et al: EMG analysis of the scapular muscles during shoulder rehabilitation program, *Am J Sports Med* 20(3):128, 1992.
60. Murray T et al: *J Shoulder Elbow Surg* 11(1): 19, 2002.
61. Neer CS: Anterior acromioplasty for the chronic impingement syndrome in the shoulder: a preliminary report, *Am J Bone Joint Surg* 54:41, 1972.
62. Neer CS: Impingement lesions, *Clin Orthop* 173:70, 1983.
63. Neer CS, Welsh RP: The shoulder in sports, *Orthop Clin North Am* 8:583, 1977.
64. Nelson MC et al: Evaluation of the painful shoulder, *Am J Bone Joint Surg* (suppl) 73:707, 1991.
65. Neviaser RJ, Neviaser TJ, Neviaser JS: Concurrent rupture of the rotator cuff and anterior dislocation of the shoulder in the older patient, *Am J Bone Joint Surg* 70:1308, 1988.
66. Osternig LR et al: Differential responses to proprioceptive neuromuscular facilitation stretch techniques, *Med Sci Sports Exerc* 22(1):106, 1990.
67. Rathburn JB, Macnab I: The microvascular pattern of the rotator cuff, *J Bone Joint Surg Br* 45:540, 1970.
68. Rockwood CA Jr, Williams GR: The shoulder impingement syndrome: management of surgical treatment failures, *Orthop Trans* 16:739, 1992.
69. Roger B et al: Imaging findings in the dominant shoulder of throwing athletes: comparison of radiography, arthrography, CT arthrography, and MR arthrography with arthroscopic correlation, *AJR Am J Roentgenol* 172:1371-1380, 1999.
70. Rothman RM, Parke WW: The vascular anatomy of the rotator cuff, *Clin Orthop* 41:176, 1965.
71. Roye KP, Grana WA, Yates CK: Arthroscopic subacromial decompression: two to seven year follow up, *Arthroscopy* 11:301, 1995.
72. Ryu RK: Arthroscopic subacromial decompression: a clinical review, *Arthroscopy* 8:141, 1992.
73. Seitz WH, Froimson AI, Shapiro JD: Chronic impingement syndrome: the role of ultrasonography and arthroscopic anterior acromioplasty, *Orthop Rev* 18:364, 1989.
74. Severud E et al: All-arthroscopic versus mini-open rotator cuff repair: A long-term retrospective outcome comparison, *Arthroscopy* 19(3): 234, 2003.
75. Shields JR: *Manual of sports surgery,* New York, 1987, Springer-Verlag.
76. Smith RH, Brunolti J: Shoulder kinesthesia after anterior glenohumeral joint dislocation, *Phys Ther* 69:106, 1989.
77. Stollsteimer GT, Savie FH III: Arthroscopic rotator cuff repair: current indication, limitations, techniques and results. In Cannon WD, editor: *Instructional course lectures 47,* Rosemont, IL, 1998, American Academy of Orthopaedic Surgeons.
78. Sullivan PE, Markos PA, Minor MD: An integrated approach to therapeutic exercise, theory and clinical application, Reston, VA, 1982, Reston Publishing Company.
79. Tauro JC: Arthroscopic rotator cuff repair: analysis of technique and results at 2 year and 3 year follow-up, *Arthroscopy* 14(1):45, 1998.
80. Tibone JE et al: Shoulder impingement syndrome in athletes treated by anterior acromioplasty, *Clin Orthop* 134:140, 1985.
81. Trott PH: *Differential mechanical diagnosis of shoulder pain.* Proceedings of the Manipulative Therapists Association of Australia, 1985.
82. Walch G et al: Impingement of the deep surface of the supraspinatus tendon on the posterosuperior glenoid rim: an arthroscopic study, *J Shoulder Elbow Surg* 1:238, 1992.
83. Warner J et al: Arthroscopic versus mini-open rotator cuff repair: A cohost comparison study, *Arthroscopy* 21 (3): 328, 2005.
84. Weber S: *Arthroscopic vs. mini-open rotator cuff repairs. A prospective study.* Paper presented at the 64th Annual American Academy of Orthopaedic Surgeons, San Francisco, 1997.
85. Weber SC: Arthroscopic debridement and acromioplasty versus mini-open repair in the treatment of significant partial-thickness rotator cuff tear, *Arthroscopy* 15:126-131, 1999.
86. Wilk KE, Arrigo CA: An integral approach to upper extremity exercises, *Orthop Phys Ther Clin North Am* 9(2):337, 1992.

87. Wilk KE, Arrigo CA: Current concepts in the rehabilitation of the athletic shoulder, *J Orthop Sports Phys Ther* 18(1):365, 1993.
88. Wilk KE et al: Stretch-shortening drills for the upper extremity, theory and clinical application, *J Orthop Sports Phys Ther* 17(5):225, 1993.
89. Wiley AM: Arthroscopy for shoulder instability and a technique for arthroscopic repair, *Arthroscopy* 1:30, 1988.

CHAPTER 6

Superior Labral Anterior Posterior Repair (SLAP Repair)

Timothy F. Tyler
Craig Zeman

INTRODUCTION

Superior labral anterior posterior (SLAP) lesions were not realized until the advent of shoulder arthroscopy. Andrews, Carson, and McLeod[1] were the first to describe labral tears of the biceps anchor; however, Synder[55] was the first to classify them, outline their treatment, and describe four basic types of lesions: I to IV (Fig. 6-1). Since then, several other variants have been described. So as to not get caught up in the subtleties of the classifications, SLAP lesions can best be understood by how they are treated and by the patient's concurrent diagnosis. The two major ways that a SLAP lesion can be treated are by débridement and repair. SLAP lesions are seen in patients who either have instability or impingement, and the kind of rehabilitation patients receive is determined by which factors they have.

Overall, nonoperative management has proven unsuccessful for a large number of patients with unstable SLAP lesions.[1,46,56] In many studies, patients underwent diagnostic arthroscopy at an average of 12 to 30 months from their initial symptoms. In one study, patients had an extended trial of activity modification and rehabilitation exercises.[43] Most patients had been treated with rest, physical therapy, steroid injections, and nonsteroidal anti-inflammatory drugs (NSAIDs) without relief of their symptoms before diagnostic arthroscopy. As the surgical equipment and understanding of SLAP lesions continue to evolve, more effective surgical treatment has become available.[24,34,44,50,65] Treatment of these lesions is directed according to its type.* In general, type I and III lesions are débrided, whereas type II and many type IV lesions are repaired.[49,56] After all SLAP repairs, rehabilitation plays an integral part in the patient's outcome.[54]

*Tables detailing the rehabilitation guidelines for SLAP repair can be found on the CD.

SURGICAL INDICATIONS AND CONSIDERATIONS

Cause

The superior labral is part of the attachment of the long head of the biceps.[12,44,46,65] The role of the long head of the biceps is to be a humeral head depressor and an anterior stabilizer.[24,50] The SLAP area is in continuity with the anterior and posterior labrum. Therefore a tear in the superior labrum can affect the entire labrum, and conversely a tear in the anterior or posterior labrum can disrupt the superior labrum. The classic mechanism to develop a SLAP lesion is force, which either pushes the humeral head over or pulls the humeral head away from the superior labrum.[34] The humeral head will pull on the superior labrum and the biceps anchor tearing them away from the glenoid. In addition, a tear of the anterior or posterior labrum from a dislocation can extend into the superior labrum. Repetitive overhead lifting, which can pinch the superior labrum and pull on it in a downward fashion, can also cause degenerative SLAP tears. In the deceleration phase of pitching, the biceps fires to stop the elbow from hyperextending, which causes a force to be placed across the superior labrum. It is this repetitive action that is felt to cause SLAP lesions in pitchers.

Clinical Evaluation

The therapist should look in the patient's history for an injury that placed an upward shear force across the shoulder—a fall on a outstretched arm that was overhead or that placed a traction force across the arm, a sudden grab and pull on something, having the arm pulled forcefully (e.g., the shoulder getting pulled on while water-skiing)—as well as mild instability in the shoulder with the repetitive throwing motion. Some patients can develop

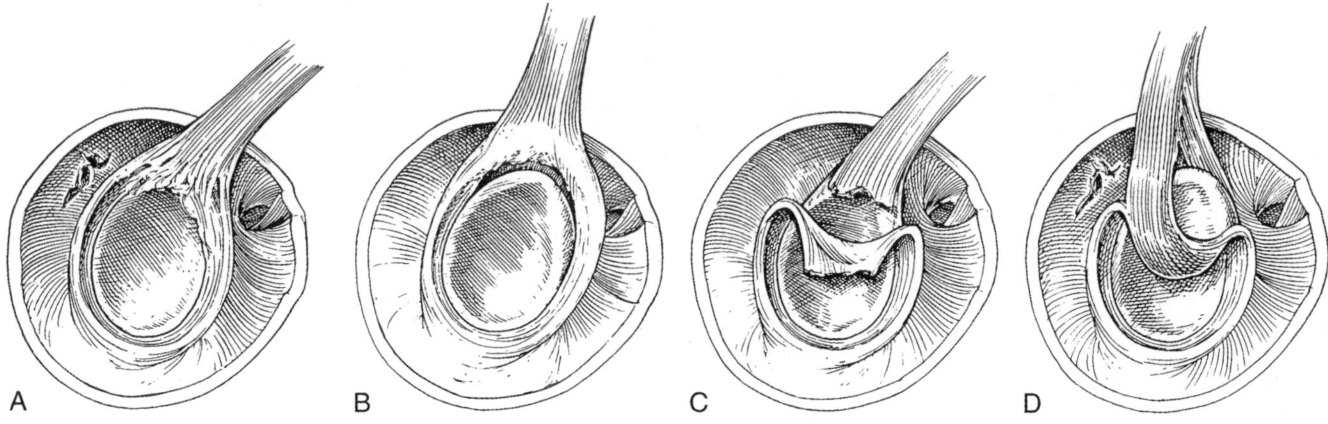

Fig. 6-1 SLAP lesions classifications. A: Type I; B: Type II; C: Type III; D: Type IV. (From Snyder SJ et al: SLAP lesions of the shoulder, *Arthroscopy* 6:274, 1990.)

SLAP lesions with no apparent cause. In questioning for cause, it is important to ask about repetitive overhead lifting and throwing activities. The patient complaints can range from instability to a vague ache in the shoulder. Many patients can show signs of impingement, and some have symptoms of locking, popping, and catching. No classic symptom pinpoints a SLAP lesion. Many physical exam tests have been described to help diagnose a SLAP lesion.[19,49,54,56] The two most common are the Speeds test and O'Brien's test, which are modified supraspinatus isolation tests and therefore can be positive if the patient has impingment.[41] The problem with diagnosing a SLAP lesion is that it is usually found in combination with either impingement or instability.

Diagnostic Testing

Plain radiographs are of little use in evaluating a SLAP lesion. A magnetic resonance imaging (MRI) with gadolinium is probably the best way to see a SLAP lesion.[11,27,57] An MRI without gadolinium is not useful. The problem with an MRI is that it can be too sensitive and tends to "over-read" the lesion. A computerized tomography (CT) scan with contrast and three-dimensional (3-D) reconstruction can also be used to see labral tears, but once again it can be too sensitive. A glenolabral cyst can be seen on both MRI and CT scan and can be commonly caused by a SLAP lesion.[18]

SURGICAL PROCEDURE

The treatment of SLAP lesions is an arthroscopic procedure. It is very difficult if not impossible to treat a SLAP lesion open. Most SLAP lesions are found on diagnostic arthroscopy; therefore the surgeon must be prepared to treat a SLAP lesion at the time of surgery.

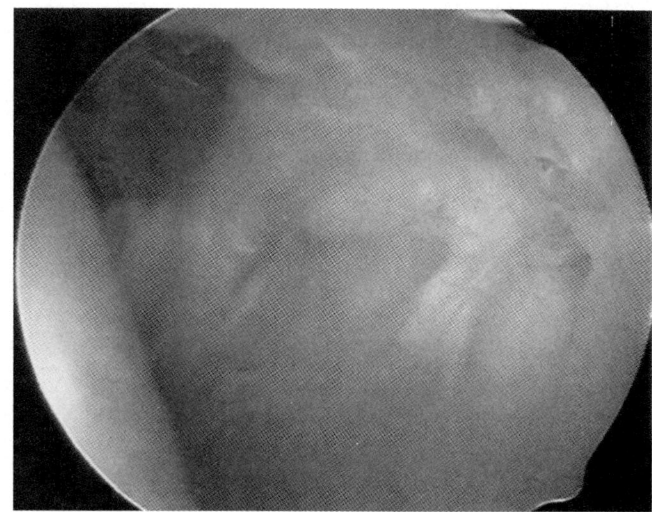

Fig. 6-2 SLAP type I lesion. Fraying of the superior labrum.

Type I

These lesions are simple fraying of the superior labrum without any significant detachment of the labrum from the superior glenoid (Fig. 6-1, A, Fig. 6-2). The frayed area usually covers a portion of the superior glenoid; however, no gross instability of the labral tissue exists. This lesion is commonly seen in patients with impingement or rotator cuff tears. It is not usually seen in patients with instability and it does not seem to cause capsular laxity. These lesions are simply débrided down to the attached base of the superior labrum with an arthroscopic shaver (Fig. 6-3).

Type II

These lesions have an unstable attachment of the superior labrum. The base of the labrum is pulled away from the superior glenoid and is highly mobile (Fig. 6-1, B, Fig. 6-4, A). If the labrum pulls away from the superior glenoid more than 3 to 4 mm when traction is applied to

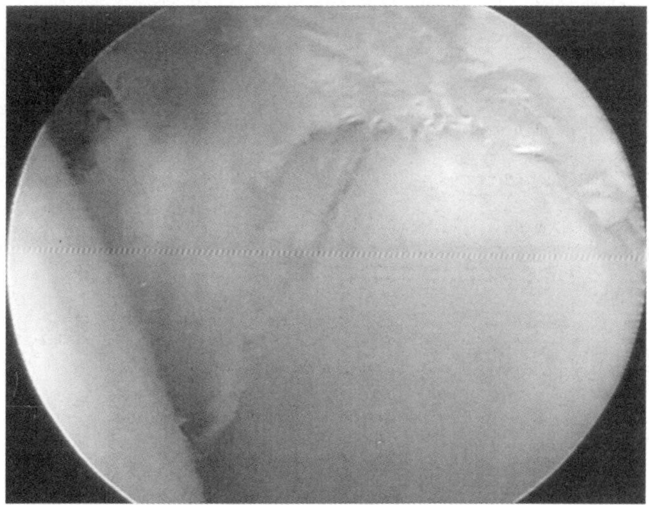

Fig. 6-3 SLAP type I Lesion after débridement.

the biceps tendon, the tear is considered unstable.[53] When the labrum is reduced, one will usually see a reduction in the capsular volume and a change in the position of the anterior and posterior labrum to a more upright position (Fig. 6-4, B). A type II lesion needs to be surgically reduced (Fig. 6-5, A and B). It is done through three portals: one posterior and two anterior. Some type of anchor with suture attached will be used to repair the tear. The detached labrum will be reattached to its anatomic position on the glenoid.

Once the portals have been established, a burr is used to débride the bone of the superior glenoid under the torn labrum. This exposes a bleeding bed of bone that will aid in the healing process. Any loose or frayed ends of the labrum are débrided down to a stable base, and an anchor is placed into the prepared bone through the superior portal. The next task is to pull the two suture ends through the torn labral tissue. This can be done in a multitude of ways; the general concept is as follows: A devise with a loop on the end is passed through the torn labral tissue. One end of the suture is then placed into this loop, which is then pulled back through the labral tissue pulling the suture through the labrum. This process is repeated again so that both ends of the suture are passed through the labrum. Using arthroscopic tying techniques, the torn labrum is firmly reattached back down to the bone of the glenoid (Fig. 6-6). Depending on the size of the tear, more anchors may need to be used to get a secure repair.

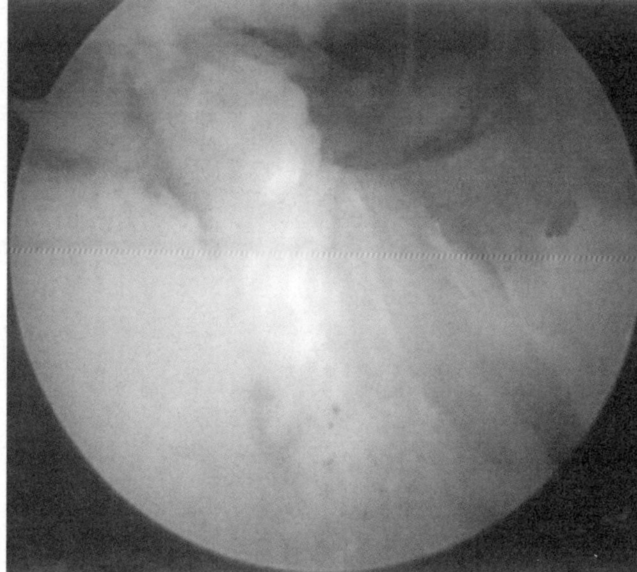

A

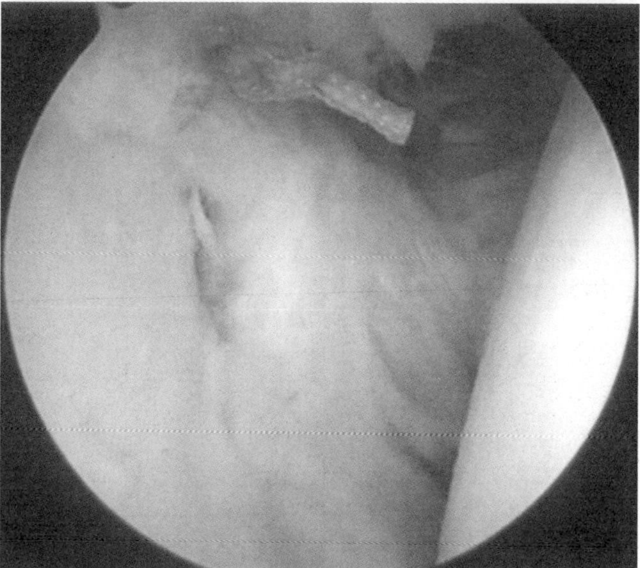

B

Fig. 6-4 **A,** SLAP type II lesion. Base of labrum pulled away from the glenoid. **B,** SLAP type II lesion (repaired).

Type III

A type III SLAP can be thought of as a *bucket handle tear of the labrum* (Fig. 6-1, C, Fig. 6-7, A and B). The unstable handle portion floats around inside the glenohumeral (GH) joint, getting caught between the humeral head and the glenoid during shoulder range of motion (ROM). This pulls on the labral and capsular tissue, producing pain in the shoulder. The portion of the labrum not involved in the tear is normally firmly attached to the glenoid; therefore the symptomatic part is the bucket handle tear, which can simply be débrided down to a stable base like a meniscus tear in the knee.

Type IV

This lesion involves a bucket handle tear of the labrum, which extends into the biceps tendon (Fig. 6-1, D, Fig. 6-8, A-C). Treatment of these lesions depends on the extent of the tear and the age and activity level of the patient. If at least 30% of the biceps remains and the remaining portion of the labrum is stable, the torn part

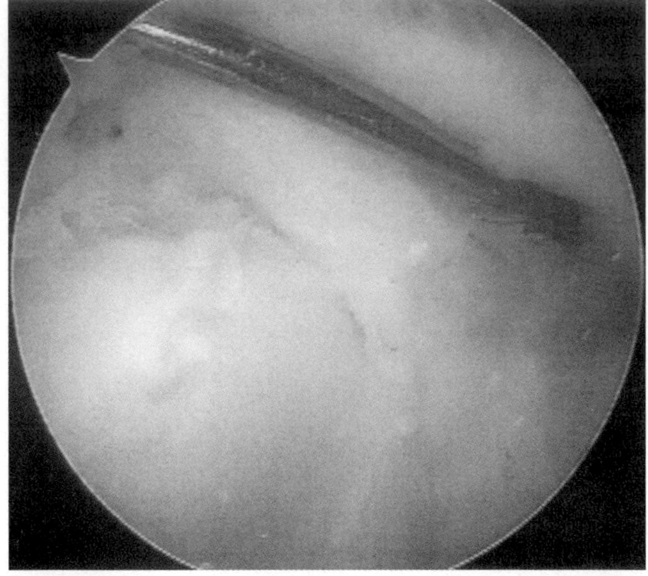

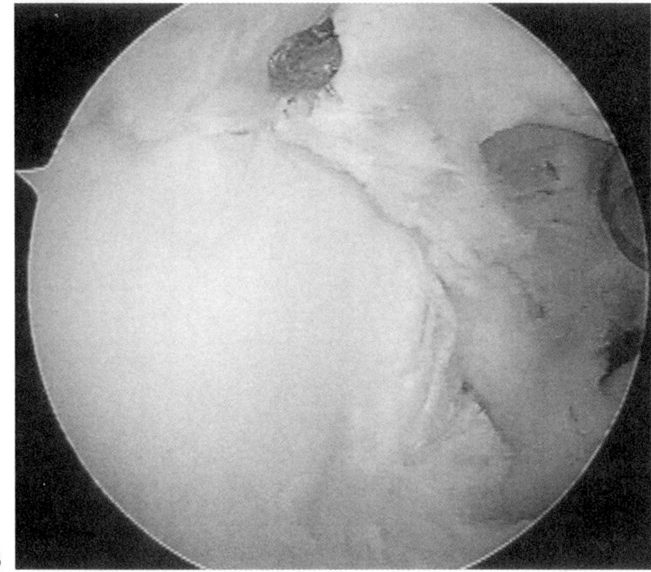

Fig. 6-5 **A,** SLAP type II lesion (repeat of tear probe picture RS). **B,** SLAP type II lesion (repaired).

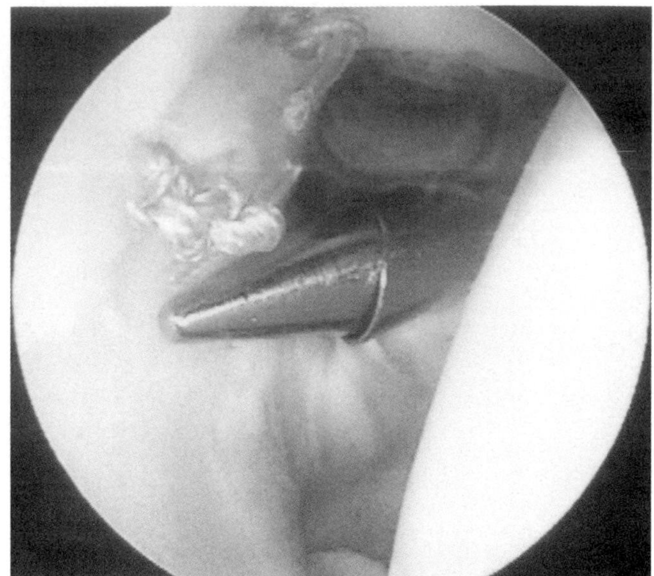

Fig. 6-6 SLAP type II Lesion (repaired using sutures).

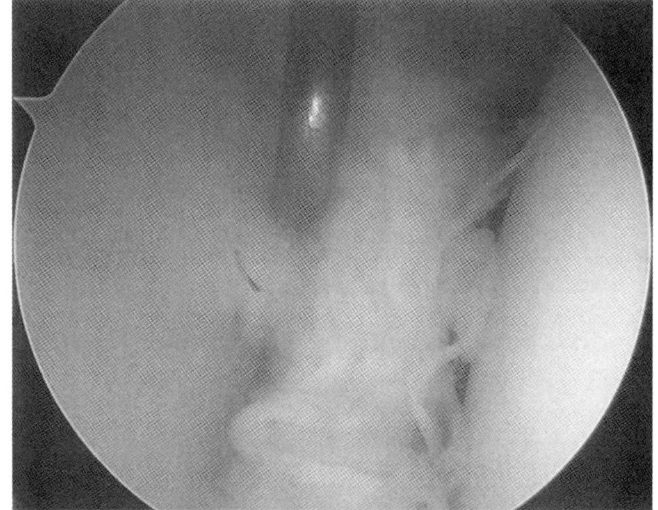

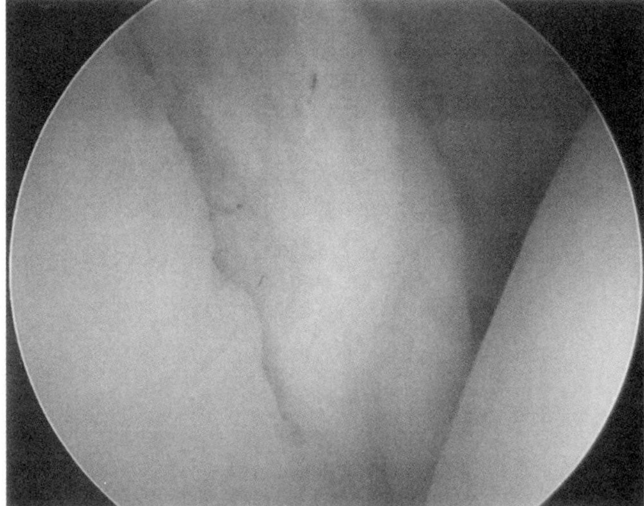

Fig. 6-7 **A,** SLAP type III tear (unstable bucket handle tear). **B,** SLAP type III tear débrided much like resolving a bucket handle tear in the knee meniscus.

can be débrided down to stable tissue. The surgical options are much more complicated if more than 30% of the biceps is torn. In a less active individual, a good option would be to débride the tear and perform a biceps tenodesis. In a throwing athlete, the best option might be to stabilize the labral tear like a type II lesion and repair the tendon of the biceps. A repair would help stabilize an unstable shoulder.

Combined lesions

SLAP lesions can be seen with anterior and posterior labral tears and with impingement and rotator cuff tears. All other surgical lesions should be treated at the same time as the SLAP repair. More times than not, the therapist

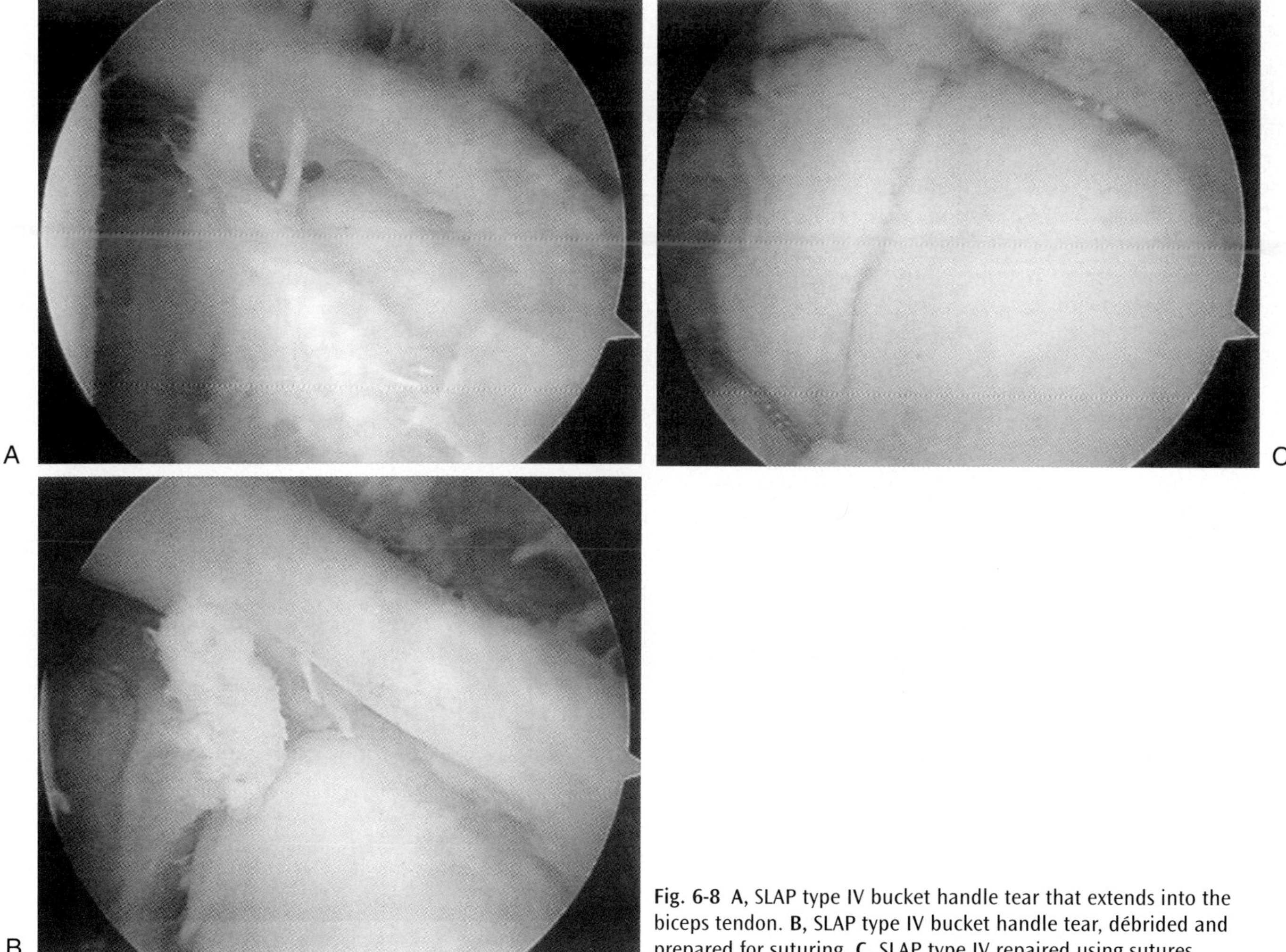

Fig. 6-8 **A**, SLAP type IV bucket handle tear that extends into the biceps tendon. **B**, SLAP type IV bucket handle tear, débrided and prepared for suturing. **C**, SLAP type IV repaired using sutures.

will be rehabilitating patients who have undergone multiple procedures.

It is important to understand everything that has been done to the patient so that a proper treatment plan can be designed.

OUTCOMES

Overall the operative treatment of SLAP lesions has been successful, but conservative care has not.[67] Short-term improvement can be seen in patients with just simple débridement, but at long-term follow-up, the patients had a high failure rate.[13] This failure is probably because the underlying instability was not addressed. Early treatment with staple fixation yields good to excellent results in 80% of the patients.[67] The first reports of suture anchor repair had 100% success.[19] A review of later reports using various techniques of fixation have seen a success rate of about 85%.[49,54] Stetson et al[56] reported on patients who had SLAP repairs and no other procedures for whom an 82% success rate was achieved. Properly performed treatment of SLAP lesions is a reliable procedure.

THERAPY GUIDELINES FOR REHABILITATION

Postoperatively, the shoulder is placed in a sling without a swathe for 2 to 4 weeks to minimize biceps muscular activity and protect any additional structures addressed during the surgical procedure. The position of the arm is in internal rotation (IR) slightly anterior to the frontal plane. Because the early labral tensile strength is weak, the early rehabilitation program is more conservative than other open-stabilization procedures.[11,19,67]

The main focus of the early protective postoperative period (zero to 4 weeks) is to maintain proximal and distal strength and mobility, provide pain relief, and prevent selective hypomobility of sections of the capsule as a result of iatrogenic change from the surgery. During this period, elbow ROM and gripping exercises are encouraged. The authors have found that instructing patients to sleep with a pillow under their elbow to support the shoulder may take stress off the labrum and reduce discomfort. Modalities can be useful tools in providing pain relief. The level of pain, postoperative swelling and type of SLAP tear that was surgically addressed will determine progression of the patient.[27,57] As the treating clinician, good communication with the surgeon is essential to proper care.[27] Understanding the specific procedure, concomitant injuries and tissue quality may also affect the level of progression.

The rehabilitation process will focus on four keys to success:

1. Regaining ROM
2. Providing scapular stabilization
3. Restoring posterior shoulder extensibility
4. Returning rotator cuff strength

Phase I (Early Protective Phase)

TIME: zero to 4 weeks after surgery
GOALS: Protect surgical procedure, educate patient on procedure and therapeutic progression, regulate pain and control inflammation, initiate ROM and dynamic stabilization, neuromuscular re-education of external rotators and scapulothoracic muscles

Q Sally is a 42-year-old female who arrives at the clinic 4 days after a SLAP repair. In passing, she tells the therapist that she has not been feeling well since surgery; she reports feeling "rundown" with a low-grade fever and fatigue the last few days. She is also complaining of severe aching around the shoulder joint. She notes her pain as 10 out of 10, and nothing she can do to will make it better. "It even hurts when I don't move, and it often wakes me up." Upon inspection the therapist notices that the entire area around the shoulder is red, swollen, and has moderate wound seepage. The area surrounding the incision is hot to the touch, and the skin is very firm. What is the most likely cause of the patient's pain and discomfort?

Initial Postoperative Exam

Outpatient physical therapy can begin as early as 3 days after SLAP repair. At this time the mobility of the sterno-clavicular (SC) joint, acromioclavicular (AC) joint, and scapulothoracic joint are addressed and mobilized if indicated. Initial evaluation documentation should include the observation of the portal sites, atrophy, swelling, posture, and functional difficulties. Observation and documentation of ROM and general willingness to move the shoulder and neurovascular measurements should be documented. Care should be taken to avoid contracting the biceps (active elbow flexion) until week 2. Tests to

A Sally is exhibiting signs of a postoperative sepsis infection. A feeling of general malaise and low-grade fever are signs of systematic infection. Sally should be referred back to her physician immediately.

Q Tom is a 52-year-old male who arrives at the clinic 4 weeks after a SLAP repair. By recommendation of his physician, Tom has worn a sling religiously for the past 4 weeks. Upon the therapist's initial evaluation, it is noted that Tom has painful and severely restricted motion in all planes. What is the most likely cause of Tom's ROM deficit, and how would this deficit be treated most successfully?

assess shoulder instability or labral pathology at this point would be inappropriate.

Early Protective Postoperative Rehabilitation

Once the milestone of mobility of the proximal joints is obtained, manual scapular stabilization is initiated. In the side-lying position, manual resistance can be given to the scapula to resist elevation, depression, protraction, and retraction (Fig. 6-9). Pain can be a limiting factor for starting scapular stabilization and rotator cuff isometrics; however, submaximal pain-free alternating isometrics for IR and external rotation (ER) may begin as early as 7 days after surgery (Fig. 6-10). Because the rotator cuff muscles are not violated, this exercise can begin with the arm at the side. Early mobilization exercises like the Pendulum's are recommended for pain relief and could prevent adhesions from forming. Pendulum's have been shown to produce very little muscular activity and are considered to be a safe exercise during this period for most shoulder surgeries.[18] **However, some surgeons feel the arm hanging in a dependent position may put unwanted stress on the repaired labral.** Initiation of active assistive range of motion (A/AROM) using a pulley for sagittal plane flexion and scapular plane elevation is advised. In addition, a cane, golf club, or umbrella can be used to assist with regaining flexion, abduction, adduction, and ER at zero and 30 degrees of abduction (or where the surgeon sets the shoulder during surgery). Gentle mobilization (grades I and II) consisting of posterior glides can be performed at this time for pain relief.

Contraindications

- No ER past the set point for 3 weeks
- No ER in the 90/90-degree position for 6 weeks to avoid the peel-back mechanism
- No active biceps contraction for 4 weeks

Early strengthening of the serratus anterior muscle is also encouraged if it is maintained slightly below 90 degrees of

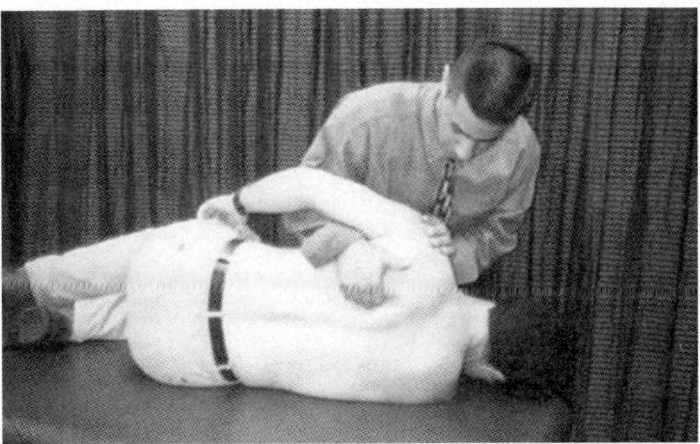

Fig. 6-9 Mobilization and rhythmic stabilization position for the scapula.

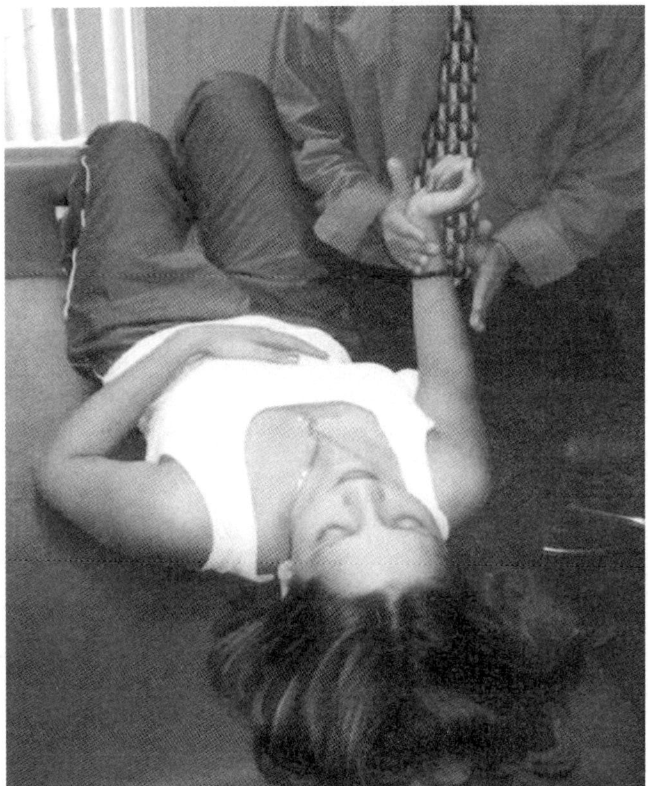

Fig. 6-10 Rhythmic stabilization exercise for internal rotation (IR) and external rotation (ER) in zero degrees of abduction.

shoulder flexion and is pain free. Subsequent atrophy of the serratus anterior muscle, as a result of immobilization, may allow the scapula to rest in downwardly rotated position, causing inferior border prominence. Decker et al[16] used EMG to determine which exercises consistently elicited the greatest maximum voluntary contraction (MVC) of the serratus anterior. It was revealed that the serratus anterior punch, scaption, dynamic hug, knee

A Tom most likely has some iatrogenic GH adhesive capsulitis (i.e., frozen shoulder). Because he is still in the tissue-healing phase of his rehabilitation, the therapist cannot use grade III or IV mobilizations to normalize arthrokinematic motion because it may disrupt the repair. Tom's treatment should be with PROM and A/AROM to decrease and prevent further loss of ROM secondary to adhesive capsulitis. He should be encouraged to remove his sling several times a day and perform pendulum exercises to provide distraction and gentle ROM.

Q Terry is a 33-year-old softball player who had a SLAP repair 5 weeks ago. He states his shoulder feels great but that he is feeling deconditioned. Terry asks the therapist if he can start running. Is running recommended at this stage in his rehabilitation?

push-up with a plus, and push-up plus exercises consistently elicited over 20% of MVC. Most importantly, it was determined that the push-up with a plus and the dynamic hug exercises maintained the greatest MVC, as well as maintained the scapula in an upwardly rotated position (Fig. 6-11). Although it would be too early in the rehabilitation process to perform these later exercises, Decker et al[16] highlighted the serratus anterior punch as a valuable exercise. Performed in a controlled, supervised setting, this is an excellent choice to initiate early serratus anterior strengthening. Transition to the more challenging serratus anterior exercises should occur after 8 weeks and be based on logical exercise progression.

A fine line exists between pushing patients too hard and progressing them as planned. Often patients may feel better than expected during this early protective phase, so therapists must always respect the laws of tissue healing. Three milestones to achieve for progression to the next phase of rehabilitation are (1) to educate the patient on the procedure he or she had and what to expect during the rehabilitation, (2) to provide some pain relief so that the patient is able to tolerate submaximal isometrics of the rotator cuff muscles at zero-degrees abduction, and (3) to attain symmetrical mobility of the SC, AC, and scapulothoracic joints, as well as the ability to protract, retract, elevate, and depress the scapula against submaximal manual resistance. A/AROM goals include achieving flexion to 110 to 130 degrees, abduction to 70 degrees, scapula plane IR to 60 degrees, and scapula plane ER to set point.

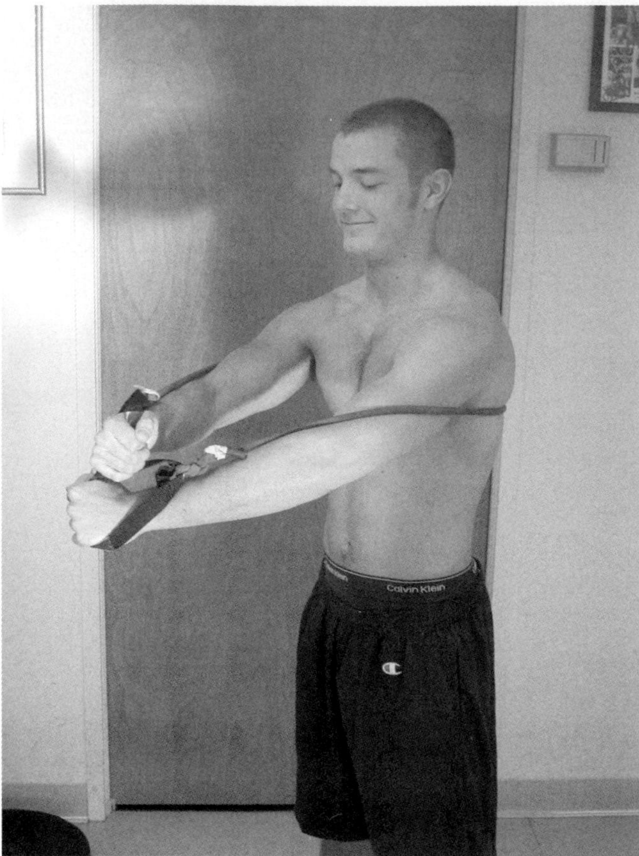

Fig. 6-11 Dynamic hug exercise.

A It would be best if Terry refrained from running until 6 to 8 weeks after surgery. Because running forces the humeral head anterior, it may stress the repair. A stationary bike or Stairmaster may be a good alternative.

Phase II (Intermediate Phase)

TIME: 5 to 8 weeks after surgery

GOALS: Normalize arthrokinematics, gains in neuromuscular control, normalization of posterior shoulder flexibility

During weeks 5 to 8, three visits per week should focus on the return of scapular stability and GH ROM. Later in this period, rotator cuff isotonic strengthening is initiated. During this period, the patient removes the sling, and more aggressive A/AROM exercises are initiated. These exercises may include the use of a pulley or cane to assist in forward elevation in the plane of the scapula and IR. Initially, ER stretching is performed in the guarded neutral position with the arm at the side, and then it is progressed into the scapular plane. While progressing through rehabilitation, the therapist should always consider patients' morphology, understanding if they are hypermobile by nature and returning motion quickly and easily; if so, they do not need to be pushed. **Patients with excessive joint laxity or generalized joint hypermobility must be progressed under a watchful eye.**[61] Excessively stretching ER in the 90/90-degree position in these patients too early during their postoperative care may jeopardize the end result. Burkhart and Morgan[7] discovered the peel-back mechanism, which can occur during rehabilitation when ER is forced passively in the 90/90-degree position before healing has occurred. Kuhn et al[30] demonstrated failure of the biceps superior labral complex in 9 of 10 cadaveric shoulders when the biceps was tensioned in the cocking position. The peel-back phenomenon occurs when the biceps-labral complex is abducted and externally rotated causing a posterior biceps vector, and shearing the biceps anchor repair off its origin.

One therapeutic intervention that can assist in decreasing tension in the biceps-labral complex is restoring posterior extensibility. By restoring posterior capsule extensibility, it allows the humeral head to centralize in the glenoid fossa and not be forced anterior. A tight posterior capsule forces the humeral head anterior, creating unwanted tension in the biceps-labral complex as the phenomenon occurs. Stretching and mobilization of the posterior capsule should be emphasized, because tightness of the posterior shoulder structures has been linked to a loss of IR ROM.[63] Loss of mobility can potentially limit progress, considering a tight posterior capsule is thought to cause anterior-superior migration of the humeral head with forward elevation of the shoulder, possibly contributing to a SLAP tear.[21] If posterior shoulder tightness and a decrease in IR ROM is observed, careful assessment must be undertaken. The Tyler test for posterior shoulder tightness can be performed to determine if posterior shoulder tightness is present (Fig. 6-12).[64,63] To further determine if the loss of IR is due to capsular contracture, a posterior glide must be performed (Fig. 6-13). An effective method of stretching this area is to stabilize the patient's scapula at the inferior angle manually while the patient provides a cross-chest adduction force in the supine position (Fig. 6-14). Further stretch may be felt by having the patient add slight pressure into IR by pressing inferiorly on the dorsal aspect of the hand or wrist. **Passive range of motion (PROM) of ER and abduction should be limited to 65 degrees and 70 degrees, respectively, as to not put stress on the healing biceps-labral complex.** Initial ROM goals are to achieve within 10 degrees of full IR and 150 to 165 degrees of passive flexion in the plane of the scapular. The goal is to maintain available mobility and prevent excessive scarring. Similar to Burkhart and Morgan[5] and Burkhart, Morgan, and Kibler,[5,10] isotonic strengthening exercises are initiated for abduction, scaption, IR, and ER in the scapular plane.[17] In addition, rhythmic stabilization at the end ROM can be performed at this time. To have normal scapulohumeral rhythm, dynamic scapula stability of this joint needs to be restored. Scapula exercises are encouraged in this phase of rehabilitation to counteract scapulohumeral dissociation and provide a stable base of support for active range of

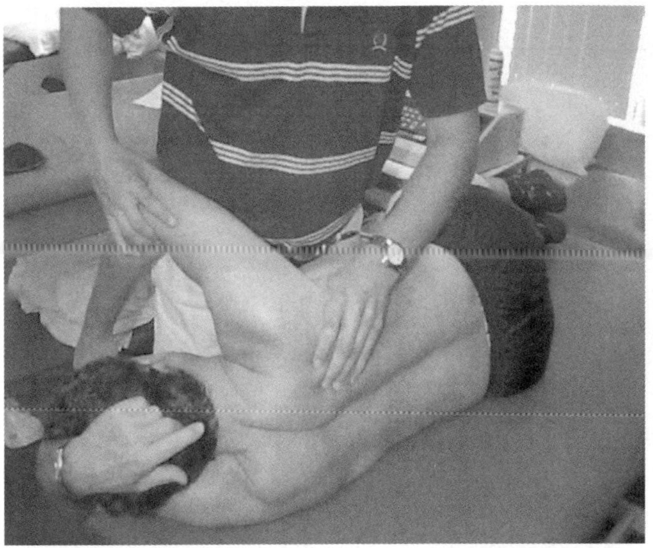

Fig. 6-12 The Tyler test for posterior shoulder tightness.

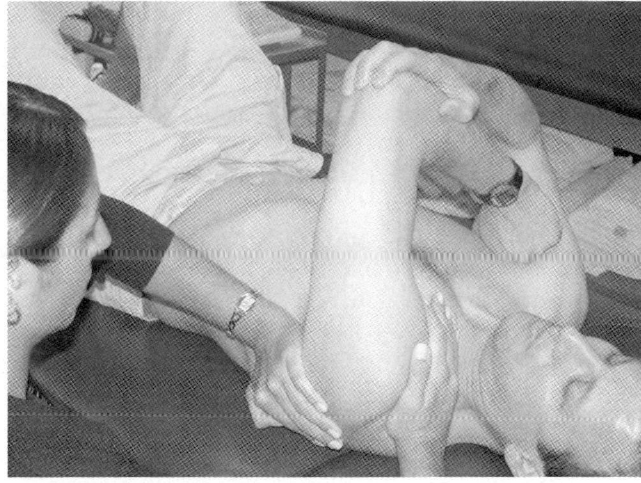

Fig. 6-14 Supine scapula stabilized assisted posterior shoulder stretch.

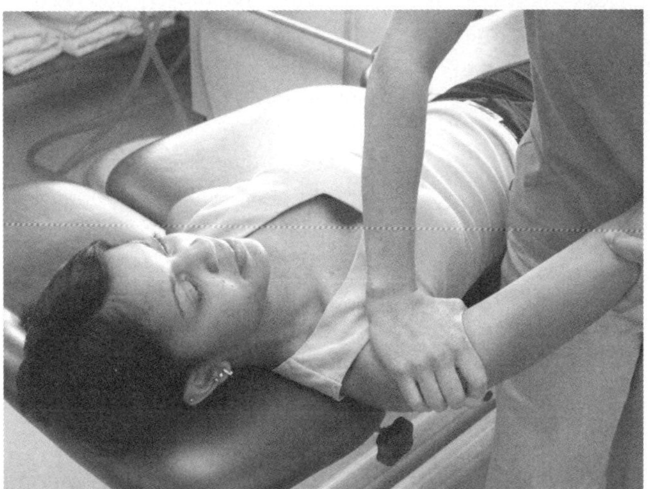

Fig. 6-13 A posterior glide in the plane of the scapula to distinguish posterior capsule tightness.

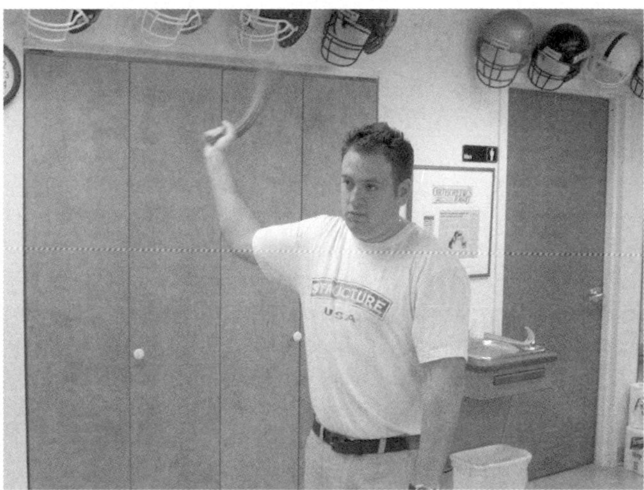

Fig. 6-15 Shoulder oscillation in the plane of the scapula keeping the wrist, elbow, and shoulder steady.

motion (AROM) to be performed.[28] Recently, the authors reported on the importance of scapula stability in generating shoulder rotation torque in microinstability patients. The results of the authors' study demonstrated patients with microinstability exhibited a significant decrease in peak shoulder ER and IR torque after exercise-induced fatigue of the scapular stabilizer.[62] Many authors have examined the EMG activity during scapular strengthening exercises; however, when choosing the appropriate exercise, the clinician must keep the activity pain free and protect the surgical repair.[33,36,38] Three relatively low-level exercises the authors like to use after SLAP repair are (1) elastic resistance rows (not to brake the frontal plane with the involved elbow); (2) standing scapular retraction against elastic resistance with straight arms just below 90 degrees of shoulder flexion; and (3) shoulder oscillation in the plane of the scapula, keeping the wrist, elbow, and shoulder steady (Fig. 6-15). Finally, in the later phases of rehabilitation, the patient can progress to more demanding open and closed kinetic chain scapular strengthening exercises.

Q Shannon is a 47-year-old college professor who had a SLAP repair 12 weeks ago on her dominant arm. She is compliant with physical therapy and postsurgical precautions. She comes to the clinic complaining of increased pain and discomfort when writing on the chalkboard and reaching for things. Upon assessment, the therapist finds poor scapulohumeral rhythm, a winging scapular, and the following post-manual muscle testing (MMT) grades: serratus anterior 2/5, rhomboids/midtrapezius 2/5, lower trapezius 1/5. Based on the clinical findings, what therapeutic exercise should be added to Shannon's program to resolve her complaints?

Strengthening exercises should progress to resistance training with elastic bands for IR, ER, abduction, and extension. Maintaining the GH joint in the scapular plane (30 to 45° anterior to the frontal plane) will minimize the tensile stress placed on the labral repair.[31] **The authors have found that giving verbal feedback to lift the chest up and pinch the shoulders back can facilitate scapular stabilization while training the external rotators.** Hintermeister et al[23] found shoulder elastic resistance training to have a low load on the shoulder and therefore to be safe for postoperative patients.

It is the authors' opinion that the use of free weights with the arm in a dependent position should be used accordingly during this period to minimize the potential for detrimental humeral head translation. Side-lying ER is typically initiated during the later portion of this phase (Fig. 6-16). Proper technique, weight, and ROM are important to execute this safely. Stabilizing the humerus to the thorax and not allowing the elbow to drift past the frontal plane of the body will place minimal winding on the labral repair.

At this phase, minimal weight should be used within the comfortable ROM to prevent ill-advised stress to the healing biceps-labral complex. It may also be recommended that the patient wait until the end of the intermediate postoperative period to initiate jogging or running for this same reason (the humeral head may be forcibly thrusted anteriorly). It is imperative that the therapist maintains supervision of the ROM progression during this period to protect the healing tissue.[17] Clinical milestones to progress to the next phase of rehabilitation include (1) achieving 160 degrees of flexion in the scapular plane, (2) scapular plane ER to 65 degrees, (3) ER at 90-degrees abduction to 45 degrees, (4) near full IR in the scapular plane, (5) IR at 90-degrees abduction to 45 degrees, (6) 150 degrees of abduction, (7) symmetrical posterior shoulder flexibility, and (8) improved isotonic internal and external strength in available ROM.

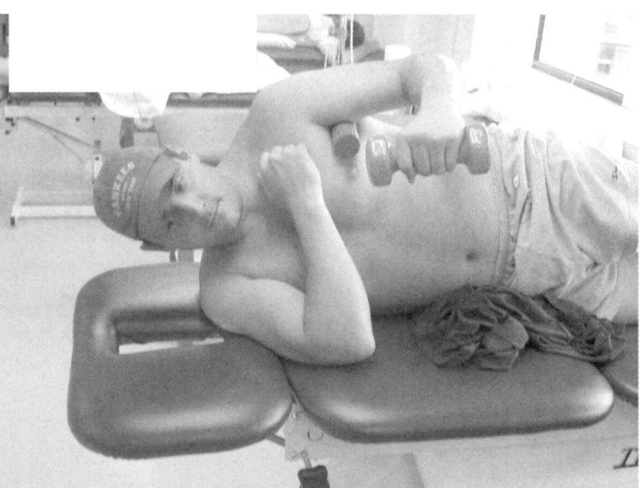

Fig. 6-16 External rotation (ER) strengthening in the side-lying position with a free weight.

> **A** The following therapeutic exercises should be added to Shannon's program: dynamic hugs, push-ups with a plus, serratus punches, scaption, and manual scapula rhythmic stabilization.

Phase III (Strengthening Postoperative Phase)

TIME: 9 to 14 weeks after surgery
GOALS: Normalize ROM, progression of strength, normalize scapulothoracic motion and strength, overhead activities without pain

> **Q** Julio is a 23-year-old male competitive weight lifter. He underwent successful type III SLAP repair. Julio has progressed as expected in ROM and strength in all planes and musculature, except for ER. Twelve weeks after surgery, Julio continues to exhibit 1/5 strength with specific testing of the infraspinatus muscle. What is the likely cause of this strength deficiency?

During weeks 9 to 14 (usually two to three treatment sessions per week), rehabilitation continues to work toward full GH ROM and dynamic stability of the humeral head in the glenoid fossa. Gaining or maintaining full AROM within 10 degrees of flexion in the sagittal plane and ER are to be achieved later during this time phase. At this time, regaining ER, abduction, and flexion does not seem to be a limiting factor for recovery. Once the patient has achieved the milestone of 70- to 80-degrees ER in the plane of the scapula, he or she will begin to acquire ER ROM at 90 degrees of abduction. Although in the past it has been expected that the patient will have full AROM 8 weeks after SLAP repair, most patients do not achieve this at 8 weeks. In the authors' experience, ER and IR ROM measured in the supine position with the GH joint abducted 90 degrees typically does not achieve full ROM until 10 to 12 weeks or longer, depending upon the patient. **It is at this point that a sleeper stretch may safely be given to a patient to regain passive IR ROM** (Fig. 6-17). This is in agreement with other authors who demonstrated a lack of full return of ROM in patients 12 weeks after SLAP repair.[5,10,14,66] In the authors' opinion, the key to a successful rehabilitation of these patients, at this phase, is finding the balance point between stretching ER and letting them naturally regain their ROM.

An arm upper body ergometer (UBE) using light resistance can be beneficial at this time to facilitate ROM and initiate active muscular control of the shoulder.

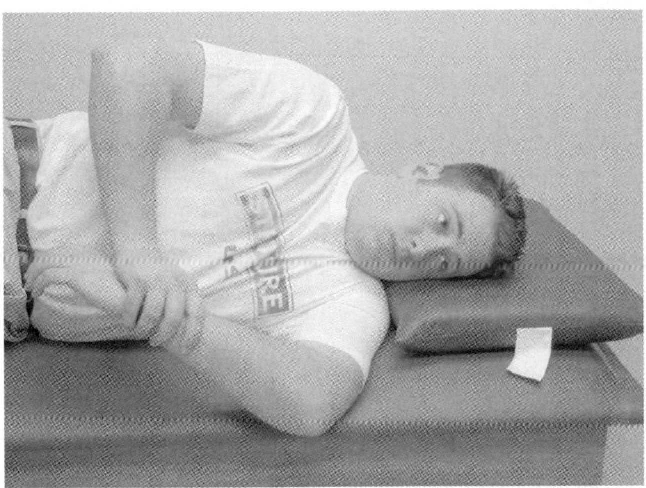

Fig. 6-17 Sleeper stretch for gaining internal rotation (IR).

A The likely cause of Julio's strength deficiency is a glenoid labral cyst leading to entrapment of the suprascapular nerve. A thorough history reveals preoperative MRI showing a labral cyst. Postoperative follow-up shows a decrease EMG and nerve conduction velocity of the infraspinatus muscle. The physical therapy prescription from physician did not note these conditions.

Q Chance arrives at the clinic 11 weeks after having a type II SLAP repair. He has followed normal progression guidelines for rehabilitation of SLAP repair and continues to have increased pain with overhead reaching. Pain is increased with increased shoulder flexion. Flexion ROM is 140 degrees with end-range pain, and resisted motion above 110 degrees is painful. He has decreased horizontal adduction on the involved arm (decreased ER at 45 degrees for this stage of rehabilitation). Chance has a positive apprehension test, and a positive relocation test (decreased pain). What is the reason that he is not progressing through the rehabilitation guidelines? What associated pathology could be present? What could be the reason for his problems, assuming that the surgical procedure was fine?

The axis of rotation of the UBE should remain below the level of the shoulder joint so as not to force forward flexion above 80 degrees. To avoid stress to the biceps-labral complex, the patient should be positioned at a distance from the axis of rotation that does not allow the elbow to move posterior to the frontal plane when performing ergometer revolutions. This exercise is not initiated earlier, because the amount of stress placed on the biceps-labral complex during the use of an UBE is unknown.

When designing the strengthening program, it is important to match patients' needs with their limitations and goals. A properly designed strengthening program will address their needs by attempting to get the most benefit from each exercise prescription. Previous EMG studies have set forth which shoulder exercises activate particular muscles, and these should be considered as the clinician prescribes a program.[16,18,36,38,61] The authors have combined many of these programs to address generalized specific weaknesses. From these studies, the authors have developed the "prone program plus" to address scapular stability and generalized weakness. The prone program plus, can be started in this phase of the rehabilitation if the exercises are pain free. The prone program plus includes prone GH horizontal abduction with GH IR (thumb down), prone scapula adduction with GH ER (thumb up), prone rows, prone shoulder flexion in the scapular plane, prone 90/90-degree ER, push-ups with a plus (therapist initiates exercise in quadruped), and ball press downs. Patients can easily get into poor habits or begin performing these exercises with improper form. It is recommended that clinicians educate their patients on these exercises and allow ample time for them to develop proper form before prescribing these as part of a home program.

A The reason for the patient's problems are the following: tight posterior capsule, posterior impingement, insufficient stretching in earlier phases, and a poor posterior glide of humerus.

Q At 12 weeks after SLAP repair, Lily has 40 degrees of GH IR PROM and 45 degrees of AROM. She has been doing the sleeper stretch but has not made any gains in ROM in the last 4 weeks. How does the therapist determine if the limitation in IR ROM is capsular or muscular to ensure that the correct therapeutic exercises are prescribed.

Proprioceptive neuromuscular facilitation (PNF) can be described as movements that combine rotation and diagonal components that closely resemble the movement patterns required for sport and work activities. PNF acts to enhance the proprioceptive input and neuromuscular responses while stressing motor relearning in the post-operative phases of rehabilitation. PNF patterns are initiated with the scapula, because scapular stability is essential for total function of the shoulder. Scapular patterns are generally performed in the side-lying position, with the head and neck in neutral alignment. The coupled patterns of anterior elevation–posterior depression and anterior

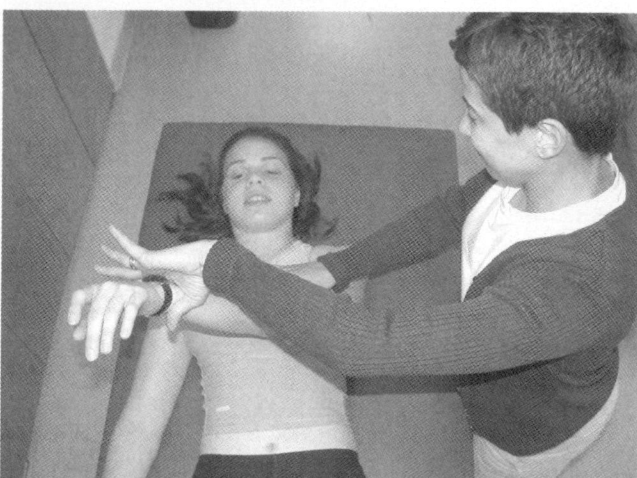

Fig. 6-18 D_2 flexion with manual resistance.

> **A** The therapist should perform a Tyler test and a posterior glide looking for side-to-side restriction. If the Tyler test is positive but the posterior glide is negative, the therapist can determine that the lack of IR is caused by muscle tightness and not capsular tightness.

depression–posterior elevation are used, respectively. Trunk rotation should eventually be combined with scapular and extremity PNF patterns to maximize combined muscular movement patterns. Techniques such as hold-relax, slow reversals, and contract-relax are used specifically to improve motion, whereas rhythmic stabilization, repeated contractions, and combination isotonics are used to enhance concentric and eccentric muscle action. Specifically, the D_2-flexion pattern combines flexion, abduction, and ER, emphasizing the posterior rotator cuff and posterior deltoid (Fig. 6-18). These neuromuscular control exercises strive to re-establish scapular positioning and stability of the humeral head in the glenoid.[28]

As the patient progresses through the program, periodical re-evaluation of the scapular dyskinesis is highly recommended. The authors stress this, especially as the patient gains full ROM and may no longer be inhibited by tight soft tissue structures. The term *scapular dyskinesis*, although indicating that an alteration exists, is a qualitative collective term that does not differentiate between types of scapular positions or motions.[29] Therefore scapular evaluation and categorization is challenging. The most common techniques for objective quantification include visual evaluation, the Lateral Scapular Slide Test (LSST), and 3-D techniques. Kibler et al[29] has recently introduced a new visual technique that may help clinicians standardize categorization. This dynamic technique categorizes the dyskinesis in one of four groups:

- Type I—inferior angle prominence (horizontal plane movement)
- Type II—medial border prominence dorsally (frontal plane movement)
- Type III—shoulder shrug motion without winging (sagittal plane movement)
- Type IV—bilaterally symmetrical movement (normal movement)

Like all scapular categorization techniques, the therapist must be concerned with combined movements, a learning curve, and patient experience; however, it does present clinicians with a valuable tool that, with practice, may enhance clinical communication.

The authors also believe that exercises directed toward facilitation of functional muscular firing patterns in both the open and closed chain may provide useful input for return to function after SLAP repair. Lear and Gross[31] demonstrated scapular muscle activity increases with a wall push-up progression. **However, the strain on the biceps-labral complex is unknown and may be too great for patients after SLAP repair. This exercise should be gradually built up to and proceeded to with caution.** Clinicians should hold this exercise until the advanced strengthening postoperative phase to protect the healing tissue.

> **Q** Sydney is a 17-year-old swimmer recovering from a SLAP repair. After 13 weeks she has been making gains in strength and ROM. She comes to the clinic with complaints of increased tightness in the anterior shoulder. Upon examination, palpation reveals increased muscle tension in the upper trapezius and pectoralis. How should the therapist alter Sydney's treatment session for the day? Sydney returns 2 days later with no reports of pain and discomfort. At that time, what should the therapist reinforce in her current program to prevent further anterior shoulder discomfort?

Isotonic exercises emphasizing light resistance and increased repetitions are used for isolated and combined movement patterns of the shoulder. The authors use a progression from three sets of 10, to two sets of 15, and on to one set of 30 repetitions. If the patient can perform one set of 30 repetitions with good form and no substitution, he or she can be progressed to 1- to 2-lb weights and back down to three sets of 10 to repeat the cycle. This rationale is based on lending objectivity to the progression and the tonic nature of the rotator cuff muscles and the scapular stabilizers. Isolated exercises are used to enhance or increase the strength of a particular muscle. Combining isotonic exercises in functional-movement patterns are performed with PNF patterns using elastic resistance or the cable column to enhance coordinated movement. In the case of a swimmer, the D1 pattern with elastic resistance will lead to a carryover to his athletic function. Initiation of isokinetic strengthening at this phase may enhance the shoulder's ability to strengthen in a pain-free ROM. It is encouraged that slower speeds be used when strengthening patients with shoulder instability. Isokinetic principles suggest that faster isokinetic speeds create greater translational forces, whereas slower speeds create stronger compressive forces (which stabilize the shoulder). Milestones that should be met to move to the next rehabilitation phase include (1) within 10 degrees of full AROM in flexion, abduction, IR, and ER in the plane of the scapula; (2) normalized scapulothoracic motion and strength; (3) moderate overhead activities without pain; (4) isometric internal and external strength should be at least 50% of the uninjured side.

A The therapist provided a treatment session of moist heat and modalities followed by manual therapy (soft tissue mobilization) to the pectoralis and upper trapezius to reduce the muscle tension. The following should be recommended: pectoralis stretch, upper trapezius stretch, and using the correct technique during rows and scaption.

Q Steve is a 22-year-old collegiate baseball pitcher who the therapist has been treating for the last 23 weeks after right-sided SLAP repair (throwing arm). Steve began a throwing program that the therapist designed 3 weeks earlier, and he has been throwing without problems. However, now that the number of pitches has increased in his throwing program, he has been complaining of anterior shoulder pain that bothers him most during the "ball release" and "follow through" phases of his pitching mechanics. Ruling out a possible compromise of the SLAP repair. What else could possibly be causing Steve's pain during the late period of his throw?

Phase IV (Advanced Strengthening Phase)

TIME: 15 to 24 weeks after surgery

GOALS: Pain-free full ROM, improve muscular endurance, improve dynamic stability

After 15 weeks the patient is in the final phase of rehabilitation. Full AROM should be attained at this time. The only restriction on ROM is that ER should not be stretched beyond 90 degrees. It may be preferable to allow the athlete to regain additional degrees of ER over time rather than stress the biceps-labral complex, potentially stretching the repair. **Posterior capsule stretching is appropriate if full IR has not been obtained yet.** Performing the side-lying sleeper stretch encourages ROM for IR (see Fig. 6-17). At the onset of this phase, a thorough strength assessment is needed to evaluate the direction of strengthening needed for the particular patient. This assessment may include manual muscle testing, hand held dynamometry, and isokinetic strengthening (or a combination of these techniques). Assessment should include the primary shoulder movers, shoulder rotators, and scapula stabilizers. Results of this assessment should be addressed with a well-rounded strengthening program to include isotonic, concentric, and eccentric loading exercises. When designing these programs, consider the everyday demands of each patient. For an overhead-throwing athlete, strengthening in the throwing position is imperative (Fig. 6-19). Once this phase of rehabilitation is reached, treatment should begin to streamline toward the functional demands of the patient.[8]

Initiation of a properly designed plyometric training program is often the missing link to discharging a high-level patient. Plyometric training for the upper extremity is used to generate rapid and powerful muscular contractions in response to a dynamic stretch–inducing load to a muscle or group of muscles. It is suggested that plyo-

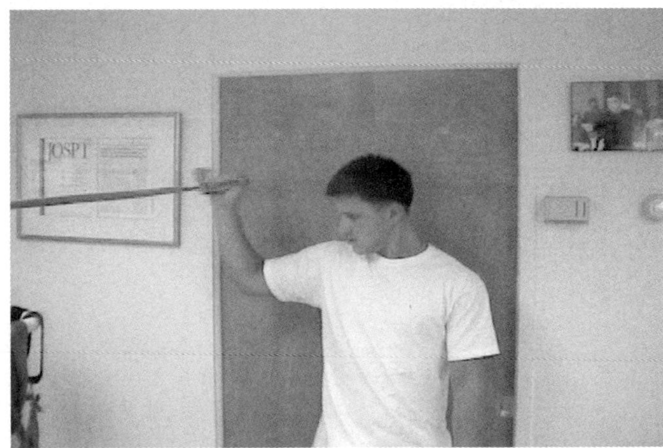

Fig. 6-19 External rotation (ER) strengthening in the 90/90-degree position with elastic resistance.

A Because the biceps acts as an elbow flexor and a forearm supinator, its functions in the late phases of throwing are to decelerate the arm and extend the elbow. Overuse of the biceps if it has not been properly strengthened can lead to bicipital tendonitis. The therapist should have Steve back off the throwing program and begin eccentric strengthening of the biceps once the inflammation of the tendonitis has subsided. In addition, Steve's rotator cuff strength should be checked, because the biceps will often be overused as a humeral head depressor if the rotator cuff is weak and not functioning properly.

metrics train the entire neuromuscular system, using the principles of stored elastic energy to use strength as quickly and forcefully as possible. The myotatic stretch reflex develops stored elastic potential. If the exercise movement is slow, such as in weight lifting, the energy is dissipated and nonproductive. However, with rapid movement, this stored elastic energy can be used to generate a force greater than that of the concentric contraction of the muscle alone. Plyometrics use the principles of progressive loading with the ultimate goal of power development. Using a trampoline will increase the EMG activity and elevate the level of eccentric loading of the shoulder rotators.[15] Therefore a progression from two-handed, side-to-side throws to overhead throws to one-handed overhead throws is encouraged to maximize the power development of the overhead athlete. A well-rounded program will address both the internal and external rotators of the shoulder, together with the core muscles of the trunk. Externally challenging the patient, by permitting stability from a naturally unstable surface, like a ball, will challenge the entire kinetic chain. Advanced exercises like the Physioball "walk outs," exemplify this concept (Fig. 6-20). As the patient walks out from the ball with the hands, core stabilizers, as well as GH stabilizers, are challenged. Milestones to progress to the final phase of rehabilitation include (1) pain-free full ROM, (2) less than 20% strength deficits for IR and ER at 90 degrees/second, and (3) 20% strength deficits in all positions.

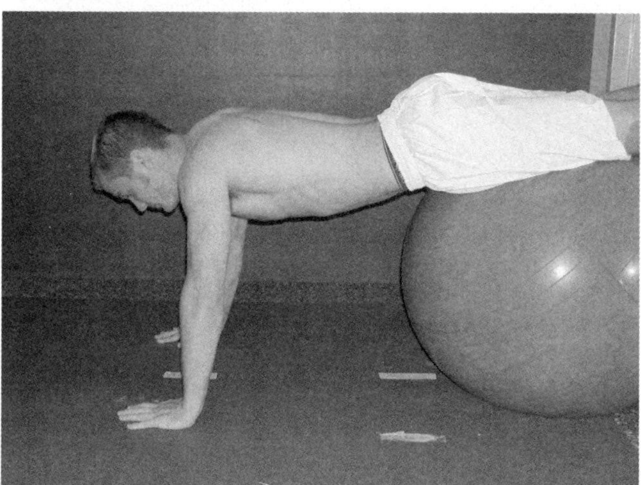

Fig. 6-20 Physioball wall walkouts.

Q Mariano arrives at the clinic after completion of an interval throwing program after 24 weeks of SLAP rehabilitation. He states his shoulder hurts after he is done throwing. After taking a history, the therapist feels that he is having some mechanical impingement. What are three likely causes of this impingement?

Phase V (Return-to-Activity and Sport Phase)

TIME: 4 to 6 months after surgery

GOALS: Pain-free full ROM, normalized strength, return to sport or activity program

This is the phase of rehabilitation at which very few therapists have the opportunity to discharge patients. All too often patients loose interest, exhaust insurance coverage, or just neglect the importance to fine-tune their shoulders before fully returning to their lifestyle. This stage is designed to prepare patients to return, without hesitation, to full participation in all activities. Milestones to successfully complete this phase include (1) total confidence in the shoulder, (2) pain-free full ROM, (3) isokinetic or hand held dynamometry less than 10% deficit in all positions.[35]

Exercises in this phase continue to emphasize functional positions, including the plyometric program (isokinetic strengthening at 90 degrees of abduction). A gradual return to sport is permitted once the patient is pain free, has nearly full ROM in all planes, confidence in the shoulder, and 85% to 90% of the strength of the opposite side on isokinetic testing at 90 degrees, 180 degrees, and 300 degrees/second for the motions of IR and ER. Confidence is achieved by the ability to perform pain-free functional movement in the patient's sport. The authors' experience has demonstrated that the throwing athlete requires an additional 1 to 2 months to allow the shoulder to accommodate to the motion. Patients also report that it takes up to 1 year before the shoulder feels "normal" after SLAP repair. The authors currently are using the *American Shoulder and Elbow Surgeons Shoulder Evaluation Form* to standardize the documentation of pain, motion, strength, stability, and function. Although it remains difficult to gather enough data to determine a criterion score for return to sport, once 6 months have passed and clinical milestones have been met, the athlete is cleared for full throwing. This time frame is in agreement with other authors' findings[45] (Table 6-1).

A Three likely caused of this impingement are (1) poor scapular stability, (2) tight posterior shoulder structure, and (3) weak external rotator.

Summary

Considerations must be given if additional procedures are performed for reattachment of labrum, ligaments, or the biceps tendon. However, stronger fixation techniques have allowed the rehabilitation to progress more rapidly with these procedures. These guidelines are a continuum of rehabilitation phases based on the effect the surgery has on the tissue and the surrounding structures. Scientific rationale is applied whenever possible; however, as surgical procedures evolve, so must the rehabilitation.

Table 6-1 Time to Return to Sports After SLAP Surgery[42]

Study	Year	Surgery	Type of SLAP	Population	Return to Sports*	Full Throwing
Yoneda et al[67]	1991	Repair	Type II	Athletes	ND	ND
Resch et al[48]	1993	Repair	Type II	Not specified	6 months	ND
Cordasco et al[13]	1993	Débridement	Type II	Not specified	ND	ND
Pagnani et al[43]	1995	Repair	Types II & IV	Not specified	4 months	6 months (not specified)
Field & Savoie[19]	1993	Repair	Types II & IV	Not specified	ND	ND
Berg & Ciullo[3]	1997	Repair	Types II & IV	Not specified	ND	ND
Segmuller et al[52]	1997	Repair	Types II & IV	Not specified	6 months	ND
Morgan et al[37]	1998	Repair	Type II	Athletes & nonathletes	4 months	7 months
Samani et al[51]	2001	Repair	Type II	Athletes & nonathletes	ND	ND
O'Brien et al[41]	2002	PAL, repair	Type II	Athletes & nonathletes	ND	ND
Jazrawi et al[25]	2003	Repair with ATCS	Type II	Athletes	3-4 months	11.2 months

ATCS, Arthroscopic thermal capsular shift; *ND*, not documented; *PAL*, partial anterolateral acromioplasty.
*In most papers, *time to return* refers to the initial return, not to full return.

These guidelines are by no means set in stone, and all exercises are not distinct to particular phases. The goals and exercises need to be modified based on the performer, the pathology, and the performance demands. Exercise prescriptions should not be viewed as protocol but as guidelines upon which to base rehabilitation. These rehabilitation guidelines are outlined in Box 6-1.

SUGGESTED HOME MAINTENANCE FOR THE POSTSURGICAL PATIENT

The home maintenance program needs to be adjusted for each patient depending on status and abilities. Refer to page 110 for the suggested home maintenance program.

TROUBLESHOOTING

Hypomobility and Hypermobility of Glenohumeral Joint

In the process of rehab after a SLAP repair, it is not uncommon to have difficulty restoring a patients normal ROM. With these hypomobile patients, it is necessary to begin early mobilization and stretching to regain normal arthrokinematic and osteokinematic motion. Using grade III and IV mobilizations can help to increase capsular pliability, especially in the posterior and inferior directions. **The therapist should avoid stretching patients into the apprehension position without applying a posterior "relocation" force, because this may cause impingement internally.**

After SLAP repair, some patients will experience a hypermobility issue. Often times this is due to generalized ligament laxity that affects all joints. This is tested by thumb-to-forearm, MCP and DIP extension, as well as elbow and knee recurvatum. These patients will regain normal ROM on their own as they progress to doing functional movements of the shoulder. Therefore it is necessary for the therapist to mobilize and stretch the GH complex. It is important to progress these patients more slowly and allow them to regain the motion on their own.

Poor Scapular Stabilization

Scapular dyskinesis, or poor scapulohumeral rhythm, is often a problem that patients and therapists face after SLAP repair surgery. Poor scapular stability may have been a precursor that helped lead to the SLAP tear, or it may be a direct result of the disuse after surgery and wearing a sling. In these cases it is necessary to establish a stable base by working the rhomboids, middle and lower trapezius, and the serratus muscles in an endurance fashion. Because normal motion requires these muscles to be tonically active, it is necessary to work them to fatigue. Failing to establish this stable base will lead to the peal-back mechanism occurring when the arm is in the 90/90-degree position. Winging of the scapula causes an increased anterior force on the humeral head that will increase the traction force on the long head of the biceps as the arm moves up into the throwing motion. It is important to avoid rotator cuff strengthening in the 90/90-degree position until scapulohumeral motion has been normalized.

Posterior Shoulder Extensibility

The throwing athlete has been known to have an increase in ER ROM and a decreased/limited IR ROM. Not maintaining total ROM with a severe loss of IR ROM may lead to a SLAP tear. The cause of the IR ROM loss may be a tight posterior capsule and musculature. If the therapist is lucky enough to see the patient before surgery, this can be addressed. In fact, the surgeon may do a posterior capsule release during the SLAP repair.

Box 6-1 Rehabilitation Guidelines for SLAP Repair

I. Early protective phase (0-4 weeks)

A. Goals:

- Protect surgical procedure
- Educate patient on procedure and therapeutic progression
- Regulate pain and control inflammation
- Initiate ROM and dynamic stabilization
- Neuromuscular re-education of external rotators and scapulothoracic muscles

B. Treatment plan (0-2 weeks):

- Sling immobilization for 2-4 weeks
- Gripping exercises
- Elbow, wrist, and hand ROM
- Pendulum exercises
- Shoulder PROM F/ABD/IR/ER* Do not go beyond the position set at time of surgery for ER (progress flexion to A/AROM)
- IR and ER proprioception training (controlled range)
- Initiate gentle alternating isometrics for IR and ER in zero-degrees abduction to scapular plane
- Initiate passive forward flexion to 90 degrees
- Initiate scapular mobility

C. Treatment plan (2-4 weeks):

- ROM progression
  Forward flexion to 110-130 degrees
  ER in scapular plane to 35 degrees (position set at time of surgery)
  IR in scapular plane to 60 degrees
- Progress submaximal alternating isometrics for IR and ER in scapular plane
- Initiate scapular strengthening
  Manual scapula retraction
  Resisted band retraction
  (Note: No shoulder extension past trunk)
- Deltoid isometrics in all directions
- Biceps-triceps strengthening
- Initiate light band work for IR and ER

D. Milestones for progression:

- Forward flexion to 90 degrees
- Abduction to 70 degrees
- ER in scapular plane to 30 degrees
- IR in scapular plane to 20 degrees
- Tolerance of submaximal isometrics
- Knowledge of home care and contraindications
- Normalize mobility of related joints (AC, SC, ST)

II. Intermediate phase (5-8 weeks)

A. Goals:

- Normalize arthrokinematics
- Gains in neuromuscular control
- Normalization of posterior shoulder flexibility
- Limit PROM of ER/ABD to 65-70 degrees to protect the healing biceps/labral complex

B. Treatment plan:

- ROM progression
  Flexion in the scapula plane passively 150-165 degrees
  ER in the scapula plane to 65 degrees
  IR in the scapula plane, full or to within 10 degrees
- Initiate joint mobilizations as necessary
- Initiate posterior capsular stretching
- Progress strengthening
  IR/ER (with GH in the scapula plane) with elastic band
  Side-lying ER
  Scaption full can (no weight if substitution patterns)
  CW/CCW ball against wall
  Body Blade at neutral or rhythmic stabilization

C. Milestones for progression:

- Forward flexion to 160 degrees
- ER in scapular plane to 65 degrees
- Full IR in scapular plane
- Symmetrical posterior capsule mobility
- Progressing isotonic strength with IR and ER in available range

III. Strengthening phase (9-14 weeks)

A. Goals:

- Normalize ROM
- Progression of strength
- Normalize scapulothoracic motion and strength
- Overhead activities without pain

B. Treatment plan:

- ROM progression; stretching ER at 90 degrees of GH abduction
  Within 10 degrees of full AROM in all plans
- Progression of scapular retractors and stabilizers
  Prone program; LT, MT, Rhmd
  LT; scapular depression
- Progress strengthening
  Challenging rhythmic stabilization
  UBE
  Initiate isokinetic IR and ER in scapular plan
  Initiate IR and ER at 90 degrees of GH abduction
  Isotonic strengthening; flex, abduction
  Closed kinetic chain exercise

C. Milestones for progression:

- Within 10 degrees of full active range in scapular plane
- Isometric strength IR and ER less than 50% deficit
- Less than 30% strength deficits; primary shoulder muscles and scapular stabilizers

IV. Advanced strengthening phase (15-24 weeks)

A. Goals:

- Pain-free full ROM
- Improve muscular endurance
- Improve dynamic stability

Box 6-1 Rehabilitation Guidelines for SLAP Repair, cont'd

B. Treatment plan:

- Maintain flexibility
- Progress strengthening
  Advanced closed kinetic chain exercise
  Wall push-ups; with and without ball
  Continue with overhead strengthening
  Continue with isokinetic IR and ER strengthening; 90 degrees of GH abduction
  Advance isotonic strengthening
  Advance rhythmic stabilization training in various ranges and positions
- Initiate plyometric strengthening
  Chest passes
  Trunk twists
  Overhead passes
  90/90-degree position single-arm plyometrics

C. Milestones for progression:

- Pain-free full ROM
- Strength deficits less than 20% for IR and ER at 90 degrees of GH abduction
- Less than 20% strength deficits throughout

V. Return-to-activity and sport phase (4-6 months)
A. Goals:

- Pain-free full ROM
- Normalized strength
- Return to sport or activity program

B. Treatment plan:

- Continue isokinetic training
- Continue with stability training
- Advance plyometric training
- Continue with closed kinetic chain exercise

C. Milestones for activity:

- Confidence in shoulder
- Strength deficits less than 10% throughout
- Pain-free full ROM
- Completion of return to sport or activity program

PROM, Passive range of motion; *A/AROM,* active assistive range of motion; *IR,* internal rotation; *ER,* external rotation; *AC,* acromioclavicular; *SC,* sternoclavicular; *ST,* scapulothoracic; *CW,* clockwise; *CCW,* counter-clockwise; *AROM,* active range of motion; *LT,* lower trapezius; *MT,* middle trapezius; Rhmd, rhomboid; *UBE,* upper body ergometer; GH, glenohumeral.

More often the posterior shoulder tightness needs to be treated after the surgery by the physical therapist. Focusing on the posterior shoulder will ensure recovery of total ROM.

Impingement Symptoms during Return-to-Activity Phase

Sometimes after SLAP repair, a patient will report back to the physical therapist with shoulder pain after returning to activity. It is not uncommon for an athlete to forget about the home exercise program or fail to complete rehabilitation. The athlete commonly complains of mechanical shoulder impingement symptoms. If this is the case it is helpful to closely examine ER strength in the 90/90-degree position, posterior shoulder strength, and scapulohumeral rhythm. It is more than likely that one or all of these parameters have not been normalized before the patient returned.

SUGGESTED HOME MAINTENANCE FOR THE POSTSURGICAL PATIENT

Because the patient spends only an estimated 2 to 3 hours per week with the physical therapist, it is what the patient does on his or her own that influences the eventual outcome. Physical therapists are teachers; they intervene manually when necessary but direct the rehabilitation based on the basic science of healing tissue. Adherence to a home exercise program is crucial for a successful outcome after SLAP repair. The home program for any patient must be individualized based on the patient's postoperative condition, age, nutritional status, limitations, and individual needs. Frequency, sets, and repetitions are determined based on the therapist's professional opinion of the expected outcome.

1. Early (0-4 weeks)
- ◆ Shoulder and elbow A/AROM flexion
- ◆ Pendulums
- ◆ No active biceps activity
- ◆ Isometric ER at zero-degrees abduction
- ◆ Scapula pinches, gripping exercises

2. Intermediate (5-8 weeks)
- ◆ Isotonic ER at 45 degrees of abduction with Theraband
- ◆ Rows with Theraband (not to break the frontal plane with the involved elbow)
- ◆ Wall crawls
- ◆ Side-lying ER with soup can
- ◆ Golf club ER stretch at 45 degrees (limit ROM of ER/ABD to 65-70 degrees)
- ◆ Scaption
- ◆ Biceps curls, elbow supported (no support later, 6-8 weeks)
- ◆ Ball proprioception

3. Dynamic strengthening (9-14 weeks)
- ◆ ER at 90 degrees abduction with Theraband
- ◆ Sleeper stretch
- ◆ UE stabilization in quadriplegic
- ◆ Door stretch
- ◆ Thrower's ten
- ◆ Eccentric biceps curls, shoulder unsupported with supination
- ◆ PNF D1, D2 pattern with Theraband
- ◆ Mirroring exercise—Stand in front of mirror, flex good arm to 45 degrees, copy motion with bad arm and eyes closed

4. Return to sports
- ◆ ER 90/90-degree position with Theraband, three sets to fatigue
- ◆ Definitions of fatigue
  Failure to complete full ROM (zero-90 degrees)
  Upper arm breaking the frontal plane
  Dropping of elbow
- ◆ Maintain Full IR at 90/90-degree position
- ◆ Sleeper stretch
- ◆ Push-ups with a plus
- ◆ Rows
- ◆ Horizontal ABD, front raises, lateral raises, posterior raises
- ◆ Completion of interval throwing program

A/AROM, Active assistive range of motion; *ER*, external rotation; *UE*, upper extremity; *PNF*, proprioceptive neuromuscular facilitation; *ABD*, abduction.

References

1. Andrews JR, Carson WG Jr, McLeod WD: Glenoid labrum tears related to the long head of the biceps, *Am J Sports Med* 13:337-341, 1985.
2. Barthel T et al: Anatomy of the glenoid labrum, *Orthopade* 32(7):578-585,2003.
3. Berg EE, Ciullo JV: The SLAP lesion: a cause of failure after distal clavicle resection, *Arthroscopy* 13(1):85-89, 1997.
4. Burkart A, Imhoff AB: The suspension sling for arthroscopic fixation of SLAP lesions, *Arthroscopy* 18(6):E33, 2002.
5. Burkhart SS, Morgan C: SLAP lesions in the overhead athlete, *Orthop Clin North Am* 32(3):431-441, 2001.
6. Burkart A et al: Biomechanical tests for type II SLAP lesions of the shoulder joint before and after arthroscopic repair, *Orthopade* 32(7):600-607, 2003.
7. Burkhart SS, Morgan CD: The peel-back mechanism: its role in producing and extending posterior type II SLAP lesions and its effect on SLAP repair rehabilitation, *Arthroscopy* 14(6):637-640, 1998.
8. Burkhart SS, Morgan CD, Kibler WB: Shoulder injuries in overhead athletes. The "dead arm" revisited, *Clin Sports Med* 19(1):125-158, 2000.
9. Burkhart SS, Morgan CD, Kibler WB: The disabled throwing shoulder: spectrum of pathology. I. Pathoanatomy and biomechanics, *Arthroscopy* 19(4):404-420, 2003.
10. Burkhart SS, Morgan CD, Kibler WB: The disabled throwing shoulder: spectrum of pathology. II. Evaluation and treatment of SLAP lesions in throwers, *Arthroscopy* 19(5):531-539, 2003.
11. Chandnani VP et al: Glenoid labral tears: prospective evaluation with MR imaging, MR arthrography, and CT arthrography, *AJR Am J Roentgenol* 161:1229-1235, 1993.
12. Cooper DE et al: Anatomy, histology, and vascularity of the glenoid labrum: an anatomical study, *J Bone Joint Surg Am* 74:46-52, 1992.
13. Cordasco FA et al: Arthroscopic treatment of glenoid labral tears, *Am J Sports Med* 21:425-431, 1993.

14. Cordasco FA et al: Arthroscopic treatment of glenoid labral tears, *Am J Sports Med* 21(3):425-430, 1993.
15. Cordasco FA et al: An electromyographic analysis of the shoulder during a medicine ball rehabilitation program, *Am J Sports Med* 24(3):386-392, 1994.
16. Decker MJ et al: Serratus anterior muscle activity during selected rehabilitation exercises, *Am J Sports Med* 27:784-791, 1999.
17. Diederichs S, Harndorf M, Stempfle J: Follow-up treatment with physiotherapy after arthroscopic reconstruction in SLAP lesions, *Orthopade* 32(7):647-653, 2003.
18. Ellsworth AA et al: *Electromyography of selected shoulder musculature during unweighted and weighted pendulum exercises.* Proceedings of the American Physical Therapy Association Combined Sections Meeting, Nashville TN, February 17, 2004.
19. Field LD, Savoie FH III: Arthroscopic suture repair of superior labral detachment lesions of the shoulder, *Am J Sports Med* 21:783-790, 1993.
20. Gartsman GM, Hammerman SM: Superior labrum, anterior and posterior lesions. When and how to treat them, *Clin Sports Med* 19(1):115-124, 2000.
21. Harryman D et al: Translation of the humeral head on the glenoid with passive glenohumeral motion, *J Bone Joint Surg* 72A(9):1334-1343, 1990.
22. Healey JH et al: Biomechanical evaluation of the origin of the long head of the biceps tendon, *Arthroscopy* 17(4):378-382, 2001.
23. Hintermeister RA et al: Electromyographic activity and applied load during shoulder rehabilitation exercises using elastic resistance, *Am J Sports Med* 26(2):210-232, 1998.
24. Itoi E et al: Stabilizing function of the biceps in stable and unstable shoulders, *J Bone Joint Surg Br* 75:546-550, 1993.
25. Jazrawi LM, McCluskey GM III, Andrews JR: Superior labral anterior and posterior lesions and internal impingement in the overhead athlete, *Instr Course Lect* 52:43-63, 2003.
26. Johnston TB: The movements of the shoulder-joint: a plea for the use of the "plane of the scapula" as the plane of reference for movements occurring at the humero-scapular joint, *Br J Surg* 252-260, 1937.
27. Karzel RP, Snyder SJ: Magnetic resonance arthrography of the shoulder: a new technique of shoulder imaging, *Clin Sports Med* 12:123-136, 1993.
28. Kibler WB: Shoulder rehabilitation: principles and practice, *Med Sci Sports Exerc* 4S:40-50, 1998.
29. Kibler WB et al: Qualitative clinical evaluation of scapular dysfunction: a reliability study, *J Shoulder Elbow Surg* 11(6):550-556, 2002.
30. Kuhn JE et al: Failure of the biceps superior labral complex: a cadaveric biomechanical investigation comparing the late cocking and early deceleration positions of throwing, *Arthroscopy* 19(4):373-379, 2003.
31. Lear LJ, Gross MT: An electromyographical analysis of the scapular stabilizing synergists during a push-up progression, *J Orthop Sports Phys Ther* 28(3):46-156, 1998.
32. Linke RD, Burkart A, Imhoff AB: The arthroscopic SLAP refixation, *Orthopade* 32(7):627-631, 2003.
33. McCann P et al: A kinematic and electromyographic study of shoulder rehabilitation exercises, *Clin Orthop Relat Res* 288:179-187, 1993.
34. Maffet MW, Gartsman GM, Moseley B: Superior labrum-biceps tendon complex lesions of the shoulder, *Am J Sports Med* 23:93-98, 1995.
35. McFarland EG et al: Results of repair of SLAP lesion, *Orthopade* 32(7):637-641, 2003.
36. McMahon PJ et al: Comparative electromyographic analysis of shoulder muscles during planar motions: anterior glenohumeral instability versus normal, *J Shoulder Elbow Surg* 2:118-123, 1996.
37. Morgan CD et al: Type II SLAP lesions: three subtypes and their relationships to superior instability and rotator cuff tears, *Arthroscopy* 14(6):553-565, 1998.
38. Moseley JB et al: ECG analysis of scapular muscles during a shoulder rehabilitation program, *Am J Sports Med* 20:128-134, 1994.
39. Musgrave DS, Rodosky MW: SLAP lesions: current concepts, *Am J Orthop* 30(1):29-38, 2001.
40. Nam EK, Snyder SJ: The diagnosis and treatment of superior labrum, anterior and posterior (SLAP) lesions, *Am J Sports Med* 31(5):798-810, 2003.
41. O'Brien SJ et al: A new and effective test for diagnosing labral tears and AC joint pathology, *J Shoulder Elbow Surg* 6:175, 1997 (abstract).
42. O'Brien SJ et al: The trans-rotator cuff approach to SLAP lesions: technical aspects for repair and a clinical follow-up of 31 patients at a minimum of 2 years, *Arthroscopy* 18(4):372-377, 2002.
43. Pagnani MJ et al: Arthroscopic fixation of superior labral lesions using a biodegradable implant: a preliminary report, *Arthroscopy* 11(2):194-198, 1995.
44. Pal GP, Bhatt RH, Patel VS: Relationship between the tendon of the long head of biceps brachii and the glenoidal labrum in humans, *Anat Rec* 229:278-280, 1991.
45. Park HB et al: Return to play for rotator cuff injuries and superior labrum anterior posterior (SLAP) lesions, *Clin Sports Med* 23(3):321-334, 2004.
46. Prodromos CC et al: Histological studies of the glenoid labrum from fetal life to old age, *J Bone Joint Surg Am* 72:1344-1348, 1990.
47. Rames RD, Karzel RP: Injuries to the glenoid labrum, including slap lesions, *Orthop Clin North Am* 24(1):45-53, 1993.
48. Resch H et al: Arthroscopic repair of superior glenoid detachment (the SLAP lesion), *J Shoulder Elbow Surg* 2:147-155, 1993.
49. Resch H et al: Arthroscopic repair of superior glenoid labral detachment (the SLAP lesion), *J Shoulder Elbow Surg* 2:147-155, 1993.
50. Rodosky MW, Harner CD, Fu FH: The role of the long head of the biceps muscle and superior glenoid labrum in anterior stability of the shoulder, *Am J Sports Med* 22:121-130, 1994.
51. Samani JE, Marston SB, Buss DD: Arthroscopic stabilization of type II SLAP lesions using an absorbable tack, *Arthroscopy* 17(1):19-24, 2001.
52. Segmuller HE, Hayes MG, Saies AD: Arthroscopic repair of glenolabral injuries with an absorbable fixation device, *J Shoulder Elbow Surg* 6(4):383-392, 1997.
53. Snyder SJ: *Shoulder arthroscopy*, New York, 1994, McGraw-Hill, pp 31-33, 122.

54. Snyder SJ, Banas MP, Karzel RP: An analysis of 140 injuries to the superior glenoid labrum, *J Shoulder Elbow Surg* 4:243-248, 1995.
55. Snyder SJ et al: SLAP lesions of the shoulder, *Arthroscopy* 6(4):274-279, 1990.
56. Stetson WB et al: *Long term clinical follow-up of isolated SLAP lesions of the shoulder.* Paper presented at the 65th Annual Meeting of the American Academy of Orthopaedic Surgeons, New Orleans, March 23, 1998.
57. Tirman PFJ et al: Magnetic resonance arthrography of the shoulder, *Magn Reson Imaging Clin N Am* 1:125-142, 1993.
58. Tirman PFJ et al: Association of glenoid labral cysts with labral tears and glenohumeral instability: radiologic findings and clinical significance, *Radiology* 190:653-658, 1994.
59. Tischer T, Putz R: Anatomy of the superior labrum complex of the shoulder, *Orthopade* 32(7):572-577, 2003.
60. Townsend H et al: Electromyographic analysis of the glenohumeral muscles during a baseball rehabilitation program, *Am J Sports Med* 19:264-272, 1991.
61. Tyler TF et al: Electrothermally assisted capsulorrhaphy (ETAC): a new surgical method for glenohumeral instability and its rehabilitation considerations, *J Orthop Sports Phys Ther* 30(7):390-400, 2000.
62. Tyler TF et al: *Effect of scapular stabilizer fatigue on shoulder external and internal rotation strength in patients with microinstability of the shoulder.* Paper presented at the AOSSM Annual Meeting, 2005.
63. Tyler TF et al: Reliability and validity of a new method of measuring posterior shoulder tightness, *J Orthop Sports Phys Ther* 29:262-274, 1999.
64. Tyler TF et al: Quantification of posterior capsule tightness and motion loss in patients with shoulder impingement, *Am J Sports Med* 28(5):668-673, 2000.
65. Vangsness CT Jr et al: The origin of the long head of the biceps from the scapula and glenoid labrum: ananatomical study of 100 shoulders, *J Bone Joint Surg Br* 76:951-954, 1994.
66. Warner JJ, Kann S, Marks P: Arthroscopic repair of combined Bankart and superior labral detachment anterior and posterior lesions: technique and preliminary results, *Arthroscopy* 10(4):383-391, 1994.
67. Yoneda M et al: Arthroscopic stapling for detached superior glenoid labrum, *J Bone Joint Surg Br* 73:746-750, 1991.

CHAPTER 7

Total Shoulder Arthroplasty

Chris A. Sebelski
Carlos A. Guanche

CLINICAL EVALUATION

History

The most common complaint in patients with advanced osteoarthritis (OA) of the shoulder is pain. Most often, the pain is insidious in its onset, although an occasional patient will report acute symptomatology only to discover severe osteoarthritic changes in the glenohumeral (GH) joint. In many cases night pain is a major problem; specifically, difficulty with lying on the affected side is a common complaint.[11]

A careful history should be taken with respect to prior injuries and prior surgical procedures. For a total shoulder replacement to be viable and functional, an intact rotator cuff is necessary. In certain patients with long-standing rotator cuff disruption, the first clinical signs are the progressive pain that comes with the developing secondary arthropathy.[61]

Another area of concern is whether the patient has undergone any prior stabilization procedures. The important principle to remember with this population is the incidence of preferential wear of certain parts of the glenoid in long-standing cases that have undergone excessive capsular-tightening procedures.[15] In addition, in certain types of stabilization procedures a variety of bony transfer procedures are performed, including a lateralization of the lesser tuberosity and a transfer of the coracoid transfer. This is important to note preoperatively, because the surgical exposure involved in these cases can be difficult because of the distorted anatomy.

Physical Examination

The most important predictor of the outcome of a total shoulder replacement is the preoperative range of motion (ROM).[35,50]

It is therefore incumbent on the physician to document all directions of the patient's motion and to discuss the implications of lack of mobility on the overall outcome.

Another important aspect is the integrity of the rotator cuff; a successful standard replacement depends very heavily on the presence of an intact cuff. The supraspinatus, the infraspinatus and teres minor complex, and the subscapularis should be carefully examined. If any doubt exists as to the function of the cuff, magnetic resonance imaging (MRI) is indicated. In cases in which a rotator cuff disruption coexists with severe OA, a determination should be made as to the possibility of repairing the cuff. In those cases in which significant chronicity of the cuff is noted, either by history or MRI examination, a simple hemiarthroplasty or a reverse total shoulder replacement (in cases in which pseudoparalysis of the arm exists) should be considered.[31]

SURGICAL INDICATIONS AND CONSIDERATIONS

Those patients with refractory pain and limitation of motion that do not respond to conservative methods of treatment (i.e., a trial of physical therapy, anti-inflammatory medications, activity modification, avoidance of inciting factors, and intra-articular corticosteroid injections) are candidates for shoulder replacement. Ideally, the patient's age should also fit within the acceptable parameters for a joint replacement. Although the ideal patient should be over the age of 65 and have a relatively limited activity level, the reality is that many patients do not fit such criteria.

In cases in which the patient's age is significantly under 65 years or the activity level is not commensurate with age, avoiding the surgery should be considered (in some of these patients, a case can be made for fusion of the joint). In addition, a spectrum of replacement procedures can be used, including a partial humeral replacement (classically termed a *hemiarthroplasty*), a hemiarthroplasty with a biologic resurfacing of the joint, and a standard total shoulder replacement; in more severe cases of patients with concurrent unrepairable rotator cuff tears, a reverse total shoulder can be used.

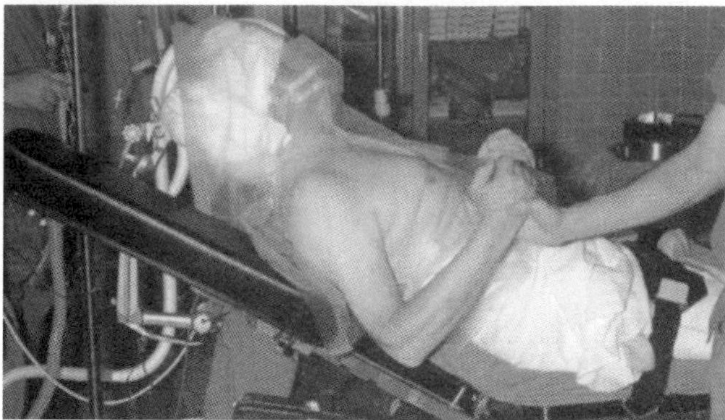

Fig. 7-1 Position for total shoulder arthroplasty (TSA), ensuring that the arm can be positioned for the insertion of the humeral device.

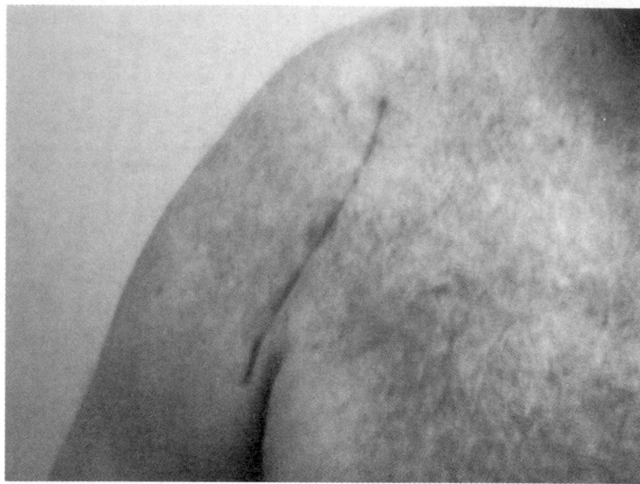

Fig. 7-2 Standard incision along the anterior aspect of the shoulder. The typical incision is about 4 inches long.

SURGICAL PROCEDURE

The choice of anesthesia depends on the clinical experience of the surgeon and anesthesiologist. Ideally, the anesthesia would include an interscalene block, either by itself or as a supplement to a general anesthetic. The use of such blocks has been shown to significantly affect the patient's postoperative course in a very positive manner.[17] In cases in which interscalene anesthesia is not used, the pre-emptive administration of a long-acting anesthetic (Marcaine) is also well-founded in the literature and has been shown to positively affect recovery.[1]

The standard approach to a shoulder replacement operation includes positioning the patient in a semi-recumbent (beach chair) position, with a small bolster under the scapula to effectively stabilize the glenoid for exposure. In addition, the operative shoulder should be examined under anesthesia with all of the directions of motion measured and documented. Finally, it is important to ensure that the operative arm can be extended and rotated appropriately for delivery of the humeral head and subsequent resection during the surgical procedure (Fig. 7-1). This is called the *ability to shotgun the arm into this position.*

The standard incision is a deltopectoral approach that is typically centered immediately lateral to the coracoid process of the scapula and extends down the proximal arm, avoiding the axilla (Fig. 7-2). It is important to allow for distal exposure of the wound should the need arise for a more complex humeral approach, such as in complications associated with humeral shaft fractures upon prosthetic insertion.

The exposure includes identification of the deltopectoral interval with identification of the cephalic vein and subsequent medial retraction. The pectoralis tendon is identified laterally and, in severe cases, released for a distance of 1 to 2 cm for improved GH joint exposure. In addition, the deltopectoral interval is exposed in its entirety from the leading edge of the clavicle to the lower end of the pectoralis muscle. Commonly, significant subdeltoid adhesions need to be released for proper delivery of the humeral head out of the wound.

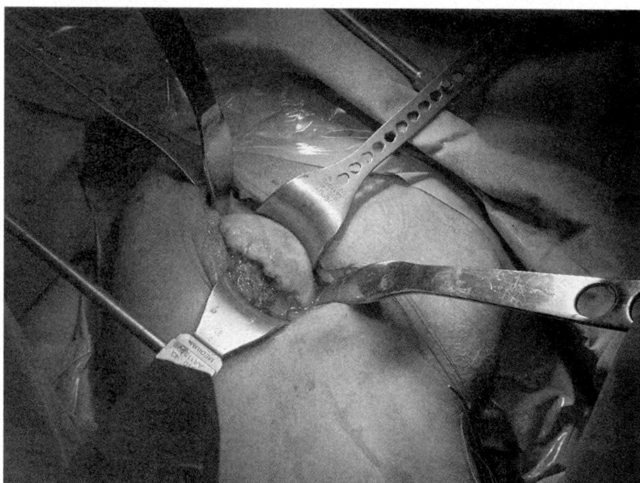

Fig. 7-3 Right humeral head exposed through the wound. The complete absence of normal cartilage on the surface and the peripheral osteophytes around the articular margin should be noted.

After complete exposure of the deltopectoral interval, the conjoint tendon is identified and released at its proximal portion for a distance of 1 cm, then the medial retractor is placed behind the tendon. Care should be taken to protect the musculocutaneous nerve when performing this maneuver.

The subscapularis tendon is now identified and released from superior to inferior, beginning at its lateral corner. The tendon is released directly off the lesser tuberosity and retracted medially. The release continues inferiorly, cauterizing the vascular leash consisting of the anterior inferior humeral circumflex vessels and proceeding along the inferior humeral head, while externally rotating the humerus (Fig. 7-3). The extent of the release is variable.

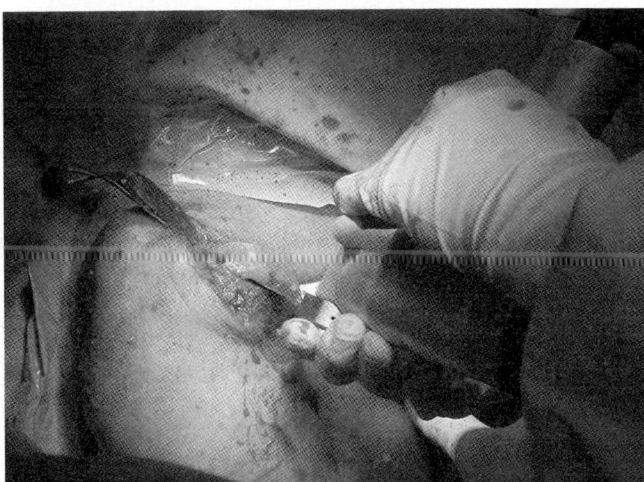

Fig. 7-4 Resection of the humeral head after removal of the peripheral osteophytes and the normal anatomic reference is found.

However, the requirement is that the entire humeral head can be delivered for resection and that adequate glenoid can be obtained if a resurfacing of that portion is being performed.

Once the exposure is complete, a variety of humeral resection techniques can be used, depending on the manufacturer's individual surgical protocol. The design the author uses involves resection of the humeral head at its anatomic base. Before completing this cut, the head must be exposed and all peripheral osteophytes should be removed to appropriately resect the head in an anatomic fashion (Fig. 7-4).

After resection of the head, the humeral canal is prepared for the prosthetic device being implanted. A series of reamers are inserted down the medullary canal, stopping when the appropriate-sized device is used. The size is typically judged from templates that measure the size of the medullary canal based on their radiographic dimension. However, ultimately the choice is made intraoperatively, based on the surgeon's experience as he or she advances the device down the shaft.

The humeral metaphysis is then prepared with a series of broaches that contour the proximal humerus for insertion of the actual component. The type of implant varies, with two major types being available: (1) cemented and (2) cementless. A cementless device uses the body's ability to grow bone into some of its surfaces; these surfaces are often prepared with a sintered metal (Fig. 7-5). In a cemented device, the prosthesis is implanted using polymethylmethacrylate cement for immediate fixation of the device. The theoretical advantages of one device over another are beyond the scope of this chapter; the reader is directed to the appropriate references.[48,51,56]

Attention is now directed to the glenoid. The important principle here is to be able to access the entire area of the glenoid from anterior to posterior and superior to inferior

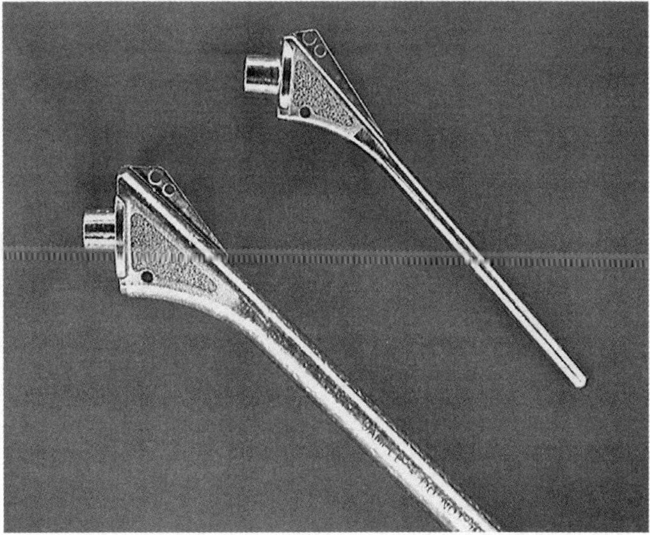

Fig. 7-5 Typical shoulder (humeral) components. These are standard components with a porous metal interface at that proximal portion to promote bony ingrowth.

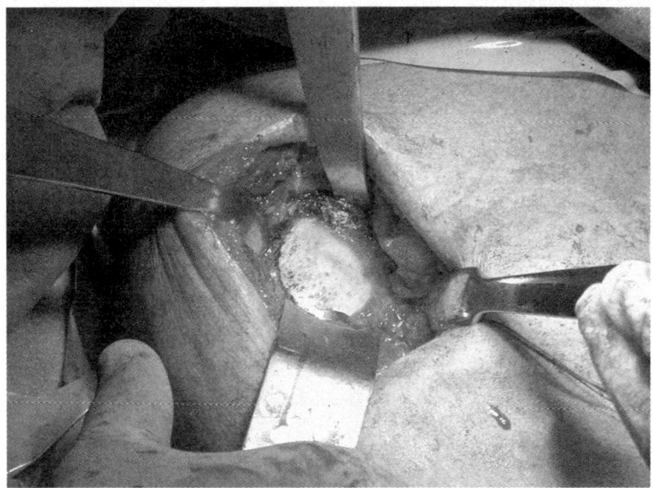

Fig. 7-6 Glenoid exposure after soft tissue resection circumferentially around the joint.

to effectively prepare the bony surface for the resurfacing device being implanted. The capsule of the joint is excised, beginning with the most anterior superior portion and extending inferiorly and posteriorly as far as necessary to allow for adequate exposure (Fig. 7-6). Once the exposure has been obtained, the central point of the glenoid is identified; then the surface is prepared for accepting the actual component. Finally, the device is cemented into position using polymethylmethacrylate cement.

The final decisions that need to be made include choosing the appropriately sized humeral head component to allow a relatively normal passive range of motion (PROM) with minimal to no instability before closure of

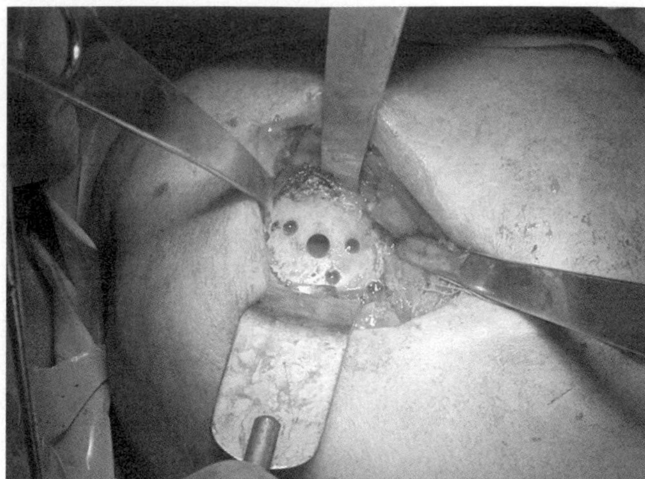

Fig. 7-7 Prepared glenoid face after drilling of central canal and preparation of face.

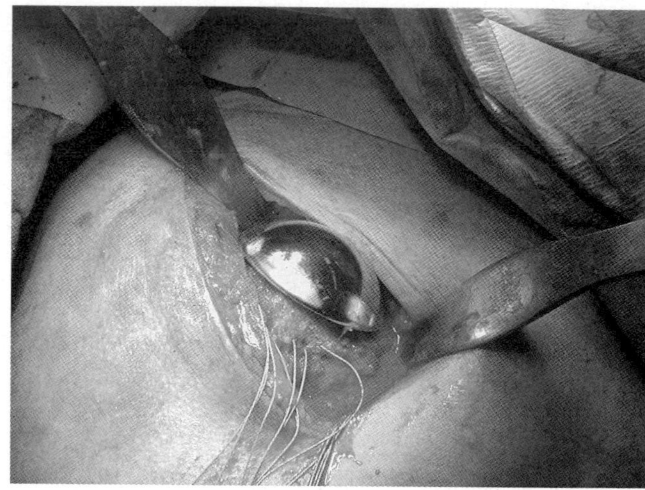

Fig. 7-9 Prepared proximal humerus with sutures through the lesser tuberosity in preparation for reattachment of the subscapularis tendon.

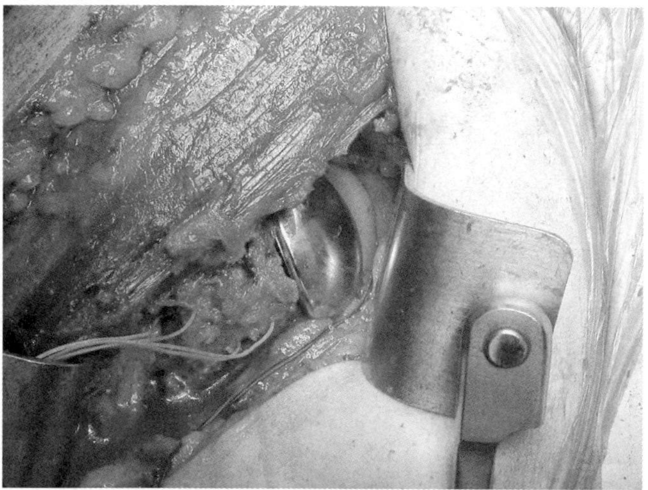

Fig. 7-8 Final view of humeral and glenoid implants before closure of the subscapularis tendon.

the subscapularis muscle tendon (Fig. 7-7). Once the appropriate head is chosen and implanted, the subscapularis muscle tendon is reapproximated to the lesser tuberosity with the use of sutures that have been prepositioned through the bone before implantation of the humeral component (Figs. 7-8 and 7-9). The repair of the subscapularis is the critical element that needs attention in the first postoperative weeks because of the importance of the subscapularis for component stability and overall shoulder girdle strength. Moreover, a disruption of the repair is notoriously difficult to diagnose in the early phases and extremely difficult to salvage when a chronic diagnosis is made.

The closure is done in layers, with a subcuticular skin closure protected by Steri-Strips being the final step. In some cases a drain may be exteriorized via a separate stab wound incision. This is typically removed on the first postoperative day. The final and perhaps most important part of the surgical procedure occurs at this time. The surgeon takes the arm through a PROM to assess the overall total motion possible without joint instability of disruption of the subscapularis tendon repair. This ROM will be used to guide the limits that will be allowed in the first phases of rehabilitation. Final radiographs are typically obtained immediately postoperatively to ensure an appropriate position of all the components and also to ascertain that no intraoperative complications such as a humeral shaft fracture have occurred (Fig. 7-10).

THERAPY GUIDELINES FOR REHABILITATION

In the United States, total shoulder arthroplasty (TSA) is performed less frequently than hip or knee total joint replacements.[57] Evidence shows that a decreased hospital stay and a higher likelihood of discharge to home may be associated with patients treated in surgical centers who have a higher volume of total shoulder arthroplasties.[32,39] No attempts have been made to correlate the patient's functional limitations and impairments on discharge with length of stay or "successful discharge." Therefore the clinician is limited when choosing evidence-based guidelines for in-hospital stay or outpatient rehabilitation.

Successful rehabilitation of a TSA depends in large part on the collegial communication between the surgeon and the therapist. Appropriate rehabilitation needs to recognize and address the preoperative history and impairments, the surgical technique, prosthetic type, and the surgeon's assessment of the tissue status on finalization of the repair.

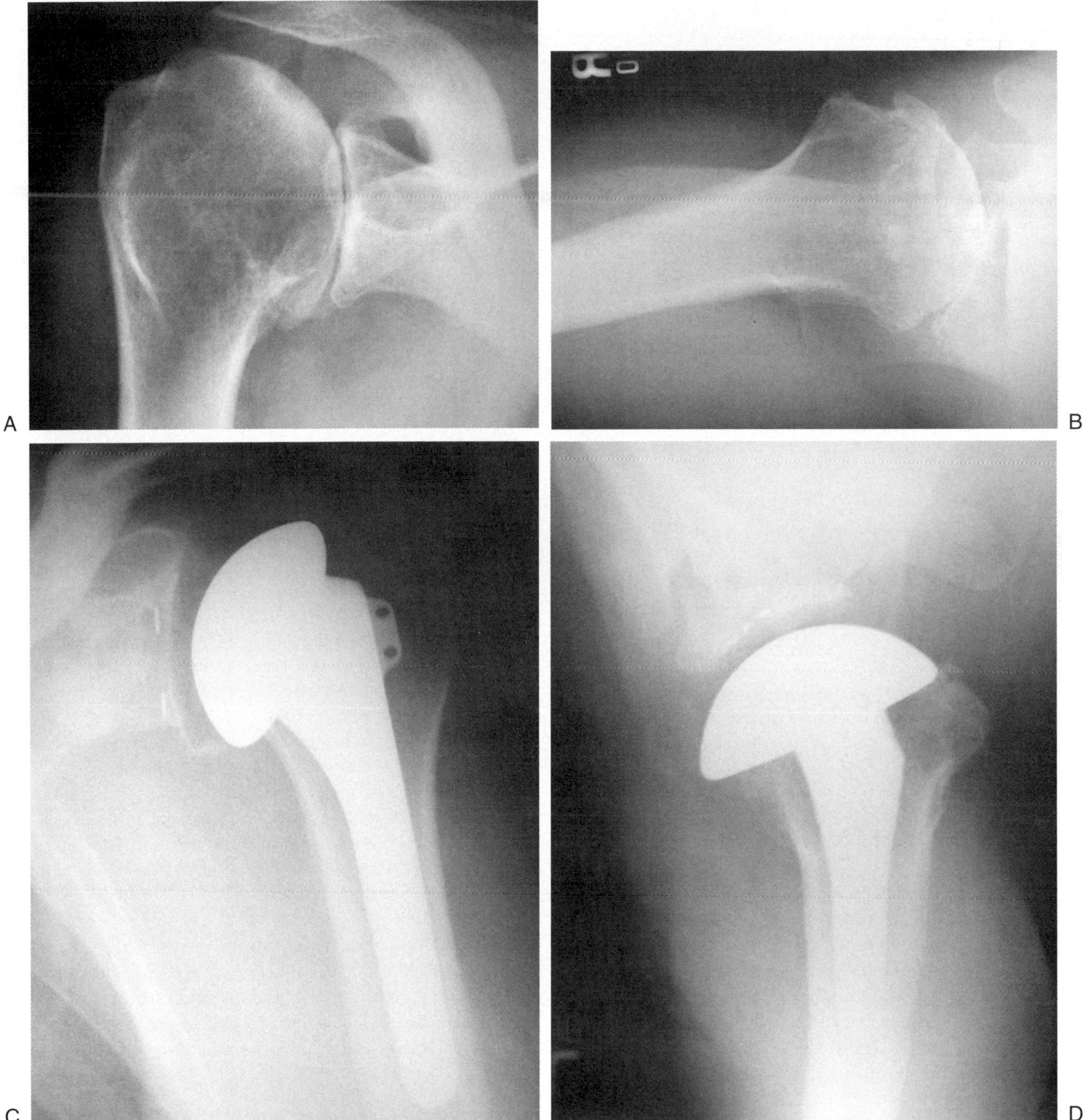

Fig. 7-10 **A**, Preoperative anteroposterior radiograph of severe glenohumeral (GH) arthritis. The lack of space between the humerus and glenoid and the peripheral osteophytes should be noted. **B**, Axillary view showing GH relationship with no joint space. **C**, Final anteroposterior radiograph of total shoulder replacement. **D**, Final axillary view of the total shoulder arthroplasty.

The majority of these issues dictate the postoperative precautions and guidelines placed on the rehabilitation timeline to ensure that protection of the prosthesis and appropriate tissue healing occurs (Box 7-1).

The patient and therapist must be aware that the primary goal for nontraumatic TSA is pain relief. Overall functional outcomes (including improvement of ROM), although often interlinked with pain relief, are not as well substantiated in the literature as the successful achievement of decreased pain.[50] Functional use of the upper extremity (UE) after TSA because of primary OA is a more likely result than TSA completed because of trauma or rheumatoid arthritis (RA), capsulorrhaphy arthropathy, or rotator cuff arthropathy (Box 7-2).[33]

Box 7-1 Potential Preoperative Impairments for Primary Total Shoulder Arthroplasty (TSA) Caused by Osteoarthritis (OA)[4]

Pain with attempted activities
- Loss of elevation range of motion (ROM)
- Loss of external rotation (ER) ROM
- Inability to complete overhead activities
- Inability to complete activities of daily living (ADLs)
- Interrupted sleep patterns caused by pain

Box 7-2 Preoperative Factors for Better Outcomes After Total Shoulder Arthroplasty (TSA)*

Better Outcomes	Worse Outcomes
No previous surgery	Surgery because of rheumatoid arthritis (RA) or trauma
Higher level of preoperative function[48]	Severe loss of passive range of motion (PROM)
Minimal rotator cuff pathology	Increased number of comorbidities
Overall well-being of the patient before surgery[33]	Radiographic evidence of humeral head subluxation
Surgery because of primary osteoarthritis (OA)	Loss of posterior glenoid bone
	Significant rotator cuff pathologic damage
	Increased fatty degeneration of the infraspinatus, subscapularis[41]

*The information for this box was compiled from multiple sources. References 5, 9, 33, 41, 49, and 50.

Attempts to prognosticate functional outcomes including achievement of active range of motion (AROM) against gravity should include the patient's prior surgical history; duration of impairments before surgery; presence and severity of a preoperative rotator cuff tear[33]; the underlying cause for use of the surgical technique; and finally, the postoperative ROM outcome while under anesthesia. These factors can help the clinician predict the maximal outcome that may be achieved. Both the patient's status before surgery and the underlying causative factors leading to surgery can be obtained in the subjective exam. The surgical information, including comments on ROM and the condition of the repaired tissue, may be obtained from communications with the surgeon (including the surgical report).

Rehabilitation progression may further be guided by precautions and recommendations directly from the surgeon (Box 7-3). **These may vary from the significantly to mildly restrictive. Some possibilities include passive range of motion (PROM) restriction for up to 6 weeks,**

Box 7-3 Common Postsurgical Precautions

Passive range of motion (PROM) for up to 6 weeks
- Abduction pillow for up to 8 weeks
- External rotation (ER) limited to 30 degrees with humerus at degree of adduction
- Sling to be worn for comfort

placement of the patient in an abduction pillow for up to 4 weeks, no external rotation (ER) greater than 30 to 40 degrees with the humerus in neutral adduction, and placement of the patient in a sling for comfort for 2 weeks or more.

PROM restrictions and placement of the UE with an abduction pillow indicates the status of tissue healing present or predicted by the surgeon. Frequently, patients with a history of RA or a long history of rotator cuff pathology may require positioning that decreases the mechanical stresses placed on the healing structures. If the UE is allowed to hang at the side without support or without the tissues placed in a shortened position, then healing time may be extended. **An ER restriction of less than 30 to 40 degrees is typical for protection of the healing subscapularis and the anterior capsule that is disrupted during placement of the prosthetic. This restriction may last up to 6 weeks.**[13,36,38] Sling use for comfort is a common recommendation.

Literary support indicates a longer immobilization period increases the risk of a contracture of the deltoid and the rotator cuff. This soft tissue imbalance is theorized to be one of the reasons for revision surgery of a TSA. Other reasons for surgical revision include glenoid loosening, rotator cuff tear, humeral head subluxation, proximal humeral head migration, and GH instability.[35,38,50] **Therefore to decrease the influence of faulty rehabilitation on these complications, the following guidelines should neither supersede the communications from the surgeon nor override sound clinical judgment to create an independent plan of care based on the patient's comorbidities, physical health, and functional needs.**

Initial Postoperative Exam

Patient examination after surgery typically occurs on day 0 (i.e., day of surgery) or on postoperative day 1. The therapist will note intravenous lines for postsurgical fluid intake, sanguineous drains, postoperative dressing, and the UE in a sling for comfort. Physical exam should include cognitive testing to orientation of name, time, place, and reason, as well as vital sign assessment on the noninvolved extremity in supine, sitting, and standing positions. Testing specific to the involved UE should adhere to the postoperative restrictions according to the patient's chart.

Neural screening should be completed within the postsurgical restrictions including myotome, dermatome, and deep tendon reflex (DTR) testing. AROM of the cervical spine, thoracic spine, elbow, wrist, and fingers should be assessed. PROM of the shoulder should be assessed with the patient in supine (understanding that some limitation in mobility may be attributable to the dressing or intravenous lines). Girth measurements may be noted distally for comparison with the uninvolved extremity. **Functional mobility assessment should include instructions cautioning against direct pushing or pulling of the involved UE during transfers (supine-sit-stand).** The patient must be assessed for independent mobility from supine to sit to stand and vice versa. Once standing is achieved, balance must be assessed for single limb support without loss of balance. Frequently, postoperative day 0 or day 1 will require the patient to use a temporary single UE support (e.g., intravenous pole or single-point cane) because of anxiety, deconditioning, and postanesthesia effects. Monitoring of vitals and orientation during the transfer and gait assessment is necessary because of the risk of hypotensive episodes. The therapist should encourage use of cough and incentive spirometer throughout the hospital stay because of the greater level of inactivity after surgery intervention.

Phase I (Hospital Phase)

TIME: 2 to 6 days after surgery
GOALS: Protection of healing structures; pain control; independent functional mobility for transfers, dressing, and ambulation; education and institution of a home exercise program within the surgical restrictions (Table 7-1)

Treatment during the hospital phase of rehabilitation focuses on the achievement of appropriate pain control, independent functional mobility for transfers, dressing and ambulation, education, and the institution of a home exercise program within the surgical restrictions. Length of hospital stay depends on multiple factors, including the hospital's volume and the surgeon's experience with the total shoulder procedure. Other factors including home support, comorbidities, and demographic features play a smaller role. Common discharge goals regarding functional limitations, pain control, and impairment objective measurements have not been established in the literature.[32,39]

Typically, PROM is initiated on day 0 or 1; then the patient is progressed to self-assisted ROM exercises, including pendulum or tabletop activities.

The home exercise program should be completed multiple times per day for short durations with each exercise bout limited to 5 minutes maximum.[13] **A PROM restriction will require the education of a caregiver or family member to institute the home program.** The helper must understand all postsurgical restrictions that limit ROM. Self-assisted ROM exercises can be based on patient comfort or surgeon preference.

Pendulum exercises involve forward flexion of the trunk and movement of the hips and trunk to drive the dangling UE into multiple, different planes motion (Fig. 7-11). The benefits of this activity for a recent TSA patient include addition of traction to the joint, stretching of the capsule, and **avoidance of active muscular contraction at the shoulder joint.**[46] Overall, the goal is prevention of soft tissue contracture and possible modulation of pain via the rhythmic movement of the UE through a PROM.[16,36]

Table 7-1 Total Shoulder Replacement

Rehabilitation Phase	Criteria to Progress to this Phase	Anticipated Impairments and Functional Limitations	Intervention	Goal	Rationale
Phase I (Hospital Phase) Postoperative 2-6 days	Things to watch out for: ◆ Hypotension ◆ Neurologic deficits	◆ Edema ◆ Pain ◆ Inadequate ROM	◆ ROM of proximal and distal joints to surgical site ◆ Balance activities of trunk ◆ Development of home exercise program CKC versus OKC discussion	◆ Modified independent bed-to-sitting transfers ◆ Modified independent sit-to-stand transfers ◆ Instruction on sleeping positions ◆ Independent with home exercise program ◆ Controlled pain	◆ Maintain ROM of proximal and distal joints to sugical site ◆ For trunk activation ◆ Continue to progress with home exercises

ROM, Range of motion; *CKC,* closed kinetic chain; *OKC,* open kinetic chain.

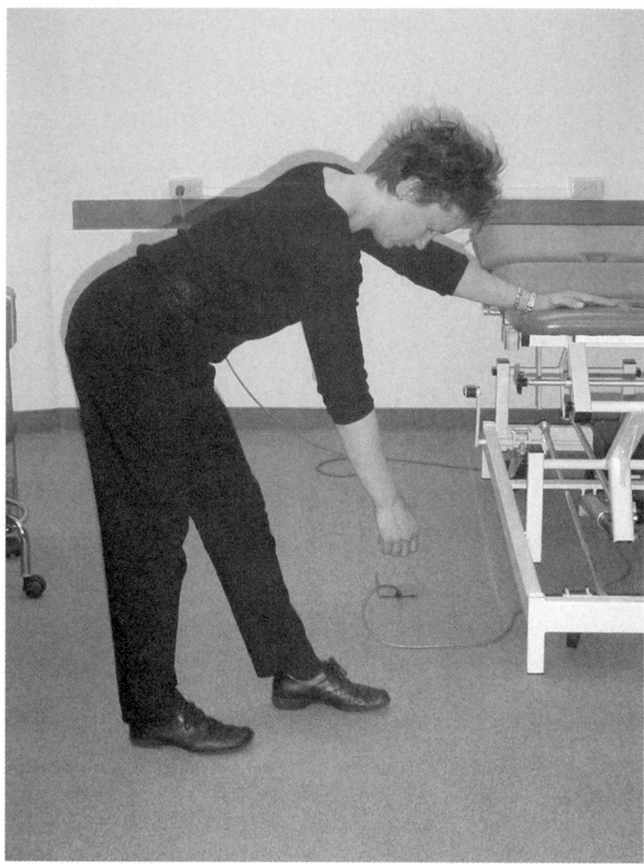

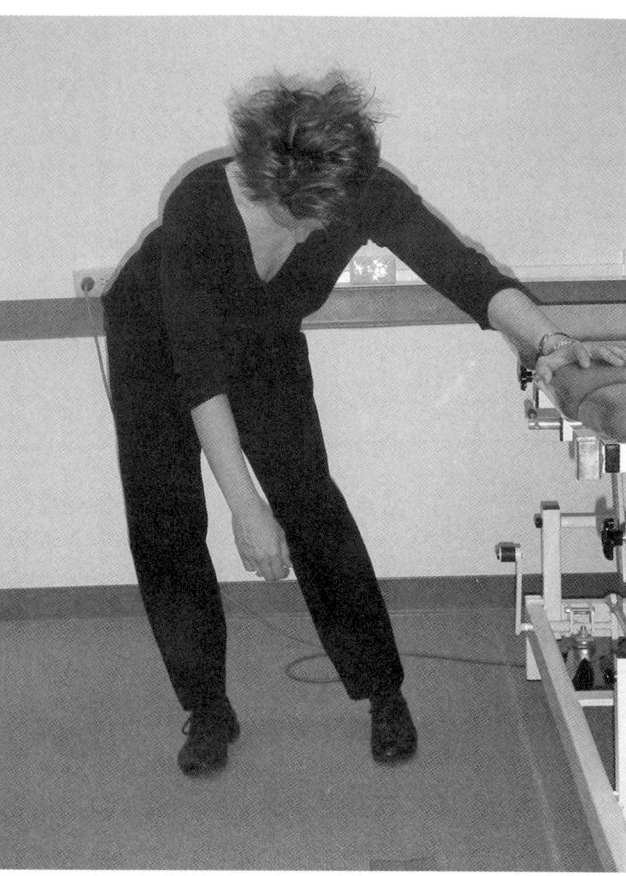

Fig. 7-11 **A,** Sagittal plane pendulum I. Patient should use shifting of body via movement of the hips and trunk to facilitate passive motion at the shoulder. Pushing the hips and trunk posterior via the noninvolved arm will facilitate shoulder flexion. Pushing the hips and trunk anterior via the noninvolved arm will facilitate shoulder extension. **B,** Frontal plane pendulum I. Pushing the hips and trunk laterally via the noninvolved arm will facilitate shoulder adduction. Pushing the hips and trunk medially or toward the noninvolved arm will facilitate shoulder abduction.

The challenges to this exercise as it applies to the patient with a recent TSA include the tendency for inappropriate performance of the exercise, recruiting excessive muscular action at the deltoid and rotator cuff versus motion from the hips and trunk; the poor mechanical alignment of the scapula on the thorax, with promotion of abduction and rotation; and lastly, excessive and unopposed stretching of the recently repaired musculature and tissues from the surgical procedure.

The Neer protocol for TSA[49] placed wall slides in the same phase as pendulum activities with literary evidence of low muscular activity about the healing structures.[46] Modification of this position to a lower gravitational–demanding position would be self-assisted ROM using the tabletop. This modification is frequently used before wall slides during this early intervention phase. The patient stands at a tabletop with bilateral UEs resting at a comfortable placement. The hands maintain a static position, and ROM is attained by lower extremity (LE) stepping into the various planes of motion (Figs. 7-12 through 7-16).[36] The benefits of weight bearing with the ROM attained via LE motion include mobility of the proximal segments (scapula) over the distal segments (hands) promoting scapula and thorax interaction in preparation for later stages of rehabilitation. The patient is able to control the excursion of the ROM of the shoulder via decreasing the step size. The supported position of the shoulder via the hand decreases the unopposed stress on the healing tissue of the open kinetic chain position. Closed kinetic chain activities at the shoulder reap similar benefits as stated for other extremities including muscular cocontraction, decrease of shear forces, increased joint compression, and increased stability about the joint.[7,62]

The home exercise program should require AROM of the cervical and thoracic spines through the cardinal planes, as well as active movement of the elbow, wrist, and hand. **Flexion of the elbow should occur only with the humerus supported to decrease the strain on the biceps tendon at its insertion.** Frequent bouts of exercise for short durations are recommended for the earlier stages of rehabilitation.

The home exercise program contains education for PROM, self-assisted ROM, or both at the shoulder, as well as AROM for proximal and distal structures and education

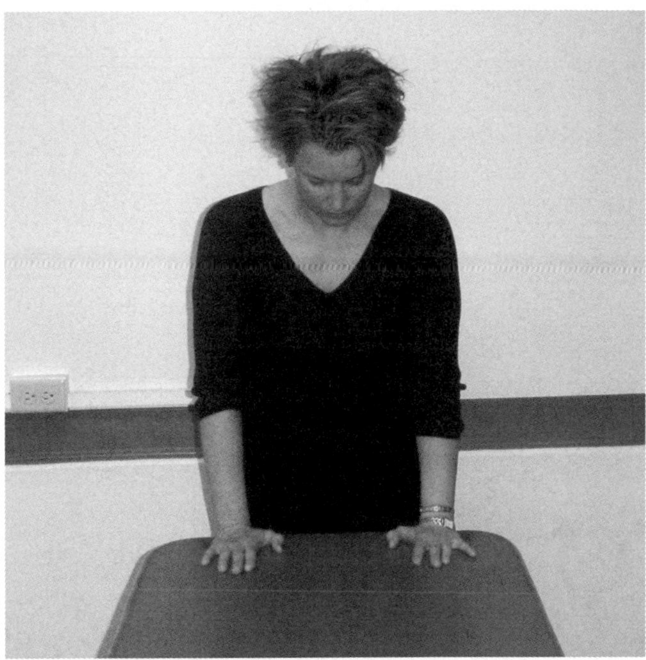

Fig. 7-12 Starting tabletop. Weight bearing on involved shoulder to patient tolerance.

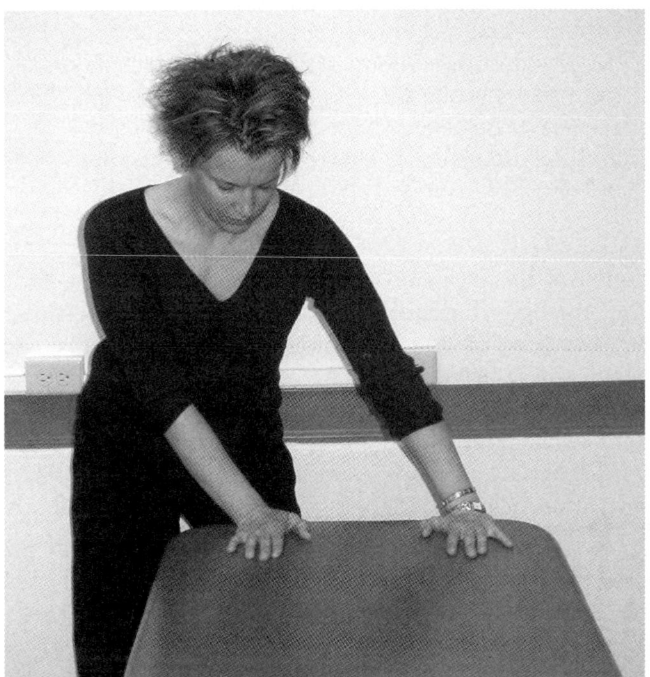

Fig. 7-13 Tabletop abduction. The involved extremity is the left upper extremity (UE). Frontal plane movement away from the involved extremity will facilitate abduction, and lateral stepping toward the involved extremity will facilitate shoulder adduction.

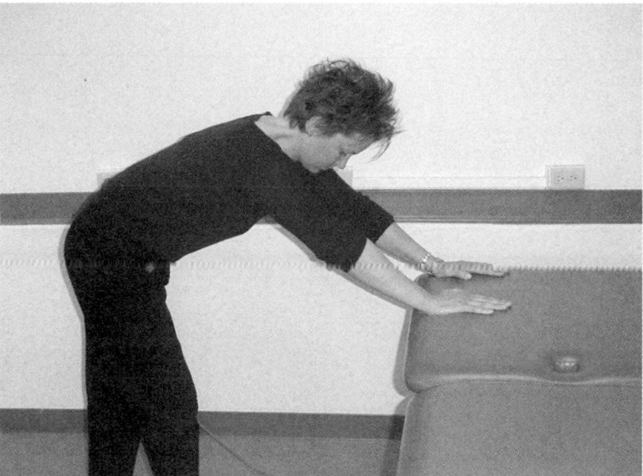

Fig. 7-14 Tabletop flexion. Incremental backward stepping away from the weight-bearing upper extremities (UEs) facilitates shoulder flexion.

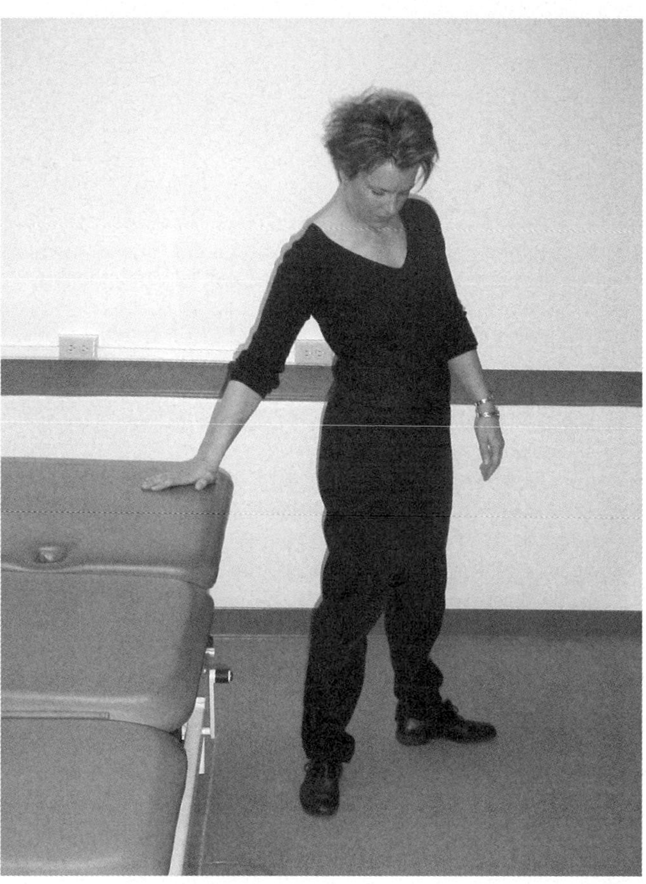

Fig. 7-15 Tabletop external rotation (ER). Stepping posterior lateral with the contralateral lower extremity (LE) will facilitate shoulder ER at the involved shoulder.

on sleeping postures. This should include positional support via the use of pillows or an immobilizer to support the healing structures during the night. The encouragement of experimentation to attain the best possible sleeping posture should be discussed. Anecdotally, after shoulder surgery patients feel better sleeping in a semireclined posture with the involved UE supported by pillows or bolsters (Fig. 7-17).

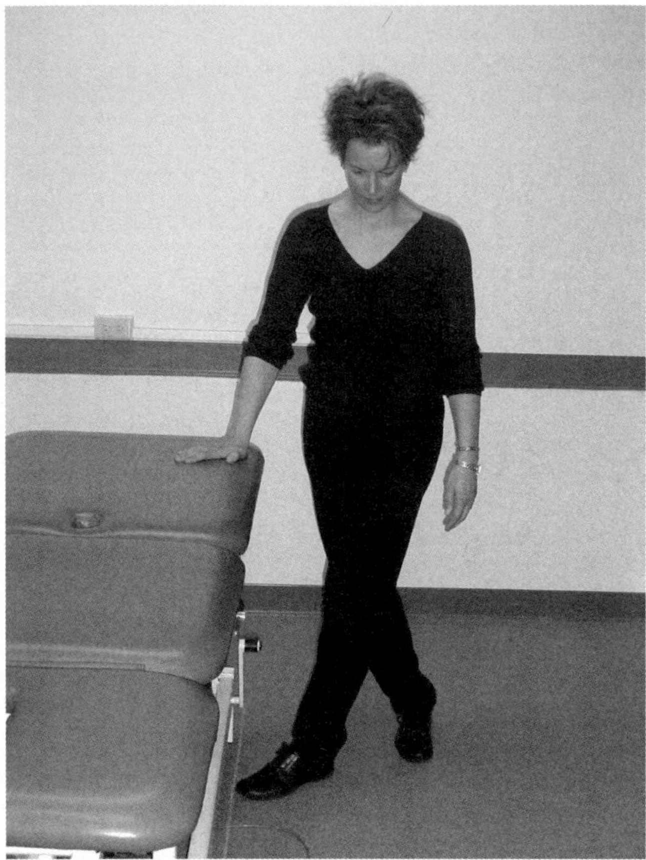

Fig. 7-16 Tabletop internal rotation (IR). Stepping anterior medial with the contralateral lower extremity (LE) will facilitate shoulder external rotation (ER) at the involved shoulder.

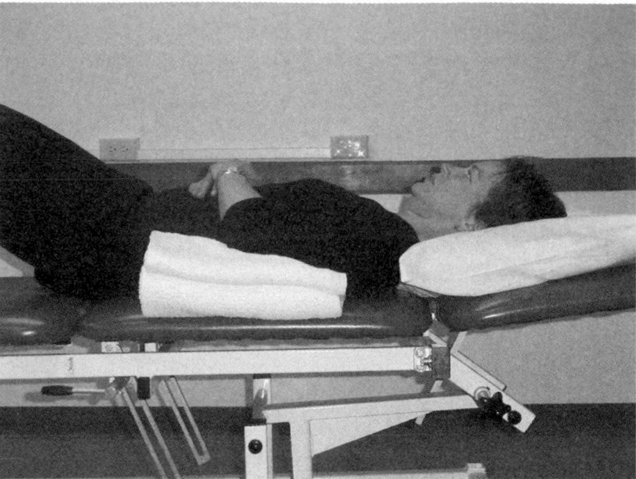

Fig. 7-17 Supine elbow support picture. Elbow supported via towels or bolster to align the humerus into the plane of the glenoid or scapula. This assists with avoidance of shoulder extension.

> **Q** Susan is a 72-year-old woman who slipped and fell 7 days ago, sustaining a four-part humerus fracture. Surgical intervention resulted in TSA. She is currently 1 day postoperative and has a compression dressing over the surgical site. The surgical team has requested that she be cleared for discharge by this evening, if possible. What functional assessments must be completed to ensure a safe discharge home?

Phase II (Outpatient Rehabilitation: Early Range of Motion)

TIME: 0 to 6 weeks after surgery

GOALS: Protection of healing structures, pain control, uninterrupted sleep pattern, normalized circumference measurements between UEs, mobilization of scar, ability to demonstrate normalized posture and increased ROM (Table 7-2)

Outpatient rehabilitation begins as a progression of the home exercise program given during the hospital stay. The focus of the first 6 weeks of rehabilitation is twofold: (1) protect the healing structures and (2) progress the ROM for prevention of muscular contracture and joint capsule stiffness. The literature supports a multitude of different intervention plans used during this first phase.[10,13,14,34] Adherence to postsurgical precautions is paramount. Treatment of the postsurgical impairments of pain, edema, and scar mobility will naturally lead to gain in shoulder ROM.

Pain control should be assisted via medications prescribed by the surgeon and alleviating positions used by the patient. Use of the sling should be gradually removed as the patient progresses through this phase. Control of pain will also be gained via the interventions to address the postsurgical inflammation and edema, as well as those interventions used to progress the limited functional use of the UE. Edema may be present in the distal UE, and ecchymosis may be present in the thorax from the overload of the lymphatic system after surgery. Modality use including ice, elevation, and electrical stimulation (ES) are appropriate for edema management.[6] Localized lymphatic massage techniques beginning at the proximal segments of the thorax and axilla and progressing distally in sequential order may also be used for effective management.

Sleeping postures should be recommended to include positional support of the humerus via the use of pillows or a bolster. Although anecdotally patients typically prefer sleeping in a semireclined posture after shoulder surgery, the therapist should encourage them to experiment.

The ER limitation is in place to promote soft tissue healing and protect those structures injured during the surgical procedure. Understanding the surgical injury to the subscapularis, therapists should consider early and gentle soft tissue mobilization for potential improvement of muscular flexibility into ER within postsurgical

Table 7-2 Total Shoulder Replacement

Rehabilitation Phase	Criteria to Progress to this Phase	Anticipated Impairments and Functional Limitations	Intervention	Goal	Rationale
Phase II (ROM) Postoperative 0-6 weeks	◆ Progression to next stage, physician clearance of tissue healing Things to watch for: ◆ Quick achievement of ROM before 8-12 weeks ◆ Excessive ER with UE at side ◆ Sustained edema in the distal UE greater than 4 weeks	◆ Edema ◆ Pain ◆ Inadequate ROM	◆ ROM of proximal and distal joints to surgical site ◆ Balance activities ◆ Soft tissue mobilization when adequate healing has occurred (subscapularis, posterior cuff, biceps tendon) ◆ PROM (performed in functional planes of movement and respecting postsurgical limitations)—Shoulder flexion, shoulder abduction, and ER (no greater than 30 degrees) ◆ ROM activities of the involved extremity ◆ Wand versus Codman's exercises (see Fig. 7-21, A + B) ◆ Closed kinetic chain (see Figs. 7-12 through 7-16) ◆ Modalities—Ice, ES for pain control ◆ Lymphatic massage ◆ Scapular mobility (see Fig. 7-18) ◆ MWM, PNF patterns versus cat-camel (many patients will require scapular adduction, upward rotation, and elevation because of typical postural dysfunction of scapular abduction and downward rotation secondary to sling posture)	◆ Protection of healing structures ◆ Pain control ◆ Uninterrupted sleep pattern ◆ Normalized circumference measurements between UEs ◆ Mobilization of scar when appropriate ◆ Ability to demonstrate normalized posture ◆ Increased shoulder ROM—Flexion=0-140 degrees 0-30 degrees, ER 0-70 degrees, IR 0-110 degrees, abduction	◆ Maintain ROM of proximal and distal joints ◆ Activation for trunk ◆ Realignment of scar tissue and collagen (to allow more unrestricted ROM) ◆ Prevent joint contractures (pain modulation) ◆ Joint traction (stretching to capsule, pain modulation) ◆ Proprioception training (proximal segment over distal segment promotes scapula and thorax interaction, cocontractions around a joint increase stability of the joint) ◆ Modalities for pain control ◆ Lymphatic massage for lymphatic drainage ◆ Prepares connective tissue around the scapula for future ROM

ROM, Range of motion; *ES,* electrical stimulation; *MWM,* mobilizations with movement*; *PNF,* proprioceptive neuromuscular facilitation.
*From Brian R. Mulligan, FNZSP (Hon), Dip MT, Mulligan Concept–Manual Therapy. Mobilizations with movement: A new approach. Available at: http://www.rptmulligan.com.

limitations. Soft tissue mobilization to this muscle promotes change to the myofascia via proposed realignment of the scar tissue and collagen. The best patient position for improvements to the subscapularis length is approximately 45 degrees of humeral abduction. Slow, deep strokes to the myofascia of the subscapularis for 7 minutes to assist in improvement of ER ROM and overhead reach are recommended.[29]

Progression of ROM may be elicited via soft tissue mobilization. Soft tissue mobilization, a form of massage, has the support of an animal model for potential cellular changes.[44] Initiation of soft tissue mobilization techniques at the posterior cuff and the deltoid will promote appropriate muscular length. Because of the probable postsurgical hypersensitivity, care should be taken at or near the surgical scar. For each of these techniques, the UE position should be adjusted to ensure the muscle or area of skin being addressed is relaxed and in a protected posture. Beginning with the soft tissue in a position of a passively shortened length will decrease sensitivity and spasm at the introduction of this type of intervention.

> **A** Because of Susan's history of falls, patient mobility safely from bed to chair, sit to stand, and ambulation must be assessed. After TSA, patients typically self-limit weight bearing to avoid full or strenuous weight bearing immediately postoperatively; therefore the patient must be assessed for independent mobility with limited use of the involved UE.

Consideration of the other joints of the shoulder complex should be initiated during this phase. During the hospital stay, the patient is instructed in cervical and thoracic AROM. Distally, the elbow and hand are used during functional activities, limiting the potential of distal disuse atrophy. Realization of the influence of the scapulothoracic juncture on GH motion can assist with restoration of this motion early in rehabilitation.

Protective posturing from the postsurgical sling typically places the scapula in an abducted and down-rotated position. Lack of humeral motion in all of the planes through the initial weeks of rehabilitation leads to further disuse of the scapula and its contribution to shoulder ROM. Scapular mobilization on a stable thorax with the GH joint in open pack position prepares the scapula and its connecting tissue for future shoulder ROM (Fig. 7-18). Because of the typical postural dysfunction of scapular abduction and down rotation, many patients will require facilitation of adduction, upward rotation, and elevation. The lack of a true joint capsule about the scapula places this type of intervention into a mobilization of the myofascial connections.

PROM via a family member in gravity-eliminated position of supine or self-assisted ROM during tabletop

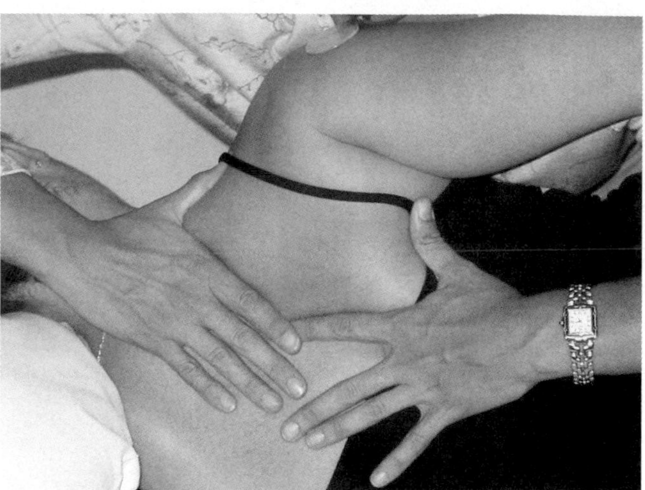

Fig. 7-18 Scapular mobilization. Therapist hand placement should be at the cranial medial border of the scapula and caudal medial border; thumb placement should be at the caudal lateral border. Facilitation of adduction, elevation, and depression can occur with the humerus in neutral adduction. Progression of the humerus to approximately 30 degrees of abduction is necessary for facilitation into up rotation, down rotation, and abduction.

weight bearing will be the primary method to promote ROM during this time. Progression should be dictated by pain report. PROM performed by the therapist, patient, or caregiver should not exceed any precautions or restrictions given by the surgeon. A tip for improved pain tolerance for motion of the UE is to favor the plane of the scapula over pure sagittal plane flexion.[21] A recommendation for moving into passive ER is alignment of the humerus perpendicular to the center of the glenoid. This occurs at approximately 30 degrees of abduction, ensuring that the capsular structures will relax and achieving a better outcome.[13]

Self-assisted activities for ROM can be varied by direction, surface, and patient position. These types of exercise promote the mobility of the proximal segments over the involved UE in a stable position. The trunk may move away from the UE in various directions to promote the cardinal planes.[14] For example, in the early stages when the patient may still be most comfortable in the sling or supported position, relative ER and facilitation of scapular control may be achieved via contralateral trunk rotation and a return to neutral (Figs. 7-19 and 7-20).[42] In an advanced stage of self-assisted exercises, the involved UE may rest on a stability ball and the patient rolls the stool away from the stability ball in the frontal plane, promoting self-assisted abduction of the involved extremity. On the other hand, the patient may progress to gravity-dependent positions using the wall as the support and the trunk moving under the body to facilitate various planes of motions (e.g., wall slides to encourage shoulder flexion).

Q It is 6 weeks after surgery for a left TSA secondary to progressive degeneration, and the patient arrives at his sixth week of therapy with increased swelling in his involved UE. The therapist is concerned about possible infection. What special questions should the therapist ask, and what signs and symptoms should they look for?

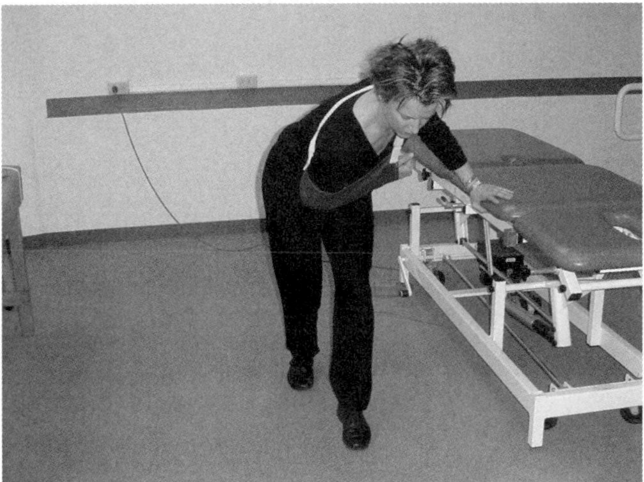

Fig. 7-19 Patient in sling facilitating internal rotation (IR). Movement of the trunk over the contralateral lower limb facilitates relative trunk, and thereby shoulder IR, while the upper extremity (UE) is supported in the sling.

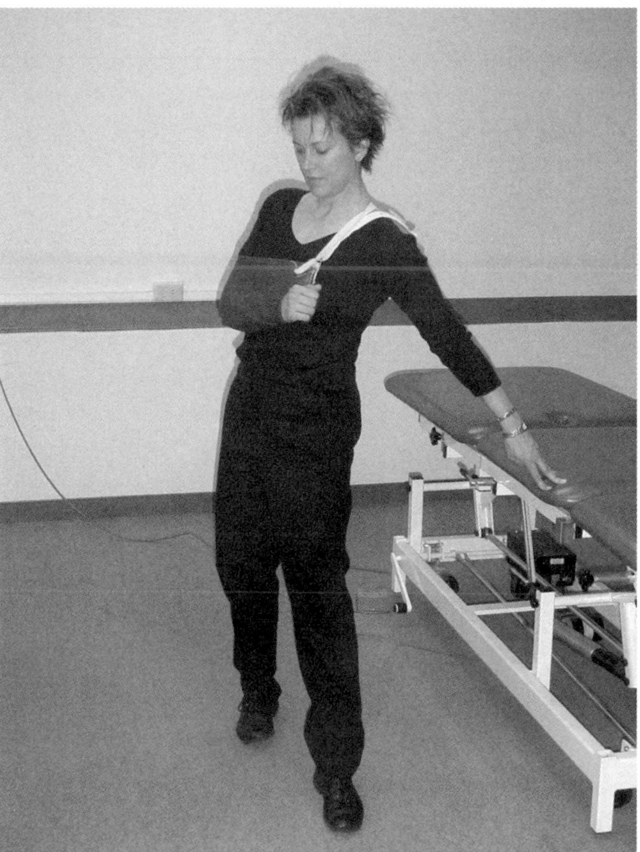

Fig. 7-20 Patient in sling facilitating external rotation (ER). Movement of the trunk over the ipsilateral lower limb facilitates relative trunk, and thereby shoulder ER, while the upper extremity (UE) is supported in the sling.

Other self-assisted activities that have been recommended during this time include wand activities and pulley stretches (Figs. 7-21 and 7-22).[10,13,14,34] Examination of pulley and wand activities compared with therapist-assisted exercises[20] indicated that therapist activities elicit less muscular activity of the supraspinatus, infraspinatus, anterior deltoid, and trapezius muscles. This would indicate that therapist-assisted activities should be used initially during this phase, with a progression to wand or pulley activities as pain or surgical restrictions allow.[12,13,14,34]

Progression from the initial outpatient phase to late ROM phase is listed in Box 7-4.

The most significant requirement is physician clearance for AROM. Many patients' restrictions will be lifted by approximately weeks 2 to 3, thereby blurring the activities of phases II and III. The therapist should monitor the patient's ROM to assist with "staging" the patient's rehabilitation. Exercises and activities should be performed with the correct mechanics and without symptoms before progression to the next phase.

Complications

Several signs and symptoms should alert the therapist for possible complications (Box 7-5). Sustained edema in the distal UE may indicate systemic complications. Excessive ER or quick achievement of ROM may indicate compromised muscular integrity. Biceps tendonitis indicates an overuse of the biceps for shoulder motion or stabilization. The biceps has an active role as a humeral depressor, and with postsurgical muscular inhibition of the rotator cuff, successful accomplishment of shoulder flexion may rely on the biceps as the primary humeral depressor.[43] As a patient successfully progresses through the different stages of rehabilitation, pain is expected to plateau, decrease, or alter to one of more muscular fatigue or muscular soreness. Progressively increasing pain is often thought of as an indicator of serious pathology.

Phase III (Outpatient Rehabilitation: Late Range of Motion and Early Strengthening)

TIME: 6 to 12 weeks after surgery
GOALS: Return to activities below 90 degrees of shoulder flexion, increased ROM, improved muscle flexibility, improved neuromuscular control, increase in strength, protection of healing structures (Table 7-3)

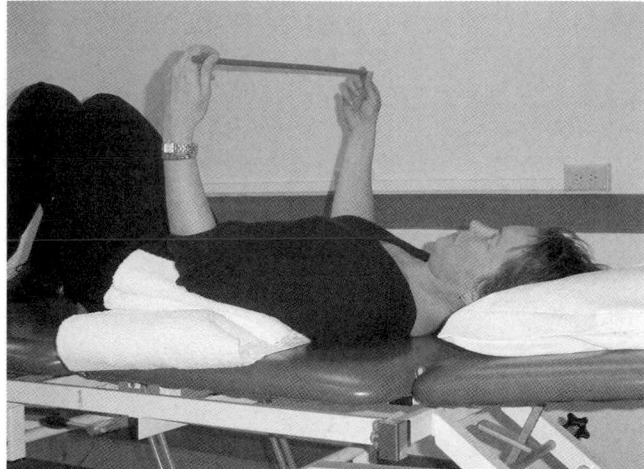

A

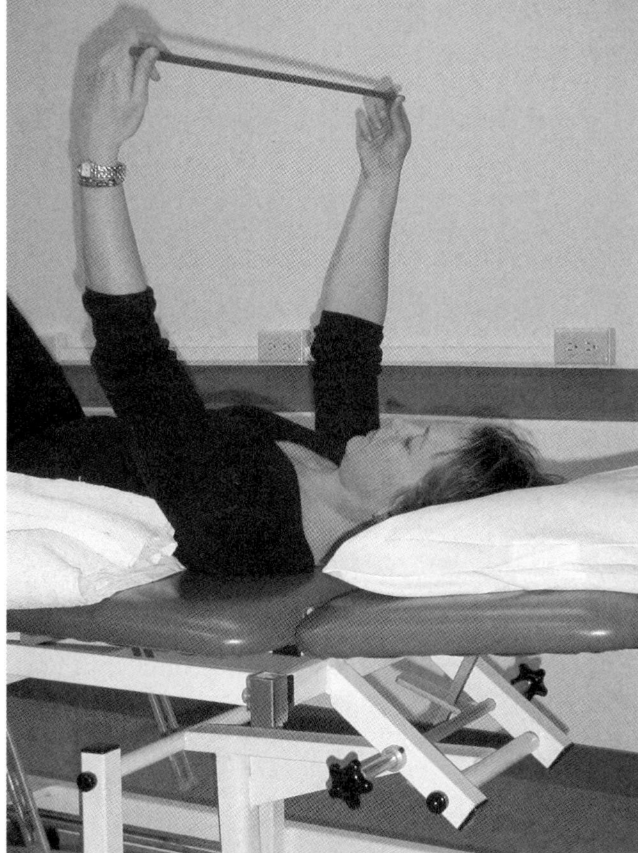

B

Fig. 7-21 A, Starting position for wand activities. Patient should have humerus supported into scaption plane. Hand support should be wide to facilitate scaption plane. Forearms should be in neutral to facilitate neutral positioning of the humerus. B, Scaption plane for wand activities. The position of the hands and the forearms should be noted.

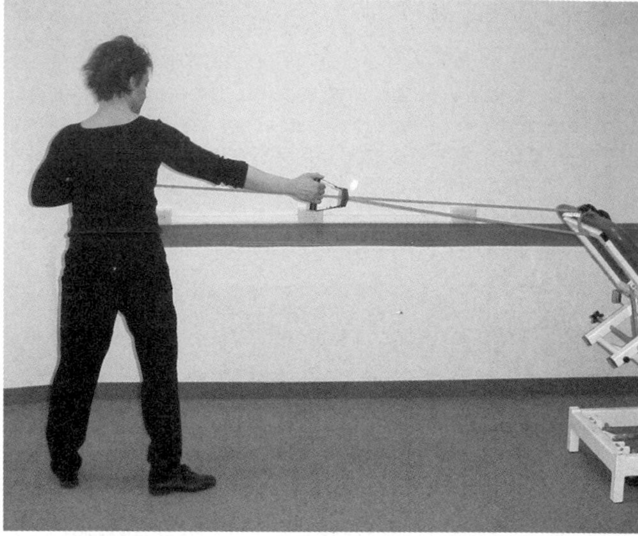

A

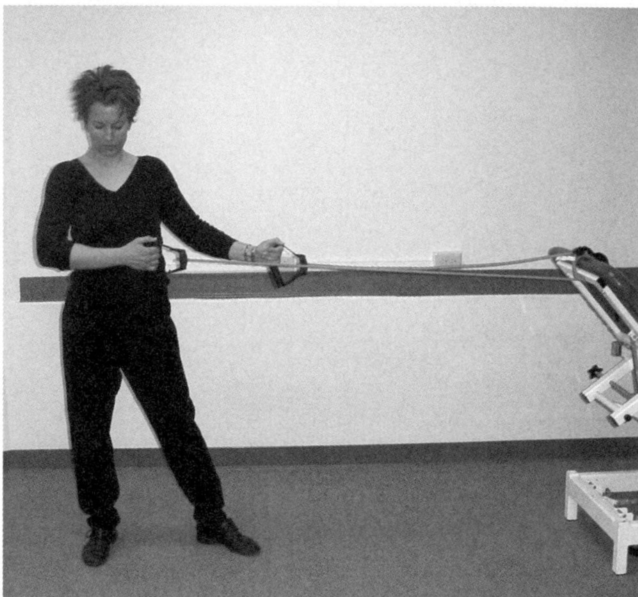

B

Fig. 7-22 A and B, Horizontal pulley. This is an alternate position for pulley activities that allows for facilitation of movement from the trunk and lower extremities (LEs). This will also allow the patient to avoid provocation of impingement symptoms and facilitation of normal scapular mechanics at a position approaching 90 degrees.

Box 7-4 Goal of Passive Range of Motion (PROM) Expected for Phase II (Supine)[30]

Flexion: 140 degrees
External rotation (ER): 30 to 45 degrees
Internal rotation (IR): greater than 70 degrees
Abduction: 110 degrees

As the patient's ROM progresses, he or she will enter a mixed phase of continued stretching to gain motion and strengthening. Choice of exercises should continue to protect the healing tissue structures. **This may include protection of the anterior joint capsule and the subscapularis via limitation of ER at the side and limitation of hyperextension of the humerus when positioned in supine for resting or exercise positioning.**[13,14] Communication with the surgeon will assist with determining which restrictions need to be maintained.

Box 7-5 Cautionary Signs and Symptoms during Early Range of Motion (ROM)

Sustained edema in the distal upper extremity (UE) greater than 4 weeks
Excessive external rotation (ER) (greater than 30 degrees) with UE at side
Quick achievement of ROM before 8 to 12 weeks
Biceps tendonitis
Progressively increasing pain

A Loss of ROM with pain or increasing pain would be associated with a potential infection after TSA. Although pain and loss of ROM may be the most objective sign during therapy, the therapist should be alert for drainage, warmth at the site, erythema, and effusion. Other subjective questions regarding possible night sweats, fever, chills, remote sites of infection, or any recent invasive procedures should be asked.[47] Early intervention in the acute phase of the infection yields the best result; therefore the therapist should recommend a return visit to the physician for blood laboratory testing.[44] Infection may present in up to 15% of all total shoulder cases[45] and may occur more than 1 year after the surgical procedure.[46]

Q Anthony is a 68-year-old man who is currently in therapy and is 9 weeks post TCA. His pain complaints have recently moved to the anterior proximal biceps area especially with attempts to move his shoulder into flexion. What may be one of the structures contributing to this pain?

The emphasis of this phase is the use of the ROM and progression to muscle strengthening. Interventions to address muscular flexibility of the rotator cuff, deltoid, and scapular stabilizers should be continued from the previous phase. Pain has been found to inhibit muscular strength and therefore can be a limitation for achievement of AROM.[37] Consideration that the source of pain may be from structures other than the traumatized muscle tissue will provide options for other interventions. Gentle joint mobilizations to the GH joint may be used to decrease possible capsular adhesions and nociceptor input.[13,14]

Considerable discussion has occurred regarding the most appropriate exercises to begin to initiate strengthening activities after a TSA. Literary support of certain exercises for effectiveness is limited, and a comparison of exercises does not exist for this particular patient population. One should always consider how the mobility is achieved and the movement patterns adopted during this time. The patient is at risk of developing faulty movement patterns that may later impede the ability to achieve AROM in gravity-resisted positions. The therapist is strongly encouraged to instruct the patient in activities that promote the separation of movement of the scapula and the humerus during the initial phases of flexion and abduction.

Isometric training is supported for early strength training, especially in cases in which muscular contraction is desired yet the patient lacks sufficient strength for mobility through a ROM.[14]

Significant muscular contraction can be elicited during isometric contraction exercises; therefore these exercises may be inappropriate during a healing phase (in which maximum tissue protection is required).[46] Initiation of isometric training of the deltoids with a contraction of the rotator cuff establishes a muscular cocontraction or force couple that is required for motion (Fig. 7-23).

Eccentric training of the scapular stabilizers, deltoid, and rotator cuff from a prone position is an option for introduction of strength training below 90 degrees of shoulder flexion. A slow lowering toward the floor after a passive preposition into horizontal abduction at 90 degrees will activate each of these key muscles. Introduction of concentric flexion and abduction may be introduced by progressively tilting supine positioning toward upright with and without weights (Fig. 7-24).[38]

If significant difficulty to perform an active contraction of targeted muscles exists and a neurologic injury has been ruled out, neuromuscular electrical stimulation (NMES) may be used. Although specific parameters are outside the scope of this chapter, dual-channel stimulation to provide for the deltoid activation and the scapular rotation necessary to achieve shoulder motion greater than 90 degrees is recommended. The therapist can stimulate scapular rotation via the lateral rotator cuff muscles on the scapula or by stabilizing the scapula by stimulating muscles off the medial border of the scapula. Electrode size and placement is a key point for effective use of NMES.[5]

Progression to the final phase requires an improvement in PROM and AROM. The patient must be able to perform all home exercises with the correct form and minimal correction by the therapist (Box 7-6).

Phase IV (Outpatient Rehabilitation: Late Phase Strengthening)

TIME: 12 weeks and more after surgery
GOALS: Return to normal activities including overhead, increased ROM, improved neuromuscular control and strength, full potential of function achieved between 6 and 12 months (Table 7-4)[36]

The goal of this phase of rehabilitation is strengthening for use of AROM and establishment of a home exercise

Table 7-3 Total Shoulder Replacement

Rehabilitation Phase	Criteria to Progress to this Phase	Anticipated Impairments and Functional Limitations	Intervention	Goal	Rationale
Phase III (Late ROM to strengthening) Postoperative 6-12 weeks	◆ No signs of infection ◆ No increase in pain or loss of ROM and physician clearance to progress	◆ Movement dysfunction—Early/unopposed shoulder elevation ◆ Inadequate strength ◆ Inadequate ROM	◆ Continue STM ◆ Joint mobility at GH joint if painful (greater than I-II) ◆ NMES—Rotator cuff and deltoid ◆ Isometric exercises (initially submaximal) progress to walkaways (see Fig. 7-21) ◆ Progression of table dusting to wall washing ◆ Progression of CKC from weight bearing at table to wall to floor (see Fig. 7-12) ◆ Pseudo CKC to OKC with UE supported but moving through ROM (angled table position [see Fig. 7-24, A-C]) ◆ Eccentric shoulder strengthening for flexion, abduction, and functional planes (assisted elevation of arm to shoulder height then have patient slowly lower arm)	◆ Return to activities below 90 degrees of shoulder flexion ◆ Increased AROM of the shoulder in supine: flexion 0-140 degrees, abduction 0-120 degrees, ER 0-40; with shoulder abducted to 90 degrees, then ER 0-40 degrees ◆ AROM sitting flexion 0-120 degrees ◆ Improved muscle flexibility ◆ Improved neuromuscular control ◆ Increase in strength ◆ Protection of healing structures	◆ Realignment of scar tissue and collagen (to allow more ROM with less soft tissue restrictions) ◆ Decrease possible capsular adhesions ◆ Decrease nocioceptor input ◆ Targeting for specific muscles ◆ Promote muscle contractions ◆ Benefits of CKC exercises as stated before ◆ Progression for antigravity strengthening ◆ Eccentric strengthening ◆ Progression to next stage

ROM, Range of motion; *STM,* soft tissue massage; *GH,* glenohumeral; *NMES,* neuromuscular electrical stimulation; *AROM,* active range of motion; *CKC,* closed kinetic chain; *OKC,* open kinetic chain; *UE,* upper extremity.

A Acute inflammation of the biceps tendon indicates an overuse of the biceps during attempts at shoulder motion. The patient will experience pain during AROM, especially with flexion and abduction. He may also demonstrate limited shoulder extension secondary to irritation as the biceps tendon is stretched. MMT of the biceps activates this muscle for its role as an elbow flexor and forearm supinator; therefore it may be pain free and strong despite the irritation at the proximal tendon. Presentation of biceps tendonitis indicates overuse of this muscle and therefore implicates inadequate contribution from the rotator cuff. Beyond the modality intervention for the inflammation of the biceps tendon, evaluation of the function of the rotator cuff should be considered.

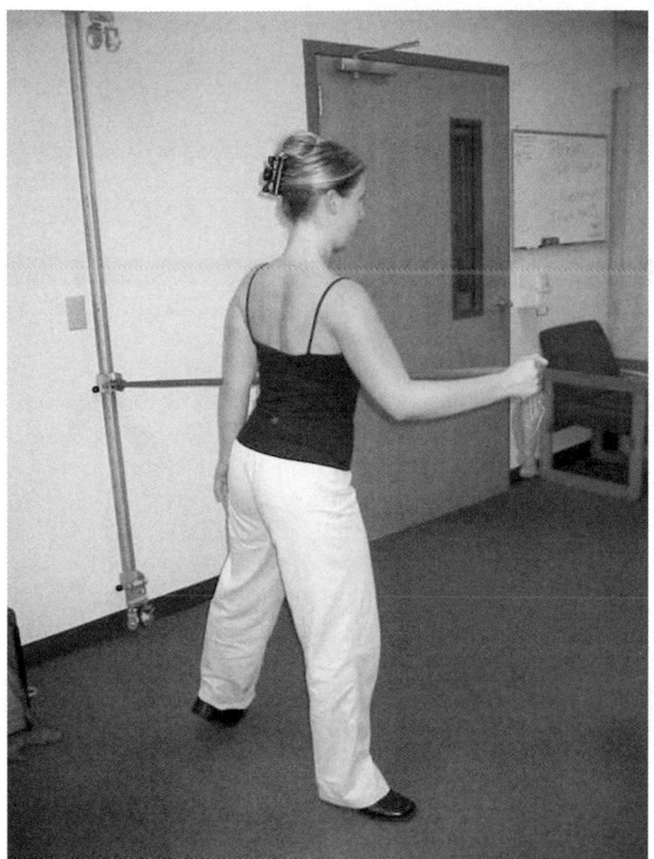

Fig. 7-23 Isometric walkaways. Patient is facilitating an isometric contraction of the deltoid via static abduction and isometric contraction of the external rotators via neutral forearm and humeral position. The resistance gradually increases with lateral stepping.

program that promotes continued strengthening. Interventions addressing pain control, edema, and underlying impairments that impede AROM should be progressively phased out; strengthening activities should address the dynamic-stabilization system necessary for overhead movement.

The primary challenge of the later stages of total shoulder rehabilitation is the functional use of the AROM. Several continuing underlying impairments might be limiting the patient's ability to demonstrate appropriate shoulder motion when attempting to raise the arm above shoulder height. If factors affecting rehabilitation have been considered adequate, including appropriate and timely surgical intervention, noncomplicated rehabilitation course, and appropriate motivation by the patient, then the typical impairment implicated for continued limitations in active overhead ROM is weakness of the deltoid or rotator cuff musculature (or weakness of both).[10,36] If the AROM demonstrated in supine is approaching the ROM goals for therapy but the patient is unable to demonstrate similar range in sitting, then weakness should be considered (Box 7-7).

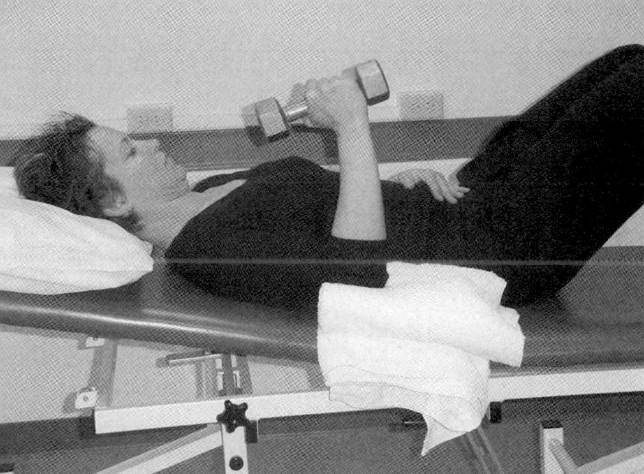

A

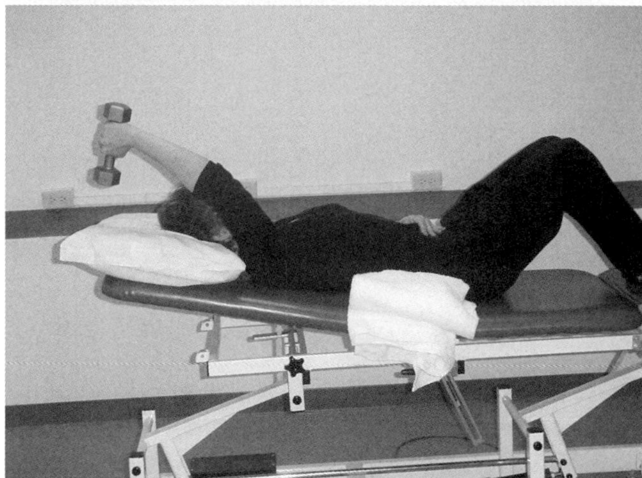

B

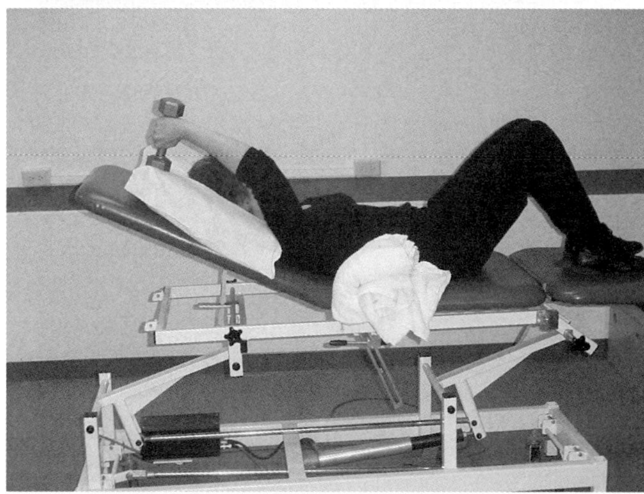

C

Fig. 7-24 A and B, Supine progressive tilt start and finish. Patient begins supine with low degree of tilt of the head of the plinth. Movement of the weight (or without weight) can be into any plane. C, Supine progressive tilt start and finish. Increasing the tilt of the head of the plinth moves the patient toward a more upright or gravity-dependent position.

Although specific rehabilitation parameters for those patients exhibiting weakness because of neural injury are not included in this discussion, this impairment should be considered as a possible contribution to a continued movement dysfunction. Typically, neural injury associated with the trauma predating the surgery or from surgical intervention is difficult to identify because of the amount of trauma to the area. Neural injury may be identified via atrophic changes to the muscle, inability of the patient to elicit an isometric contraction of the muscle with the humerus positioned in neutral, and possible sensory changes in the UE. Isolated neural injuries after shoulder arthroplasty are considered a low risk because of the transient nature of the injuries and the tendency for resolution without operative intervention.[9] When denervation of shoulder musculature is present before surgery, most likely the patient will be placed in a limited-goals category.[49] This category is discussed later in this chapter.

Box 7-6 Goals of Range of Motion (ROM) Expected for Phase III

Full passive range of motion (PROM) in supine
- Active range of motion (AROM) flexion in supine: 140 degrees
- AROM abduction in supine: 120 degrees
- AROM external rotation (ER) in supine at side: 40 degrees
- AROM ER in supine at 90-degrees abduction: 40 degrees
- Active sitting flexion: 120 degrees

Q Ralph is a 68-year-old man who underwent a right TSA 18 weeks ago. His course has been uncomplicated thus far; however, during observation of shoulder flexion, Ralph demonstrates a shoulder hike. What impairments should the therapist continue to assess to alter the treatment plan?

Evaluation of weakness in patients with adequate innervation of the shoulder musculature should include manual muscle testing (MMT) and the identification of balance of two of the force couples that move the shoulder, including the deltoid and rotator cuff, the scapular stabilizers, and the deltoid. Both of these force couples must have a balanced contraction to facilitate flexion and abduction without impingement of the humerus at the subacromial arch.[52]

Strengthening of the shoulder is the primary intervention during this phase. A progression of the eccentric training initiated in the previous phases should occur. The patient should be able to complete an overhead wand activity, with a release of the involved UE from the wand once the arm is overhead (with a slow lowering of the involved extremity back toward the waist).[12] This type of training can also be initiated for strengthening into adduction.

Box 7-7 Cautionary Signs and Symptoms During Later Stages of Rehabilitation[51]

Loss of motion
- Progressively increasing pain
- "Clunk" felt during range of motion (ROM)

Table 7-4 Total Shoulder Replacement

Rehabilitation Phase	Criteria to Progress to this Phase	Anticipated Impairments and Functional Limitations	Intervention	Goal	Rationale
Phase IV (Late Phase strengthening) Postoperative 12 weeks after surgery to discharge from therapy	◆ No increase in pain or loss of ROM and physician clearance to progress Things to watch for: ◆ Excessive ER with UE at side ◆ Sustained edema in the distal upper extremity	◆ Movement dysfunction—Early/unopposed shoulder elevation ◆ Inadequate strength ◆ Inadequate ROM	◆ Continue STM ◆ Joint mobility strengthening continues (both OKC and CKC) ◆ Progression to terminal end ROM and home exercise program	◆ Return to activities including overhead ◆ Increased ROM ◆ Improved strength ◆ Improved neuromuscular control	◆ Realignment of scar tissue and collagen (to allow more ROM with less soft tissue restrictions) ◆ Decrease possible capsular adhesions ◆ Decrease nocioceptor input ◆ Increase strength ◆ Increase endurance ◆ Improve function ◆ Progression to discharge

STM, Soft tissue massage; *OKC,* open kinetic chain; CKC, closed kinetic chain; *ROM,* range of motion.

Typically, patients should be discouraged from heavy loading of the shoulder either for recreation or work demands. The concern is the risk of glenoid wear or loading of the glenoid rim leading to instability or component loosening.[36,54] Surgical methods and placement of the prosthesis during total joint surgery are thought to contribute to these complications. Direct effect of various therapy interventions beyond monitoring the load on the shoulder may not be apparent. Changes in the GH translations and loading mechanics can be attributed to an imbalance of muscular forces either from length or strength impairments and the mobility of the joint capsule.[40] A therapist may believe that loading of the patient during the late phases of rehabilitation elicits strength gains without ensuring appropriate resolution of joint mobility, extremity alignment, and muscular balance. He or she may also believe that this practice might contribute to the development of complications and poorer outcomes.

A lack of understanding of the forces about the shoulder and the effect of an external load on potential outcomes forces the therapist to consider indirect information when determining the intensity of the load for the patient with a TSA. The outcome tools used postsurgically may assist the therapist with guidelines for how to load the shoulder. The simple shoulder test, a commonly used evaluation tool for function includes the ability to lift 1 lb to shoulder height, the ability to lift 8 lb to shoulder level, and the ability to carry an item weighing 20 lb.[30,45]

Additional assistance for decision making may be found considering studies of external moments about the shoulder during activities of daily living (ADLs). The average external moments to reflect loading of the shoulder during several ADLs, including picking up a 5 kg box, moving a 10 kg suitcase, and transferring from sit to stand have been evaluated. They have been found to represent a large proportion of UE strength in normal men and women.[2] Patients who receive a TSA must be considered to possess less than normal strength, especially during the rehabilitation process. **Therefore current caution for heavy loading of the shoulder for strength training demonstrates appropriate concern by the therapist for the external moments created by these lifts, thereby protecting the prosthesis and its design. Limiting the intensity prescribed to the patient for strength training exercises should be examined. Discussion with the referring surgeon may give the therapist more specific guidelines for possible lifting restrictions.**

Resolution of functional limitation in ADLs and ROM goals should guide the determination of timely discharge. AROM goals are listed in Table 7-5. **The therapist should not predict attainment of full ROM as evidenced by multiple studies on total shoulder procedures, regardless of the presence or lack of underlying pathologies or comorbidities.**[22,28] Additionally, both patient and therapist should be aware that functional improvements continue beyond the discharge of therapy up to approximately 1 year after surgery.[36]

A

Weakness of the deltoid, scapular stabilizers, and rotator cuff must be assessed. Additional impairments contributing to this movement dysfunction may include inadequate transverse plane ROM, inadequate length of the scapulohumeral musculature, inadequate mobility of the GH joint capsule, and inadequate mobility of the scapula on the thorax. Determination of the primary impairment limiting this motion will guide the plan of care to eliminate the shoulder hike.

Table 7-5 Range of Motion (ROM) Goals to Advance to the Next Phase of Rehabilitation*

	In Hospital[34]	Early Rehabilitation[30]	Late Rehabilitation	Phase IV[36]
Flexion	PROM supine 140 degrees	PROM supine 140 degrees	Full PROM in supine AROM supine 140 degrees, sitting 120 degrees	Full PROM in supine AROM sitting 145-150 degrees[53]
Abduction	n/a	PROM supine 110 degrees	AROM supine 120 degrees	n/a
ER at side	PROM supine 40 degrees	PROM supine 30-45 degrees	AROM supine 45 degrees	AROM sitting 45-60 degrees[38]
ER at 90-degrees abduction	n/a	n/a	AROM supine 45 degrees	n/a
IR at side	n/a	PROM supine greater than 70 degrees	AROM supine greater than 70 degrees	AROM supine greater than 70 degrees
IR at 90-degrees abduction	n/a	PROM supine greater than 30 degrees	AROM supine greater than 70 degrees	AROM supine greater than 70 degrees

ER, External rotation; *IR*, internal rotation; *PROM*, passive range of motion; *AROM*, active range of motion; *n/a*, not available.
*The information for this table was compiled from multiple sources. See references 30, 34, 36, and 38.

Box 7-8 Limited-Goals Category[12,16]

For patients with tissue insufficiency, rheumatoid arthritis (RA)
- Goal is joint stability
- Initiation of motion delayed
- Joint mobilizations delayed
- Active range of motion (AROM) delayed until after 8 weeks

Box 7-9 Limited-Goals Category Range of Motion (ROM) Achievement*

- Flexion: 75 to 90 degrees
- Abduction: 70 to 80 degrees
- External rotation (ER): 30 degrees
- Internal rotation (IR): Hand behind back to L5

*The information for this box was compiled from multiple sources. See references 10 and 53.

LIMITED-GOAL CATEGORY FOR TOTAL SHOULDER ARTHROPLASTY

Neer, Watson, and Stanton[49] first mentioned the limited-goals category after TSA in 1982. Criteria for inclusion into the limited-goals category included evaluation of the rotator cuff and the stability of the implant. Patients were placed into a limited-goals category if the rotator cuff was detached and not capable of recovery secondary to denervation or irreversible contracture, or if the stability of the implant was problematic as evaluated by the surgeon during the procedure (Boxes 7-8 and 7-9). Specific diagnosis typically associated in this category includes RA, massive rotator tear, component malposition, septic arthritis, or neurovascular injury.[41]

Specific ROM goals are seldom mentioned when preparing a patient for a TSA. This is true whether a patient is placed in the standard-goals category versus the limited-goals category. The primary focus for those patients in the limited-goals category is pain relief with a decreased emphasis on ROM gains. This group will achieve less than satisfactory gains in functional ROM.[41]

TOTAL SHOULDER SECONDARY TO TRAUMA

Comparison of expected goals and outcomes of patients with a TSA secondary to trauma versus degeneration notes pain relief and resumption of daily function in both patient populations. Two important preoperative factors influence postrehabilitation function. The first is the timing of the surgery in relation to the injury. The longer the delay before surgery, the worse the outcome. The second factor is the skill of the surgeon regarding positioning of the tuberosities. This also correlates to the earlier presentation of improved outcomes with larger surgery centers and higher-volume surgeons.[47] The most common complication is superior migration of the humeral head that may occur for a variety of reasons, including failure of the rotator cuff, muscular imbalance, or glenoid loosening (Box 7-10). For patients with TSA secondary to trauma, rehabilitation may be initiated by prescribing a longer period of immobilization with PROM only to ensure appropriate bony healing about the prosthesis. Additional time spent in a sling with limited AROM might last up to 6 weeks, further delaying the potential resumption of ROM.[47]

Box 7-10 Common Complications After Total Shoulder Arthroplasty (TSA)[51]

Glenoid loosening
- Glenohumeral (GH) joint instability
- Infection
- Neurologic injury
- Recurrent cuff tear
- Periprosthetic fracture

SUGGESTED HOME MAINTENANCE FOR THE POSTSURGICAL PATIENT

A home maintenance program is provided on page 135. These are general guidelines; however specific guidance and details need to be addressed by the physical therapist. Consideration must be given according to the status and capabilities of the patient.

TROUBLESHOOTING

Stiffness

Stiffness of GH joint after TSA presents a complex problem. The origin of the stiffness may be caused by inadequate intraoperative tissue release, intense healing inflammatory response postsurgery, or slow rehabilitation. Communication with the referring surgeon and the history of the patient's ROM impairment before surgical intervention may help the therapist decide how to decrease the risk of stiffness after surgery. Initiating therapy with good pain control immediately postoperatively may prevent the development of pathologic stiffness. Presentation of stiffness later in the rehabilitation process must be evaluated for the primary contributing impairments. Consideration should be given to the GH joint capsule, the flexibility of the scapulohumeral muscles, and the separation of scapular motion from humeral motion.

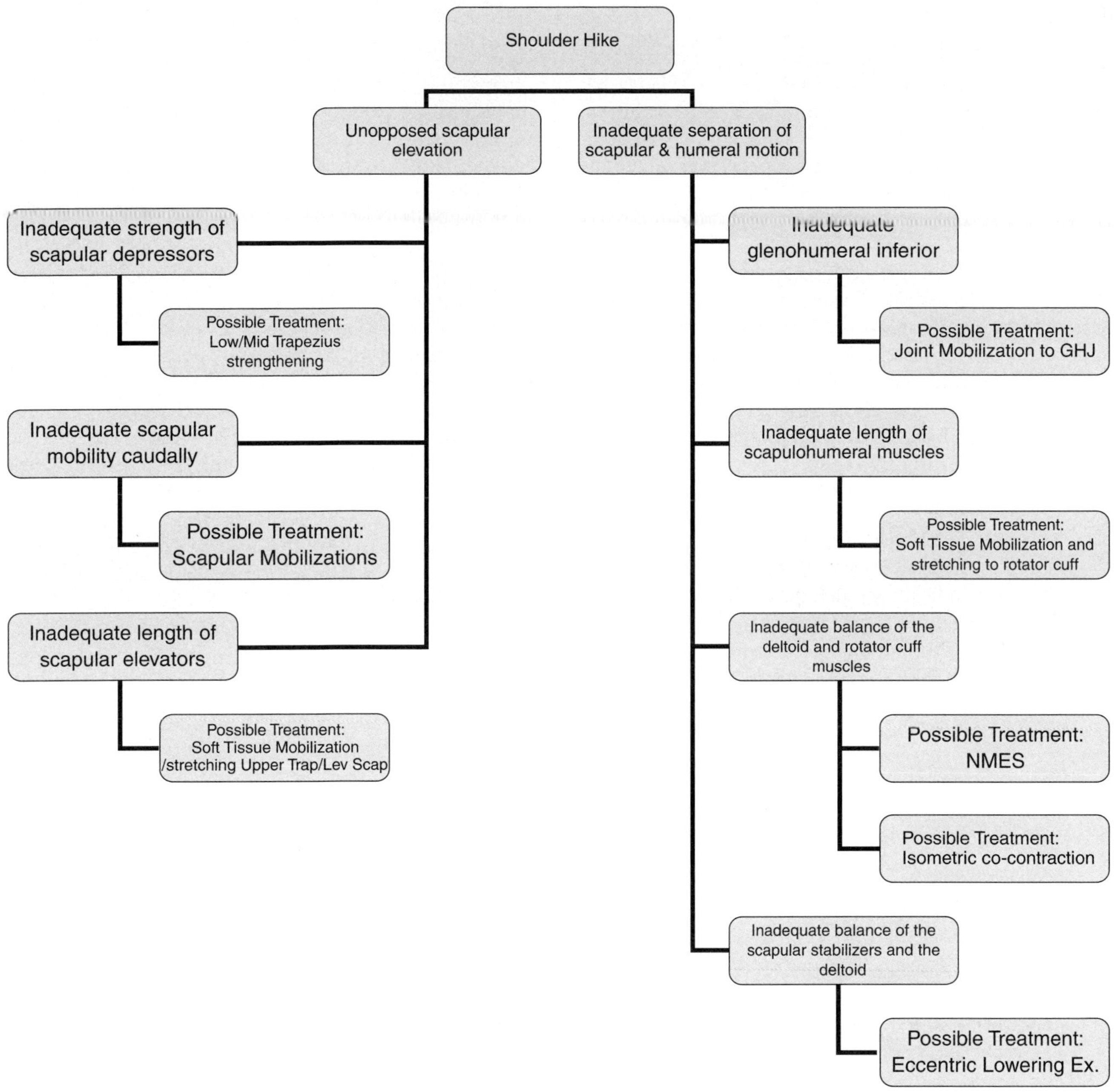

Fig. 7-25 Problem-solving the movement dysfunction of shoulder hike.

Shoulder Hike

The most common observable movement dysfunction is a shoulder hike with attempts at raising the arm in either frontal or sagittal plane of motion. The movement dysfunction of a shoulder hike could be renamed *unopposed scapular elevation* or *inadequate separation of scapular and humeral motion.* A therapist must determine which of the resources necessary to accomplish flexion or abduction without a shoulder hike is limiting the appropriate movement pattern. Weakness is only one of the impairments that may contribute to shoulder hiking. Additional impairments contributing to this movement dysfunction include inadequate transverse plane ROM, inadequate length of the scapulohumeral musculature, inadequate mobility of the GH joint capsule, and inadequate mobility of the scapula on the thorax. Determination of the primary impairment limiting this motion will guide the plan of care to eliminate the shoulder hike (Fig. 7-25).

> **Q** Michael recently underwent a total shoulder surgery. Surgical indications included a significant loss of motion, interrupted sleep, and pain secondary to the RA. His questions during his session relate to the expected ROM goals. Because of his presentation, what should the therapist predict regarding ROM?

Infection

After TSA a patient with decreasing ROM despite continued physical therapy sessions and compliance to home exercise program in conjunction with pain or increasing pain should alert the clinician to possible infection.[19] Infection may present in up to 15% of all total shoulder cases[18] and may occur more than 1 year after the surgical procedure.[59] Although pain and loss of ROM may be the most objective sign during therapy, the therapist should be alert for drainage, warmth at the site, erythema, and effusion. Other subjective questions regarding possible night sweats, fever, chills, remote sites of infection, or any recent invasive procedures should be asked.[8] Early intervention in the acute phase of the infection yields the best result; therefore the therapist should recommend a return visit to the physician for blood laboratory testing.[19]

A Michael would have a higher chance of being placed in the limited-goals category. He has several of the indications, including a medical history of RA. A limited-goals category means that expected ROM at the shoulder is conservatively estimated to reach flexion (75 to 90°), abduction (70 to 80°), ER (30°), and IR (hand behind back to L5).

Biceps Tendon Tendonitis

Biceps tendon tendonitis is a preventable complication during the postrehabilitation process. Acute inflammation of the tendon indicates an overuse of the biceps during attempts at shoulder motion. The patient will experience pain during AROM, especially with flexion and abduction. He or she may also demonstrate limited shoulder extension secondary to irritation as the biceps tendon is stretched. MMT of the biceps activates this muscle for its role as an elbow flexor and forearm supinator; therefore it may be pain free and strong despite the irritation at the tendon. Attempts at special tests for the tendonitis may be inconclusive because of the surgical trauma to the area and the patient's inability to attain the necessary positions. The biceps also has a role in shoulder flexion and is a primary humeral depressor.[43] **After total shoulder surgery, the rotator cuff typically demonstrates muscular inhibition, thus increasing the demand on the biceps as the primary humeral depressor during shoulder motion.** Presentation of the biceps tendon tendonitis indicates continued overuse of this muscle, therefore implicating inadequate contribution from the rotator cuff. Beyond the modality intervention for the inflammation of the biceps tendon, evaluation of the function of the rotator cuff should be considered.

SUGGESTED HOME MAINTENANCE FOR THE POSTSURGICAL PATIENT

Early phase: 0-6 weeks

GOALS FOR THE PERIOD: Aware of sleeping positions, independent with home exercise program, control pain, maintain range of motion (ROM) of proximal and distal joints, protect healing structures

Exercises:
1. Instruct the patient on sleeping positions and encourage experimentation (usually semireclined with upper extremities [UE] supported by pillows or bolster).
2. When appropriate, initiate passive range of motion (PROM) or self-assisted ROM at the shoulder (avoid ER beyond 40°).
3. Wear a sling for comfort.
4. Have the patient perform active range of motion (AROM) of the wrist and hand, elbow flexion only with humerus supported to decrease strain on biceps tendon, and AROM of cervical spine and thoracic spine through the cardinal planes.

Midphases: 6-12 weeks

GOALS FOR THE PERIOD: Increase shoulder ROM, initiate strengthening, increase functional activities

Exercises:
1. Continue previously mentioned ROM exercises.
2. Initiate submaximal isometrics (being careful not to irritate the healing subscapularis muscle).
3. Perform active assistive range of motion (A/AROM) exercises in supine, then progress to AROM in supine, and finally AROM in sitting as able (the patient must perform exercise correctly).

Late phases: 13 weeks to discharge

GOALS FOR THE PERIOD: Return to activities (including overhead activities), increase ROM, improve strength, improve neuromuscular control

Exercises:
1. Continue with previously mentioned exercises as needed.
2. Use AROM for concentric and eccentric strengthening at the shoulder.
3. Perform rotator cuff strengthening (elevation exercises must be performed correctly).

References

1. Aida S et al: Involvement of presurgical pain in preemptive analgesia for orthopaedic surgery: a randomized double-blind study, *Pain* 84:169-173, 2000.
2. Anglin C, Wyss UP: Arm motion and load analysis of sit to stand, stand to sit, cane walking and lifting, *Clin Biomech (Bristol, Avon)* 15:441-448, 2000.
3. Antuna SA et al: Shoulder arthroplasty for proximal humeral malunions: long term results, *J Shoulder Elbow Surg* 11:122-129, 2002.
4. Arntz CT, Jackins S, Matsen FA III: Prosthetic replacement of the shoulder for the treatment of defects in the rotator cuff and the surface of the glenohumeral joint, *J Bone Joint Surg* 75-A(4):485-491, 1993.
5. Baker LL, Parker K: Neuromuscular electrical simulation of the muscles surrounding the shoulder, *J Am Phys Ther Assoc* 66(12):1930-1937, 1986.
6. Baker LL et al: *Neuromuscular electrical stimulation: a practical guide,* Downey, CA, 2000, Los Amigos Research & Education Institute Inc, p 66.
7. Beynnon BD: Anterior cruciate ligament strain behavior during rehabilitation exercises in vivo, *Am J Sports Med* 23(1):24-34, 1995.
8. Bishop JY, Flatow, EL: The failed arthroplasty: options for revision. In Warner JJ, Iannotti JP, Flatow EL, editors: *Complex and revision problems in shoulder surgery,* Philadelphia, 2005, Lippincott Williams & Wilkins, p 533.
9. Boardman ND III, Cofield RH: Neurologic complications of shoulder surgery, *Clin Orthop Relat Res* 368:44-53, 1999.
10. Boardman ND et al: Rehabilitation after total shoulder arthroplasty, *J Arthroplasty* 16(4):483-486, 2001.
11. Bonutti PM, Hawkins RJ: Rotator cuff disorder, *Baillieres Clin Rheumatol* 3:535-550, 1989.
12. Brems JJ: Rehabilitation following shoulder arthroplasty. In RJ Friedman, editor: *Arthroplasty of the shoulder,* New York, 1994, Thieme, pp 103, 108-109.
13. Brems JJ: Rehabilitation following total shoulder arthroplasty, *Cin Orthop Relat Res* 307:70-85, 1994.
14. Brown DD, Friedman RJ: Postoperative rehabilitation following total shoulder arthroplasty, *Orthop Clin North Am* 29(3):535-547, 1998.
15. Buscayet F et al: Glenohumeral arthrosis in anterior instability before and after surgical treatment: incidence and contributing factors, *Am J Sports Med* 32:1165-1172, 2004.
16. Calliet R: *Shoulder pain,* Philadelphia, 1991, FA Davis, pp 76-78.
17. Casati A et al: Interscalene brachial plexus anesthesia and analgesia for open shoulder surgery. A randomized double-blind comparison between levobupivacaine and ropivacaine, *Anesth Analg* 96:253-259, 2003.
18. Cofield RH, Edgerton BC: Total shoulder arthroplasty: complications and revision surgery, *Instr Course Lect* 39:449-462, 1990.
19. Coste JS et al: The management of infection in arthroplasty of the shoulder, *J Bone Joint Surg Br* 86-B:65-69, 2004.

20. Dockery ML, Wright TW, LaStayo PC: Electromyography of the shoulder: an analysis of passive modes of exercise, *Orthopedics* 21(11):1181-1184, 1998.
21. Duralde XA: Total shoulder replacements. In RA Donatelli, editor: *Physical therapy of the shoulder,* Philadelphia, 2004, Churchill Livingstone.
22. Edwards TB et al: The influence of rotator cuff disease on the results of shoulder arthroplasty for primary osteoarthritis, *J Bone Joint Surg* 84-A:2240-2248, 2002.
23. Edwards TB et al: A comparison of hemiarthroplasty and total shoulder arthroplasty in the treatment of primary glenohumeral osteoarthritis: results of a multicenter study, *J Shoulder Elbow Surg* 12:207-213, 2003.
24. Fehringer EV et al: Characterizing the functional improvement after total shoulder arthroplasty for osteoarthritis, *J Bone Joint Surgery* 84-A:1349-1353, 2002.
25. Franklin JL et al: Glenoid loosening in total shoulder arthroplasty. Association with rotator cuff deficiency, *J Arthroplasty* 3:39-46, 1988.
26. Gartsman GM, Roddey TS, Hammerman SM: Shoulder arthroplasty with or without resurfacing of the glenoid in patients who have osteoarthritis, *J Bone Joint Surg* 82-A(1): 26-34, 2000.
27. Gill TJ et al: Complications of shoulder surgery, *Instr Course Lect* 48:359-374, 1999.
28. Godeneche A et al: Prosthetic replacement in the treatment of osteoarthritis of the shoulder: early results of 268 cases, *J Shoulder Elbow Surg* 11:11-18, 2002.
29. Godges JJ et al: The immediate effects of soft tissue mobilization with proprioceptive neuromuscular facilitation on glenohumeral external rotation and overhead reach, *J Orthop Sports Phys Ther* 33:713-718, 2003.
30. Goldberg BA et al: The magnitude and durability of functional improvement after total shoulder arthroplasty for degenerative joint disease, *J Shoulder Elbow Surg* 10:464-469, 2001.
31. Goutallier D et al: Shoulder surgery: from cuff repair to joint replacement. An update, *J Bone Joint Surg,* 70A:422-432, 2003.
32. Hammond JW et al: Surgeon experience and clinical and economic outcomes for shoulder arthroplasty, *J Bone Joint Surg* 85A(12):2318-2324. 2003.
33. Hetterich CM et al: Preoperative factors associated with improvements in shoulder function after humeral hemiarthorplasty, *J Bone Joint Surgery* 86A(7):1446-1451, 2004
34. Hugh M, Neers CS II: Glenohumeral joint replacement and postoperative rehabilitation, *Phys Ther* 55(8):850-858, 1975.
35. Iannotti JP, Norris TR: Influence of preoperative factors on the outcome of shoulder arthroplasty for glenohumeral arthritis, *J Bone Joint Surg* 85A(2):251-258, 2003.
36. Iannotti JP, Williams GR: *Disorders of the shoulder: diagnosis and management,* Philadelphia, 1999, Lippincott, Williams & Wilkins, pp 524, 538-539, 591.
37. Itoi E et al: Isokinetic strength after tears of the supraspinatus tendon, *J Bone Joint Surg Br* 79-B(1):77-82, 1997.
38. Jackins S: Postoperative shoulder rehabilitation, *Phys Med Rehabil Clin N Am* 15(3):643-682, 2004.
39. Jain N et al: The relationship between surgeon and hospital volume and outcomes for shoulder arthroplasty, *J Bone Joint Surg* 86A(3):496-505. 2004.
40. Karduna AR et al: Glenohumeral joint translations before and after total shoulder arthroplasty: a study in cadavera, *J Bone Joint Surg* 79-A(8):1166-1174, 1997.
41. Kelley MJ, Leggin BG: Rehabilitation. In Williams GR et al, editors: *Shoulder and elbow arthroplasty,* Philadelphia, 2005, Lippincott Williams & Wilkins, p 254.
42. Kibler WB, McMullen J, Uhl T: Shoulder rehabilitation strategies, guidelines and practice, *Orthop Clin North Am* 32(3):527-538. 2001.
43. Kido T et al: The depressor function of the biceps on the head of the humerus in shoulders with tears of the rotator cuff, *J Bone Joint Surg* 82-B:416-419, 2000.
44. Langevin HM et al: Dynamic fibroblast cytoskeletal response to subcutaneous tissue stretch ex vivo and in vivo, *Am J Physiol Cell Physiol* 288:747-756, 2005.
45. Matsen FA III et al: Correlates with comfort and function after total shoulder arthroplasty for degenerative joint disease, *J Shoulder Elbow Surg* 9:465-469, 2000.
46. McCann PD et al: A kinematic and electromyographic study of shoulder rehabilitation exercises, *Clin Orthop Relat Res* 288:179-188, 1993.
47. Mighell MA et al: Outcomes of hemiarthroplasty for fractures of the proximal humerus, *J Shoulder Elbow Surg* 12:569-577, 2003.
48. Mileti J et al: Monoblock and modular total shoulder arthroplasty for osteoarthritis, *J Bone Joint Surg* 87B:496-500, 2005.
49. Neer CS, Watson DC, Stanton FJ: Recent experience in total shoulder replacement, *J Bone Joint Surg* 64A 3:319-337, 1982.
50. Norris TR, Iannotti JP: Functional outcome after shoulder arthroplasty for primary osteoarthritis: a multicenter study, *J Shoulder Elbow Surg* 11:130-135, 2002.
51. Norris TR, Lachiewicz PF: Modern cement techniques and the survivorship of total shoulder arthroplasty, *Clin Orthop Relat Res* 328:76-85, 1996.
52. Oatis CA, editor: Mechanics and pathomechanics of muscle activity at the shoulder complex. In *Kinesiology: the mechanics & pathomechanics of human movement,* Philadelphia, 2004, Lippincott, Williams & Wilkins, pp 165-166.
53. Orafaly RM et al: A prospective functional outcome study of shoulder arthroplasty for osteoarthritis with an intact rotator cuff, *J Shoulder Elbow Surg* 12:214-221, 2003.
54. Parsons IM IV, Millett PJ, Warner JJP: Glenoid wear after shoulder hemiarthroplasty, *Clinical Orthop Relat Res* 421:120-125, 2004.
55. Rozencwaig R et al: The correlation of comorbidity with function of the shoulder and health status of patients who have glenohumeral degenerative joint disease, *J Bone Joint Surg* 80A(8):1146-1453, 1998.
56. Skiruing AP: Total shoulder arthroplasty—current problems and possible solutions, *J Orthop Sci,* 4:42-53, 1999.
57. Smith KL, Matsen FA III: Total shoulder arthroplasty versus hemiarthroplasty: current trends, *Orthop Clin North Am* 29:491-506, 1998.
58. Sojberg JO et al: Late results of total shoulder replacement in patients with rheumatoid arthritis, *Clin Orthop Relat Res* 366:29-45, 1999.
59. Sperling JW et al: Infection after shoulder arthroplasty, *Clin Orthop Relat Res* 382:206-216, 2001.

60. Trail IA, Nuttall D: The results of shoulder arthroplasty in patients with rheumatoid arthritis, *J Bone Joint Surg* 84B:1121-1125, 2002.
61. Visotsky JL et al: Cuff tear arthropathy: pathogenesis, classification and algorithm for treatment, *J Bone Joint Surg* 86A:35-40, 2004.
62. Yack HJ, Collins CE, Whieldon TJ: Comparison of closed and open kinetic chain exercise in the anterior cruciate ligament-deficient knee, *Am J Sports Med* 21(1):49-54, 1993.

CHAPTER 8

Tennis Elbow: Extensor Brevis Release and Lateral Epicondylectomy

James H. Calandruccio
Douglas N. Calhoun
Kelly Akin Kaye
Kristen Griffith Lowrance

A pathologic condition of the wrist extensor tendons at their elbow origin is commonly termed *lateral epicondylitis* or *tennis elbow*. However, the syndrome of lateral elbow pain is neither exclusively inflammatory nor always related to athletic activity.[22] The lack of inflammatory cells in the tissue removed from patients during surgical intervention makes the term *lateral epicondylitis* a misnomer, and *lateral epicondylosis* is probably more appropriate. Moreover, many patients who have focal tenderness just distal and anterior to the lateral epicondyle and localized pain in the same region do not play tennis.

SURGICAL INDICATIONS AND CONSIDERATIONS

Etiology

Injury to the extensor tendons at the elbow often can be attributed to repetitive trauma or overuse, leading to mechanical fatigue or biomechanical overload. Some literature reports the possibility of exostosis in the area of the extensor tendons or a degenerative process that causes pain at the lateral epicondyle.[7] Symptoms may be described as an ache at the elbow, with sharp pain that often radiates to the dorsal forearm and occasionally to the middle and ring fingers with attendant loss of grip strength.[25]

The most frequently involved tendon is that originating from the extensor carpi radialis brevis (ECRB). It is responsible for the static wrist extension required for certain tasks and stabilizes the wrist while grasping. Lesions can occur at the extensor digitorum communis, extensor carpi ulnaris, extensor digiti minimi, and supinator tendon. According to the current literature, microtraumatic ECRB tendon tears may propagate to include the common extensors.[22] Plancher, Halbrecht, and Lourie[22] report that gross tendon rupture is noted in a large number of patients at the time of surgical intervention.

Microtears can result from repeated sprains, repetitive forceful wrist extension and gripping, and suboptimal mechanics in hitting. Inadequate racquet size or improper tool grip size also can predispose to injury. Other factors that may influence the onset of symptoms are inadequate strength, endurance, and flexibility of the forearm musculature, changes in regular activity, increasing age, and hormonal imbalance in women.[25] The incidence is equal in men and women during the fourth and fifth decades, with 75% of all cases involving the dominant arm.[22] Among the older population, the insult is predominantly work related, in contrast to the sports-related injuries seen in the younger population.

Lateral epicondylitis can be managed successfully nonsurgically in 90% of patients with a combination of activity modification, nonsteroidal anti-inflammatory drugs (NSAIDs), functional and counter-force bracing, various therapeutic modalities, and injection therapy. A small percentage of patients with persistent and disabling symptoms require surgical intervention.[3] Lesions caused by overuse during job-related activities are more likely to require surgical intervention secondary to an inability to stop the aggravating activity.

Indications for surgery are individualized according to patient demands and activity level. The period of disability and previous conservative management must be considered before surgical management is chosen. No absolute indications exist for surgical intervention to treat lateral epicondylitis, and the clinician must exercise caution in cases in which secondary gain may be important.

The most important factors in considering surgical intervention are the intensity, frequency, and duration of disability caused by pain. Constant and unrelenting focal lateral elbow discomfort is not tolerated well by active individuals. Most patients treated surgically have symptoms for 1 year, but special consideration may be given to patients in whom other therapies have failed after 6 months of aggressive attempts. When symptoms are present for more than 12 months, they will rarely respond to further therapeutic management. Although cortisone injections are reserved for significant cases of tennis elbow, the failure of three or more injections to produce relief is another indication for surgery. These injections are usually delivered over a 6- to 12-month period. In addition, attempts have been made at injection of autologous blood and lidocaine in hopes of promoting healing via a cytokine-mediated response.

Calcification around the lateral aspect of the elbow portends a less favorable outcome to conservative measures. Calcification seen on radiographic examination may occur in as many as 20% of cases and may indicate surgical intervention before the 1-year period ends.

SURGICAL PROCEDURES

Modified Nirschl Method

Numerous surgical procedures to treat lateral epicondylitis have been described, and no single technique has been or will be adopted by all surgeons. The common denominator for all procedures, however, is the alleviation of traction on the diseased ECRB origin. Hypervascular granulation tissue is characteristically found on the undersurface of the ECRB attachment to the lateral epicondyle and appears as tan-gray degenerative regions. A limited approach that is commonly used consists of resection of the diseased section of the tendon combined with a limited lateral epicondylectomy.

A 5 cm-long, gently curved incision is centered over the lateral epicondyle. The extensor fascia is identified through this opening (Fig. 8-1, A). The anterior edge of the ECRB tendon origin is clearly developed by elevating the posterior border of the extensor carpi radialis longus, which at this level is muscular and partially overrides the ECRB origin. The extensor digitorum communis origin partially obscures the deeper portion of the ECRB (Fig. 8-1, B). The ECRB portion of the conjoined tendon is elevated at the midportion of the lateral epicondyle, distally in line with the forearm axis. The abnormal-appearing ECRB tendon is sharply dissected from the normal-appearing Sharpey's fibers. The diseased tissue may appear fibrillated and discolored and can contain calcium deposits.

Occasionally the disease process also involves the extensor digitorum communis origin. No reason exists to enter the joint itself unless preoperative evaluation indicates an intra-articular process, such as loose bodies, degenerative joint disease, effusion, or synovial thickening.

The lateral 0.5 cm of the lateral epicondyle is decorticated with a rongeur or osteotome, with the surgeon taking care not to enter the joint and damage the articular cartilage or compromise the lateral ulnar collateral ligament (Fig. 8-1, C). The ECRB is intimately associated with the annular ligament just proximal to the radial head, thereby limiting distal migration of the ECRB tendon. However, the remaining normal ECRB tendon may be sutured to the fascia or periosteum or attached with nonabsorbable sutures through drill holes in the epicondyle.

The extensor carpi radialis longus and extensor digitorum communis interval is closed with absorbable

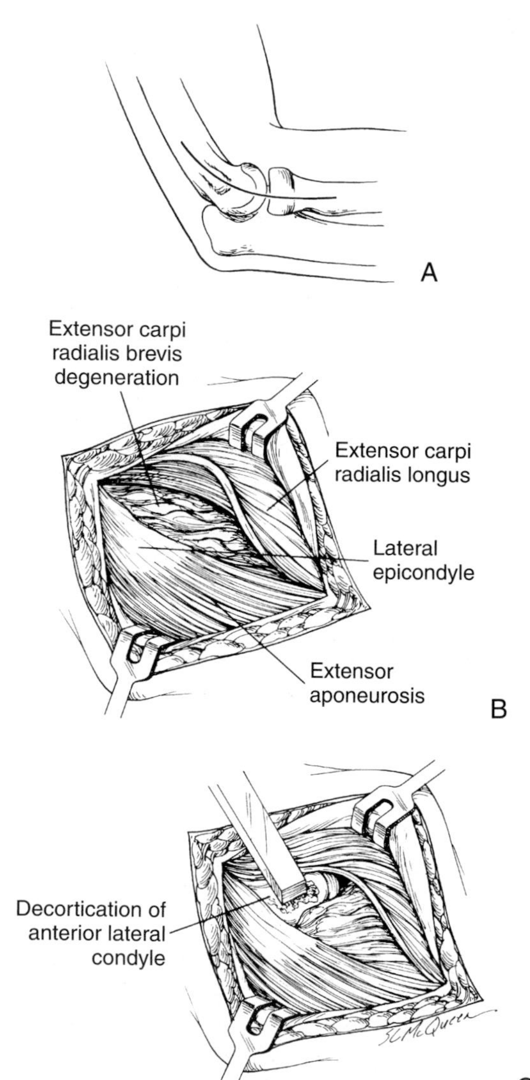

Fig. 8-1 Surgical technique for correction of tennis elbow. **A,** Skin incision, **B,** Identification of the origins of the extensor carpi radialis longus and extensor digitorum communis. **C,** Osteotome decortication.

(Redrawn from Nirschl RP, Pettrone F: The surgical treatment of lateral epicondylitis, *J Bone Joint Surg* 61A:832, 1972. In Canale ST, editor: *Campbell's operative orthopedics,* St Louis, 1998, Mosby.)

sutures. The skin incision may be closed with subcuticular nylon (4-0) sutures and adhesive strips.

Arthroscopic Release

The elbow joint is distended with 30 ml of saline using an 18-gauge needle through a straight lateral approach. A proximal medial portal is established 2 cm proximal and 2 cm anterior to the medial epicondyle using a 2- to 3-mm skin incision. Next, using a blunt trochar, either a 2.7-mm or a 4.0-mm 30-degree arthroscope is introduced into the joint. The proximal lateral portal is then established under direct visualization approximately 2 cm anterior and 2 cm proximal to the lateral epicondyle. Next, a thorough joint inspection is carried out and any intra-articular pathology is addressed.

Viewing through the proximal medial portal, the lateral capsule and undersurface of the ECRB tendon is visualized and evaluated. A 4.5-mm resector is inserted through the proximal lateral portal, and the capsule is débrided to reveal the undersurface of the ECRB tendon. The tendon release is begun at the site of pathology and carried to the insertion on the lateral epicondyle. Next, a burr is used to decorticate the lateral epicondyle and the distal portion of the lateral condylar ridge in the area of the ECRB origin.

After completion, the arthroscope is removed and the portals closed using a single nylon suture material or subcuticular suture and adhesive strips. The elbow is then placed in a soft dressing and sling for 2 to 3 days.

SURGICAL OUTCOMES

According to Nirschl and Ashman,[16] 85% of patients were able to return to all previous activities without pain. Pain that occurred during aggressive activities was noted in 12% of the cases observed, and no improvement was apparent in 3% of the cases. Reasons for failure include misdiagnosis or the concomitant diagnosis of entrapment of the posterior interosseous nerve, intra-articular disorders, and lateral elbow instability. Poor prognostic factors include poor initial response to cortisone injections, numerous previous cortisone injections, bilateral lateral epicondylitis, other concomitant associated disorders, and smoking.

Differences in the outcomes between open and arthroscopic release of tennis elbow is currently being debated. The long-term results do not appear to be significantly different between the two groups. Although not statistically significant, it does appear, however, that patients treated with arthroscopic release returned to work earlier than patients treated with open release, and they may require less postoperative therapy.

THERAPY GUIDELINES FOR REHABILITATION

Phase I

TIME: 1 to 14 days after surgery
GOALS: Achieve full range of motion (ROM) of adjacent joints, promote wound healing, control edema and pain, increase active range of motion (AROM) of the elbow (Table 8-1)

After surgery, the therapist instructs the patient concerning the need to elevate the site to avoid edema and initiates gentle AROM exercises for the hand and shoulder. The patient is to remain immobilized in the postoperative splint with the elbow positioned at 90 degrees.

On the fifth day after surgery the postsurgical dressing and splint are removed, and therapy is initiated to the elbow. In this phase the patient's wounds are kept clean and dry until the sutures are removed 10 to 14 days after surgery. After the operative site has been exposed, other forms of edema control can be used, including ice, pneumatic intermittent compression (performed at a 3:1 on-off ratio at a pressure of 50 mmHg), and high-voltage galvanic stimulation (HVGS). The recommended settings for the use of HVGS to prevent edema are negative polarity with continuous modulation at 100 intrapulse microseconds and intensity to the sensory level.[9] The patient also can be fitted with a light elastic compression wrap or stockinette (such as Coban or Tubi-Grip) to wear intermittently throughout the day and at night for continued edema control at home (Fig. 8-2). AROM exercises also are initiated for the elbow, forearm, and wrist after the postoperative dressing is removed.[15] **Passive range of motion (PROM) and joint mobilization of the elbow and forearm are contraindicated at this time.**

Some surgeons prefer to keep the elbow immobilized in a removable posterior elbow splint until the second week after surgery. This splint is typically fabricated from a low-temperature plastic with the elbow positioned at 90 degrees; it is worn between exercise sessions and at night (Fig. 8-3).

Pain can be managed using HVGS at the same settings as those used for edema control; the physician also may prescribe oral medications.

The first postoperative visit is a good time to begin patient education regarding activity modification and proper mechanics during work- and sports-related activities. **Patients should be taught to avoid forceful static grip, repetitive wrist extension, and resistive supination.** The primary mode of lifting should be a bilateral underhanded or neutral forearm approach (Fig. 8-4).

During this initial phase the therapist should closely monitor the patient's reports of pain and tolerance to ROM exercises, noting any sympathetic changes that may

Table 8-1 Extensor Brevis Release and Lateral Epicondylectomy

Rehabilitation Phase	Criteria to Progress to this Phase	Anticipated Impairments and Functional Limitations	Intervention	Goal	Rationale
Phase 1 Postoperative 1-2 weeks	◆ Postoperative	◆ Postoperative pain ◆ Postoperative edema ◆ Limited UE mobility ◆ Unable to grasp and reach	◆ Monitoring of incision site ◆ Instruction of client in activity modification ◆ Cryotherapy ◆ Pneumatic intermittent compression ◆ HVGS ◆ Elastic compression wrap or stockinette ◆ Fabrication of removable splint ◆ PROM-AROM—Shoulder (all ranges, maintaining elbow in neutral position) ◆ AROM—Hand (finger flexion/extension); wrist (flexion/extension); elbow (flexion/extension pronation/supination after operative dressing is removed)	◆ Prevent infection ◆ Decrease stress on surgical site ◆ Decrease pain ◆ Control and decrease edema ◆ Protect surgical site ◆ Maintain ROM of joints proximal and distal to the surgical site ◆ Full AROM of neighboring joints ◆ Elbow ROM to 60% (extension will be more limited)	◆ Prevention of postoperative complications ◆ Decrease stress on the common extensor tendons ◆ Pain control ◆ Edema management ◆ Prevent associated joint stiffness and dysfunction of neighboring joints and muscles ◆ AROM to assist with pain control an promote edema management ◆ Improve ROM of elbow (sutures are usually removed at 10 to 14 days)

UE, Upper extremity; *HVGS,* high-voltage galvanic stimulation; *ROM,* range of motion; *PROM,* passive range of motion; *AROM,* active range of motion.

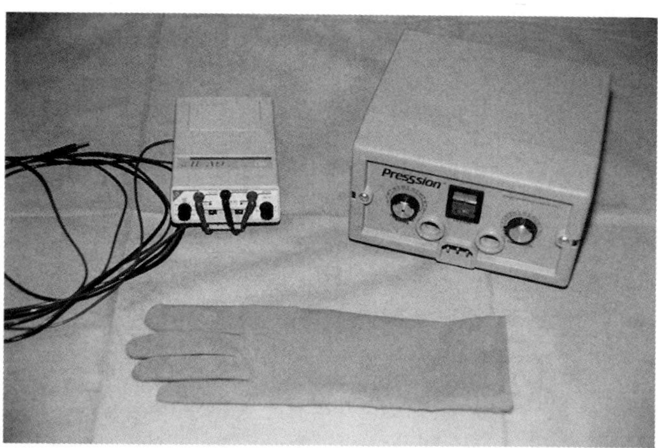

Fig. 8-2 Edema control. Portable high-voltage galvanic stimulation (HVGS) unit, portable intermittent compression unit, and compressive garment (Isotoner glove).

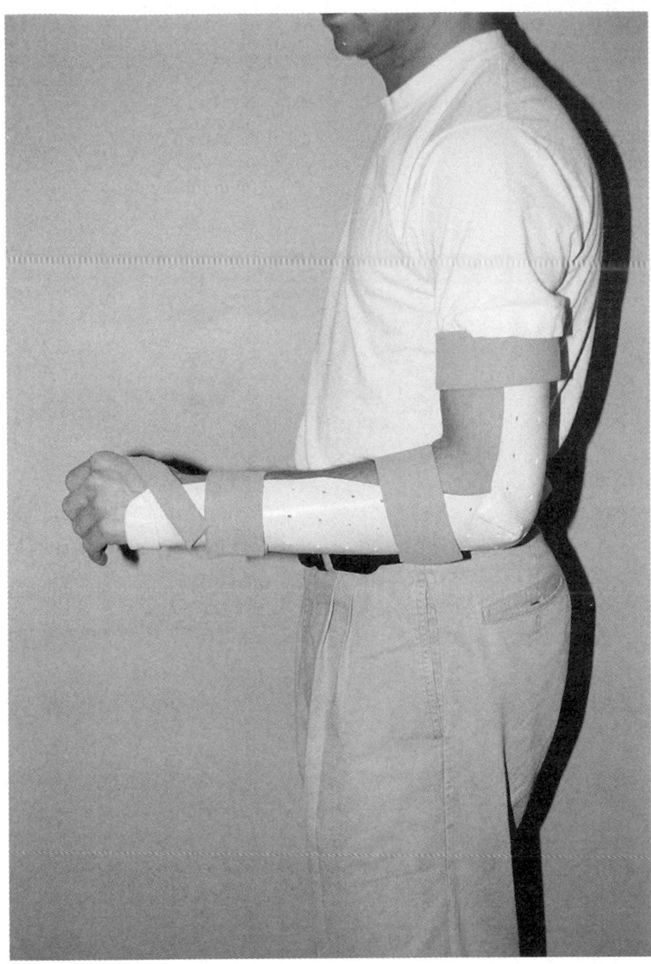

Fig. 8-3 Posterior elbow splint.

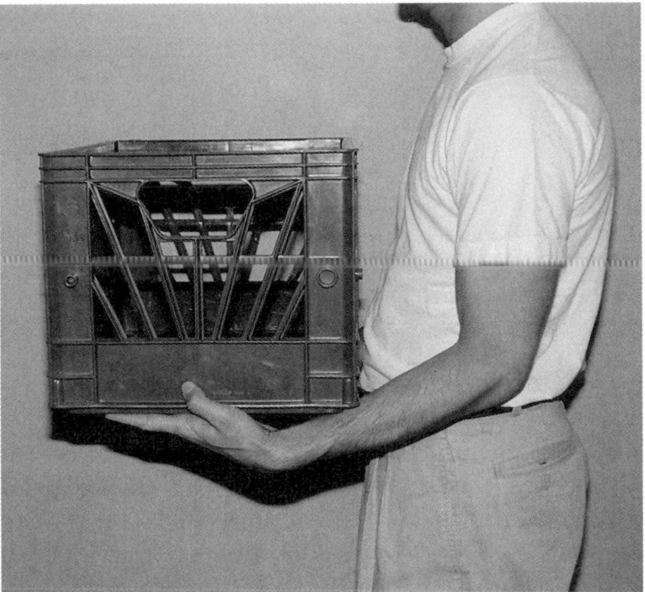

Fig. 8-4 Underhanded-lifting technique.

lead to a complex regional pain syndrome. Signs and symptoms to be noted are as follows:

- Pain out of proportion to the stimulus
- Excessive edema
- Temperature and color changes
- Excessive joint stiffness

Q Cindy is a 60-year-old housewife who had arthroscopic release of her right tennis elbow 3 weeks ago. She is now complaining about right shoulder pain. She does not remember any injury to this region. She states that although she is working on her elbow motion regularly, she wears her arm sling for comfort during the day. On exam, her active and passive motion of her right shoulder is painful and somewhat limited. What should be added to her therapy program, and what instructions should she be given?

Phase II

TIME: 15 days to 4 to 5 weeks after surgery
GOALS: Control edema and pain, achieve full elbow PROM, maintain full ROM of adjacent joints, promote mobility of the scar tissue (Table 8-2)

After the immobilization phase, the therapist should initiate gentle AROM exercises for the patient's elbow three to four times each day.[12] During the first ROM phase, the therapist should emphasize the importance of complying with the home exercise program, as well as attending the regular therapy sessions.

ROM exercises to be included are as follows:

- Elbow extension and flexion
- Wrist extension and flexion
- Forearm supination and pronation

The patient should avoid positions that place maximal stress on the common extensor tendons, such as elbow extension with extreme wrist flexion (Fig. 8-5).[25] Perform elbow flexion and extension with wrist in neutral to slightly extended position, and perform wrist flexion and extension exercises with elbow flexed. **To prevent reinjury, progressive resistive exercises also should be avoided at this time.**

Stanley and Tribuzi[25] recommend isometric exercises with the wrist in a neutral position or at no more than 30 degrees of extension or flexion in preparation for further resistive training. Exercises should be performed three to four times daily with 15 to 20 repetitions being sufficient. **Isometrics should be performed with submaximal effort only.**

Table 8-2 Extensor Brevis Release and Lateral Epicondylectomy

Rehabilitation Phase	Criteria to Progress to this Phase	Anticipated Impairments and Functional Limitations	Intervention	Goal	Rationale
Phase II Postoperative 3-5 weeks	◆ Incision well healed with no signs of infection ◆ Improving PROM of elbow ◆ No increase in pain or edema	◆ Continued pain and mild edema ◆ Limited UE mobility ◆ Unable to grasp and reach for functional use	Continuation of edema and pain management techniques as in Phase I: ◆ Soft tissue massage ◆ Retrograde massage with elevation ◆ Scar desensitization after sutures are removed and incision is healed ◆ Silicon gel sheet for scar pad ◆ PROM—Elbow flexion/extension (within pain tolerance) ◆ Isometrics (with wrist in neutral position, between 30-degrees (flexion/ extension); wrist (flexion/extension)	◆ Intermittent pain ◆ Manage edema ◆ Encourage limited ADLs ◆ Promote scar mobility and proper remodeling ◆ Promote full elbow PROM	◆ Management of edema and pain with progression to self-management ◆ Improvement of soft tissue mobility ◆ Use of compression to remodel scar ◆ Promotion of normal joint arthrokinematics ◆ Preparation of muscles for further resistive training ◆ Encourage quality muscle contraction

PROM, Passive range of motion; *UE,* upper extremity; *ADLs,* activities of daily living.

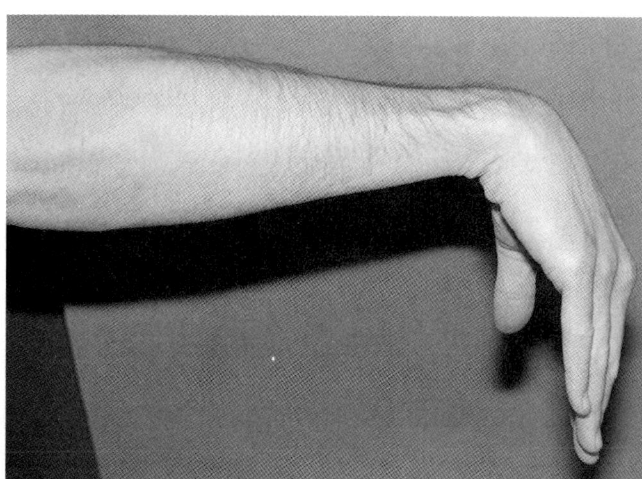

Fig. 8-5 Extreme wrist flexion with elbow extension.

A Cindy has developed an early adhesive capsulitis of her shoulder and should be instructed to stop wearing her arm sling. She should also be started on a shoulder program to work on her ROM. This could begin with Codman's exercises and a PROM program followed by AROM and strengthening.

Q Marvin is a 50-year-old diabetic who had extensor brevis release and lateral epicondylectomy 14 days ago. His sutures were removed, and he was taken out of the postoperative splint 2 days ago. He has full shoulder, forearm, and hand mobility with elbow AROM of 45 to 110 degrees. His pain remains 3 or 4 out of 10 even at rest, and moderate edema is localized to the elbow and proximal one third of the forearm. His incision shows mild dehissence with small amounts of exudate. What is appropriate intervention for his continued pain, edema, and suspicious wound?

As ROM progresses, the therapist should carefully monitor the patient's edema. The management of edema is specific to the patient, and only one technique may be required. The following technique can be used for mild edema:

1. Ice and elevation for 10 minutes at the end of treatment
2. Compression wraps and stockinette
3. HVGS for 15 minutes

Moderate edema is treated with the following:

1. Retrograde massage
2. Intermittent pneumatic compression with elevation
3. HVGS with elevation and ice for 20 to 30 minutes

A The therapist should begin by ruling out infection. The patient's basal and elbow surface temperatures should be assessed, and he should be checked for redness or streaking near the elbow and forearm. If the patient shows no temperature or color change and exudate is clear, Steri-Strips should be applied to the incision and the patient's physician should be contacted. Once infection is ruled out, the following should be done: edema control using retrograde massage (avoiding the area of incision), HVGS and elevation (or both), PROM, and A/AROM to the elbow for flexion and extension. Scar remodeling should be delayed until the incision is well closed.

After the sutures are removed and the incision has healed appropriately, scar management is needed. This includes both desensitization and scar remodeling. Because hypersensitivity can limit functional use, desensitization should begin during the patient's first therapy session after suture removal.[12] Scar remodeling consists of using massage (when appropriate) to help maintain mobility of the scar by freeing restrictive fibrous bands, increasing circulation, and allowing the pressure to flatten and smooth the scar site (Fig. 8-6).[12] The therapist also may consider using a silicone gel sheet or other silicone-based putty mix as a pad over the scar to assist in remodeling.

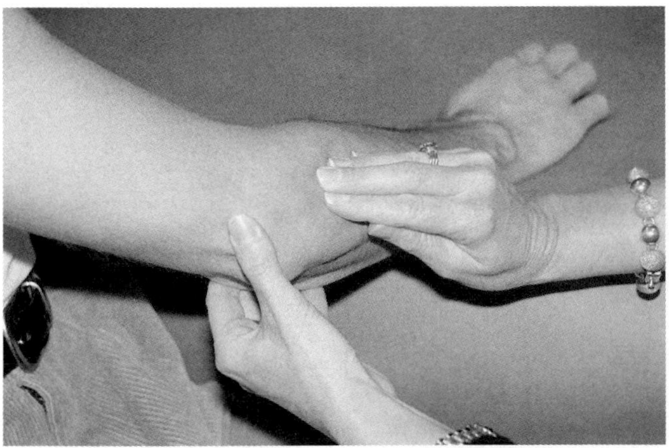

Fig. 8-6 Scar remodeling by manual massage technique.

The therapist should instruct the patient to rub the sensitive area for 2 to 5 minutes three to four times daily with textures such as fur, yarn, rice, Styrofoam, or corn. Other useful textures include towels, clothing, dry beans, and rice.[12]

Patients will be limited to lifting no more than 10 lb after surgery. On grip strength testing, patients typically demonstrate a 50% deficit when the operative hand is compared with the nonoperative one.

Q Jim is 34 years old. Approximately 7 weeks ago he had an extensor brevis release and lateral epicondylectomy performed. He is anxious to recover quickly so that he can play softball on the weekends. Mild resisted exercises were initiated 1 week ago, and Jim is performing them at home. His pain level has noticeably increased over the past 4 days. However, he can control the pain with ice and anti-inflammatory medication. Should Jim's exercise program be altered? If so, how should it be altered?

Phase III

TIME: Between 4 to 6 weeks to 6 months after surgery

GOALS: Control pain, maintain full elbow and forearm ROM, strengthen upper extremity (UE), regain normal forearm flexibility (Table 8-3)

Between 4 to 6 weeks after surgery the therapist should initiate a progressive strengthening program.[12] At this point in the rehabilitative process, the patient should have full ROM of the hand, wrist, and elbow, and the focus should be on building strength and training for endurance with the goal of returning the patient to work or sports.

The goal of the strengthening program is to promote conditioning of the UE, particularly the forearm, to prevent reinjury caused by overstretching or overloading. To ensure that maximal strengthening is achieved, eccentric exercises are recommended for the extrinsic forearm muscles.[25] At this time it is appropriate to initiate extrinsic forearm stretching.

Each patient's conditioning program is formulated according to activity tolerance, previous activity level, and requirements for return to work or sports. If the patient can perform active exercises without pain, then he or she is well enough to begin resistive and light work or sports-related activities using free weights and a work stimulator such as the Baltimore Therapeutic Equipment (BTE) or Lido (Fig. 8-7). The key is to continue educating the patient and training him or her to lift with the forearm in a neutral position and avoid postures that stress the extensor muscles.

Table 8-3 Extensor Brevis Release and Lateral Epicondylectomy

Rehabilitation Phase	Criteria to Progress to this Phase	Anticipated Impairments and Functional Limitations	Intervention	Goal	Rationale
Phase III Postoperative 6-24 weeks	◆ PROM full and AROM near full ◆ Pain and edema controlled/self-managed ◆ No decrease in strength since last phase	◆ Minimal, intermittent pain and edema ◆ Minimal mobility limitations in elbow ◆ Unable to grasp and reach for functional use	Continue pain and edema management as indicated: ◆ Patient education regarding activity modification and performance of activities with good mechanics ◆ PREs—Putty exercises, finger pinch and grip ◆ Isotonics—Shoulder (see Chapter 3); elbow (flexion, extension, pronation, supination); wrist (flexion, extension, radial, ulnar deviation) ◆ Work simulator (12-16 weeks) ◆ Return to sport program (refer to Appendix A) (12-16 weeks)	◆ Self-manage pain ◆ Prevent flare-up with progression of functional activities ◆ Grip strength to 85% of uninvolved side ◆ Symmetric strength of shoulder and scapula region ◆ Wrist strength to within 80% ◆ Return to previous activity/work level	◆ Avoidance of postures that place stress on the extensor musculature ◆ Promotion of return to functional activities without flare of symptoms ◆ Increased strength and endurance for return to work or sport ◆ Strengthening of upper quarter to ensure optimal functional use of UE ◆ Monitoring of wrist isotonics to ensure safe maximal strengthening ◆ Simulation of work/sport loads in the clinic to train muscles to allow safe return to sport or work

PROM, Passive range of motion; *AROM,* active range of motion; *PREs,* progressive resistance exercises; *UE,* upper extremity.

A 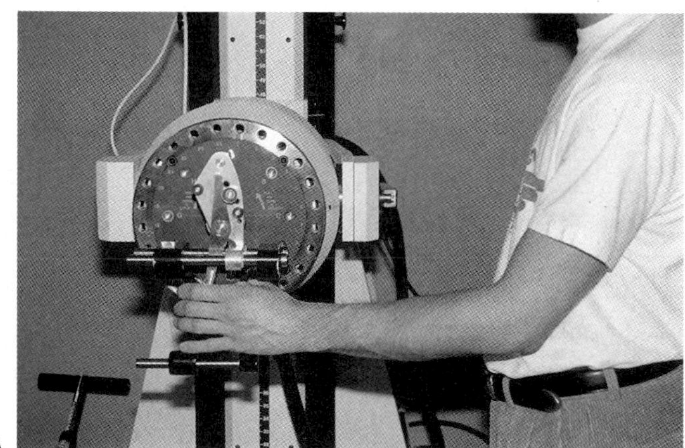

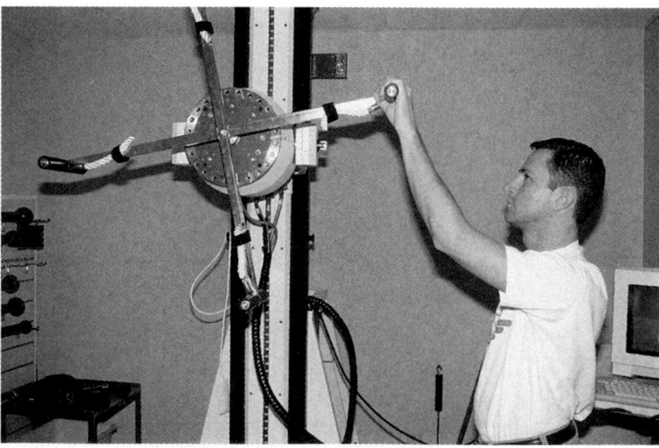 B

Fig. 8-7 A, Baltimore Therapeutic Equipment work simulator for grip strengthening. **B,** Simulated work activity.

A

Jim is aggravating his symptoms with the exercises. He also may be doing the home exercises too aggressively. The primary goal should be to alleviate pain and swelling. After pain and swelling are under control, gradual strengthening can be initiated in small doses with more rest periods than before. Treatment soreness should be minimal and controllable with the administration of ice packs. The amount of exercise and resistance should be gradually increased.

Q

Sharon is 45 years old. She works as a computer programmer and had extensor brevis release and lateral epicondylectomy 14 weeks ago. She is performing a home exercise program of progressive resistive exercises and intrinsic stretches for the forearm and elbow four times a week and has returned to work full time. She now complains of pain at the end of the day, with mildly noticeable swelling at the lateral elbow. She attends therapy once a week. What should the therapist evaluate at this week's appointment? What are the right recommendations?

The components of the program are as follows:

- Hand (grip and pinch) strengthening
- Forearm strengthening
- Upper-arm strengthening
- Shoulder strengthening
- Endurance training

Initiate grip strengthening with resistive putty (very light to light consistency) two to three times daily, progressing from 2- to 5-minute sessions; increase putty resistance as pain and strength allow. It is also advised to begin a functional grip activity such as sustained gripping. Have patient "dig" into putty using a 1-lb weight, beginning with 2 minutes, working up to 5 minutes, and increasing putty resistance per patient response. Begin progressive resistive exercises for the forearm and wrist with 1-lb weights once daily for one set of 10 repetitions, progressing to 5 to 8-lb up to three sets of 15 repetitions, and decreasing frequency to three to four times weekly. These exercises include wrist flexion and extension and forearm pronation and supination. Use of a "wrist stick" with a weighted ball on string incorporates wrist flexion and extension eccentric training. Ball weights generally begin at 2 oz and progress to 2 lb. Biceps, triceps, and shoulder girdle initial resistance depends on the patient's general health, age, sex, and activity level before surgery. Males and athletes will tolerate heavier weights than females or older adults. Intrinsic stretches should be performed three to four times daily for five to six repetitions, holding each 15 to 20 seconds.

Work simulation and sport-related activities are initiated postoperatively. Begin with movement patterns that do not elicit pain and partial ranges progressing to full range motions as the patient tolerates. Athletes may return to sport practice 1 hour daily. It is important to review proper mechanics, which may require a desk setup or sport equipment evaluation.

Normally a return to activity can be anticipated by the fourth month after surgery.[15]

A

The therapist should assess the patient's grip strength and forearm, elbow, and shoulder girdle strength as compared with the uninvolved side and previous week's values. Elbow mobility and edema (via palpation girth measurements) should also be checked. The patient should be asked to fill out a pain questionnaire or visual analog scale for pain. If strength values show a decrease of 10% or are less than 85% of the uninvolved side, the patient might have returned to work too early. If strength values are within desired limits but the patient shows significant edema and increased pain, she should be encouraged to decrease the weight with progressive resistive exercises and begin using ice packs for 10 to 15 minutes at the end of her work day. Stretching technique should be reviewed to make sure that the patient is not overstretching, as well as proper mechanics and activity modification while at work. The patient should be asked to wear a counterforce brace while at work (for up to 6 months postoperatively).

SUGGESTED HOME MAINTENANCE FOR THE POSTSURGICAL PATIENT

An exercise program has been outlined at the various phases. The home maintenance box on page 149 outlines the rehabilitation the patient is to follow. The physical therapist can use it in customizing a patient-specific program. Consideration of the patient's age, needs, and capabilities guides the rate of progression, intensity, and type of treatment provided.

TROUBLESHOOTING

Problems encountered after lateral epicondylectomy include pain, recurrence of symptoms, edema, inadequate ROM or stiffness, and scar expansion.

Increase in Pain Level or Recurrence of Symptoms

The therapist should carefully monitor the patient's pain level throughout the rehabilitation process. The Magill

Pain Questionnaire can aid in monitoring changes in levels or characteristics of pain. Exercise progression should occur based on the patient's reports of pain. In some cases of severe pain, the physician may prescribe a transcutaneous electrical nerve stimulation (TENS) unit. If the pain persists or occurs at the end of the rehabilitative process, then the therapist may consider the use of a counterforce brace to allow the patient to return to the previous level of activity.

Persistent Edema

Edema control involves ice, elevation, HVGS, pulsed ultrasound, compression wraps, retrograde massage, and lymphatic massage. Continuous passive-motion machines have been used intermittently throughout the day and at night with some success to reduce edema. Decreasing the activity level or suspending the use of resistive exercises also may be necessary.

Q Janet is a 35-year-old accountant. She had an extensor brevis release and lateral epicondylectomy after various attempts at conservative treatment failed. At 7 weeks after surgery, Janet's elbow extension ROM is –15 degrees. What type of treatment may be effective at this stage for increasing her elbow extension?

Inadequate Range of Motion or Stiffness in Adjacent Areas

The most common mobility problem involves loss of full elbow extension. By 6 to 8 weeks after surgery, the therapist can talk to the surgeon about using static progressive or dynamic splints to improve extension. Static splinting is achieved by using custom-made low-temperature plastic material molded to the patient at the available end ROM and adjusting it weekly. Dynamic splints are available commercially. For hand and finger stiffness, use of a flexion glove or composite flexion stretching with a Coban or elastic (Ace) wrap is usually successful (Fig. 8-8).

A The patient should be placed in a dynamic splint or in a static progressive splint at night to gain full extension.

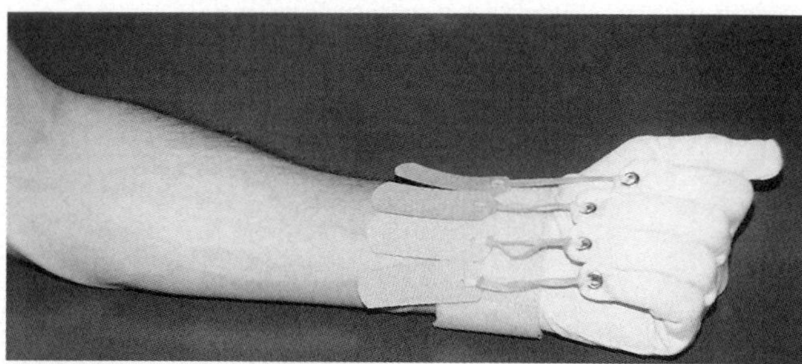

A

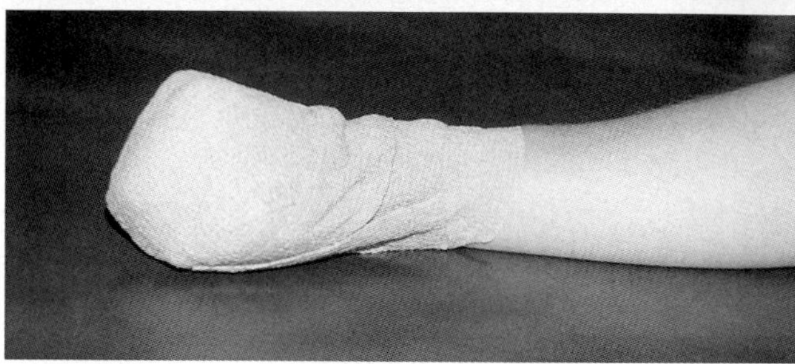

B

Fig. 8-8 **A**, Commercially available finger flexion glove for hand stiffness. **B**, Composite finger flexion using Coban.

Increase in or Painful Scar

If the scar management techniques detailed earlier do not produce the desired result, additional methods may be used:

- Ultrasound
- Mechanical vibration
- Compressive dressings or garments to prevent scar adherence

(Note: Circumferential desensitization using fluidotherapy also may be considered.)

SUGGESTED HOME MAINTENANCE FOR THE POSTSURGICAL PATIENT

Days 1-5

GOALS FOR THE PERIOD: Promote wound healing and control edema

1. Elevation
2. Active range of motion (ROM) of hand and shoulder

Days 6-14

GOALS FOR THE PERIOD: Promote wound healing, control edema, and begin ROM

1. Elevation
2. Compression wrap
3. Active range of motion (AROM) exercises for hand and shoulder
4. Gentle active flexion and extension of elbow
5. Gentle active supination and pronation of forearm

Day 15-week 5

GOALS FOR THE PERIOD: Improve ROM, provide scar management, and control edema

1. Scar massage
2. Desensitization
3. Use of scar pad
4. Compression wrap
5. AROM of hand, wrist, and shoulder
6. Gentle AROM of elbow and forearm

Weeks 6-18

GOALS FOR THE PERIOD: Strengthen muscles, increasing ROM if limited

1. Scar management
2. Compression wrap for edema if needed
3. AROM and passive range of motion (PROM) of hand, wrist, elbow, forearm, and shoulder
4. Gentle progressive exercises of wrist, elbow, and forearm, including wrist curls, forearm rotation, and biceps and triceps strengthening

Months 4-6

GOAL FOR THE PERIOD: Return to activity

1. Isotonic shoulder exercises as needed
2. Continue progressive exercises of the wrist, elbow, and forearm

References

1. Brotzman SB: *Clinical orthopaedic rehabilitation,* St Louis, 1996, Mosby.
2. Brown M: The older athlete with tennis elbow. Rehabilitation considerations, *Clin Sports Med* 14:1, 1995.
3. Canale ST: *Campbell's operative orthopaedics,* ed 9, St Louis, 1998, Mosby.
4. Doran A et al: Tennis elbow. A clinicopathologic study of 22 cases followed for 2 years, *Acta Orthop Scand* 61:6, 1990.
5. Ernst E: Conservative therapy for tennis elbow, *Br J Clin Pract* 46:1, 1992.
6. Foley AE: Tennis elbow, *Am Fam Physician* 48:2, 1993.
7. Gellman H: Tennis elbow (lateral epicondylitis), *Orthop Clin North Am* 23:75, 1992.
8. Green S et al: Non-steroidal anti-inflammatory drugs (NSAIDS) for treating lateral elbow pain in adults, *Cochrane Database Syst Rev* (2):CD003686, 2002.
9. Hayes KW: *Manual for physical agents,* ed 4, NJ, 1993, Appleton & Lange.
10. Hong QN, Durand MJ, Loisel P: Treatment of lateral epicondylitis: where is the evidence? *Joint Bone Spine* 71:5, 369-373, 2004.
11. Hubbard TJ, Denegar CR: Does cryotherapy improve outcomes with soft tissue injury, *J Athl Train* 39(3):278-279, 2004.
12. Hunter JM, Mackin EJ, Callahan AD: *Rehabilitation of the hand: surgery and therapy,* ed 4, St Louis, 1995, Mosby.
13. Jerosch J, Schunck J: Arthroscopic treatment of lateral epicondylitis: indications, technique and early results, *Knee Surg Sports Traumatol Arthrosc* 14(4):379-382, 1996.
14. Morrey BF: *The elbow and its disorders,* ed 2, Philadelphia, 1993, WB Saunders.
15. Jobe FW, Ciccotti MG: Lateral and medial epicondylitis of the elbow, *J Am Acad Orthop Surg* 2:1, 1994.
16. Nirschl RP, Ashman ES: Elbow tendinopathy: tennis elbow, *Clin Sports Med* 22:4, 813-836, 2003.
17. Noteboom T et al: Tennis elbow: a review, *J Orthop Sports Phys Ther* 19:6, 1994.
18. Ollivierre CO, Nirschl RP: Tennis elbow. Current concepts of treatment and rehabilitation, *J Sports Med* 22:2, 1996.
19. Ollivierre CO, Nirschl RP, Pettroe FA: Resection and repair for medial tennis elbow: a prospective analysis, *J Sports Med* 23:2, 1995.
20. Owens BD, Murphy KP, Kuklo TR: Arthroscopic release for lateral epicondylitis, *Arthroscopy* 17:6, 2001.
21. Peart RE, Strickler SS, Schweitzer KM: Lateral epicondylitis: a comparative study of open and arthroscopic lateral release, *Am J Orthop* 33(11):565-567, 2004.
22. Plancher KD, Halbrecht J, Lourie GM: Medial and lateral epicondylitis in the athlete, *Clin Sports Med* 2:283, 1996.
23. Schnatz P, Steiner C: Tennis elbow: a biomechanical and therapeutic approach, *J Am Osteopath Assoc* 93(7):778, 1993.

24. Solveborn SA, Oelrud C: Radial epicondylalgia (tennis elbow): measurement of range of motion of the wrist and elbow, *J Orthop Sports Phys Ther* 22:4, 1996.
25. Stanley BG, Tribuzi SM: *Concepts in hand rehabilitation,* Philadelphia, 1992, FA Davis.
26. Stasinopoulis D, Johnson MI: Cyriax physiotherapy for tennis elbow/lateral epicondylitis, *Br J Sports Med* 38:6, 675-677, 2004.
27. Verhaar J et al: Lateral extensor release for tennis elbow. A prospective long-term follow-up study, *J Bone Joint Surg Am* 75:7, 1993.
28. Weir S: Corticosteroid injections for tennis elbow, *J Fam Pract* 43:3, 1996.

CHAPTER 9

Reconstruction of the Ulnar Collateral Ligament with Ulnar Nerve Transposition

Kevin E. Wilk
Michael M. Reinold
Mark T. Bastan
Wendy J. Hurd
James R. Andrews

The ulnar collateral ligament (UCL) is the elbow's primary stabilizer to valgus stress within a functional range of motion (ROM). For the overhead-throwing athlete, throwing motions promote valgus stress at the elbow that exceeds the ultimate tensile strength of the UCL. Repetitive throwing motions produce cumulative microtraumatic damage and may eventually cause the ligament to overstretch and create symptomatic medial elbow instability. To correct this, both surgical intervention and a carefully coordinated rehabilitation program are required if the athlete is to return to full, pain-free function. This chapter describes the way the anatomy and biomechanics of the elbow can be applied to a scientifically based rehabilitation program for use after UCL reconstruction.

SURGICAL INDICATIONS AND CONSIDERATIONS ANATOMY

Bony Structures

The elbow joint has three articulations: the humeroulnar, humeroradial, and superior radioulnar joints. Collectively these joints may be classified as *trochoginglymoid*[27] and are enclosed by a single joint capsule.

The humeroulnar joint is a single-axis diarthrodial joint with 1 degree of freedom—flexion and extension. The bony structures of the joint include the distal humerus and proximal ulna (Fig. 9-1). The distal humerus flares to form the medial and lateral epicondyles, which are directly above the capitellum and trochlea, respectively. The medial epicondyle is much more prominent than the lateral epicondyle; the UCL and flexor-pronator muscle group attach to it (Fig. 9-2). The flat, irregular surface of the lateral epicondyle serves as the attachment site for the lateral collateral ligament and the supinator-extensor muscle groups. Just posterior to the medial epicondyle is the cubital tunnel, or ulnar groove, a key depression that protects and houses the ulnar nerve. Immediately above the anterior articular surface of the humerus is a bony depression called the *coronoid fossa.* The olecranon process of the ulna glides into this concavity during flexion. The olecranon fossa, located on the posterior aspect of the humerus, accepts the large olecranon process during extension. The proximal ulna provides the major articulation of the elbow and is responsible for its inherent stability. The trochlear ridge is a bony projection running from the olecranon posteriorly to the coronoid process anteriorly. The trochlear notch is a concave surface located on either side of the trochlear ridge; it forms a close articulation with the humeral trochlea.

The proximal radius and distal lateral aspect of the humerus articulate to form the humeroradial joint, which is also a single-axis diarthrodial joint. Similar to the humeroulnar joint, the humeroradial joint contributes to flexion and extension movements by gliding around the coronal axis. However, the humeroradial articulation also pivots around a longitudinal axis with the superior radioulnar joint to perform rotational movements. The proximal radial head is mushroom shaped,[9] with a central

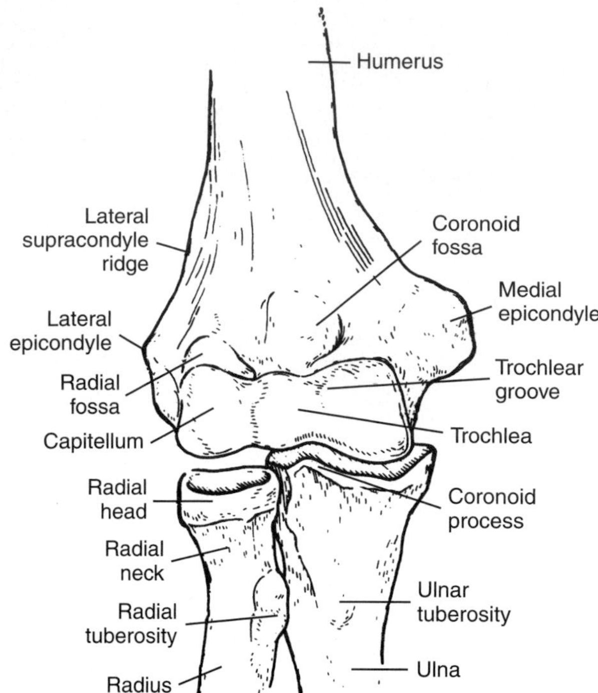

Fig. 9-1 The osseous anatomy of the elbow complex.
(From Stoyan M, Wilk KE: The functional anatomy of the elbow, *J Orthop Sports Phys Ther* 17:279, 1993.)

depression located above it. The radial head narrows distally to form the radial neck. The head and neck are not colinear, with the shaft of the radius forming an angle of approximately 15 degrees. Further distal is the radial tuberosity, where the biceps tendon attaches. In the distal humerus the capitellum is almost spherical. A groove (the capitotrochlear groove) separates the capitellum from the trochlea. The rim of the radial head articulates with this groove throughout the arc of flexion and during pronation and supination.

The superior and inferior radioulnar joints function as single-axis diarthrodial joints that allow the elbow to pronate and supinate. Proximally, the convex medial rim of the radial head articulates with the concave radial ulnar notch. During supination and pronation, the radial head rotates within a ring formed by the annular ligament and radial ulnar notch. An interosseous membrane connects the shafts of the radius and ulna to form a syndesmosis. Distally, the ulnar head with the radial ulnar notch forms the inferior radioulnar joint articulation. This joint is *L*-shaped and has an articular disc between the lower ends of the radius and ulna. During supination and pronation, the ulnar notch and articular disc swing on the ulnar head.

Ligamentous Structures

A single joint capsule surrounds the elbow joint and is lined by a synovial membrane. Specialized thickenings of the medial and lateral capsule form the collateral ligament complexes.

The UCL is traditionally described as having three portions: the anterior, posterior, and transverse bundles (Fig. 9-3).[9] The anterior bundle of the UCL is the strongest and most discrete component, coursing from the medial

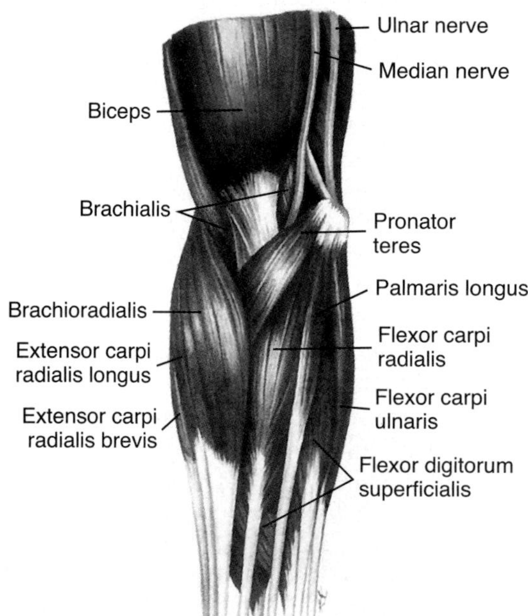

Fig. 9-2 The medial epicondyle serves as the attachment site for the ulnar collateral ligament (UCL) and flexor pronator group.
(From Stoyan M, Wilk KE: The functional anatomy of the elbow, *J Orthop Sports Phys Ther* 17:279, 1993.)

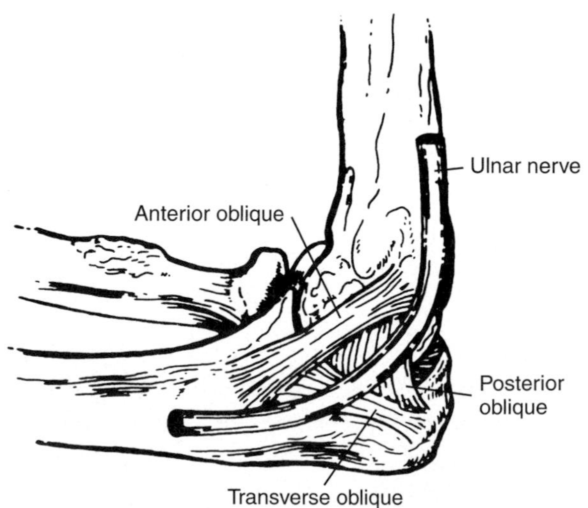

Fig. 9-3 The ulnar collateral ligament (UCL) complex of the elbow consists of three bundles: anterior, posterior, and transverse oblique.
(From Stoyan M, Wilk KE: The functional anatomy of the elbow, *J Orthop Sports Phys Ther* 17:279, 1993.)

epicondyle to the sublime tubercle on the medial coronoid margin. The anterior bundle consists of two layers: (1) a thickening within the capsular layers and (2) an added complex superficial to the capsular layers.[29] The anatomic design of this ligament makes pathologic conditions in the central portion of the anterior bundle (as seen in a chronic, attenuated state) difficult to see during arthroscopic surgery. Functionally, the UCL is subdivided into two bands: (1) the anterior band, which is tight in extension, and (2) the posterior band, which is taut in flexion.[1] The anterior oblique bundle of the UCL is the primary stabilizer to valgus stress at the elbow. Compromise of this structure causes gross instability in all elbow positions except full extension. The fan-shaped posterior bundle runs from the medial epicondyle to the middle margin of the trochlear notch. This band becomes especially taut in flexion beyond 60 degrees,[19,34] but sectioning the posterior oblique ligament does not significantly affect medial elbow stability.[26] The transverse ligament (also known as *Cooper's ligament*) has an ulnar-to-ulnar attachment and contributes minimally to elbow stability.[189]

The anatomy of the lateral collateral ligament complex can vary significantly.[18,20] Typically four components are found: (1) the radial collateral ligament (RCL), (2) the annular ligament, (3) the lateral UCL, and (4) the accessory lateral collateral ligament (Fig. 9-4). The RCL originates from the lateral epicondyle and terminates on the annular ligament. It provides varus stability by maintaining close approximation of the humeral and radial articular surfaces.[18] The annular ligament is a strong band of tissue encompassing and stabilizing the radial head in the radial ulnar notch. The anterior part of this ligament becomes taut with extreme supination and the posterior portion with extreme pronation.[15] The lateral UCL originates at the midportion of the lateral epicondyle, passes over the annular ligament, and attaches to the tubercle of the supinator. This ligament is analogous to the anterior band of the UCL and is the primary lateral stabilizer of the elbow, preventing posterolateral rotary instability.[20] Finally, the accessory lateral collateral ligament extends proximally from the inferior margin of the annular ligament and attaches distally on the tubercle of the supinator crest. It further stabilizes the annular ligament during varus stress.[15,16,1920]

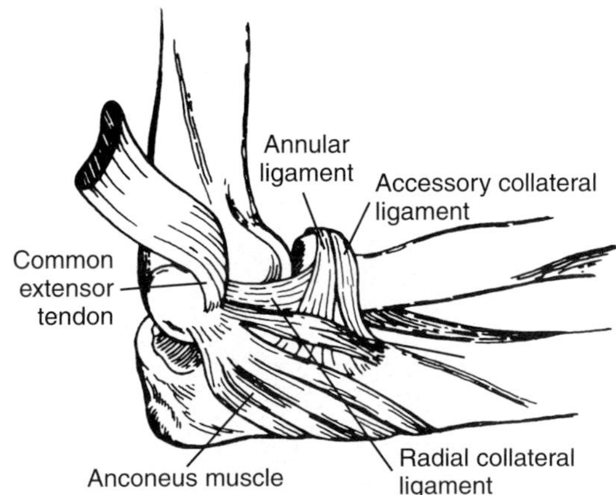

Fig. 9-4 The lateral collateral ligament complex of the elbow consists of the radial collateral ligament (RCL), annular ligament, and lateral ulnar collateral ligament (UCL).
(From Stoyan M, Wilk KE: The functional anatomy of the elbow, *J Orthop Sports Phys Ther* 17:279, 1993.)

Muscular Structures

The musculature surrounding the elbow joint may be divided into four main groups:

1. The elbow flexors
2. The elbow extensors
3. The flexor-pronator group
4. The extensor supinator group

The *flexor group* is located anteriorly and comprises the biceps brachii, brachialis, and brachioradialis muscles. The biceps brachii acts both as a major elbow flexor and as a supinator of the forearm (primarily with the elbow flexed), with a distal insertion at the radial tuberosity and bicipital aponeurosis, which attaches to the anterior capsule of the elbow. The brachioradialis originates at the proximal two thirds of the lateral supracondylar ridge of the humerus and attaches distally at the base of the styloid process of the radius, giving it the greatest mechanical advantage of the elbow flexors. The cross-sectional area of the brachialis is the largest of the elbow flexors, but this has no mechanical advantage because it crosses so closely to the axis of rotation. As the brachialis crosses the anterior capsule, some muscle fibers insert into the capsule and help retract the capsule during flexion.

The anconeus and triceps brachii perform elbow extension and are located posteriorly. The triceps brachii has three heads (long, lateral, and medial) proximally that converge distally to form a single insertion at the posterior olecranon. The much smaller anconeus originates at the posterior aspect of the lateral epicondyle and inserts on the dorsal surface of the proximal ulna. Besides extending the elbow, the anconeus may be a lateral joint stabilizer.

The flexor-pronator muscles, which all originate completely or in part at the medial epicondyle, include the pronator teres, flexor carpi radialis, palmaris longus, flexor carpi ulnaris, and flexor digitorum superficialis. The primary role of these muscles is in hand and wrist function, but they also act as elbow flexors and dynamically stabilize the medial aspect of the elbow.

Finally, the extensor supinator muscles include the brachioradialis, extensor carpi radialis brevis and longus, supinator, extensor digitorum, extensor carpi ulnaris, and extensor digiti minimi. Each of these muscles originates near or directly onto the lateral epicondyle of the humerus and provides dynamic support over the lateral aspect of the elbow.

Neurologic Structures

The relationship of neurologic structures coursing through the elbow to their surrounding features can be crucial to function, pathologic conditions, and treatment (Fig. 9-5). The radial nerve descends anterior to the lateral epicondyle, behind the brachioradialis and brachialis muscles. At the antecubital space the nerve divides into superficial and deep branches, with the superficial branch continuing distally in front of the lateral epicondyle and running under the brachioradialis muscle while on top of the supinator and pronator teres muscles. The deep branch pierces the supinator, travels around the posterolateral radial neck, and emerges distally 8 cm below the elbow joint to the terminal motor branches.

The median nerve follows a straight course into the medial aspect of the antecubital fossa, medial to the biceps tendon and brachial artery. From the antecubital fossa, the median nerve continues under the bicipital aponeurosis and usually passes between the two heads of the pronator teres, then travels below the flexor digitorum superficialis.

The musculocutaneous nerve innervates the major elbow flexors of the anterior brachium, then passes between the biceps and brachialis muscles to pierce the brachial fascia lateral to the biceps tendon. It continues distally to terminate as the lateral antebrachial cutaneous nerve, providing sensation over the lateral forearm.

Finally, the ulnar nerve travels anterior to posterior in the brachium through the arcade of Struthers. It then extends around the medial epicondyle and through the cubital tunnel. The cubital tunnel is the most frequent site for ulnar nerve injury; length changes in the medial ligament structures during elbow flexion can lead to significant reduction of the volume of the cubital tunnel, resulting in ulnar nerve compression.[11] This compression occurs as the cubital retinaculum, which forms a roof over the cubital tunnel, tightens with elbow flexion.[17] Absence of the cubital tunnel retinaculum has been associated with congenital ulnar nerve subluxation. After passing through the cubital tunnel, the ulnar nerve enters the forearm by traveling between the two heads of the flexor carpi ulnaris.

Cause

Injury to the UCL and resultant medial elbow instability are secondary to valgus loads that exceed the ultimate tensile strength of the ligament. Although excessive valgus loads may be secondary to trauma, as with an elbow dislocation caused by a fall or playing a sport such as football or wrestling, the most common mechanisms of injury are associated with repetitive overhead activities, such as baseball, javelin throwing, tennis, swimming, and volleyball. The single largest patient population experiencing medial elbow instability is undoubtedly overhead throwers.[37] This is secondary to the tremendous forces imparted to the elbow joint during the overhead-throwing motion.

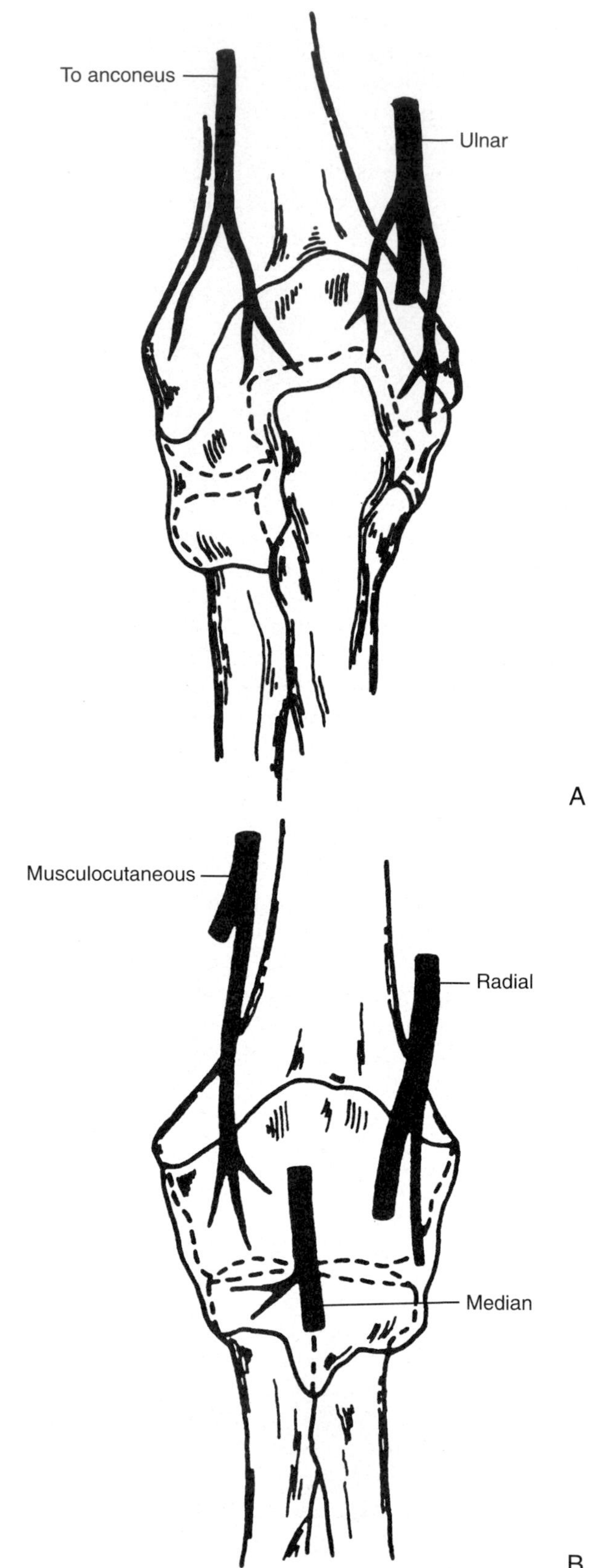

Fig. 9-5 A, Anterior view showing the neurologic innervation of the elbow. **B,** Posterior view showing the ulnar nerve of the elbow ligament.
(From Stoyan M, Wilk KE: The functional anatomy of the elbow, *J Orthop Sports Phys Ther* 17:279, 1993.)

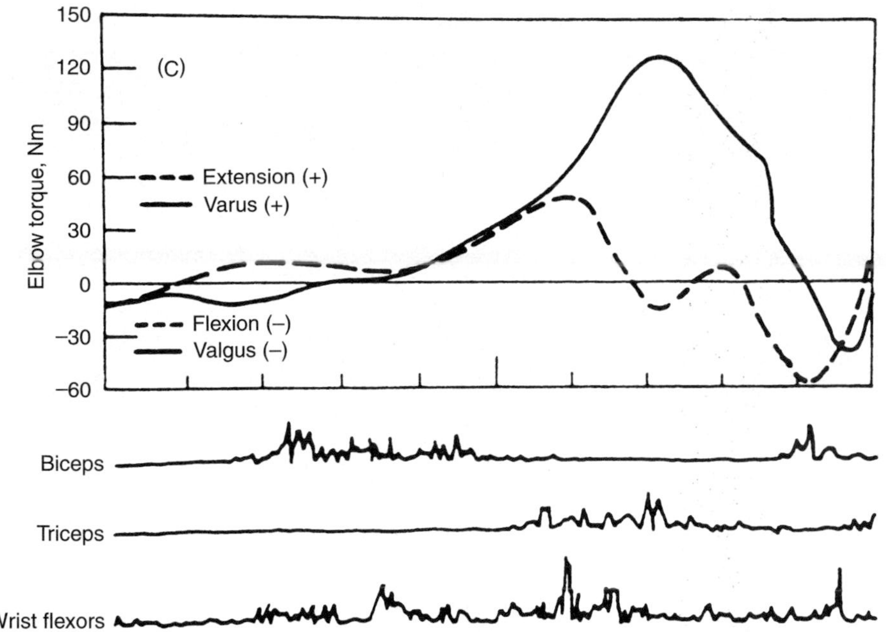

Fig. 9-6 Resting tensile strength of the ulnar collateral ligament (UCL) is measured at 33 nm but demands associated with pitching have been measured at 35 nm. (From Werner SL et al: Biomechanics of the elbow during baseball pitching, *J Orthop Sports Phys Ther* 17:274, 1993.)

The initiation of valgus stress occurs at the conclusion of the arm-cocking stage. The thrower's shoulder is abducted, extended, and externally rotated about 130 degrees, with the elbow flexed at about 90 degrees. In transition from cocking to acceleration, the shoulder then internally rotates and the elbow flexes another 20 to 30 degrees; this further increases the valgus load on the medial elbow. As the arm continues to accelerate, the elbow extends from about 125 to 25 degrees of flexion at ball release.[21,35] Dillman, Smutz, and Werner[7] report that mean ultimate valgus torque measured from cadaveric testing was 33 N∑m (newton-meters) (Fig. 9-6). During analysis of the dynamic demands of the pitching motion, Fleisig et al[8] estimate that 35 N∑m of valgus torque is placed on the UCL. The flexor carpi ulnaris and flexor digitorum superficialis muscles are located directly over the anterior band of the UCL and assist in combating medial joint distraction forces during the throwing motion. With any increased load transmitted to the UCL—whether with improper mechanics, warm-up, or conditioning—the structural integrity of the primary medial stabilizer of the elbow may be compromised.

Injuries to the UCL are described as either *acute* or *chronic*. An acute rupture of the UCL is frequently associated with a "pop," a feeling of pain during late acceleration or at ball release; it is often accompanied by swelling. More commonly, chronic injuries to the ligament are seen in the overhead-throwing athlete.[10] This occurs from the accumulated repetitive microtrauma of overloading the ligament with throwing and can result in symptomatic medial elbow instability.[6] Accurate identification of medial instability is often difficult with clinical examination alone, because laxity is only slightly increased. In addition, performing valgus laxity assessment is often difficult because of humeral rotation. Often magnetic resonance imaging (MRI) is used to confirm diagnosis. Timmerman, Schwartz, Andrews[31] believe that use of saline-enhanced MRI improves the results when a UCL tear is suspected. The authors of this chapter have found a typical leakage of contrast fluid around the ulnar insertion of the UCL when an undersurface tear is present, which has been called the *T-sign*.[24]

Surgical reconstruction of the UCL is indicated in athletes who have persistent medial elbow pain, cannot throw or participate in desired sports, show documented valgus laxity, and fail a 6-month conservative course of treatment.

SURGICAL PROCEDURE

The goal of reconstruction is to restore the static stability of the anterior bundle of the UCL. The surgical procedure used at the authors' center by Dr. James Andrews is a modification of an earlier technique.

The presence or absence of the palmaris longus must be documented before surgery because it is the preferred donor tendon. If it is not present, then alternate donor sites must be evaluated, including the contralateral palmar longus, the plantaris tendon, and the extensor tendon from the fourth toe.

Surgery to correct for valgus instability is initiated with a brief arthroscopic evaluation. The procedure itself begins with arthroscopic examination to assess the integrity of the intra-articular structures and valgus instability. After that is completed, a medial incision is made with subcutaneous ulnar nerve transposition. The incision is centered over the medial epicondyle and extends about

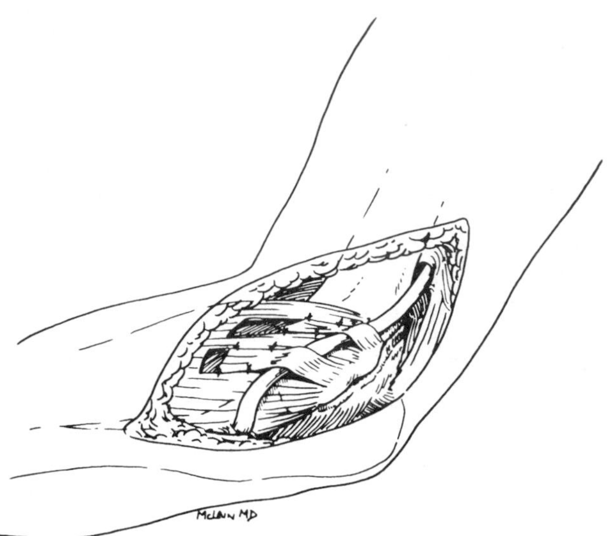

Fig. 9-7 To begin the reconstruction procedure, a medial incision is made in the elbow for ulnar collateral ligament (UCL) reconstruction and ulnar nerve transposition.
(From Andrews JR et al: Open surgical procedures for injuries to the elbow in throwers, *Oper Tech Sports Med* 4(2):109, 1996.)

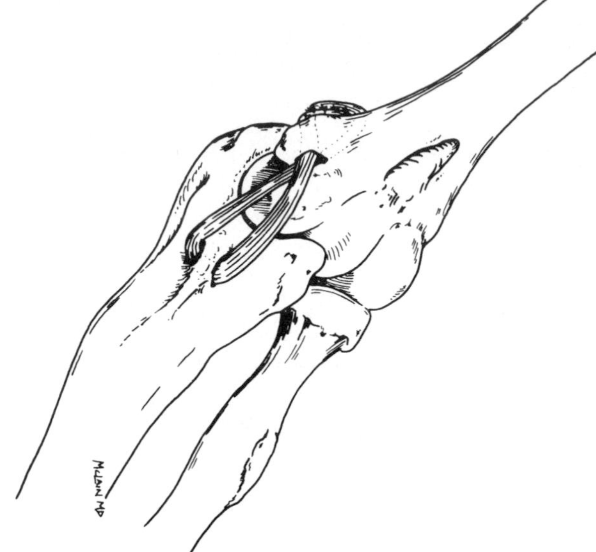

Fig. 9-8 Figure-eight reconstruction of the ulnar collateral ligament (UCL) using an autogenous graft.
(From Andrews JR et al: Open surgical procedures for injuries to the elbow in throwers, *Oper Tech Sports Med* 4[2]:109, 1996.)

3 cm proximally and distally (Fig. 9-7). The medial antebrachial cutaneous nerve is identified, preserved, and protected during the procedure to avoid neuroma development. After elevating the skin flaps to expose the deep fascia covering the flexor pronator muscles, the surgeon identifies the ulnar nerve. Anterior transposition of the ulnar nerve must be performed before the medial ligament complex is explored. To do so, the cubital tunnel is first incised to mobilize the nerve. Proximally, the mobilization continues to include the arcade of Struthers, and a portion of the intermuscular septum is excised to prevent impingement of the nerve as it is transposed anteriorly. Distally, the flexor carpi ulnaris is incised along the course of the nerve. The ulnar nerve is then transposed anteriorly and preserved throughout the remainder of the procedure.

To complete visualization of the UCL, the split in the flexor carpi ulnaris is followed down to the insertion of the anterior band of the UCL on the sublime tubercle of the ulna. Starting at the insertion of the ulna, the surgeon develops the interval between the UCL and flexor muscle mass, extending proximally to the medial epicondyle. The flexor muscles are then retracted anteriorly to provide full exposure to the ligament, at which point the pathologic condition can be assessed. In a complete rupture, the joint is exposed. If the external surface appears normal, then a longitudinal incision is made in line with the fibers of the anterior bundle. This incision may reveal pathology, including tissue discoloration, fraying of the tissue, and detachment from the bony insertion on the ulna indicative of an undersurface tear, as described by Timmerman and Andrews.[30]

The remnants of the ligament are preserved and augmented with the tendon graft. After the donor tendon has been secured, muscle is stripped off the graft, the ends are trimmed, and a nonabsorbable suture is placed at each end with a locking stitch to help graft passage. Two drill holes are made at right angles just anterior and posterior to the sublime tubercle at the level of insertion of the anterior bundle. The drill holes are then connected with curettes and a towel clip. Proximally, two convergent tunnels are drilled to meet at the insertion of the ligament on the medial epicondyle. The graft is then passed through the ulna and crossed in a figure eight across the joint. Each end is then brought out through the two tunnels at the humerus end. If the graft is long enough, then one end is passed through a second time. The graft tension is adjusted with the elbow in 30 degrees of flexion and by application of a varus stress. The graft is then secured with nonabsorbable 2-0 sutures over the medial epicondyle. The remaining ligament is sutured to the graft for added stability, and the flexor carpi ulnaris is loosely closed (Fig. 9-8).

Ulnar nerve transposition is now completed. An incision is made in the flexor pronator fascia, leaving attachments at the medial epicondyle; these flaps are about 3 cm long and 1 cm wide. Muscle is dissected away from the fascia, and the defect is closed to prevent herniation. The nerve is then transferred subcutaneously and anteriorly to lie under the fascial flaps. The flaps are reattached loosely to provide a sling to keep the nerve in position without compressing it. A drain is placed subcutaneously, and the skin is closed with an absorbable 3-0 subcuticular suture.

THERAPY GUIDELINES FOR REHABILITATION

Rehabilitation after UCL reconstruction should match the surgery used and meet the needs of the patient. The following guidelines are based on the procedure just described and are geared to the overhead-throwing athlete. The complete rehabilitation program is outlined in the home maintenance box.

Q The patient is a 16-year-old female tennis player who had UCL reconstruction 16 weeks ago. She has full ROM and has been progressing with her isotonic strengthening program. She expresses that she is ready to start playing. What types of intervention still need to be incorporated in her program before she can begin sporting activities, and what is the rationale for doing so?

Phase I

TIME: 1 to 3 weeks after surgery
GOALS: Decrease pain and inflammation, retard muscle atrophy, protect healing tissues (Table 9-1)

Table 9-1 Ulnar Nerve Transposition

Rehabilitation Phase	Criteria to Progress to this Phase	Anticipated Impairments and Functional Limitations	Intervention	Goal	Rationale
Phase I Postoperative 1-3 weeks	◆ Postoperative	◆ Postoperative pain ◆ Postoperative edema ◆ Arm immobilized in postoperative dressing ◆ Limited elbow and wrist ROM ◆ Limited UE strength ◆ Limited reach, grasp, and lift capacity of UE	◆ Posterior splint with elbow at 90 degrees of flexion (see Fig. 9-9) ◆ Remove splint at 7 days after surgery and place in a hinged elbow brace set at −30 degrees of extension and 100 degrees of flexion ◆ Brace ROM progressed by 10 degrees of extension and 10 degrees of flexion each week ◆ Cryotherapy ◆ Compression dressing (5-7 days) ◆ Isometrics—Submaximal shoulder flexion/extension, abduction, and IR (no ER) (at 2 weeks add wrist flexion/extension) ◆ After 2 weeks add AROM for wrist flexion and extension	◆ Protect surgical site ◆ Increase elbow ROM ◆ Improve tolerance to elbow ROM ◆ Control pain ◆ Manage edema ◆ Improve UE strength and muscle contraction ◆ Improve active ROM of wrist	◆ Soft tissue healing without irritating surgical site ◆ Hinged brace to avoid valgus stress ◆ Gradual addition of stress to surgical site allowing ROM progression on a graduated basis ◆ Self-management of pain and edema ◆ Prevention of associated UE muscle atrophy without stressing UCL (avoiding ER) ◆ Nonpainful, safe strengthening of wrist musculature ◆ Increase in available active ROM gradually as function and strength progress

ROM, Range of motion; *UE,* upper extremity; *UCL,* ulnar collateral ligament; *ER,* external rotation.

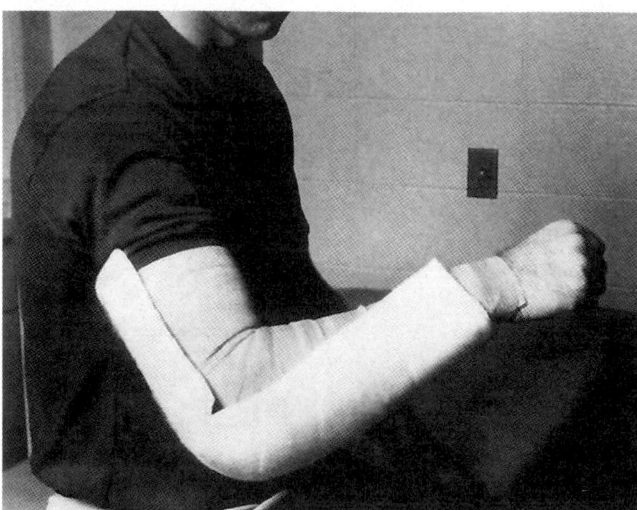

Fig. 9-9 A postoperative posterior elbow splint is used to protect healing tissues.

The patient should be placed in a posterior elbow splint at 90 degrees of flexion (Fig. 9-9), which allows initial healing of the UCL graft and soft tissue healing of the fascial slings for the transferred ulnar nerve.[36] Edema and pain are managed with frequent gripping exercises, cryotherapy, and a bulky dressing. The dressing is applied immediately after surgery and is removed between postoperative days 5 and 7.

The therapist initiates submaximal shoulder isometrics (except internal rotation [IR], which promotes a valgus stress at the elbow) and active wrist ROM to prevent neuromuscular inhibition.

The therapist evaluates ulnar nerve function postoperatively and frequently throughout the rehabilitation process. Paresthesia and impaired motor function occur at rates as high as 31% with intramuscular ulnar nerve transposition. The procedure described in this chapter uses fascial slings to complete transposition of the nerve, so the chance of postoperative neurologic complications is extremely low, usually less than 3%.

Compression wraps that are too tight and ill-fitting braces also may lead to transient ulnar nerve paresthesia and should be carefully assessed.

Early ROM and frequent assessment are vital in the early rehabilitative process. After 7 days the posterior splint is removed and the elbow placed in a hinged brace set at 30 to 100 degrees (Fig. 9-10). ROM is then advanced weekly by 10 degrees of extension and 10 degrees of flexion. During the third postoperative week, active range of motion (AROM) for the wrist, elbow, and shoulder may be initiated.

A

Before any overhead sporting activity such as hitting a tennis ball, it is important that the patient has progressed through a proper rehabilitation program, including isotonics, dynamic stabilization drills, a plyometric program, and an interval sport program. These exercises are essential to enhancing functional strength and dynamic joint stability, as well as preparing the upper extremity for the acceleration and deceleration forces required of her sport-specific activity.

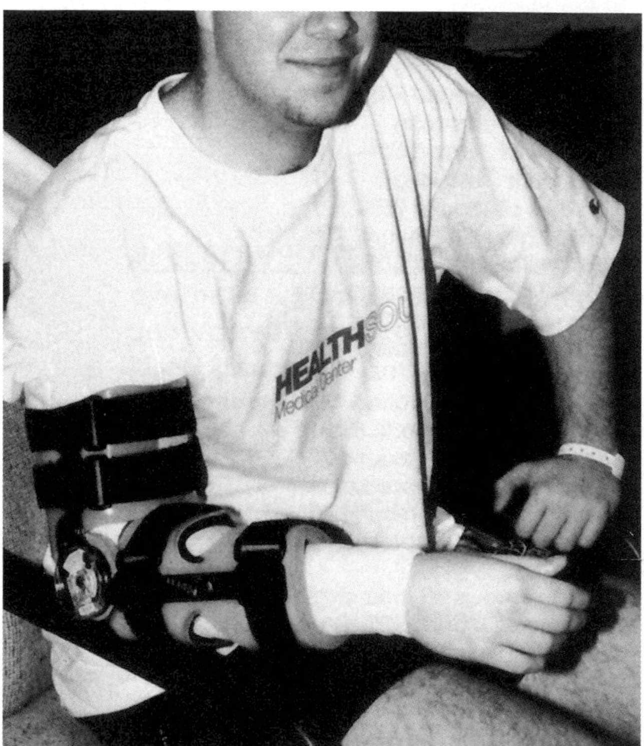

Fig. 9-10 The postoperative range of motion (ROM) brace is used to improve elbow ROM gradually while allowing soft tissue healing.

Phase II

TIME: 4 to 7 weeks after surgery

GOALS: Gradually increase ROM, heal tissues, restore muscular strength (Table 9-2)

The intermediate phase begins approximately at week 4. Advancement through the rehabilitation process is adjusted based on the response of the patient to surgery, tissue healing constraints, and a criterion-based progression.

Light wrist and elbow isotonics can be initiated during week 4, as well as rotator cuff strengthening. The therapist should advance the resistance with isotonic exercises as the patient's strength improves. Typically, the patient progresses by 1 lb per week.

Table 9-2 Ulnar Nerve Transposition

Rehabilitation Phase	Criteria to Progress to this Phase	Anticipated Impairments and Functional Limitations	Intervention	Goal	Rationale
Phase II Postoperative 4-8 weeks	◆ No sign of infection ◆ No loss of ROM ◆ No increase in pain	◆ Limited ROM ◆ Limited UE strength ◆ Limited reach, grasp, and lift capacity of UE ◆ Pain	Continue exercises as in Phase I as indicated: ◆ Elbow ROM zero-135 degrees week 5, D/C brace week 5 ◆ Isotonics (1-2 lb)—Wrist flexion, extension; forearm pronation/supination; elbow flexion/extension; rotator cuff exercises (after 6 weeks, see Box 9-2) After 6 weeks: ◆ Active ROM—Elbow flexion/extension ◆ Progression of all exercises to incorporate full body strengthening	◆ Elbow active ROM zero-145 degrees ◆ Protect elbow from unprotected valgus force ◆ Increase functional strength of UE ◆ Improve tolerance to active ROM ◆ Increase upper quarter strength ◆ Increase lift tolerance	◆ Promotion of elbow ROM ◆ Progression toward protected active ROM of elbow ◆ Advancing of UE strength and ROM in preparation to restore previous level of functioning ◆ Continued avoidance of valgus forces ◆ By 6 weeks soft tissue healing should be stable enough to tolerate valgus stress ◆ Attaining of full ROM ◆ Objective progression of exercises

ROM, Range of motion; *UE*, upper extremity; *D/C*, discharge.

Q The patient is a college baseball pitcher that had UCL surgery with ulnar nerve transposition 7 weeks ago. He is now performing some light isotonic exercises. What two muscles should the therapist target to enhance the dynamic stabilization of the medial elbow during a throwing motion?

Training the muscles in the way they are to perform with throwing is the focus. For example, the flexor carpi ulnaris and flexor digitorum superficialis muscles are located directly over the anterior band of the UCL and may contribute to dynamic stabilization of the medial elbow. Rhythmic stabilization drills in the throwing position assist in training these muscles in a similar manner. In addition, the elbow extensors act concentrically to accelerate the arm during the acceleration phase, whereas the elbow flexors act eccentrically to control the rapid rate of elbow extension during follow-through. Biasing the exercise selection appropriately for these muscle groups allows more effective strength training and provides neuromuscular training, allowing the muscles to function more efficiently when performing skilled movement patterns.

A The focus should be on training the muscles in the way they are to perform during throwing. The flexor carpi ulnaris and the flexor digitorum superficialis muscles are located directly over the anterior band of the UCL and may contribute to dynamic stabilization of the medial elbow.

Q The patient is a 20-year-old male pitcher who had UCL reconstruction 6 weeks ago. He arrives from another clinic with a 15-degree flexion contracture. What course of action should the therapist take to address this ROM deficit immediately?

During this phase the therapist should pay careful attention to the patient's ROM. One of the most common complications after UCL reconstruction is development of an elbow flexion contracture and joint stiffness. In addition, flexion contracture is common in overhead-throwing athletes. Therefore early intervention and progressive motion and stretching exercises are important preventatives against elbow flexion contracture (Box 9-1).[387]

ROM is gradually progressed to achieve zero to 135 degrees by week 5. At this time, the brace may be removed. The intimate configuration of the elbow joint is prone to develop contractures. In addition, scarring of the brachialis muscle to the capsule may further lead to loss of motion. ROM and stretching techniques are continued to ensure the prevention of motion complications. Additionally, low-load long-duration stretching may be incorporated as needed.

Box 9-1 Stretching Program to Improve Elbow Motion

1. Passive warm-up (warm whirlpool) (7 to 10 minutes)
2. Active warm-up (upper body ergometer [UBE]) (10 minutes)
3. Joint mobilization
   a. Distraction glides
   b. Posterior ulnar glide for upward elbow extension
   c. Mobilization of radial head
4. Low-load, long-duration stretching (12 to 15 minutes)
5. Manual proprioceptive neuromuscular facilitation (PNF) stretches using contract-relax technique
6. Passive stretching
7. Repeat process twice

A The patient is behind with his ROM. The elbow joint is prone to develop a flexion contracture as the result of the intimate joint congruency. In the instance of a flexion contracture, the therapist should introduce treatments designed to create a plastic response in the collagen tissue. These include a passive warm-up, followed by active warm-up, joint mobilizations (including distraction and posterior ulnar glides), low-load, long duration, as well as contract-relax and passive stretching.

Phase III

TIME: 8 to 13 weeks after surgery
GOALS: Increase strength, power, and endurance, maintain full ROM, gradually add sports activities (Table 9-3)

Table 9-3 Ulnar Nerve Transposition

Rehabilitation Phase	Criteria to Progress to this Phase	Anticipated Impairments and Functional Limitations	Intervention	Goal	Rationale
Phase III Postoperative 9-13 weeks	◆ No increase in pain ◆ No loss of ROM ◆ Steady progression of elbow and wrist ROM	◆ Limited UE strength ◆ Limited tolerance to reach, grasp, and lift activities	Continue exercises as in Phases I and II: ◆ Progress with plyometric exercises: ◆ Isotonics—Progress wrist, elbow, and shoulder exercises ◆ Initiate eccentric elbow flexion/extension exercises ◆ Plyometrics—Incorporate functional throwing position (see Fig. 9-11) ◆ PNF patterns (see Fig. 9-12) ◆ Light sporting activities (golf, swimming) ◆ Continue shoulder Thrower's Ten Program (see Box 9-2)	◆ Increase strength of UE ◆ Increase muscular control of UE ◆ Prepare for return to previous activities ◆ Improve recruitment of UE musculature ◆ Allow client to become pain free or self-manage with gradual return to activities ◆ Strengthen UE with sport-specific activities	◆ Continuation of strengthening UE and progressing resistance ◆ Training of muscles in movement patterns similar to overhead activities ◆ Preparation of UE for accelerating and decelerating activities ◆ Use of neuromuscular patterns to enhance functional strength and dynamic joint stabilization ◆ Use of cross-training to vary stresses on UE ◆ Specificity of training principle

ROM, Range of motion; *UE,* upper extremity; *PNF,* proprioceptive neuromuscular facilitation.

During this phase aggressive wrist, forearm, elbow, and shoulder strengthening are advanced with a Thrower's Ten Program (Box 9-2). The patient may begin light plyometric exercise during this phase. Plyometrics are initiated with two-hand drills, close to the body, such as a chest pass. These exercises are progressed away from the body to include side-to-side and overhead throws and finally, one-hand drills at week 12. These drills are used to develop power and explosiveness with weighted balls, often incorporating the functional throwing position (Fig. 9-11). Manual proprioceptive neuromuscular facilitation (PNF) drills such as D_2 flexion and extension encourage strengthening in functional movement patterns and facilitate dynamic joint stabilization (Fig. 9-12).

Box 9-2 Thrower's Ten Program

1. Diagonal pattern D_2 flexion and extension
2. External rotation (ER) and internal rotation (IR) tubing
3. Shoulder abduction
4. Full can
5. Side-lying ER
6. Prone: horizontal abduction, horizontal abduction at 100 degrees, row, and row into ER
7. Press-ups
8. Push-ups starting from the wall in standing
9. Elbow flexion and extension
10. Wrist extension and flexion, pronation, and supination

Phase IV

TIME: 14 to 26 weeks after surgery
GOALS: Increase strength, power, and endurance of upper extremity muscles, gradually return to sports activities (Table 9-4)

In this final phase the physical therapist should take care to return the patient to sports activities gradually; an interval sport program may help ensure that goal (Boxes 9-3 and 9-4). Other throwing programs are described in Chapter 3 and Appendix A. An interval throwing program may be initiated for an overhead thrower at 16 weeks after surgery, with throwing off the mound usually occurring around 5 to 6 months after surgery.[38] Return to competition typically occurs between 9 and 12 months. The competitive overhead athlete should participate in a year-round con-

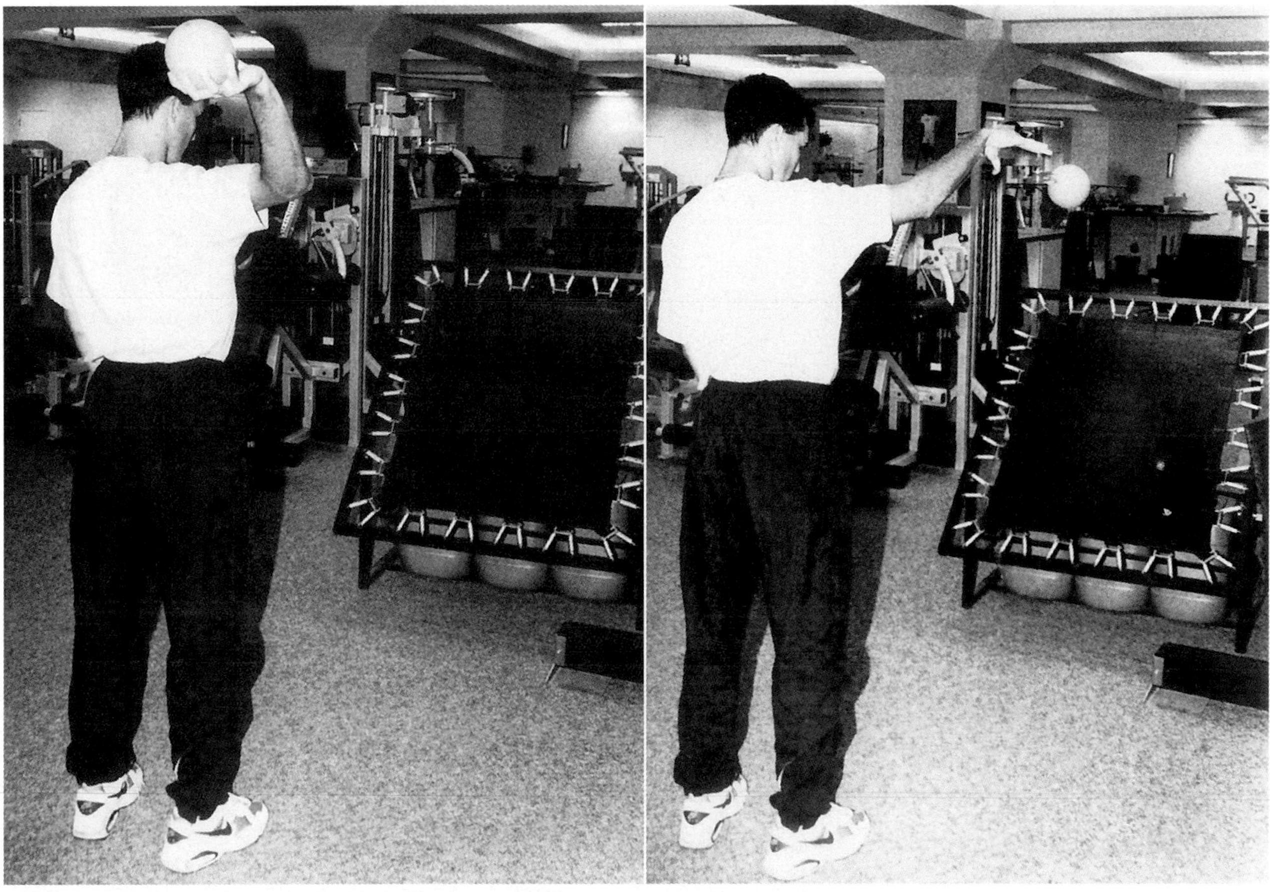

Fig. 9-11 Plyometric exercise drills develop power and explosiveness. The one-handed baseball throw to simulate throwing mechanics is shown.

ditioning program that consists of isotonic strengthening (see Box 9-2), plyometric and neuromuscular training, and a sport-specific training program. In addition, the athlete should continue flexibility exercises for the elbow, wrist, and hand. The interval throwing program emphasizes a proper warm-up, correct throwing mechanics, and a gradual progression of intensity. The therapist also must teach the athlete to "listen" to the arm: if pain is present, then the patient should not advance the program prematurely.

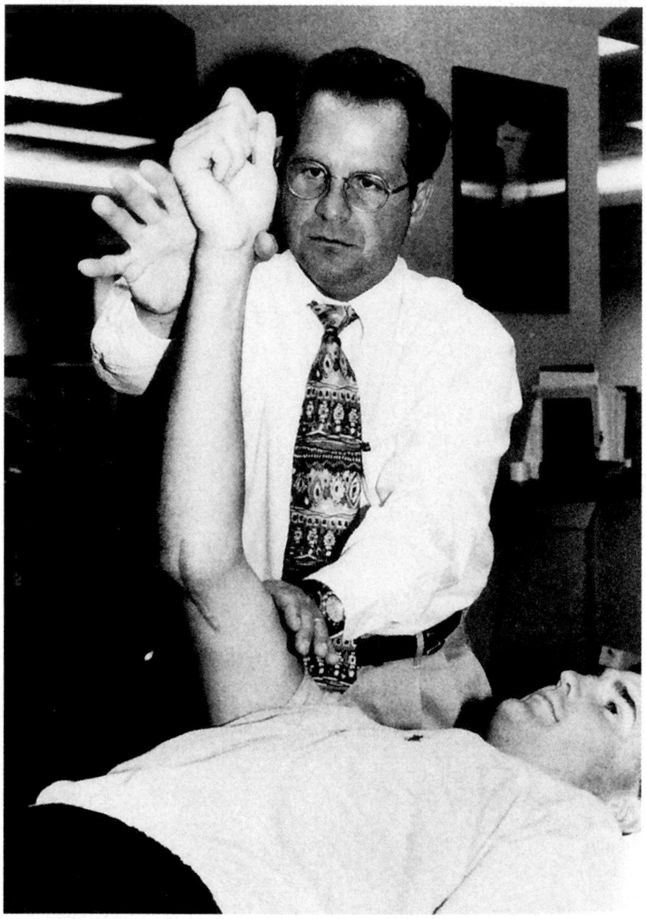

Fig. 9-12 Manual resistance proprioceptive neuromuscular facilitation (PNF) promotes strengthening in functional movement patterns and dynamic joint stabilization. This movement pattern is referred to as a *D_2 flexion and extension upper extremity pattern.*

SUGGESTED HOME MAINTENANCE FOR THE POSTSURGICAL PATIENT

The home maintenance box on page 166, as well as Box 9-2, review exercises that are commonly prescribed for the patient to perform at home. The exercises are progressed gradually to allow the tissue proper healing time, with the ultimate goal of full restoration of strength and ROM. The exercises are to be performed at home in conjunction with treatment sessions in the rehabilitation setting.

TROUBLESHOOTING

As already noted, the most common complication after UCL reconstruction is a flexion contracture or stiff joint. Factors that predispose the elbow joint to this loss of ROM include the following:

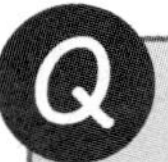

A patient who had UCL surgery 16 weeks ago wants to begin throwing. Is this appropriate?

A

Provided the patient has full ROM, good strength, and is pain free, an interval throwing program is initiated at week 16. Each stage is to be performed twice, with a day of rest in between, before moving to the next stage. Should the patient report pain or excessive soreness, he or she should move back a stage and continue from there.

Table 9-4 Ulnar Nerve Transposition

Rehabilitation Phase	Criteria to Progress to this Phase	Anticipated Impairments and Functional Limitations	Intervention	Goal	Rationale
Phase IV Postoperative 14-26 weeks	◆ No increase in pain ◆ No loss of ROM ◆ No loss of strength	◆ Limited tolerance to repetitive overhead activities ◆ Limited strength	◆ Initiate interval throwing program (see Boxes 9-3 and 9-4) ◆ Continue strengthening as in Phases I through III	◆ Symmetric UE strength ◆ Gradual return to unrestricted sport activity	◆ Normalization of UE strength to avoid reinjury with return to sport activities ◆ Gradual progression to sport

ROM, Range of motion; *UE,* upper extremity.

Box 9-3 Interval Throwing Program Phase I

45-Foot phase

Step 1
1. Warm-up throwing
2. 45 feet (25 throws)
3. Rest 15 minutes
4. Warm-up throwing
5. 45 feet (25 throws)

Step 2
1. Warm-up throwing
2. 45 feet (25 throws)
3. Rest 10 minutes
4. Warm-up throwing
5. 45 feet (25 throws)
6. Rest 10 minutes
7. Warm-up throwing
8. 45 feet (25 throws)

60-Foot phase

Step 3
1. Warm-up throwing
2. 60 feet (25 throws)
3. Rest 15 minutes
4. Warm-up throwing
5. 60 feet (25 throws)

Step 4
1. Warm-up throwing
2. 60 feet (25 throws)
3. Rest 10 minutes
4. Warm-up throwing
5. 60 feet (25 throws)
6. Rest 10 minutes
7. Warm-up throwing
8. 60 feet (25 throws)

90-Foot phase

Step 5
1. Warm-up throwing
2. 90 feet (25 throws)
3. Rest 15 minutes
4. Warm-up throwing
5. 90 feet (25 throws)

Step 6
1. Warm-up throwing
2. 90 feet (25 throws)
3. Rest 10 minutes
4. Warm-up throwing
5. 90 feet (25 throws)
6. Rest 10 minutes
7. Warm-up throwing
8. 90 feet (25 throws)

120-Foot phase

Step 7
1. Warm-up throwing
2. 120 feet (25 throws)
3. Rest 15 minutes
4. Warm-up throwing
5. 120 feet (25 throws)

Step 8
1. Warm-up throwing
2. 120 feet (25 throws)
3. Rest 10 minutes
4. Warm-up throwing
5. 120 feet (25 throws)
6. 120 feet (25 throws)
7. Rest 10 minutes
8. Warm-up throwing

150-Foot phase

Step 9
1. Warm-up throwing
2. 150 feet (25 throws)
3. Rest 15 minutes
4. Warm-up throwing
5. 150 feet (25 throws)

Step 10
1. Warm-up throwing
2. 150 feet (25 throws)
3. Rest 10 minutes
4. Warm-up throwing
5. 150 feet (25 throws)
6. Rest 10 minutes
7. Warm-up throwing
8. 150 feet (25 throws)

180-Foot phase

Step 11
1. Warm-up throwing
2. 180 feet (25 throws)
3. Rest 15 minutes
4. Warm-up throwing
5. 180 feet (25 throws)

Step 12
1. Warm-up throwing
2. 180 feet (25 throws)
3. Rest 10 minutes
4. Warm-up throwing
5. 180 feet (25 throws)
6. Rest 10 minutes
7. Warm-up throwing
8. 180 feet (25 throws)

Step 13
1. Warm-up throwing
2. 180 feet (25 throws)
3. Rest 10 minutes
4. Warm-up throwing
5. 180 feet (25 throws)
6. Rest 10 minutes
7. Warm-up throwing
8. 180 feet (25 throws)

Box 9-4 Interval Throwing Program Phase II

Stage 1: fastball only

Step 1:
Interval throwing
15 throws off mound at 50%

Step 2:
Interval throwing
30 throws off mound at 50%

Step 3:
Interval throwing
45 throws off mound at 50%

Step 4:
Interval throwing
60 throws off mound at 50%

Step 5:
Interval throwing
30 throws off mound at 75%

Step 6:
30 throws off mound at 75%
45 throws off mound at 50%

Step 7:
45 throws off mound at 75%
15 throws off mound at 50%

Step 8:
60 throws off mound at 75%

Stage 2: fastball only

Step 9:
45 throws off mound at 75%
15 throws in batting practice

Step 10:
45 throws off mound at 75%
30 throws in batting practice

Step 11:
45 throws off mound at 75%
45 throws in batting practice

Stage 3

Step 12:
30 throws off mound at 75% during warm-up
15 throws off mound; 50% breaking balls
45-60 throws in batting practice (fastball only)

Step 13:
30 throws off mound at 75%
30 breaking balls at 75%
30 throws in batting practice

Step 14:
30 throws off mound at 75%
60-90 throws in batting practice; 25% breaking balls

Step 15:
Simulated game, progressing by 15 throws per workout (use interval throwing to phase 12, No. 8 in Box 9-3 as warm-up). All throwing off the mound should be done in the presence of the pitching coach to stress proper throwing mechanics. Use speed gun to aid in effort control.

Q A patient who had UCL surgery 8 months ago is beginning to throw on mound near full effort and begins to report medial elbow pain. What should the therapist do?

1. The intimate congruency of the elbow joint complex, especially the humeroulnar joint
2. The tightness of the elbow joint capsule
3. The tendency of the anterior capsule to scar and become adhesive[23]

Box 9-1 outlines a program found to be effective in combating flexion contractures of the elbow. It includes both passive and active warm-up, joint mobilizations, and manual stretching techniques. One of the most effective components to the stretching regimen is the low-load, long-duration stretching technique. The three most important components of this technique are (1) duration of stretch (10 to 15 minutes), (2) intensity of stretch (low to moderate), and (3) frequency of stretch (5 to 6 times daily) (Fig. 9-13).

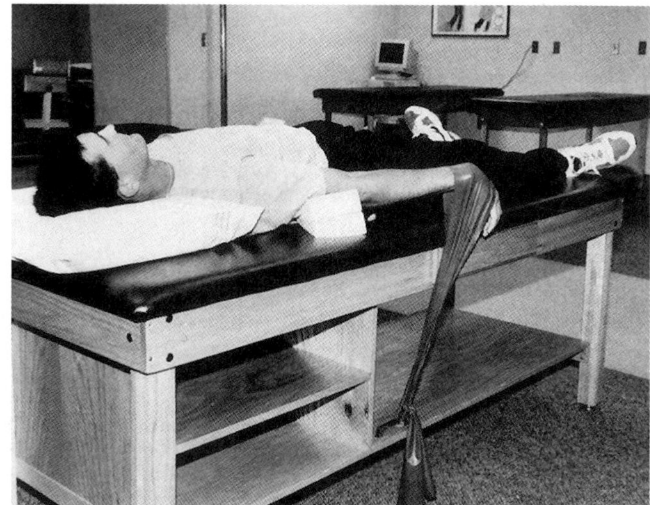

Fig. 9-13 A low-load, long-duration stretch is performed to improve elbow extension. A Theraband is secured at one end and wrapped around the patient's distal forearm.

This stretching technique may be enhanced by the use of other modalities such as moist hot packs or ultrasound. The rationale for the success of this technique is its ability to produce a plastic response within the collagen tissue, resulting in permanent elongation.[14,26,32,33]

If ROM complications persist, the therapist may want to prescribe a splint to be worn both day and night. A static splint holds the joint in a constant position, whereas a dynamic splint uses a spring to exert force and create a progressive stretch. Patients are encouraged to remove the splint daily for strengthening and stretching exercises.

During the aggressive stretching program the patient often experiences increased elbow soreness or pain. Pain control using cryotherapy, high-voltage galvanic stimulation (HVGS), transcutaneous electrical nerve stimulation (TENS), and interferential current is highly effective.

A The therapist should tell the patient to step back to a partial effort for a week and treat the pain symptoms. If the patient continues to feel pain when progressing, then he or she may need to see a physician and potentially stop throwing to allow time to heal while continuing with exercises.

Q A patient had UCL surgery 3 days ago and has been unable to adduct his thumb, abduct or adduct his fingers, and has weakness in flexor carpi ulnaris. He also reports numbness in the fifth digit. What is the assessment? Is this cause for concern?

Other complications include hand and grip weakness, ulnar neuropathy, rotator cuff tendonitis, and UCL failure. Intrinsic weakness of the hand may be avoided by initiating gripping exercises immediately after surgery and increasing intensity as rehabilitation progresses. Ulnar neuropathy generally develops immediately after surgery. Transposition of the ulnar nerve may cause sensory changes of the little finger and ulnar half of the ring finger. Motor deficits may include the inability to adduct the thumb, weakness of the finger abductor and adductors, adduction of the little finger, and weakness of the flexor carpi ulnaris. The most frequent patient complaint is paresthesia through the ulnar nerve sensory distribution, but this is usually transient and should resolve within 7 days.

Inactivity can lead to rapid deterioration of rotator cuff strength and a subsequent inability to stabilize the glenohumeral (GH) joint during the throwing motion. Integrating a Thrower's Ten Program with the emphasis on rotator cuff strengthening several weeks before throwing greatly reduces the chances of developing tendonitis.

A These signs and symptoms are consistent with an ulnar neuropathy, which is common after ulnar nerve transposition. The therapist can check for tight-fitting wraps or ill-fitting braces, but typically these complications resolve within 7 days after surgery.

UCL failure is the most serious of all postoperative complications. Graft failure or poor bone quality with inadequate graft stabilization necessitates subsequent surgery or the cessation of overhead activities. Fortunately, with advanced surgical and rehabilitation techniques, successful outcomes are much more likely than failures. Andrews and Timmerman[2] found 78% of professional baseball players returning to their previous level of play after UCL reconstruction.

SUGGESTED HOME MAINTENANCE FOR THE POSTSURGICAL PATIENT

Weeks 1-3

GOALS FOR THE PERIOD: Protect healing tissues, decrease pain and inflammation, and limit muscle atrophy

Week 1:

1. Posterior splint at 90-degree elbow flexion
2. Wrist assisted range of motion (AROM) extension and flexion
3. Elbow compression dressing (5 to 7 days)
4. Gripping exercises, wrist range of motion (ROM), shoulder isometrics (except shoulder external rotation [ER]), biceps isometrics, others as indicated
5. Cryotherapy

Week 2:

1. Application of functional brace 30 to 100 degrees
2. Initiation of wrist isometrics
3. Initiation of elbow flexion and extension isometrics
4. Continuation of all exercises listed previously

Week 3:

Advance brace (gradually increase ROM; 10 degrees of extension and 10 degrees of flexion per week)

Weeks 4-7

GOALS FOR THE PERIOD: Gradually increase ROM, healing tissues, and regain and improve muscle strength

Week 4:

1. Begin light resistance exercises for arm (1 lb), wrist curls, extensions, pronation, and supination, and elbow extension and flexion
2. Progress shoulder program, emphasizing rotator cuff strengthening
3. Initiate shoulder ER strengthening
4. Progress shoulder program

Week 5:

Continue as for week 4, discharge brace, full passive range of motion (PROM) week 5

Weeks 6-7:

1. ROM zero to 145 degrees
2. Progress elbow-strengthening exercises

Weeks 8-13

GOALS FOR THE PERIOD: Increase strength, power, and endurance; maintain full elbow ROM; gradually begin sports activities

Week 8:

1. Initiate eccentric elbow flexion and extension
2. Continue isotonic program for forearm and wrist
3. Continue shoulder program (Thrower's Ten Program)
4. Begin manual resistance diagonal patterns
5. Begin two-hand plyometrics

Week 9-11:

Continue as for week 8, progress strength

Weeks 12-13:

1. Continue as for week 11
2. Begin one-hand plyometrics
3. Begin light sports activities (e.g., golf, swimming)

Weeks 14-26

GOALS FOR THE PERIOD: Continue to increase strength, power, and endurance of upper extremity muscles; gradually return to sports activities

Week 14:

1. Continue strengthening program
2. Emphasize elbow and wrist strengthening and flexibility exercises

Weeks 15-21:

Continue with program

Week 16:

Begin phase I interval throwing program

Weeks 22-26:

Return to competitive sports as appropriate

References

1. Andrews JR: *Ulnar collateral ligament injuries of the elbow in throwers.* Paper presented at the Injuries in Baseball Course, Birmingham, AL, January 28, 1990.
2. Andrews JR, Timmerman LA: Outcome of elbow surgery in professional baseball players, *Am J Sports Med* 23(4):407, 1995.
3. Azar FM et al: Operative treatment of ulnar collateral ligament injuries of the elbow in athletes, *Am J Sports Med* 28(1): 2000.
4. Cain EL et al: Elbow injuries in throwing athletes: a current concepts review, *Am J Sports Med* 31(4):621-35, 2003.
5. Chen FS, Rokito AS, Jobe FW: Medial elbow problems in the overhead-throwing athlete, *J Am Acad Orthop Surg* 9(2):99-113, 2001.
6. Conway JE et al: Medial instability of the elbow in throwing athletes, *Am J Bone Joint Surg* 74:67, 1992.
7. Dillman C, Smutz P, Werner S: Valgus extension overload in baseball pitching, *Med Sci Sports Exer* 23:S135, 1991.
8. Fleisig GS et al: Kinetics of baseball pitching with implications about injury mechanisms, *Am J Sports Med* 23(2):233, 1995.
9. Guerra JJ, Timmerman LA: Clinical anatomy, histology, and pathomechanics of the elbow in sports, *Sports Med Arthrosc Rev* 3(3):160, 1995.
10. Hyman J, Breazeale NM, Altchek DW: Valgus instability of the elbow in athletes, *Clin Sports Med* 20(1):25-45, 2001.
11. Jobe FW, Fanton GS: Nerve injuries. In Morrey BF, editor: *The elbow and its disorders,* Philadelphia, 1985, WB Saunders.
12. Jobe FW, Kvitne RS: Elbow instability of the athlete, *Instr Course Lect* 40:17, 1991.
13. Jobe FW, Stark H, Lombardo SJ: Reconstruction of the ulnar collateral ligament in athletes, *J Bone Joint Surg* 68:1150, 1986.
14. Kottke FJ, Pauley DL, Ptak RA: The rationale for prolonged stretching for correction of shortening of connective tissue, *Arch Phys Med Rehabil* 47:345, 1968.
15. Martin BJ: The annular ligament of the superior radioulnar joint, *J Anat* 52:473, 1958.
16. Martin BJ: The oblique of the forearm, *J Anat* 52:609, 1958.
17. Morrey BF: Anatomy and kinematics of the elbow. In Tullos HS, editor: *American Academy of Orthopaedic Surgeons instructional course lectures 40,* St Louis, 1991, Mosby.
18. Morrey BF: Anatomy of the elbow joint. In Morrey BF, editor: *The elbow and its disorders,* Philadelphia, 1993, WB Saunders.
19. Morrey BF, An RN: Articular and ligamentous contributions to the stability of the elbow joint, *Am J Sports Med* 11:315, 1983.
20. O'Driscoll SW, Bell DF, Morrey BF: Posterolateral rotary instability of the elbow, *Am J Bone Joint Surg* 73:440, 1991.
21. Pappas A, Zawack RM, Sullivan TJ: Biomechanics of baseball pitching: a preliminary report, *Am J Sports Med* 13(4):216, 1985.
22. Petty DH et al: Ulnar collateral ligament reconstruction in high school baseball players, *Am J Sports Med* 32(5):1158-1164, 2004.
23. Reinold MM et al: Interval sports programs: guidelines for baseball, tennis and golf, *J Orthop Sports Phys Ther* 32(6):293-298, 2002.
24. Safran MR: Ulnar collateral ligament injury in the overhead athlete: diagnosis and treatment, *Clin Sports Med* 23(4):643-663, 2004.
25. Sapega AA et al: Biophysical factors in range of motion exercise, *Arch Phys Med Rehab* 57:122, 1976.
26. Schums GH et al: Biomechanics of elbow stability: role of the medial collateral ligament, *Clin Orthop* 146:42, 1980.
27. Steindler A: *Kinesiology of the human body,* Springfield, IL, 1955, Charles C. Thomas.
28. Timmerman LA, Andrews JR: Arthroscopic treatment of posttraumatic elbow pain and stiffness, *Am J Sports Med* 22(2):230, 1994.
29. Timmerman LA, Andrews JR: Histology and arthroscopic anatomy of the ulnar collateral ligament of the elbow, *Am J Sports Med* 22(5):667, 1994.
30. Timmerman LA, Andrews JR: Undersurface tear of the ulnar collateral ligament in baseball players: a newly recognized lesion, *Am J Sports Med* 22(1):33, 1994.
31. Timmerman LA, Schwartz ML, Andrews JR: Preoperative evaluation of the ulnar collateral ligament by magnetic resonance imaging and computed tomography arthrography, *Am J Sports Med* 22(1):26, 1994.
32. Warren CB, Lehman JF, Koblanski JN: Elongation of cat-tail tendon: effect of load and temperature, *Arch Phys Med Rehab* 52:465, 1971.
33. Warren CG, Lehman JF, Koblanski JN: Heat and stretch procedures: an evaluation using cat-tail tendon, *Arch Phys Med Rehab* 57:122, 1976.
34. Warwick R, Williams PL: *Gray's anatomy, descriptive and applied,* ed 35, Philadelphia, 1980, WB Saunders.
35. Werner SL, Fleisig GS, Dillman CJ: Biomechanics of the elbow during baseball pitching, *J Orthop Sports Phys Ther* 17:274, 1993.
36. Wilk KE, Arrigo CA, Andrews JR: Rehabilitation of the elbow in the throwing athlete, *J Orthop Sports Phys Ther* 17:305, 1993.
37. Wilk KE, Azar FM, Andrews JR: Conservative and operative rehabilitation of the elbow in sports, *Sports Med Arthrosc Rev* 3:237, 1995.
38. Wilk KE et al: Rehabilitation following elbow surgery in the throwing athlete, *Oper Tech Sports Med* 4(2):69, 1996.
39. Williams RJ III, Urquhart ER, Altchek DW: Medial collateral ligament tears in the throwing athlete, *Instr Course Lect* 53:579-586, 2004.

CHAPTER 10

Surgery and Rehabilitation for Primary Flexor Tendon Repair in the Digit

Linda J. Klein
Curtis A. Crimmins

SURGICAL INDICATIONS AND CONSIDERATIONS

Flexor tendon injuries have a long history of challenging the hand surgeon and therapist. Surgical and rehabilitation techniques have evolved significantly since Bunnell[2] suggested that tendon lacerations over the proximal phalanx not be repaired, but ultimately grafted. This basic premise went unchallenged until early mobilization techniques were developed in an attempt to prevent tendon adhesions during the healing process. In the 1960s multiple investigators were able to document that primary flexor tendon repair was superior to delayed tendon grafting.[10,13,27]

Despite dramatic improvement in outcome over the past 25 years, research has continued with both clinical and laboratory investigations at a breakneck pace. Biomechanical studies of human cadaver tendons have been extraordinarily useful. Investigators have established how much force is applied to a tendon during rehabilitation motions and during normal hand activities.[26] The most recent repair techniques have greater tensile strength,[19] which has allowed early postrepair motion to advance from passive flexion to controlled active flexion. The results are fewer adhesions, with better active motion and functional outcomes.

Tendon Healing Stages

Tendon healing occurs in three general stages. The inflammatory phase lasts about 1 week and begins with a fibrin clot at the repair site. Macrophages and other inflammatory cells begin work by removing nonviable material and attracting fibroblasts. Epitenon cells bridge the repair site to restore the gliding surface. The active repair phase lasts from 1 to 2 months. Collagen bundles form and reorient to strengthen the bond between the tendon ends. The tendon begins to revascularize primarily from the intrinsic supply of the proximal stump. The remodeling phase follows until the collagen is mature along the lines of tension and the repair site strength is maximized. The maturation phase, as with all healing tissue, lasts a number of months.[9]

SURGICAL PROCEDURE

The principles of flexor tendon repair are well established and must be rigorously applied to achieve consistently good results. The first step is to educate the patient about the inherent complexity of the injury. They should not only understand the demanding technical nature of the injury but also the extraordinarily demanding rehabilitation. The patient must accept that a successful outcome will depend in large part on their commitment to and involvement in the rehabilitation protocol. If possible, the patient should be counseled by a hand therapist preoperatively to establish rapport and discuss the therapy protocol. Finally, every patient must be informed that a perfect outcome is unusual and multiple surgical procedures may be necessary.

Flexor tendon repairs should be done in the operating room by experienced hand surgeons within 1 week of the injury. Precise surgical technique is rewarded by better outcomes. Tendon ends usually retract after being cut, and an adequately large surgical incision is generally needed to locate and retrieve the tendon ends. Incisions require careful planning to allow adequate exposure without compromising the vascularity of the skin flaps. Zigzag or midaxial approaches are preferred to prevent scar contracture (Fig. 10-1).

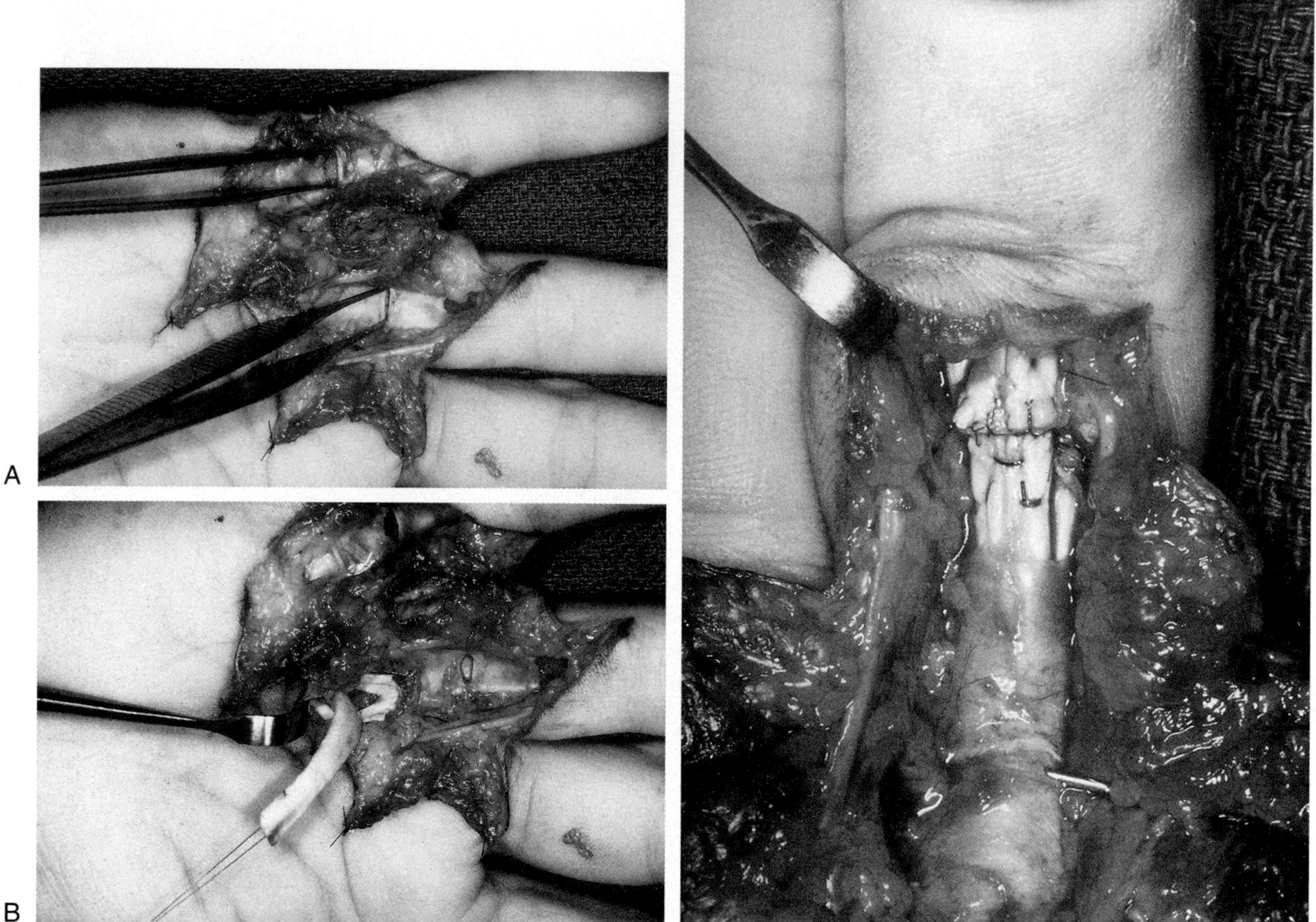

Fig. 10-1 Repair of lacerated flexor tendons in the ring and small fingers. **A,** Sheaths are empty, because flexor tendons have retracted into the digit and palm. Flexor digitorum profundus (FDP) and superficialis tendons are retrieved from the palm. **B,** The profundus tendon is rethreaded through the chiasm of Camper of the superficialis tendon before repair. **C,** Completed repair of flexor tendons, now placed within the sheath and pulley system, repaired between the A2 and A4 pulleys.
(Courtesy of Curtis Crimmins.)device.

The hallmark of successful flexor tendon repair surgery is atraumatic handling of the soft tissue, especially of the tendon itself. Flexor tendons almost always retract and must be retrieved and advanced back through the flexor sheath. This may well be the most difficult part of the operation. Great care must be exercised to avoid injury to the delicate synovial lining of the fibro-osseous sheath or the epitenon of the flexor tendon. Damage of one or the other may increase the probability of adhesion formation and a poor outcome.

Once the tendon ends have been located and threaded back through the sheath and pulleys as carefully as possible, the tendons are repaired through a window between the pulleys, while maintaining the anatomic relationship of the profundus and superficialis tendons. The flexor digitorum superficialis tendon divides into two slips over the proximal phalanx, then it merges again, creating a buttonhole type opening referred to as the *chiasm of Camper*, just before inserting on the middle phalanx. The flexor digitorum profundus (FDP), which lies deep to the superficialis until this point, emerges through the chiasm of Camper, continuing distally, to insert on the distal phalanx of the digit (Fig. 10-2). When both tendons are lacerated over the proximal phalanx, the surgeon must be certain to re-establish this special relationship. Furthermore, each divided slip of the superficialis has a tendency to derotate 180 degrees as it retracts. This must also be corrected as the tendon is repaired. Only restoration of normal anatomic relationships will allow excellent return of function after repair of lacerated flexor tendons.

The actual suturing of the flexor tendons has been a major focus in the evolution of stronger repairs. The current state of the art suggests that suture repair achieve adequate strength to allow early active-flexion rehabilitation protocols. To achieve this, the repair must ensure secure knots, provide a smooth juncture of tendon ends at the repair site, prevent gapping, maintain tendon vascularity, and be relatively straightforward to perform. Biomechanical studies have definitively shown that multistrand core suture techniques can withstand forces encountered during active motion protocols. In general, at least four strands of 3-0 or 4-0 sutures are needed to cross the repair site to ensure adequate strength for an early active motion protocol. Numerous suture techniques to achieve a repair of at least four strands are described in the literature. The authors prefer a double Kessler suture to produce the four strands of suture crossing the repair site, with a running epitendinous suture (Fig. 10-3).[20]

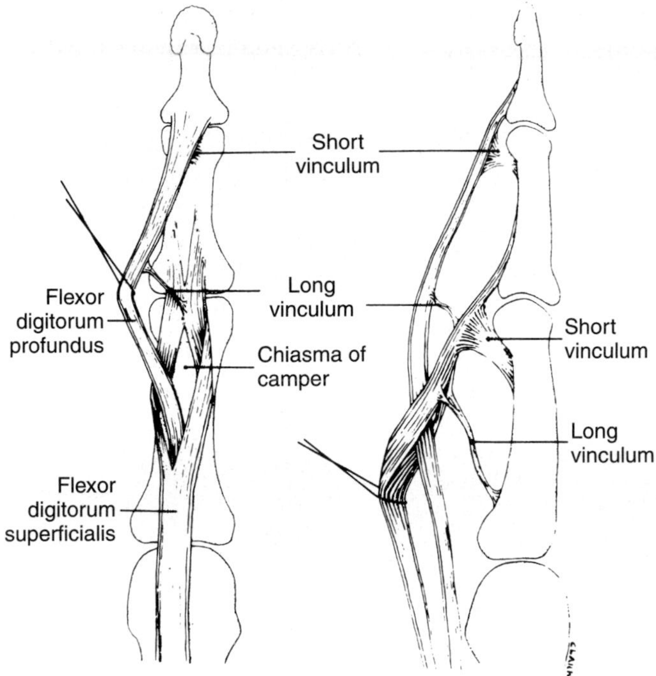

Fig. 10-2 The flexor digitorum superficialis lies volar to the flexor digitorum profundus (FDP) as the tendons enter the sheath. At the level of the proximal phalanx, the superficialis divides and the two slips pass around the profundus tendon, merging and splitting again before inserting on the middle phalanx (chiasm of Camper). (From Schneider LH: *Flexor tendon injuries,* Boston, 1985, Little, Brown.)

During the process of repairing the flexor tendons, it is important to preserve as much of the flexor tendon sheath and pulley system as possible. The surgeon must attempt to preserve the A2 and A4 pulleys to prevent tendon bowstringing (Fig. 10-4).

A tendon injury at the level of either of these pulleys is technically demanding. Even repairs at other levels must be technically precise to allow gliding of the repair under preserved portions of the flexor sheath. Suture knots should be placed to minimize impingement of the flexor tendon repair as it passes through the pulley system. Current techniques meet these requirements, and results are expectedly good, with 75% or more tendon repairs falling consistently within the excellent to good categories.

Recent and future trends in flexor tendon surgery research include investigations of the ability of substances such as hyaluronic acid and 5-flourouracil to enhance tendon healing.[17] Polyvinyl alcohol shields and anti-adhesion gels have been proposed and studied with some success to decrease adhesions.[13] As these trends continue, we must stay abreast of current developments to maximize functional outcomes for patients after flexor tendon injury.

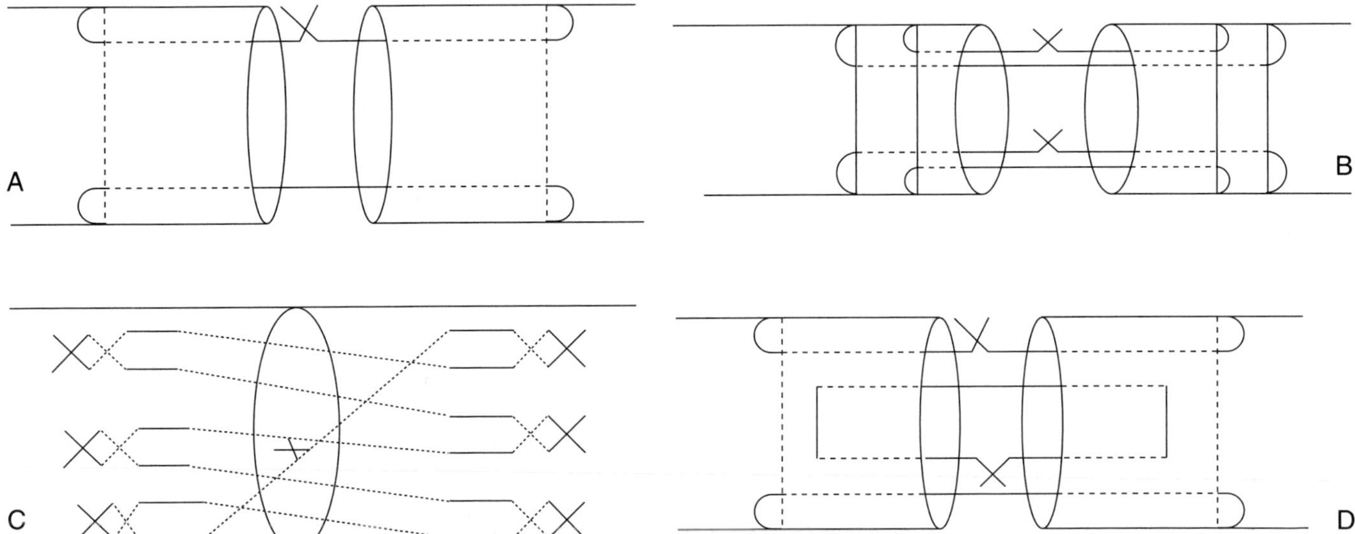

Fig. 10-3 Types of flexor tendon repairs demonstrating different amount of suture strands crossing the repair. **A,** Modified Kessler is a two-strand repair. **B,** Double Kessler is a four-strand repair. **C,** Savage is a six-strand repair. **D,** Indiana is a four-strand repair. (From Shaieb MD, Singer DI: Tensile strengths of various suture techniques, *J Hand Surg* 22B(6):765, 1997.)

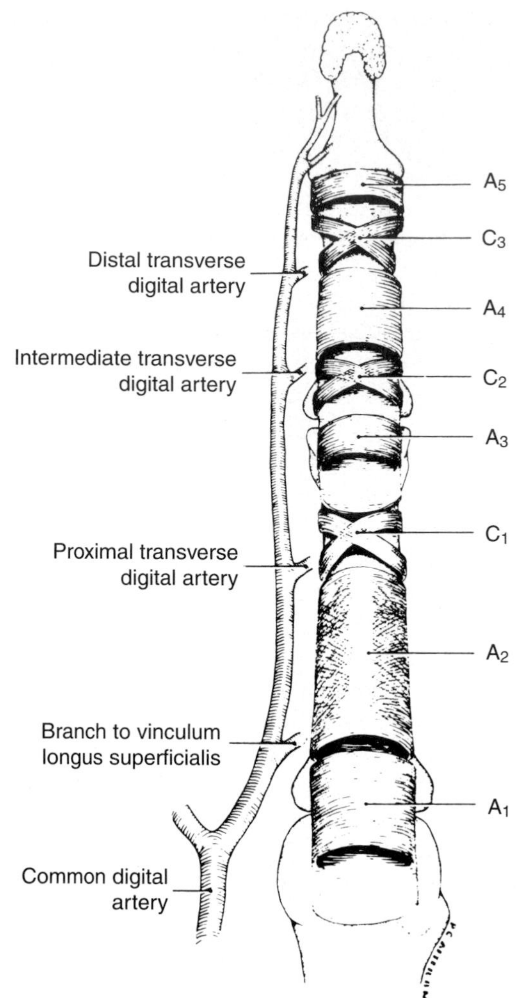

Fig. 10-4 The fibro-osseous sheath or pulley system has five annular pulleys (A1 to A5) and three cruciform pulleys (C1 to C3). The A2 and A4 pulleys must be preserved to prevent bowstringing of the flexor tendons.
(From Schneider LH: *Flexor tendon injuries*, Boston, 1985, Little, Brown.)

THERAPY GUIDELINES FOR REHABILITATION

Flexor tendon repairs in the hand require a special rehabilitation effort. Flexor tendons will heal if positioned without tension or stress; however, adhesions to surrounding tissue will prevent tendon gliding necessary to allow active flexion once the tendon has healed. Thus the need to move a flexor tendon early in the healing process has been evident since repair of flexor tendons has begun. **After repair it takes approximately 12 weeks for a flexor tendon to regain enough tensile strength to avoid rupture with normal strong use of the hand required to grasp, hold, or lift objects during daily activities.** A variety of protocols for flexor tendon rehabilitation have been developed over the past 50 years, making the choice of which protocol to use difficult. No exact method exists to determine the strength of a tendon repair during the healing process; therefore the therapist and surgeon rely on general guidelines regarding tendon healing, as well as factors that affect rate of healing to determine advancement of the patient within a flexor tendon rehabilitation protocol. The factors that are considered include the type of injury; status of the tendon, sheath, and vessels at the time of repair; injury to surrounding structures; patient health issues such as diabetes; and lifestyle factors such as smoking, which decreases oxygen to the tissues; and ability to comply with the rehabilitation program. Consideration of these factors and clear communication with the surgeon are necessary to determine the most appropriate approach to choose for each particular patient. Before describing the variety of guidelines from which to choose for flexor tendon rehabilitation, it is important to understand how exercise concepts are modified for flexor tendon repair rehabilitation.

CONCEPTS OF HEALING AND EXERCISES FOR FLEXOR TENDON REPAIR

Role of Adhesions After Flexor Tendon Repair

Adhesions occur very early in many cases, often within 1 week after surgery, preventing gliding of the flexor tendon needed to flex the digit. The end result of dense adhesions can be a digit that does not flex any further than it did before the tendon repair was performed, but with the additional pain, discomfort, and cosmetic changes caused by extensive surgical incisions in the digit, as well as many weeks of lost use of the hand while rehabilitation is attempted. Adhesions are the most difficult to deal with in zones I and II of the hand. Zones I and II extend from the distal palmar crease of the hand to the distal phalanx, and they incorporate the area of the digit in which the flexor tendons pass under a very tight pulley system, encompassed within a tendon sheath filled with synovial fluid that allows the tendon to glide under the tight pulleys (see Fig. 10-4). When adhesions form within the sheath-pulley system in zones I and II of the digit, they are very difficult (in many cases impossible) to overcome, and the result is a digit that is limited in active flexion. Historical perspectives on tendon healing help clinicians understand the reasoning behind current approaches to flexor tendon surgery and rehabilitation. Before the 1960s, flexor tendons were allowed to heal by immobilization for the first few weeks because it was thought that the tendon could not heal without nutrition from the surrounding scar tissue.[22] This immobilization for the first few weeks resulted in dense adhesions, especially with repairs in zones I and II, with inability to actively flex the digit. This led to the development of immediate passive-flexion

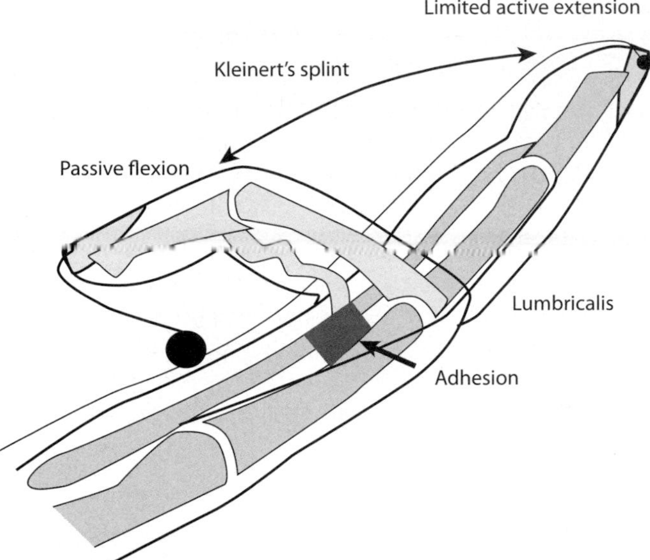

Fig. 10-5 Theoretical basis of passive flexion and limited active motion of interphalangeal (IP) joints do not always move the suture site of the digital flexor tendon. Passive flexion makes the distal segment of the tendon kink, which can be stretched by active extension of IP joints, without moving the suture site.
(From Tajima T: Indication and techniques for early postoperative motion after repair of digital flexor tendon particularly in zone II. In Hunter JM, Schneider LH, Mackin EJ (eds): *Tendon and nerve surgery in the hand: a third decade,* St Louis, 1997, Mosby, p 330.)

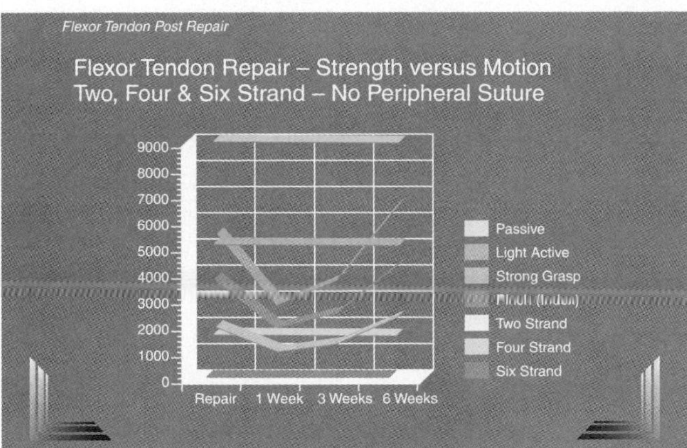

Fig. 10-6 Tensile strengths of flexor tendon repairs compared with the tension developed within the tendon with use of the hand. The comparison shows that at its weakest point after surgery, a two-strand repair is not strong enough to tolerate light gripping; however, four or more strand repairs have adequate tensile strength to tolerate light gripping.
(From Strickland JW, Cannon NM: Flexor tendon repair—*Indiana method, Indiana Hand Center Newsl* 1:4, 1993.)

protocols. The goal was that by passively flexing the digit and allowing partial, protected extension, the flexor tendon would glide far enough under the pulley system to prevent dense restricting adhesions and allow active motion when the tendon was adequately healed. However, in many cases, tendinous adhesions still developed. Research has shown that proximal gliding of the FDP tendon is inconsistent during passive flexion.[21] The flexor tendon, when the digit is passively flexed, is thought in some cases to kink, or bunch up, between the pulleys, rather than passively glide through the pulley system (Fig. 10-5). To ensure proximal gliding of the flexor tendon, an active contraction of the muscle is needed to pull the tendon proximally through the pulley system. Because ongoing research has shown that tendons do heal intrinsically without surrounding adhesions,[1,14,15] an effort to actively flex the repaired flexor tendon immediately after repair was initiated to prevent the onset of dense adhesions. To avoid rupture of the flexor tendon with active motion immediately after surgery, however, stronger suture techniques had to be developed.

Understanding Repair Strength

Flexor tendon surgery has undergone an evolution over the past 10 to 15 years. This evolution has resulted in the development of stronger suture repair techniques that will withstand the tension placed on the repair with controlled active flexion immediately after the repair. These new and stronger tendon repair techniques, as discussed in the earlier portion of this chapter, allow immediate controlled active motion without rupture, preventing the formation of dense adhesions. In general, the more strands of suture material that cross the tendon repair, the stronger the repair (Fig. 10-6).[20,24,25]

Traditional surgical procedure, using a two-strand repair, will tolerate passive motion, but is not shown to be sufficiently strong enough to tolerate active motion immediately after repair. A four-strand repair will tolerate gentle active motion. A six-strand repair (or more) will certainly tolerate active motion; however, it is technically demanding and may become so bulky as to not glide under the pulleys, creating friction, possible wearing, and eventual rupture. Thus a four-strand repair technique is frequently chosen for which to apply an immediate active motion protocol.

After the traditional two-strand repair, it is safe to perform immediate *passive-flexion* protocols (described later in the chapter), or where necessary by patient limitation, immobilization. Immediate *active-flexion* protocols are generally not applied to the tendon with a traditional two-strand technique, but require a stronger four-strand technique and must be discussed with the surgeon. It is extremely important for the therapist to understand the type of suture repair that was done for a flexor tendon repair, to ensure that the protocol chosen for a particular patient stays within the tension limits of the repair.

Edema Control and Scar Management After Flexor Tendon Repair

Elevation is essential in the early phase after flexor tendon repair, because other forms of edema control are limited by the continuous splinting. Shoulder, elbow, and cervical motion exercises are performed to help with lymphatic function and circulation. In the intermediate and late phases of flexor tendon healing, use of a light compressive wrap at night is appropriate. **This should not be used during the day, because compressive wraps will increase resistance to the flexor tendon during active flexion.** The therapist initiates massage of the scar (for firmness) and edema massage after sutures are removed; the patient can continue this process at home when made feasible by the presence of the splint. Commercially available scar management pads may be placed or formed over the scar, applied at night only, if scars become thickened or raised. Because the splint is worn full time in the early phase of the rehabilitation programs, it is difficult for the patient to safely apply the scar management pads at night, and they are often applied beginning in the intermediate phase for this reason.

> **Q** A new patient is scheduled for splint fabrication, evaluation, and treatment after repair of flexor tendons. No further information is available on the prescription. What steps should the therapist take before beginning the first session?

Passive-Flexion Exercises After Flexor Tendon Repair

Passive flexion of the digits is performed through all the phases of flexor tendon rehabilitation. Passive flexion of the digit after a flexor tendon repair places the repaired tendon on slack. Very little tension develops within the flexor tendon during passive flexion of the digit, as long as the patient is truly relaxed and not actively assisting the passive flexion.[18] After flexor tendon repair, a finger will become stiff because of swelling, incisional scarring, and pain if passive flexion is not performed within 1 week after the procedure. If passive flexion remains limited after sutures are removed, then other therapy techniques may be used to assist in regaining passive flexion, such as heat combined with stretch into flexion before manual passive flexion within the patient's pain tolerance.

Wrist Tenodesis Exercises After Flexor Tendon Repair

Wrist tenodesis exercises use wrist motion to assist in moving the flexor tendons. The wrist is flexed to comfortable tolerance, and the fingers allowed to gently straighten at all three joints. This will give the tendon slack at the wrist and glide the tendon distally during the finger extension. Next, the fingers are relaxed, the wrist is extended to 30 degrees, and the fingers are gently flexed. The wrist extension pulls the flexors slightly proximally and gives slack to the finger extensors, allowing the flexors to glide proximally (Fig. 10-7). The wrist tenodesis exercise

> **A** The therapist should contact the physician to determine the following:
>
> - The type of repair performed (to determine whether immediate passive- or immediate active-flexion approaches should be considered)
> - The surgeon's preference of elastic traction or static IP positioning in the splint
>
> If the surgeon is not available, the therapist should begin an immediate passive-flexion approach. If passive flexion is limited, then therapy should begin with the elastic traction splint. If passive flexion is 50% or better, then the therapist may consider the static IP positioning splint.

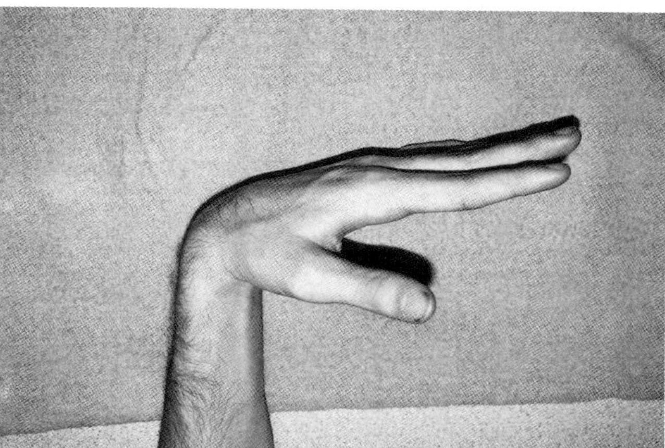
A

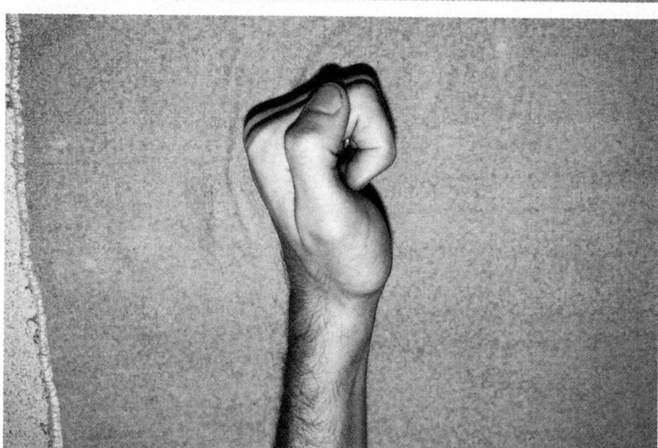
B

Fig. 10-7 **A,** The patient performs wrist tenodesis exercises by relaxing the wrist into flexion and extending the fingers to assist in gliding the flexor tendon distally. **B,** The wrist is then extended to 20 to 30 degrees while the fingers are gently flexed, to assist in gliding the flexor tendon proximally.
(Courtesy of Linda Klein.)

is started in the intermediate phase of rehabilitation after a two-strand repair, because it creates tension in the tendon. It is started within 3 days after surgery within an immediate active-flexion approach after a four-strand repair (unless otherwise directed by the physician).

Active Extension of the Fingers After Flexor Tendon Repair

Full extension of all three finger joints at the same time must be limited immediately after flexor tendon repair, to avoid pulling the repair apart by stretch. Extension is limited in the early phase of tendon healing by positioning within the dorsal blocking splint that places the metacarpophalangeal (MP) joints in flexion. However, interphalangeal (IP) extension is very important to obtain shortly after the repair in zones I and II, because the proximal interphalangeal (PIP) and distal interphalangeal (DIP) joints contract into flexion very quickly after repairs in these zones. All flexor tendon protocols emphasize attaining full IP extension immediately after surgery, unless a digital nerve has been lacerated or another injury prevents placement of the IP joints in full extension, as directed by the surgeon. When a digital nerve has been repaired in the digit, the PIP joint is generally allowed to extend to 15 degrees less than full extension. **Composite extension of all three finger joints at the same time will place adverse stretch effect on the flexor tendon repair in zone I or II initially after surgery, but it can be tolerated at 4 weeks after surgery with the wrist in flexion. Wrist and full finger extension are not performed at the same time until the late stage of tendon healing.**

Passive Finger Extension After Flexor Tendon Repair

Passive extension of the fingers is potentially more dangerous than active extension, because if done over aggressively, it may stretch the tendon repair apart. It is also possible for the patient to have some tension within the flexor tendon during the passive extension, resulting in resistance to the repaired tendon and possible rupture. **In the early phase of tendon healing, passive IP extension is only performed when active IP extension is limited (in the presence of PIP or DIP joint flexion contractures).** When IP joint flexion contractures appear early, passive IP joint extension can be performed carefully, with the flexor tendon in a protected position and ensuring that the patient's hand is fully relaxed. The protected position for a flexor tendon is with all other joints supported in flexion while one joint is extended. For instance, to treat a PIP flexion contracture 3 weeks after repair, the therapist flexes the wrist and MP joints as far as can be tolerated, then passively extends the PIP joint by applying pressure under the middle phalanx into extension. The DIP is not passively extended at the same time as the PIP joint to avoid stressing the tendon across two joints in the early phase of tendon healing.

> **Q** A new patient is being seen for the first time in therapy after repair of both flexor tendons at the level of the proximal phalanx of a single digit. During the initial visit, the patient begins to sweat, becomes light-headed, and has significant pain with gentle passive flexion. The patient is unable to tolerate more than 30 degrees of passive flexion at each of the IP joints of the injured finger. What can the therapist do to maximize tendon gliding and joint motion within the first week after surgery in the immediate passive- or immediate active-flexion approaches?

Active Finger Flexion After Flexor Tendon Repair

Active flexion introduces significantly increased tension in the repaired flexor tendon. Traditional approaches using immediate passive flexion or immobilization for the early phase of tendon healing introduce active flexion of the repaired digit in the intermediate phase of healing (4 weeks postoperatively). An assessment of flexor tendon gliding is done to determine what type of active flexion is appropriate. To assess flexor tendon gliding, passive flexion is compared with active flexion. **The initial assessment of active flexion is done cautiously, with the wrist in 20 to 30 degrees of extension** (Fig. 10-8). When a significant difference exists between passive flexion of the repaired digit, and active flexion (40- to 50-degree difference), it indicates the presence of adhesions, limiting tendon gliding. When flexor tendon adhesions limit active flexion significantly more than passive 4 weeks after surgery, active tendon-gliding exercises are initiated. Tendon gliding can be achieved by performing a sequence of three fists: hook fist, straight fist, and composite fist (Fig. 10-9). A hook fist is similar to a claw position, flexing the PIP and DIP joints with the MPs extended. This type of fist results in the largest differential gliding of the FDP and flexor digitorum superficialis and should be initiated cautiously. A straight fist results in the most excursion of the flexor digitorum superficialis. A composite fist results in the most excursion of the FDP tendon.

Active flexion is begun in the early phase of tendon healing when the patient is placed in an immediate active motion flexor tendon rehabilitation approach. At the first postoperative physician or therapy visit 2 to 3 days after surgery, a controlled method of active flexion termed *place-hold* is begun. Place-hold flexion uses the therapist's or patient's other hand to passively place the fingers into a light fist; then the patient holds the fingers actively in the light-fist position as the other hand is removed. This

A This patient is likely to have significant difficulty because of stiffness and adhesions unless he or she becomes more comfortable with passive motion of the digit within a few days. The patient's understanding of the cause of the pain and what to expect in the next few days is crucial at this point. A reassuring, gentle approach at the first appointment is important. The therapist should emphasize the following points:

- Most of the initial pain is related to a fresh incision, and swollen and sore joints need to be moved.
- Although the digit is very painful during the first attempts at motion, if performed to a tolerable level on a frequent basis (every 1½ to 2 hours), then the pain should be minimal within a few days.
- The finger motion may be permanently limited to the level of motion that is achieved within the first 1 or 2 weeks, because adhesions develop within this time. Explaining how a tendon glides and the way in which adhesions can limit this gliding helps motivate the patient to passively flex the digit to full tolerance. If allowed to be in an immediate active approach, then the position of active hold in flexion can only improve as passive flexion improves.

This patient may be best placed in an elastic traction approach between exercises, because the elastic traction will hold the digits in flexion at a tolerable level, gradually increasing flexion as resistance of the tissue decreases. The next session should be scheduled for the next day, because the patient is usually feeling better and can tolerate motion and better understand directions. If the pain level continues to significantly limit the initial exercises, then the therapist may perform slow, gentle passive flexion to demonstrate the methods to be used at home. Ongoing frequent therapy visits may be needed in the early phase of tendon healing if improvement is not seen quickly.

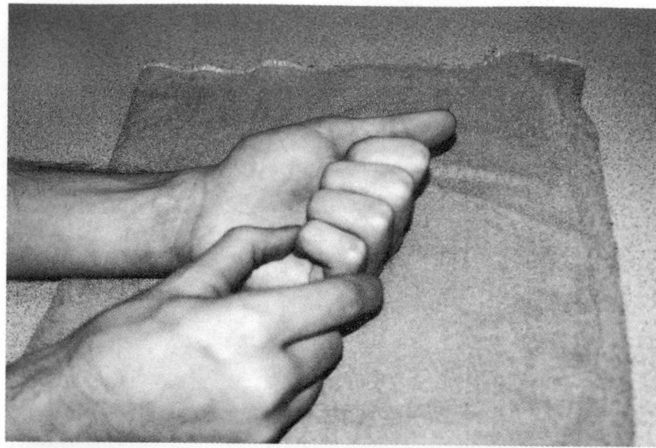
A

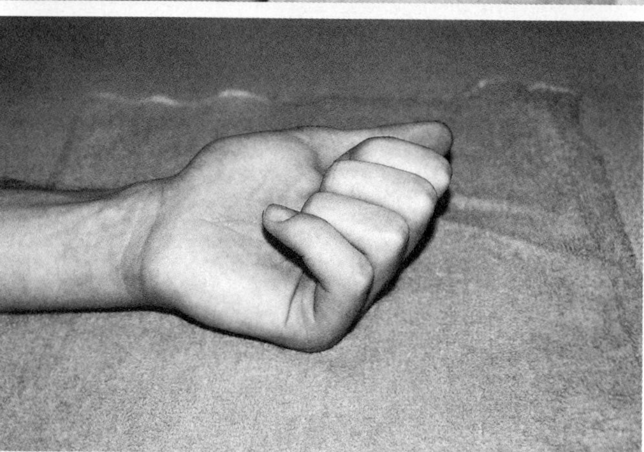
B

Fig. 10-8 The therapist assesses flexor tendon gliding by comparing passive flexion of the repaired digit (**A**) to active flexion (**B**). When a large difference exists between active and passive flexion, with passive flexion 40 or 50 degrees more than active, it signifies the presence of significant flexor tendon adhesions that limit active flexion.
(Courtesy of Linda Klein.)

requires an active muscle contraction and flexor tendon gliding in a proximal direction to keep the finger in a flexed position actively. The place-hold exercise is believed to result in less tension on the repaired tendon than if the finger were actively flexed without the assistance of the patient's opposite hand or the therapist's hand. **Within an immediate active motion approach, the three types of fists described earlier are not performed until the intermediate phase of tendon healing if flexor tendon adhesions develop in spite of early active motion attempts.**

There are three ways of making a fist:

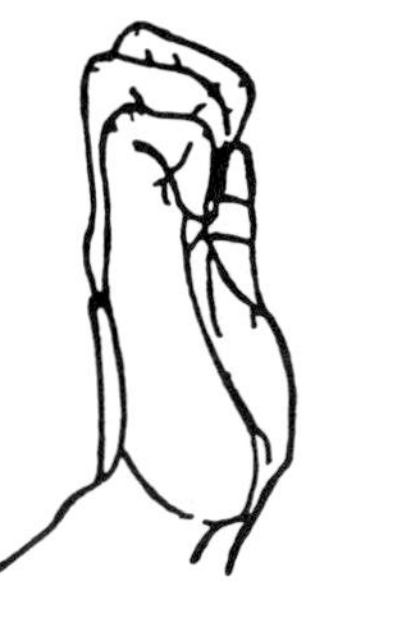

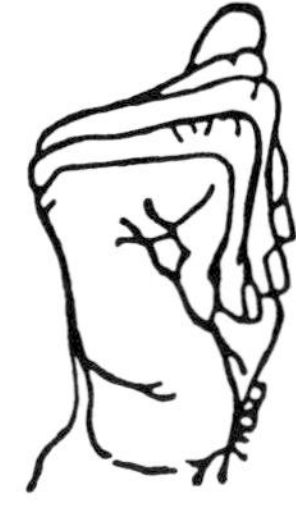

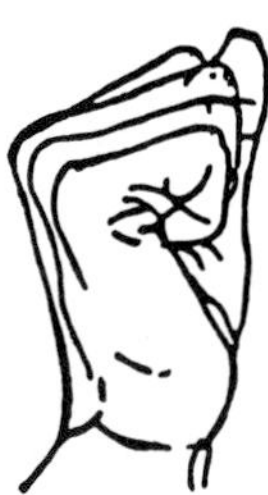

Fig. 10-9 Active flexor tendon gliding exercises consist of three positions: hook fist, straight fist, and full or composite fist.
(From Stewart Pettengill K, van Strien G: Postoperative management of flexor tendon injuries. In Mackin EJ et al, editors: *Rehabilitation of the hand,* ed 5, St Louis, 2002, Mosby, p 440.)

Postoperative Guidelines

In general, three types of flexor tendon rehabilitation guidelines exist. These are (1) immobilization, (2) immediate passive flexion, and (3) immediate active-flexion approaches. The reasoning for choosing one approach over another is based on the complexity of injury, the age of the patient, patient compliance, patient health factors, and the suture repair technique. The choice of which set of guidelines within which to place a patient is best determined in conjunction with the referring surgeon, with the final decision resting with the surgeon.

Within each approach the patient progresses through three general levels or phases: early, intermediate, and late phases. The decision of when to advance a patient to the next level within each approach is determined by the amount of flexor tendon adhesion that limits the tendon gliding and the amount of time after repair. To determine the level of flexor tendon adhesion, the therapist compares passive flexion to active flexion. When a large discrepancy exists between passive and active flexion, with passive flexion significantly better than active flexion (40- to 50-degrees difference), it signifies the presence of flexor tendon adhesions. When adhesions limit gliding of the flexor tendon (active flexion more limited than passive), *and* the time period after repair is adequate to allow increased tension on the tendon, the patient is progressed to the next level of the rehabilitation approach. **The tendon that does not have limiting adhesions is more at risk for rupture than the tendon with strong adhesions that surround the tendon repair site.** When tendon adhesions limit active flexion significantly more than passive flexion, the tendon can tolerate more tension before rupture, and thus can be advanced to the next level sooner than the tendon without limiting adhesions. Flexor tendon adhesions are assessed on a continual basis to determine the level of the rehabilitation program that is appropriate for the patient at that time. The time after surgery, combined with the level of flexor tendon adhesion, determines the placement of the patient in the program. When adhesions prevent gliding of the flexor tendon, it is appropriate to advance the patient to the next phase of rehabilitation to encourage tendon gliding, with surgeon approval. When flexor tendon gliding is adequate, the patient is kept in the current level of the program until the number of weeks after surgery dictates that the repair is strong enough to tolerate the increased tension of the next phase of the treatment protocol.

The appropriate choice of which guideline to use and advancement of the patient within the chosen guideline requires in depth knowledge of flexor tendon healing and tensile strength guidelines at various times after repair, awareness of the type of repair and the patient's compliance level, as well as communication with the referring surgeon.

IMMOBILIZATION APPROACH

Indications for Immobilization

Immobilization is rarely used after a flexor tendon repair; however, some situations call for its application. Immobilization is used for young children, who are unable to adhere to a motion protocol with its specific precautions. Children younger than age 12 are most often placed in immobilization for the first 3 to 4 weeks, but each child should be evaluated related to their maturity level. Other population types that may be placed in immobilization after a flexor tendon repair would be those that have cognitive limitations (e.g., Alzheimer's disease, noncompliant patients). It is sometimes difficult to know the patient's compliance ability at the first therapy session. When a patient demonstrates inability to appropriately comply with the precautions and exercises within a certain approach, it may become necessary to change the rehabilitation approach to one with less early motion, or a cast may be needed instead of a removable splint in the first 4 to 5 weeks after surgery. When a concomitant fracture or significant loss of skin requiring a skin graft occurs, a period of immobilization may be necessary to allow the bone or skin to heal adequately before beginning motion. Not all fractures require immobilization. Stable fractures or those that have had open reduction internal fixation may tolerate immediate controlled motion, as determined by the surgeon. Few sets of guidelines exist for therapy after immobilization of the repaired flexor tendon because of dense adhesion formation. The most frequently sited guideline, described as follows, encourages motion and light resistance to facilitate tendon gliding after the initial phase of tendon healing.[4,23]

Immobilization Guidelines

Phase I (Early)

TIME: 0 to 4 weeks
GOALS: Prevent joint stiffness, avoid tension on tendon repair, prevent flexion contractures, patient and family education regarding tendon protection, manage edema, full active range of motion (AROM) of upper extremity (UE) joints proximal to the wrist

Splinting

When used, the immobilization approach will place the patient's hand in a dorsal blocking cast (or in a dorsal blocking splint wrapped securely in place, with instructions not to remove the splint at home). The position of the cast or splint in the early phase of immobilization is 20- to 30-degrees wrist flexion, and 40- to 50-degrees MP flexion, with IP extension. This position keeps the flexor tendons on slack, yet prevents the most difficult joint problems (e.g., PIP flexion contractures). The cast or splint will stay in place for 3 to 4 weeks.

Exercises

With exercises in phase I (zero to 3 or 4 weeks after surgery) the patient generally remains immobilized in the dorsal blocking splint or cast. When referred to therapy during the early phase, the therapist may perform passive flexion to prevent joint stiffness and a significant other, such as a parent, may be taught to perform passive flexion at home if he or she is reliable. Goals in the early phase of the immobilization approach include protecting the repaired flexor tendon(s) from rupture with full time splinting and patient education, obtaining passive flexion when allowed, edema control, and obtaining full active motion of the UE proximal to the wrist.

> **Q** A patient had flexor tendons repaired in a digit 3 weeks ago. During active IP extension exercises, the patient is lacking 30 degrees of PIP extension and 10 degrees of DIP extension. What steps can be taken to improve IP extension?

Phase II (Intermediate)

TIME: 3 or 4 weeks to 6 weeks
GOALS: Improve joint mobility (full flexion passive range of motion [PROM], partial flexion AROM, full IP extension), patient and family education, scar management, splinting to prevent tendon repair rupture between exercises

Exercises

With phase II exercises, the splint position is adjusted to bring the wrist to neutral. The splint is removed for exercises hourly. Passive flexion is initiated first, to loosen stiff joints created by immobilization, swelling, and scarring. After passive flexion, wrist tenodesis is initiated as described previously, to begin gentle tendon gliding (see Fig. 10-7). Tendon-gliding exercises are initiated, with three types of fisting exercises (i.e., straight fist, hook fist, and composite fist; see Fig. 10-9), as described previously. Assessment of flexor tendon adhesions is performed after 3 to 4 days of these exercises by comparing passive flexion to active flexion of the digit or digits. When active flexion is significantly more limited than passive flexion (50 or more total degree difference between passive and active flexion of the finger joints), blocking exercises of the PIP and DIP joints are added. Additional flexor tendon gliding can be obtained with isolated tendon gliding exercises. The therapist can isolate the FDP tendon by blocking the MP and PIP in extension while performing active DIP flexion. The flexor digitorum superficialis (FDS) tendon is isolated with blocking of the FDP tendon by holding all other fingers in complete extension and allowing the injured finger to flex at the PIP joint. If improvement is noted in tendon gliding 1 week later, then these exercises are continued until 6 weeks postoperatively.

If no improvement occurs in active flexion with blocking and tendon gliding exercises, then light resistance of gripping with very soft putty is initiated at 5 weeks after surgery. Resistance is initiated in the intermediate phase of healing only in the presence of flexor tendon adhesions that limit active flexion significantly more than passive flexion. Extension of the fingers is performed with the wrist flexed. When PIP flexion contractures are present, limiting the PIP joints, DIP joints, or both from full extension, they are splinted in a volar extension splint at night, beginning at 4 or 5 weeks postoperatively. Goals in the intermediate phase of the immobilization approach include obtaining full passive flexion and partial active flexion, full IP extension, and protecting the repaired tendon from rupture with appropriate splinting between exercises and patient education, as well as scar management.

> **A** In therapy, *gentle* PIP joint mobilization (i.e., accessory glides and gentle passive PIP extension) can be considered with the flexor tendon in the protected position of full wrist and MP flexion. The patient *must* be relaxed, with no tension in the flexor tendons during the passive flexion, to avoid resisting the repaired flexor tendons.
>
> The therapist should emphasize the IP extension portion of the home exercise program. Full passive MP flexion assists IP extension. The patient should be instructed to passively flex the MP joint of the involved finger fully using the other hand while actively extending the IP joints. A dynamic IP extension splint should not be considered in this early phase of flexor tendon healing.

Phase III (Late)

TIME: 6 to 12 weeks
GOALS: Normalize PROM and AROM, improve strength to allow a "light fist," patient and family education to avoid tendon repair rupture

Exercises

This phase generally lasts from 6 to 12 weeks after surgery. All protective splinting is discontinued. When passive flexion continues to be limited by joint stiffness and swelling, therapeutic techniques such as heat and PROM are continued. Active flexion, joint blocking, and tendon gliding exercises continue, to attempt to bring active flexion to match the level of passive flexion. Resistance can be introduced or advanced during this phase. Light resistance can be provided with putty or light manual resistance of the therapist, and it can be advanced to light grippers in the middle of the late phase of tendon healing.

If flexor tendon adhesions are minimal, then resistance is initiated at 8 weeks after surgery, gently at first, with strong resistance restricted until after 12 weeks after surgery. Goals in the late phase of the immobilization approach include obtaining full passive and active flexion and extension of the injured finger or fingers, increasing strength to obtain a light fist, and protecting the repaired tendon from rupture with patient education.

Regardless of the goals, active motion after use of an immobilization approach is frequently limited because of adhesion formation. Limited active flexion of the repaired digit, especially the DIP joint, is frequently seen, and there may be difficulty actively flexing the adjacent digits because of the common muscle belly of the FDP to the last three digits (i.e., quadregia effect). Grip strength will be diminished secondary to loss of active flexion. It is common for flexor tendons with adhesions to require a more prolonged time of therapy, with a strong emphasis on a home program of blocking exercises and resistance even longer than the 12-week healing period, to continue to facilitate tendon gliding during the long remodeling process. Further surgical procedures are available for the repaired flexor tendon with significant adhesions that limit functional use of the hand, which are most often performed between 3 and 6 months after repair.

IMMEDIATE PASSIVE-FLEXION APPROACH

Immediate passive-flexion approaches apply passive flexion to the fingers, beginning within 3 or 4 days after surgery. These guidelines are appropriate for, and have been traditionally applied to, the patient with a two-strand repair of their flexor tendon. No active contraction of the repaired flexor muscle and tendon unit occurs; therefore limited proximal gliding of the flexor tendon occurs in the early phase of tendon healing within this approach. The benefits of an immediate passive-flexion approach are that the finger does not become overly stiff, and a limited amount of gliding of the repaired tendon occurs. Results vary widely regarding results of the immediate passive-flexion approach and tendinous adhesions. Two main categories encompass all the immediate passive-flexion guidelines. These two categories are approaches that use either elastic traction or static-positioning splints during the early phase of tendon healing. Both approaches use a dorsal blocking splint with the wrist at 20 to 30 degrees of flexion and the MPs at 50 to 60 degrees of flexion, with the IPs allowed full extension within the splint. The difference between the two approaches (the positioning of the fingers in either dynamic flexion or static IP extension in the early phase of healing) will be described within each guideline.

The static-positioning guideline follows the modified Duran and Houser[6,23] rehabilitation program, while the elastic traction guideline is patterned after the modified Kleinert,[12] Washington[5] or Chow[3] rehabilitation programs. These guidelines will be generalized in the following paragraphs.

Immediate Passive Flexion with Static-Positioning Guidelines

Patients are placed into an immediate passive-flexion approach that does not use elastic traction to the fingers when it is the preference of the surgeon and therapist or when elastic traction is contraindicated. These **contraindications include questionable soft tissue tolerance to prolonged flexion, early development of IP flexion contractures, or presence of a concomitant injury such as a fracture that would not tolerate passive flexion.**

Phase I (Early)

TIME: 0 to 4 weeks
GOALS: Attain full passive flexion, full active IP extension, minimize edema, prevent rupture of flexor tendon by splinting and patient education, full AROM of UE joints proximal to the wrist

Splinting

A dorsal blocking splint is fabricated and applied within the first 5 days after surgery. The wrist is placed in 20 to 30 degrees of flexion, the MP joints are placed in approximately 50 degrees of flexion, and the IP joints are straight (Fig. 10-10). The patient is instructed to remain in the splint at all times for the first 4 weeks after surgery. It is removed in therapy for cleansing of the skin and splint, as well as skin assessment for pressure and fit.

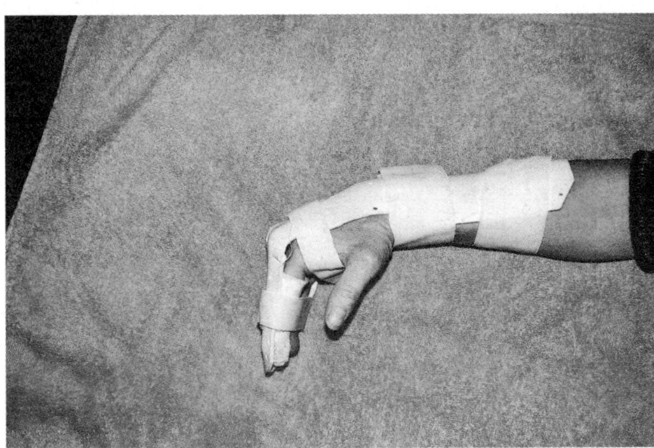

Fig. 10-10 Dorsal blocking splint with the wrist and metacarpophalangeal (MP) joints flexed keeps the repaired flexor tendon on slack during the early healing phase. It is used for the immobilization protocol and the immediate passive-flexion protocols that do not use elastic traction.
(Courtesy of Linda Klein.)

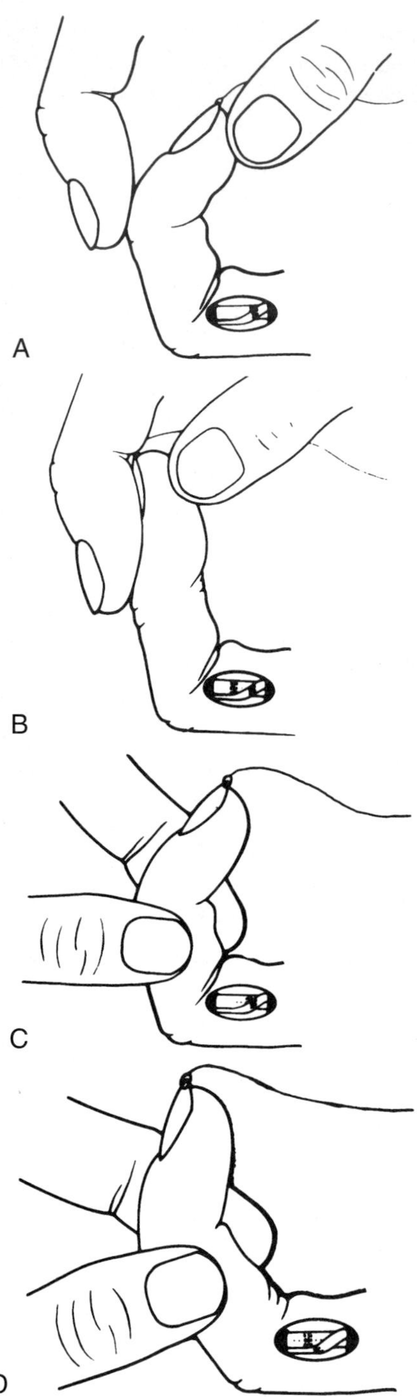

Fig. 10-11 Specific passive exercises described by Duran and Houser. With the metacarpophalangeal (MP) and PIP joints flexed (**A**), the distal phalanx is passively extended (**B**). This moves the flexor digitorum profundus (FDP) tendon distally away from the flexor digitorum superficialis tendon. The next step is with the DIP and MP flexed (**C**), the PIP joint is passively extended (**D**). This moves both repairs distally away from the site of repair and any surrounding tissues to which they may adhere.
(From Stewart Pettengill K, van Strien G: Postoperative management of flexor tendon injuries. In Mackin EJ et al, editors: *Rehabilitation of the hand, ed 5,* St Louis, 2002, Mosby, p 443.)

Exercises

Exercises should be performed in therapy and at home, 10 repetitions every hour. Within the splint, passive PIP flexion to tolerance, passive DIP flexion to tolerance, and then composite passive flexion of MP, PIP, and DIP joints to tolerance. Duran and Houser[23] described specific passive exercises (Fig 10-11). Active IP extension exercises to the hood of the dorsal blocking splint are also performed.

Q A patient had the flexor tendons repaired 5 weeks ago and has been advanced to the intermediate phase of an immediate passive approach, including gentle active motion. At this appointment, the patient shows a sudden decrease in active DIP flexion compared with the previous session, with trace to no visible active flexion noted by the therapist. What should the therapist consider?

Phase II (Intermediate)

TIME: 4 to 7 weeks
GOALS: Attain partial active flexion (at least 50%) of the injured digit, full passive flexion, full active extension, protect flexor tendon from rupture with splinting between exercises and patient education

Exercises

Exercises continue to be performed in therapy and at home, 10 repetitions every hour. Remove splint at home for exercises and bathing. Begin with wrist tenodesis exercises, and place-active hold flexion. Advance to gentle active-flexion exercises. If flexor tendon adhesions are noted (active flexion significantly more limited than passive flexion), then begin blocking exercises for PIP and DIP flexion. Active finger extension is performed with wrist flexed until 6 weeks, then with the wrist neutral. Passive IP extension is begun if PIP or DIP flexion contractures exist, with the tendon in a protected position.

A Whenever a sudden complete loss of flexion of the DIP joint occurs, a rupture of the FDP tendon must be considered. The therapist should have the patient make an appointment with the referring surgeon as soon as possible, because some surgeons consider immediate repair. Other surgeons wait for maturation of the healing process and consider later tendon grafting if a rupture occurs. The therapist should discuss the patient's activity level to determine if he or she has used the hand actively, which would place the patient at risk for rupture. The therapist should check tendon integrity by blocking the PIP joint in extension while the patient attempts to actively flex the DIP joint. Any active DIP flexion indicates that the FDP tendon is intact.

Phase III (Late)

TIME: 7 to 12 weeks

GOALS: Attain full active and passive flexion and extension of digits, light grip strength, protect repaired tendon from rupture with patient education

Discontinue use of splint. Continue with active motion exercises. If flexor tendon adhesions are present, then begin light resistive exercises. Dynamic IP extension splinting after 8 weeks is initiated if flexion contractures persist. At 12 weeks after surgery, the patient is allowed to perform normal activities.

IMMEDIATE PASSIVE FLEXION WITH ELASTIC TRACTION APPROACH

Indications

Elastic traction was added to the early phase of the passive-flexion guidelines described previously in an attempt to increase proximal tendon gliding by placement of the fingers in flexion between exercises, in part by allowing more time for the tendon to be resting proximally in relation to the repair site and to the pulley system. It also decreases stiffness of the digits in the direction of flexion by applying passive flexion for a greater portion of time. **Placement in passive flexion with elastic traction to the fingers between exercises also decreases the potential for even inadvertent active flexion of the fingers in the early phase of flexor tendon healing, protecting the tendon from rupture.** The negative effect of elastic traction is the increased potential to develop IP flexion contractures, as well as the increase in complexity perceived by the patient by having a dynamic splint on the hand (as opposed to a less complicated static splint). Patients are placed into this approach by preference of the surgeon-therapist team (those patients that are not showing signs of IP flexion contracture, those that can be compliant with the rehabilitation program, and those who have no soft tissue healing complication).

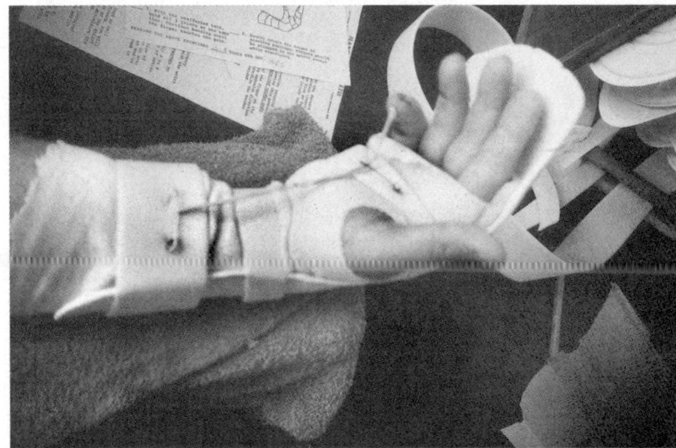

A

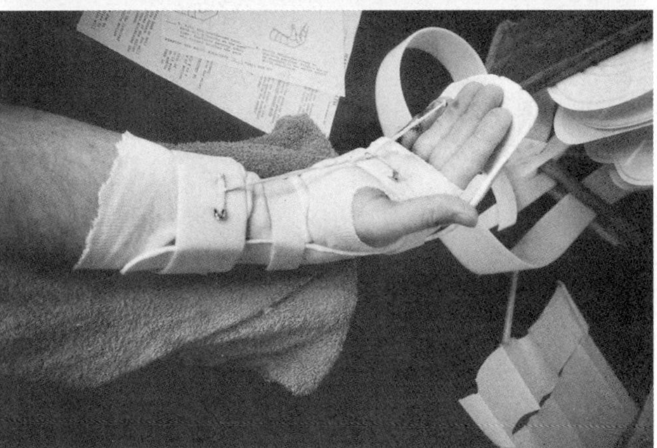

B

Fig. 10-12 A, Dorsal blocking splint with elastic traction places the metacarpophalangeal (MP) joints and wrist in partial flexion and attaches an elastic band to the fingertip of the injured finger. B, Exercises are to fully passively flex the digit and to actively extend the IP joints to the hood of the splint.
(Courtesy of Linda Klein.)

Immediate Passive Flexion with Elastic Traction Guidelines

Phase I (Early)

TIME: zero to 4 weeks

GOALS: Attain full passive flexion, full active IP extension, minimize edema, prevent rupture of flexor tendon with splinting and patient education, full AROM of UE joints proximal to the wrist

Splinting

The splint applied for this approach is the same dorsal blocking splint base as described for the static position approach, with the addition of elastic traction applied from the fingertip of the injured finger or fingers, which passes under a distal palmar pulley and is connected at the midforearm level to the proximal splint strap on the volar forearm (Fig. 10-12, A). The wrist is in 20 to 30 degrees flexion, the MP joints in 50 to 60 degrees flexion, and the IP joints straight. The elastic traction may consist of rubber bands, rubber band and monofilament line combination, or other elastic thread. It can be attached to the tip of the finger by a suture placed by the surgeon through the fingernail or an attachment such as a dress hook glued to the fingernail. Some therapists have also used self-adhesive moleskin or other fabric with a hole for the elastic traction attachment applied to the fingertip. The line is threaded through a pulley at the level of the distal palmar crease and attached at the level of the forearm, generally to the proximal splint strap, around a safety pin. The distal palmar pulley concept is important, because it achieves passive DIP flexion. A safety pin in the strap across the palm is a simple method to obtain the distal palmar pulley. Other methods of designing a distal palmar pulley include line guides or D rings embedded in splint material that is brought across the palm.

It is important to assess IP extension on an ongoing basis because of increased potential for PIP and DIP flexion contractures (a result of the increased time in flexion during the day). Most therapists instruct the patient to remove the proximal attachment of the elastic traction at night, to allow the fingers to be strapped to the dorsal hood of the splint. The splint is worn full time for the first 4 weeks. It is removed in therapy for skin and splint cleansing and for skin assessment of pressure areas.

Exercises

Exercises should be performed in therapy and at home, 10 repetitions every hour. Passive flexion of the fingers is performed within the splint. Full passive PIP flexion, DIP flexion, and composite finger flexion are performed passively to the strap across the palm. Full active PIP and DIP extension are performed within the splint, to the dorsal hood of the splint (Fig. 10-12, B). It is important to maintain full IP extension, especially within this protocol, unless a digital nerve repair has been made. Goals in the early phase of the immediate passive-flexion approaches include attaining full passive flexion and active IP extension, tendon gliding as possible within these exercises, edema control, protecting the repaired flexor tendon from rupture with appropriate splinting and patient education, and attaining full UE motion proximal to the wrist.

Phase II (Intermediate)

TIME: 4 to 7 or 8 weeks
GOALS: Attain partial (at least 50%) active flexion of the injured digit, full passive flexion, full active extension, protect repaired tendon from rupture with splinting between exercises and patient education

Exercises

Exercises should continue as in phase I, and the patient can remove the splint for exercises and bathing. In therapy and at home, active flexion is initiated. Begin with wrist tenodesis exercises and gentle place-active hold in flexion exercises. Advance to active flexion and composite finger extension with the wrist flexed. At 6 weeks, discontinue protective splinting and begin active extension of the fingers with the wrist in neutral. **If flexor tendon adhesions are noted (passive flexion is significantly better than active flexion), then blocking exercises are initiated for PIP and DIP flexion.** Goals in the intermediate phase of the immediate passive-flexion programs include attaining at least half range of active flexion of the injured digit, full passive flexion, full active finger extension, and protecting the repaired tendon from rupture with appropriate splinting between exercises and patient education.

Phase III (Late)

TIME: 7 or 8 to 12 weeks
GOALS: Full active and passive flexion and extension, light grip strength, protect repaired tendon from rupture with patient education

Splinting is discontinued and light active use is initiated. If flexor tendon adhesions are present, then advance to light resistive exercises at 8 weeks after surgery. **If good tendon gliding is evidenced by equal or nearly equal active and passive flexion, then delay resistance until 10 to 12 weeks after surgery and advance gradually.** If IP flexion contractures are present, then passive IP extension exercises and dynamic IP extension splinting may be initiated with surgeon approval. Goals in the late phase of the immediate passive-flexion approaches include full active and passive flexion and extension, regaining light grip strength, and protecting the repaired tendon from rupture with patient education. Full grip and pinch strength can be performed as part of a home exercise program after 12 weeks after surgery, at which time the repaired flexor tendon is considered to be strong enough to tolerate normal daily activities.

In general, when a digit with a repaired flexor tendon demonstrates good active flexion within the first 5 or 6 weeks after surgery, advancement to resistance is delayed, because minimal additional support of adhesions to the repair site exists. When flexor tendon adhesions limit active flexion significantly more than passive flexion, the digit can be advanced through the phases listed previously at the earlier of the times indicated, as the tendon has the support of surrounding adhesions and can tolerate the additional tension applied within the advancing phases of treatment with less chance of rupture. The decision to advance a patient with a flexor tendon injury to the next phase of treatment is best done in conjunction with the referring surgeon, because advancing the partially healed flexor tendon to active flexion, passive extension, and most significantly, resistance, creates an increase in tension at the repair site.

Full passive flexion and nearly full extension of the injured finger or fingers should be the expected result of use of an immediate passive-flexion approach (however, active DIP flexion may be limited). Extension is occasionally limited as well. When composite extension of the wrist and digits is limited in the late phase of tendon healing, a resting pan splint in maximum composite extension, worn at night, will help distal gliding of the tendon to allow composite extension. A finger-length splint may be used if just the IP joints are contracted in flexion.

Functional deficits in motion or strength present after 12 weeks can be treated with any traditional therapy approaches, including modalities and dynamic splinting for stiffness or contractures, AROM and PROM, joint mobilization, blocking exercises, and strengthening.

IMMEDIATE ACTIVE-FLEXION APPROACH

Indications

Development of immediate active-flexion guidelines is the most recent advancement in rehabilitation after flexor tendon repairs. These guidelines have been developed after the onset of surgical advancements of stronger repair techniques described earlier in this chapter. Active-flexion approaches have been developed to minimize flexor tendon adhesions in the early phase of tendon healing and have been very successful in improving outcomes of flexor tendon repairs.[7,11,20,26] Immediate active-flexion approaches are reserved for patients who have had a strong enough surgical repair to tolerate the additional stress placed on the tendon by active flexion, as well as those who can be compliant to the splinting and exercise program. **The presence of severe edema, joint stiffness, or health factors that would slow tendon healing would prohibit placement of a patient in an active-flexion approach.** It is important to minimize the stress on the tendon, especially in the early phase of tendon healing, to prevent rupture.

Minimizing Tension on a Tendon Within Immediate Active-Flexion Approaches

Because active flexion results in an increase in tension within the flexor tendon, it is important to minimize this tension in the early phase of tendon healing, to prevent rupture. Edema and stiffness both present increased resistance to active flexion, thereby requiring the flexor muscles to pull harder on the tendon, increasing the work of flexion within an immediate flexion protocol. *Work of flexion* is a term that describes the amount of tension created within the tendon during active flexion.[8] Work of flexion increases with swelling, stiffness, or any internal friction encountered by the tendon caused by bulk of repair, tight pulleys, or swelling of the tendons, in addition to the tension normally developed during active flexion. The therapist's goal is to minimize the work of flexion, thereby minimizing stress on the repaired tendon, when active motion is initiated immediately after repair. The therapist does this by minimizing edema and joint stiffness and using optimal joint positions that minimize the amount of tension developed within the tendon during active flexion. Studies have shown that the wrist position that results in the least tension within the flexor tendon during active flexion is partial wrist extension and MP flexion.[18] **When the wrist is flexed, a significantly increased amount of work is required by the flexor muscles to flex the fingers, compared with when the wrist is slightly extended. By placing the wrist in slight extension, the extensor tendons are given slack at the wrist, allowing the fingers to relax into partial flexion.** It requires only a slight pull by the muscle to further flex the digits actively into a light fist. Thus most immediate active-flexion protocols use a position of wrist neutral to slightly extended during the active-flexion exercises, and avoid active digit flexion with the wrist flexed. Attaining the end ranges of active flexion also significantly increases tension within the flexor tendon, and achieving a light fist with at least 45 degrees of DIP flexion is the main goal in the early phase of tendon healing. More than 45 degrees of DIP flexion is allowed if attained easily by the patient, without excessive effort, when the surgeon has performed a four-strand (or more) repair. Education of the patient placed in this protocol is very important, because those patients that attempt to do more than allowed are much more likely to rupture.

Immediate Active-Flexion Guidelines

Phase I (Early)

TIME: 0 to 4 or 5 weeks
GOALS: Attain full passive flexion, ability to actively hold the fingers in a light fist, minimize edema, protect flexor tendon from rupture with splinting and patient education, attain full UE motion proximal to the wrist

Splinting

A large variety of splints have been developed to apply when he or she is placed in an immediate active-flexion approach. The splint design was changed to bring the wrist into an optimal position, as described previously, during the exercises that are done at home. The wrist position in the traditional protocols (immobilization and passive-flexion protocols) was that of flexion, to place the repaired flexor tendon on slack and prevent tension on the tendon at rest. During active digit flexion, however, the wrist is better placed in a position of slight extension, as described earlier, to prevent excessive tension within the tendon during active flexion. A few of the most commonly used splints will be described; however, additional options are sure to exist, because splinting and guidelines are evolving constantly.

The Indiana protocol uses a wrist hinge splint that allows 30 degrees of wrist extension and full wrist flexion, applied for exercises only (Fig. 10-13, A and B).[26] A static dorsal blocking splint with the wrist and MPs flexed is worn at all times between the active exercises in the early phase of tendon healing. This requires that the patient be trusted to change splints at home for exercises without inadvertent stretch applied to the tendon, or use of the hand while the splint is removed. The wrist hinge splint, worn for exercises, maximizes use of the wrist tenodesis exercises and ideal wrist position of partial extension during active flexion of the fingers.

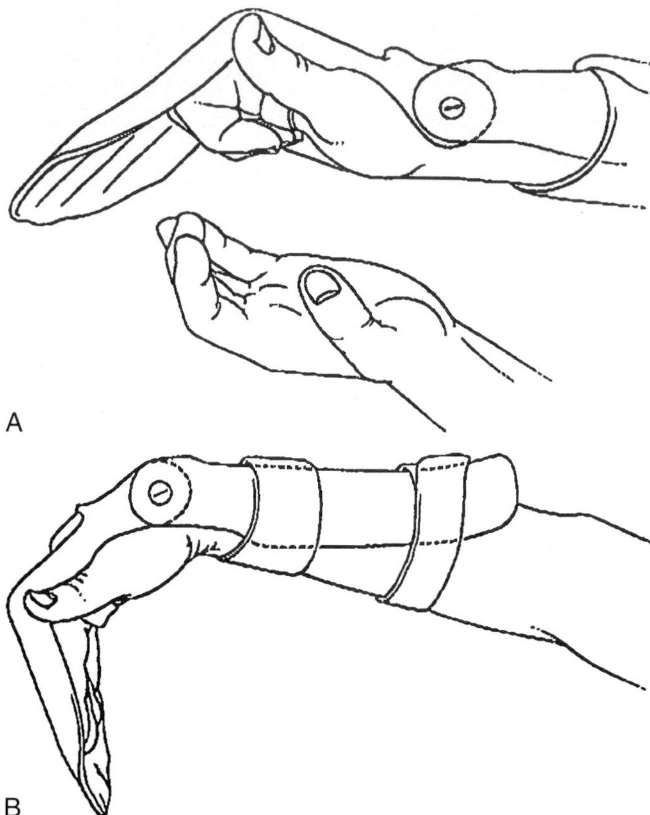

Fig. 10-13 The wrist hinge splint, designed at the Indiana Hand Center, allows 30 degrees wrist extension while performing place-hold flexion (**A**) and wrist flexion with IP extension (**B**).
(From Cannon N: Post flexor tendon repair motion protocol, *Indiana Hand Center Newsl* 1:13, 1993.)

Silfverskiold and May[20] use a cast (with the wrist neutral) that is worn at all times, for both exercises and at rest between exercises. Elastic traction is applied to all four fingers regardless of the number of injured fingers, and the elastic traction is removed or loosened for the active-flexion exercises. This concept eliminates the need for the patient to change splints at home, yet achieves the need to bring the wrist out of the flexed position for exercises. This author has used this wrist-neutral concept for both splinting and exercises.[11] The author's preferred splint is a dorsal blocking splint with the wrist in neutral, MP joints flexed to 50 degrees, and the IP joints allowed full extension unless a digital nerve has been repaired. The use of elastic traction with this splint is optional. When IP flexion contractures are beginning, the fingers may simply be strapped to the dorsal hood of the splint between exercises. If desired, then elastic traction is applied to all four fingers (or if the thumb flexor tendon was repaired, then elastic traction is applied to the tip of the thumb only), through a palmar pulley, attached on the proximal strap of the forearm (Fig. 10-14, A). The splint is not allowed to be removed at home by the patient in the early phase of tendon healing, but it is removed in therapy for splint and skin cleansing and assessment of skin for pressure areas, as well as for wrist tenodesis exercises. The author's preferred approach for a flexor tendon injury with a four-strand repair follows.

Exercises

Exercises should be performed in therapy and at home, 10 repetitions every hour. The splint is worn at all times. Passive flexion of the digits to the palm is initiated. Active extension of the IP joints is performed fully unless a digital nerve has been repaired (Fig. 10-14, B). The active-flexion portion of the exercises is performed with place-active hold in flexion of the fingers. This is performed by gently, passively flexing the fingers to the palm using the patient's other hand or the therapist's hand. After placing the fingers into gentle flexion, the other hand is removed, while the patient actively holds the fingers of the injured hand in the fist (Fig. 10-14, C and D). It is important to attain DIP flexion during this exercise to ensure FDP gliding. **The patient should not place pressure on the palm or squeeze the palm with any fingertips to avoid increasing tension within the tendon.** The place-active hold flexion portion of the exercise is the main difference between the immediate active and immediate passive-flexion guidelines. When the patient is successful in maintaining the actively flexed position of the digits without the repaired digit being trapped or overly supported by the adjacent digit, proximal gliding of the repaired tendon through the pulley system and the area of surgery has been achieved. This place-active hold exercise of the digits is important to obtain within the first 5 days after surgery, or flexor tendon adhesions are much more likely to limit the ability to gain full active flexion at a later time. If active flexion and passive flexion are nearly equal, then it indicates good to excellent flexor tendon gliding. If good flexor tendon gliding occurs, the patient is continued in this phase longer than six weeks because increased tension within the well-gliding tendon is more likely to cause a rupture than in the adherent tendon (where the tendon is supported by the surrounding scar tissue). If IP flexion contractures develop, then passive PIP extension may be performed with the wrist and MP supported in flexion, as described in the previous discussion of passive IP extension exercises. **Avoid pushing on the DIP joint while performing passive PIP extension in the early phase of tendon healing.** Goals in the early phase of an immediate active-flexion rehabilitation program include attaining full passive flexion, ability to actively hold in a light fist including at least 75 degrees of PIP and 45 degrees of DIP flexion, full PIP and DIP extension, edema control, protecting the flexor tendon from rupture with appropriate splinting and patient education, and attaining full UE motion proximal to the wrist.

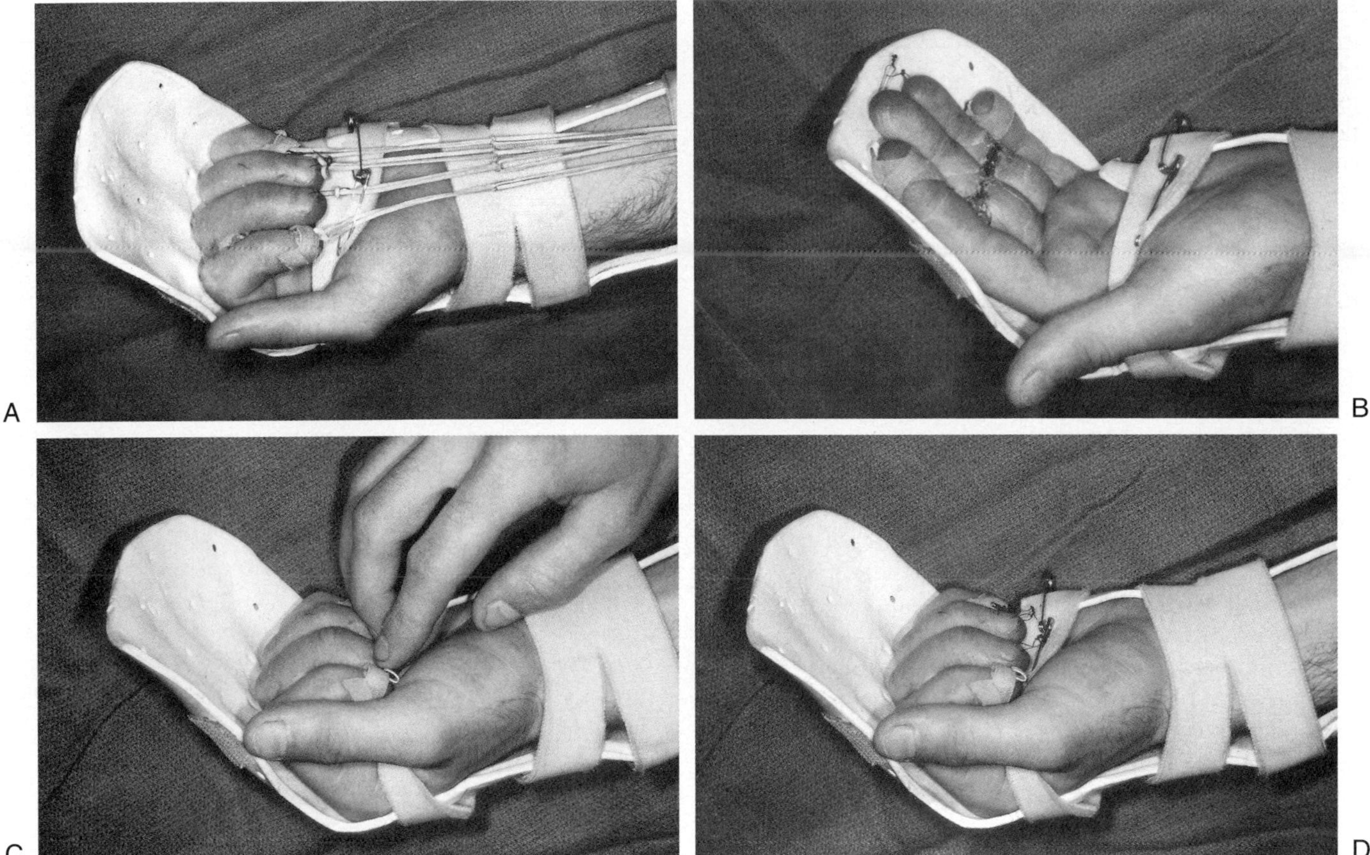

Fig. 10-14 Wrist-neutral dorsal blocking splint with elastic traction used in an immediate active-flexion protocol. Elastic traction is applied to all fingertips between exercises in this option (**A**). Exercises consist of active extension to the hood of the splint with elastic traction released (**B**) and place-active hold in flexion (**C** and **D**). The fingers are gently placed in flexion with the other hand and actively held in flexion when the supporting hand is removed. This requires proximal gliding of the flexor tendon, minimizing potential adhesions in the early phase of healing in an immediate active-flexion protocol after a four-strand or stronger repair technique.
(Courtesy of Linda Klein.)

Q A patient had flexor tendon repair 7 weeks ago. The finger has 30 degrees active DIP flexion when the PIP is blocked in extension by the therapist but no active DIP flexion when all finger joints are flexed into a fist. What does this mean?

Phase II (Intermediate)

TIME: 4 to 5 weeks to 8 weeks
GOALS: Attain full passive and active flexion and full finger extension, protect the repaired flexor tendon from rupture with splinting between exercises and patient education

Exercises

The splint is removed at home for bathing and exercises. If elastic traction was used in the early phase, then it is discontinued at this time and the static splint is worn between exercises to protect the patient against inadvertent resistance to the well-gliding tendon. Exercises continue as in the early phase, with the addition of full finger extension with the wrist flexed, gradually bringing the wrist to neutral with the fingers extended within the intermediate phase. **Active finger flexion is added during this phase, but no resistance is allowed.** Wrist tenodesis exercises are performed, allowing wrist extension as tolerated with the fingers relaxed in flexion and wrist flexion as tolerated. Some protocols discontinue the protective splint in the intermediate phase; however, with a well-gliding flexor tendon, it is possible to rupture the repaired tendon when resistance is encountered during normal daily activities. Most patients are not able to predetermine how much resistance each activity they perform with the hand will cause, and this author prefers to **continue splinting during the intermediate phase unless flexor tendon adhesions are present.** If flexor tendon adhesions limit active flexion more than passive flexion, then blocking exercises are initiated. If IP extension is limited, then passive IP extension is performed with the MPs held in flexion. Goals in the intermediate phase of the immediate active-flexion guideline include full passive and active flexion, full composite finger extension, and protecting the flexor tendon from rupture with appropriate splinting between exercises and patient education.

> **A** The FDP tendon has adhesions. When the finger is held in extension at the MP and PIP joints, it takes only a small amount of glide of the FDP tendon to result in partial DIP joint flexion. However, when the MP and PIP joints are flexed, such as in a composite fist, the FDP tendon must glide much further to pick up the slack created in the tendon by flexion of the first two joints of the finger before it can then flex the DIP joint. Adhesions limit full gliding of the tendon. The therapist should consider increasing the exercises of blocking, gradually increasing the amount of flexion at which the MP and PIP joints are blocked. The surgeon should be contacted to discuss the potential of adding ultrasound or light resistance to minimize adhesions.

Phase III (Late)

TIME: 8 to 14 weeks

GOALS: Full active flexion and extension of the fingers, prevent or minimize intrinsic tightness, prevent flexor tendon from rupture with splinting during resistive activities and patient education

The splint is removed except for activities that require pinching, lifting, or strong grip. Resistance to DIP flexion (e.g., hook grasp with resistance or squeezing with the tips of the fingers) is prohibited with a well-gliding flexor tendon that demonstrates flexion in the good to excellent range according to the Strickland-Glogovac formula.[26] **A small hand-based dorsal blocking splint is used to prevent the patient from performing this type of activity while at work or during heavier home management tasks.** Exercises are performed as previously described, adding intrinsic stretches with the wrist flexed. If flexor tendon adhesions are present (active flexion more limited than passive flexion), then resistance may be added during this phase, consisting of light gripping and blocking exercises. At 12 weeks after surgery, the patient is released to normal activities and instructed to avoid maximal resistive activities for another 2 weeks, gradually increasing tolerance to normal activities during this period. Goals in the late phase of the immediate active motion approach include full active flexion and extension of the fingers, prevention of intrinsic tightness, and light functional use of the hand. **Prevention of flexor tendon rupture with appropriate splinting during tip pinch, strong grip and hook fist, or lifting activities, as well as patient education is emphasized.**

Regaining full grip, pinch, and full UE strength is appropriate after the 12- to 14-week flexor tendon healing process (through traditional strengthening exercises and activities).

REPAIRS IN ZONES PROXIMAL TO ZONE II

The question often arises regarding guidelines for flexor tendon repairs in other zones of the hand and distal forearm. This author uses the same guidelines described previously for all zones. Less complications of flexor tendon adhesions occur when the tendons are repaired in the midpalm, where no tight pulley system and synovial sheath is found in which to become adherent. At the wrist and distal forearm, however, there remains the problem of adhesions to the flexor retinaculum and the carpal tunnel. These areas respond more easily to efforts at regaining tendon gliding in the intermediate and late phases of tendon healing and rehabilitation than does the digit. When the repair is anywhere other than the digit itself, IP flexion contractures are much less common.

EVALUATING THE RESULTS OF A FLEXOR TENDON REPAIR

Adding flexion of the IP joints and subtracting any loss of extension is the method used to evaluate the motion of a finger in which a flexor tendon has been repaired in the hand. Although a number of formulas exist, Strickland and Glogovac's formula[27] is commonly used (at bottom of page).

$$\frac{(\text{PIP} + \text{DIP flexion}) - (\text{loss of PIP extension} + \text{loss of DIP extension})}{175} \times 100 = \%\text{ of normal}$$

To clarify the formula, add PIP flexion + DIP flexion (measured in full-fist composite flexion). From this total, subtract any loss of extension of the PIP and DIP joints, measured in full composite extension. Divide the result by 175, and multiply by 100 to determine the percent of normal motion. The normal amount of PIP and DIP flexion is 175 degrees, and zero is the normal loss of extension of the IP joints. Thus if the total active PIP and DIP flexion equals 175 degrees and no loss of extension of the IP joints occurs, then the patient would have 100% of motion after the flexor tendon repair. Classification includes excellent results as 85% to 100%, good as 70% to 84%, fair as 50% to 69%, and poor as less than 50% of normal motion.

An example is a patient whose final composite motion measurements are MP zero to 85 degrees, PIP 10 degrees loss of extension to 80 degrees of flexion, and DIP 5 degrees loss of extension to 40 degrees of flexion. The formula applied would be as follows:

$$\frac{(80 + 40) - (10+5)}{175} \times 100\% \text{, which is}$$

$$\frac{120 - 15}{175} \times 100\% = 60\%$$

Sixty percent would be classified as a fair result according to this classification. MP motion is not used in this formula, because it is infrequently affected by tendon repairs in zones I or II. Results in the good and excellent categories are considered functional, without need for further intervention. Fair and poor results may need further surgery or therapeutic intervention to regain function of the hand, depending on individual patient needs for ADLs and work.

SUMMARY

The amount of information available regarding flexor tendon rehabilitation is overwhelming, and the task of determining what approach to use for which patient is daunting. Patient and injury variables require the therapist to be aware of immobilization, immediate passive flexion, and immediate active-flexion guidelines for treatment of a flexor tendon repair. Within each hand treatment facility, it is typical to use one approach from the immediate passive-flexion group and one approach from the immediate active-flexion group for most patients. Then, depending on the type of surgical repair, the recommendation of the surgeon and patient compliance, placement of the patient within immediate passive- or immediate active-flexion approach is less complex. It is good, however, to be familiar with other options, because some patients will do better with elastic traction than others. Most of this author's patients are placed in the immediate active flexion with elastic traction program as described previously, because the referring surgeons are all performing four-strand repairs of the flexor tendon.

For those therapists whose patients have traditional two-strand flexor tendon repairs, it is important to choose from the passive-flexion guidelines. If active flexion is performed with these patients in the early phase, then it is done very gently through partial range of flexion (and only under the supervision of the therapist).[7]

It is important to keep in mind the occasional need to place a patient in an immobilization approach, as well. Individualization of each of the guidelines is necessary. A young child may not advance as quickly as the immobilization guideline described in this chapter indicates. Discussion with the referring surgeon is necessary at each advancement point.

Understanding the concepts of flexor tendon healing in the hand and the tensile strengths of the healing tendon compared with tension demands of motion and use is important. Education of the patient regarding importance of compliance with the instructions within the guidelines and the type of activity that is likely to result in rupture is important. Study of literature and supervised experience in treating patients with this diagnosis is strongly recommended whenever possible.

References

1. Becker H et al: Intrinsic tendon cell proliferation in tissue culture, *J Hand Surg* 6:616-619, 1981.
2. Bunnell S: Repair of tendons in the fingers and description of two new instruments, *Surg Gynecol Obstet* 26:103-110, 1918.
3. Chow JA et al: A splint for controlled active motion after flexor tendon repair. Design, mechanical testing and preliminary clinical results, *J Hand Surg* 15A:645, 1990.
4. Cifaldi Collins D, Schwarze L: Early progressive resistance following immobilization of flexor tendon repairs, *J Hand Ther* 4:111, 1991.
5. Dovelle S, Kulis Heeter P: The Washington regimen: rehabilitation of the hand following flexor tendon injuries, *Phys Ther* 69:1034, 1989.
6. Duran RJ et al: Management of flexor tendon lacerations in zone 2 using controlled passive motion postoperatively. In Hunter JM et al, editors: *Rehabilitation of the hand*, ed 3, St Louis, 1990, Mosby, pp 410-413.
7. Evans RB, Thompson DE: The application of force to the healing tendon, *J Hand Ther* 6:266-284, 1993.
8. Halikis MN et al: Effect of immobilization, immediate mobilization, and delayed mobilization on the resistance to digital flexion using a tendon injury model, *J Hand Surg* 22A:464-472, 1997.
9. Joyce ME, Lou J, Manske PR: Tendon healing—molecular and cellular regulation. In Hunter JM, Schneider LH, Mackin EJ, editors: *Tendon and nerve surgery in the hand—a third decade*, St Louis, 1997, Mosby, pp 286-296.
10. Kessler I, Nissim F: Primary repair without immobilization of flexor tendon division within the digital sheath: an experimental and clinical study, *Acta Orthop Scand* 40:587-601, 1969.
11. Klein L: Early active motion flexor tendon protocol using one splint, *J Hand Ther* 16(3):199-206, 2003.
12. Kleinert HE et al: Primary repair of lacerated flexor tendons in "no man's land," *J Bone Joint Surg* 49:577, 1967.
13. Kobayashi M, Oka M, Toguchida J: Development of polyvinyl alcohol-hydroget (PV-H) shields with a high water content for tendon injury repair, *J Hand Surgery* 26B(5):436-440, 2001.
14. Lundborg G, Rank F: Experimental intrinsic healing of flexor tendons based upon synovial fluid nutrition, *J Hand Surg* 3(1)3:21-31, 1978.

15. Manske PR, Lesker PA: Biochemical evidence of flexor tendon participation in the repair process-an in vitro study, *J Hand Surg* 9B(2):117-120,1984.
16. Moran S et al: Effects of 5-fluorouracil on flexor tendon repair, *J Hand Surg* 25A(2):242-251, 2000.
17. Savage R: The influence of wrist position on the minimum force required for active movement of the interphalangeal joints, *J Hand Surg* 13B:262-268, 1988.
18. Schuind F et al: Flexor tendon forces: in vivo measurements, *J Hand Surg* 17A(2):291-298, 1992.
19. Shaieb MD, Singer DI: Tensile strengths of various suture techniques, *J Hand Surg* 22B (6):764-767, 1997.
20. Silfverskiold KL, May EJ: Flexor tendon repair in zone II with a new suture technique and an early mobilization program combining passive and active flexion, *J Hand Surg* 19A:53, 1994.
21. Silfverskiold KL, May EJ, Tornvall AH: Flexor digitorum profundus tendon excursions during controlled motion after flexor tendon repair in zone II: a prospective clinical study, *J Hand Surg*17A:122-133, 1992.
22. Skoog T, Persson B: An experimental study of the early healing of tendons, *Scand J Plast Reconstr Surg* 13:384-399, 1954.
23. Stewart Pettengill K, van Strien G: Postoperative management of flexor tendon injuries. In Mackin EJ et al, editors: *Rehabilitation of the hand*, ed 5, St Louis, 2002, CV Mosby, pp 431-456.
24. Strickland J: Development of flexor tendon surgery: twenty-five years of progress, *J Hand Surg* 25A:214-235, 2000.
26. Strickland JW, Cannon NM: Flexor tendon repair—Indiana method, *Indiana Hand Center Newsl* 1:1-12, 1993.
27. Strickland JW, Glogovac SV: Digital function following flexor tendon repair in zone II: a comparison of immobilization and controlled passive motion techniques, *J Hand Surg* 5:537-543, 1980.
28. Verdan CE: Practical considerations for primary and secondary repair in flexor tendon injuries, *Surg Clin North Am* 44:951-970, 1964

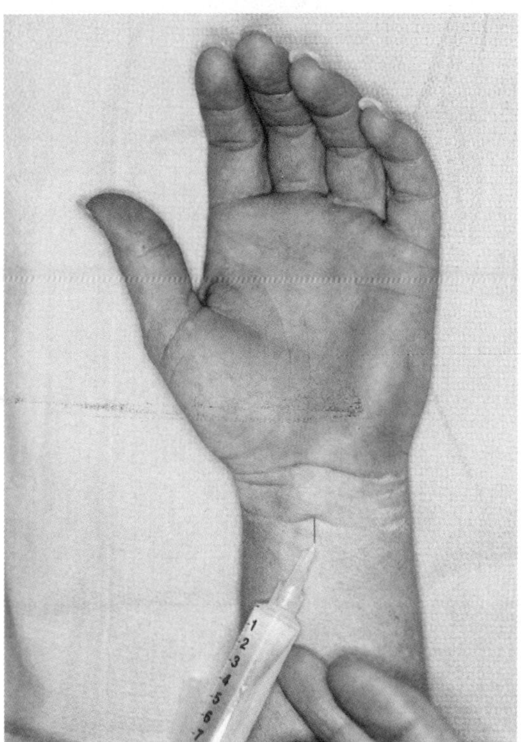

Fig. 11-1 Local anesthesia using 1% plain lidocaine is infiltrated into the operative area through a 25-gauge needle.

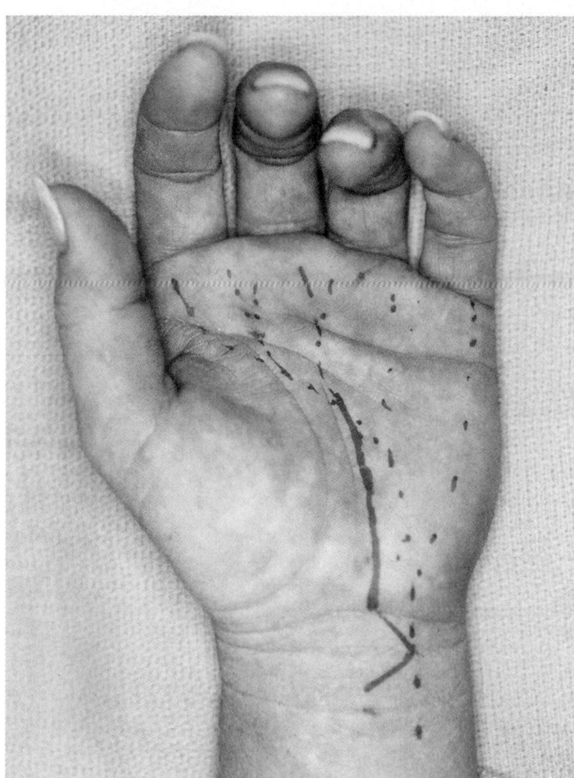

Fig. 11-2 Exposure of the carpal canal is performed through an incision represented by the solid line. Dashed lines represent the course of the ulnar artery and its branches (common digital and proper digital arteries) that must be preserved during exposure.

Proximally, the incision crosses the distal wrist crease in a zigzag fashion, just ulnar to the ulnar border of the palmaris longus tendon (Fig. 11-2). The incision is made sharply and deepened through the subcutaneous tissue of the palm and the palmar fascia, thereby exposing the transverse carpal ligament (Fig. 11-3). The ligament is then divided sharply under direct visualization, with the surgeon taking care to avoid damage to the underlying median nerve and tendons. After the ligament is divided, the nerve is carefully examined (Fig. 11-4). The wound is then irrigated with saline and the incision closed by reapproximating the skin edges with interrupted monofilament nonabsorbable sutures (Fig. 11-5). Sterile dressings are placed over the incision, and a wrist splint is applied with the wrist in slight extension, leaving the metacarpal-phalangeal and interphalangeal joints free.

The splint is left in place for approximately 10 days, after which it is taken off and the sutures are removed. Patients are instructed in any necessary local wound care, which is usually minimal, and encouraged to resume use of the hand gradually.

THERAPY GUIDELINES FOR REHABILITATION

Postoperative Rehabilitation

The frequency and duration of treatment is highly variable after a carpal tunnel release. All patients referred to therapy are instructed in a home exercise and ergonomic program appropriate to the phase of recovery and their individual needs.

In general, patients tend to do quite well after carpal tunnel release. However, because the extent of the damage to the median nerve cannot fully be known before surgery, predicting the exact outcome of carpal tunnel release is difficult. Patients with mild to moderate symptoms can expect full recovery of sensation and resolution of the numbness and tingling caused by entrapment of the nerve. Patients with more advanced disease who have significant sensibility loss and muscle weakness usually achieve significant improvement of their condition. Patients with muscle atrophy can expect a halt to progression of muscle wasting and in some cases can regain muscle mass.

The recovery of the median nerve directly relates to the success of the surgery. Ultrasonography postoperatively may be beneficial in identifying the initial beneficial morphological changes. However, the nerve conduction studies could take as long as 3 to 6 months to change.[13] Patients must understand that they may have some element of incisional pain after surgery, which can last as long as 3 to 6 months. They must also be informed that they will temporarily lose some strength in the hand, which usually improves after 3 to 6 months.

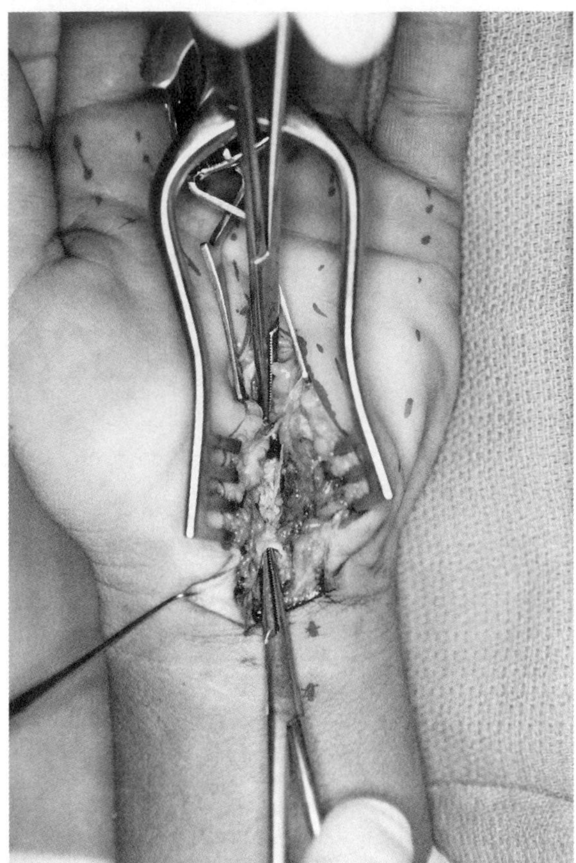

Fig. 11-3 The transverse carpal ligament has been exposed and is being tented proximally and distally by hemostats.

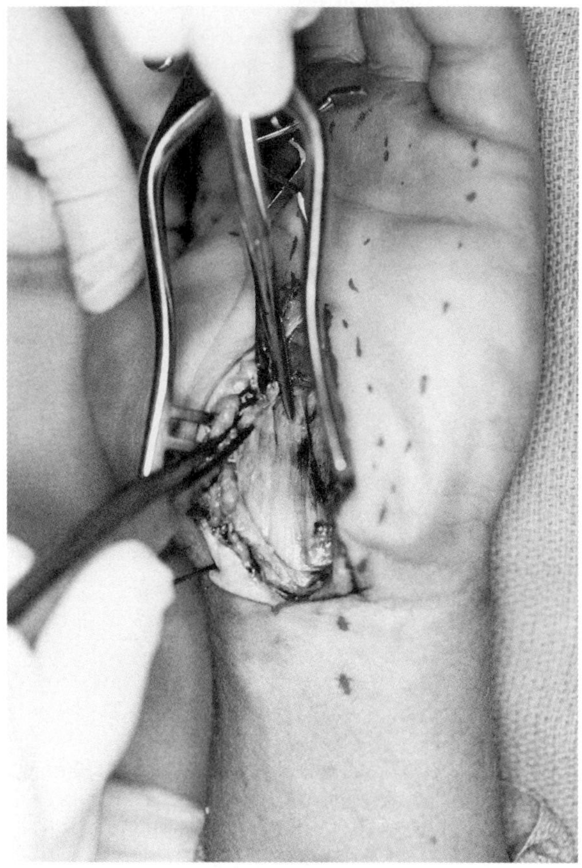

Fig. 11-4 The transverse carpal ligament has been divided, and the contents of the underlying carpal canal are exposed. The median nerve is demonstrated at the tip of the dissecting scissors.

Postoperative Evaluation

In general, patients may be referred to therapy anywhere from 1 to 3 weeks. The timing of the first visit will dictate which tests are appropriate to perform and which should be deferred until a later time. The comprehensive evaluation after carpal tunnel release includes the following:

- Patient history
- Subjective pain report
- Finger dexterity assessment
- Edema measurement
- Grip and pinch measurements

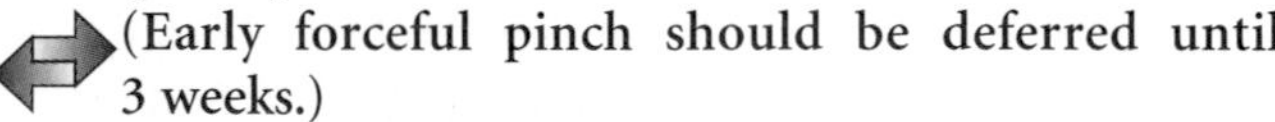

(Early forceful pinch should be deferred until 3 weeks.)

- Manual muscle testing (MMT)

(On appropriate muscles, flexors should be deferred until risk of bowstringing has passed [generally 3 to 6 weeks].)

- Active range of motion (AROM) measurements

(On appropriate motions, flexion should be deferred until 3 to 6 weeks to avoid the risk of bowstringing.)

- Sensibility testing
- Wound and scar assessment

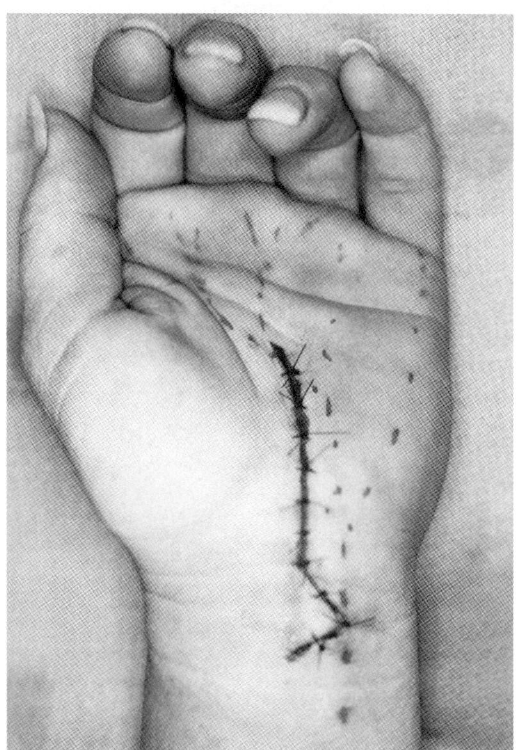

Fig. 11-5 Skin closure is achieved with the use of simple interrupted monofilament nonabsorbable suture.

- Nerve tension testing
- Documentation of the patient's previous and present functional status

The patient's history is obtained by patient interview. Information to be noted in the history includes age, gender, hand dominance, cause of CTS, type and date of the carpal tunnel release, occupation, avocational interests, onset and description of symptoms before surgery, and notes regarding whether symptoms were unilateral or bilateral.

The patient is asked to quantify the pain on a scale from 0 (representing no pain) to 10 (indicating severe pain requiring medical attention). The patient is asked to rate the pain both at rest and with use. The quality of the patient's pain is obtained by documenting the descriptive terms the patient uses when discussing the symptoms.[21]

Finger dexterity is generally evaluated on a nine-hole peg test. The nine-hole pegboard is positioned on the table with the end containing the pegs on the same side as the hand being tested. The score is recorded as the total time in seconds to put the nine pegs into the board one at a time and remove the pegs one at a time for the dominant and nondominant hand. A comparison of the time required for the patient's postoperative hand is made with the hand that was not operated on or with the norms established in 1985 by Mathiowetz and colleagues.[31]

Edema of the hand is recorded either by volumetric or circumferential measurements. If edema is profuse throughout the hand, then volumetric measurements are preferred provided that stitches have been removed and the patient has no open wounds. The volumetric assessment should be administered following the American Society of Hand Therapists (ASHT) guidelines: The thumb should be oriented toward the spout of the volumeter and the hand lowered into the volumeter so that the web space between the middle and ring fingers rests on the bar. The displaced water is measured in milliliters and recorded for both hands.[22] If edema is minimal or the stitches have not yet been removed, then circumferential measurements recorded in centimeters should be obtained at the distal wrist crease and the distal palmar crease (DPC).

Grip strength is recorded using a dynamometer with the handle positioned at the second setting[2,3] per American Society of Surgery of the Hand (ASSH) and ASHT guidelines. **If the patient is seen before day 21 after surgery, then grip strength testing may be deferred.** To perform a grip test the patient should be "seated with the shoulder adducted and neutrally rotated, elbow flexed to 90 degrees, forearm in neutral position" and unsupported.[16,17] The therapist may support the dynamometer to prevent dropping. However, the dynamometer should not be allowed to rest on the table. The therapist should document three grip measurements alternating the right and left hands,[29] unless repetitive grasping of the dynamometer would increase the discomfort in the patient's hand. Several authors have published normal values for grip strength. However, because of the high standard deviation[11] and inconsistencies in the studies "comparison of grip scores to the contralateral extremity or longitudinal comparison to earlier values for each patient is recommended by ASSH and ASHT."[3,17,30]

Two types of pinch are recorded using a pinch meter. Finger positioning for three-point pinch is performed with the index and middle finger on the top of the pinch meter and the thumb on the bottom. Lateral pinch positioning is performed with the pinch meter held between the radial side of the index finger and the thumb on the top of the meter. **Early forceful pinch is contraindicated and should be deferred until 3 weeks after surgery.**

The hand is assessed for obvious atrophy of the thenar eminence after which MMT of the upper quarter is performed. As mentioned previously, care is taken to avoid undo stress on the flexor tendons until at least 3 weeks after surgery. In assessing the function of the Median nerve, the "abductor pollicis brevis is the muscle of choice for clinical assessment because it is superficial, solely innervated by the median nerve, and the earliest affected."[28,36]

AROM measurements are obtained using a goniometer for the wrist and forearm. Individual finger AROM measurements may not be necessary when motion limitations are minimal. A global measurement of finger flexibility is obtained by measuring composite finger flexion to the DPC. The distance from the middle of the fingertips to the DPC is measured in centimeters for each finger. Functional thumb opposition is recorded as the ability to oppose the thumb to each fingertip, as well as the ability to touch the thumb to the base of the small finger. The therapist should record any inability in centimeters. **To prevent bowstringing (i.e., subluxing of the flexor tendons through the healing transverse carpal ligament) wrist flexion measurements should be deferred until 3 weeks after surgery.**

"Sensibility testing is the evaluation of the ability to feel or perceive a stimulus applied to an area."[42] Sensibility assessment is completed using the Semmes-Weinstein pressure aesthesiometer kit (a five-filament kit is adequate). This type of sensory test is a pressure threshold test. The patient is seated comfortably for testing with the forearm supinated and the hand supported on a towel roll. The therapist should occlude the patient's vision during the test and instruct the patient to report when a finger is stimulated and which finger feels the stimulus. The volar fingertips and thumb pulp are tested starting with the 2.83 monofilament. "Each monofilament is applied perpendicular to the skin for 1.5 seconds and lifted for 1.5 seconds."[42] The therapist should apply monofilaments 2.83 and 3.61 three times to the same spot, and apply monofilaments 4.31 through 6.65 once. The lowest-numbered monofilament felt for each digit should be recorded on the evaluation form.[42] Full hand mapping is rarely required after a carpal tunnel release. "Two point discrimination values are most often normal in CTS, and if they are abnormal it indicates advanced disease."[19] The therapist should complete two-point discrimination testing if the patient demonstrates significant deficits on the Semmes-Weinstein Monofilament Test. Two-point discrimination is an innervation density test.[19] The difference between the pressure threshold test and an innervation density test is the sensitivity of the pressure threshold test to gradual loss or improvement in nerve function versus an all-or-none response on an innervation density test. The difference can be explained by the comparison of a light bulb having a dimmer switch versus being on or off.

Tinel's testing is helpful in evaluating a patient before surgery. However, the authors of this chapter do not recommend Tinel's testing after surgery to avoid aggravating an irritable healing nerve.

The surgical incision or scar is evaluated for its stage of healing. The therapist should document whether the scar is raised or flat, tough or soft, mobile or adherent. The color of the scar also is noted. Upper-limb tension testing of the median nerve is appropriate to determine whether the patient has restrictions in nerve gliding.

The patient's present functional status is documented in the areas of grooming, dressing, bathing, cooking, home care, work, avocational activities, and driving. The patient is re-evaluated monthly or before returning to the doctor.

Phase I (Inflammatory Phase)

TIME: 1 to 6 weeks after surgery
GOALS: Decrease pain, manage edema, improve AROM of UE, initiate self-management and patient education

Treatment of the patient after carpal tunnel release is based on the phases of wound healing. Phase I (inflammatory phase) is from the day of surgery through day 21 after surgery[4] (Table 11-1).

Postoperative care of the patient in phase I is divided into pre- (Ia) and post- (Ib) suture removal. During phase Ia a postoperative dressing is usually worn for 7 to 10 days after surgery. The patient should be instructed to elevate the hand above the heart and ice frequently to help decrease edema. Exercises during phase Ia consist of AROM to the shoulder, elbow, and digits. The patient is instructed in tendon-gliding exercises (Fig. 11-6) to prevent adhesion of the tendons and nerves through the carpal tunnel and decrease edema.[47] AROM exercises are performed three times per day for 10 repetitions each. The patient at this time will most likely not require a formal therapy program and, after instruction, can perform exercises as a home program.

Table 11-1 Carpal Tunnel Release

Rehabilitation Phase	Criteria to Progress to this Phase	Anticipated Impairments and Functional Limitations	Intervention	Goal	Rationale
Phase Ia Postoperative 1-10 days	◆ Postoperative	◆ Edema ◆ Pain ◆ Limited ROM of UE ◆ Limited functional use of UE	◆ Instruct on surgical site protection and monitor for drainage ◆ Elevate and ice hand and wrist ◆ AROM—Shoulder (all ranges), elbow (all ranges), forearm (pronation, supination), fingers (tendon-gliding thumb AROM all ranges)	◆ Prevent infection and postoperative complications ◆ Manage edema ◆ Decrease pain ◆ Full AROM of shoulder, elbow, forearm ◆ Increase AROM of fingers within limits of postoperative dressing	◆ Catch infection early to prevent further complications ◆ Begin to have patient self-manage edema and pain ◆ Restore ROM to prepare UE for functional use ◆ Limit scar adhesions to tendons and nerves

ROM, Range of motion; *UE,* upper extremity; *AROM,* active range of motion.

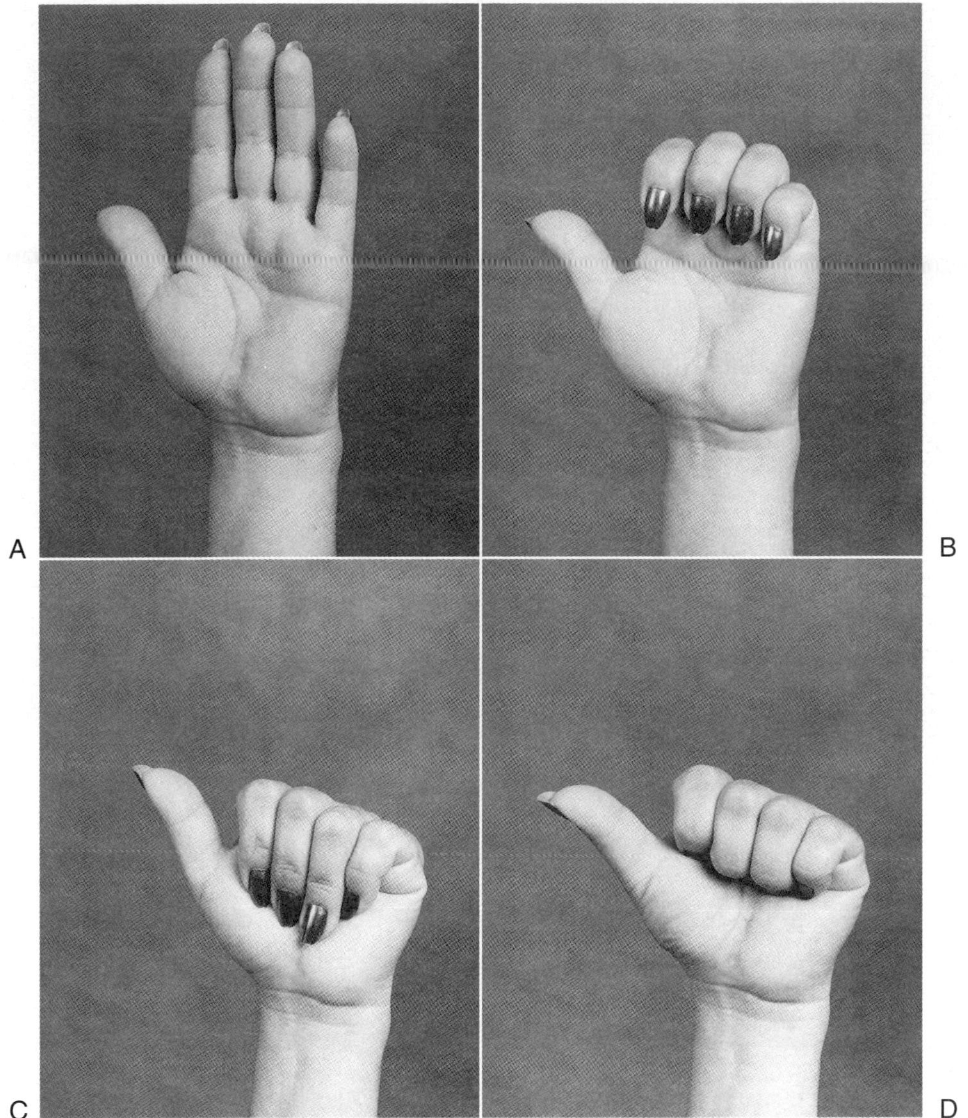

Fig. 11-6 Tendon-gliding exercises. **A**, Tendon-gliding exercises are initiated in full finger extension. The patient then completes 10 repetitions in the hook fist (**B**), straight fist (**C**), and full fist (**D**) to maximize differential tendon gliding and full excursion of the tendons through the carpal tunnel.
(From Wehbe M: Tendon gliding exercises, *Am J Occup Ther* 41:164, 1987.)

Q Yvonne is a 48-year-old grocery checker who has been diagnosed with intermediate CTS; she has constant numbness and paresthesia but no thenar atrophy. She had surgery 3 weeks ago for a carpal tunnel release, and the edema is persistent. What are some treatment techniques that may be helpful for decreasing her edema at this point?

Phase Ib begins when the sutures are removed and the patient is referred for formal therapy (Table 11-2). Modalities are used to decrease pain, cocontraction of muscles, and edema. Modalities also are used to increase elasticity of tissues and promote tissue healing.[44]

Moist heat by itself or in conjunction with transcutaneous electrical nerve stimulation (TENS) or interferential current is used for pain control before exercise. Severe pain is rare, but patients experiencing it may consider renting a home unit for a few weeks. The modalities of phonophoresis,[32] iontophoresis,[44] and high-voltage galvanic stimulation (HVGS)[44] are helpful in reducing the local swelling and pain experienced by patients after carpal tunnel release. Phonophoresis using a 3 MHz head[32] is performed over the closed, healing incision and the thenar and hypothenar eminences. The ultrasound intensity is set between .30 and .50 w/cm^2 for 5 minutes.

Iontophoresis is the modality of choice for decreasing local edema about the incision site.[44] However, the

Table 11-2 Carpal Tunnel Release

Rehabilitation Phase	Criteria to Progress to this Phase	Anticipated Impairments and Functional Limitations	Intervention	Goal	Rationale
Phase Ib Postoperative 11-21 days	◆ No signs of infection ◆ Sutures removed	◆ Edema ◆ Pain ◆ Limited functional use of UE ◆ Limited AROM of hand and wrist ◆ Limited strength of hand and wrist ◆ Scar sensitivity, adhesions, and thickening ◆ Persistent paresthesia, especially at night ◆ Limited hand function ◆ Limited patient knowledge of neutral wrist positioning	◆ Hot pack ◆ ES ◆ Ultrasound, phonophoresis ◆ Iontophoresis ◆ Cryotherapy ◆ Retrograde massage ◆ Initiate pain-free isometrics—Wrist (flexion, extension), careful to avoid pain ◆ AROM—Progress exercises as indicated and add wrist extension, radial deviation, and ulnar deviation ◆ Finger AROM-PREs (maintaining the wrist in a neutral position), paper crunches, rice gripping ◆ No AROM for wrist flexion until 3 weeks post surgery ◆ Wrist splint worn at night as needed ◆ Scar desensitization: gentle manual massage, mini-vibrator massage, add different textures ◆ Mobilization of the median nerve Instruct patient in the following: ◆ Proper use of hand protection while performing self-care ◆ Neutral wrist positioning ◆ Nerve-gliding techniques ◆ Fabricate scar conformer	◆ Decrease postoperative pain by 50% ◆ Manage edema ◆ Increase strength and facilitate gross grasp and wrist stabilization ◆ Full AROM of shoulder, elbow, and forearm ◆ AROM—Wrist (extension 45 degrees, radial deviation 20 degrees, ulnar deviation 30 degrees), thumb (opposition to tip of small finger), finger (flexion to 1 cm of DPC) ◆ Decrease sensitivity of scar ◆ Increase mobility of scar ◆ Decrease scar adhesion to flexor tendons, skin, and median nerve ◆ Decrease paresthesia ◆ Promote independent self-care ◆ Maintain neutral wrist position during exercises ◆ Encourage self-management of exercise program ◆ Fatten and or soften scar	◆ Modalities to manage edema and decrease pain; help in preparation for stretching and strengthening ◆ Massage to facilitate lymphatic return ◆ Increased wrist stabilization strength ◆ Promote full return of UE AROM, continuation of tendon-gliding exercises to decrease scar adhesion ◆ Wrist flexion exercises are contraindicated until 21 days after surgery to prevent bowstringing of tendons ◆ Strengthening and improvement of endurance of wrist and hand while maintaining neutral position ◆ Encouragement of wrist extension with finger flexion ◆ Neutral position to minimize pressure on median nerve ◆ Organized sensory input normalizes sensory interpretation ◆ Early motion organizes collagen development in scar and limits scar from restricting median nerve ◆ Initiation of self-management ◆ Minimizing of development of pillar pain ◆ Incorporation of neutral position during exercises and ADLs to prevent complications ◆ Pressure applied over a scar organizes collagen

UE, Upper extremity; *AROM*, active range of motion; *ES*, electrical stimulation; *PREs*, progressive resistance exercises; *DPC*, distal palmar crease; *ADLs*, activities of daily living.

incision must be completely healed and able to tolerate the stimulation.

Cryotherapy administered after exercises for 10 minutes may be helpful for managing edema and pain. Light retrograde massage also may facilitate lymphatic return. Patients with persistent edema may benefit from wearing a compression glove in conjunction with other edema-controlling modalities. The glove should be worn almost continuously at first and then worn only at night as edema decreases. Splinting the wrist in a neutral position may be beneficial for patients experiencing moderate to severe surgical discomfort or persistent paresthesia.

A Light retrograde massage may facilitate lymphatic return. Patients with persistent edema may benefit from wearing a compression glove in conjunction with other edema-controlling modalities. Initially the glove should be worn almost continuously. As the edema decreases, the patient only needs to wear the glove at night.

The therapist should initiate scar desensitization when the surgical incision is closed. The desensitization process is initiated gently and can be performed in many ways. These methods include manual self-massage of the scar or the use of a mini-vibrator, gripping of different textured particles, and rubbing the scar with different textures such as a towel.[46] Scar massage is initiated with minimal force, and the force is increased as the incision increases in tensile strength (Fig. 11-7). Scar massage is done for 1 to 3 minutes five times per day. Performing scar massage with the mini-vibrator can be especially helpful for patients with bilateral involvement.

Q Yvonne tends to heal quickly after having surgery. In fact, she had difficulty regaining full knee ROM after knee surgery because adhesions quickly formed around the joint. Limiting the development of scar adhesions also is important in the patient who has had carpal tunnel release. What are some problematic areas Yvonne may have after her carpal tunnel release? What types of treatment can be used to limit scar adhesions in this area?

Limiting the development of scar adhesion to tendons, skin, and nerves is another important aspect of scar management after carpal tunnel release surgery. Tendon-gliding exercises are continued to move the flexor tendons differentially in the carpal tunnel. Nerve-gliding techniques are helpful in maintaining mobility of the median nerve after a carpal tunnel release.[4] The patient's initial home program for median nerve gliding begins with the arm held at the side of the body, the elbow extended, and the forearm and wrist in neutral position. The patient is instructed to extend the wrist from a neutral position in a pumping action for three sets of four repetitions, three times per day. The patient should be cautioned not to be overzealous with these exercises and to inform the therapist if symptoms increase.

When the incision is fully closed, a scar conformer can be fabricated from silicone elastomers[4] or cut from silicone gel sheets (Fig. 11-8). Because the scar conformer works by applying pressure over the scar, it needs to be held firmly in place. The therapist should use a self-adherent wrap such as Coban to secure the conformer over the scar. The patient should be instructed not to wrap the scar conformer too tightly with the Coban because tight wrapping will cause edema and pain in the hand. An

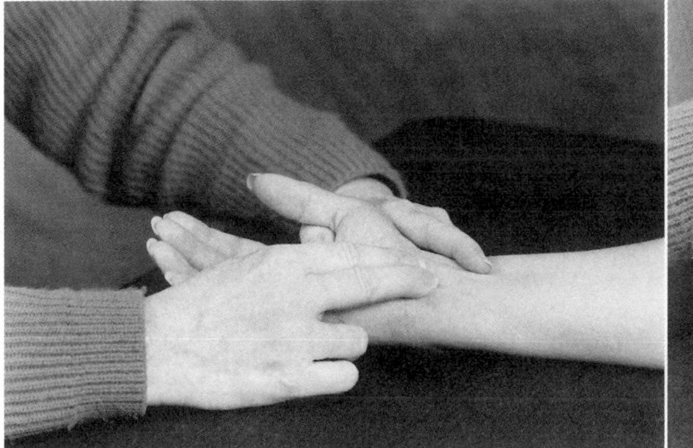

A

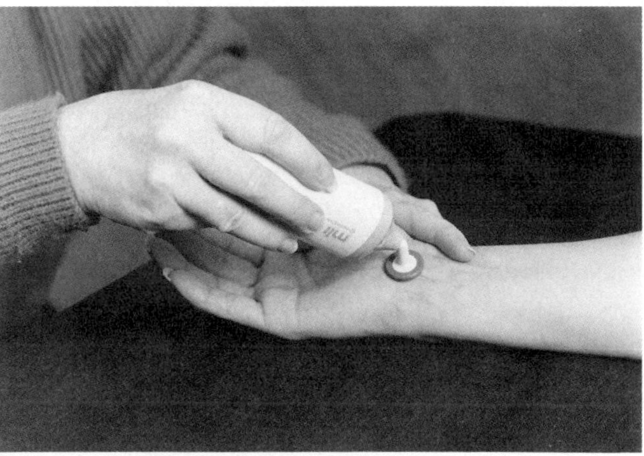

B

Fig. 11-7 Scar massage is initiated using manual techniques to decrease scar adhesion to the underlying tissues (**A**) and progressed with a mini-vibrator (**B**).

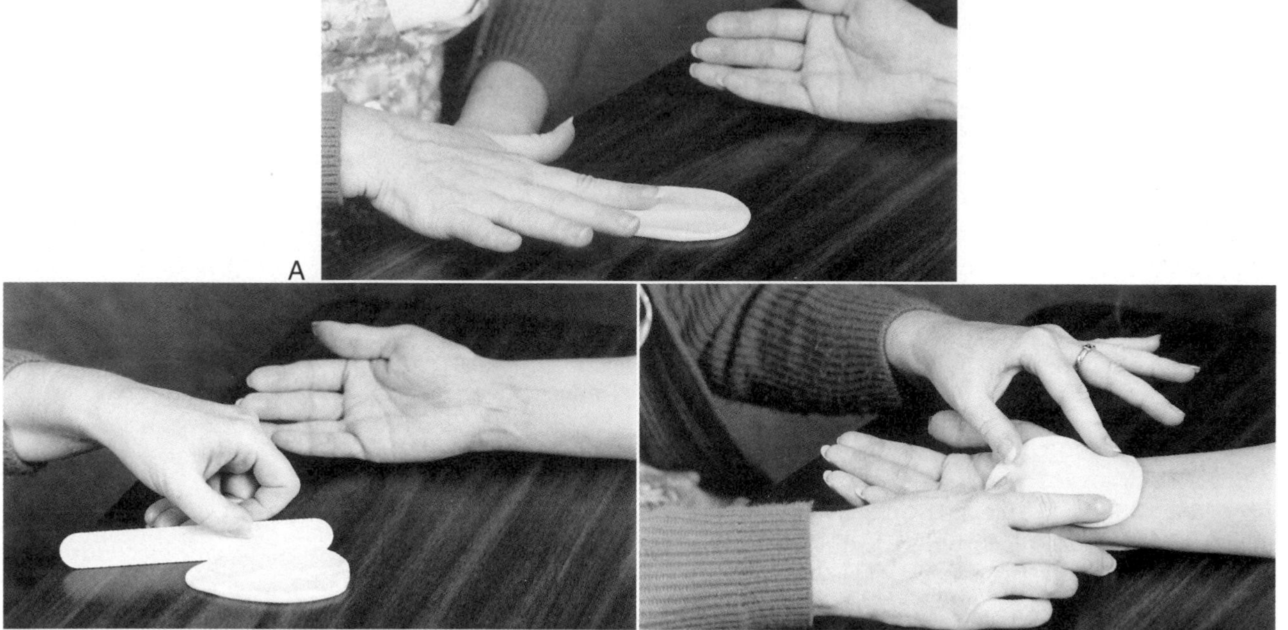

Fig. 11-8 **A,** The clinician fabricates an elastomer scar conformer by mixing the base in the hands and then forming the scar conformer on the table to ensure a smooth back. **B,** A tongue depressor is used to shape the edges while the scar conformer partially sets up. **C,** The scar conformer is molded to the patient just before setting up is completed.

explanation should be given to the patient regarding the purpose and importance of wearing the scar conformer properly at night for at least 3 months. The patient should wash the scar conformer daily to prevent skin irritation and replace the scar conformer if it becomes worn or soiled. The patient should observe the skin closely for signs of skin maceration or heat rash. If these problems occur, then the patient should stop using the scar conformer and inform the therapist. Decreasing the amount of wear time or placing a light gauze or tissue between the scar conformer and the skin may control skin maceration and heat rash.

> **A** Limiting the development of scar adhesion to tendons, skin, and nerves is another important aspect of scar management in the patient after carpal tunnel release surgery. Tendon-gliding exercises are continued to move the flexor tendons differentially in the carpal tunnel. Nerve-gliding techniques are helpful in maintaining mobility of the median nerve after a carpal tunnel release.

The exercises given in phase Ia are continued, and wrist exercises are added. Wrist AROM exercises should be limited to extension, radial deviation, and ulnar deviation. **Flexion of the wrist is avoided until 21 days after surgery to prevent bowstringing of the flexor tendons through the healing carpal ligament.**

Paper crunches and rice gripping are two beneficial activities to facilitate the development of gross grasp, maintain a neutral wrist position, and increase finger and wrist extensor endurance. Fig. 11-9 provides instructions for the paper crunch exercise. Rice gripping is beneficial for scar site desensitization and encouragement of wrist extension with finger flexion. The exercise is performed with the patient standing at a table with the container of rice stabilized on the table. The patient grasps the rice while extending the wrist and releases it into the same container. Wrist flexion is avoided in this phase. Grasping endurance is built up to 3 minutes and is continued as a home exercise two times per day.

The therapist should then initiate isometric strengthening exercises for wrist extension and flexion. Wrist isometrics are performed in a neutral wrist position.[23] The patient applies enough resistance with the opposite hand to create a muscle contraction, which is held for 5 seconds without increasing pain. Isometric exercises should be performed for five repetitions three times per day. The exercises can be progressed by increasing resistance and repetitions. Instruction on ways to maintain a neutral wrist position during functional use of the hand is emphasized with paper crunch activity and isometric strengthening exercises. This education is further emphasized with ergonomic instruction in phase II.

The patient should be encouraged to use the affected hand for self-care while avoiding wrist flexion, forceful repetitive grip, and lifting more than 3 pounds. Tasks that

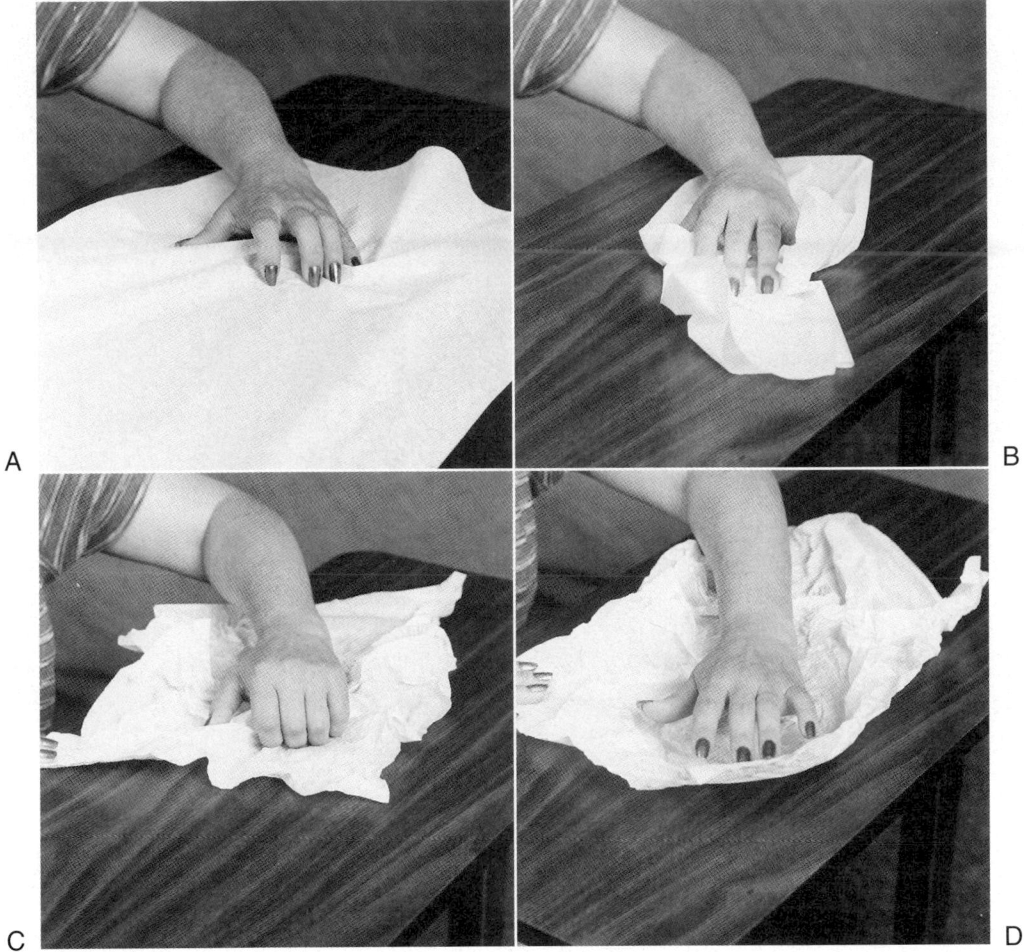

Fig. 11-9 Paper crunches. **A,** A 22-inch square of examination table paper is placed on a table with the patient sitting in a straight-back chair, elbow at about 90 degrees, and the wrist positioned in neutral. **B,** The patient starts at one corner of the paper and crumples it into a ball using the involved hand. **C,** The patient then stabilizes the paper with the uninvolved hand and makes a fist with the involved hand with the forearm and wrist in neutral 2 inches above the paper. **D,** The patient rapidly extends the digits, pushing the paper open while maintaining a neutral wrist position. The process of fisting and extending the digits is repeated until the paper is opened fully. The paper crunches are progressed from one to three repetitions per session as the patient tolerates.

require forceful grip such as vacuuming, handling wet laundry, putting fitted sheets on the bed, yard work, tool use, lifting, and pushing should be avoided for 6 to 8 weeks to allow healing.

Phase II (Proliferation Phase)

TIME: 4 to 6 weeks after surgery
GOALS: Complete self-management of symptoms and home maintenance program; return to full-time work activities

Phase II focuses primarily on strengthening and education (Table 11-3). It begins on day 22 after surgery and continues until day 42 (6 weeks after surgery). Phase Ib modalities are continued for edema and pain control. Moist heat is continued before exercises. Scar desensitization is continued with scar massage, and the patient may progress to use of a larger vibrator for desensitization. Texture desensitization techniques are continued, especially as part of the home program. Use of a gel shell to pad the sensitive palm may increase comfort for performing self-care and light home care. Tendon-gliding and nerve-gliding exercises and scar massage are continued to decrease scar adhesions. The pressure used for scar massage is increased in intensity for manual massage. Use of the scar conformer is continued at night to soften and flatten the scar.

The patient can add active wrist flexion exercises after 21 days with the expectation of full wrist flexion by the end of the sixth week after surgery. Rice gripping (Fig. 11-10) and paper crunches are continued. However, the patient transfers the rice to a second container, focusing on wrist extension when gripping the rice and wrist flexion when dropping the rice into the second container.

Table 11-3 Carpal Tunnel Release

Rehabilitation Phase	Criteria to Progress to this Phase	Anticipated Impairments and Functional Limitations	Intervention	Goal	Rationale
Phase II Postoperative 4-6 weeks	◆ Pain controlled ◆ No loss of ROM ◆ No loss of strength ◆ Well-healed incision	◆ Mild edema ◆ Mild pain ◆ Limited AROM of wrist, fingers, and thumb ◆ Scar sensitivity ◆ Scar adhesion ◆ Scar raised or thickened ◆ Limited UE strength ◆ Limited ability to perform light ADLs involving gripping and twisting ◆ Limited knowledge of proper work environment organization (ergonomics) ◆ Limited tolerance to repetitive finger and hand use	◆ Continuation of modalities as indicated from Phase Ib Continuation of the following: ◆ Scar desensitization techniques ◆ Retrograde massage ◆ AROM and PREs ◆ Scar conformer at night ◆ Progress firmness of manual scar massage and use large vibrator to massage scar Add the following: ◆ PROM (stretches)—Pectoralis Composite motions of the following: 1. Wrist flexion, forearm pronation, and elbow extension 2. Wrist extension, forearm pronation, and elbow extension 3. Wrist extension, forearm supination, and elbow extension ◆ AROM—Wrist flexion ◆ Putty exercises (light resistive putty)—Finger pinch, finger grip ◆ Isotonics—Upper-quarter exercises as in Table 5-3 (using 1 or 2 lb weights); wrist (weight well—flexion, extension [begin with 0-2 lb and progress as indicated]); forearm (pronation supination [progress as indicated]) ◆ Patient education regarding body mechanics, joint protection, and modification of ADLs using adaptive equipment (grip assistive devices) ◆ Ergonomic evaluation ◆ Work-simulated exercises, emphasizing neutral position of the wrists and pacing tasks; may need handwriting retraining	◆ As in Tables 11-1 and 11-2 ◆ Resolve edema in fingers ◆ Decrease pain by 70% ◆ Decrease sensitivity of scar and increase scar mobility ◆ Decrease scar adhesion to flexor tendon, skin, and median nerve ◆ Increase tolerance of UE to reaching away from body ◆ AROM of Wrist—Extension 60 degrees, radial deviation 25 degrees, ulnar deviation 35 degrees ◆ Make a full fist to DPC ◆ Thumb to DPC at base of small finger ◆ Grip strength 30%-50% of uninvolved hand ◆ Wrist strength 80%-90% ◆ Proximal strength greater than 85% ◆ Lift and carry 3-5 lb with involved hand ◆ Independence with ADLs using assistive devices as necessary and limiting exposure to heavy grasping activities ◆ Organize work environment to decrease potential for reinjury and maximize efficiency ◆ Work simulation for 10 minutes, alternating tasks	◆ As in Tables 11-1 and 11-2 ◆ Decrease reliance on modalities and increase patient's ability to self-manage edema and pain ◆ Continuation of exercises as indicated to allow progression of program as tolerated by patient response to treatment ◆ Scar should now be able to handle increased mobilization techniques ◆ UE stretches to elongate muscle tendon units for increased function ◆ Healing of transverse carpal tunnel ligament is adequate to prevent bowstringing of the flexor tendons (Note: Monitor triggering of one or more digits, stop gripping exercises, and treat per physician's orders) ◆ Upper-quarter strengthening as a functional unit ◆ Initiate exercises with low repetitions to prevent development of tenosynovitis and pillar pain ◆ Use appropriate assistive device to prevent reinjury and increase independence with ADLs; avoiding heavier gripping activities such as vacuuming, laundry, and yard work; use forearms to carry versus finger grip (e.g., groceries in paper bags versus plastic) ◆ Promote self-management of symptoms and prevent reinjury in the work environment ◆ Prepare for return to work

ROM, Range of motion; *AROM,* active range of motion; *UE,* upper extremity; *ADLs,* activities of daily living; *PREs,* progressive resistance exercises; *PROM,* passive range of motion; *DPC,* distal palmar crease.

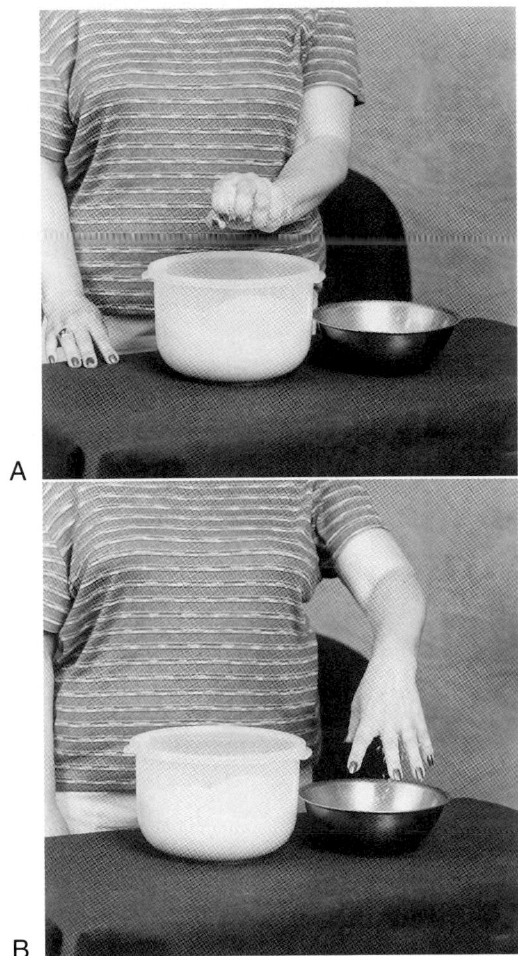

Fig. 11-10 A, The clinician initiates rice gripping by grasping the rice and extending the wrist. B, During phase II the patient is allowed to flex the wrist while transferring the rice into a separate bowl.

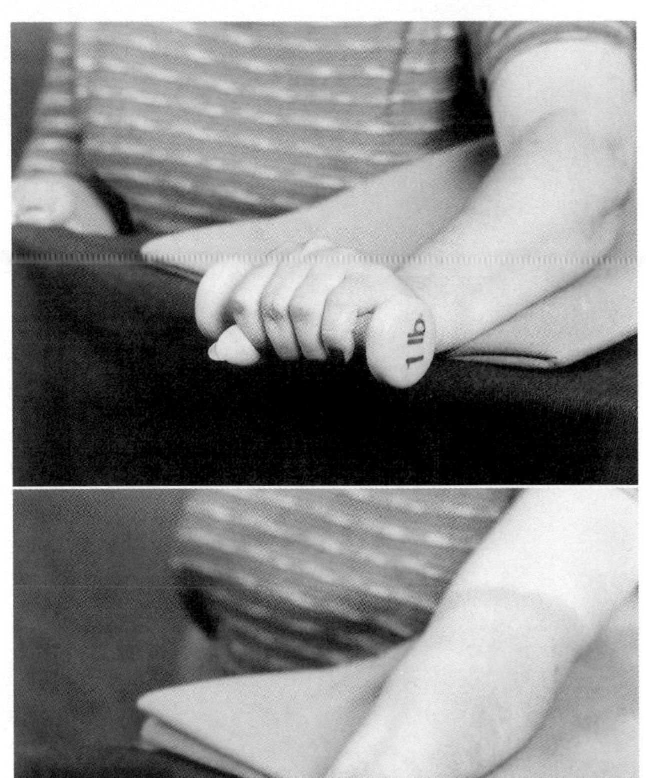

Fig. 11-11 Progressive resistance exercises (PREs) are important to strengthen the wrist extensor (A) and flexor (B) musculature. The table is padded with a towel to prevent excessive pressure on the median and ulnar nerves.

Full UE stretching exercises are added at this time. UE stretches include composite motions of (1) wrist flexion, forearm pronation, and elbow extension; (2) wrist extension, forearm pronation, and elbow extension; and (3) wrist extension, forearm supination, and elbow extension.[35]

Resistive gripping and pinching exercises with light resistive putty may be started 28 days after surgery. Initially, putty exercises should be limited to 3-minute sessions two times per day. Putty exercises must be comfortably tolerated before moving to more resistive putty. Clinically the authors of this chapter have noted that the overuse of repetitive gripping with putty increases the chance of developing pillar pain. Pillar pain is described as pain in the thenar or hypothenar eminence and is distinguished from local scar tenderness.[7,8,27] The therapist should instruct the patient that the maximum use of putty is two times a day for 5 minutes and tell him or her to stop using the putty and notify the therapist if the pain increases significantly.

Wrist isometric exercises are continued along with the initiation of grip isometric exercises. The patient can perform grip isometric exercises by squeezing a towel roll in the hand. Light progressive resistance exercises (PREs) are added when pain is controlled. PREs are added for both wrist extension and flexion (Fig. 11-11).[23] Resistance should begin at ½ to 1 pound and progressed to 3 pounds as the patient tolerates. **The abductor pollicis longus and the extensor pollicis brevis are prone to tenosynovitis at the first dorsal extensor compartment, so specific strengthening in radial deviation is not done.**

Wrist and grip strengthening are progressed to using a weight well or computerized work simulator (Fig. 11-12). The patient starts on the weight well with no weight or on the work simulator at minimal torque and progresses as tolerated.

Proximal muscle strengthening of the forearm, elbow, shoulder, and shoulder girdle are started on day 28 after surgery. Forearm rotation can be strengthened using a

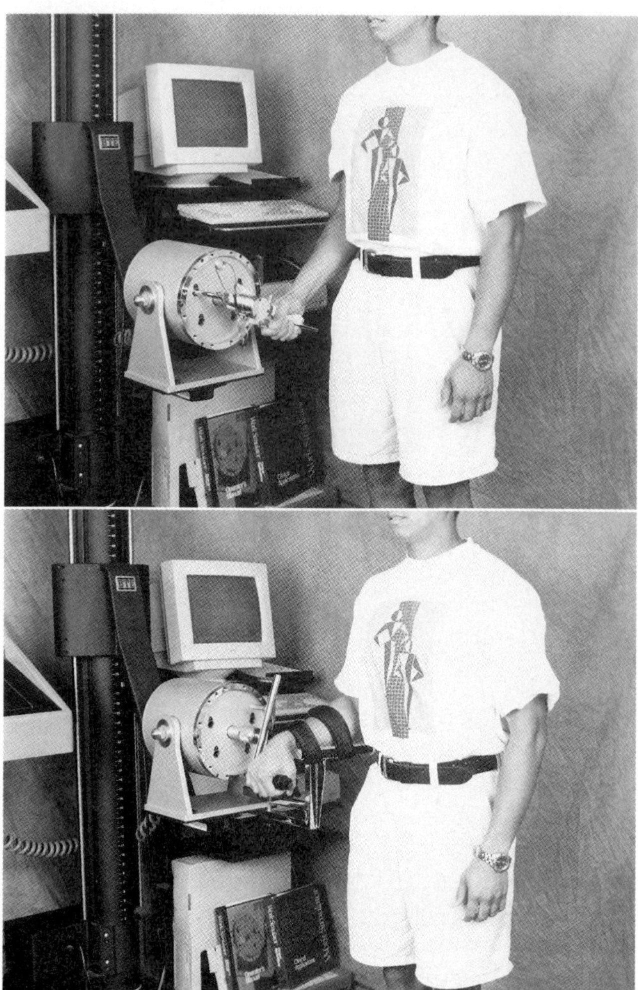

Fig. 11-12 Computerized equipment is an effective way of simulating many work tasks and strengthening muscles; it requires a relatively small area in the clinic.

16 oz hammer held with the elbow flexed at 90 degrees and stabilized against the side of the body. The therapist should ask the patient to rotate the forearm from the neutral position into supination and then return to neutral. After completing the desired repetitions, the patient repeats the exercise into pronation. Simply moving the hammerhead away from the hand to increase resistance or toward the hand to decrease resistance can change the resistance of the exercise. Biceps curls and elbow extension exercises can be performed with dumbbells beginning at 1 or 2 pounds and progressing as the patient tolerates. Shoulder and shoulder girdle exercises beginning with 1 to 2 pounds are important and are performed for flexion, abduction, internal and external rotation, and scapular retraction. The patient should be monitored closely during the advancement of the proximal strengthening program to prevent the development of other cumulative trauma disorders such as shoulder impingement syndrome, lateral epicondylitis, or de Quervain's syndrome.

> **Q** Lupe is returning to work (as a receptionist) 8 weeks after carpal tunnel release. Her symptoms have resolved but she is still tender over the incision. What ergonomic recommendations should be made?

Treatment of the patient after carpal tunnel release surgery also must include instruction on ergonomic principles, proper posture, and body mechanics for lifting to prevent recurrence of CTS or the development of other repetitive stress injuries. Instruction should include general topics for all patients and job-specific teaching for those returning to highly repetitive or heavy-labor jobs.

Ergonomic Recommendations

Patients with jobs involving computers should be instructed in workstation setup. A good chair is important. An ergonomic chair should include (1) an adjustable height, (2) a proper seat depth (two to three fingers' clearance from the front edge of the seat pan of the chair to the back of the knees), and (3) an adjustable back height with lumbar support.[12] The keyboard should be placed directly in front of the patient and the height of the chair adjusted so the patient's elbows are flexed to 90 degrees or a little less with wrists in a neutral position over the keyboard. A keyboard tray may need to be added to the desk to achieve proper positioning. A footrest is used for patients whose feet do not reach the floor after the chair height is properly adjusted. Using ergonomic keyboards or negatively tilting the keyboard also may be useful for maintaining a neutral wrist position. When a wrist rest is used, the patient should be instructed not to press on it during typing but to use it to support the UEs when scanning the monitor screen. The monitor should be positioned with the top at eye level and approximately 18 in away from the patient.[35] When typing from text, the patient should position the work next to the monitor and at the same height and use a monitor stand to decrease cervical and shoulder strain. He or she also should position the mouse at the same height as the keyboard and within forearm length. The therapist should try as many ergonomic adjustments as possible in the clinic and encourage patients to evaluate other options at a local computer store and pick items that are most comfortable for their individual work stations.

Patients in highly repetitive jobs (such as assembly workers) or those involved in heavy labor present other problems. Patients in these fields are constantly using their wrists and hands for turning screwdrivers, using wrenches, swinging hammers, and using power equipment. These activities generate high torque, pressure, and vibration on the carpal tunnel. Therefore they should be instructed to perform their job tasks using a neutral wrist position. Various ergonomic tools or a change to a power tool may assist the patient with achieving the most ergonomically correct position. Patients may be encouraged to go to their local hardware store to evaluate tools for comfort and applicability to their work. The use of work splints and antivibration gloves also may provide benefits by decreasing pain, providing support, and decreasing hypersensitivity. The patient should wear the gloves only when performing heavy or highly repetitive tasks.

Patients with sedentary jobs are usually discharged to a home program by the end of phase II. Heavy laborers generally progress to phase III at 6 to 8 weeks after surgery, where more emphasis is placed on increasing strength, endurance, and return to work activities.

> **A** In general, a worksite evaluation should be made. Close attention should be paid to the degree of wrist extension (should be less than 20 degrees), and postural setup (i.e., head on neck, shoulder, elbow, and overall spine and pelvis position while seated) as it relates to her monitor and job duties.

Phase III (Remodeling and Maturation Phase)

Phase III begins at 43 days (6 weeks) after surgery and ends when the scar is mature (Table 11-4). This phase can last for 1 year or longer. The patient is normally discharged by day 84 (after 12 weeks). The types of patients who progress to phase III are heavy laborers, construction workers, mechanics, and assembly workers. These patients should be able to progress from local heating modalities such as hot packs to aerobic exercise using a bicycle, treadmill, or UE ergometer. The stretching program and scar management program from phase II is continued. Scar massage also continues, with the patient wearing the scar conformer until the scar color is no longer reddened. Scar maturation can take as long as 1 year. Phase II strengthening exercises should be continued and progressed as tolerated. Large muscle group exercises using gym equipment or free weights are appropriate at this time for general body conditioning.

Work activity simulation is an important aspect of the phase III therapy protocol. These activities can include using a pipe tree or assembly boards and learning lifting and carrying techniques. The use of work simulation equipment can be helpful for strengthening and simulation of specific work activities (see Fig. 11-12).

Clearly, CTS affects patients physically, financially, and psychologically. Comprehensive management of the patient recovering from surgery for CTS optimizes the potential to return to ADLs, work, and avocational activities.

SUGGESTED HOME MAINTENANCE FOR THE POSTSURGICAL PATIENT

The home maintenance section outlines the shoulder rehabilitation the patient is to follow. The physical therapist can use it in customizing a patient-specific program.

Table 11-4 Carpal Tunnel Release

Rehabilitation Phase	Criteria to Progress to this Phase	Anticipated Impairments and Functional Limitations	Intervention	Goal	Rationale
Phase III Postoperative 6-12 weeks	◆ Patients need to perform job that requires heavy lifting	◆ Limited UE and grip strength ◆ Limited UE and grip endurance	◆ Continuation of exercises and stretches in Phases I and II as indicated ◆ Progress UE strengthening exercises, emphasizing endurance for return to work activities ◆ Functional capacity evaluation ◆ Work-simulated activities	◆ Decrease number of exercises and stretches ◆ Adequate strength to return to work activities full time ◆ Self-management of symptoms	◆ Increase efficiency of home exercises in self-management of condition ◆ Promote muscle balance of UE ◆ Assess potential to return to work ◆ Initiate appropriate program (work hardening, work conditioning, or supervised gym program)

UE, Upper extremity.

SUGGESTED HOME MAINTENANCE FOR THE POSTSURGICAL PATIENT

Days 1-10

GOALS FOR THE PERIOD: Decrease pain, manage edema, improve active range of motion (AROM) of upper extremity (UE), initiate self-management and patient education

1. Protect incision
2. Elevate the hand above the heart
3. Ice frequently
4. AROM exercises for shoulder, elbow, forearm, and thumb
5. Tendon-gliding exercises

Days 11-21

GOALS FOR THE PERIOD: Decrease pain, manage edema, improve AROM of UE, initiate self-management and patient education

1. Moist heat
2. Retrograde massage when incision has closed
3. Scar massage when incision has closed
4. Continue tendon-gliding exercises
5. Nerve-gliding exercises
6. Continue AROM exercises for shoulder, elbow, forearm, and thumb
7. Add AROM exercises for wrist extension, radial deviation, and ulnar deviation (avoid wrist flexion)
8. Paper crunches
9. Rice gripping (into same container)
10. Isometric exercises for wrist extension and flexion
11. Use scar conformer at night
12. Use splint at night as needed to control persistent paresthesias
13. Ice as necessary

Days 22-42

GOALS FOR THE PERIOD: Decrease pain, manage edema, improve AROM of UE, initiate self-management and patient education

1. Continue all previous exercises and modalities as indicated
2. Add wrist flexion AROM
3. Rice gripping (transferring rice to a second container)
4. Add UE stretching exercises
   a. Wrist flexion, forearm pronation, and elbow extension
   b. Wrist extension, forearm pronation, and elbow extension
   c. Wrist extension, forearm supination, and elbow extension
5. Add putty gripping and pinching exercises with light resistive putty (only two times a day for 5 minutes)
6. Add grip isometric exercises by squeezing a towel roll
7. Add progressive resistance exercises (PREs) for wrist extension and flexion with ½ to 1 pounds
8. Add PREs for shoulder girdle, shoulder, elbow with 1 to 2 pounds
9. Add forearm strengthening using a 16 oz hammer
10. Continue to use scar conformer at night
11. Practice ergonomic principles

Days 43-84

GOALS FOR THE PERIOD: Complete self-management of symptoms and home maintenance program, return to full-time work activities

1. Aerobic warm-up exercise using a bicycle or treadmill
2. Continue previous exercises as indicated, progressing intensity and duration as indicated

References

1. Agee J et al: Endoscopic release of the carpal tunnel: a randomized prospective multicenter study, *J Hand Surg* 17A:987, 1992.
2. American Society for Surgery of the Hand: *The hand: examination and diagnosis*, Aurora, CO, 1978, The Society.
3. American Society for Surgery of the Hand: *The hand: examination and diagnosis*, ed 2, New York, 1983, Churchill Livingstone.
4. Baxter-Petralia PL: Therapist's management of carpal tunnel syndrome. In Hunter JM et al, editors: *Rehabilitation of the hand: surgery and therapy*, ed 3, St Louis, 1990, Mosby.
5. Beckenbaugh RD: Carpal tunnel syndrome. In Cooney WP, Linsscheid RL, Dobyns JH, editors: *The wrist: diagnosis and operative treatment*, St Louis, 1998, Mosby.
6. Boz C et al: Individual risk factors for carpal tunnel syndrome: an evaluation of body mass index, wrist index and hand anthropometric measurements, *Clin Neurol Neurosurg* 106(4):294-299, 2004.
7. Brown RA et al: Carpal tunnel release: a prospective, randomized assessment of open and endoscopic methods, *J Bone Joint Surg* 75A:1265, 1993.
8. Buchanan RT et al: Method, education and therapy of carpal tunnel patients, *Hand Surg Quarterly*, Summer 1995.
9. Bureau of Labor Statistics: *Survey of occupation injuries and illness in 1994*, Washington, DC, 1996, US Department of Labor.
10. Cosgrove JL et al: Carpal tunnel syndrome in railroad workers, *Am J Phys Med Rehabil* 81(2):101-107, 2002.

11. Crosby C, Wehbe M, Mawr M: Hand strength: normative values, *J Hand Surg* 19A:665, 1994.
12. Donkin S: *Sitting on the job, how to survive the stresses of sitting down to work—a practical handbook*, Boston, 1989, Houghton Mifflin.
13. El-Karabaty H et al: The effect of carpal tunnel release on median nerve flattening and nerve conduction, *Electromyogr Clin Neurophysiol* 45(4):223-227, 2005.
14. Evangelista S, Reale V: Fibroma of tendon sheath as a cause of carpal tunnel syndrome, *J Hand Surg* 17A:1026, 1992.
15. Eversmann WW Jr: Entrapment and compression neuropathies. In Green DP, editor: *Operative hand surgery*, ed 3, New York, 1993, Churchill Livingstone.
16. Fess EE, Morgan C: *Clinical assessment recommendations*, Indianapolis, 1981, American Society of Hand Therapists.
17. Fess EE: Grip strength. In American Society of Hand Therapists, editors: *Clinical assessment recommendations*, ed 2, Chicago, 1992, The Society.
18. Frymoyer J, Bland J: Carpal tunnel syndrome in patients with myxedematous arthropathy, *J Bone Joint Surg* 55A:78, 1973.
19. Gelbrman R et al: Sensibility testing in peripheral-nerve compression syndromes, an experimental study in humans, *J Bone Joint Surg* 65A(5):632, 1983.
20. Gell N et al: A longitudinal study of industrial and clerical workers: incidence of carpal tunnel syndrome and assessment of risk factors, *J Occup Rehabil* 15(1):47-55, 2005.
21. Gretchen L, Jezek S: Pain assessment. In American Society of Hand Therapists, editors: *Clinical assessment recommendations*, ed 2, Chicago, 1992, The Society.
22. Jaffe R, Farney-Mokris S: Edema. In American Society of Hand Therapists, editors: *Clinical assessment recommendations*, ed 2, Chicago, 1992, The Society.
23. Kasch M: Therapists evaluation and treatment of upper extremity cumulative trauma disorders. In Hunter JM, Mackin EJ, Callahan AD, editors: *Rehabilitation of the hand: surgery and therapy*, ed 4, St Louis, 1995, Mosby.
24. Kerwin G, Williams CS, Seilier JG III: The pathophysiology of carpal tunnel syndrome, *Hand Clin* 12(2):243, 1996.
25. Liu CW et al: Relationship between carpal tunnel syndrome and wrist angle in computer workers, *Kaohsiung J Med Sci* 19(12):617-623, 2003.
26. Louise DS et al: Carpal tunnel syndrome in the work place, *Hand Clin* 12(2):305, 1996.
27. Ludlow KS et al: Pillar pain as a postoperative complication of carpal tunnel release: a review of the literature, *J Hand Ther* 10(4):277, 1997.
28. MacDermid J: Accuracy of clinical tests used in the detection of carpal tunnel syndrome: a literature review, *J Hand Ther* 4(4):169, 1991.
29. Macmermid J et al: Interrater reliability of pinch and grip strength measurements in patients with cumulative trauma disorders, *J Hand Ther* 7(1):10, 1984.
30. Mathiowetz V et al: Grip and pinch strength: normative data for adults, *Arch Phys Med Rehabil* 66:69, 1985.
31. Mathiowetz V et al: Adult norms for the nine hole peg test of finger dexterity, *Occup Ther J Res* 5:24, 1985.
32. Michlovitz SL: Use of ultrasound in upper extremity rehabilitation. In Hunter JM, Mackin EJ, Callahan AD, editors: *Rehabilitation of the hand: surgery and therapy*, ed 4, St Louis, 1995, Mosby.
33. Muller M et al: Effectiveness of hand therapy interventions in primary management of carpal tunnel syndrome: a systematic review, *J Hand Ther* 17(2):210-228, 2004.
34. Nathan PA, Istvan JA, Meadows KD: A longitudinal study of predictors of research-defined carpal tunnel syndrome in industrial workers: findings at 17 years, *J Hand Surg [Br]* 30(6):593-598, 2005.
35. Pascarelli E, Quilter D: *Repetitive strain injury, a computer user's guide*, New York, 1994, John Wiley & Sons.
36. Phalen GS: The carpal tunnel syndrome: seventeen years experience in diagnosis and treatment of six hundred and fifty-four, *J Bone Joint Surg* 48:211, 1966.
37. Robbins H: Anatomical study of the median nerve in the carpal tunnel and etiologies of the carpal tunnel syndrome, *J Bone Joint Surg* 45A:953, 1963.
38. Rosecrance JC et al: Carpal tunnel syndrome among apprentice construction workers, *Am J Ind Med* 42(2):107-116, 2002.
39. Sailer SM: The role of splinting and rehabilitation in the treatment of carpal and cubital tunnel syndromes, *Hand Clin* 12(2):223, 1996.
40. Spindler H, Dellon A: Nerve conduction studies and sensibility testing in carpal tunnel syndrome, *J Hand Surg* 7:260, 1982.
41. Steinberg DR: Surgical release of the carpal tunnel, *Hand Clin* 18(2):291-298, 2002.
42. Stone J: Sensibility. In American Society of Hand Therapists, editors: *Clinical assessment recommendations*, ed 2, Chicago, 1992, The Society.
43. Tanaka S et al: Prevalence and work-relatedness of self-reported carpal tunnel syndrome among US workers: analysis of the occupational health supplement data of 1988 National Health Interview Survey, *Am J Ind Med* 27:451, 1995.
44. Taylor Mullins PA: Use of therapeutic modalities in upper extremity rehabilitation. In Hunter JM, Mackin EJ, Callahan AD, editors: *Rehabilitation of the hand: surgery and therapy*, ed 4, St Louis, 1995, Mosby.
45. Viera AJ: Management of carpal tunnel syndrome, *Am Fam Physician* 15;68(2):265-272, 2003.
46. Waylett-Rendall J: Desensitization of the traumatized hand. In Hunter JM, Mackin EJ, Callahan AD, editors: *Rehabilitation of the hand: surgery and therapy,* ed 4, St Louis, 1995, Mosby.
47. Wehbe M: Tendon gliding exercises, *Am J Occup Ther* 41:164, 1987.
48. Weiss ND et al: Position of the wrist associated with the lowest carpal-tunnel pressure: implications for splint design, *J Bone Joint Surg* 77A(11):1695, 1995.
49. Werner RA, Franzblau A, Gell N: Randomized controlled trial of nocturnal splinting for active workers with symptoms of carpal tunnel syndrome, *Arch Phys Med Rehabil* 86(1):1-7, 2005.
50. Werner RA et al: Incidence of carpal tunnel syndrome among automobile assembly workers and assessment of risk factors, *J Occup Environ Med* 47(10):1044-1050, 2005.

SPINE

PART 3

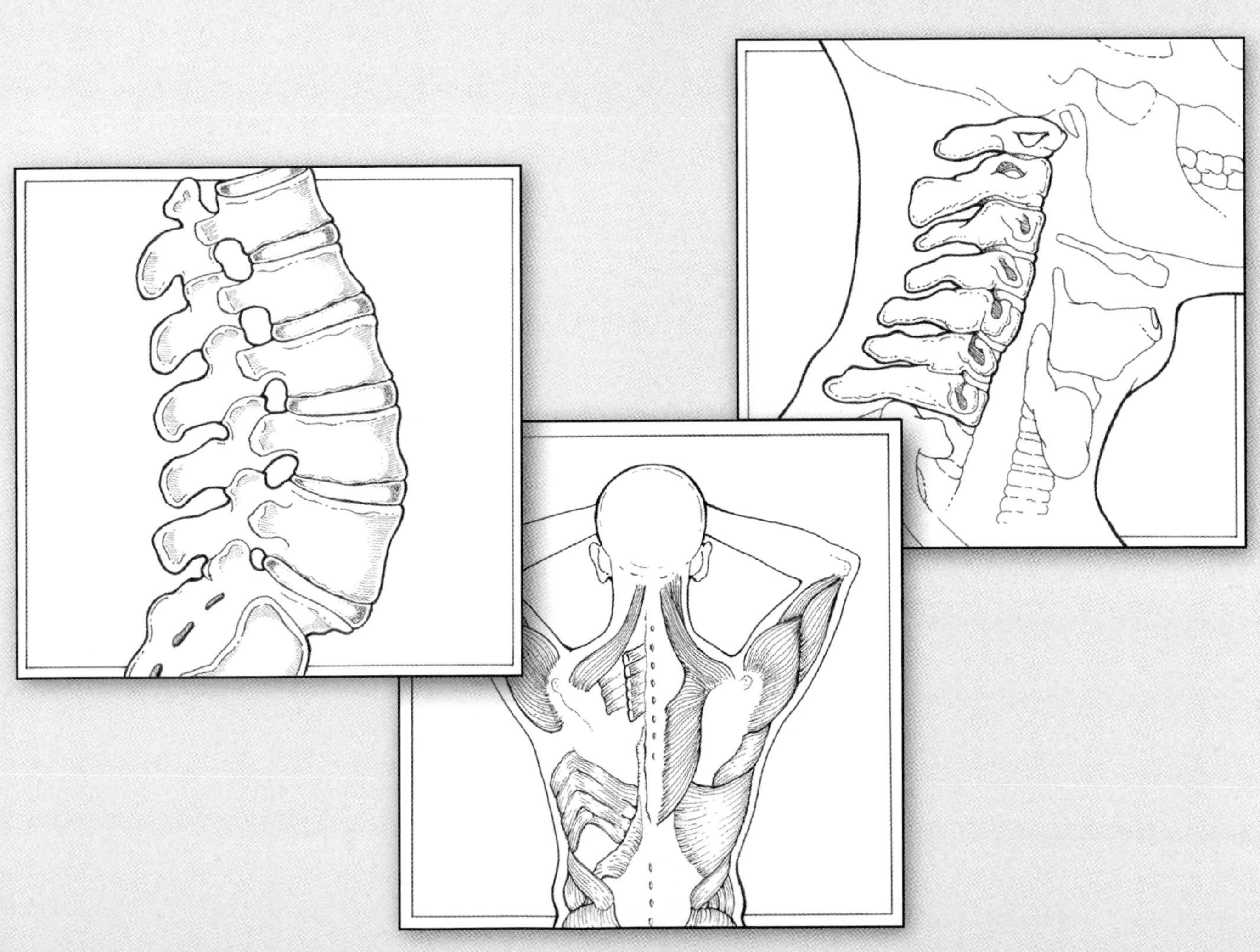

CHAPTER 12

Anterior Cervical Discectomy and Fusion

Erica V. Pablo
Ben B. Pradhan
Derrick G. Sueki
Rick B. Delamarter
Jason T. Huffman

Degenerative disc disease, lumbar or cervical, is common in the adult population and has a number of different presentations. Cervical degenerative discs may present as purely axial neck pain, as neck stiffness, or as headaches. In cases of disc herniation or osteophyte formation, radicular symptoms in the upper extremities (UEs) may be present. Progressive cervical degeneration may lead to the development of cervical spondylotic myelopathy (Figs. 12-1 and 12-2). Studies of the natural history of degenerative disc disease demonstrate that the majority of cases of neck pain and radiculopathy will resolve without surgical treatment. Myelopathy, however, tends to slowly progress.

SURGICAL INDICATIONS AND CONSIDERATIONS

Causes

Cervical disc degeneration is a progressive process similar to the degenerative cascade that occurs in other joints. Annular tears or incompetence and biochemical changes in the nucleus can lead to decreased water content in the disc, shrinking or herniation of nuclear tissue, and disc collapse. This places increased stress on the annulus and associated facet and uncovertebral joints, causing them in turn to degenerate, which can then lead to axial pain and stiffness. In addition, this can lead to the formation of bony spurs and disc herniations that may encroach on the neuroforamina, resulting in radiculopathy.[9] This entire process can be accelerated by an acute injury such as a cervical sprain in a motor vehicle accident.

The clinical presentation of cervical disc degeneration can vary and must be distinguished from other causes of neck pain, including muscular pain referred from the shoulders or viscera. Nonmechanical neck pain (i.e., pain at rest, without activity) is less likely to be related to disc disease, and other sources including tumor and infection must be considered. Mechanical neck pain caused by disc disease will often be exacerbated by neck extension and rotation to the affected side (affected side is loaded or squeezed). In contrast, muscular neck pain is often exacerbated by neck flexion and rotation away from the more painful side (muscle in affected side is stretched). In cases of lower cervical degenerative disease, the pain often radiates to the shoulder, upper arm, or infrascapular areas, and upper cervical disease may present as temporal pain and retro-orbital headaches. Associated radiculopathy presents as pain and paresthesias in a single or multiple nerve root distribution. *Spurling's sign* is a reproduction of radicular pain caused by extending the neck and rotating the head to the symptomatic side, which leads to further decreased caliber of the neuroforamina. Axial compression and the Valsalva maneuver may also reproduce symptoms. The *shoulder abduction sign* is the reduction of radicular symptoms by placing the hand of the affected arm on top of the head, which should decrease the stretch on the nerve roots.[10]

Other diagnostic tests, including imaging and electromyographic (EMG) or nerve conduction studies can be used to enhance the causative workup. Plain radiographs, including anteroposterior, lateral, oblique, and lateral flexion and extension views, can demonstrate developmental stenosis, disc space narrowing, loss of normal alignment, dynamic instability, and osteophyte formation. Findings on radiographs may be the cause of the clinical

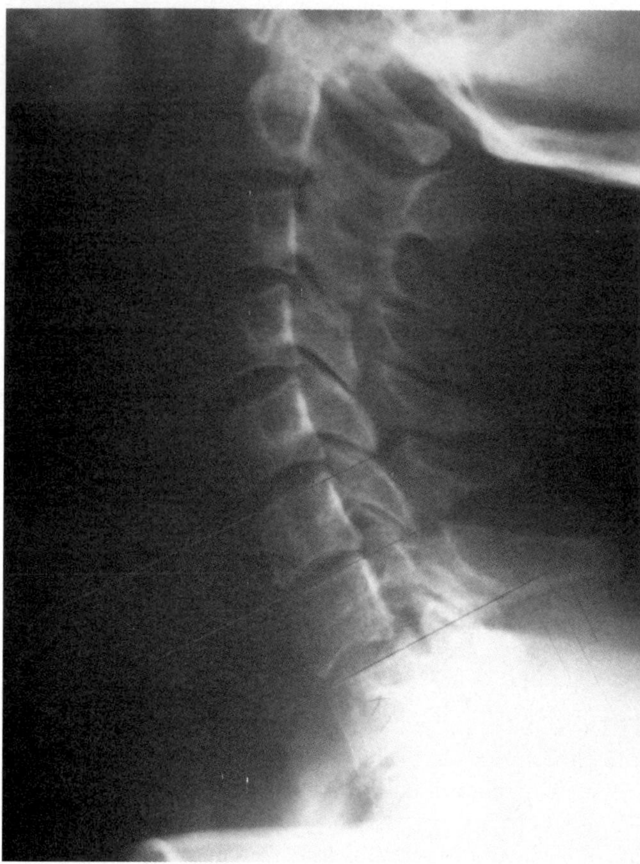

Fig. 12-1 Preoperative lateral radiograph demonstrating a small bony spur formation and disc height loss at C6-7.

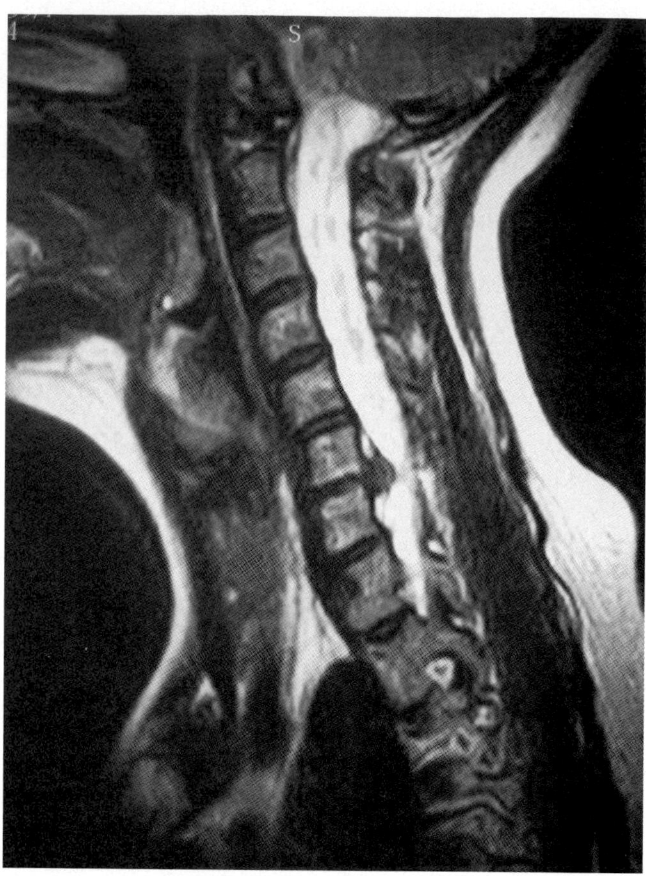

Fig. 12-2 Preoperative sagittal magnetic resonance image (MRI) showing C6-7 disc degeneration and a large herniation.

picture or may also be representative of normal age-related degenerative changes. When surgical intervention is being considered, magnetic resonance imaging (MRI) is usually obtained. MRI is the most sensitive modality for demonstrating spinal cord morphology in relation to the surrounding bony and soft tissue structures (Fig. 12-3). Cervical myelogram followed by computed tomography (CT) is a superior study for demonstrating foraminal stenosis and cortical bony margins, but it is invasive and does have a small risk of complications.[43] EMG and nerve conduction studies can help distinguish between nerve root compression and a peripheral neuropathy, and they are useful in patients with an unclear diagnosis. In cases of mechanical neck pain without radiculopathy, several studies support the use of provocative discography to confirm a discogenic origin of the pain and to clarify which disc levels are appropriate to treat.[20,48]

The majority of patients with axial neck pain can be expected to experience acceptable resolution of symptoms without surgical intervention. Cervical radiculopathy also tends to resolve, but many patients progress to experience recurrent or persistent symptoms.[35] Nonoperative treatment recommendations vary, however, and few good studies demonstrate the superiority of one modality over another. Activity modification and a brief period of soft collar use are often recommended, but prolonged inactivity may lead to deconditioning. Medical treatment usually begins with nonsteroidal anti-inflammatory drugs (NSAIDs) or acetaminophen. In cases of severe acute pain, narcotic analgesics may be used. Paraspinal muscle spasm may be relieved with muscle relaxants but is often improved with a soft collar alone. Occasionally a brief course of oral corticosteroids is tried.[15] All medications should be prescribed only with careful regard for the potential adverse reactions and interactions with other medications that the patient is taking. Physical therapy is a part of many practitioners' treatment programs and may include modalities such as traction and heat and cold therapy, as well as an isometric neck and shoulder stabilizing exercise program. The specifics of a physical therapy program are often left up to the discretion of the particular therapist.

Surgical intervention for patients with cervical radiculopathy is indicated when the symptoms are persistent or recurrent (despite appropriate conservative care), or they are severe or debilitating enough to merit surgery.[50] A more prolonged conservative course is recommended for treatment of axial neck pain alone. If surgery is being considered for axial neck pain and a workup has failed to

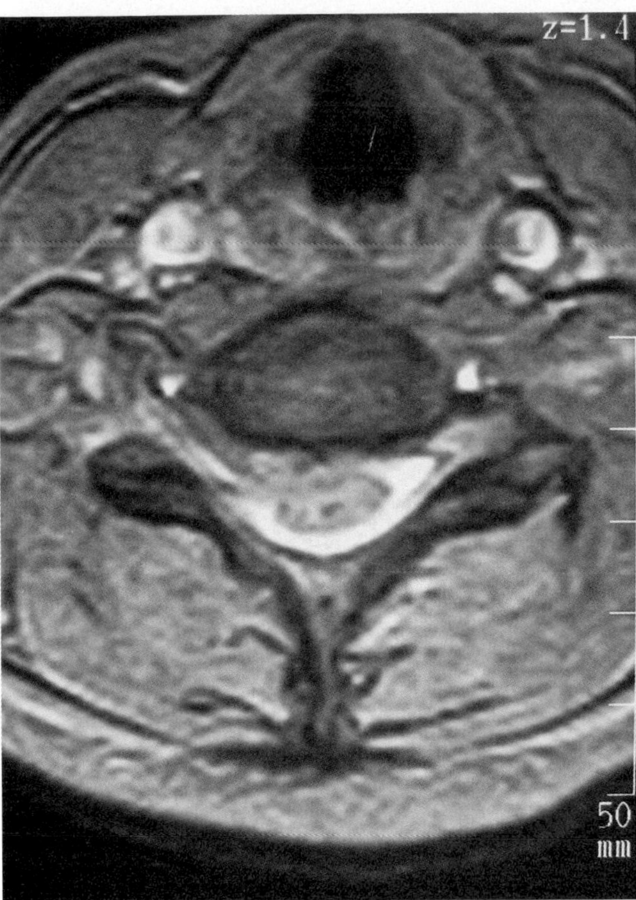

Fig. 12-3 Preoperative axial magnetic resonance image (MRI) showing large right-sided disc herniation at C6-7.

identify the specific level responsible for the pain, then a discogram is obtained to avoid fusing asymptomatic levels. As with any elective surgical procedure, appropriate patient expectations and selection should be considered before any surgical intervention is undertaken (Box 12-1). In general workers' compensation patients and those involved in litigation can be expected to have worse outcomes even after successful fusion surgery.[11,17]

Box 12-1 Indications for Anterior Cervical Discectomy and Fusion (ACDF) in Cervical Disc Disease

Strong indications:

1. Progressive cervical myelopathy
   Relative indications:
   a. Radiculopathy that has failed to respond to conservative treatment regimen of at least 6 weeks
   b. Recurrent radiculopathy
   c. Progressive neurologic deficit
   d. Severe, incapacitating axial neck pain that fails to respond to prolonged course of conservative treatment with consistent exam and diagnostic studies

SURGICAL PROCEDURE

Single-level cervical disc disease is most commonly treated with anterior cervical discectomy and fusion (ACDF). For one or more adjacent levels, some surgeons choose to perform a corpectomy of the intervening vertebral bodies instead of multilevel ACDF. After the disc is removed, graft choices include harvested iliac crest bone graft or allograft, usually a fibular ring or strut. Currently, most surgeons use an anterior cervical plate fixed to the adjacent vertebral bodies to prevent graft displacement anteriorly and to provide stability while the fusion matures. In cases of severe stenosis or instability, intraoperative neuromonitoring is often used in an attempt to prevent injury and assess adequacy of decompression.

Surgery begins with the induction of general endotracheal anesthesia. The patient is then placed in the supine position on a radiolucent operative table to allow imaging in both the anterior-posterior and lateral planes. A soft bump is placed transversly beneath the scapula, and a cervical traction collar is placed beneath the patient's chin and occiput; gentle traction is then applied. In addition, gentle skin traction is applied with wide tape on the shoulders pulling toward the foot of the bed. The anterior neck is then prepped and draped, with care taken not to restrict the surgical field. Palpating the bony landmarks (or alternatively by using a radio-opaque skin marker and a lateral radiograph) determines the level of the skin incision. A transverse incision is then made through the skin and subcutaneous fat, and bleeding is controlled using electrocautery. The platysma muscle is carefully cut in line with the incision to avoid cutting the large superficial veins just beneath it. Beneath the platysma muscle, the deep cervical fascia is identified and divided laterally to the anterior boarder of the sternocleidomastoid muscle where it is dissected inferiorly and superiorly off of the muscle belly. A finger is then used for blunt dissection between the carotid sheath laterally and the trachea and esophagus medially down to the prevertebral fascia. A hand-held Cloward retractor is then used to retract the midline structures, allowing direct visualization of prevertebral fascia and underlying longus colli muscles and disc spaces. When a disc space is identified, a short needle is inserted into the disc space and a radiograph is obtained to confirm that the appropriate level has been approached.

When the appropriate level is confirmed, the longus colli muscles are dissected off of bone laterally and a self-retaining retractor is placed, exposing the disc space to the uncovertebral joints. The operating microscope, sterilely draped, is then brought into the field (Fig. 12-4). Under direct visualization using the microscope, the disc is incised with a scalpel and the anterior portion is removed using a pituitary forceps and an angled curette. A high-speed drill may be used to complete the discectomy and expose the posterior longitudinal ligament (PLL).

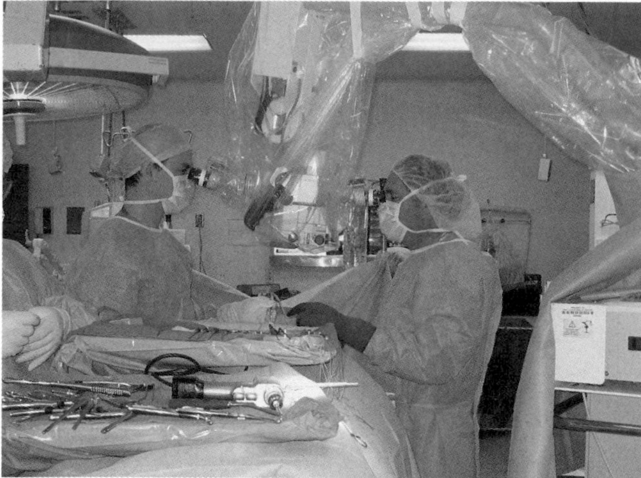

Fig. 12-4 Intraoperative photo showing primary surgeon and assistant using the microscope during discectomy.

After exposure the PLL is elevated off of the posterior aspect of the vertebral bodies using a small 4-0 forward-angled curette; it is then excised using 1 mm and 2 mm Kerrison rongeurs. The PLL does not need to be routinely removed if no nuclear protrusion or extrusion is found, but this has to be carefully explored. The posterior aspect of the uncinate process is then excised using the 3-0 curette, followed by the 1 and 2 mm Kerrison rongeurs. The foramina can be probed with the 90-degree angled nerve hook to confirm adequate decompression or any remaining loose disc fragments.

When the discectomy and foraminotomies are complete, the disc space is measured and an appropriately sized graft is chosen. While increased traction is applied on the halter traction device, the graft is gently impacted into position. When it is adequately positioned, all traction is removed. An appropriate-sized plate is then chosen and applied on the anterior aspect of the cervical spine. Care is taken when drilling screw holes to choose a length that will be contained in the vertebral body and to parallel the endplate of the disc space. When the plate is in position, a lateral radiograph is obtained and graft and hardware positioning is checked (Figs. 12-5 and 12-6).

After instrumentation is complete, the wound is copiously irrigated and thoroughly checked for hemostasis. Often a drain is used even if the wound appears very dry, because a postoperative hematoma may cause significant morbidity. The platysma muscle and subcutaneous tissue are then closed with interrupted absorbable sutures. A running subcuticular layer of suture may follow this closure, or Steri-Strips alone may be applied followed by a sterile dressing. The patient is then placed into a rigid cervical orthosis such as an Aspen collar before moving or extubation.

In the immediate postoperative period the head of the patient's bed is maintained in an elevated position to decrease swelling in the neck. The patient should be able to walk, void, swallow liquids, and tolerate a diet before discharge. Most patients are discharged the day after surgery. Patients commonly complain of sore throat and pain with swallowing in the first few days after surgery. If these complaints seem more severe than usual, then a single dose or short course of oral corticosteroids may be given in an attempt to minimize swelling.

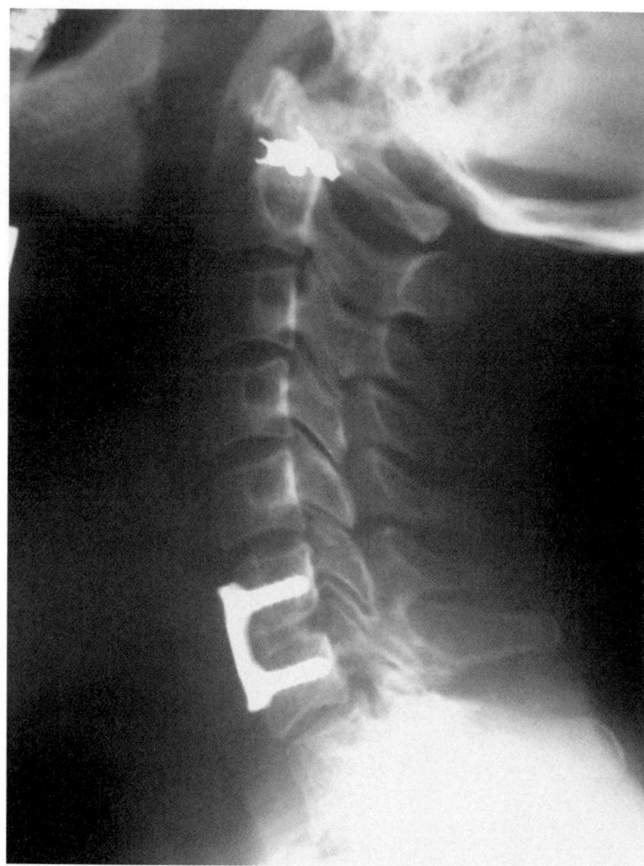

Fig. 12-5 Postoperative lateral radiograph showing solid fusion of C6 and C7 with anterior cervical plate and screws.

Outcomes

Patients with radicular symptoms will often note immediate relief of symptoms after surgery. Most patients report a change in the quality of their axial neck pain to one more typical of postoperative pain. Generally patients treated for radicular symptoms achieve greater than 90% satisfactory results, whereas those treated for axial neck pain generally achieve about 80% satisfactory results.

One concern in the postoperative period is overactivity before fusion is achieved. Solid consolidation of fusion often requires 6 to 12 weeks, so excessive motion and loading are discouraged during this period. Often patients are maintained in a cervical collar for 6 to 12 weeks to restrict their activities, but patients frequently recover from their surgery much sooner and desire to remove

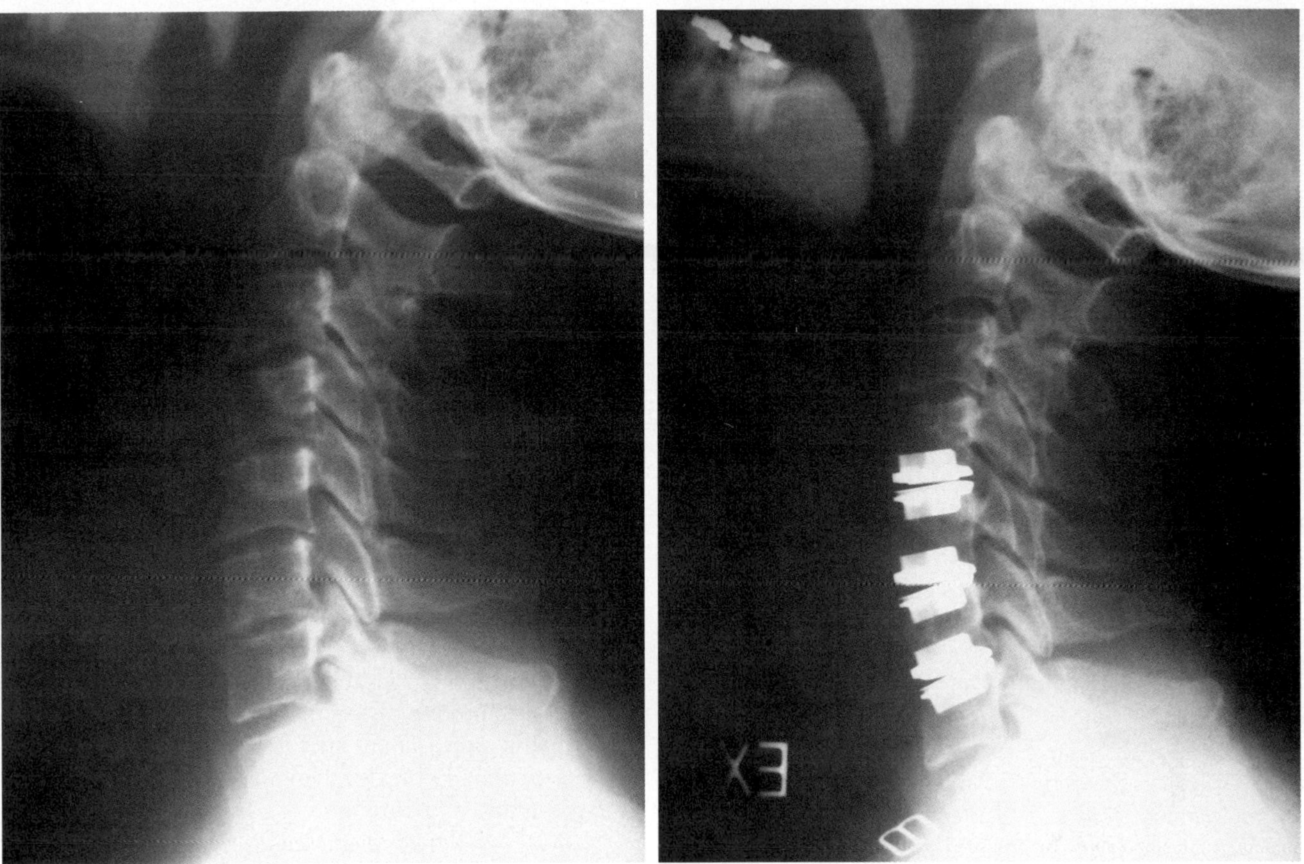

Fig. 12-6 **A,** Preoperative lateral radiograph showing multilevel cervical disc degeneration. **B,** Postoperative lateral radiograph of the same patient after three-level cervical disc replacement.

the orthosis and resume activities. Months of relative immobilization can result in significant deconditioning, which can be a challenge to the therapist. In the early period of return to activity and therapy, it is important to avoid injury caused by overly strenuous exercises or an overzealous patient.

Future Directions

Spinal fusion in general has had less satisfying results than some other commonly performed orthopaedic surgeries, leading medical researchers to search for alternative treatments. Recently the first lumbar disc replacement prosthesis gained Food and Drug Administration (FDA) approval in the United States (Charite lumbar artificial disc) with another pending (ProDisc-L lumbar artificial disc), and cervical disc replacements (e.g., ProDisc-C, Bryan, Prestige artificial cervical discs) have also completed clinical trials.[12-14,23,24] Further research is underway in the field of biologic disc replacement or rejuvenation. These treatments have the potential of offering shorter recovery times and more rapid return to activity and may help prevent the progression of spondylosis at adjacent levels.

THERAPY GUIDELINES FOR REHABILITATION

Rehabilitation after a surgery is a *science* and an *art*. The science of rehabilitation relies on a firm understanding of the body's normal response to injury and trauma. The art of rehabilitation rests in the clinician's ability to interpret the individual patient's unique signs and symptoms. The ability to formulate a plan of care that maximizes an individual's healing potential relies on the ability to blend the science and the art of rehabilitation. The initial portion of this chapter is designed to provide the clinician with an understanding of the role that tissue healing plays in the development of a rehabilitation program. This will serve as a scientific foundation upon which a clinician can base his or her clinical reasoning process. This tissue-healing model will then be placed in the context of ACDF. The activities and precautions of each phase of the rehabilitation process will be rooted in current understanding of the phases of tissue healing. Specific treatment options are provided throughout the chapter, but these should only serve as a guide to treatment and should not replace sound clinical reasoning or judgment when rehabilitating after ACDF.

Q Angel is a 45-year-old woman who has arrived at the outpatient clinic for an initial evaluation status after ACDF. The surgery was 4 weeks ago. Her chief complaint is stiffness and soreness in her neck with difficulty sleeping at night. She also notes continued difficulty swallowing and complains of a dry mouth. She asks the therapist's opinion regarding whether she should see her doctor. What should the therapist tell her?

The decision to operate on the cervical spine may be driven by localized tissue damage and subsequent focal pain, but the majority of spinal surgeries are initiated because of damage to (or threat of damage to) the neural network of the body. Myelographic CT and MRI studies have all demonstrated that 20% to 30% of people who have disc herniation and stenosis do not have radicular symptoms, and many of these people do not have neck pain.[42] It has also been shown that under anesthesia, only nerves that are inflamed will produce radicular symptoms when compressed or tractioned. Therefore although the intervertebral disc or stenosis can be the source of neck pain, it is generally injury to the nerve that drives the decision to undergo surgery. Protecting the nervous system from further damage and providing an environment in which the nerve can heal are primary goals of the surgery and rehabilitation thereafter.

Within the spine, injury or damage to the nerve often occurs at the spinal nerve root or the dorsal root ganglia. Anatomically, differences in the nerve root make it more susceptible to injury than at other regions of the peripheral nerve. The nerve root is not as well protected, less able to withstand deformation, and less able to repair itself than the remainder of the peripheral nerve. The other structure within the intervertebral foramen that is susceptible to damage is the dorsal root ganglia. The position of the dorsal root ganglia is not constant and can be found inside the foramen, outside the foramen, or in the spinal canal, which can increase the likelihood that it will be injured. In addition, unlike the spinal nerve root and peripheral nerve, the dorsal root ganglia do not have a blood-nerve barrier, which is necessary to prevent foreign substances from invading the nerve. These anatomic differences predispose the dorsal root ganglia to edema and mechanical compression.[42,44,45]

Nerves must also be able to move and glide within the tissue. For this to occur, some slack in the system must exist. The spinal cord changes length by 7 cm from flexion to extension. Studies in the arm show that a 7 mm excursion occurs in the nerves with movement. In addition to compression, increased tension of the nerve can result in nerve damage. **More specifically, tension in nerves causing a 20% to 30% increase in length will cause the nerve to break. Therefore exercises that place undue stress and tension on the nerves should be avoided.**[5]

Neurons are incapable of dividing and migrating; therefore regeneration occurs only through existing neurons. If the connective tissue sheathing remains intact, then a potential for nerve regrowth exists. If the sheath is disrupted, then the potential for regrowth diminishes. Initially, like any tissue, an inflammatory process is seen within the nerve. Within hours after injury, the nerves start to grow back from the distal stump at 1 to 2 mm per day. In addition to transmitting nerve impulses, the axon of the nerve functions to transmit nutrients and chemicals down its lumen. These axons are filled with axoplasm, which is necessary for nerve health and survival. Axoplasm is a viscous substance and is thixotropic, which means that it needs constant agitation or it will gel.[42,44,45] **Thus care must be taken to encourage movement and gliding of the nerve, but at the same time, positions that place tension on the nerve should be avoided.**

A Angel is likely experiencing dysphagia, which is a common short-term side effect to the surgery. The therapist should ask the patient for further information on the duration and intensity of the symptoms. Mild symptoms of dysphagia may be expected, although increased symptoms related to cardiovascular signs such as difficulty breathing, shortness of breath, or symptoms of sleep apnea would warrant a physician consultation.

ACDF surgery affects the sternocleidomastoid, platysma, anterior scalene, middle scalene, and the longus colli muscles. It also requires the resection of the anterior longitudinal ligament, PLL, joint capsule, and synovium.[1,26,27,51] After the trauma incurred during surgery, the body is only capable of repairing small muscle lesions with regeneration of muscle tissue. Large lesions fill with dense connective tissue. Although dense connective tissue can function to re-establish tissue continuity, it lacks the contractile elements of normal muscle tissue and the tensile strength of normal ligament and tendon tissue. Therefore the ability to generate contractile forces or resist tensile loading through the region of repair is compromised.[18,19,40,41]

Bone grafts from the iliac crest are often used within the disc space, between two vertebral bodies, to aid in the mineralization and fixation of the region. The iliac crest is used as the primary source of graft material because of its cancellous bone composition. Cancellous bone has a greater potential for revascularization and osteogenesis than grafts from denser cortical bone sources. Healing after a cortical bone graft can take up to two times longer than its cancellous bone graft counterpart.[18,19] As will become apparent later in the chapter, the healing and mineralization of bone at the site of fusion is a major factor driving progression through the rehabilitation process.

Q Ned is a 41-year-old man who was involved in a motor vehicle accident 2 years ago. His primary pain symptoms because of the accident included paresthesias and a burning sensation throughout his right UE. He underwent ACDF surgery 4 weeks ago and continues to have neural paresthesias in his right arm. What interventions should be administered?

Phase I (Inflammation)

The inflammation phase is the first phase of tissue healing. It begins with injury to the tissue, reaches its peak within the first 72 hours after injury, and is generally completed within 14 days. During these first 14 days, several events occur. Vascular structures in the immediate area constrict to prevent blood loss, and vascular tissues in the surrounding areas dilate to provide conduits through which healing materials can enter the injured site. Cells and chemical mediators are brought into the area to remove all foreign debris and dead or dying tissue and are responsible for the closure of the wound. Both of these actions are important in the prevention of infection.[18,19] During the inflammation phase in bone healing, a hematoma is formed at the site of the surgery. This begins immediately after surgery and is usually completed within 7 days. The hematoma will form around the graft and fusion site, and granulation tissue will fill any open space between the graft, the vertebral bodies, and the instrumentation.[18,19,40,41] Clinically, rehabilitation during the inflammation phase of tissue and bone healing should focus on the prevention of blood loss, reduction of inflammation, and managing the pain that accompanies tissue damage (Table 12-1).

A Possible interventions include gentle UE AROM exercises to the elbow in flexion and extension (as well as to the wrists and fingers) below 90 degrees of shoulder elevation to allow the nerves to glide. The therapist should encourage the patient to move the arms below shoulder level and advise the patient not to lift and move his arms excessively above 90 degrees.

Phase II (Reparative)

The reparative phase is the second phase of tissue healing. This phase begins almost immediately after injury and is completed in 21 days. The primary function of this phase is the formation of the dense connective tissue needed to repair the wound and re-establish structural continuity of the affected region. The process of repairing the tissue into its original state is a time-consuming process, and little evidence supports the notion that tendons, ligaments, or large muscle injuries heal by regenerating into their original tissue. Thus the re-establishment of structural continuity and integrity of tendons, ligaments, and large muscle lesions is completed through the creation of dense connective tissue. Reparation with dense connective tissue patches or *scar tissue* is a fast process that can allow for quicker recovery of the tissue. Angioblasts and fibroblasts begin to enter the injured region within 5 days of the injury. These cells begin the process of tissue repair and the revascularization of the region. Most of the actual dense connective tissue development is completed by day 21. During bone healing at this time, a synthesis and organization of collagen is seen in the hematoma. Once the hematoma is organized, blood vessels invade the area. This allows osteoblasts to migrate into the region and form woven bone, which is known as a *soft callus*.[18,19,40,41] Clinically, the goal of rehabilitation in this phase should be to promote the development of the new dense connective reparative tissue and woven bone (see Table 12-1).

Table 12-1 Soft Tissue and Bone Healing Time Frames

Phase	Events	Time Frame
Phase I Inflammation	Vasoconstriction in immediate area Vasodilation in surrounding areas Wound closure Removal of foreign and necrotic tissue Hematoma formation in the bone	0-14 days
Phase II Reparative	Fibroblasts enter region to create dense connective tissue scars Angioblasts enter region for revascularization Soft callus formation in the bone	0-21 days
Phase IIIa Remodeling	Dense connective tissue is converted from cellular to fibrous Hard callus formation in the bone	22-60 days
Phase IIIb Remodeling	Dense connective tissue is strengthened Bone is remodeled and strengthened	61-84 days
Phase IIIc Remodeling	Dense connective tissue is strengthened Bone is remodeled and strengthened	85-360 days

Q Sam is a 54-year-old man who underwent ACDF 12 weeks ago. He started outpatient physical therapy services 6 weeks ago and has made significant improvements in his upper-quarter ROM and strength. Recently, Sam has begun a gym exercise program as he prepares for discharge from physical therapy. However, after approximately 2 weeks at the gym, Sam reports feeling soreness in his neck and shoulders after performing the following exercises: seated scapular rows, latissimus pull-downs, biceps curls, inclined bench press, and an introductory spinning or cycling class for aerobic conditioning. Which of the previously mentioned exercises may be causing Sam's symptoms?

Phase III (Remodeling)

The remodeling phase is the last phase of the tissue healing process. The purpose of this phase is to strengthen the newly formed scar tissue. Two subphases make up tissue remodeling: (1) consolidation and (2) maturation. During the consolidation subphase, tissue is undergoing conversion from a cellular type to one that is fibrous in nature. The actual size of the scar stops growing by 21 days, although the scar will continue to strengthen in response to stress. This subphase lasts from 22 to 60 days. During this phase of bone remodeling, the soft callus phase begins to mineralize and form a hard callus. Variations in mineralization time exist, but generally mineralization is completed by day 64. Mineralization of the callus is used diagnostically as a marker for when it is appropriate to begin rehabilitation. The patient will not be referred for rehabilitation until radiographic evidence indicates that the callus has mineralized.[18,19,40,41] Clinically, rehabilitation should address protection and prevention of excessive motion through the fusion site. **Excessive motion at the fusion site can lead to excessive callus formation and delay of the reparative process. The goal of rehabilitation in this phase should be the strengthening of the newly formed connective tissue. Care must be taken during this phase not to exceed the mechanical limits of the newly formed tissue, because overstress of the tissue will result in tissue injury and delay healing.**

The maturation subphase occurs from day 60 to 360 when the tissues are fully fibrous in nature. For this reason, a progression in the strengthening of the affected tissues may begin. For bone remodeling, the hard callus begins to adapt to the stresses placed upon it. These stressors can be internal and external and include low serum calcium levels, skeletal microdamage, and changes in mechanical stress. The bone-remodeling process generally takes 6 months from initiation to completion, but it can take up to 4 years.[18,19,40,41] Clinically, rehabilitation programs must provide appropriate levels of stress to the bone to encourage bone strengthening and remodeling without creating or exacerbating tissue injury (see Table 12-1).

A The introductory spinning or cycling class may be the cause of Sam's pain symptoms because of the cervical positioning this type of bike provides. This style of bike usually places the cervical spine in hyperextension and the thoracolumbar spine in flexion, causing Sam to feel soreness after maintaining this extreme position for the duration of the class. Use of a stationary upright bike may place the cervical spine in a more comfortable position and relieve Sam's symptoms. In addition, it would be prudent for the therapist to advise Sam to postpone latissimus pull-downs at this time. They can be started later in the rehabilitation process; however, at this time it is not wise to complete resisted activities above shoulder level. Finally, the therapist should assess the amount of weight the patient is using.

Summary

Although guidelines can provide generalized time frames for healing and recovery, it is important to realize that a firm grasp of the factors listed previously will enable the clinician to individualize the rehabilitation program for each patient. No two patients are identical. Therefore no two rehabilitation programs should be identical. Solid clinical reasoning regarding the patient and the nature of the injury and surgery will ultimately drive the rehabilitation process.

Certain key components should be kept in mind during each phase of the rehabilitation process for ACDF.

Phase I:

The initial goal of rehabilitation should be the reduction of inflammation, closure of the wound, and reduction in pain.

Phase II:

The surgical site should be protected until dense connective tissue is formed and the bone shows evidence of mineralization.

Movement of the UEs below shoulder levels to promote nerve mobility and healing should be encouraged.

Phase III:

Gliding of the neural tissue through the surgical site to prevent the formation of adhesions should be promoted.

The therapist should begin placing stress on the soft tissue and bone in graded increments to promote proper soft tissue and bone growth and development.

Q Sherry is a 50-year-old woman who had ACDF surgery 6 weeks ago and has just recently removed her cervical collar and returned to work as an accountant. She has a forward head posture, rounded and slumped shoulders, and bilateral scapular winging. She also continues to have numbness and tingling in her right UE, and her pain level reaches a 6 out of 10 (10 being the worst) by lunchtime. She is worried that the fusion has been unsuccessful. What is the therapist's response?

DESCRIPTION OF REHABILITATION AND RATIONALE FOR USING INSTRUMENTATION

Phase I (Inflammatory Phase)

TIME: 1 to 2 weeks after surgery (days 0 to 14)
GOALS: Protect the surgical site, decrease pain and inflammation, maintain UE flexibility, initiate patient education regarding neutral cervical spine mechanics (Table 12-2)

During the initial phase of rehabilitation, the primary focus of physical therapy is to protect the surgical site and make sure that the patient is educated on the mechanics of maintaining a proper neutral cervical spine (Fig. 12-7). Hospitalization after ACDF in most cases will be for 1 to 2 days. During this time the patient will be given a cervical collar to wear to immobilize the neck and encourage soft tissue and bone healing. Instructions regarding the frequency of collar wear will be determined by the physician and may differ on a case-by-case basis. Physical evaluation during this time may include wound assessment and the assessment of bed mobility and gait. **Because of the fragility of the wound and fusion sites, assessment of cervical range of motion (ROM) and UE strength are not appropriate in this phase.** The primary physical impairments that the patient is likely to experience are pain, limited cardiovascular endurance, and limited tolerance to upright activities. During this time the injured vasculature around the wound begins to close and the noninjured vessels dilate, which may lead to increased warmth and redness around the incision site. This may be accompanied by neck pain and a sore throat. Oral analgesics may be given by the physician to manage the pain and inflammation.

The inflammatory phase lasts approximately 2 weeks. During this time activities should center on resuming normal daily activities. Ambulation to and from the restroom should begin immediately, with assistance as needed, and progress until the patient is independent. The patient should be encouraged to increase the daily

Table 12-2 Anterior Cervical Discectomy and Fusion

Rehabilitation Phase	Criteria to Progress to this Phase	Anticipated Impairments and Functional Limitations	Intervention	Goal	Rationale
Phase I Acute inflammatory phase Postoperative weeks 1-2 (days 0-14)	• Postoperative	• Pain • Edema • Limited neck ROM • Limited nerve mobility • Limited tolerance to upright activities • Limited cardiovascular endurance	Patient education regarding the following: • Proper use of cervical support • Protection of surgical site • Correct body mechanics and maintenance of neutral cervical spine • Daily walking program	• Decrease pain and edema • Protection of surgical repair (soft tissue and bone) • Restoration of UE ROM • Understand the time frame for healing structures • Understand correct body mechanics and maintenance of neutral cervical spine • Gradual increase in walking speed and duration	• Encourage self-management of pain and edema • Prevent adhesions of neural tissue • Prevent reinjury with patient education on body mechanics and maintenance of neutral cervical spine with activity • Gradually improve cardiovascular endurance

ROM, Range of motion; *UE*, upper extremity.

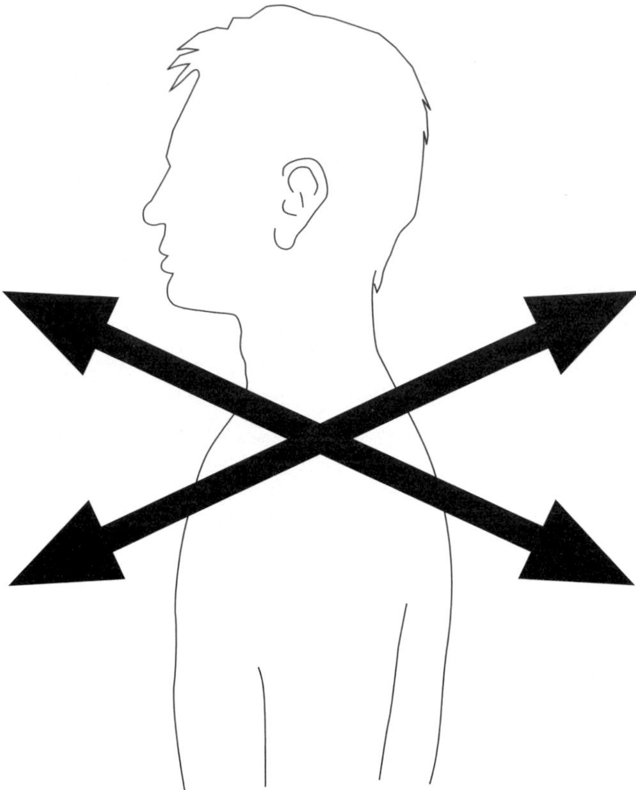

Fig. 12-7 Neutral cervical spine. Proper alignment of the cervical, thoracic, and lumbar spine in which stress to the joints, muscles, and vertebrae is minimized.

Box 12-2 Discharge Instructions after Anterior Cervical Discectomy and Fusion (ACDF) Surgery

- Wear cervical collar as instructed.
- Do not pick up or carry anything heavier then a gallon of milk.
- Do not sleep with arms over head.
- Do not lift anything above shoulder level.
- Sleep on a firm pillow to help support the neck.
- Avoid sitting or standing for prolonged periods of time. Change positions frequently.
- Get plenty of rest, but do not spend all of your time in bed.
- Gradually increase walking time. Do not get overtired.
- Avoid strenuous exercise or activities.
- Keep incision dry. Showering is allowed 10 days after surgery if wound is not red or draining.
- You may sleep in any position that is comfortable, except on your stomach or with arms over head.
- Do not drive until approved by your physician.
- Notify your doctor if any of the following occur:
- Temperature greater than 10° F
- Redness or swelling around your incision
- Any drainage from your incision
- Separation of wound edges
- Any new bruising around the wound
- New numbness or tingling in your hands or fingers
- Increased pain in neck, shoulders, or arms
- New weakness of either arm, hands, or legs

sitting tolerances. Pain and fatigue should guide the progression. Once discharged from the hospital, the patient will be instructed to protect the cervical region. The cervical collar issued earlier should be worn 24 hours a day unless otherwise ordered by the physician. **Before discharge from the hospital, it is important that the therapist educate the patient on proper cervical spine mechanics during activity, as well as the need to restrict large amounts of movement in the neck to prevent soft tissue and bone injury.** (Refer to Box 12-2 for specific patient guidelines to follow after discharge.) Because of the many muscular attachments of the shoulder girdle to the cervical spine, the patient should be advised to refrain from heavy lifting and from activities above shoulder level. Before discharge, the need to continue a home walking program and use of the cervical collar should also be addressed.

A

In this case patient education on the need for proper posture throughout the spine appears warranted. The explanation should address proper ergonomic positioning in the workplace to provide the neck and spine an optimal position for work-related activities. In addition, an explanation concerning the effects and stress her posture imposes on nerves and soft tissues will put her at ease. Tight musculature of the pectoralis major and other anterior tissues may be pinching on the brachial plexus, or the nerve roots may be affected secondary to the forward posturing. Interventions to improve her posture should be initiated to relieve undue stresses, and light strengthening of weakened muscles from the upper-cross syndrome can be addressed as tolerated. The patient should also be advised to take regular breaks while at work to allow her to change positions and prevent prolonged static postures. The therapist should encourage the patient to lie down or sit in a reclined position during these breaks, to allow the postural stabilizers of the neck to rest.

Phase II (Reparative Phase)

TIME: 3 weeks after surgery (days 0 to 21)
GOALS: Understand neutral spine concepts, increase UE soft tissue mobility and flexibility, improve upright tolerance, improve activities of daily living (ADLs), increase cardiovascular function (Table 12-3)

> **Q** Angela underwent ACDF surgery to C5-C6 8 weeks ago. She started outpatient physical therapy last week. Her chief complaint is of decreased neck mobility. She also reports that she is experiencing a nagging pain in her right anterior superior iliac crest. This is where the graft for the cervical fusion was harvested. Angela wants to know if the hip pain is normal and whether it will resolve. How should the therapist respond?

In many instances, phase II of the rehabilitation process will take place independently in the patient's home. Home therapy is rarely indicated; therefore education regarding patient progression through the first month after surgery is an important aspect of hospital care. The patient will be progressed to phase III once sufficient radiographic evidence of callus formation and mineralization is seen. During the reparative phase of tissue and bone healing, the body begins to form and lay down scar tissue at the surgical site, enhancing the integrity of the musculature to withstand gradual increases in loads to the tissues. Within the bone fusion site, callus formation is nearing completion. Rehabilitation throughout this phase should be a continuation of phase I, and a broadening of the focus to include the restoration of UE ROM to shoulder level and independence with self-care skills while protecting the surgical site (Fig. 12-8). At this time in the rehabilitation process, the patient may begin active range of motion (AROM) exercises of the shoulders. Nerves and soft tissue require movement to heal properly. Movement also prevents the formation of scar tissue adhesions between the nerve and the healing tissue surrounding the surgery. Therefore movement of the arms below shoulder level should be encouraged.

Exercises incorporating flexion and extension of the elbow, wrist, and fingers should also be implemented at this time.

Motion above shoulder level should still be avoided. Throughout all activities and exercises, the patient should be encouraged to maintain a neutral cervical spine. As neck pain and inflammation begin to subside in this phase and the patient continues to progress in activity level, trunk stabilization exercises may be introduced to allow the patient to achieve the overall neutral spine concept. Trunk stabilization exercises will allow loads to be properly distributed along the spine so as not to

Table 12-3 Anterior Cervical Discectomy and Fusion

Rehabilitation Phase	Criteria to Progress to this Phase	Anticipated Impairments and Functional Limitations	Intervention	Goal	Rationale
Phase II Reparative phase Postoperative week 3 (days 15-21)	◆ No signs of infection ◆ Incision site is healing well	◆ As in Phase I ◆ Limited upper-body strength ◆ Limited upper-body ROM ◆ Limited tolerance to prolonged sitting or standing positions	Continue interventions in Phase I with the following: ◆ Initiate gentle stretching of chest (corner stretch) ◆ Gentle UE AROM ◆ Trunk-bracing techniques in multiple planes ◆ Progress walking program to 15-20 minutes as tolerated	Same goals as Phase I with the following: ◆ Improve upright tolerance ◆ Restore functional ROM to UEs ◆ Restore patient independence with self-care skills ◆ Improve upper-body standing/ sitting posture ◆ Improve ADLs while protecting surgical site ◆ Increase cardiovascular function ◆ Independent with home exercise program	◆ Restore UE ROM and tissue tension to allow for proper movement mechanics ◆ Reduce stiffness in surrounding joints ◆ Prepare patient to be independent in self-care skills ◆ Restore proper posture throughout trunk to allow patient to achieve overall neutral spine concept ◆ Improve cardiovascular endurance

ROM, Range of motion; *UE,* upper extremity; *AROM,* active range of motion; *ADLs,* activities of daily living.

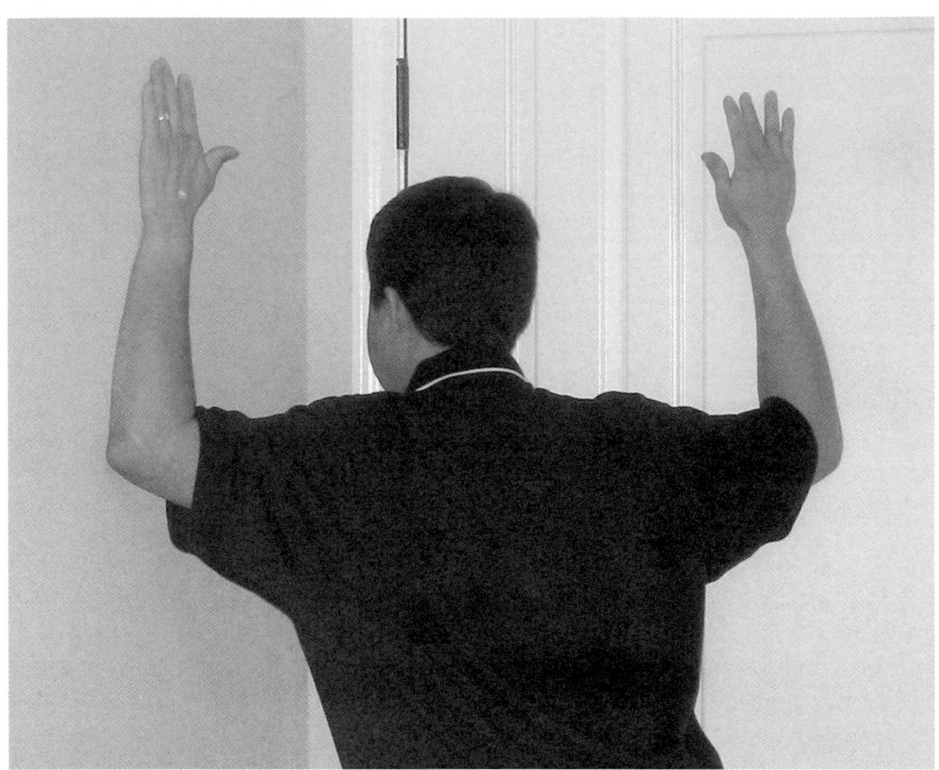

Fig. 12-8 Corner stretch. The patient stands facing a corner with the arms placed on the wall and elbows bent 90 degrees. The patient leans the entire body forward with the knees slightly bent.

adversely increase loads to the cervical region during activities. Moreover, improved trunk stability and overall neutral spine will contribute to improving tolerance to upright postures.

A At approximately 8 weeks after surgery, bone is undergoing a transformation from a soft callus to a hard callus. Although mineralization of bone may have been completed in the cervical region based on radiographs, the affected hip rarely undergoes a series of radiographs before outpatient physical therapy is initiated. Generally, no contraindications exist to physical therapy for hip pain. The harvest site may be tender for several months after the graft removal because of the trauma of surgery and bone-remodeling process, but the pain should gradually abate. Occasionally the lateral femoral cutaneous nerve may be affected by the graft harvest. If this is the case, then the patient will experience numbness or paresthesias down the lateral aspect of the thigh. Recovery of the nerve will depend on whether the nerve was cut during the surgery or simply compressed by inflammation. If it was excised, then recovery potential is poor. If it is simply compressed, then function of the nerve should return once the source of the compression is removed.

Q Stacey is a 52-year-old woman who underwent ACDF 8 weeks ago. She has been attending physical therapy for the last 2 weeks but continues to complain that her neck motion is limited. Although she is not currently working, she is worried that she will not be able to resume her position as a bus driver because she is unable to turn her head to look for oncoming traffic. How should the therapist address this problem?

Phase IIIa (Remodeling Phase)

TIME: 4 to 8 weeks after surgery (days 22 to 60)
GOALS: Enhance nerve healing and mobility, prevent scar tissue formation, increase UE strength and endurance, improve thoracic spine mobility (Table 12-4)

During this period of recovery, the patient (along with the soft tissues and bone of the surgical site) begins to experience numerous changes. Between the end of the fourth week and up to the sixth postoperative week, the physician will reassess the patient. Generally this reassessment will include a new radiographic study.

Protection of the surgical site and proper immobilization should continue until the physician has seen evidence of mineralization and callus formation of the bone graft. Once the surgical site has sufficiently

Table 12-4 Anterior Cervical Discectomy and Fusion

Rehabilitation Phase	Criteria to Progress to this Phase	Anticipated Impairments and Functional Limitations	Intervention	Goal	Rationale
Phase IIIa Remodeling phase (consolidation) Postoperative weeks 4-8 (days 22-60)	◆ Patient understanding of neutral spine concepts ◆ No increase in pain symptoms ◆ No increase in nerve-related symptoms	◆ Limited nerve mobility ◆ Limited UE strength ◆ Limited ability to perform overhead activities ◆ Limited mobility in thoracic region ◆ Limited cardiovascular endurance	Continue with Phase II interventions as needed with the following: ◆ PROM to shoulder above 90 degrees ◆ Begin gentle AROM of cervical spine as tolerated ◆ Begin neuromobility techniques ◆ Begin strengthening deep neck flexors ◆ Begin PRE program of the UEs below 90 degrees of shoulder elevation (biceps curls, isometric shoulder exercises) ◆ Trunk stabilization exercises with cocontraction of scapular stabilizers ◆ Begin gentle soft tissue mobilization of thoracic region ◆ Begin gentle thoracic spine mobilizations to the mid or lower T/S only ◆ Thoracic AROM exercises (wall angels, scapular retractions) ◆ Walking tolerance to 30 minutes	Same as Phase II with the following: ◆ Enhance nerve healing and mobility ◆ Prevent scar tissue formation ◆ Increase UE muscular strength and endurance ◆ Increase coordination in activating trunk and scapular stabilizing muscles ◆ Improve mobility of thoracic spine ◆ Improve aerobic capacity	◆ Prevent soft tissue adhesions at surgical site ◆ Prevent neural adhesions ◆ Increase stabilization while performing daily activities to prevent reinjury ◆ Decrease joint stiffness to allow proper movement with decreased pain ◆ Independence with self-care activities

UE, Upper extremity; *PROM*, passive range of motion; *AROM*, active range of motion.

mineralized, the physician may permit additional rehabilitation.

Postural Rehabilitation

Rehabilitation specialists should expect to see patients in an outpatient setting at approximately 6 weeks after ACDF. Upon initial evaluation, observation of the patient's posture will give the physical therapist (PT) a significant amount of information concerning weakness, elongation, and strength of specific musculature, as well as the patient's ability to maintain a neutral cervical spine. According to Janda,[28] a common postural alignment seen in people with upper-quarter pathology is known as the *upper-cross syndrome* (Fig. 12-9). Regardless of the cause, this alignment will consist of an upper-quarter muscle pattern in which certain muscles will be weakened and lengthened and others will be strong and shortened, resulting in an increased thoracic kyphosis, increased midcervical lordosis, and increased upper cervical extension. Protraction of the scapula will often accompany this postural deviation. More specifically, a weakening and lengthening of the rhomboids, middle and lower trapezius, deep neck flexors, supraspinatus, infraspinatus, and the deltoid musculature occurs. This is combined with a tightening and shortening of the pectoralis major and minor, levator scapulae, upper trapezius, scalenes, subscapularis, and sternocleidomastoid

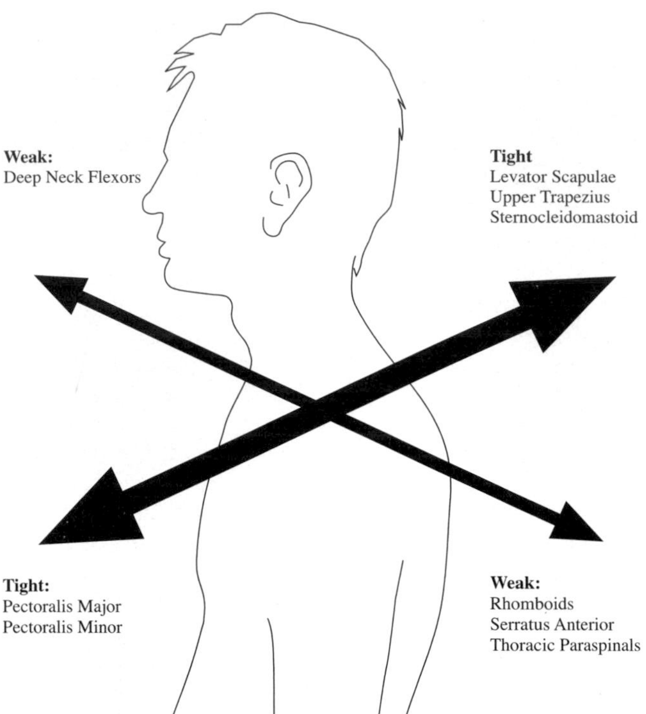

Fig. 12-9 Upper-cross syndrome. An imbalance of shortened and weak musculature that are in opposition in the cervical spine region. Tightened muscles are generally upper trapezius, sternocleidomastoid, pectoralis major and minor, and levator scapulae. Weakened muscles include rhomboids major and minor, deep neck flexors, middle and lower trapezius and the serratus anterior.
(Courtesy of Tamiko Murakami.)

muscles. Thus knowledge of how each muscle has been affected after surgery is necessary to guide the rehabilitation program. Postural rehabilitation should be implemented, and interventions should focus on the stretching of shortened musculature, strengthening of the weakened muscles of the trunk and neck, and performing UE movements while maintaining neutral cervical spine (Fig. 12-10).

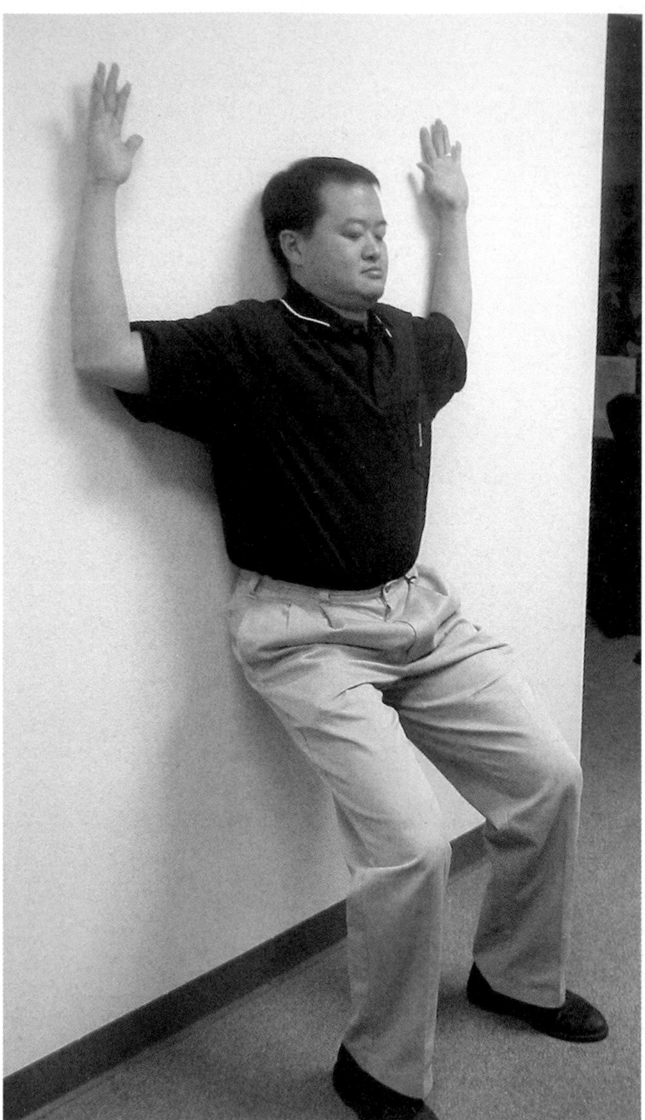

Fig. 12-10 Wall angels. The therapist has the patient stand with the head, back, and arms against the wall, knees slightly bent, chin tucked, and shoulders slightly abducted. The patient continues to elevate the arms against the wall and bring them down, making the shape of angel wings.

A At 8 weeks after surgery, the patient can begin active cervical ROM exercises in all planes. Stacey should be instructed in how to perform these motions beginning in neutral cervical spine position. She should also be told monitor her symptoms and only move her head until she feels the muscles stretching. Pain should be avoided when completing cervical ROM exercises. This may be added to the patient's home exercise program, but she should be advised that if she experiences increased pain during or after the exercises, then she should stop them until she has an opportunity to talk with her PT.

Q Daniel is a 40-year-old man who underwent C5-6 ACDF surgery 10 weeks ago. He has made improvements with his active cervical ROM but is still unable to fully side bend or rotate his head in either direction without moving his trunk. He lacks full shoulder elevation in the sagittal and coronal plane. He also notices difficulty and discomfort while driving slightly longer distances. What form of intervention should the therapist follow?

Cervical Stability

ACDF surgery requires the partial resection of the longus colli muscle.[1] From a functional recovery perspective, the longus colli has an important role in maintaining cervical stability. Although research is lacking regarding cervical stability, numerous studies have been conducted on the role of lumbar stability to control motion and stabilize spinal segments.[56] Richardson and associates[47] performed a series of studies on the ability of deep lumbar muscles to stabilize spinal segments in patients with lumbar pain. Their findings suggest that deep muscle activation is a necessary component in the re-establishment of spinal control after a low back injury. Subjects that did not re-establish segmental control continued to experience low back pain. Recently, the same group has turned their attention to the cervical spine.[29] They suggest that deep cervical muscles are necessary for normal cervical spine stability. The role may be even greater than that seen in the lumbar region because of the large role cervical spine muscles play in the maintenance and control of a region designed to provide mobility. Thus exercises designed to recruit deep neck flexors will be imperative to provide adequate stability of a highly mobile region. These exercises can include supine chin tucks in a neutral spine using a rolled towel or pillow if necessary, progressing to an inclined position and eventually a sitting position (Fig. 12-11). Jull[29] has proposed the use of a blood pressure cuff behind the neck as a means of monitoring the amount of cervical muscle recruitment (Fig. 12-12 and Box 12-3).

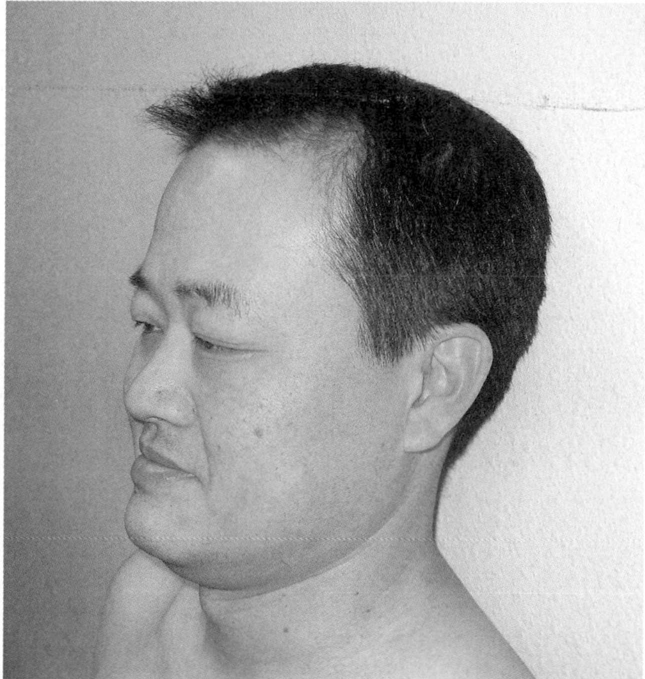

Fig. 12-11 Chin tucks. In a sitting or standing posture, the patient tucks in the chin and extends the cervical spine.

A progressive resistance exercise (PRE) program for the UEs may be initiated during this phase with light weights. Biceps curls, triceps extensions, wrist and hand exercises, and isometric shoulder exercises are all appropriate at this time.

The strengthening program should still be carried out below 90 degrees of glenohumeral (GH) elevation to ensure that the musculature of the neck is not being overstressed. Each patient will need to begin at a different level after taking into account his or her present functional status and familiarity with the exercises. The focus should be on the use of light weights to build endurance of

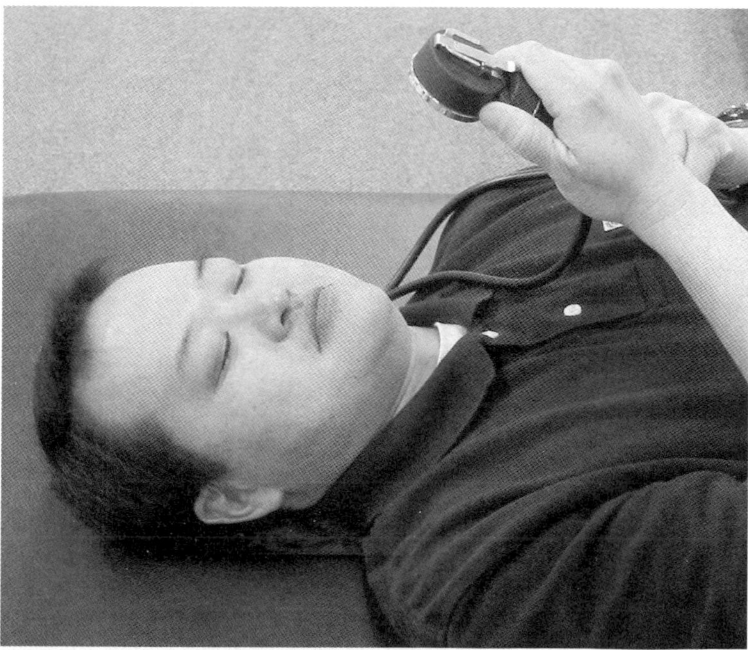

Fig. 12-12 Blood pressure cuff technique. The patient lies supine, with the blood pressure cuff placed under the neck and inflated to 20 mm Hg and the display held in front to monitor the dial. The patient nods or retracts the head to raise the pressure 2 mm Hg. Once the patient is able to maintain this pressure without fatigue, he or she may progress and increase the pressure by 2 mm Hg.

Box 12-3 Strengthening and Retraining of Deep Cervical Flexors Using Blood Pressure Cuff

Patient position:

- Patient is supine in hook-lying position.
- The head is placed in a neutral position.
- Towels may be placed beneath the patient's head to achieve neutral cervical position.
- The patient's chin may need to be tucked in and down to achieve a neutral cervical spine.

Procedure:

- A pressure biofeedback unit or blood pressure cuff is placed beneath the patient's neck.
- Inflate pressure biofeedback unit or blood pressure cuff to 20 mm Hg.
- The patient holds the display in one hand and gently retracts or nods the upper cervical region until pressure rises to 22 mm Hg.. This process is repeated for 24 mm Hg, 26 mm Hg, 28 mm Hg, and 30 mm Hg. Above 30 mm Hg is not relevant. The pressure that the patient can hold for several seconds without activation of the superficial neck muscles is the beginning exercise value.
- The patient is instructed to retract or nod until target pressure is achieved. This amount of force is held for 10 seconds and repeated ten times.
- When the patient can contract for the designated duration and repetitions without fatigue or discomfort, it is appropriate to increase pressure 2 mm Hg.
- To discourage substitution with the superficial neck muscles, the patient can be instructed to place the tongue on the roof of the mouth with lips together and teeth just separated when completing the exercise.

Adapted from Jull G: Management of cervicogenic headaches. In Grant R: *Physical therapy of the cervical and thoracic spine*, St Louis, 2002, Churchill Livingstone.

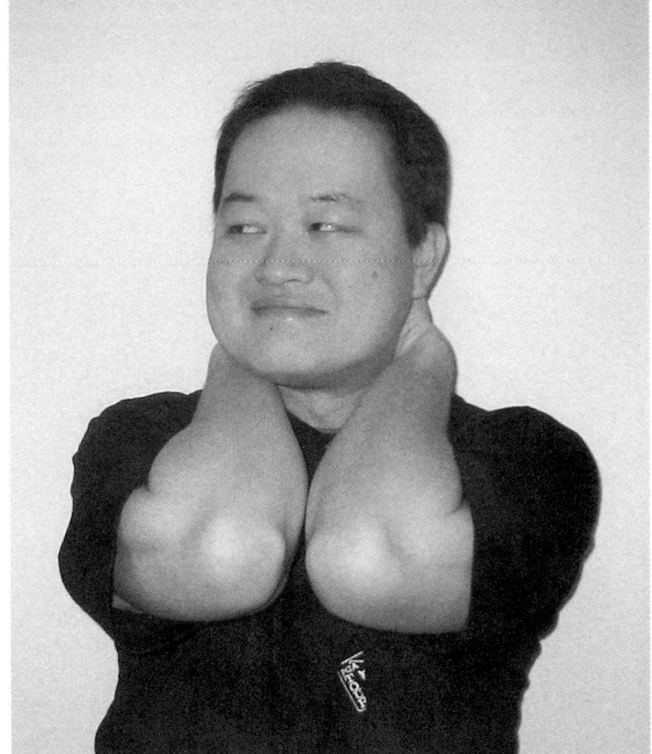

A

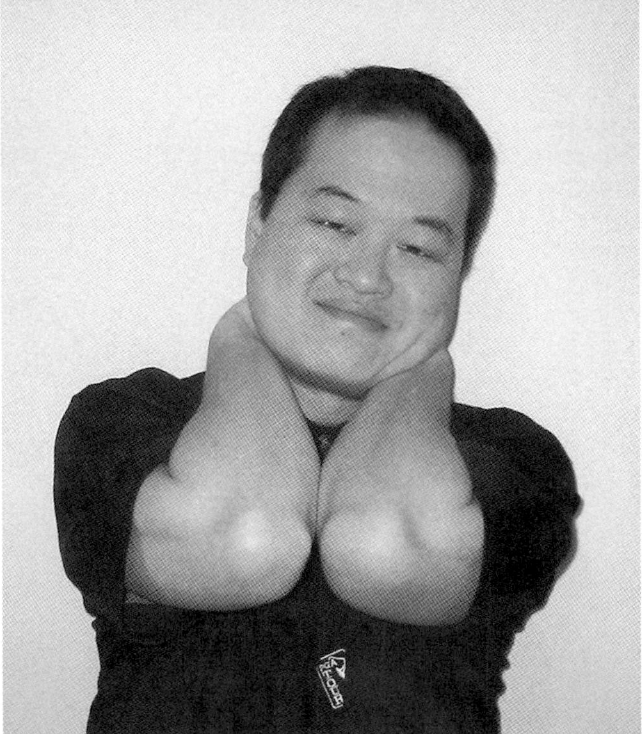

B

Fig. 12-13 Active cervical range of motion (ROM). The patient is placed in a comfortable sitting position and asked to complete each cervical ROM movement slowly through the full ROM.

the musculature initially to assist with return-to-work activities and maintenance of prolonged postures.

Joint Mobilization

Decreased flexibility in thoracic spine segments and the soft tissue of the thoracic region may prevent proper body alignment, including full GH ROM. Thus treatment should include soft tissue mobilization to the mid- and lower thoracic spine. Later mobilization to the mid-thoracic spine can be included with the authorization of the physician.

It is appropriate to begin AROM and passive range-of-motion (PROM) activities at this time (Fig. 12-13). The clinician should keep in mind that the biomechanics of the cervical spine will be altered by cervical fusion surgery. An understanding of how it will be affected is critical in assessing a patient's progress and ultimate outcome. The cervical vertebrae are the smallest and most mobile of all spinal vertebrae. The cervical region functions to provide mobility for the head on the trunk. It also functions to protect vital structures, such as the spinal cord, as they route distally down the body. In total, the functional units of the cervical region must work together

Table 12-5 Approximate Range of Motion (ROM) for the Three Planes of Movement for the Joints of the Craniocervical Region

Joint or Region	Flexion/Extension (Degrees)	Axial Rotation—Unilateral (Degrees)	Lateral Flexion—Unilateral (Degrees)
Atlanto-occipital	Flexion: 5 Extension: 10 Total: 15	Negligible	Approximately 5
Atlantoaxial	Flexion: 5 Extension: 10 Total: 15	40-45	Negligible
Midcervical	Flexion: 35 Extension: 70 Total: 105	45	35
Total cervical	Flexion: 45 to 50 Extension: 85 Total: 130 to 135	90	Approximately 40

Adapted from Neumann D: Axial skeleton: osteology and arthrology. In Neumann D: *Kinesiology of the musculoskeletal system—foundations for physical rehabilitation,* St Louis, 2002, Mosby.

to provide 45 to 50 degrees of flexion and 85 degrees of extension, for a total of 130 to 135 degrees of total sagittal plane motion. In the horizontal plane, the cervical spine must be able to provide 90 degrees of unilateral motion and 180 degrees of total rotational motion. Finally, 40 degrees of unilateral frontal plane motion occurs—or 80 degrees in total (Table 12-5).[2,39] Segmentally, two adjacent spinal vertebrae and the intervertebral disc between the two comprise a functional motion segment. Each functional spinal unit provides varying degrees to the total motion seen in the cervical region. The fusing of one or several of the functional motion segments will alter the mechanics of adjacent segments. The body will eventually accommodate; the end result is transitional degeneration. **Therefore initially a fusion to the C5-6 motion segment may result in a loss of 10 to 15 degrees of unilateral rotation.[30,56] Therefore the objective goal of rehabilitation should not be to attain 90 degrees of unilateral rotation. Instead normal unilateral rotation after fusion to C5-6 would be 65 to 70 degrees of motion.**

Mobilization techniques are a mainstay of physical therapy. In practice, they are used to increase ROM within targeted regions by moving specific joints or specific muscles. Care must be taken in choosing the appropriate time to begin implementation of soft tissue and particularly passive joint mobilization techniques because of the potential translational effect they may have on the cervical spine at the region of the fusion. Although studies are lacking in the area of mobilization of the cervical spine, several studies have addressed the effects of mobilization in the lumbar region. Researchers[31-34] studied the effects of a posterior to anterior force placed on the spinous process of L3. Their study showed a force at L3 could result in movement as far away as T8; in a follow-up study by the same group, the same posterior to anterior force resulted in an anterior rotation of the sacrum. The implications of these findings for the patient after a cervical fusion is that even mobilizations to distant segments may have a translatory effect on the fusion site. Therefore mobilization of the spine should not be initiated until the fusion site itself has shown radiographic evidence of sufficient mineralization and callus formation. This information and the authorization of mobilization to the cervical spine should come from the surgeon. Moreover, research has revealed transitional degeneration in the segments directly above and below the fusion. Once this is found, proper mobilization and joint forces may be added to begin stimulating proper formation and modeling of bone tissue.

Although it is difficult to imagine an instance when direct mobilization to the fusion site would be warranted, mobilization to adjacent structures and segments is justified to increase spinal ROM and decrease the demands placed upon the fusion site.

However, therapists should be wary of applying mobilization techniques close to the fusion site. Research has revealed transitional degeneration in the segments directly above and below the fusion.[7] Transitional degeneration is a common long-term complication after a spinal fusion, particularly in multilevel fusions. It consists of segmental articular degeneration and spondylytic changes in the spine. It has been hypothesized that these changes are the result of the increased stress placed on these segments because of the decreased mobility of the fusion spinal segments. Goffin and colleagues[22] studied 120 patients after ACDF surgery and at a mean follow-up period of 98 months. They found that 92% of the patients demonstrated segmental degenerative changes. Eventually, when dense connective tissue and bone has been adequately strengthened and stabilized, then distant spinal segments can be mobilized when needed.

A Daniel's loss of ROM is normal after ACDF. His cervical rotation ROM will likely continue to improve given that C1-2 is a major source (accounting for up to 50%) of rotation. The therapist should keep in mind that AROM expectations for the cervical spine are less than full (65 to 70° of unilateral rotation versus 90°). The fact that he also has limits in shoulder elevation may indicate a thoracic spine mobility issue. Soft tissue mobilization techniques to the upper- and midthoracic segments may relieve the tension on the shoulder and neck, allowing for increases in AROM. Improved posture should also follow, allowing a better distribution and absorption of forces while driving.

Q Joe is a 49-year-old man who has been referred to the clinic by his physician 5 months after undergoing ACDF to C4-5 and C5-6. His primary impairments include numbness and tingling in his left UE, decreased cervical ROM, and poor cardiovascular function. After 1 month of physical therapy, Joe has increased his neck ROM and aerobic capacity but still complains of numbness and weakness in his left arm. He asks if the numbness will resolve. What should the therapist tell him?

Neural Mobilization and Neural Dynamics

Neural mobility techniques should also be progressed in this phase to prevent neural adhesions to the surrounding tissue. Scar tissue has the ability to restrict joints; scar tissue can adhere to nerves and affect their mobility. **Because the patient is likely to have experienced nerve-related symptoms as a contributing factor before undergoing surgery, it is important not to aggravate or overstretch the neural tissue, because a strong likelihood exists that soft tissue restrictions may be limiting the ability of the nerve to glide properly.** Neurodynamics is the concept that a relationship exists between the nervous system and associated connective tissues. Neurodynamic testing of the upper limb enables the clinician to assess the movement capabilities of neural tissues in relation to the soft tissue structure that surrounds them. Elvy[16] developed the upper-limb neurodynamic tests (ULNTs) as a method for differentiating potential sources of cervicobrachial symptoms. Upper-limb neurodynamic test 1 (ULNT 1) (Fig. 12-14) was designed to assess the movement capabilities of neural tissues associated with the median nerve. Given the mechanical continuity of the nervous system, it has recently been recognized that all upper-quarter neural tissues are stressed during ULNT 1; however, components of the test

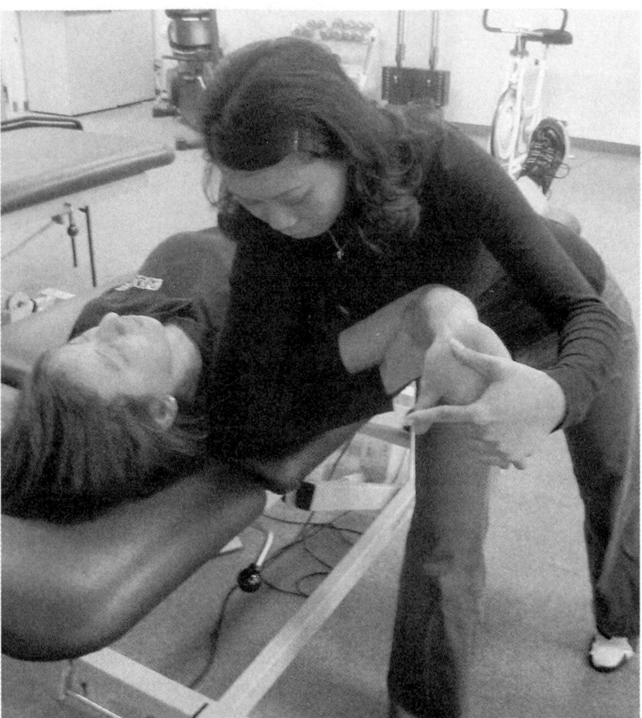

Fig. 12-14 ULNT 1 technique.

are specifically biased toward the median nerve trunk and C5-7 nerve roots[6] (Table 12-6). Although originally designed to test the median nerve, clinicians are using it as a general clearing test for UE neuromobility, because all three major peripheral nerves in the UE are stressed by the ULNT 1 position (Box 12-4).

Treatments using the ULNTs have generally been a point of confusion for clinicians. A positive test is indicative of restricted mobility in the nerve being tested. Therefore using the test position to stretch the nerve and release any adhesions along the course is a common treatment philosophy. What is overlooked is the fact that nerve tissue is different from muscle tissue. Muscles have the potential to elongate and stretch, whereas neural tissue is not as elastic and responds adversely to stretching. **Therefore treatment should address the gliding and not stretching of nerves** (Fig. 12-15). **Soft tissue structures along the course of the nerve can be mobilized to allow for nerve mobility. Movement of the UE can be combined with small movements of the neck to encourage gliding of the nerve rather then stretching. Finally, communication with the patient is essential, because radicular pain or paresthesias are indications that the nerve is being stretched and potentially irritated. The patient and therapist should work in ROMs that do not reproduce the patient's radicular symptoms.**

To facilitate the return-to-work transition in this phase, cardiovascular endurance should be continued. A daily walking program should be continued and progressed as tolerated.

Table 12-6 Upper-Limb Nerve Testing (UNLT) Positions

Test	Nerve Assessed	Test Position
ULNT 1	General	Supine—Leg straight and uncrossed Spine in midline position Stabilization of shoulder girdle Shoulder abduction Wrist and finger extension Forearm supination Shoulder lateral rotation Elbow extension Cervical lateral flexion away Cervical lateral flexion toward
ULNT 2a	Median	Supine—Leg straight and uncrossed Spine in midline position Stabilization of shoulder girdle Shoulder girdle depression Elbow extension Whole-arm lateral rotation Wrist and finger extension Shoulder abduction
ULNT 2b	Radial	Supine—Leg straight and uncrossed Spine in midline position Stabilization of shoulder girdle Shoulder depression Elbow extension Whole-arm internal rotation (IR) Wrist flexion
ULNT 3	Ulnar	Supine—Leg straight and uncrossed Spine in midline position Stabilization of shoulder girdle Wrist extension Forearm pronation Elbow flexion Shoulder lateral rotation Shoulder girdle depression Shoulder abduction

Adapted from Butler D: *The sensitive nervous system,* Adelaide, Australia, 2000, Noigroup Publications.

Box 12-4 Testing Procedure for Upper-Limb Neurodynamic Test 1 (ULNT 1)

1. First, establish the patient's baseline resting symptoms. Remember to reassess baseline symptoms, resistance, and ROM with the addition of each new component.
2. The patient is positioned in supine near edge of table.
3. Therapist position:
   a. The therapist takes a stride-stance position facing the patient's head.
   b. Next, the therapist uses *a pistol grip* handhold on the fingers of the limb to be tested. It is important to maintain finger extension and thumb abduction during the procedure.
   c. The therapist will then lean his or her elbow on the table for support and stabilize the patient's shoulder girdle in neutral.
   d. Alternatively, the clinician may stabilize the patient's shoulder girdle by pushing his or her fist vertically downward on the examination table with the shoulder girdle in neutral.
4. Procedure:
   a. The shoulder is abducted in the neutral coronal plane to 100 to 130 degrees. Care must be taken to prevent any shoulder girdle elevation.
   b. Next, the therapist adds wrist extension, finger extension, and forearm supination.
   c. Add shoulder lateral rotation.
   d. Add elbow extension.
5. Sensitizing maneuvers include:
   a. Contralateral cervical lateral flexion
   b. Ipsilateral cervical lateral flexion
   c. Release of wrist extension

Adapted from: Butler D: *The sensitive nervous system,* Adelaide, Australia, 2000, Noigroup Publications.

Phase IIIb (Remodeling Phase)

TIME: 9 to 12 weeks after surgery (days 61 to 84)
GOALS: Restoration of strength to the cervical spine, maintenance of neutral spine for prolonged periods of time with concurrent UE movement, improvement in scapulothoracic mechanics (Table 12-7)

Progression to this phase of rehabilitation should begin once the patient is able to tolerate the exercises of phase IIIa without an increase in neck or arm symptoms. Interventions from the previous phase have focused on loading the upper and lower body without directly loading the cervical spine. The purpose of this precaution is to prevent overstressing newly healed structures. This particular stage in the rehabilitation process will slowly begin to incorporate direct treatment to the cervical spine structures and therefore should not be started until the patient has adequately demonstrated tolerance to the loads placed on the neck. The patient should also be able to demonstrate proper neutral cervical spine concepts.

The thoracic spine musculature such as the rhomboids and middle and lower trapezius can be further challenged from the previous phase by adding resistance with light weights on a seated or standing rowing machine or through the use of resistance tubing (Figs. 12-16 and 12-17). Proprioceptive neurofacilitation techniques may also be used to strengthen thoracic paraspinals and scapulothoracic musculature. PREs may be increased in weight, sets, and repetitions as tolerated. Exercises above 90-degree shoulder elevation may be initiated to further strengthen cervical musculature. Isometric cervical spine strengthening may begin in all planes. Attention should be given to complete these exercises in neutral cervical spine to strengthen the musculature of the cervical spine to allow for proper

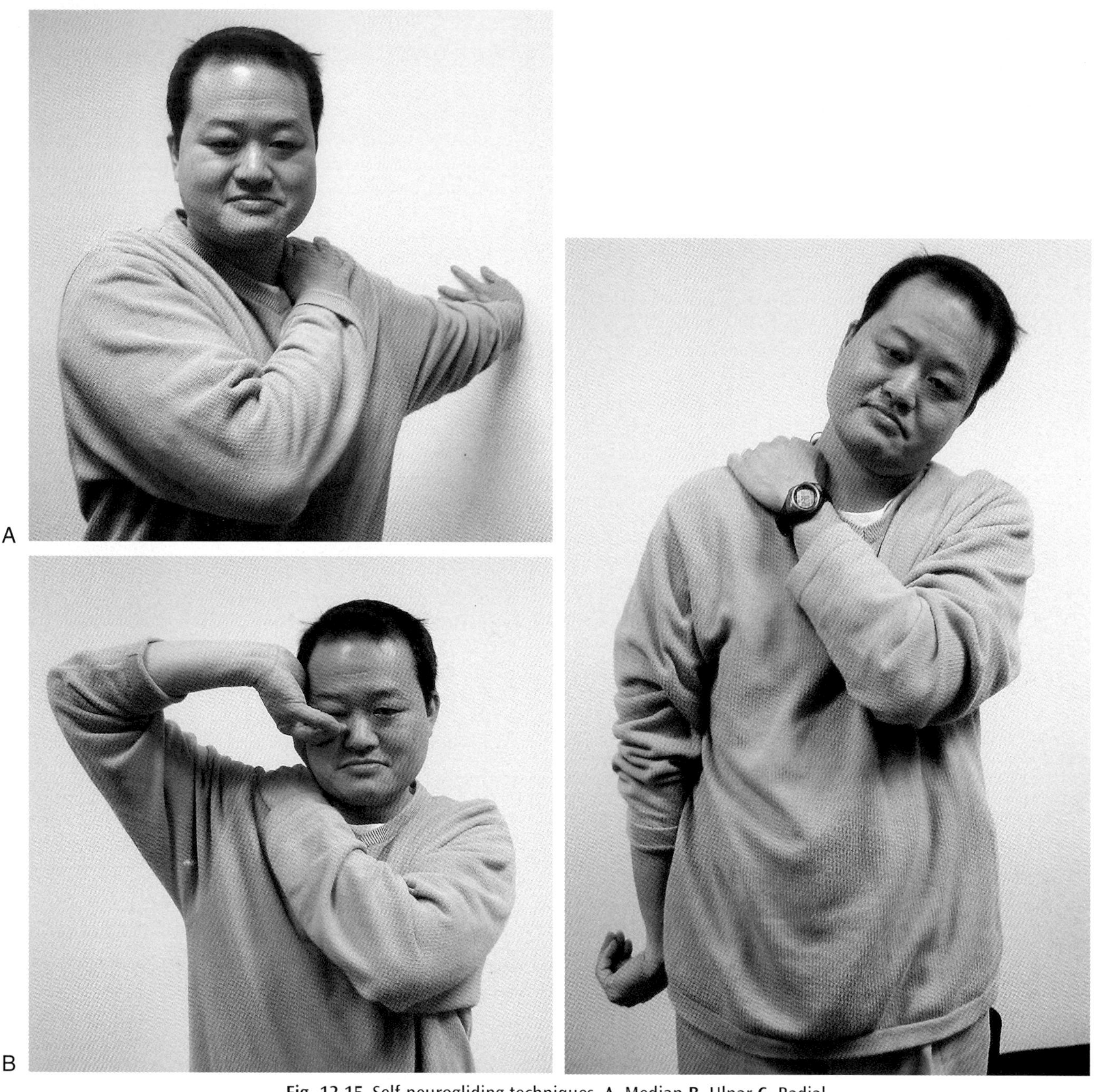

Fig. 12-15 Self-neurogliding techniques. **A**, Median **B**, Ulnar **C**, Radial.

posture and force production of these muscles. The patient is placed in a comfortable sitting position. For flexion, the patient places both hands on the forehead and brings the forehead into the hands without moving. In extension, the patient places both hands on the back of the head and brings the head backwards into the hands without moving (Fig. 12-18). During the side bend, the patient places one hand on the side of the head and attempts to bring the ear to the shoulder without moving. In rotation, the patient places one hand to the side of the head in front of the ear and looks over the shoulder without allowing movement. Strength and trunk control can be further challenged through the addition of an unstable base of support such as a half foam roller placed under the feet or the use of a stabilization ball. A therapist or assistant should be assisting the patient at all times during these exercises. Synchronized UE movements, such as biceps curls while balancing on an unstable support, will further challenge the trunk and neck complex simultaneously. Placing the patient in positions such as quadruped or prone on the stabilization ball should warrant caution and be delayed if the patient has yet to demonstrate deep neck flexor strength or the ability to maintain a neutral cervical spine in an antigravity position.

Table 12-7 Anterior Cervical Discectomy and Fusion

Rehabilitation Phase	Criteria to Progress to this Phase	Anticipated Impairments and Functional Limitations	Intervention	Goal	Rationale
Phase IIIb Remodeling phase (maturation) Postoperative weeks 9-12 (days 61-84)	◆ Surgical site has healed ◆ No increase in pain symptoms ◆ Patient demonstrates neutral spine concepts	Same as Phase II with the following: ◆ Limited ability to perform activities in a prolonged sitting/standing position ◆ Patient is not fully independent with ADLs	Continue with Phase II interventions as needed with the following: ◆ Begin isometrics of the cervical spine ◆ Begin gentle UE strengthening above 90 degrees of shoulder elevation ◆ PREs—Shoulder shrugs, triceps push-down, wall push-ups ◆ Scapulothoracic and thoracic paraspinal strengthening using PNF techniques ◆ Thoracic exercises—Scapular retractions with resistance ◆ Progress abdominal strengthening exercises in different positions—Standing, quadruped ◆ Initiate upper-body exerciser as tolerated in neutral spine	◆ Restore strength to cervical spine ◆ Improve scapulothoracic mechanics ◆ Maintenance of neutral spine in various positions/planes with concurrent UE movement	◆ Independent with self-care and ADLs ◆ Prevent reinjury with increase in dynamic activities ◆ Knowledge of pain-relieving strategies/positions during prolonged activities

UE, Upper extremity; *ADLs,* activities of daily living; *PREs,* progressive resistance exercises; *PNF,* proprioceptive neuromuscular facilitation.

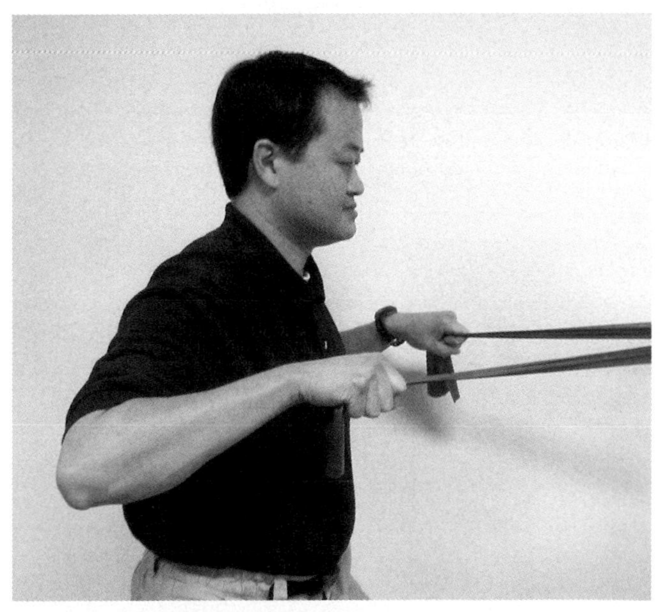

Fig. 12-16 Scapular retractions using resistance tubing. The patient sits or stands (with knees slightly bent) with resistance tubing secured in front. He or she pulls the tubing simultaneously to the sides by retracting the scapula and bending the elbows. The patient is instructed to relax the shoulders and pinch the shoulder blades together.

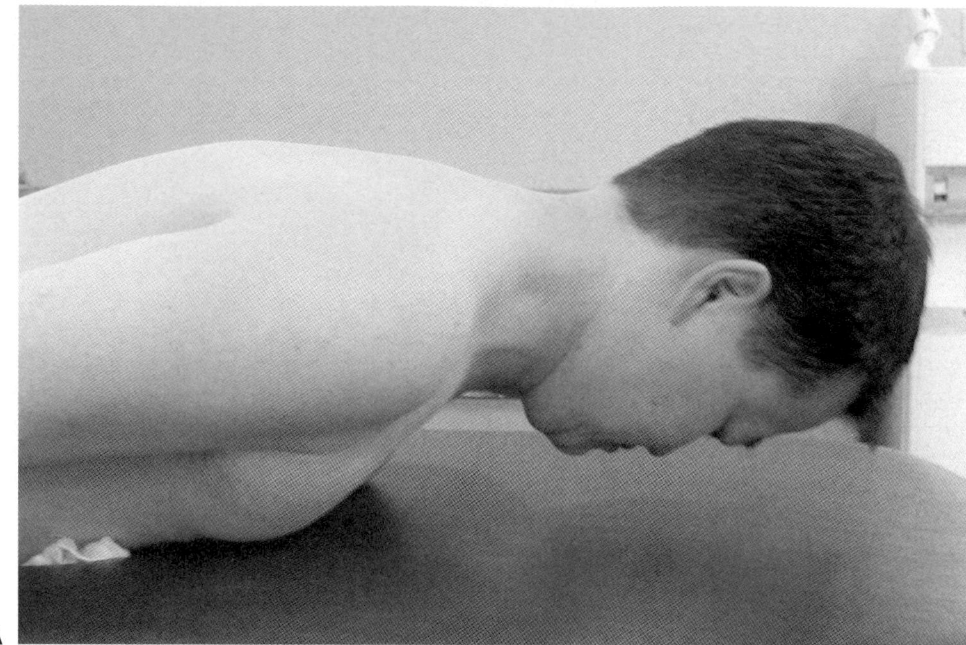

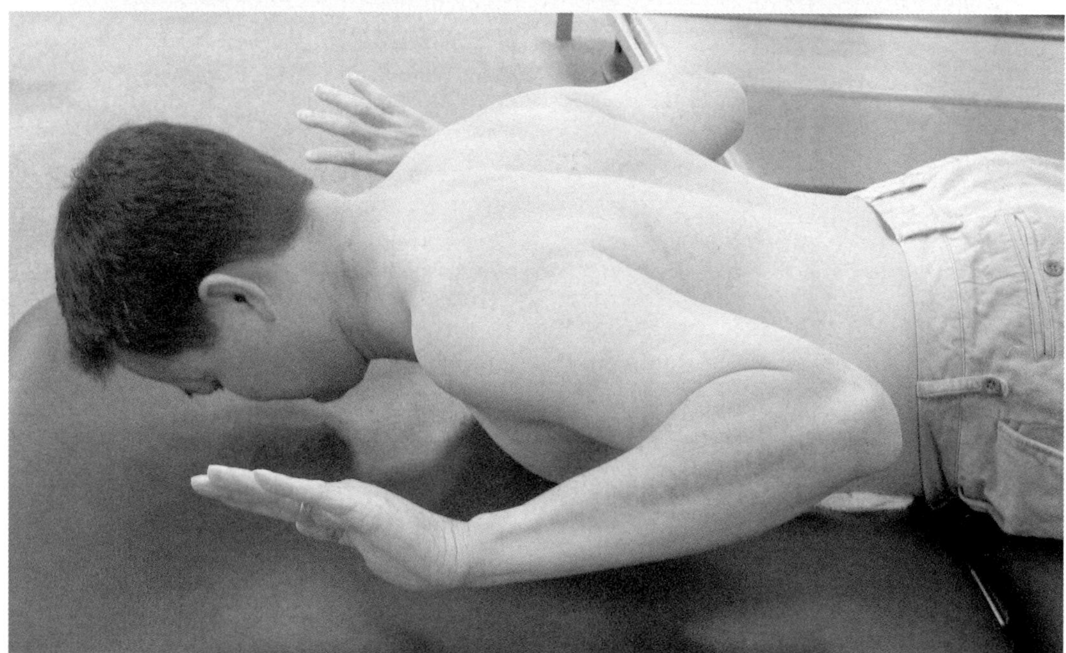

Fig. 12-17 Prone scapular retraction progression. The patient is placed in a prone position on the table with the arms at the sides. The therapist instructs the patient to lift the forehead off the table, keeping the chin tucked in a neutral cervical spine position. The patient can then perform scapular retraction exercises.

Proper neck alignment should be maintained during execution of all therapeutic activities.

At this stage of rehabilitation, the patient may find it difficult to perform activities that require prolonged sitting or standing postures. It is important to assist the patient in recognizing methods or activities that have the ability to relieve some of the pain or soreness. It is also important that he or she be assisted in the development of strategies to increase muscle endurance so that the patient may gradually build a tolerance to these positions. Strategies may include limiting the time spent in any one position, the use of cryotherapy to the neck, or active cervical ROM exercises to relieve stiffness and soreness. Cardiovascular endurance and strength should continue during this phase, and the use of an upper-body exerciser may be initiated for short amounts of time.

Phase IIIc (Remodeling Phase)

TIME: 13 to 52 weeks after surgery (days 85 to 360)
GOALS: Return to presurgical strength and endurance, return to prior level of functioning, pre-

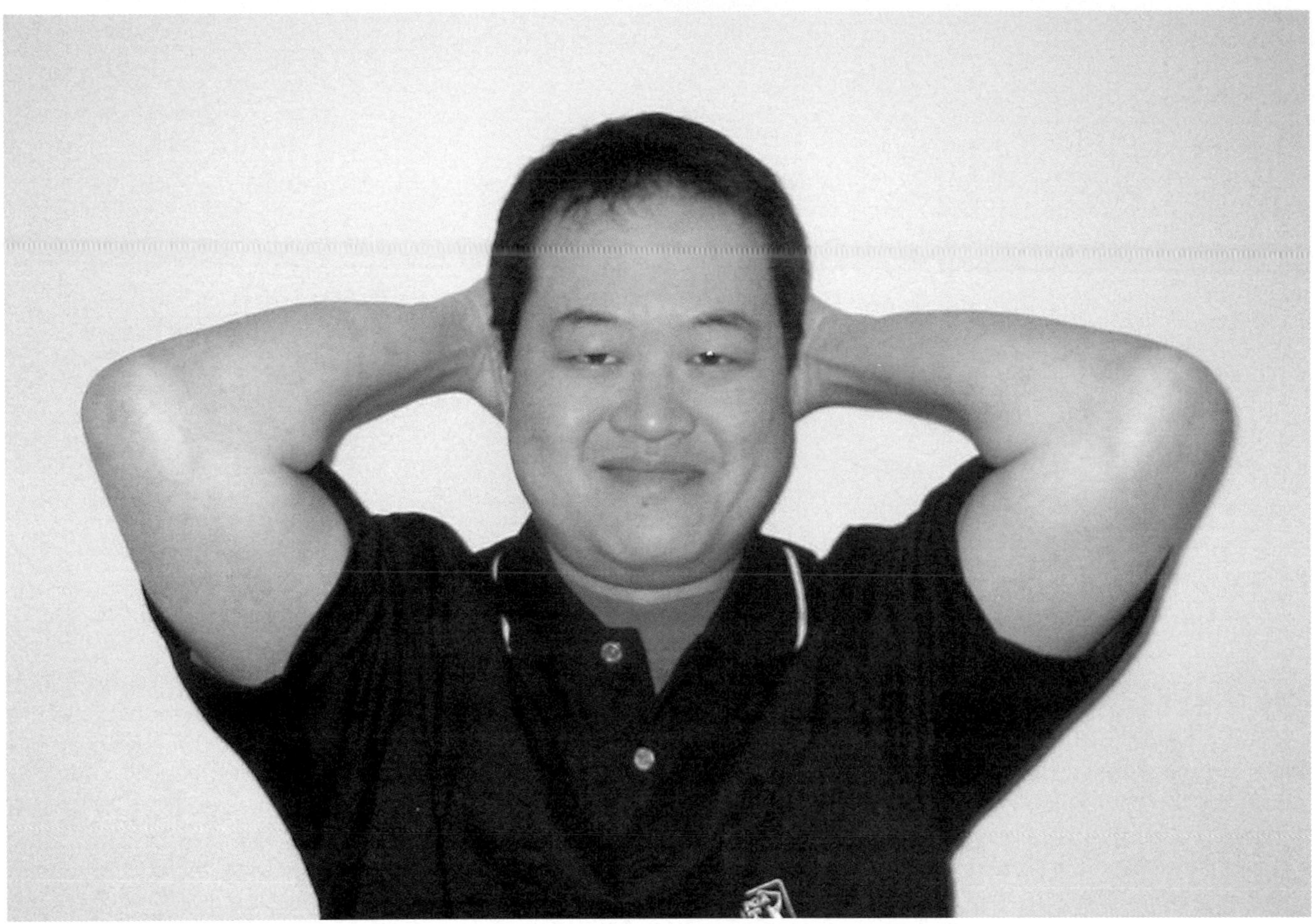

Fig. 12-18 Extension: The patient places both hands on the back of the head and brings the head backwards into the hands without moving.

A

Several categories of nerve injury are based on the amount of tissue damage occurring at the nerve. A neuropraxia is local conduction block of the nerve. It usually occurs with compression injuries in which the nerve lumen is compressed and neural and chemical transition down the nerve axon is impaired. The axon and surrounding neurium tissue remains intact. *Axontomesis* refers to a condition in which a loss of axon continuity occurs. The neurium tissue remains intact, but because of the loss of axon continuity, degeneration of distal nerve occurs. This condition can be the result of traction to the nerve or severe compression. Neurotomesis is the loss of axon continuity in which the neurium tissue is damaged. Similar degeneration of distal nerve occurs, as seen in axontomesis; however, because no neurium tissue exists, the nerve has very little chance to heal. This type of injury generally occurs with injuries in which the nerve is severed. Recovery will depend on whether the nerve axon can regrow back to its distal muscular attachment before scar tissue infiltrates the region and blocks axon growth. When the axon and neurium are damaged, little potential exists for full recovery of the nerve. Therefore the therapist should advise the patient that after 6 months, resolution of numbness and weakness is unlikely to occur. Strength can continue to increase, but this is generally the result of muscle hypertrophy and not from innervation of muscle tissue.

pare for discharge from physical therapy (Table 12-8; see also Suggested Home Maintenance Box)

The remaining phase of the rehabilitation process centers on regaining presurgical strength and endurance. By the end of this phase, the patient should be able to function independently at home and in the workplace. As the patient progresses through the rehabilitation process, functional retraining of work- or sport-specific activities should be assessed. Activities that require increased loads on the cervical spine should be evaluated; pending physician approval, rehabilitation geared toward functional training can be initiated. Return to activities or sports that require contact between players or heavy lifting will require the physician's approval. At this time the PT may

Table 12-8 Anterior Cervical Discectomy and Fusion

Rehabilitation Phase	Criteria to Progress to this Phase	Anticipated Impairments and Functional Limitations	Intervention	Goal	Rationale
Phase IIIc Remodeling phase (maturation) Postoperative weeks 13-24 (days 85-168)	◆ Patient able to self-manage pain ◆ No decrease in functional ability	◆ Difficulty lifting heavy objects ◆ Difficulty maintaining prolonged postures	◆ Progress sets and repetitions of UE-resisted exercise program as tolerated by patient ◆ Functional retraining activities (work or sport related per physician approval)	◆ Return to prior level of functioning ◆ Return to presurgical level of strength and endurance ◆ Prepare patient for discharge	◆ Improve patient's ability to manage work-related schedule ◆ Promote continuance of proper postures and home maintenance program after discharge from physical therapy

UE, Upper extremity.

implement a gym- or home-based exercise program to assist in maintenance of proper strength and muscle function. Discharge of the patient should occur once the patient, physical therapist, and physician have all determined that the patient has reached his or her functional goals and is able continue the rehabilitation process safely and independently.

SUGGESTED HOME MAINTENANCE FOR THE POSTSURGICAL PATIENT

The contents of the home exercise program (found on page 234) will vary depending on the patient, their status, their abilities, their age, etc. The therapist must curtail the program to fit the needs of the patient.

TROUBLESHOOTING

Red Flags

The majority of postoperative complications and red flags will occur within the first several weeks after surgery. PTs should be aware of these complications and should educate the patient to notify his or her physician immediately if any of the following complications should occur. Although the majority of the red flags will occur before a patient's release to outpatient rehabilitation, the outpatient clinician should be cognizant of any drastic changes that would warrant communication with the physician for further assessment and testing.

Infection

The risk of infection after cervical spine surgery is difficult to determine. Postoperative infection rates of 0% to 6% have been reported. Several factors affect a patient's risk for acquiring an infection, including a patient's age, duration of surgical procedure, and the patient's preoperative physical condition.[55] Obesity is also a risk factor for infection, because adipose tissue is poorly vascularized. Uncontrolled diabetes also increases the risk of infection. Signs and symptoms of infections include erythema, edema, purulent wound drainage, tenderness, fever, and increased pain.

Dysphagia

The incidence of dysphagia in patients after ACDF has been reported as high as 28%.[36,54] Additional studies have noted that 51% of patients will have swallowing difficulty at 1 month after surgery, 31% at 2 months, and 15% at 6 months.[58] Therefore speech and swallowing problems after ACDF is not uncommon, although dysphagia is one of the primary symptoms accompanying plate and screw loosening. Therefore persistent symptoms should be cause for further examination by the physician.

Esophageal Injury

Esophageal injury is rare but can occur up to 1 year after surgery.[25] The mechanism behind the injury has been attributed to laceration or pressure necrosis of the esophagus by graft displacement. Signs and symptoms of an esophageal injury include increased neck and throat pain, odynophagia, erythema, swelling, tenderness, crepitus, subcutaneous emphysema, unexplained tachycardia, sepsis, and difficulty swallowing.

Neural Injury

The recurrent laryngeal nerve is susceptible to nerve injury after ACDF surgery. Incidence of injury has been reported to be between 0.07% and 11%.[3] Injury to the recurrent laryngeal nerve may be the result of endotracheal tubing that may compress and damage the nerve. Symptoms of nerve injury include vocal cord paralysis. Spinal cord injury secondary to ACDF is 0.4%.[59] Most often the source of the spinal cord injury is posterior displacement of the bone graft. Nerve root injury is also low at 0.6%. The most affected nerve root is C5. Most incidence of injury resolved in 6 weeks.

Vascular Complications

The exact prevalence of vascular complications after ACDF is unknown. Most studies report values in the neighborhood of 0.6% or less for vertebral artery injury after ACDF surgery.[37,52] Signs and symptoms of vertebral artery injury include dizziness, dysphagia, dysarthria, diplopia, and drop attacks.

Cervical Spine Bracing

Skin breakdown and soft tissue injuries are common with the long-term use of cervical bracing. In addition, muscle atrophy, dysphagia, and gastrointestinal dysfunction have also been reported. Signs and symptoms of pressure sores or swallowing dysfunction must be monitored.[55]

Graft Failure

Graft failure after ACDF may be caused by the following: graft displacement, nonunion, instrumentation failure, host factors including osteoporosis or extreme kyphosis, and technical factors such a short or long graft. Graft failures are highest with multilevel fusions at 60%, and graft dislodgement has been reported in 5% to 50% of multilevel surgeries without instrumentation. Nonunion rates are higher in iliac crest allografts (60%) versus autografts (17%), although they are the same rate at 5% for single level fusions.[53] Clinical symptoms for patients who are symptomatic from nonunion include increasing neck pain and worsening axial pain 6 months after surgery. Patients may have difficulty swallowing and breathing after an anterior graft displacement. Patients who experience a worsening of pain and symptoms should be referred to the physician for additional evaluation and testing procedures.

Chronic Pain

Changes in the peripheral and central nervous system occur almost immediately after an injury. Some of these changes are reversible, and other changes are nonreversible. Many of these changes have been proposed as the pathomechanisms behind the chronicity of pain. It is beyond the scope of this chapter to describe all the neural changes that occur with injury; however, from a clinician's viewpoint it is important to realize that not all patients will have full resolution of symptoms after surgery. Surgery may have addressed the structures that were originally the source of the patient's symptoms, but the adaptations that have occurred in the central and peripheral nervous system may not be reversible. Rehabilitation after ACDF has 80% to 90% satisfactory results. There remain an elusive 10% to 20% of patients who continue to experience pain despite the fact that the offending structures have been addressed through removal or fixation. As a clinician it is important to realize that not all pain is a reflection of actual tissue damage. Some pain is the result of tissue changes, and this will affect the ability to rehabilitate patients.[5,21,49,57]

SUMMARY

Rehabilitation of a patient after ACDF surgery is unique in terms of the close relationship the neck has with the shoulder region and its neural network. Unlike other regions of the body such as the shoulder and the wrist, complete immobilization of the cervical spine is difficult, which can affect the healing potential of the fusion site. Therefore educating the patient on the need to adhere to surgical protection guidelines immediately after surgery is important. Protection of the surgical site is the key aspect of early rehabilitation, and stressing of the fusion site should not begin before mineralization of the callus. Moreover, the shoulder girdle and UE, unlike the hip and lower extremity (LE), rely on coordinated muscle actions to maintain function and stability. Many of these muscles have their proximal attachments at the cervical spine. Therefore protection of the fusion must also address limiting UE activity until the surgical site is fully healed. Finally, because radicular pain and UE paresthesias are often the symptoms driving the decision for ACDF, the prevention of neural adhesions and promotion of nerve healing should be addressed appropriately.

SUGGESTED HOME MAINTENANCE FOR THE POSTSURGICAL PATIENT

The patient can use the following home maintenance program during the rehabilitation process. The contents of the home maintenance program may change, depending on the patient's tolerance and ability to complete the exercises properly and without the onset of pain symptoms.

Weeks 1-3

GOALS FOR THE PERIOD: Protection of the surgical site, decrease pain and edema, understanding of proper body mechanics and posture, increase walking speed and endurance

1. Protection of the surgical incision
2. Proper use of the cervical collar per physician
3. Knowledge of correct body mechanics and cervical neutral spine during activities
4. Increase upright sitting tolerance
5. Daily walking program as tolerated

Weeks 4-8

GOALS FOR THE PERIOD: Increase upper-extremity (UE) range of motion (ROM), improve thoracic spine mobility, begin mild weight training

1. Continue use of collar per physician
2. Continue proper body mechanics and maintenance of neutral spine
3. Progress walking program
4. Active UE ROM in flexion, abduction, horizontal abduction, and adduction
5. Wall angels
6. Scapular retractions
7. Begin biceps curls using light weights
8. After removal of collar, patient may begin active range of motion (AROM) to tolerance of cervical spine in rotation, side bend, flexion, and extension (with physician approval)

Weeks 9-12

GOALS FOR THE PERIOD: Increase cervical strength, UE strength, independence with activities of daily living (ADLs)

1. Continue with previous exercises and progress repetitions, weight, or sets as tolerated
2. Scapular retractions with light resistance tubing
3. Wall push-ups
4. Chin tucks in sitting position
5. Triceps push-down using light resistance tubing
6. Latissimus pull-downs using light resistance tubing
7. Home neural mobility exercises

Weeks 13-24

GOALS FOR THE PERIOD: Return to previous functional level and review home conditioning program

1. Continue previous exercises and progress as tolerated
2. Develop independent gym exercise program
   a. Seated or standing rows
   b. Latissimus pull-downs
   c. Triceps push-downs
   d. Biceps curls
3. Patient may perform previously mentioned exercises while sitting on stabilization ball and using resistance tubing
4. Self-resistance to cervical spine: isometrics
   a. Flexion
   b. Extension
   c. Side bend
   d. Rotation

References

1. Albert T: Surgical approaches to the cervical spine. In Emery S, Boden S: *Surgery of the cervical spine,* Philadelphia, 2003, Saunders.
2. Bogduk N: Biomechanics of the cervical spine. In Grant R: *Physical therapy of the cervical and thoracic spine,* St Louis, 2002, Churchill Livingstone.
3. Bohler J, Gaudernak T: Anterior plate stabilization for fracture dislocation of the lower cervical spine, *J Trauma* 20:203-205, 1980.
4. Bolesta M, Viere R: Surgical complications. In Emery S, Boden S: *Surgery of the cervical spine,* Philadelphia, 2003, Saunders.
5. Butler D: *The sensitive nervous system,* Adelaide, Australia, 2000, Noigroup Publications.
6. Butler D: Upper limb neurodynamic test: clinical use in a "big picture" framework. In Grant R: *Physical therapy of the cervical and thoracic spine,* St Louis, 2002, Churchill Livingstone.
7. Clark C: Complications of anterior cervical plating. In Clark C: *The cervical spine,* Philadelphia, 2005, Lippincott Williams & Wilkins.
8. Cleland J et al: Immediate effects of thoracic manipulation in patients with neck pain: A randomized clinical trial, *Man Ther* 10:127-135, 2005.
9. Connell MD, Wiesel SW: Natural history and pathogenesis of cervical disc disease, *Orthop Clin North Am* 23:369-380, 1992.
10. Davidson R, Dunn E, Metzmaker J: The shoulder abduction test in the diagnosis of radicular pain in cervical extradural compressive monoradiculopathies, *Spine* 6:441-446, 1981.
11. DeBerard MS et al: Outcomes of posterolateral lumbar fusion in Utah patients receiving workers' compensation, *Spine* 27:738-747, 2001.
12. Delamarter RB, Bae HW, Pradhan BB: Clinical results of ProDisc-II lumbar total disc replacement: Report from the United States clinical trial, *Orthop Clin North Am* 36(3):301-313, 2005.
13. Delamarter RB, Pradhan BB: Indications for cervical spine prostheses, early experiences with ProDisc-C in the USA, *SpineArt* 1:7-9, 2004.
14. Delamarter RB et al: Artificial total lumbar disc replacement: Introduction and early results from the United States clinical trial, *Spine* 28:S167-175, 2003.
15. Dillin W, Uppal G: Analysis of medications used in the treatment of cervical disc degeneration, *Orthop Clin North Am* 23:421, 1992.
16. Elvey R: Treatment of arm pain associated with abnormal brachial plexus tension, *Aust J Physiother* 32:225-230, 1986.
17. Franklin GM et al: Outcome of lumbar fusion in Washington State workers' compensation, *Spine* 17:1897-1903, 1994.
18. Frenkel S, Grew J: Soft tissue repair. In Spivak J et al: *Orthopaedics—a study guide,* New York, 1999, McGraw-Hill.
19. Frenkel S, Koval K: Fracture healing and bone grafting. In Spivak J et al: *Orthopaedics—a study guide,* New York, 1999, McGraw-Hill.
20. Garvery TA et al: Outcome of anterior cervical discectomy and fusion as perceived by patients treated for dominant axial-mechanical cervical spine pain, *Spine* 27:1887-1894, 2002.
21. Gifford L, Butler D: The integration of pain sciences in clinical practice, *J Hand Ther* 10:86-95, 1997.
22. Goffin J et al: Long-term results after anterior cervical fusion and osteosynthetic stabilization for fractures and/or dislocations of the cervical spine, *J Spinal Disord* 8:499-508, 1995.
23. Goffin J et al: Intermediate follow-up after treatment of degenerative disc disease with the Bryan Cervical Disc Prosthesis: Single-level and bi-level, *Spine* 28:2673-2678, 2003.
24. Guyer RD et al: Prospective randomized study of the Charite artificial disc: Data from two investigational centers, *Spine J* 4:252S-259S, 2004.
25. Hanci M et al: Oesophageal perforation subsequent to anterior cervical spine screw/plate fixation, *Paraplegia* 33:606-609, 1995.
26. Heller J: Surgical treatment of degenerative cervical disc disease. In Fardon D et al: *Orthopaedic knowledge update: Spine 2,* Rosemont, IL, 2002, American Academy of Orthopaedic Surgeons.
27. Heller J, Pedlow F, Gill S: Anatomy of the cervical spine. In Clark C: *The cervical spine,* Philadelphia, 2005, Lippincott, Williams & Wilkins.
28. Janda V: Muscles and motor control in cervicogenic disorders. In Grant R: *Physical therapy of the cervical and thoracic spine,* St Louis, 2002, Churchill Livingstone.
29. Jull G: Management of cervicogenic headaches. In Grant R: *Physical therapy of the cervical and thoracic spine,* St Louis, 2002, Churchill Livingstone.
30. Kapandji I: *The physiology of the joints,* vol 3, New York, 1995, Churchill Livingstone.
31. Lee M: Effects of frequency on response of the spine to lumbar posteroanterior forces, *J Manipulative Physiol Ther* 16:439, 1993.
32. Lee M, Gal J, Herzog W: Biomechanics of manual therapy. In Dvir Z: *Clinical biomechanics,* St Louis, 2000, Churchill Livingstone.
33. Lee M, Kelly D, Steven G: A model of spine, ribcage and pelvic responses to a specific lumbar manipulative force in relaxed subjects, *J Biomech* 28:1403, 1995.
34. Lee M, Lau T, Lau H: Sagittal plane rotation of the pelvis during lumbar posteroanterior loading, *J Manipulative Physiol Ther* 17:149, 1994.
35. Lees F, Turner J: Natural history and prognosis of cervical spondylosis, *Br Med J* 2:1607-1610, 1963.
36. Lowery G, McDonough R: The significance of hardware failure in anterior cervical plate fixation. Patients with 2 to 7 year follow up, *Spine* 23:181-186, 1998.
37. Mann D et al: Anterior plating of unstable cervical spine fractures, *Paraplegia* 28:564-572, 1990.
38. Marco R, An H: Anatomy of the spine. In Fardon D et al: *Orthopaedic knowledge update: Spine 2,* Rosemont, IL, 2002, American Academy of Orthopaedic Surgeons.
39. Neumann D: Axial skeleton: Osteology and arthrology. In Neumann D: *Kinesiology of the musculoskeletal system—foundations for physical rehabilitation,* St Louis, 2002, Mosby.

40. Nitz A: Bone injury and repair. In Placzek J, Boyce D: *Orthopaedic physical therapy secrets,* Philadelphia, 2001, Hanley and Belfus.
41. Nitz A: Soft tissue injury and repair. In Placzek J, Boyce D: *Orthopaedic physical therapy secrets,* Philadelphia, 2001, Hanley and Belfus.
42. Olmarker K, Rydevik B: Nerve root pathophysiology. In Fardon D et al: *Orthopaedic knowledge update: Spine 2,* Rosemont, IL, 2002, American Academy of Orthopaedic Surgeons.
43. Penning L et al: CT myelographic findings in degenerative disorders of the cervical spine: Clinical significance, *Am J Neuroradiol* 7:119-127, 1986.
44. Posner M: Compression neuropathies. In Spivak J et al: *Orthopaedics—a study guide,* New York, 1999, McGraw-Hill.
45. Posner M: Nerve lacerations: Acute and chronic. In Spivak J et al: *Orthopaedics—a study guide,* New York, 1999, McGraw-Hill.
46. Ricci J: Tissue anatomy. In Spivak J et al: *Orthopaedics—a study guide,* New York, 1999, McGraw-Hill.
47. Richardson C et al: *Therapeutic exercise for spinal segmental stabilization in low back pain—scientific basis and clinical approach,* Edinburgh, 1999, Churchill Livingstone.
48. Roth DA: Cervical analgesic discography: A new test for the definitive diagnosis of the painful disc syndrome, *J Am Med Assoc* 235:1713-1714, 1976.
49. Shacklock M: Neurodynamics, *Physiotherapy,* 81:9-16, 1995.
50. Sidhu K, Herkowitz H: Surgical management of cervical disc disease: Surgical management of cervical radiculopathy. In Herkowitz H et al, editors: *The spine,* Philadelphia, 1999, WB Saunders, pp 497-511.
51. Singh K, Vaccaro A: Surgical approaches to the cervical spine. In Devin V: *Spine secrets,* Philadelphia, 2003, Hanley and Belfus.
52. Swank M et al: Anterior cervical allograft arthrodesis and instrumentation: Multilevel interbody grafting or strut graft reconstruction, *Eur Spine J* 6:138-143, 1997.
53. Thongtrangan I, Balabhadra R, Kim D: Management of strut graft failure in anterior cervical spine surgery, *Neurosurg Focus* 15:3, 2003.
54. Vaccaro A: Point of view, *Spine* 23:186-187, 1998.
55. Wakefield A, Benzel E: Complications of cervical surgery. In Fardon D et al: *Orthopaedic knowledge update: Spine 2,* Rosemont, IL, 2002, American Academy of Orthopaedic Surgeons.
56. White A, Panjabi M: *Clinical biomechaincs of the spine,* ed 2, Philadelphia, 1990, JB Lippincott.
57. Winkelstein B, Weinstein J: Pain mechanisms: Relevant anatomy, pathogenesis, and clinical implications. In Clark C: *The cervical spine,* Philadelphia, 2005, Lippincott, Williams & Wilkins.
58. Winslow C, Winslow T, Wax M: Dysphonia and dysphagia following the anterior approach to the cervical spine, *Arch Otolaryngol Head Neck Surg* 127:51-55, 2001.
59. Zeigman S, Ducker T, Raycroft J: Trends and complications in cervical spine surgery: 1989-1993, *J Spinal Disord* 10:523-526, 1997.

CHAPTER 13

Posterior Lumbar Microscopic Discectomy and Rehabilitation

Haideh V. Plock
Ben B. Pradhan
Rick B. Delamarter
David Pakozdi

Lumbar herniated nucleus pulposus (HNP) falls within the spectrum of degenerative spinal conditions and can occur with little or no trauma. Lumbar disc abnormalities increase with age.[5,130] The actual incidence of lumbar disc herniations is unknown, because many people with herniations are asymptomatic.[5,7,41] Approximately 90% of lumbar herniations occur at the L4-L5 and L5-S1 levels.[5,17,31] More than 200,000 discectomies are performed in the United States each year, and this number is likely increasing.[14] The success of this procedure, as with all surgical procedures, depends vastly on proper patient selection and to a lesser extent on surgical technique. However, it is incumbent on the spinal surgeon to be absolutely meticulous with intraoperative technique once the decision for surgery is made. To this end, the use of a microscope is recommended for lumbar discectomy. Once the learning curve has been mastered, the microscope not only offers advantages over loupes but also forces one to think at a much higher level of clarity about what and where root encroachment pathology is present.[18] More importantly, the patient has less morbidity and an earlier hospital discharge compared with standard or limited discectomy.*

SURGICAL INDICATIONS AND CONSIDERATIONS

Pathophysiology

Intervertebral discs cushion and tether the vertebrae, providing both flexibility and stability. The normally gelatinous nucleus pulposus is surrounded by the ligamentous annulus fibrosis. In the young and healthy disc, the nucleus and annulus blend. Degenerative or pathologic changes can cause separations of the two entities, as well as compromise the integrity of the annulus, such that a sufficient load can cause nuclear fragments to migrate and impinge on neural elements.[131] Lumbar disc herniations may occur with little or no trauma, although patients frequently report a bending or twisting motion as the inciting event, causing the onset of symptoms. Common causes of lumbar herniations include falls, car accidents, repetitive heavy lifting, and sports injuries of all types.

*References 11, 17, 59, 101, 103, 110, 111.

Diagnosis

The radiographic diagnosis of lumbar disc herniation has been made rather simple with magnetic resonance imaging (MRI). The clinical diagnosis is frequently straightforward as well. A patient with a lumbar herniation generally has some element of low back pain with radiation into the buttocks, thigh, leg, and foot. The leg radiation almost always follows a dermatomal distribution. Patients frequently complain of numbness, tingling, or weakness in the affected dermatome. Lying down may relieve the symptoms. Whereas sitting, walking, and standing may exacerbate them. Complaints of bowel and bladder dysfunction may signal a cauda equina syndrome, and may necessitate emergent workup and treatment.

Physical Examination

Visual inspection may reveal lumbar muscle spasm, fasciculations, and postural changes, including listing to the side and a forward flexed position. Gait observation can reveal a listing antalgic walk. Weakness can give a dropped foot type gait (anterior tibialis) or buckling of the leg (quadriceps). Range of motion (ROM) testing may be limited secondary to pain. Neurologic testing is extremely important and should include motor, sensory, and reflex testing. Lumbar herniations may cause varying degrees of dermatomal weakness, sensory deficits, and reflex changes. Straight leg raises (SLRs) are a good indicator of nerve root impingement in lower lumbar herniations, and a positive femoral stretch can indicate an upper lumbar herniation.

Imaging and Other Tests

MRI is clearly the imaging study of choice to diagnose a lumbar disc herniation (Fig. 13-1, A and B). Plain radiographs should always be obtained to evaluate overall alignment, bony integrity, and stability. Patients who cannot obtain an MRI can be diagnosed using computed tomography (CT), CT myelogram, or CT discogram. These imaging tests are so sensitive that discectomy is not indicated if a disc is not found to be herniated by one of these techniques. Other tests can include an electromyogram (EMG) or nerve conduction study (NCS).

Management

It is important to understand that most patients with symptomatic herniated lumbar discs will get better over time, regardless of the type of treatment. Weber's classic study[120] reported that sciatica from HNP would improve 60% of the time with nonsurgical methods, and 92% of the time with surgery at 1 year. By 4 years out, no statistical difference was found between the two groups, and no difference at 10-year follow-up. In the absence of cauda equina syndrome, progressive or significant neurologic deficits, most practitioners attempt at least 4 to 8 weeks of conservative care before suggesting surgical intervention.

Nonoperative Treatment

Nonoperative treatment may include:

1. Modified activity
2. Modified bed rest for 2 to 3 days (prolonged bed rest should be avoided)[20,46,115]
3. Analgesic, anti-inflammatory medication (e.g., nonsteroidal anti-inflammatory drugs [NSAIDs], steroids), or both
4. Physical therapy (as tolerated) or external support (e.g., corset, brace)
5. Epidural steroid injections (the authors recommend up to three)

Indications for Surgery

Surgical indications, as currently recommended by the North American Spine Society (NASS), include a definite diagnosis of ruptured lumbar intervertebral disc and the following:[9,21]

A

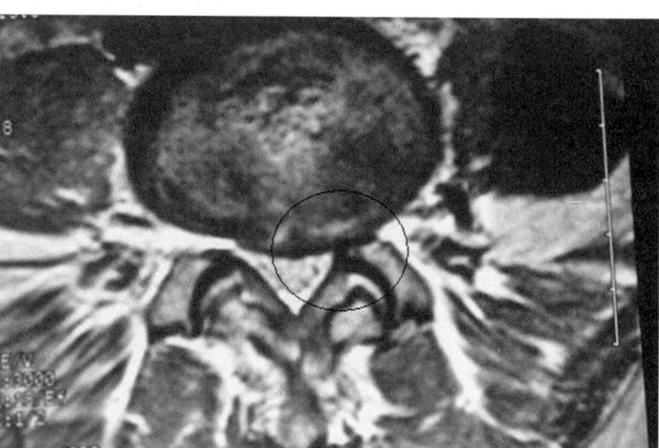

B

Fig. 13-1 **A,** Sagittal magnetic resonance imaging (MRI) showing herniated discs at the bottom two lumbar discs, at L4-5 and L5-S1. **B,** An axial cut of a lumbar spine MRI revealing a left-sided broad-based paracentral disc herniation effacing the thecal sac, causing left-sided lateral recess, foraminal stenosis, and neural compression.

1. Failure of conservative treatment
2. Unbearable or recurrent episodes of radicular pain (or both)
3. Significant neurologic deficit
4. Increasing neurologic deficit (absolute indication)
5. Cauda equina syndrome (absolute indication)

Conservative treatment consists of nonoperative management and careful observation for at least 4 to 8 weeks. Some may benefit from a short trial of nonoperative treatment even after 8 weeks if no prior care was given. Failed conservative treatment is the most common indication for lumbar discectomy. Those who have not improved sufficiently and are not experiencing continued improvement might then be offered treatment by surgical excision of the disc. Such patients should be advised that this is an elective operation but that delay for longer than 3 to 6 months in the face of persistent and severe symptoms may compromise the best ultimate result.[21,62]

The other indications (2 to 5) are exceptions to the 4- to 8-week rule. Excruciating pain may not be relieved by nonoperative means and may require earlier surgical decompression. Recurrent sciatica should also receive consideration for surgery: the chance of recurrent sciatica after the second episode is 50% and after the third episode is almost 100%.[62] An example of a significant neurologic deficit may be a foot drop or weakness that prevents normal posture, gait, or affects the patient's profession or a particular skill. Any definite progression of neurologic deficit is an absolute indication for surgery. Cauda equina syndrome is relatively rare, being reported in 1% to 3% of patients with confirmed disc herniations,[45,99] which is an orthopedic or neurosurgical emergency. Features include rapid progression of neurologic signs and symptoms, bilateral leg pain, caudal sensory deficit, bladder overflow incontinence or retention, and loss of rectal sphincter tone with or without fecal incontinence.

Contraindications for Discectomy

NASS and the American Academy of Orthopaedic Surgeons (AAOS) have identified the following factors as absolute or relative contraindications for discectomy[21,30]:

1. Lack of clear clinical diagnosis, anatomic level of lesion, and radiographic evidence of HNP
2. Lack of trial of nonoperative treatment (with the exceptions mentioned previously)
3. Disabilities with major nonorganic components (i.e., multifocal, nonanatomic, or disproportionate signs and symptoms)
4. Systemic disease processes that can negatively influence outcome of surgery (e.g., diabetic neuropathy)
5. Medical contraindications to surgery (e.g., major co-morbidities, unfavorable survival)
6. Disc herniation at a level of instability (may need additional stabilization)

SURGICAL PROCEDURES

One only has to review the natural history of lumbar disc disease to realize that spinal surgeons play a palliative role in the management of HNP.* Surgical procedures as treatment for lumbar HNP include the following:

1. Lumbar discectomy (microscopic or standard open technique)
   a. Hemilaminotomy and discectomy
   b. Laminectomy and discectomy
2. Minimally invasive percutaneous techniques
   a. Chemonucleolysis
   b. Percutaneous discectomy (suction, shaver, laser, endoscopic tools)

Use of an Operating Microscope

The attempt to improve visualization and illumination has led many spine surgeons to use loupes and a headlight. The authors believe the magnification and illumination built into the microscope offer many surgical advantages, the most important of which is reduced wound size and decreased tissue manipulation. The surgeon can limit the amount of tissue dissection by working through a small exposure directly over the pathology to be removed. Microsurgical techniques can also be used to preserve the ligamentum flavum and epidural fat to minimize postoperative epidural fibrosis and improve clinical results by preserving natural tissue planes.[15,18] With this approach, the disc herniation can be easily removed, lateral recess stenosis can be decompressed, and nerve root manipulation is kept to a minimum. The senior author has used this technique since 1986 for most lumbar disc herniations and has found the approach to be safe, with fewer dural tears and nerve root injuries and less postoperative epidural fibrosis than with standard discectomy.[17,18,59,63]

However, the microscope is not without its disadvantages. Peripheral vision is lost, with the field of vision limited to approximately 4 to 5 cm. Because of this, the surgeon needs to know detailed anatomy of the spine. The line of vision is fixed through the microscope. To look over structures (to overcome tissue overhang), the patient or microscope has to be adjusted during the surgery. This can be avoided by proper retraction or dissection of tissue away from the line of vision. Researchers reported increased disc space infection after microsurgery.[126,127] This was most likely caused by contamination from unsterile parts of the microscope during surgery; although no one has looked at the potential for an increased infection rate when two surgeons with loupes and headlights bump heads over the wound! Recent reports by those who have experience with the microscope do not show any increased infection rates.[17,59,94,111]

*References 22, 23, 29, 57, 121.

Lumbar Microdiscectomy

Microscopic discectomy (microdiscectomy) has become the *gold standard* for operative treatment of lumbar disc herniations, and the latest minimally invasive percutaneous techniques have not been shown to be more effective.[16,18,55] Although no statistical differences can be shown in the ultimate long-term outcomes of microscopic versus standard open discectomies,* the microscope provides improved illumination and magnification, and patients have less morbidity and earlier hospital discharge when compared with standard discectomies (Fig. 13-2).†

Operative Setup

General anesthesia is preferable because of patient comfort, as well as airway and sedation control. Another advantage is the option of hypotensive anesthesia. The procedure can also be done under epidural or local anesthesia with sedation, although this is not the authors' preference. The patient's position is always prone with the abdomen free, thus relieving pressure on the abdominal venous system and, in turn, decreasing venous backflow through Batson's venous plexus into the spinal canal. This has the effect of decreasing bleeding from the epidural veins intraoperatively. Several frames are available for this, but the authors prefer a Wilson frame on a regular operating table because of the ease of setup.

Identification of Level and Side

A preincision lateral radiograph or fluoroscopy image, with a radio-opaque skin marker placed according to preoperative radiographs and anatomic landmarks, will identify the appropriate incision location for the disc space to be exposed. This is best done by placing a spinal needle as straight vertically as possible, approximately 2 cm from midline contralateral to the side of surgery. The side of surgery is usually the more symptomatic side, although occasionally a midline HNP can be approached from either side.

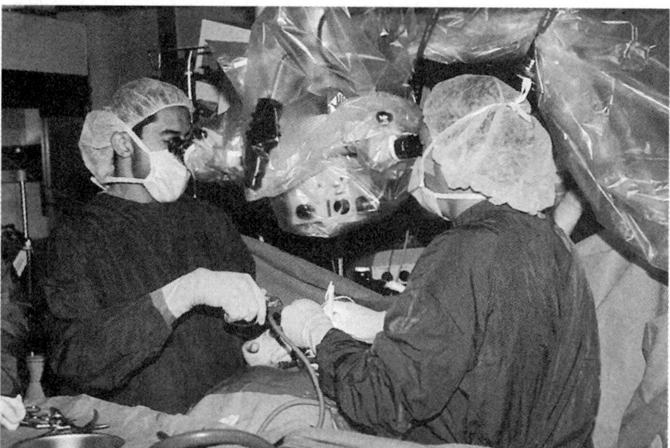

Fig. 13-2 A surgeon and an assistant surgeon using the operative microscope with a high-intensity light source and microscopic magnification. The two surgeons can work hand-in-hand with unobstructed view of the operative field.

Skin Incision and Interlaminar Space Exposure

A 2- to 3-cm incision is made midline or up to 1 cm lateral to the spinous process on the symptomatic side, at a level directly over the disc space based on the localizing lateral radiograph. At L5-S1 this incision tends to be directly over the interlaminar space, but as one moves up the lumbar spine, this incision will be progressively over the cephalad lamina. The dissection is carried down to the lumbodorsal fascia, which is sharply incised. The fascial incision is placed carefully, just lateral to the spinous processes to avoid damage to the supraspinous and interspinous ligament complex. The subperiosteal muscle dissection and elevation are confined to the interlaminar space and approximately half of the cephalad and caudad lamina. The facet capsules are carefully preserved. A Cobb elevator and Bovie cautery are used. A framed retractor is then placed. The surgeon should expose the lateral border of the pars as a landmark for preserving enough of the pars during laminotomy to prevent fracture.

At this time another localizing lateral radiograph should be obtained to confirm the proper level. A forward-angled curette can be placed underneath the cephalad lamina of the interspace. With this intraoperative radiographic verification, wrong-level surgery is impossible. The radiograph will also indicate how much of the cephalad lamina needs to be removed to expose the disc space. The microscope is then brought into position.

Spinal Canal Entry

After exposure of the interlaminar space and placement of the retractor, a high-speed burr is used to remove several millimeters of the cephalad lamina and 2 to 3 mm of the medial aspect of the inferior facet (Fig. 13-3). Once the cephalad lamina and medial aspect of the inferior facet have been removed, the ligamentum flavum is easily seen as its bony attachments are exposed. The ligamentum attaches at the very cephalad edge of the lower lamina, but approximately halfway up the upper lamina, and it attaches to the medial aspect of the superior facet. Thus the high-speed burr can be used relatively safely on top of the bottom half of the superior lamina, as well as the medial aspect of the inferior facet.

Free Ligamentum Flavum

The ligamentum flavum is then released from the medial edge of the superior facet with a forward-angled curette. It can also be released from the undersurface of the upper and lower lamina (Fig. 13-4). It is safest to start the curette

*References 1, 4, 57, 101, 106, 110, 111.

†References 17, 11, 59, 101, 103, 110, 111.

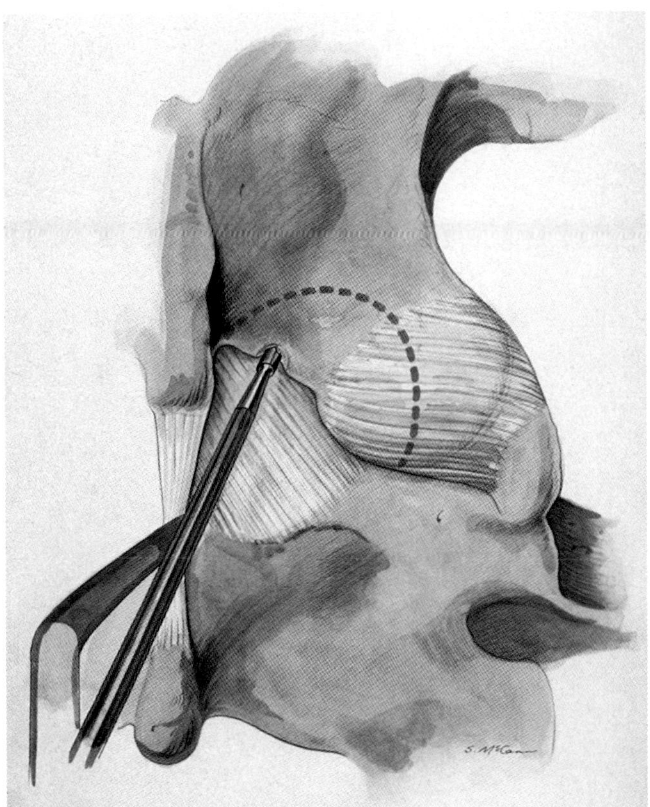

Fig. 13-3 After skin exposure and subsequent subperiosteal elevation, the retractor in position reveals the interlaminar interval, with exposure of the upper and lower laminae. Several millimeters of the cephalad lamina and 2 to 3 mm of the medial edge of the inferior facet are removed with the high-speed burr. This bone can be safely removed because the undersurface is protected by the ligamentum flavum.

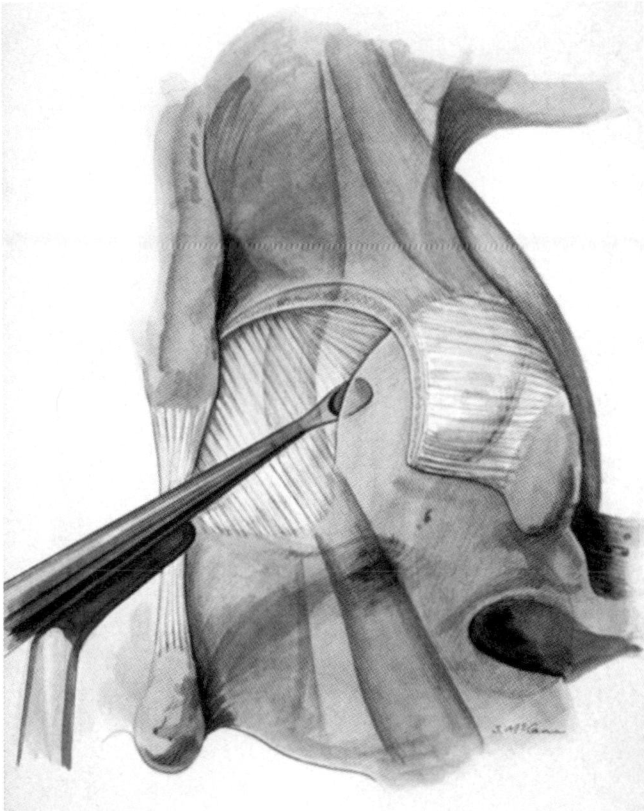

Fig. 13-4 A small, forward-angled curette frees the ligamentum flavum from its attachment to the medial edge of the superior facet. The ligamentum flavum also can be freed from the undersurface of the upper and lower laminae.

inferolaterally toward the superior aspect of the pedicle (caudal aspect of the foramen).

A ligamentum- and epidural fat-sparing approach, by creating a flap of the ligamentum as described previously, decreases postoperative epidural fibrosis and can improve results.[15,18] However, this can make it more difficult to get a good view of the nerve root. Certainly this is easier with a microscope than without one. The less-experienced surgeon may perform partial removal of these tissues. The ligamentum flap is also not recommended for large midline disc herniations (with or without cauda equina syndrome) and severely stenotic canals, because the ligamentum itself occupies more room in the already severely compromised spinal canal and would also interfere with direct visualization for the delicate manipulation of the thecal sac.

Lateral Recess Exposure

After release of the ligamentum flavum, the medial edge of the superior facet is resected with 2- to 4-mm Kerrison rongeurs. This resection goes from the lower pedicle to the tip of the superior facet (Fig. 13-5). This medial facet resection decompresses any lateral recess stenosis at the level of the pedicle and up into the foramen, and it allows easy access to the lateral disc space. If needed, some of the lateral ligamentum flavum, particularly into the foramen, can be removed with the Kerrison rongeurs.

Nerve Root and Ligamentum Retraction

Bipolar cautery can be used at this time to cauterize any epidural bleeding over the lateral disc space, directly cephalad to the pedicle. The authors recommend finding the pedicle and then using it as a guide to release the epidural non-neural tissues above the disc space. At this point a nerve root retractor can be placed on the disc space, and the ligamentum flavum, epidural fat, and nerve root are retracted toward the midline, generally exposing the herniation (Fig. 13-6). Again, the bipolar can be used to cauterize any epidural veins over the disc herniation. Any free large fragments of disk can now be removed (Fig. 13-7). If needed, a forward-angled curette can be used to scrape the inferior and posterior bony margins of the foramen, using a unidirectional pulling motion. Using the bony pedicle as a starting point ensures that the end

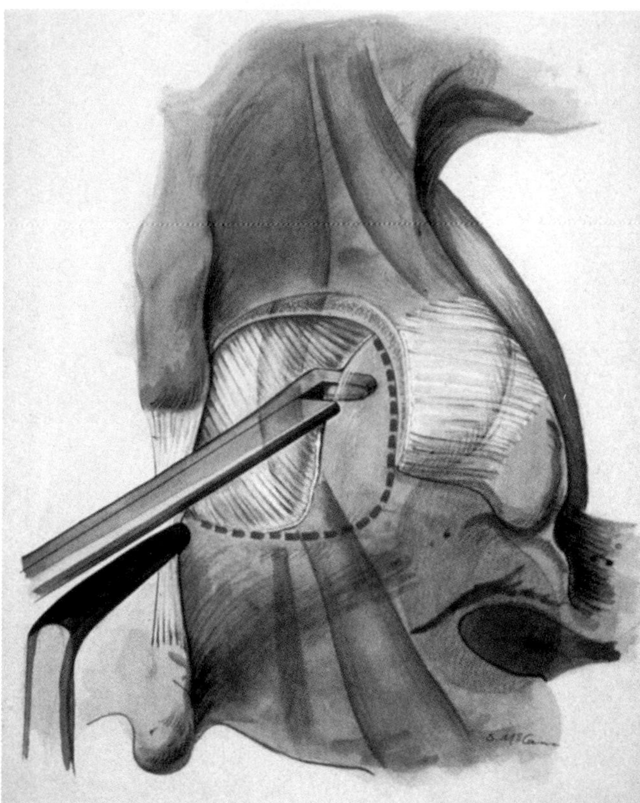

Fig. 13-5 A 3-mm or 4-mm Kerrison rongeur is used to remove the lateral recess (subarticular) stenosis (i.e., the medial edge of the superior facet) back to the pedicle of the lower vertebra and cephalad to the top of the superior facet. This bony resection removes the lateral recess (subarticular) stenosis and allows exposure of the lateral disc space.

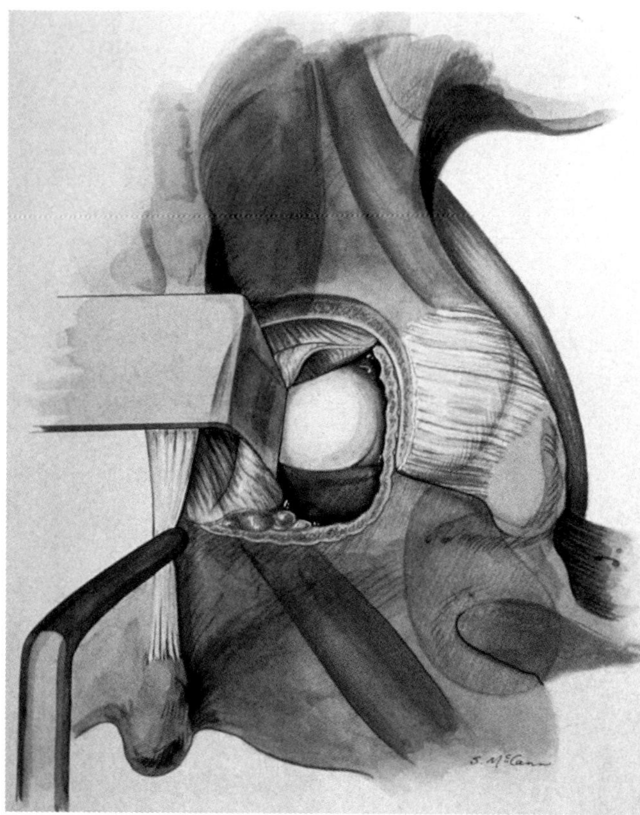

Fig. 13-6 A nerve root retractor is used to retract the ligamentum flavum, nerve root sleeve, and epidural fat toward midline over the herniated disc. Bipolar cautery can be used to cauterize the epidural plexus over the disc herniation.

of the curette does not include any neural tissue before scraping.

Discectomy

Frequently the annular defect of the disc herniation is all that is necessary to allow cleaning out of any loose nucleus pulposus inside the disc space, although the annulotomy can be enlarged with a No. 11 blade. The herniated nuclear material is then cleaned out with straight or angled pituitary rongeurs and small back-angled curettes. Care should be taken not to damage or curette the endplates. The annulotomy can be performed in various shapes, which are not discussed in detail here.[84,126]

One unresolved issue is how much disc to remove from the discal cavity. Removal of as much disc as possible implies curettage of the interspace, including possible removal of the cartilaginous endplates. Critics of this approach point out that no matter how long the surgeon works, it is impossible to remove all disc material in this fashion. They also argue that this method increases risk of damage to anterior visceral structures and increases risk of chronic back pain induced by conditions such as sterile disciitis and instability. Although some surgeons believe that extensive intradiscal débridement decreases the rate of recurrent HNP, others refute that position.* In the end, the only reasonable prospective controlled study is Spengler's,[104] which suggests that limited disc excision is all that is necessary. The advantages of limited disc excision are less trauma to endplates and less dissection, less nerve root manipulation, a lower prevalence of infection, reduced risk of damage to structures anterior to disc space, and less disc space settling postoperatively (theoretically reducing the incidence of chronic back pain).

Disc Space Irrigation

After the HNP and any remaining loose material is removed, the disc space is irrigated under some pressure with a long angiocatheter; then the pituitary rongeur is again used to remove any loose fragments. The spinal canal is then palpated underneath the nerve root and across the vertebral bodies above and below for any residual fragments. In doing the limited disc excision, one must also be sure to probe under the posterior annulus (both

*References 78, 92, 125, 126.

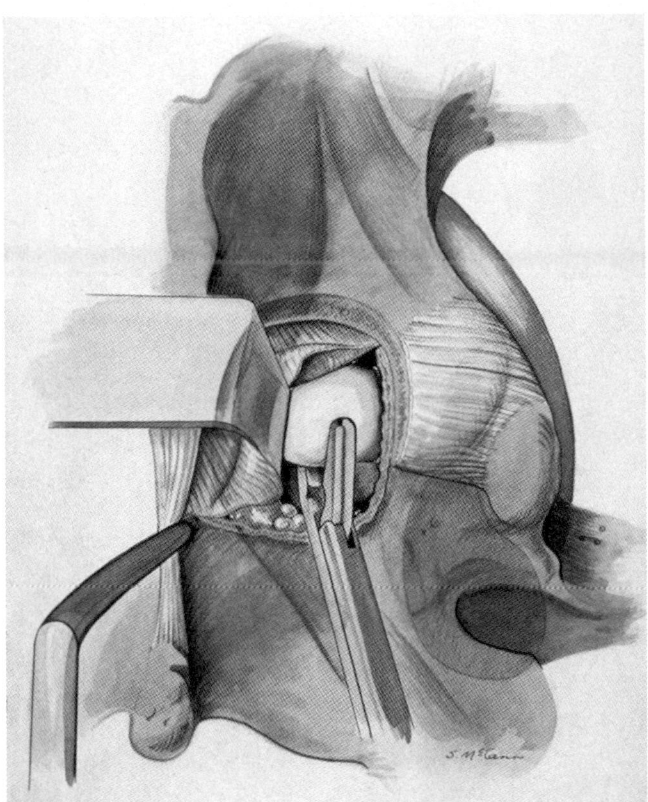

Fig. 13-7 After exposure of the disc herniation, large free fragments can be removed with a pituitary rongeur, the natural annulotomy from the disc herniation can be enlarged with a No. 11 blade, or both can be done.

medially and laterally) for loose fragments. This is an important step to ensure that no displaced or sequestered fragments are missed. Residual disc material will feel rough, whereas the native dural surface is quite smooth. In the end the patient must be left with a freely mobile nerve root. The preoperative MRI should be carefully studied for displaced fragments, but it is important to keep in mind that fragments may have moved since the MRI was taken.

Closure

Once the decompression is complete, the entire surgical wound is thoroughly irrigated with antibiotic-containing irrigant. Any final bleeding is controlled with bipolar cautery, thrombin-soaked gel foam, or FloSeal hemostatic gel. After complete hemostasis and removal of all gel foam, the closure is performed in layers. Many attempts have been made to design substances to seal the laminotomy defect and prevent scar formation, including fat grafts, hydrogel, silicone, Dacron, and steroids.[64] The authors simply prefer the ligamentum flap (Fig. 13-8).[17,18,62] The dorsal lumbar fascia is closed with No. 1-0 sutures, the subcutaneous layer with 2-0 sutures, and the skin with 3-0 subcuticular sutures. Using this ligamentum flavum–sparing approach, blood loss should be no more than 10 to 20 cc. With good hemostasis, drainage of the surgical wound is not necessary.

Postoperative Course

Many microdiscectomy procedures can be done on an outpatient basis.[6,73,103,133] Most patients are encouraged to walk as tolerated. Sitting is also tolerated, but may be more limited. Many return to work within 5 to 10 days, especially those with desk type of work. All patients are required to participate in lumbar physical therapy, primary stabilization, and mobilization beginning at around 4 weeks after surgery. Most athletes return to their normal athletic activities within 8 weeks after surgery. However, the postoperative course is variable, and return to normal activities depends on the patient's overall medical condition, as well as neurologic and overall recovery.[10,118,120]

Unusual Disc Herniations

Herniated Nucleus Pulposus at High Lumbar Levels (L1-L2, L2-L3, L3-L4)

High lumbar HNPs are uncommon (5%). When they occur they are likely to be foraminal or extraforaminal.[61,62] Important skeletal anatomy in the higher lumbar spine for the spinal surgeon to be aware of includes the following: (1) the pars are narrower, and facet integrity is easily lost with excessive laminotomy; (2) the laminae are broader; (3) the interlaminar window is narrower; (4) the inferior border of the lamina overhangs more of the disc space; (5) at L1-L2, the conus cannot be retracted like the cauda equina at lower levels; (6) the nerve roots exit more horizontally and are less mobile; and (7) epidural veins may be more prevalent. At these levels, because of limited size of the interlaminar space, ligamentum excision rather than sparing is recommended.

Recurrent Disc Rupture

The incidence of recurrent HNP is 2% to 5%.[17,52,81] The microscope is especially valuable in this scenario, because of the scar between tissue planes, including neural elements. Adequate time must be spent carefully teasing the tissues apart with a blunt instrument (e.g., bipolar, curette, Penfield) before forcefully mobilizing the nerve root. The incidence of complications is understandably higher in revision discectomies.

Cauda Equina Syndrome

The classic teaching in cauda equina syndrome is that (1) it is an orthopedic emergency, and (2) a wide decompression through a bilateral approach is necessary. The authors agree with the first point, but not the second. Few disc herniations are too big to be addressed microsurgically. A wider hemilaminectomy may be needed. The microscope is invaluable when working in the severely stenotic canal.

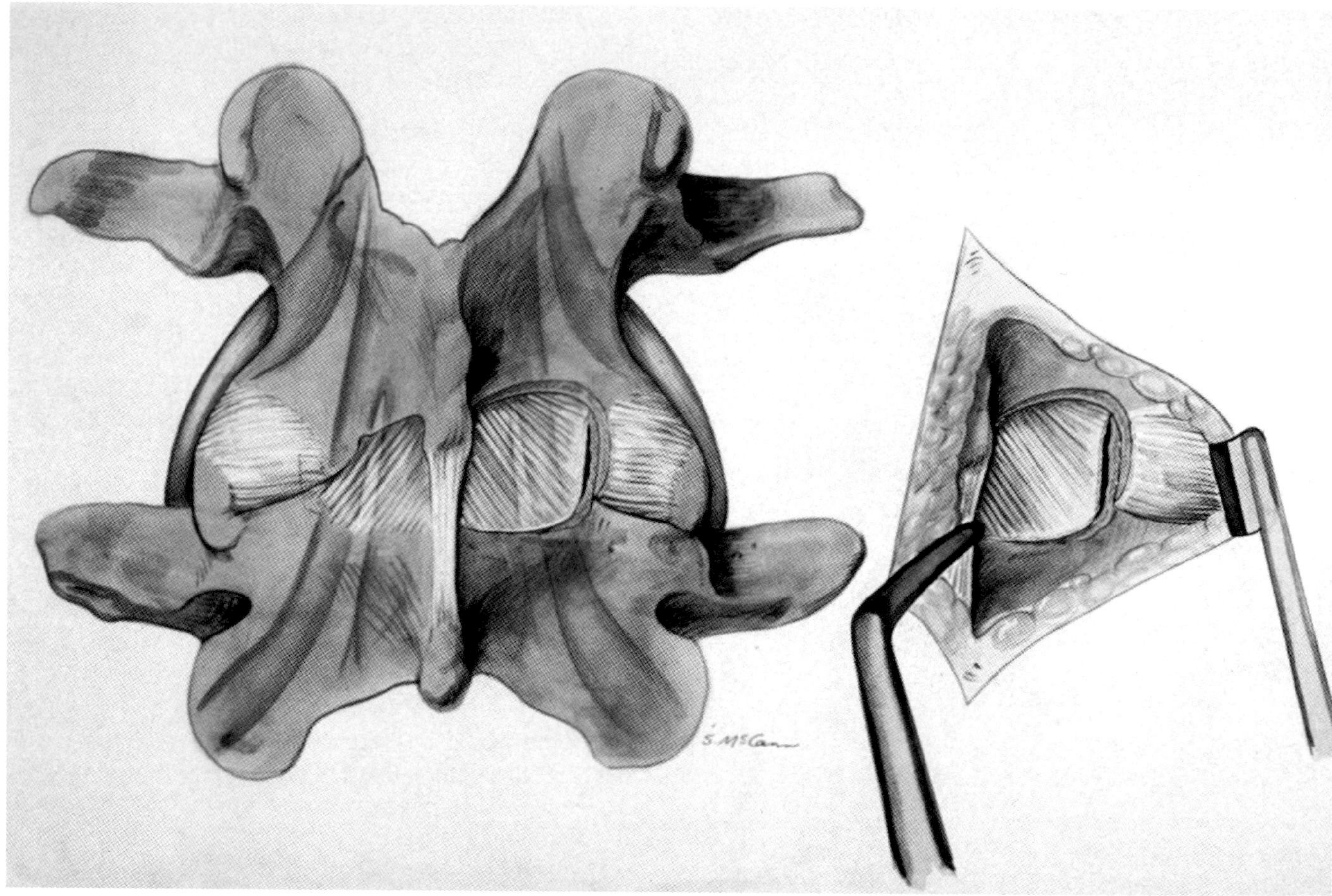

Fig. 13-8 After thorough irrigation, the nerve root retractor is released, allowing the ligamentum flavum and nerve root sleeve to return to their normal anatomic positions.

If the disc cannot be easily or totally excised unilaterally, then bilateral hemilaminotomies may be done.[45,99]

Herniated Nucleus Pulposus in the Adolescent Patient

The risk for recurrence of HNP after surgical excision is higher in adolescents than in adults. Because of the high proteoglycan content in adolescent discs and the prevalence of disc protrusions rather than disc extrusions, some have recommended percutaneous chemonucleolysis rather than surgical intervention in this age group.[25,51,62] Studies have been published with controversial results for surgical discectomy in this patient population.[19,83,102] Chemonucleolysis may have merit in the treatment of symptomatic disc protrusions, but discectomy is necessary in the setting of an extruded or sequestered disc causing significant or progressive neurologic deficit or pain. These extruded or sequestered fragments are frequently heavily collagenized.[21,75]

Complications

Complications for the discectomy procedures include dural tears, neural injury, visceral injuries, postoperative infection, recurrence of herniation, inadequate decompression, and iatrogenic instability.

Dural tears occur in 1.0% to 6.7% of cases, although the incidence decreases with experience.* If possible, then repair should be done by direct suture (5-0 to 7-0 silk, nylon, or polypropylene) with or without a dural patch.[60] The patient should be kept flat for a few days after surgery to lower the hydrostatic pressure in the lumbar thecal sac while the repair seals.

Neural injuries are rare, although the risk is greater with unusual disc herniations as described previously. Visceral injuries occur when an instrument penetrates the anterior annulus. Among these, vascular injuries are the most common.[60,91] If these are recognized, then immediate laparotomy for surgical repair is indicated.

Postoperative disciitis occurs in 1% of cases or less in experienced hands, although clearly a learning curve exists in developing facility with the microscope. Higher infection rates (up to 7%) have been reported with the use of a microscope during surgery, although in experienced hands

*References 17, 60, 94, 98, 107, 120.

this has been shown not to be true.[60] An MRI is the best diagnostic imaging tool. An image-guided needle biopsy may be performed to assist in appropriate antibiotic selection. Reoperation may not be necessary unless the patient develops root compression, cauda equina syndrome, or an epidural abscess.

The literature reports recurrent HNP occurring anywhere from 2% to 5% after lumbar discectomy.[62,122] When reoperating for a recurrent HNP, it is important to get adequate exposure of the dural sac above and below the disc space. Then using a combination of blunt (nerve hook, Penfield, bipolar) and sharp (Kerrison) dissection, the dural sac and nerve root are exposed and mobilized above the HNP.

Iatrogenic mechanical instability is fortunately a rare occurrence after discectomy, even if a decompressive laminectomy was required for a stenotic canal or to excise a large disc.[31] Symptomatic mechanical treatment may require surgical stabilization. Suboptimal results after discectomy surgery can be the result of several other problems that, unfortunately, do not have a straightforward medical or surgical treatment. Although very rare, these can include epidural fibrosis, arachnoiditis, and complex regional pain syndrome.[60]

Discussion

Most modern studies using microscopic techniques for treatment of herniated lumbar discs report 90% to 95% success rates.* A multicenter, prospective trial has proved what cannot be repeated often enough: If the therapist selects patients with dominant radicular pain (compared with back pain), with neurological changes and painful SLRs, and with a study confirming a disc rupture, then he or she can anticipate a high level of success for discectomy, with or without a microscope.[1] The rate of successful outcome drops significantly as more of these inclusion criteria are not met. Persistent back pain occurs in up to 25% of patients who undergo microdiscectomy.[98,107] This has led to the opinion that it is important to save the supraspinous and intraspinous ligament complex, remove as little lamina as possible, save the ligamentum flavum as a flap, and do a limited discectomy. These steps theoretically reduce iatrogenic instability, epidural fibrosis, sterile disciitis, and loss of disc height. All of these steps are facilitated by the use of a microscope, but no proof exists that these steps reduce the incidence of back pain.

The most frequent cause of poor result from lumbar disc surgery is faulty patient selection because of erroneous or incomplete diagnosis. Technical errors such as wrong-level surgery, incomplete decompression, and intraoperative complications explain a small percentage of failures. A 1981 study assigned the following frequency of missed diagnoses as sources of failure: lateral spinal stenosis 59%, recurrent or persistent herniation 14%, adhesive arachnoiditis 11%, central canal stenosis 11%, and epidural fibrosis 7%. Finally, the results of repeat surgery are not as good as primary surgery, regardless of the reason or whether a microscope was used, because of scar tissue, higher incidence of complications, or larger dissections.

In the past decade, a substantial increase in interest in minimally invasive procedures has occurred in all areas of medicine, particularly for spinal disorders. Several methods to remove HNP have been proposed as alternatives to standard open discectomy. Injected chymopapain can dissolve much of the central nucleus, but is not likely to act on extruded or sequestered fragments, which are often heavily collagenized.[21,25,75] Likewise, percutaneous suction discectomies and removal of nucleus (either mechanically or by laser from the center of the disc) may reduce intradiscal pressure but are unlikely to influence the effects of extruded or sequestered disc material. Therefore although alternative minimally invasive techniques hold considerable promise, lumbar microdiscectomy is still the gold standard for surgical treatment of lumbar HNP with radiculopathy. However, the skills and technology to remove herniated discs by such alternatives are evolving.*

*References 4, 11, 15, 17, 18, 22, 52, 94, 98, 101, 103, 106, 110, 111, 122, 127, 128.

*References 16, 21, 24, 55, 76, 77.

THERAPY GUIDELINES FOR REHABILITATION

Postoperative spine rehabilitation allows for a safer and faster return to functional activities. The early return to *appropriate* activities has been encouraged after surgeries of the extremities for many years. The same approach should be applied to the spine. Careful instruction and frequent re-evaluation enable a therapist to progress the patient's functional activities to premorbid levels safely. The therapist should apply a functionally appropriate and suitably aggressive postoperative protocol to the patient recovering from lumbar microdiscectomy.

Lumbar disc herniations can do more than compromise the nerve root. Compensatory movement patterns, altered mechanics of the motion segment, and muscle splinting may result in misleading referred pain patterns (e.g., myofascial trigger points). Furthermore, the literature suggests that abnormal changes in paraspinal muscle activity occur after a HNP.[28,68] Triano and Schultz[108] found a high correlation between the absence of the flexion-relaxation phenomenon (i.e., the relaxation of the lumbar paraspinal muscles at terminal flexion in standing) and poor results on the Oswestry Pain Disability Scale (Box 13-1).

Box 13-1 Oswestry Low Back Pain Disability Questionnaire

This questionnaire has been designed to give your physical therapist (PT) information as to how your back pain has affected your ability to manage in everyday life. Please answer every question by marking the *one* box that applies. We realize you may consider that two of the statements in any one section relate to you, but please just mark the box that most closely describes your problem.

Name: ____

Date: ______________ Initial Interim/Discharge

1. Pain intensity
   - ☐ I can tolerate the pain I have without having to use painkillers.
   - ☐ My pain is bad, but I manage without taking painkillers.
   - ☐ Painkillers give me complete relief from my pain.
   - ☐ Painkillers give me moderate relief from my pain.
   - ☐ Painkillers give me very little relief from my pain.
   - ☐ Painkillers have no effect on my pain, and I do not use them.
2. Personal care
   - ☐ I can look after myself normally without causing extra pain.
   - ☐ I can look after myself normally, but it causes extra pain.
   - ☐ It is painful to look after myself, and I am slow and careful.
   - ☐ I need some help, but I manage most of my personal care.
   - ☐ I need help every day in most aspects of self-care.
   - ☐ I do not get dressed, wash with difficulty, and stay in bed.
3. Lifting
   - ☐ I can lift heavy objects without causing extra pain.
   - ☐ I can lift heavy objects, but it gives me extra pain.
   - ☐ Pain prevents me from lifting heavy weights off the floor, but I can manage light to medium objects if they are conveniently positioned.
   - ☐ I can lift only very light objects.
   - ☐ I cannot lift anything at all.
4. Walking
   - ☐ Pain does not prevent me from walking any distance.
   - ☐ Pain prevents me from walking more than 1 mile.
   - ☐ Pain prevents me from walking more than $\frac{1}{2}$ mile.
   - ☐ Pain prevents me from walking more than $\frac{1}{4}$ mile.
   - ☐ I can only walk using a cane or crutches.
   - ☐ I am in bed most of the time and have to crawl to the toilet.
5. Sitting
   - ☐ I can sit in any chair as long as I like.
   - ☐ I can sit only in my favorite chair as long as I like.
   - ☐ Pain prevents me from sitting more than 1 hour.
   - ☐ Pain prevents me from sitting more than $\frac{1}{2}$ hour.
   - ☐ Pain prevents me from sitting more than 10 minutes.
   - ☐ Pain prevents me from sitting at all.
6. Standing
   - ☐ I can stand as long as I want without extra pain.
   - ☐ I call stand as long as I want, but it gives me extra pain.
   - ☐ Pain prevents me from standing more than 1 hour.
   - ☐ Pain prevents me from standing more than $\frac{1}{2}$ hour.
   - ☐ Pain prevents me from standing more than 10 minutes.
   - ☐ Pain prevents me from standing at all.
7. Sleeping
   - ☐ Pain does not prevent me from sleeping well.
   - ☐ I can sleep well only by taking medication for sleep.
   - ☐ Even when I take medication, I have less than 6 hours' sleep.
   - ☐ Even when I take medication, I have less than 4 hours' sleep.
   - ☐ Even when I take medication, I have less than 2 hours' sleep.
   - ☐ Pain prevents me from sleeping at all.
8. Sex life
   - ☐ My sex life is normal and gives me no extra pain.
   - ☐ My sex life is normal but causes some extra pain.
   - ☐ My sex life is nearly normal but is very painful.
   - ☐ My sex life is severely restricted by pain.
   - ☐ My sex life is nearly absent because of pain.
   - ☐ Pain prevents any sex life at all.
9. Social life
   - ☐ My social life is normal and gives me no extra pain.
   - ☐ My social life is normal but increases the degree of pain.
   - ☐ Pain has no significant effect on my social life apart from limiting my more energetic interests, such as dancing.
   - ☐ Pain has restricted my social life, and I do not go out as often.
   - ☐ Pain has restricted my social life to my home.
   - ☐ I have no social life because of pain.
10. Traveling
    - ☐ I can travel anywhere without extra pain.
    - ☐ I can travel anywhere, but it gives me extra pain.
    - ☐ Pain is bad, but I manage journeys over 2 hours.
    - ☐ Pain restricts me to journeys of less than 1 hour.
    - ☐ Pain restricts me to short, necessary journeys of less than $\frac{1}{2}$ hour.
    - ☐ Pain prevents me from traveling except to the doctor or hospital.

Microdiscectomy is designed to decompress neural tissues by removing the disc material that is causing the neurologic signs and symptoms not alleviated through aggressive conservative care.[58] Surgery *cannot* correct poor posture and body mechanics, relieve myofascial pain syndromes, or remedy faulty motor patterns of synergistic activity accompanying muscle substitution that occur in many patients with low back pain. Additionally, Hides, Richardson, and Jull[33,34] have found that the lumbar multifidi, a primary segmental stabilizer, do not spontaneously recover after low back pain, so it is doubtful that they will spontaneously recover after the trauma of spine surgery. The loss of these crucial active segmental stabilizers may lead to recurrent lumbar pain syndromes. To avoid this and aid the patient's rehabilitation after spinal surgery, the therapist must tirelessly question and reassess, using a problem-solving approach.

The following guidelines are not intended to be a substitute for sound clinical reasoning. Rather they are intended as a guide for the successful postoperative rehabilitation of patients after lumbar microdiscectomy. The primary goals after a lumbar microdiscectomy are the reduction of pain, prevention of recurrent herniation, maintenance of dural mobility, improvement of function, and early return to appropriate activities. Each patient's program must be individualized to attain these goals for the following reasons:

1. Patients have slightly different pathoanatomic abnormalities and surgical procedures.
2. Patients have different levels of strength, flexibility, and conditioning after surgery.
3. Patients' goals vary.
4. Patients have varying psychosocial factors.
5. Patients possess different levels of kinesthetic-proprioceptive coordination that affect their rate of motor learning.

Each patient must therefore receive care in accordance with individual needs. To this end the guidelines should be *progressed as tolerated,* and the therapist should *not* try to keep the patient "on schedule."

Increasing lower extremity (LE) symptoms, progressive neurologic deficit, and incapacitating pain are obvious "red flags" that require prompt re-evaluation. Although the therapist must not ignore pain, an acceptable level of discomfort is reasonable if the patient is increasing functional activities and progressing in the program as anticipated. Pain should be monitored in three parameters, with the therapist carefully noting the pain pattern (e.g., left lateral thigh to knee), observing the frequency (e.g., constant, intermittent, rare), and having the patient rate the intensity (0 to 10). This allows close tracking of changes in pain with exercise and activity so that the program can be progressed or modified accordingly.

Finally, any successful spinal rehabilitation program must not ignore psychosocial factors that negatively affect the program. It has been suggested that the greatest indicator for postoperative results is preoperative psychologic testing, not MRI or clinical signs.[95-97] Additionally, patients who have active litigation or workers' compensation claims have been shown to return to activity later than patients who do not.[43,85] These factors must be considered in evaluating patients, progressing exercise programs, and assessing clinical results.

Q

Rick is 41 years old. He has had progressing back pain episodes over the past 2 years. An MRI shows a herniated disc at L4-L5. Rick also has intermittent complaints of left radicular leg pain. He had microdiscectomy surgery 2 weeks ago and has come to outpatient physical therapy for evaluation and treatment. How should a spinal evaluation be altered to assess a patient who has recently had microdiscectomy surgery?

Phase I (Protective Phase)

TIME: 1 to 3 weeks after surgery

GOALS: Protect the surgical site to promote wound healing, maintain nerve root mobility, reduce pain and inflammation, educate patient to minimize fear and apprehension, establish consistently good body mechanics for safe and independent self-care (Table 13-1)

The first postoperative week typically consists of protective rest, progressive ambulation, and appropriately limited activities. Activity tolerance is the result of progressive activity, not rest. The patient should be encouraged to walk at a comfortable pace for short distances several times a day. Patients are usually allowed to shower 7 days after surgery, depending on wound healing. **Driving is usually not allowed for 1 to 2 weeks, although this may be extended if the right LE is significantly compromised.** Typically patients can return to office work within 1 week. Because the patient in phase I has difficulty tolerating sustained positioning, he or she may require support during driving, sitting, and lying postures. Additionally, patients may need to be directly educated in changing positions frequently. Patients may have significant incisional pain, especially with flexion movements. **The therapist must avoid all loaded lumbar flexion in patients in phases I and II.** The patient can apply cold packs to the surgical site for 15 to 20 minutes several times a day to help control pain, muscle spasm, and swelling.

The therapist may begin outpatient physical therapy as soon as the patient can comfortably come to the clinic, usually in the second or third week. Treatment begins only after the patient is evaluated to ascertain the following:

- A thorough history of the condition, including previous treatments or surgeries and time out of work

Table 13-1 Microdiscectomy

Rehabilitation Phase	Criteria to Progress to this Phase	Anticipated Impairments and Functional Limitations	Intervention	Goal	Rationale
Phase I Postoperative 1-3 weeks	◆ Postoperative	◆ Edema ◆ Pain ◆ Limited tolerance to transfers ◆ Limited tolerance to sustained positions ◆ Limited ADLs ◆ Limited nerve mobility ◆ Limited LE ROM ◆ Limited trunk and LE strength ◆ Limited mobility of neighboring regions ◆ Limited walking ◆ Limited cardiovascular endurance	◆ Cryotherapy ◆ ES ◆ Supportive corset or brace as indicated ◆ Body mechanics training—Maintenance of lumbar lordosis and avoidance of trunk flexion with the following: 1. Sitting and driving (supported as appropriate) 2. Sleeping (supported as necessary, avoiding fetal position) 3. Standing and walking (limit based on symptoms) 4. Transfers—Supine to sit-stand, in and out of car, and floor to stand 5. Self-care 6. Avoid lifting 7. Bending using hip hinging and neutral spine method ◆ Supine dural mobilization ◆ Prone dural mobilization ◆ PROM stretches—Hip (flexion [knee bent], SLR [gently], ER, standing gastrocnemius-soleus) ◆ Joint mobilization of hip and thoracic spine as indicated ◆ Progressive walking program on treadmill or flat surfaces ◆ Begin progressive exercise program (unloaded positions only) ◆ Pelvic rocks ◆ Supine pelvic rocks	◆ Manage edema ◆ Control pain ◆ Decrease pain with upright postures ◆ Prevent complications and reinjury ◆ Good understanding and use of proper body mechanics ◆ Sit up to 20 minutes ◆ Resume driving after 2 weeks ◆ Improve sleep patterns ◆ Use "log roll" technique with transfers ◆ Independent with self-care ◆ Improve nerve mobility ◆ Prevent adhesions that limit nerve mobility ◆ Restore ROM to LE ◆ Improve mobility of restricted joints ◆ Increase tolerance to walking level surfaces for 30 minutes ◆ Establish a healthy environment for the disc ◆ Good neutral control of lumbar spine while supine and prone ◆ Increased LE strength	◆ Promote self-management of edema and pain ◆ Provide abdominal support and decompression ◆ Initiate education to prepare patient for independence with ADLs, avoiding reinjury ◆ Maintain lordosis and avoid flexion postures to avoid excessive elongation tension on surgical site ◆ Promote protective rest and resumption of limited activities ◆ Transfer while avoiding unnecessary stress on surgical site ◆ Avoid lifting to prevent risk of reinjury ◆ Decrease stress on surgical site ◆ Prevent nerve fibrosis and dural adhesions ◆ Improve LE flexibility to decrease stress on the lumbar spine ◆ Avoid irritating sciatic nerve ◆ Maintain and improve proximal and distal mobility to reduce stress on the surgical site

Table 13-1 Microdiscectomy—Cont'd

Rehabilitation Phase	Criteria to Progress to this Phase	Anticipated Impairments and Functional Limitations	Intervention	Goal	Rationale
			(midrange lumbar flexion AROM) ◆ Side-lying pelvic rocks (midrange lumbar lateral flexion) ◆ Quadruped pelvic rocks (midrange lumbar AROM) ◆ Prone pelvic rocks (midrange lumbar extension AROM) ◆ Supine abdominal bracing (isolated transverse abdominis contraction) ◆ Supine abdominal bracing with arms behind head, progressed to alternating arm raises ◆ Prone abdominal bracing with alternating arm raises, progressed to bilateral arm raises ◆ Partial squatting to 60 degrees		◆ Prepare patient to resume ADLs and promote good cardiovascular conditioning ◆ Controlled lumbar movements are beneficial after microdiscectomy secondary to hydrostatic changes of the disc to promote vascularity ◆ Increase strength of trunk musculature to stabilize and protect the spine from injury ◆ Increase tolerance to upright postures ◆ Help with maintaining good body mechanics

ADLs, Activities of daily living; *ES*, electrical stimulation; *LE*, lower extremity; *ROM*, range of motion; *PROM*, passive range of motion; *SLR*, straight leg raises; *ER*, external rotation; *AROM*, active range of motion.

◆ The present pain pattern (intensity and frequency) plus activities or postures that alter these symptoms
◆ The status of the wound site
◆ Anthropometric data and postural and body mechanics assessment
◆ Limited mechanical testing **(Standing motion testing and end-of-range movements are not assessed until after the fifth week postoperatively.)**
◆ Neurologic status (Examination includes neural tension testing.)
◆ Baseline core strength testing in nonaggravating position (i.e., supine)

The therapist must take care during the initial evaluation to avoid any testing that may injure an already compromised patient. The authors of this chapter typically include Waddell signs[113] late in the rehabilitation process to help delineate nonorganic physical signs (Box 13-2).

The mechanical examination must be very limited in the phase I and phase II patient. It is intended to elicit symptomatic and mechanical responses that suggest mechanical problems and so dictate the treatment course.

Box 13-2 Waddell Signs

1. Superficial tenderness to light touch in the lumbar region or widespread tenderness to deep palpation in nonanatomic distributions
2. Increased symptoms with simulated axial loading or simulated rotation tests
3. Inconsistent supine and sitting straight leg raising (SLR) tests
4. Regional weakness or sensory abnormalities that are not myotomal or dermatomal
5. Physical overreaction or disproportionate verbalization during assessment

Because weight-bearing motion testing and end-of-range movements are typically not performed until after the fifth week postoperatively, the therapist uses responses to positioning and midrange movements in prone, supine, and side-lying positions to determine mechanical problems in the initial weeks.

Hip muscle strength testing should be postponed in the early stages of healing to prevent stressing inflamed lumbosacral tissues. Neural tension testing is an integral part of the lumbar evaluation. Therefore the therapist should have the patient perform the SLR, Cram's test, femoral nerve stretch test (prone knee flexion), and supine dural stretch and do the appropriate measuring, recording, and comparison with the opposite limb.

Slump testing should not be performed until after the fourth or fifth week postoperatively. Core strength testing may be performed in a variety of ways; however, Lee[48] describes a nice functional approach based on grouping core musculature into *slings*. A good understanding of soft tissue healing rates, spinal mechanics, and the specific surgical procedure helps avoid needless soft tissue trauma. For further evaluation of the patient's physical limitations and guidance toward appropriate functional training, the therapist can use the Modified Low Back Pain Oswestry Questionnaire[40] (see Box 13-1) or the Roland-Morris Functional Disability Questionnaire.[92] These are easily administered and helpful. The therapist should document the patient's perceived disability status before treatment and at predetermined intervals to monitor functional progress and determine the appropriate direction of functional training exercises.

After evaluation the therapist thoroughly explains the existing problems and the treatment plan to the patient. Therapist and patient should work together to reach mutual agreement on realistic goals. Patient education is crucial to achieving positive results, because the patient ultimately treats himself or herself several hours each day with a home exercise program and self-treatment techniques. *Furthermore, avoiding reinjury is perhaps the single most important postoperative factor responsible for a rapid progression in the program and ultimately full recovery.* Through patient education, a safe and relatively rapid return to activities can occur. The physical therapist (PT) educate should the patient regarding proper postures, home exercises, self-care techniques, and body mechanics for the safe performance of activities of daily living (ADLs). Proper postures and body mechanics are crucial during the postoperative healing phase. Ideally the therapist should instruct the patient before surgery, but if this does not occur, then the first postoperative task is to teach the patient correct postures and body mechanics.

> **A** Mechanical testing should be limited (standing motion testing and end-of-range movements are not assessed until 5 weeks after surgery). Hip muscle strength testing should be postponed in the early stages of healing to prevent stressing inflamed lumbosacral tissues. Slump testing is not performed until much later. A good understanding of soft tissue healing rates, spinal mechanics, and the specific surgical procedure helps avoid needless soft tissue trauma.

Proper Postures

The PT teaches the patient to maintain normal lumbar lordosis.

Patients should avoid lumbar flexion in standing or sitting, because intradiscal pressures are increased and excessive shear forces occur. Intolerance to prolonged postures is typical in phase I, and frequent movement breaks are recommended. The concept of abdominal bracing should be taught early. The therapist also should investigate the ergonomics of the patient's workstation to avoid potential problems.

Sitting and driving. The therapist should do the following:

- **Caution the patient to never slouch while sitting.**
- Instruct the patient in the use of a lumbar roll or similar device to maintain lordosis during sitting and driving.
- Advise the patient to try to always sit on firm, straight-back chairs **and never sit on soft sofas or chairs.**
- **Caution the patient to avoid all backless seating.** If the patient eventually will need to sit in bleachers or similar backless seating, then a Nada-Chair (Nada Concepts, Inc., Minneapolis, MN) or a similar device should be recommended that supports the lumbar spine during this type of sitting.
- Encourage frequent movement breaks. Instruct the patient to avoid sitting longer than 20 minutes at a time for the first 2 weeks. This increases in subsequent weeks, depending on tolerance to pain.
- Allow patients to return to driving for short periods after about 1 to 2 weeks. Remind the patient that safety is a priority—not a convenience.

Sleeping. The therapist should do the following:

- Teach the patient to sleep in supported supine, supported side lying, or supported prone three-quarter lying with the spine straight (see Fig. 14-7, A through C). **Instruct the patient to avoid sleeping in the fetal position because of the prolonged lumbar flexion. Have the patient avoid unsupported prone three-quarter lying positions because of the rotational component.**
- Caution the patient to avoid lying on soft mattresses or sofas.

Standing and walking. The therapist should do the following:

- Advise patients to limit standing at the kitchen sink or bathroom counter to short periods and avoid bending at the waist.
- Encourage the patient to maintain lumbar lordosis during standing and walking while performing an abdominal brace.

> **Q** Verlyn is a 40-year-old woman. She had microdiscectomy surgery for the L5 disk 6 weeks ago. Back pain is minimal. LE flexibility and strength is gradually improving. Trunk strength also is progressing. She is now seeing a PT for treatment. Previous treatments have included modalities for pain control, LE flexibility exercises, trunk and general strengthening, cardiovascular conditioning, and body mechanics. Verlyn is concerned about the intermittent radicular pain in her right leg. Prolonged sitting, walking, or standing aggravates her right leg. She reports reproduction of calf pain with hamstring stretching. What treatment technique should be used to decrease calf pain frequency and intensity?

Body Mechanics

To allow the patient to progress rapidly, the therapist should do everything possible to avoid reinjury. Minor setbacks may delay progression of the program, and a major setback may be irreparable. The therapist should pay close attention to the patient's movements. Patients may say they understand correct mechanics but display incorrect movement patterns. Frequent and critical observation allows the therapist to evaluate the patient's spinal mechanics and determine whether the patient has integrated the correct postures and mechanics. A checklist of basic functional movements (i.e., rising from lying, rising from sitting, sitting in neutral, reaching over head, bending to knee level) is helpful to record the performance of these skills and whether they require cues to complete the task.

Transfers. The therapist should do the following:

- Teach the patient to move correctly from supine to sitting (see Fig. 14-4), from standing to lying on the floor (see Fig. 14-6), and from sitting to standing (see Fig. 14-5). Rolling in bed as a unit and rising from bed must be performed correctly. In addition, give instruction on entering and exiting a car.

  Remember that all twisting motions are prohibited. Instruct them to move their feet to turn instead.

Dressing. The therapist should do the following:

- Instruct the patient in the correct way to put on pants, socks, and shoes in the supine position. Slip-on shoes are the easiest to handle in the first 2 weeks. Tying shoes can later be performed safely by putting the foot on a stool or chair.

Hygiene. The therapist should do the following:

- Explain that showering can begin after the second week. Have the patient shave her legs in the standing position, with the foot on the tub or shower seat, avoiding lumbar flexion.

Lifting. The therapist should do the following:

- Remember that correct lifting techniques should be taught early (see Fig. 14-11), and instruct patients to try to avoid all lifting in phase I. "Swoop lifting" is usually a safe and well-tolerated technique for light lifting in phase II. The patient performs it by making a long stride forward to the kneeling position (i.e., lunge) and then reaching to lift a light object. The exercise is then performed in reverse.

Bending. The therapist should do the following:

- **Advise the patient to avoid all bending at the waist. Lumbar flexion with loading is arguably the most hazardous movement in the first two phases.** The interdiscal pressures are significantly increased, and tension on the healing posterior annulus compounds the problem. Prolonged or repetitive bending is especially injurious.[32]
- Remember that, on occasion, limited bending is necessary. Teach the patient the correct way to bend and instruct him or her to avoid lumbar flexion while bending. The patient can safely bend by simultaneously flexing at the knees and hips ("hinge at the hips"), while maintaining a neutral spine and an abdominal brace. This is easy to teach by placing a 4-foot wooden pole (1 to 2 inches in diameter) along the spine with contact at the thoracic and sacral regions (see Fig. 14-9). By flexing slowly at the hips and knees while maintaining a neutral spine position and viewing themselves in a mirror, patients can practice this important movement.

Occasionally, patients with low back pain possess poor kinesthetic-proprioceptive coordination. A simple technique to improve the patient's sense of lumbar movement and position involves the use of tape. First, the therapist places the patient on all fours and has him or her assume a neutral spine position. The therapist places a 12 to 18 cm long piece of tape on the paraspinals parallel to the spine (Fig. 13-9), while avoiding placing the tape directly over the incision site. The therapist then asks the patient to make small movements into flexion and extension, always returning to neutral. The additional feedback from the tape pulling or wrinkling will assist the patient in learning spinal proprioception. Various postures can then be tried, including kneeling, side lying, sitting, and standing, with small motions of the lumbar spine while in each position.

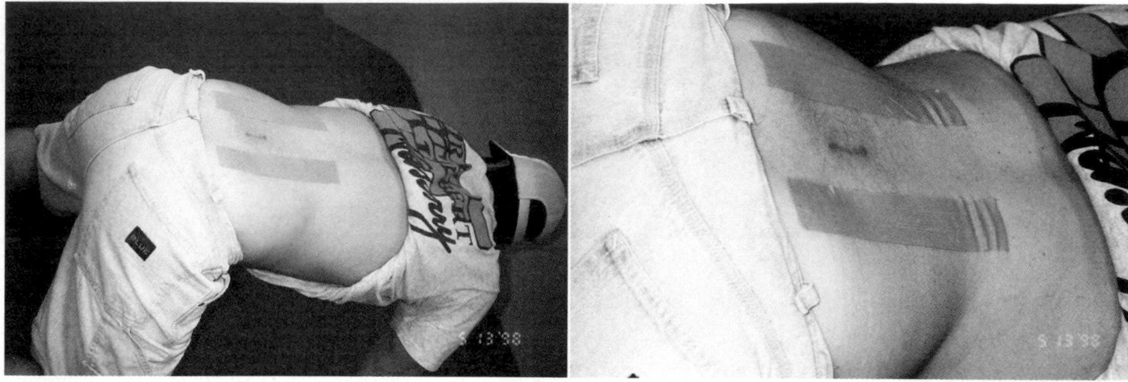

Fig. 13-9 Patient assumes a quadruped position, while the therapist places a 12- to 18-cm strip of tape on the paraspinals adjacent to the spine. The therapist should take care to avoid the incision site. **A**, Appearance of tape in squatting position. **B**, Close-up view of tape with return to standing position.

> **A** Verlyn tested positive for adverse neural tension in the right leg. After several treatments of mobilization to the nervous system, complaints of pain decreased significantly in intensity and frequency.

The patient then progresses to functional movements (e.g., transfers, walking, bending).

Exercise

Dural stretching (i.e., mobilization of the nervous system, neurodynamic exercise, nerve root gliding, neural tension exercises) should begin as soon as possible in the first week. The preoperative neural compromise and the postoperative inflammation in and around the epidural space contribute to neural fibrosis and dural adhesions. They are occasionally problematic and are easily preventable. An excellent presentation of neural mobilization principles and techniques can be found in Butler.[8]

Technique. The therapist should do the following:

- Supine dural stretching (lower lumbar neural mobilization)—Have the patient lie supine on a firm surface with both knees extended. While the patient holds the back of the thigh with both hands, he or she slowly extends the knee with the ankle dorsiflexed to the point of stretch. He or she then slowly flexes and relaxes the limb. Any symptoms and the maximal amount of knee extension attained should be recorded to monitor progress.
- Prone dural stretching (upper lumbar neural mobilization)—Have the patient lie prone on a firm surface with both knees extended. Initially the patient may use a pillow under the abdomen for comfort if needed. Have the patient slowly flex the knee to the point of stretch, then slowly extend the knee and relax. Make sure the patient maintains the abdominal brace throughout the exercise to stabilize the lumbar spine. Alternate legs.

Dural stretching should be done several times a day. The therapist must caution the patient that this exercise may provoke neural symptoms, and that he or she must allow the pain or tingling to resolve to baseline levels before beginning the next repetition. The patient should not overstretch the neural tissues. As with any exercise, self-mobilization of the nervous system at home is inappropriate until a positive response has been established from repeated movements in the clinic. The dural stretches are progressed as tolerated to include other components of the affected nerve (e.g., ankle dorsiflexion, hip internal rotation [IR]). Eventually (in phase III) the patient can perform neural stretches while sitting ("sitting slump stretch").

The early initiation of a progressive spinal-stabilization program is crucial to the eventual tolerance of more strenuous functional activities and sports skills. Because the lumbar spine is inherently unstable around the neutral zone, the trunk musculature must be sufficiently strong and coordinated to stabilize and protect the spine from injury.[44,79] The stabilization program progresses from unloaded spinal positions to partially loaded and eventually fully loaded functional training. The posterior pelvic tilt exercise is the *least* desirable exercise to obtain active lumbar stability.[44,86,89,90] The transversus abdominis must be isolated from the remaining abdominal musculature because it has consistently been shown to be active before the other abdominal muscles or the primary movers during limb motions, regardless of direction.[37,129] In addition, the transversus abdominis can become dysfunctional in patients with low back pain.[37] Therefore the transversus abdominis possesses a superior ability to stabilize the lumbar spine actively and locally.[38] Although the more superficial abdominal muscles (the obliques) are important in lumbar stability, they are trained later in the program for their rotational contribution to limit lateral shear and torsional stresses and create trunk rotation. Early in phase II the lumbar multifidi are isolated and trained because of their ability to stabilize segmentally.[3,66] More recent literature has investigated the importance of the pelvic floor musculature in stabilizing the lumbar spine.[72,95] Evidence shows that the pelvic floor muscles cocontract with the transverse abdominus; therefore recruiting the pelvic floor muscles should be considered when instructing in bracing. Eventually a cocontraction of transversus abdominis, multifidus, and pelvic floor (abdominal bracing) is performed during all exercises and functional activities. All the exercises should focus on control and technique and be progressed as tolerated to improve endurance of these primary stabilizers.

The PT should instruct the patient in the *neutral spine* concept and help the patient find the neutral spine position in various postures. The patient can then be taught to control the transverse abdominus with electromyographic (EMG) biofeedback or pressure biofeedback (Stabilizer, Inc., Chattanooga, TN) in several positions (e.g., supine, all fours, prone). After that, the patient can progress the postures to include sitting and standing and increase the duration of the contractions to 60 seconds.

Based on the information obtained in the history, the responses to various positions, and the limited clinical testing performed during the initial evaluation, the therapist determines which midrange lumbar movements are tolerated and are indicated for exercise. Correct and controlled lumbar movements are beneficial to the patient after microdiscectomy, because hydrostatic changes of the disc promote improved vascularity.[39,112] To this end the therapist teaches *pelvic rocks* in pain-free positions (e.g., all fours, prone). A pelvic rock is a repetitive and continuous pelvic tilt from an anterior to a posterior position. A bias toward lumbar extension is typical in the patient who has undergone microdiscectomy, because lumbar extension reduces tangential stress posteriorly. A flexion bias is usually not recommended because the surgical entry is into the posterior disc and flexion positions tend to create stress to this area and tension on the incision. A healthy respect for soft tissue healing periods is essential.

The therapist instructs the patient in most of the following exercises in phase I, but he or she should not prescribe any exercise or position for the home program until repeated trials in the clinic have proven painless. Stabilization, flexibility, coordination, and spinal mobility exercises are included in an attempt to address all parameters. The exercise sequence is important and should be considered by the PT when adding exercises. Good technique and control of movement are essential. No exercise should increase the pain pattern or cause lingering pain. Clearly some muscular soreness may accompany the program, but this should be well tolerated and transient. The typical patient should be able to contract the transversus abdominis for 60 seconds in various positions within approximately 1 week after the initial visit.

The following exercises are taught in phase I:

1. Abdominal bracing on all fours (i.e., isolated transverse abdominis contraction, lumbar multifidus and pelvic floor cocontraction) progressed to quadruped abdominal bracing with alternate arm raises
2. Quadruped pelvic rocks (i.e., midrange lumbar active range of motion [AROM])
3. Supine dural stretching (or prone dural stretching for upper lumbar disorders)
4. Supine abdominal bracing (isolated transverse abdominis contraction, lumbar multifidus, and pelvic floor cocontraction)
5. Supine pelvic rocks (i.e., midrange lumbar flexion AROM)
6. Supine abdominal bracing with arms behind head progressed to abdominal bracing with alternating arm raises
7. Supine gluteal, hip external rotator, and hamstring stretches to correct myofascial limitations; actively holding neutral spine during these low-load, long-hold exercises is important (Fig. 13-10)
8. Side-lying pelvic rocks (i.e., midrange lumbar lateral flexion AROM)
9. Prone pelvic rocks (i.e., midrange lumbar extension AROM)
10. Prone abdominal bracing with alternate arm raises progressed to prone abdominal bracing with bilateral arm raises
11. Gastrocnemius and soleus stretching in standing position (Fig. 13-11)
12. Partial squats to 60 degrees of knee flexion while maintaining neutral spine with abdominal bracing

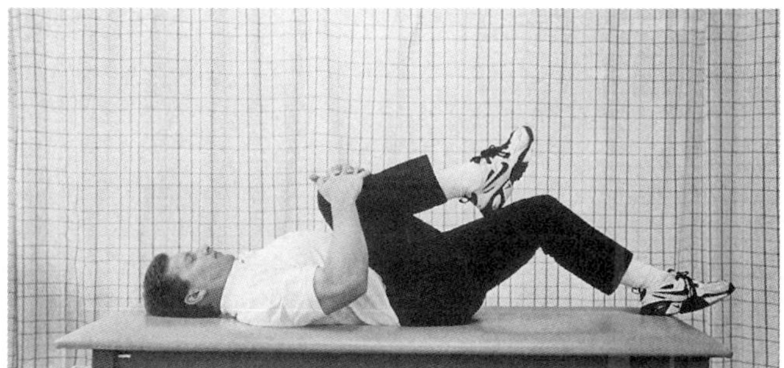

Fig. 13-10 Hip flexion is very important. When stretching the gluteals, the patient should pull the thigh toward the belly rather than toward the nose. This patient is attempting to increase the hip flexion angle rather than draw the pelvis into a posterior tilt.

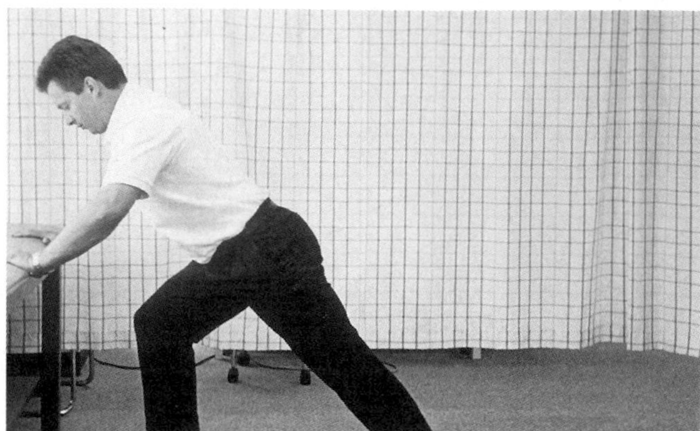

Fig. 13-11 Gastrocnemius and soleus stretching. While keeping the foot and heel of the back leg on the floor, the patient shifts the weight forward to the front leg. A stretch should be felt in the calf area. The patient should maintain the spine in neutral with an abdominal brace as the weight is shifted toward the front foot and keep the supporting thigh directly below in the frontal plane.

> **Q** Myrna had microdiscectomy 2 weeks ago. She wants to go to her son's baseball game this weekend. What should her therapist tell her?

Spinal Mobilization

Spinal mobilization of the lumbar spine is rarely used in phase I or II. Mobilization of the hips or thoracic spine may be needed and is best addressed on an individual basis. When progress is poor with active movements and deemed secondary to a hypomobile segment, mobilization to restore lumbar movement may be necessary in phase II. In phase III, mobilization can play an important role and is used frequently to reduce pain during specific lumbar motions, especially at end of range. A review of Maitland,[53] Mulligan,[69] and Paris[81] may assist in clinical reasoning.

Cardiovascular Conditioning

Cardiovascular conditioning is an important part of the rehabilitation program and is beneficial both for patients recovering from lumbar microdiscectomy and those with chronic low back pain.[54] In addition, endurance training of the LE musculature improves tolerance to prolonged standing and walking. When LE muscles fatigue, poor body mechanics soon follow. The patient typically performs aerobic training by progressive walking (on a treadmill or outdoors without hills), stationary cycling (on recumbent or upright bikes with the patient paying close attention to the maintenance of lordosis and avoidance of hip sway), or swimming (initially only the freestyle stroke with avoidance of "craning" during the breathing phase). Craning is suboccipital extension with rotation (occipitoatlantal to atlantoaxial) or cervical extension with rotation (C2 to C7). Swimming and aqua therapy are usually delayed until the second or third week after surgery to ensure complete wound healing and sufficient lumbar stabilization. The PT must caution **patients never to jump or dive into the water, but rather use the ladder or steps.** Aquatic therapy for postoperative lumbar rehabilitation is not covered in this chapter, but Watkins , Williams, and Watkins[119] present a good source for the interested clinician.

The therapist determines the patient's training heart rate and adheres to this guideline during all conditioning exercises. Patients who have no prior history of aerobic exercise or who are very deconditioned must progress slowly and be carefully monitored. Aerobic conditioning in phase I (with focus on correct postures and mechanics) may include walking, stationary cycling, and water exercises. Patients should avoid stair climbers and cross-country skiing machines until phase II, when adequate trunk stability is usually attained. In addition, rowing, running, and in-line skating should be avoided until phase III, when significant active lumbar stability has been achieved.

The progression of cardiovascular training is highly variable and depends on the patient's prior level of conditioning and present goals. He or she can usually begin with 5- to 10-minute bouts and progress at 5-minute intervals up to 30 or 60 minutes. The therapist must pay careful attention to patient position, because correct postures deteriorate as fatigue increases. Neurologic weakness of the hip flexors or abductors, quadriceps, hamstrings, ankle dorsiflexors, and plantar flexors significantly alters gait and requires modification of the aerobic program to avoid abnormal mechanical stress.

Modalities

In general, the use of passive treatment techniques alone should be avoided; however, occasionally they may be necessary to augment the functional restoration program. The therapist should use pain control modalities only as needed to support the exercise program. Cryotherapy and interferential stimulation applied to the low back for 15 to 20 minutes after an exercise session are helpful. Some therapists may prefer electric myostimulation (EMS), microstimulation, or transcutaneous electrical nerve stimulation (TENS) for muscle spasm reduction and pain control. However, EMS that is delivered too intensely in the first several weeks after surgery may unwittingly jeopardize the healing paraspinal muscle tissue and should therefore be used judiciously. The patient's posture during modalities is always important and varies depending on positional tolerance. Supported prone lying or supported supine lying (see Fig. 14-7, *A* and *C*) is usually quite comfortable in this phase.

Wound Care

Along with the patient's history, the inspection of the incision site during the initial evaluation helps determine whether extra measures are needed. Any signs of infection are a red flag that requires prompt medical intervention. Some patients desire "invisible" scars, while others are much less concerned. Because patients scar differently, the therapist should monitor their progress and offer solutions to excessive scarring or scar stretching. A compression taping technique can be used to limit hypertrophic scar formation and reduce surgical scar widening. First, the therapist folds a 10 × 6 cm Neoprene pad in half and secures it with a 2-inch wide elastic tape (Elastikon tape, Johnson & Johnson, New Brunswick, NJ) (Fig. 13-12). The pad is then affixed horizontally over the closed wound (Figs. 13-13 and 13-14) to provide both compression and approximation of the surgical scar. The patient wears the compression patch constantly for 6 to 10 weeks, removing it only to bathe. It should not be applied until the wound site is completely healed (approximately 2 weeks).

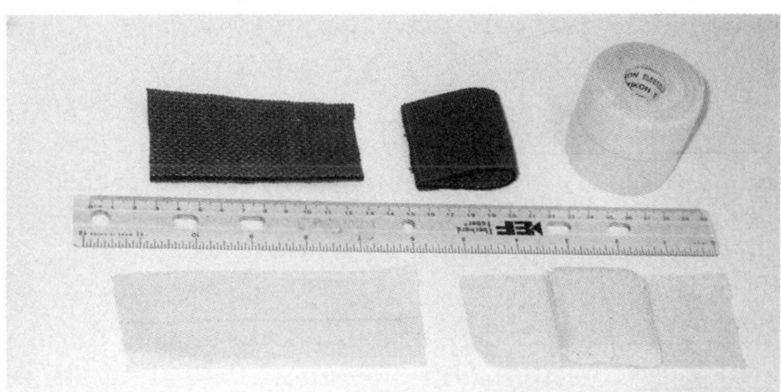

Fig. 13-12 Materials to manufacture compression patch (10 × 6 cm Neoprene pad, 2-inch elastic tape).

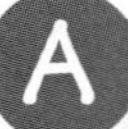

Her therapist should tell her the following:

- Caution her to avoid sitting in bleachers or on benches without any back support.
- Suggest she take some type of alternative seating device that has some back support.
- Recommend frequent changes of position (avoid sitting greater than 20 minutes at a time).
- She should avoid slouching while sitting to prevent increased intradiscal pressures and shear forces that can be caused by flexing in a sitting position.

Q

Karla has a 5-month-old daughter at home. She arrives at therapy 3 weeks after a microdiscectomy procedure. What should Karla be instructed to do immediately?

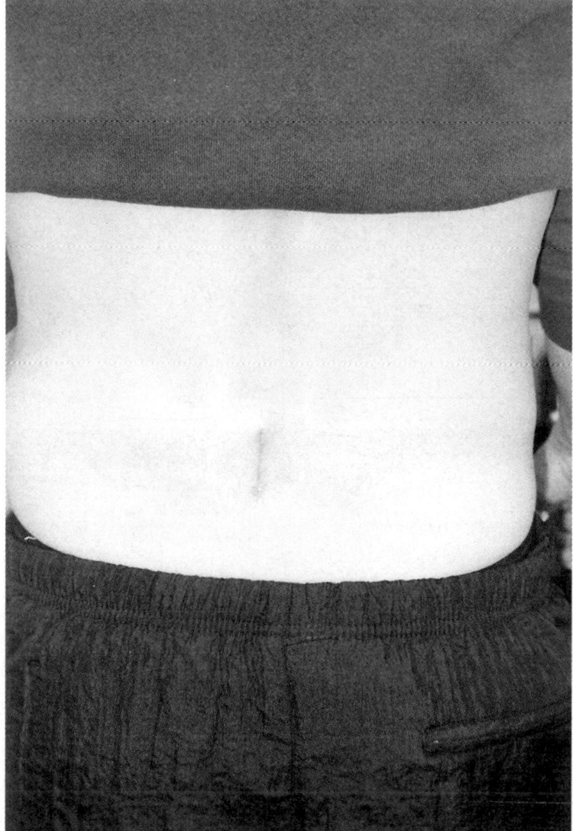

Fig. 13-13 Inspection of scar before application of compression patch.

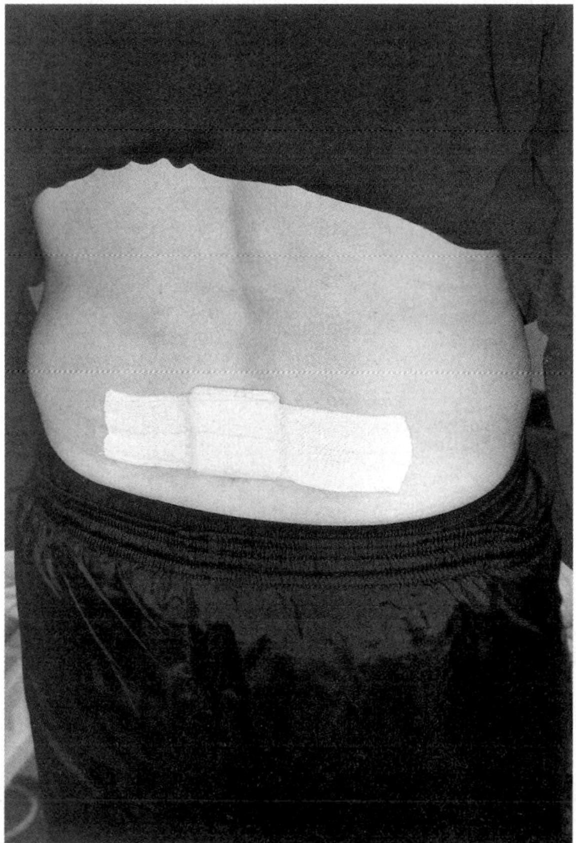

Fig. 13-14 The pad is affixed horizontally over the closed wound and held in place by 2-inch elastic tape.

Phase II (Functional Recovery Phase)

TIME: 4 to 6 weeks after surgery
GOALS: Understand neutral spine concept, improve cardiovascular condition, increase trunk strength to 80%, increase soft tissue mobility and LE flexibility and strength, maintain nerve root mobility (Table 13-2)

As surgical site pain diminishes and active spinal stability improves, the PT can increase the patient's program of functional activities and exercise. The patient in phase II should have complete wound healing, although some tenderness and paraspinal spasm may persist. Neural tension signs should be negative, but neurodynamic testing may reveal limitations. The patient should be gaining tolerance to functional activities and be able to perform all self-care with minor modifications. The patient's tolerance to aerobic exercise also should be improving. Correct body mechanics and postures should be maintained as functional activity increases. Patients should have confidence in their ability to stabilize the lumbar spine actively in all loaded positions. Pain-free lumbar AROM should be increasing to end-of-range strain only, although terminal flexion may still provoke pain. **The patient should continue to avoid loaded lumbar flexion.** Through brief re-evaluations in each treatment session, the therapist collects additional lumbar motion data. For example, if prone pelvic rocks are well tolerated, then the patient's positional tolerance to elbow lying and partial extension in lying can be assessed safely. **The therapist should avoid standing motion testing and sitting testing except for the most conditioned patients who are doing very well.**

Exercise

The therapist should instruct the patient in the correct way to contract and control the lumbar multifidus with EMG biofeedback. Special attention to the training of this important segmental stabilizer is essential.[124] Retraction of the paraspinal muscles during surgery can denervate the multifidus muscle.[100] Fortunately, lumbar microdiscectomy requires a minimal wound opening, so this complication is lessened. The patient should perform abdominal bracing (holding neutral spine with a cocontraction of the transverse abdominis, multifidus, and pelvic floor) in supine, prone, and all-fours positions, progressing to transition movements. Ultimately, the cocontraction is used to stabilize the lumbar spine during all ADLs. The therapist can progress the patient's midrange lumbar movements and spinal-stabilization program as tolerated, using Swiss ball exercises to improve balance and dynamic lumbar stabilization during sitting. *The patient should continue to avoid axial loading during end-range lumbar flexion or lateral flexion movements.* As the patient shows control and tolerance, the exercise level may be increased. Pain during exercise typically requires correction of the technique or exercise modification. In addition, muscle groups that may have been weakened by neurologic compromise (e.g., hip abductors, quadriceps, ankle plantar flexors, dorsiflexors) must be strengthened. The slow twitch fibers are most involved and are easily fatigued. The longer that neural compression and inflammation have been present, the longer the period before regeneration occurs. *Careful attention to back-protected positions during strengthening exercises is crucial to avoiding reinjury.*

Typical phase II exercises. The therapist should do the following:

1. Supine abdominal bracing with alternate SLRs, progressed to abdominal bracing with unsupported LE extension (i.e., *cycling*), progressed to abdominal bracing with unsupported upper extremity (UE) and lower extremity (LE) extension (i.e., *dying bug*) (Fig. 13-15)
2. Supine dural stretching, progressed to incorporate a belt or towel around the foot to enhance the stretch

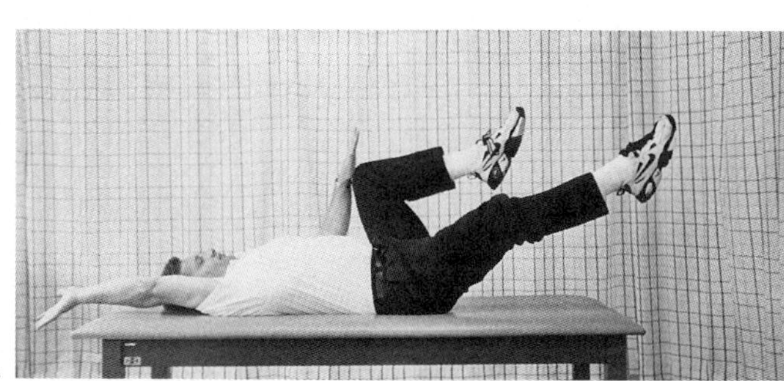
A

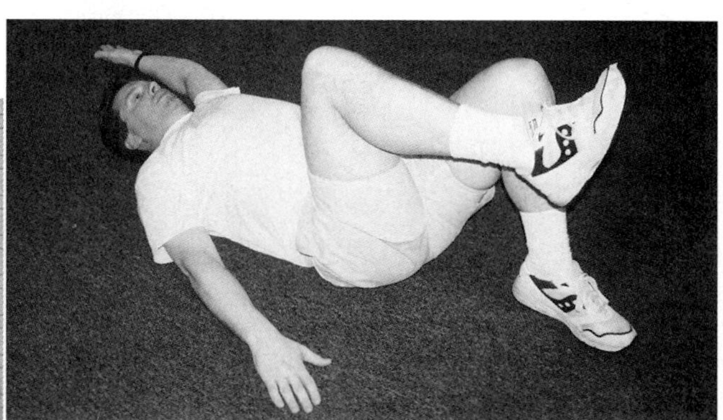
B

Fig. 13-15 A and **B**, Dying bug. This exercise teaches the patient to control extension and side bending at the same time. The patient starts with the hands touching the knees directly over the hips and then extends the same-side arm and leg slowly and deliberately. The physical therapist (PT) monitors the patient for side bending or extension. The patient can modify this exercise by moving the arms and legs in smaller increments.

Table 13-2 Microdiscectomy

Rehabilitation Phase	Criteria to Progress to this Phase	Anticipated Impairments and Functional Limitations	Intervention	Goal	Rationale
Phase II Postoperative 4-6 weeks	◆ No signs of infection ◆ No increase in pain ◆ Gradual increase in tolerance to activity ◆ Demonstration of good knowledge of body mechanics ◆ Performance of self-care with minimal modifications	◆ Pain ◆ Limited nerve mobility ◆ Limited trunk strength ◆ Limited scar mobility ◆ Limited soft tissue mobility ◆ Limited tolerance to ADLs and sustained postures ◆ Limited trunk stability and strength in numerous postures ◆ Limited mobility of lumbar spine soft tissues ◆ Poor recruitment of paraspinal muscles ◆ Limited LE ROM ◆ Limited cardiovascular endurance	◆ Continue as in Phase I and progress cardiovascular activities as appropriate ◆ Self-nerve mobilization using a belt to enhance the stretch ◆ Isometrics with AROM—Supine abdominal bracing with alternate SLRs; progressed to cycling and dying bug when appropriate ◆ Partial sit-ups with added rotation for obliques when appropriate ◆ Prone abdominal bracing with SLR (extension): Begin with single leg and progress to double leg on-elbows lying, progress to partial press-ups ◆ AROM with isometrics—All fours (abdominal bracing with single-leg raise, progress to opposite arm and leg raises); standing (abdominal bracing with squats to 60 degrees, progress to 90 degrees for 2-3 minutes); sitting on Swiss ball (abdominal bracing with hip flexion, arm flexion, and combinations of opposite arm and leg) ◆ EMG training of lumbar spine multifidus muscles ◆ PROM (stretches), then add iliopsoas and quadriceps ◆ STM	◆ Cardiovascular exercise 20 minutes ◆ Minimal to no neural tension signs ◆ Trunk strength 80% ◆ Use of neutral spine concepts in a variety of positions ◆ Avoidance of lumbar spine extension while performing hip extension ◆ Partial press-ups without pain ◆ Good neutral control of lumbar spine in a variety of postures ◆ Increased strength of LEs ◆ Improved sitting tolerance ◆ Isolated contraction of lumbar spine paraspinal muscles ◆ Increased LE flexibility ◆ Increased soft tissue mobility	◆ Improve cardiovascular fitness ◆ Restore neural-gliding mechanics ◆ Prevent neural fibrosis and dural adhesions ◆ Strengthen trunk musculature via neutral spine concepts ◆ Perform exercises in midrange of lumbopelvic mobility ◆ Stabilize and strengthen trunk while moving extremities, progressing from passive prepositioning to dynamic stabilization ◆ Restore full extension in nonweight-bearing position ◆ Strengthen paraspinals and abdominals in a neutral position ◆ Promote maintenance of a neutral spine in an upright posture to improve tolerance to compression positions ◆ Increase tolerance to upright postures ◆ Use biofeedback to improve recruitment of paraspinals ◆ Improve flexibility of LEs to decrease stress on the spine ◆ Improve myofascial interface and restore soft tissue mobility

ADLs, Activities of daily living; *AROM,* active range of motion; *SLRs,* straight leg raises; *LE,* lower extremity; *ROM,* range of motion; *EMG,* electromyographic; *PROM,* passive range of motion; *STM,* soft tissue massage.

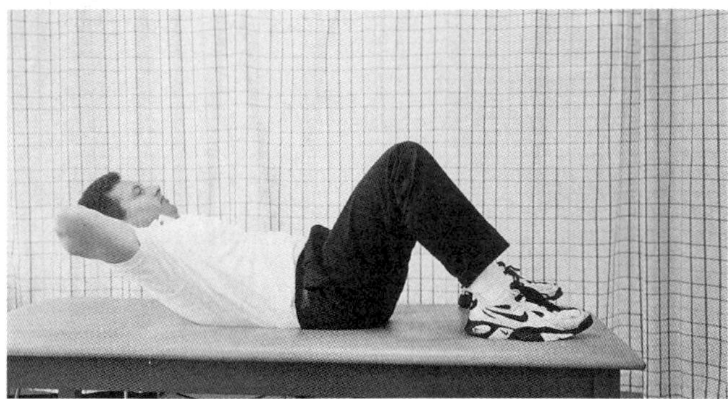

Fig. 13-16 Partial sit-ups are done in many positions. The important point is that the spine must remain in neutral, the abdominals must remain contracted throughout the exercise, and eccentric control must be emphasized. The lift is of the chest, not the head. Legs can be in extended position to bias lumbar extension.

3. Supine partial sit-ups, progressed to partial sit-ups with rotation to facilitate oblique strengthening (Fig. 13-16)
4. Double-leg bridging, progressed to single-leg bridging and then to single-leg bridging with opposite knee straight (Fig. 13-17)
5. Prone elbow lying, progressed to partial press-ups
6. Prone abdominal bracing with single-leg raises, progressed to prone double-leg raises
7. Standing repetitive squats to 60 degrees, progressed to 90 degrees for 2 to 3 minutes
8. Abdominal bracing on all fours with single-leg raise, progressed to opposite arm and leg raises (Fig. 13-18)
9. Balance board training on both limbs, progressed in duration
10. Isolated strengthening of neurologically compromised muscles
11. Swiss ball sitting exercise progression (in neutral spine with abdominal brace)
12. Stretching of the quadriceps, gluteals, hip external rotators, iliopsoas, hamstrings, and calves as required to correct myofascial limitations (Figs. 13-19 through 13-22; see also Fig. 13-11)

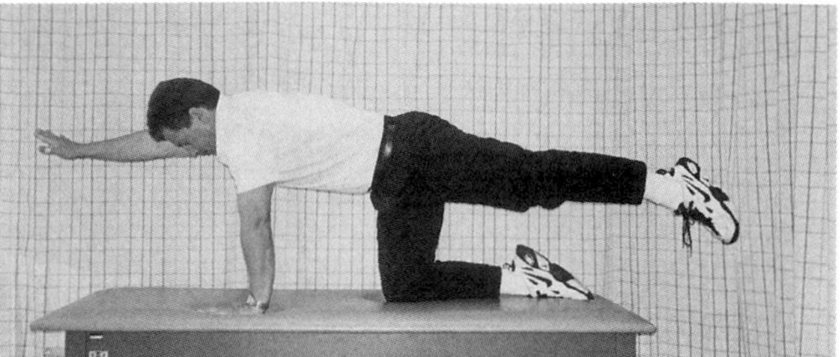

Fig. 13-18 From the quadruped position, the therapist should teach the patient to keep the hands under the shoulders and knees under the hips, extending the opposite arm and leg.

Soft Tissue Mobilization

Scarring of myofascial elements with collagen cross-fibers or fibrofatty tissue limits muscle broadening during contraction and connective tissue elasticity during movement.[27] Muscle spasm and protective guarding of the gluteals and low back musculature may persist. Soft tissue mobilization of the lumbar paraspinals and buttock musculature is frequently needed to improve muscle function and reduce spasm.[12] The PT must exercise care when performing soft tissue mobilization to the paraspinals before the third or fourth week after surgery, because the tissue healing is incomplete. The mechanical and reflexive effects of soft tissue mobilization are well suited for patients recovering from microdiscectomy, and certain techniques are particularly beneficial before paraspinal strengthening (e.g., side-lying paraspinal pull from midline). Careful questioning and soft tissue examination will uncover gluteal trigger points that can cause buttock or LE pain patterns.[108] These myofascial pain syndromes are not uncommon preoperatively and may linger postoperatively. With appropriate treatment they can be relieved so that the functional restoration program may progress. Scar massage to release adherent soft tissue also may be needed.

Spinal Mobilization

Spinal mobilization using nonthrust maneuvers may be beneficial for patients in phase II if they do not have

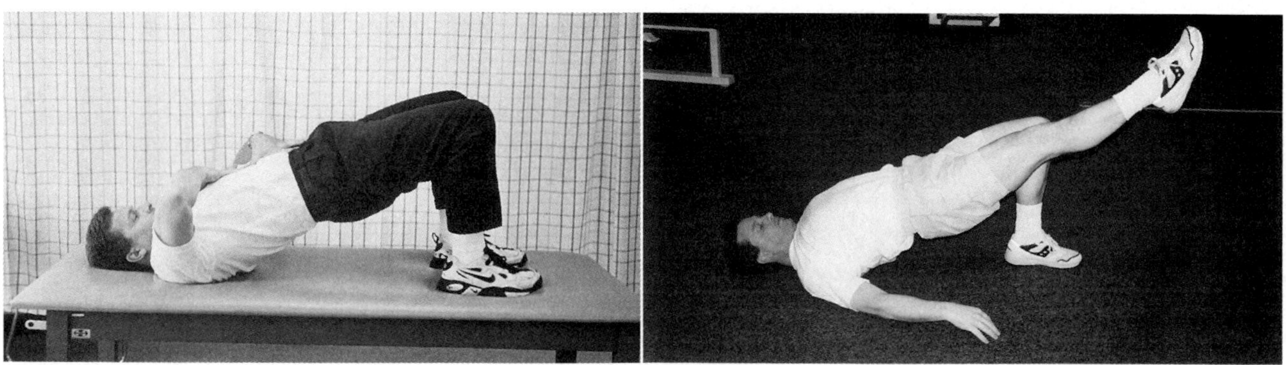

Fig. 13-17 A and B, Bridging. This exercise teaches the patient to brace the spine first, then lift the trunk as a unit. The patient is moving in and out of a hip hinge and emphasis is on coordinating the trunk and hip muscles.

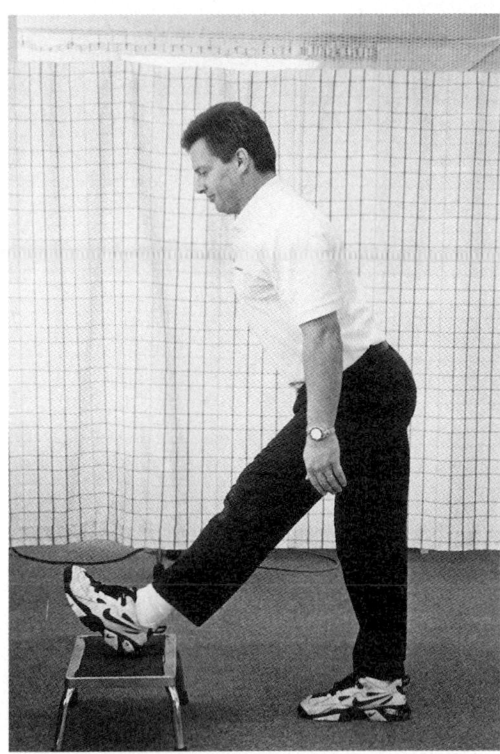

Fig. 13-19 Hamstring stretching is taught in a standing position if possible so that the patient can work on contralateral hip stability, as well as trunk control while stretching. The patient can work the foot up and down while maintaining the stretch to increase the nerve-gliding component. A slight bend in the knee with more hip hinge will move the stretch up from the musculotendinous junction into the muscle belly.

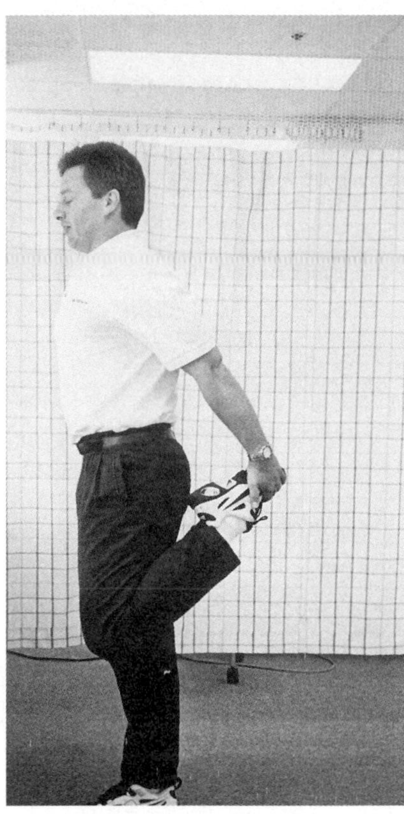

Fig. 13-20 Initially the quadriceps stretch is performed in a prone position and then is taught in standing position if possible to develop trunk control against an extension moment. If the patient does not have sufficient range of motion (ROM), then he or she should modify the stretch by placing the foot on a table. Abdominal control prevents lumbar extension.

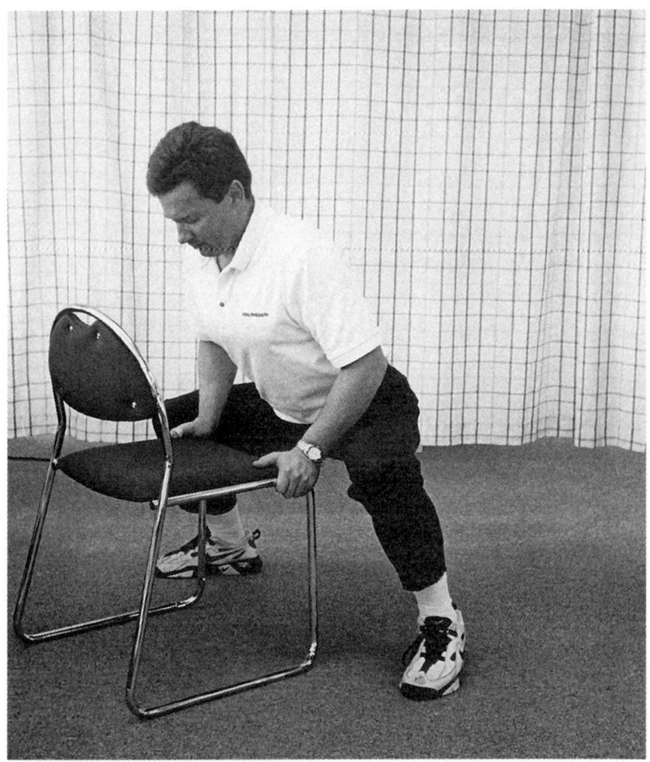

Fig. 13-21 Gracilis stretch is important for squatting to the side.

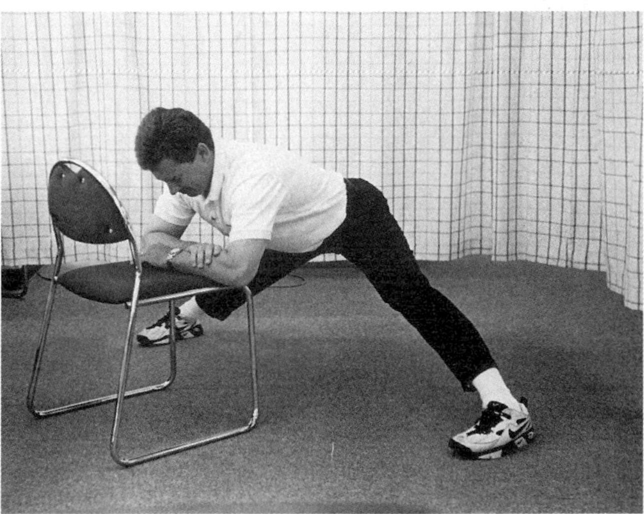

Fig. 13-22 Adductor flexibility is important for squatting. The patient can vary the trunk angle or apply pressure to the inner knee to increase the stretch.

protective muscle spasm, bone disease of the spine, or hypermobile or irritable adjacent motion segments. Muscle energy techniques are usually well tolerated and best suited for phase II.

Thrust maneuvers (grade V or high-velocity manipulations) are not indicated.

Cardiovascular Conditioning

The PT should continue to progress the cardiovascular program in intensity and duration of aerobic training. The use of cross-country ski machines, stair climbers, and swimming for aerobic exercise is allowed if sufficient trunk stability has been achieved. Patients should avoid rowing and in-line skating until phase III. **Running is not recommended until after the twelfth week after surgery because of the degree of spinal stabilization required and the repetitive axial loading sustained by the disc.**

Modalities

The therapist and patient should use modalities only as needed to support the exercise program. Cryotherapy and interferential stimulation to the low back after exercise may be beneficial.

A Karla should be instructed to do the following:

- She should avoid lifting and carrying her child as much as possible for the first 3 to 4 weeks after her surgery. This may require educating her family members that she will require assistance initially.
- She should be instructed in proper body mechanics and correct lifting techniques when lifting or carrying her daughter.
- She should be taught that hip hinging and swoop lifting are necessary when bending to pick up after her child.

Q Jason works in a warehouse where he must repeatedly carry heavy boxes and walk for most of the day. He had surgery 9 weeks ago and does not understand why his therapist has him riding a bicycle and walking on a treadmill as part of his lumbar microdiscectomy rehabilitation. If he has to do aerobic exercise, he would rather run. What is the therapist's rationale for these exercises?

Phase III (Resistive Training Phase)

TIME: 7 to 11 weeks after surgery
GOALS: Ensure patient is independent in self-care and ADLs with minimal alterations, increase tolerance to activities, progress return to previous level of function (Table 13-3)

The patient in phase III should consistently perform correct body mechanics and postures without prompting and should tolerate almost all functional activities. Prolonged positioning (e.g., unsupported sitting) may still provoke low back pain, but this should be easily relieved with change of position or simple stretching exercises. Soft tissue healing at this stage is largely complete, although some surgical site tenderness may still be present. All self-care and ADLs should be performed confidently and painlessly with minimal modifications. Patients in phase III should have good tolerance to midrange lumbar movements and sufficient spinal stabilization to perform spinal movements in loaded positions.

The resumption of lifting activities must be progressive and occur with careful instruction (see Fig. 14-11, A and B). Because approximately half of all workers' compensation claims for low back injury result from lifting objects, this patient group needs proportionally more instruction and functional training.

Because soft tissue healing is nearly complete by phase III, more extensive mechanical testing can be performed to ascertain tolerance to various lumbar movements, as well as the end range sensation. **Standing motion testing (without overpressure) and seated testing can be performed safely on most patients after 6 weeks.** The outcome of the movement testing determines to a great extent the treatment and exercise progression. Neural tension signs should be negative unless scarring has occurred. Occasionally some neurologic signs and symptoms persist into the third phase, but with monitoring and calm encouragement the PT can reassure affected patients that these symptoms will subside with continued neural stretching and time.

Researchers[109] and clinicians note that flexibility, strength (stability), and coordination return at different rates after injury. During spinal rehabilitation, flexibility should precede strength, proximal strength should precede distal strength, and strength should precede coordination. This culminates in the more rapid and fluid functional movements seen in uninjured persons. The

A The following explains the therapist's rationale:

- Cardiovascular conditioning is beneficial for patients recovering from microdiscectomy surgery.
- Jason's job requires prolonged walking; he will need endurance of his LEs to prevent fatigue of his legs, which can lead to poor body mechanics.
- Running should not be initiated until after the twelfth week of surgery, when the patient is able to stabilize his spine well and the repetitive axial loading is not as much of a concern.

Table 13-3 Microdiscectomy

Rehabilitation Phase	Criteria to Progress to this Phase	Anticipated Impairments and Functional Limitations	Intervention	Goal	Rationale
Phase III Postoperative 7-11 weeks	◆ No increase in pain ◆ No loss in mobility or function ◆ Good knowledge of neutral spine concepts during a variety of positions	◆ Limited stability of trunk in challenging positions ◆ Not totally independent with self-care ◆ Limited tolerance to prolonged positions	◆ Continuation of interventions from Phases I and II as appropriate ◆ PREs ◆ Isotonics—Progressive lifting training using change of position, rotational and overhead activities, and balance boards ◆ Cardiovascular exercise, walking progressed to running (after 12 weeks), stationary bike, or cross-country skiing (after 8 weeks) ◆ Sport- and activity-specific drills when appropriate (refer to Exercise under Phase III, Resistive Training Phase) (see criteria on p. 260) ◆ Functional capacity evaluation after 10 to 12 weeks	◆ Weaning from interventions that are no longer of benefit ◆ Consistent use of good body mechanics ◆ Independent self-care ◆ Independence with ADLs with minimal modifications ◆ Increased tolerance to physically demanding activities ◆ Return to previous level of activity as appropriate	◆ Promote self-management of condition ◆ Use of pain-easing techniques to relieve symptoms from prolonged positions ◆ Prevent reinjury ◆ Prepare for discharge ◆ Promote continuation of good cardiovascular fitness as indicated ◆ Gradually progress to previous activities ◆ Evaluate the ability to return to previous function

PREs, Passive resistance exercises; *ADLs,* activities of daily living.

PT must be sure to consider the sequence of return of these various elements, the existing limitations uncovered during mechanical testing, and the patient's realistic goals when planning the progression of the exercise program.

Exercise

Functional training exercises (i.e., sports-specific drills, work-hardening activities) typically begin in phase III. Preset goals determine the kinetic activities that are to be the focus of rehabilitation. The therapist closely supervises the progression of these activities, paying careful attention to the quality of spinal mechanics and lumbar stabilization. Functional training is focused on trunk movements that simulate activities to which the patient will return. Sports-specific training (Figs. 13-23 through 13-26) can begin if the patient has achieved sufficient active lumbar stability and spinal mobility in fully loaded positions, as well as adequate myofascial flexibility and conditioning. The therapist can use proprioceptive training with balance boards and Swiss balls. Initially, athletes who take part in running and jumping activities are most safely trained with unloading devices (e.g., Vigor Equipment, Inc., Stevensville, MI) during supervised treadmill running or jump training. These patients are typically well conditioned before surgery and have progressed postoperatively without setbacks.

Golfers need to be trained to hold the neutral spine dynamically during all five phases of the swing. The PT can incorporate specific strength, flexibility, and balance exercises to achieve a safe and mechanically sound golf swing.[119]

Work-hardening activities for medium to heavy work classifications typically begin at 8 weeks and include lift training from 25 to 50 lbs (see Fig. 14-11). Workers in these fields need special attention with regard to materials handling and should have a functional capacity evaluation 10 to 12 weeks after surgery to determine appropriate return-to-work status.

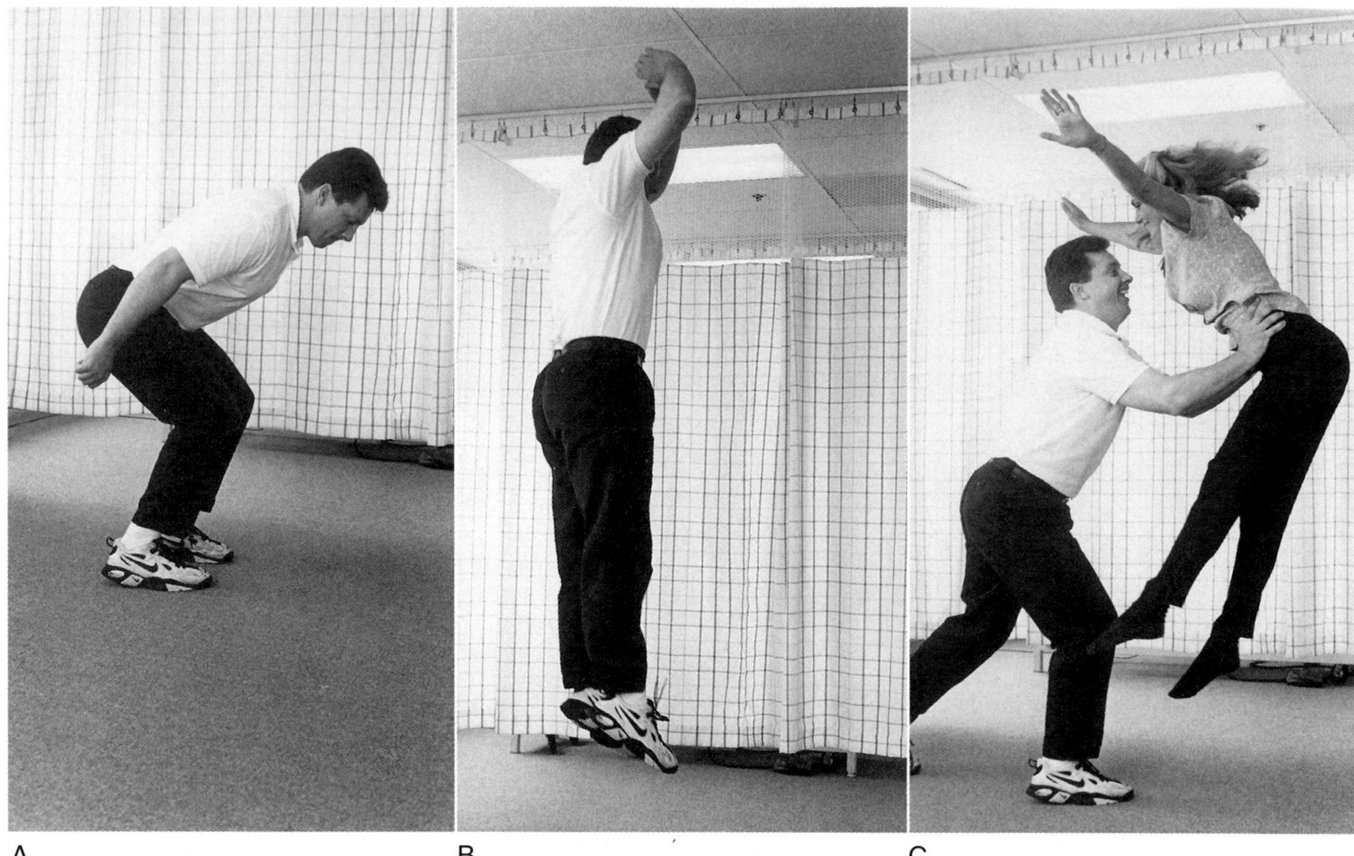

Fig. 13-23 **A,** Landing from a jump is invariably more difficult for jumping athletes. It is imperative that they learn to land in a hip hinge position and be trained to absorb as much shock as possible eccentrically through the hips, knees, and ankles, before it reaches the spine. Plyometric drills are helpful. **B,** While in the air with the arms overhead, the therapist should train the jumping athlete to perform a brace with the transverse abdominals to prevent extraosseous lumbar motion. When blocking a ball with the arms overhead (as in volleyball), the athlete should brace more intensely to resist the impact of the ball. Medicine ball drills are helpful. **C,** In some contact sports the athlete will be hit while in the air (e.g., basketball, football). For a frontal impact the athlete should give way at the hips; for a hit from an angle, he or she should learn to pivot away from the blow. Drills such as those shown here with progressively more difficult blows are helpful to train this specialized skill.

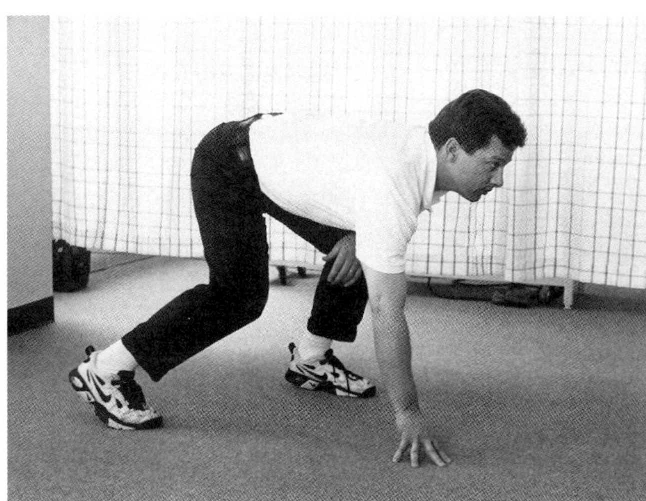

Fig. 13-24 A three-point stance is frequently used in football. It is essentially an exaggerated hip hinge. Adequate hip flexibility is essential, as well as preaction abdominal bracing.

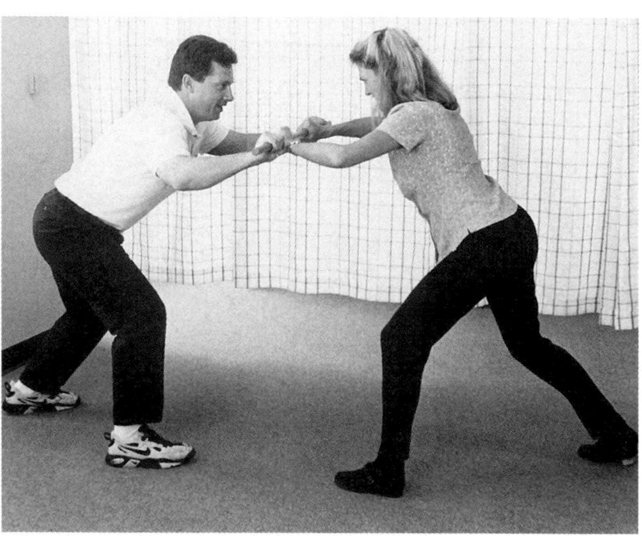

Fig. 13-25 In rugby and football, an athlete is frequently required to prevent someone from running around him or her. Stick drills such as this can teach a patient to adapt quickly to changing forces, while maintaining a neutral spine with an abdominal brace.

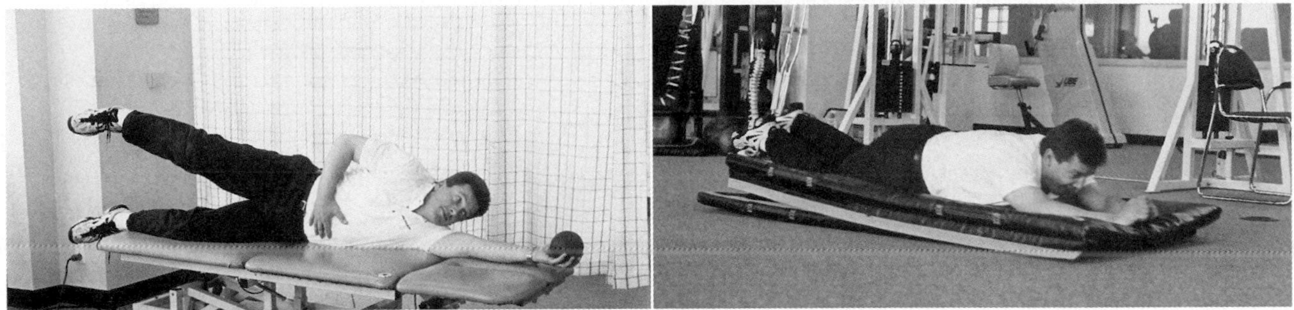

Fig. 13-26 A and B, When diving for a ball (as in baseball or volleyball), an athlete is taught to go low to the ground, stay horizontal, and land as a unit. A significant abdominal brace is required.

The exercise program progresses in intensity and difficulty to include rotational trunk stability, overhead activities, and balance training using a balance board. Training the patient in diagonal patterns in loaded positions better simulates real-life situations. A new stabilization exercise for patients in phase III challenges the obliques and transverse abdominals with minimal stress to passive tissues.[108] McGill[65] refers to this exercise as *isometric side-support* on knees or on feet (depending on the degree of difficulty). Therapists should prescribe this exercise for home performance only after proving patient tolerance during clinic sessions.

The spinal mobility program attempts to restore painless and full lumbosacral ROM. The PT should prescribe appropriate exercises and incorporate mobilization to achieve full and pain-free lumbar ROM and continue the stretching exercises needed to attain normal myofascial flexibility.

Soft Tissue Mobilization

Soft tissue mobilization should continue as needed to ensure a pliable surgical scar, proper gluteal and paraspinal muscle function, and soft tissue extensibility.

Spinal Mobilization

Spinal mobilization should be used when necessary to restore motion at hypomobile segments and reduce pain associated with movement. Because the restoration of normal spinal motion is a primary goal, the therapist must identify and correct aberrant arthrokinematics. The expanded mechanical testing in phase III will reveal limitations or provoke symptoms that require attention. Maitland,[53] Mulligan,[69] and Paris[81] can be reviewed to assist in clinical reasoning.

Cardiovascular Conditioning

Cardiovascular conditioning should continue to progress in intensity and duration. The patient's aerobic fitness program is determined by the ultimate activity goals. A typical sedentary office worker obviously does not train as intensely as a professional athlete. However, the therapist should not underestimate the aerobic demands placed on a manual laborer and should encourage appropriate endurance exercises.

Aerobic conditioning (focusing on correct postures and mechanics) may include treadmill walking, stationary cycling, the use of cross-country ski machines and stair climbers, swimming, and skating (in-line or on ice). Patients who have had previous experience with rowing may resume this exercise. Attention to proper stroke form is important, and modification to maintain lordosis may be necessary. **Patients should not start a running program until after the twelfth week postoperatively because of the high compressive and repetitive axial loads at heel strike.** A walk-run program should be initially implemented on a treadmill, with the therapist supervising and analyzing gait. When the patient does resume running, it should be in the morning hours when the disc is maximally hydrated.[119]

Modalities

Cryotherapy may still be beneficial after intensive training sessions. EMS, TENS, microcurrent, interferential stimulation, and other modalities are seldom necessary.

Discharge Planning

When the anticipated goals and desired outcomes have been attained, the patient is discharged with a home or club exercise program (or with both). The exercise program is to be maintained indefinitely. As always, the postsurgical patient should try to return to premorbid activity levels. Because goals vary dramatically among patients, some may require substantially more training than others, such as overhead lift training, plyometric jump training, or sport-specific skill training. A reasonable level of tolerance to strenuous work activities or recreational sports should be attained before these higher activity level patients are discharged.

The comprehensive lumbar evaluation performed in phase III reveals any limitations in motion, weaknesses, neural restrictions, and painful movements that still need to be addressed. The PT can obtain additional information from computerized testing devices[109] (e.g., Lumbar Motion Monitor, Chattanooga Group, Inc., Chattanooga,

TN) that provide objective data on lumbar motion speed, acceleration and deceleration, and degree of ROM. Other testing equipment, such as computerized isokinetic machines, determines objective trunk strength values at various speeds of lumbar ROM. This information can be helpful in guiding the therapist to choose appropriate exercises to remedy any weaknesses or limitations, especially in more physically active patients.

Most patients recovering from lumbar microdiscectomy progress uneventfully if properly educated and carefully rehabilitated. The PT can facilitate the systematic training program to achieve a safe and rapid return of function by applying clinical knowledge and manual skills.

SUGGESTED HOME MAINTENANCE FOR THE POSTSURGICAL PATIENT

The home maintenance program is customized to the individual patient. Patients may progress at different rates depending on age, previous level of function, goals, nerve and tissue conditions, and rate of healing.

SUGGESTED HOME MAINTENANCE FOR THE POSTSURGICAL PATIENT

Week 1

GOALS FOR THE WEEK: Protect the surgical site to promote wound healing, maintain nerve root mobility, reduce pain and inflammation, educate patient, establish consistently good body mechanics for safe and independent self-care

1. Protect the incision site.
2. Begin gentle nerve root gliding.
3. Maintain lumbar lordosis and correct body mechanics.
4. Avoid holding positions for prolonged periods and avoid all lumbar flexion.
5. Walk daily with a gradual increase in the duration and speed.
6. Use ice as needed for discomfort.

Weeks 2-3

GOALS FOR THE PERIOD: Protect the surgical site to promote wound healing, maintain nerve root mobility, reduce pain and inflammation, educate patient to minimize fear and apprehension, establish consistently good body mechanics for safe and independent self-care

1. Progress walking program to 20 to 30 minutes.
2. Maintain nerve root mobility.
3. Begin progressive exercise program (unloaded positions only):
   a. Pelvic rocks in quadruped and prone positions
   b. Abdominal bracing in several positions
   c. Supported dying bug at end of 3 weeks or when appropriate
   d. Elbow lying to partial extension in lying
   e. Prone alternating arm raises
   f. Partial squatting (to 60 degrees)
   g. Gentle stretching of hamstrings, calves, gluteals, hip adductors, and rotators as needed
4. Maintain proper postures and body mechanics.
5. Practice isolated contractions of transverse abdominal muscles used frequently during daily activities.
6. Begin scar compressive taping as needed.
7. Use ice as needed for discomfort.

Weeks 4-6

GOALS FOR THE PERIOD: Understand neutral spin concept, improve cardiovascular condition, increase trunk strength to 80%, increase soft tissue mobility and lower extremity (LE) flexibility and strength

1. Maintain nerve root mobility.
2. Progress exercise program (partially loaded positions):
   a. Partial press-ups to full press-ups
   b. Prone alternating leg raises to prone double-leg raises
   c. Unsupported dying bug
   d. Double-leg bridging progressing to single-leg bridging
   e. Partial sit-ups with rotation
   f. Side-lying double-leg raises
   g. All-fours arm and leg raises
   h. Repetitive squatting (starting at 60 degrees and progressing to 90 degrees)
3. Strengthen neurologically compromised muscles as needed (e.g., hip abductors, ankle dorsiflexors, plantar flexors, evertors).
4. Gentle stretching of hamstrings, calves, quadriceps, gluteals, hip adductors, and rotators as needed.
5. Progress aerobic conditioning (e.g., walking, swimming, cycling) to 30 to 60 minutes.
6. Practice cocontractions of transverse abdominal muscles and multifidus frequently during daily activities.
7. Use ice as needed for discomfort.
8. Massage the scar as needed.
9. Continue compressive scar care as needed.

Weeks 7-11

GOALS FOR THE PERIOD: Ensure patient is independent in self-care and activities of daily living (ADLs) with minimal alterations, increase tolerance to activities, progress return to previous level of function

1. Progress exercise program (loaded positions):
   a. Press-ups
   b. Prone "Superman" (simultaneous arm and leg raises)
   c. Dying bug with weights
   d. Single-leg bridging with weights
   e. Partial sit-ups with rotation
   f. Side-lying double-leg raises with weights
   g. Isometric side support on elbow and knees progressed to feet
   h. All-fours arm and leg raises with weights
   i. Standing rotary-torso with resistive tubing
   j. Repetitive squatting (to 90 degrees)
2. Begin functional training exercises (sports- and work-specific activities) at end of phase if able.
3. Continue LE myofascial stretching as needed.
4. Continue strengthening neurologically compromised muscles.
5. Develop and segue into final home or club exercise program (or into both).

References

1. Abramovitz JN, Neff SR: Lumbar disc surgery: results of the prospective lumbar discectomy study of the Joint Section on Disorders of the Spine and Peripheral Nerves of the American Association of Neurological Surgeons and the Congress of Neurological Surgeons, *Neurosurgery* 29:301-308, 1991.
2. Akuthota V, Nadler SF: Core strengthening, *Arch Phys Med Rehabil* 85(3 suppl 1):S86-92, 2004.
3. Barr KP, Griggs M, Cadby T: Lumbar stabilization: Core concepts and current literature. I. *Am J Phys Med Rehabil* 84(6):473-480, 2005.
4. Barrios C et al: Microsurgical versus standard removal of the herniated lumbar disc, *Acta Orthop Scand* 61:399-403, 1990.
5. Boden SD et al: Abnormal magnetic resonance scans of the lumbar spine in asymptomatic subjects: a prospective investigation, *J Bone Joint Surg* 72A:403-408, 1990.
6. Bookwalter JW, Buxch MD, Nicely D: Ambulatory surgery is safe and effective in radicular disc disease, *Spine* 19:526-530, 1994.
7. Buirski G, Silberstein M: The symptomatic lumbar disc in patients with low-back pain: Magnetic resonance imaging appearances in both a symptomatic and control population, *Spine* 18:1808-1811, 1993.
8. Butler DS: *Mobilization of the nervous system,* Melbourne, 1991, Churchill Livingstone.
9. Carragee EJ: Indications for lumbar microdiscectomy, *Instr Course Lect* 51:223-228, 2002.
10. Carragee EJ, Helms E, O'Sullivan GS: Are postoperative activity restrictions necessary after posterior lumbar discectomy? A prospective study of outcomes in 50 consecutive cases, *Spine* 21(16):1893-1897, 1996.
11. Caspar W et al: The Caspar microsurgical discectomy and comparison with a conventional standard lumbar disc procedure, *Neurosurgery* 28:78-87, 1991.
12. Cottingham JT, Maitland J: A three-paradigm treatment model using soft tissue mobilization and guided movement-awareness techniques for a patient with chronic low back pain: A case study, *J Orthop Sports Ther* 26(3):155, 1997.
13. Dai LY et al: The effect of flexion-extension motion of the lumbar spine on the capacity of the spinal canal, *Spine* 14(5):523, 1989.
14. Davis H: Increasing rates of cervical and lumbar spine surgery in the United States, 1979-1990, *Spine* 19:1117-1124, 1994.
15. De Divitiis E, Cappabianca P: Lumbar discectomy with preservation of the ligamentum flavum, *Surg Neurol* 57(1):5-13, 2002.
16. Deen HG, Fenton DS, Lamer TJ: Minimally invasive procedures for disorders of the lumbar spine, *Mayo Clin Proc* 78(10):1249-1256, 2003.
17. Delamarter RB: Lumbar microdiscectomy: microsurgical technique for treatment of lumbar herniated nucleus pulposus, *Instr Course Lect* 51:229-232, 2002.
18. Delamarter RB, McCulloch J: Microdiscectomy and microsurgical spinal laminotomies. In Frymoyer JW, editor: *The adult spine, principles and practice*, ed 2, Philadelphia, 1997, Lippincott-Raven, pp 1961-1988.
19. DeLucca PF et al: Excision of herniated nucleus pulposus in children and adolescents, *J Pediatr Orthop* 14:318-322, 1994.
20. Deyo RA et al: How many days of bed rest for acute low back pain? A randomized clinical trial, *N Engl J Med* 315:1064, 1986.
21. Errico TJ, Fardon DF, Lowell TD: Open discectomy as treatment for herniated nucleus pulposus of the lumbar spine, *Spine J* 3:45S-49S, 2003.
22. Findlay GF et al: A 10-year follow-up of the outcome of lumbar microdiscectomy, *Spine* 23(10):1168-1171, 1998.
23. Gibson JN, Grant IC, Waddell G: Surgery for lumbar disc prolapse, *Cochrane Database Syst Rev* 200(3):CD001350.
24. Gill K: Percutaneous lumbar discectomy, *J Am Acad Orthop Surg* 1(1):33-40, 1993.
25. Gogan WJ, Fraser RD: Chymopapain: a 10-year, double blind study, *Spine* 17:388-394, 1992.
26. Graves JE et al: Effect of training frequency and specificity on isometric lumbar extension strength, *Spine* 15(6):505, 1990.
27. Groslin AJ, Cantu R: *Myofascial manipulation: theory and clinical management,* New York, 1989, Forum Medicum.
28. Haig A et al: Prospective evidence for changes in paraspinal muscle activity after herniated nucleus pulposus, *Spine* 17(7):926, 1993.
29. Hakelius A: Prognosis in sciatica: a clinical follow-up of surgical and non-surgical treatment, *Acta Orthop Scand* 129(suppl):1-76, 1970.
30. Hanley EN: The surgical treatment of lumbar degenerative disease. In Vaccaro AR, editor: *Orthopaedic knowledge update: spine,* Rosemont, IL, 1997, American Academy of Orthopaedic Surgeons.
31. Hardy RW: Lumbar discectomy: surgical tactics and management of complications. In Frymoyer JW, editor: *The adult spine, principles and practice*, ed 2, Philadelphia, 1997, Lippincott-Raven, pp 1947-1959.
32. Hickey DS, Hukins DWL: Relation between the structure of the annulus fibrosus and function and failure of the intervertebral disc, *Spine* 5(2):106, 1980.
33. Hides JA, Richardson CA, Jull GA: Multifidus inhibition in acute low back pain: recovery is not spontaneous. *MPAA Conference Proceedings,* 1995;57.
34. Hides JA, Richardson CA, Jull GA: Multifidus muscle recovery is not automatic after resolution of acute, first-episode low back pain, *Spine* 21(23):2763-2769, 1996.
35. Hides JA et al: Evidence of lumbar multifidus muscle wasting ipsilateral to symptoms in patients with acute/subacute low back pain, *Spine* 19(2):165, 1994.
36. Hodges PW: Core stability exercise in chronic low back pain, *Orthop Clin North Am* 34(2):245-254, 2003.
37. Hodges PW, Richardson CA: Contraction of the abdominal muscles associated with movement of the lower limb, *Phys Ther* 77:132, 1997.
38. Hodges PW et al: Intervertebral stiffness of the spine is increased by evoked contraction of transverse abdominis and the diaphragm: in vivo porcine studies, *Spine* 28(23)2594-2601, 2003.

39. Holm S, Nachemson A: Variations in the nutrition of the canine intervertebral disc induced by motion, *Spine* 8(8):866, 1983.
40. Hudson-Cook N, Tomes-Nicholson K, Breen A: A revised Oswestry disability questionnaire. In Roland MO, Jenner JR, editors: *Back pain: new approaches to rehabilitation and education,* New York, 1989, Manchester University Press.
41. Jensen MC et al: Magnetic resonance imaging of the lumbar spine in people without back pain, *N Engl J Med* 331:69-73, 1994.
42. Johannsen F et al: Exercises for chronic low back pain: A clinical trial, *J Orthop Sports Ther* 22(2):52, 1995.
43. Karas R et al: The relationship between nonorganic signs and centralization of symptoms in the prediction of return to work for patients with low back pain, *Phys Ther* 77(4):354, 1997.
44. Kavcic N, Grenier S, McGill SM: Determining the stabilizing role of individual torso muscles during rehabilitation exercises, *Spine* 29(11):1254-1265, 2004.
45. Kostuik J et al: Cauda equina syndrome and lumbar disc herniation, *J Bone Joint Surg* 68:386, 1986.
46. Krolner B, Toft B: Vertebral bone loss: an unheeded side effect of therapeutic bed rest, *Clin Sci* 64:437, 1983.
47. Kuslich SD, Ulstrom CL, Michael CJ: The tissue origin of low back pain and sciatica, *Orthop Clin North Am* 22(2):181, 1991.
48. Lee D: *The pelvic girdle,* ed 2, Edinburgh, UK, 1999, Churchill Livingstone.
49. Lee HWM: Progressive muscle synergy and synchronization in movement patterns: an approach to the treatment of dynamic lumbar instability, *J Manual Manip Ther* 2(4):133, 1994.
50. Lindgren K-A et al: Exercise therapy effects on functional radiographic findings and segmental electromyographic activity in lumbar spine instability, *Arch Phys Med Rehabil* 74:933, 1993.
51. Lorenz M, McCulloch JA: Chemonucleolysis for herniated nucleus pulposus in adolescents, *J Bone Joint Surg* 67A:1402-1404, 1985.
52. Loupasis GA et al: Seven- to 20-year outcome of lumbar discectomy, *Spine* 24(22):2313-2317, 1999.
53. Maitland GD: *Vertebral manipulation,* ed 5, London, 1986, Butterworth-Heinemann.
54. Manniche C et al: Intensive dynamic back exercises with or without hyperextension in chronic back pain after surgery for lumbar disc protrusion, *Spine* 18(5):560, 1993.
55. Maroon JC: Current concepts in minimally invasive discectomy, *Neurosurgery* 51(5S):137-145, 2002.
56. Marras WS et al: Quantification and classification of low back disorders on trunk motion, *Eur J Phys Med Rehab* 3:218, 1993.
57. McCulloch JA: Focus issue on lumbar disc herniation: macro- and microdiscectomy, *Spine* 21(suppl 24): 45S-56S, 1996.
58. McCulloch JA: Microdiscectomy: the gold standard for minimally invasive disc surgery, *Spine: State of the Art Rev* 11(2):373, 1997.
59. McCulloch JA, Snook D, Kruse CF: Advantages of the operating microscope in lumbar spine surgery, *Instr Course Lect* 51:243-245, 2002.
60. McCulloch JA, Young PH: Complications (adverse effects) in lumbar microsurgery. In *Essentials of spinal microsurgery,* Philadelphia, 1998, Lippincott-Raven, pp 503-529.
61. McCulloch JA, Young PH: Foraminal and extraforaminal lumbar disc herniation. In *Essentials of spinal microsurgery,* Philadelphia, 1998, Lippincott-Raven, pp 383-428.
62. McCulloch JA, Young PH: Microsurgery for lumbar disc herniation. In *Essentials of spinal microsurgery,* Philadelphia, 1998, Lippincott-Raven, pp 329-382.
63. McCulloch JA, Young PH: The microscope as a surgical aid. In *Essentials of spinal microsurgery,* Philadelphia, 1998, Lippincott-Raven, pp 3-17.
64. McCulloch JA, Young PH: Wound healing and mobilization. In *Essentials of spinal microsurgery,* Philadelphia, 1998, Lippincott-Raven, pp 43-53.
65. McGill SM: Distribution of tissue loads in the low back during a variety of daily and rehabilitation tasks, *J Rehabil Res Dev* 34(4):448, 1997.
66. McKenzie RA: *The lumbar spine,* Waikanae, New Zealand, 1981, Spinal Publications.
67. Moffroid M et al: Some endurance measures in persons with chronic low back pain, *J Orthop Sports Ther* 20(2):81, 1994.
68. Moreland J et al: Interrater reliability of six tests of trunk muscle function and endurance, *J Orthop Sports Ther* 26(4):200, 1997.
69. Mulligan BR: *Manual therapy "NAGS", "SNAGS", "MWMS" etc,* ed 3, New Zealand, 1995, Plane View Services.
70. Nagata CB, Tsujii Y: Manual therapy rounds, *J Manual Manip Ther* 5(2):87, 1997.
71. Neumann P, Gill V: Pelvic floor and abdominal muscle interaction: EMG activity and intra-abdominal pressure, *Int Urogynecol J Pelvic Floor Dysfunct* 13(2):125-32, 2002.
72. Newman MH: Outpatient conventional laminotomy and disc excision, *Spine* 20:353-365, 1995.
73. Ng JK-F, Richardson CA, Jull GA: Electromyographic amplitude and frequency changes in the iliocostalis lumborum and multifidus muscles during a trunk holding test, *Phys Ther* 77(9):954, 1997.
74. Nordby EJ, Fraser RD: Chemonucleolysis. In Frymoyer JW, editor: *The adult spine, principles and practice,* ed 2, Philadelphia, 1997, Lippincott-Raven, pp 1989-2008.
75. Obenchain TG: Speculum lumbar extraforaminal microdiscectomy, *Spine J* 1(6):415-420, 2001.
76. Onik GM: Percutaneous discectomy in the treatment of herniated lumbar disks, *Neuroimaging Clin N Am* 10(3):597-607, 2000.
77. Onik GM, Kambin P, Chang MK: Minimally invasive disc surgery. Nucleotomy versus fragmentectomy, *Spine* 22(7):827-828, 1997.
78. Panjabi MM: The stabilizing system of the spine. I. Function, dysfunction adaptation and enhancement, *J Spinal Disord* 5:383, 1992.
79. Panjabi MM et al: On the understanding of clinical instability, *Spine* 19(23):2642, 1994.
80. Pappas CTE, Harrington T, Sonntag VKH: Outcome analysis in 654 surgically treated lumbar disc herniations, *Neurosurgery* 30:862-866, 1992.

81. Paris SV: Mobilization of the spine, *Phys Ther* 49:988, 1979.
82. Parisini P et al: Lumbar disc excision in children and adolescents, *Spine* 26(18):1997-2000, 2001.
83. Peacock EE Jr: Dynamic aspects of collagen biology. I. Synthesis and assembly, *J Surg Res* 7:433-446, 1967.
84. Peterson M, Wilson J: Job satisfaction and perceptions of health, *J Occup Environ Med* 38(9):891, 1996.
85. Rantanen J et al: The lumbar multifidus muscle five years after surgery for a lumbar intervertebral disc herniation, *Spine* 18(5):568, 1993.
86. Richardson C, Jull G: Muscle control-pain control. What exercises would you prescribe? *Man Ther* 1:2, 1995.
87. Richardson C, Toppenberg R, Jull G: An initial evaluation of eight abdominal exercises for their ability to provide stabilization for the lumbar spine, *Aust J Physiother* 36(1):6, 1990.
88. Richardson C et al: Techniques for active lumbar stabilization for spinal protection: a pilot study, *Aust J Physiother* 38(2):105, 1992.
89. Richardson C et al: Therapeutic exercise for spinal segmental stabilization in low back pain: scientific basis and clinical approach, 2000.
90. Roberts MP: Complications of lumbar disc surgery. In Hardy RW, editor: *Lumbar disc disease,* New York, 1992, Raven Press, pp 161-70.
91. Rogers LA: Experience with limited versus extensive disc removal in patients undergoing microsurgical operations for ruptured lumbar disc, *Neurosurgery* 22:82-85, 1988.
92. Roland M, Morris R: A study of the natural history of back pain. I. The development of a reliable and sensitive measure of disability in low-back pain, *Spine* 8:141, 1983.
93. Salvi V et al: Microdiscectomy in the treatment of lumbar disc herniation, *Chir Organi Mov* 85(4):337-344, 2000.
94. Sapsford RR et al: Co-activation of the abdominal and pelvic floor muscles during voluntary exercises, *Neurourol Urodyn* 20(1):31-42, 2001.
95. Scalzitti DA: Screening for psychological factors in patients with low back problems: Waddell's nonorganic signs, *Phys Ther* 77(3):306, 1997.
96. Schofferman J et al: Childhood psychological trauma and chronic refractory low-back pain, *Clin J Pain* 9(4):260, 1993.
97. Schutz H, Watson CPN: Microsurgical discectomy: prospective study of 200 patients, *Neurol Sci* 14:81-3, 1987.
98. Shapiro S: Cauda equina syndrome secondary to lumbar disc herniation, *Neurosurgery* 32:743-746, 1993.
99. Sihvonen T et al: Local denervation atrophy of paraspinal muscles in postoperative failed back syndrome, *Spine* 18:575, 1993.
100. Silvers HR: Microsurgical versus standard lumbar discectomy, *Neurosurgery* 22:837-841, 1988.
101. Silvers HR: Lumbar disc excisions in patients under the age of 21 years, *Spine* 19:2387-2392, 1994.
102. Singhal A, Bernstein M: Outpatient lumbar microdiscectomy: a prospective study in 122 patients, *Can J Neurol Sci* 29(3):249-252, 2002.
103. Souza GM, Baker LL, Powers CM: Electromyographic activity of selected trunk muscles during dynamic spine stabilization exercises, *Arch Phys Med Rehabil* 82(11):1551-1557, 2001.
104. Spengler DM: Lumbar discectomy: results with limited disc excision and selective foraminotomy, *Spine* 7:604-607, 1982.
105. Striffeler H, Groger U, Reulen HJ: "Standard" microsurgical lumbar discectomy vs "conservative" microsurgical discectomy, *Acta Neurochir (Wien)* 112:62-64, 1991.
106. Thomas AMC, Afshar F: The microsurgical treatment of lumbar disc protrusions, *J Bone Joint Surg* 69B:696-698, 1987.
107. Travell JG, Simmon DG: *Myofascial pain and dysfunction: the trigger point manual,* vols 1-2, Baltimore, 1992, William & Wilkins.
108. Triano JJ, Schultz AB: Correlation of objective measures of trunk motion and muscle function with low-back disability ratings, *Spine* 12(6):561, 1987.
109. Tullberg T, Isacson J, Weidenhielm L: Does microscopic removal of lumbar disc herniation lead to better results than standard procedure? *Spine* 18:24-27, 1993.
110. Tureyen K: One-level one-sided lumbar disc surgery with and without microscopic assistance: 1-year outcome in 114 consecutive patients, *J Neurosurg* 99(suppl 3): 247-250, 2003.
111. Urban JPG et al: Nutrition of the intervertebral disc, *Clin Orthop Relat Res* 170:296, 1982.
112. Vroomen PC et al: Lack of effectiveness of bed rest for sciatica, *N Engl J Med* 340(6):418-423, 1999.
113. Waddell G: A new clinical model for the treatment of low-back pain, *Spine* 12(7):632, 1987.
114. Waddell G: Evaluation of results in lumbar spine surgery. Clinical outcomes measures—assessment of severity, *Acta Orthop Scand Suppl* 251:134, 1993.
115. Waddell G et al: Non-organic physical signs in low-back pain, *Spine* 5:117, 1980.
116. Walker ML et al: Relationships between lumbar lordosis, pelvic tilt, and abdominal performance, *Phys Ther* 67(4):512, 1987.
117. Wang JC et al: The outcome of lumbar discectomy in elite athletes, *Spine* 24(6):570-573, 1999.
118. Watkins RG, Dillin WH: Lumbar spine injury in the athlete, *Clin Sports Med* 9(2):419, 1990.
119. Watkins RG IV, Williams LA, Watkins RG III: Microscopic lumbar discectomy results for 60 cases in professional and Olympic athletes, *Spine* 3(2):100-105, 2003.
120. Weber H: Lumbar disc herniation: a controlled, prospective study with 10 years of observation, *Spine* 8:131-140, 1983.
121. Weir BKA, Jacobs GA: Reoperation rate following lumbar discectomy. An analysis of 662 lumbar discectomies, *Spine* 5:366-370, 1980.
122. White T, Malone T: Effects of running on intervertebral disc height, *J Orthop Sports Phys Ther* 12:410, 1990.
123. Wilke HJ et al: Stability increase of the lumbar spine with different muscle groups, *Spine* 20(2):192, 1995.
124. Williams RW: Microdiscectomy—myth, mania, or milestone? An 18-year surgical adventure, *Mt Sinai J Med* 58:139-145, 1991.
125. Williams RW: Microlumbar discectomy: a conservative surgical approach to the virgin herniated lumbar disc, *Spine* 3:175-182, 1978.

126. Wilson DH, Harbaugh R: Microsurgical and standard removal of the protruded lumbar disc: a comparative study, *Neurosurgery* 8:422-427, 1981.
127. Wilson DH, Kenning J: Microsurgical lumbar discectomy: preliminary report of 83 consecutive cases, *Neurosurgery* 4:137-140, 1979.
128. Wohlfahrt D, Jull G, Richardson C: The relationship between the dynamic and static function of abdominal muscles, *Aust J Physiother* 39(1):9, 1993.
129. Yasuma T et al: Histologic changes in aging lumbar intervertebral discs, *J Bone Joint Surg* 72A:220-229, 1990.
130. Yasuma T et al: Histological development of intervertebral disc herniation, *J Bone Joint Surg* 68A:1066-1072, 1986.
131. Zahrawi F: Microlumbar discectomy: is it safe as an outpatient procedure? *Spine* 9:1070-1074, 1994.

CHAPTER 14

Lumbar Spine Fusion

Haideh V. Plock
Jessie Scott
Paul Slosar
Arthur White

In the early 1900s two surgeons began performing lumbar fusions. Dr. Russell Hibbs[11] and Dr. Fred Albee[2] pioneered the posterior approaches for arthrodesis. Over the subsequent decades, many surgeons improved fusion techniques, with extension of the fusion laterally to incorporate the transverse processes and the sacral ala.[4,8,39,43] The patient's autogenous iliac crest is the standard source of bone graft material.[9,10] A rapid evolution has occurred in the development and use of spinal fixation devices. Although tracing the historical evolution of these devices is beyond the scope of this chapter, they can simply be categorized as anterior or posterior fixation devices. The most common and most controversial are the pedicle screw and rod and plate systems. Anterior fixation devices include screw and rod and plate systems, as well as the recently introduced interbody cages. This chapter describes the indications for elective lumbar fusions and discusses the various methods of arthrodesis.

SURGICAL INDICATIONS AND CONSIDERATIONS

In the elective patient population, most indications for lumbar arthrodesis are based on the presence of severe, disabling back or leg pain. Post-traumatic cases of segmental instability or potential neurologic injury also may require fusions, but this chapter focuses on patients with degenerative spinal pathology.

Patients with low back pain experience symptoms resulting from tissue aggravation during the degenerative cascade.[43] Trauma or overuse causes the disc wall to begin to develop microtears; this eventually results in a loss of disc height that alters the alignment of the facet joints, and this may lead to pain with accompanying spasm and guarding. The joints begin to develop synovitis, articular cartilage degeneration, and adhesions. This alters the spinal motion mechanics at that segment, further stressing the annulus of the disc and accelerating the degenerative process of the facet. Increased wearing of the cartilage and hypermobility of the facet also occur. The superior and inferior facet surfaces begin to enlarge. As the joint becomes more disrupted, normal motion at that segment becomes impossible. The disc begins to undergo greater strain. The disc wall weakens further, begins to bulge, and can eventually herniate. The disc continues to lose fluid and height, causing narrowing of the neural foramen, or foraminal stenosis. This process is outlined in Table 14-1.

Patients with severe back pain that is refractory to conservative care may be candidates for surgical evaluation. Conservative care should include a rigorous attempt at exercise-based dynamic-stabilization training, therapeutic injections, and medications. Surgical treatment should only be discussed with the patient after a firm diagnosis has been made.

Diagnostic Tests

Spinal radiographs show osteophytes and segmental disc space narrowing in patients with degenerative spondylosis. A defect in the pars interarticularis is seen in patients with spondylolysis. Anterolisthesis, or a forward slippage of one vertebra on the next, is the hallmark radiographic finding in spondylolisthesis. Instability or excessive motion on flexion and extension films, although rare in degenerative lumbar conditions, can occasionally be observed.

Computed tomography (CT) reliably evaluates the bone or spondylosis compression against the nerves. Computer-enhanced reformatted CT images are as effective in evaluating spinal stenosis as myelography. CT scanning is more sensitive than magnetic resonance imaging (MRI) in the evaluation of bony stenosis, whereas MRI gives useful information about the health of the discs and nerves. Combining the two imaging modalities gives a very accurate, thorough picture of the lumbar spinal pathoanatomy.

Provocative discography is an essential diagnostic tool in the workup of patients with painful degenerative lumbar disc disease. Unfortunately, the practitioner cannot examine the disc directly (as a knee or hand can be observed). The lumbar discs are deep within the abdominal cavity and do not have true dermatomal pain patterns in axial discogenic cases. Overlapping sclerodermal referred pain patterns in the lumbar spine make the localization of the true pain

Table 14-1 The Degenerative Cascade

Structure	Damage at Each Stage		
	Stage 1: Dysfunction	Stage 2: Instability	Stage 3: Stability
Intervertebral disc	◆ Circumferential tears ◆ Inflammatory exudates and irritation	◆ Radial tears ◆ Loss of disc height ◆ Internal disruption ◆ Disc bulges and herniations	◆ Loss of proteoglycans and water, fibrotic resorption ◆ Sclerosis and eventual bony ankylosis
Facet joints	◆ Synovitis ◆ Minor cartilage degeneration	◆ Laxity of joint capsule ◆ Moderate cartilage degeneration	◆ Significant bony overgrowth ◆ Grossly degenerated cartilage ◆ Hypomobility
Muscles	◆ Spasm, guarding	◆ Chronic shortening and fibrosis	◆ Further shortening and fibrosis
Neural foramen	◆ Unaffected	◆ Narrowed through annular bulges ◆ Disc narrowing ◆ Bony overgrowth	◆ Significant stenosis ◆ Disc narrowing

generator difficult. Discography has evolved as a test to examine the lumbar discs morphologically and, most importantly, provocatively. On injection into the disc, the patient must communicate to the discographer if that disc is concordantly painful. Many degenerative discs are either not painful or discordantly painful. This information is essential for the surgeon and the patient contemplating lumbar arthrodesis.

Diagnosis

Among patients undergoing elective lumbar arthrodesis, painful degenerative disc disease is the most prevalent diagnosis. Confirmatory diagnostic testing often includes MRI scanning and discography. Overlap occurs among patients who have had previous surgery and have a diagnosis of "failed back surgery syndrome," a nonspecific diagnosis. Before surgery is contemplated, every effort must be made to arrive at a diagnosis that specifically isolates the source of pain.

Patients often have numerous diagnoses, each of which may be valid. For example, a 45-year-old man who had a laminotomy performed 5 years ago for a herniated nucleus pulposus comes to his physician complaining of 50% low back pain and 50% right leg pain and numbness. Diagnostic imaging is significant for L4-L5 segmental degeneration with osteophytes and narrowing of the disc space. A multiplanar CT scan reveals moderate spondylosis (bone spurs) with stenosis along the right neural foramen. Discography is concordant with pain reproduction at the L4-L5 disc. The appropriate diagnoses include painful degenerative disc disease, lumbar spondylosis with stenosis, and postlaminectomy syndrome.

The absolute requisite for a successful lumbar surgery outcome is matching concordant patient symptoms with the appropriate surgical procedure. Patients who cannot manage their pain with conservative measures and have demonstrable, concordant pathology on diagnostic testing may benefit from lumbar arthrodesis.

TYPES OF FUSIONS

Instrumentation Versus Noninstrumentation

The goal of a lumbar arthrodesis is the successful union of two or more vertebra. Controversy exists over the most efficient way to achieve this result. Instrumentation can be used to immobilize the moving segments while the fusion becomes solid. One of the original and most popular systems is the Harrington hook-and-rod construct. Although this *distraction* type of fixation immobilizes the spine in certain planes, it causes a loss of physiologic lordosis, or a "flat-back syndrome," in many patients.

Today most spine surgeons use pedicle screw constructs to immobilize the vertebrae rigidly while preserving the normal lumbar lordosis[11] (Fig. 14-1). Typically, external orthosis bracing is not needed in these cases. As well-controlled studies emerge, data support the use of internal fixation for fusion.[12] Most studies support the use of pedicle screw fixation to obtain a more reliable bony union, although complication rates tend to be higher with these devices as well.[15,17]

Some surgeons do not routinely use pedicle screws for arthrodesis. In most of these situations (when pedicle screws are used), the patient must wear a lumbar orthosis for an extended period postoperatively. To immobilize the L5-S1 motion segment effectively, an orthosis with a thigh-cuff extension must be applied. Patients with non-instrumented fusions may take an extensive amount of time to stabilize and become comfortable in their rehabilitation. Conversely, most patients with internal

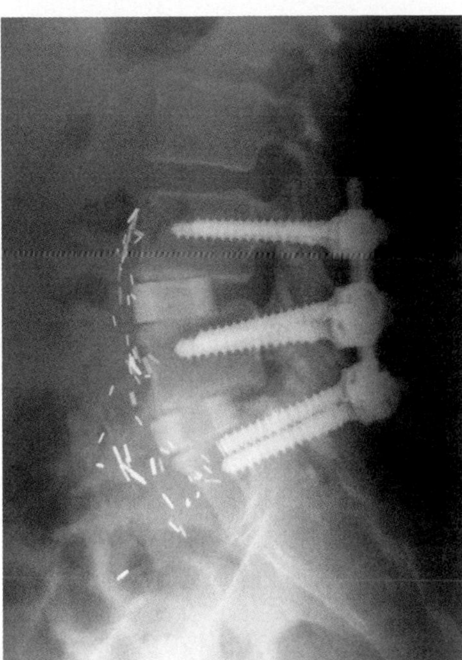

Fig. 14-1 Pedicle screw instrumentation in a circumferential lumbar fusion.

fixation become mobile and independent more rapidly, making early rehabilitation more predictable.

Posterior Fusion

Posterolateral Lumbar Fusion

Different surgeons use different techniques to perform a lumbar fusion. The traditional approach is through a midline posterior incision. If necessary, then the surgeon performs a laminectomy or laminotomy to address the pertinent pathologic conditions. Most surgeons perform a posterolateral fusion, which means that the transverse processes, pars interarticularis, and, if needed, the sacral alae are decorticated. The patient's own iliac crest bone graft is harvested and morselized. The bone graft is then placed on the decorticated surfaces, forming a fusion bed contiguous with all the surfaces to be fused. Pedicle screws and rods or plates may be placed to immobilize the motion segments rigidly and augment the formation of a solid union.

The problems with a posterolateral fusion are both mechanical and physiologic. The fusion is attempting to form at a mechanical disadvantage because of tension. Bone heals more reliably under protected physiologic loads of compression, not tension. In addition, the available area for the bone union to occur is limited to the remaining posterolateral bone surfaces. After extensive decompression of the neural elements (laminectomy), the available fusion area is reduced and often poorly vascularized. These local factors reduce the likelihood of a successful arthrodesis. Nicotine use negatively influences the formation of posterolateral lumbar fusions.

Finally, the usual source of pain in these patients is the disc itself, hence the term *discogenic*. In routine cases of posterolateral fusions, the disc is not radically resected. Biomechanical studies have shown that people bear load through the middle and posterior thirds of the disc. Several reports describe a persistently painful disc under a solid posterior fusion.[40] As surgeons recognized the biomechanical and physiologic aspects of the discs, they began performing interbody fusions.[6]

Interbody Fusion

Posterior lumbar interbody fusion. Interbody fusions evolved to address many of the drawbacks of traditional posterolateral fusions. Radical excision of the disc and anterior column support (with rigid bone grafting) are performed. The available area for successful bone union is greatly increased by using the interbody space.

Using a posterior lumbar approach, a surgeon performs a posterior lumbar interbody fusion (PLIF). After a wide laminectomy, the posterior two thirds of the disc is resected and an interbody tricortical strut is placed into the evacuated disc space. This provides anterior interbody stability through a posterior approach. PLIF is a technically demanding procedure associated with a higher incidence of postsurgical nerve injuries.

Anterior lumbar interbody fusion. Because the risks associated with PLIF were too great for routine use, many surgeons moved to anterior lumbar interbody fusion (ALIF). Using the same principles of disc excision and interbody bone grafting, many surgeons achieved excellent results. However, ALIF alone cannot withstand the forces across the grafts, so many collapse or do not fuse. Surgeons who perform ALIF have learned to protect the grafts with posterior instrumentation, leading to a predictable fusion rate and good clinical results.

From a technical standpoint, anterior lumbar surgery is most easily and safely accomplished through a retroperitoneal approach. After the anterior disc is exposed, it is relatively simple to perform a discectomy and insert the bone graft of the surgeon's choice. Posterior fusion and instrumentation can be placed through a separate posterior approach on either the same day or in a staged procedure. A circumferential fusion is accomplished in this manner (see Fig. 14-1).

Cages. Recent technologic advances have been made in interbody cages. Essentially, these devices are hollow cylinders made of titanium, carbon, or bone (Fig. 14-2). They are filled with autogenous bone graft and inserted between the vertebral bodies. The cages usually have threads along the outside edges that afford very rigid immediate fixation. This has dramatically reduced the need for posterior fixation. Research is moving rapidly to find a reliable substitute for the autogenous bone graft,

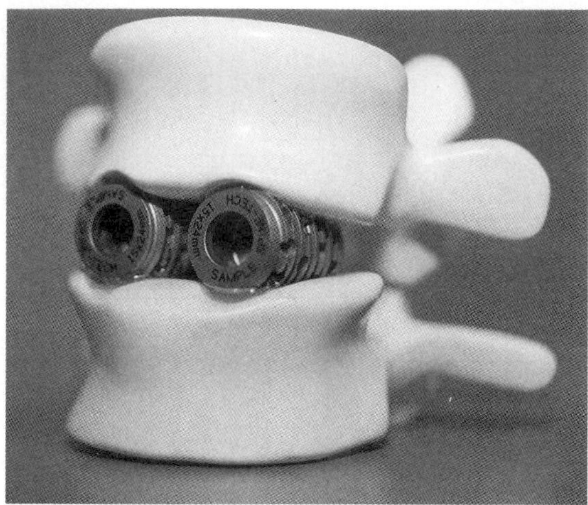

Fig. 14-2 BAK interbody cage device (Sulzer-Spine Tech, Minneapolis, MN).

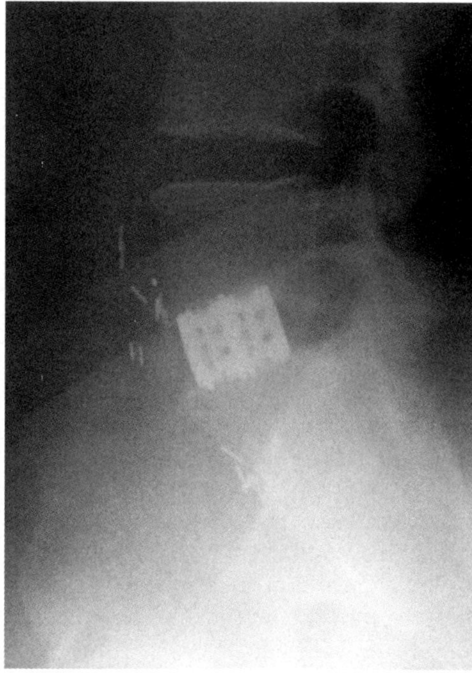

Fig. 14-3 Lumbar fusion with the BAK interbody cage (Sulzer-Spine Tech, Minneapolis, MN).

most likely with the use of bone-morphogenic protein. If medical advances could eliminate the need to harvest bone from the patient's iliac crest, then cage technology would certainly represent a minimally invasive spinal fusion (Fig. 14-3).

Most surgeons implant these devices through an anterior approach, with some using laparoscopic-assisted anterior surgery. This can potentially reduce the length of stay in hospital but can produce a slightly higher complication rate.

Most patients begin physical therapy between 6 weeks and 3 months after surgery.

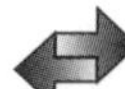

Extension-biased exercises should be avoided during the first 6 months of the postoperative recovery phase.

SURGICAL PROCEDURE

The most common lumbar fusion is the posterolateral fusion. The patient is placed in a knee-chest position, which allows the abdomen to hang free. This decompresses the lumbar epidural veins and minimizes bleeding. A skin incision is made over the operative levels, and the paraspinal muscles are stripped off the posterior elements (i.e., spinous process, lamina, transverse processes). Deep retractors hold back the muscles to allow the surgeon to expose the bone for fusion. Using small curettes or a high-speed burr, the surgeon decorticates the dorsal aspect of the transverse processes and facet joints in preparation for the bone graft placement. Through a separate fascial incision, the surgeon harvests the necessary amount of cortical and cancellous bone graft from the posterior iliac crest. This bone graft material is then carefully placed in the recipient site.

If screws are used to augment the fusion, a pilot hole is made over the entry site of the pedicle with a burr. Usually probes are placed in the pedicles, and a radiograph is taken to confirm the position of the pedicle probes. After confirmation, the pedicles are tapped and appropriate-length screws are placed into the pedicles. Again, an intraoperative radiograph is taken to confirm the position of the screws. The rods or plates are connected to the screws, and lordosis is preserved in the construct. The wound is usually irrigated with an antibiotic solution to minimize the chance of infection and closed over a deep suction drain. The drain is removed when the postsurgical drainage is minimal.

THERAPY GUIDELINES FOR REHABILITATION

An understanding of the specific procedure performed is essential for safe rehabilitation. Before beginning a rehabilitation program, the therapist must know whether the patient has had a fusion with or without instrumentation. Patients who were operated on with instrumentation can generally be progressed more aggressively in the first phase of rehabilitation. Patients who were operated on without instrumentation require more time for the bony fusion to take place. Generally a callus should form within 6 to 8 weeks; the surgeon monitors this by radiograph and usually does not refer for therapy before a callus has formed. The therapist also must know the surgical approach and the levels fused. After a motion segment is fused, increased stress is placed on the levels above and below the fusion. This creates risk for acceleration of the degenerative cascade at the adjacent levels. Obviously the more levels that have been fused, the greater the stress placed on the remaining segments. When the fusion includes the L5-S1 motion segment, abnormal forces are then translated to the sacroiliac joints. To minimize these forces, the therapist must be sure that normal motion exists at all remaining segments, including the thoracic spine and lower extremities (LEs).

During a posterior fusion, the multifidi are retracted from the spine. This partially tears the dorsal divisions of the spinal nerves, resulting in partial denervation of the multifidi.[12,43] If an anterior fusion also has been performed, then a midline skin incision will be apparent and the abdominal muscular incision is lateral. The incision passes through the obliques, also partially denervating them. For this reason the therapist should teach the patient the proper way to recruit the transverse abdominus, multifidi, and pelvic floor muscles and watch for any substitution patterns to promote proper spinal stabilization.

Description of Rehabilitation and Rationale for Using Instrumentation

Opinion about the degree of rehabilitation needed after spinal surgery ranges from the optimistic view that no rehabilitation is needed to others who argue for aggressive exercise- and education-based programs. This chapter is written from the point of view that the patient is not merely recovering from surgery but from a breakdown in the spine exacerbated by predisposing factors such as stiffness and poor muscle tone, movement habits, and proprioception.

The following guidelines are not intended to substitute for sound clinical reasoning but rather serve as a foundation on which a trained physical therapist (PT) can base the rehabilitation of a patient after spinal fusion. It is assumed that the therapist will know the basics of spinal evaluation and will monitor the patient for symptoms that require prompt re-evaluation.

Q Tom is 50 years old. He had a lumbar fusion at L4-L5 and L5-S1, 3 weeks ago. He is now in therapy. The PT gives Tom an exercise to facilitate nerve root gliding. The patient asks, "What is the significance of this exercise?" What should the therapist tell the patient?

Phase I

TIME: 1 to 5 days after surgery
GOALS: Patient education about daily movements, neural mobilization, and home care principles (Table 14-2)

Inpatient Phase

Most patients remain in the hospital for several days after fusion surgery. Physical therapy management during this phase consists of teaching patients the proper way to get in and out of bed, dress and undress, and walk (perhaps with a walker for the first 1 or 2 days). The therapist also can teach basic and simple neural mobilization for the involved level and principles for using ice at home. Patients should leave the hospital with an understanding of the home care required until they begin their outpatient physical therapy. If the physician requests bracing

Table 14-2 Lumbar Fusion and Laminectomy

Rehabilitation Phase	Criteria to Progress to this Phase	Anticipated Impairments and Functional Limitations	Intervention	Goal	Rationale
Phase I Postoperative 1-5 days	Postoperative (inpatient)	◆ Pain ◆ Limited bed mobility ◆ Limited self-care ◆ Limited activities of daily living (ADLs) ◆ Limited tolerance to prolonged postures (sit/stand) ◆ Limited tolerance to walking	Inpatient care ◆ Bed mobility training, log roll technique with supine-sit-stand ◆ ADL training with assistive devices as necessary (dressing, bathroom transfers) ◆ Body mechanics training ◆ Gait training, with walker if necessary	◆ Independent with the following: 1. Bed mobility 2. Don/doff clothing, and corset if indicated 3. Transfers 4. Gait, using assistive device as appropriate ◆ Demonstrate appropriate body mechanics with self-care and basic ADLs	◆ Promote restoration of independent function ◆ Use log roll to avoid placing stress on the surgical site ◆ Emphasize walking to improve tolerance to upright postures ◆ Use proper body mechanics to avoid reinjury

of any kind, then the patient should understand the way to get in and out of the brace and when to wear it. **Patients will be given instructions from the physician to avoid driving, prolonged sitting, lifting, bending, and twisting.** The PT should reinforce this information and teach patients the proper way to avoid these activities by hip hinging or pivoting. This information should be provided in written form, because many patients may be medicated or overwhelmed by the recent surgery and therefore have difficulty recalling or applying what they have just been taught. Most patients are referred for physical therapy 5 weeks after their discharge from the hospital.

A Local inflammation occurs after lumbar spine surgery. The body forms scar tissue in response to inflammation. The nerve root may become restricted from the scar tissue as it exits through an opening called the *intervertebral foramen.* Because of the inflammatory process, the nerve also can lose elasticity within itself. Therefore by performing movements that move the nerve within its covering (sheath), the nerve root will not develop adhesions or may free itself from adhesions, which can cause pain, numbness, tingling, and other symptoms.

Phase II

TIME: 6 to 10 weeks after surgery
GOALS: Increased activity, tissue modeling, stabilization, and reconditioning (Table 14-3)

During phase II, patients gradually increase their activity level. While taking account of soft tissue healing, the PT can safely begin to influence the direction of tissue modeling through carefully applied stress. Patients should begin to approximate normal activities while the therapist controls the intensity of movement and exercise.

Patients progressing to the latter portion of phase II increase the intensity of the stabilization program begun in the earlier stages of the phase. They may increase repetitions and level of difficulty. Patients should do 20 minutes of cardiovascular exercise daily and add stabilization exercises for the lumbar paraspinal muscles and the upper back. They can begin a light weight-training program, avoiding exercises that load the lumbar spine. Patients should no longer require assistance with most daily activities. **Common restrictions are no lifting greater than 10 lbs and no overhead lifting.** Examples of exercises for this phase are listed in the following sections.

Evaluation

Before initiating treatment the therapist should assess the physical problems that can be addressed in therapy such as strength, body mechanics, range of motion (ROM), and neuromuscular control; the therapist can then establish goals for treatment. **This evaluation should include ROM for the LEs but *not* for the lumbar spine.** A complete neurologic examination should be performed to establish a baseline and should include neural tension testing. **The therapist can perform strength testing for the LEs with the exception of testing hip flexor strength.** He or she also can check the patient's ability to stabilize or brace the lumbar spine isometrically, which is a test of the patient's ability to recruit the core trunk muscles to control the spine. Core strength testing may be performed in a variety of ways; however, Lee[19] describes a functional approach based on grouping core musculature into "slings." The patient's spontaneous body mechanics and the way the patient responds to the challenge of daily activities should be assessed. The goals of phase II are as follows:

- Consistently good body mechanics for activities of daily living (ADLs)
- Protection of the surgical site from infection and mechanical stress
- Maintenance of nerve root mobility at the involved levels
- Control of pain and inflammation
- Minimization of patient fear and apprehension
- Beginning of a stabilization and reconditioning program
- Maintenance of scar and soft tissue mobility
- Treatment for restrictions of thoracic motion and motion at the hip and LE
- Education to minimize sitting time and maximize walking time

Body Mechanics Training

If body mechanics training was provided preoperatively, then it should be reviewed after surgery. If body mechanics training is new to the patient, then the therapist should go through the entire program, which is as follows:

- In and out of bed (Fig. 14-4)
- In and out of a chair (Fig. 14-5)
- Up and down from the floor (Fig. 14-6)
- Lying postures (Fig. 14-7)
- Sitting (Fig. 14-8)
- Standing
- Dressing
- Bending (Fig. 14-9)
- Reaching
- Pushing and pulling (Fig. 14-10)
- Lifting (Fig. 14-11)
- Carrying (Fig. 14-12)

Patients must perform these activities to get dressed, use the bathroom, travel to doctor's appointments, and shop for and prepare meals. A patient who can do these activities without stressing the surgical site will heal faster and with less discomfort. Patients can accomplish all

Table 14-3 Lumbar Fusion and Laminectomy

Rehabilitation Phase	Criteria to Progress to this Phase	Anticipated Impairments and Functional Limitations	Intervention	Goal	Rationale
Phase II Postoperative 6-10 weeks	Outpatient candidate No signs of infection Cleared by physician to begin therapy	◆ Pain limited with ADLs ◆ Limited nerve root mobility ◆ Limited trunk stability ◆ Limited mobility of regions adjacent to surgical site	◆ Cryotherapy ◆ Relative rest ◆ Review of body mechanics training ◆ Nerve mobilization ◆ Passive range of motion— Lower extremity stretches— Hip flexors (gently initiate after 8 weeks with physician approval) Gluteals Hip rotators Quadriceps Hamstrings Calf ◆ Isometrics with active range of motion— Abdominal bracing with squats, transfers, and gait ◆ Spinal stabilization exercises— Bridging Dying bug (after 8 weeks, with physician approval) Quadruped Superman (after 8 weeks, with physician approval) ◆ Walking program—emphasize “tiny steps” after 8 weeks (with physician approval) ◆ Joint mobilization to upper and midthoracic spine, gentle if mobilizing lower T/S ◆ Soft tissue massage after incision is closed ◆ Patient education ◆ UBE and/or brisk walking	◆ Control pain ◆ Protect surgical site ◆ Improve or maintain nerve root mobility ◆ Improve flexibility of lower extremity musculature ◆ Improve trunk stability strength ◆ Improve walking tolerance ◆ Improve mobility of thoracic spine as indicated ◆ Decrease patient apprehension ◆ Improve cardiovascular conditioning	◆ Self-manage pain ◆ Prevent reinjury ◆ Perform ADLs without adding increased stress to the lumbar spine ◆ Prevent neural adhesions ◆ Improve mobility of lower extremities to decrease stress on the lumbar spine ◆ Initiate trunk stabilization while performing ADLs to decrease potential for reinjury ◆ Perform cardiovascular conditioning and “tiny steps” to avoid excessive lumbar spine movement during gait ◆ Improve mobility of thoracic spine to decrease stress on the lumbar spine ◆ Improve mobility of soft tissue ◆ Reduce volitional muscle guarding ◆ Perform cardiovascular conditioning

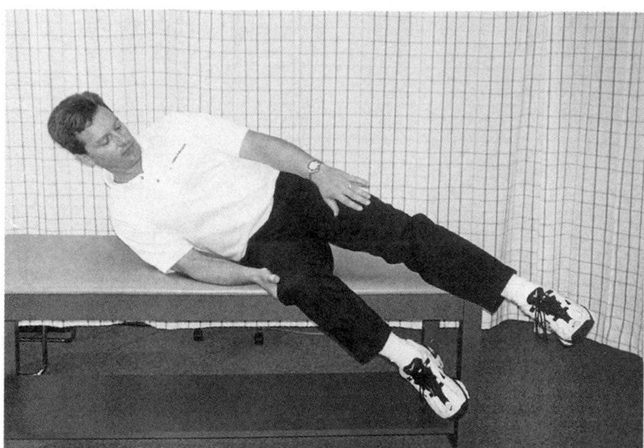

Fig. 14-4 To rise from a lying position, the patient begins with bracing to maintain a neutral spine and rolls to the edge of the bed as a unit. The patient then pivots off the elbow while throwing the legs to the ground. This momentum makes an otherwise difficult movement easier. To avoid twisting the trunk, the patient should reach toward the top foot with the top arm.

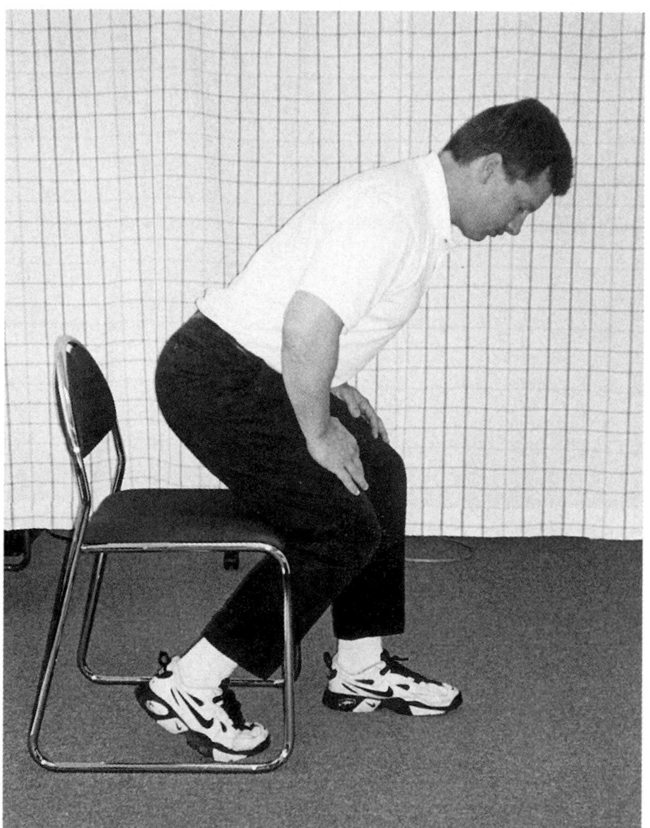

Fig. 14-5 To get out of a chair, the patient places one foot under the chair, hinges the hip, and then raises off the thigh. The hips should be the first to leave the chair and the last to land. The patient should *not* attempt to keep the back vertical, merely straight. To get into the chair the process is reversed. If no room is available to get the foot under the chair, such as in a couch, then the patient pivots on the hips until perpendicular to the chair. This offsets the feet and allows for easier rising.

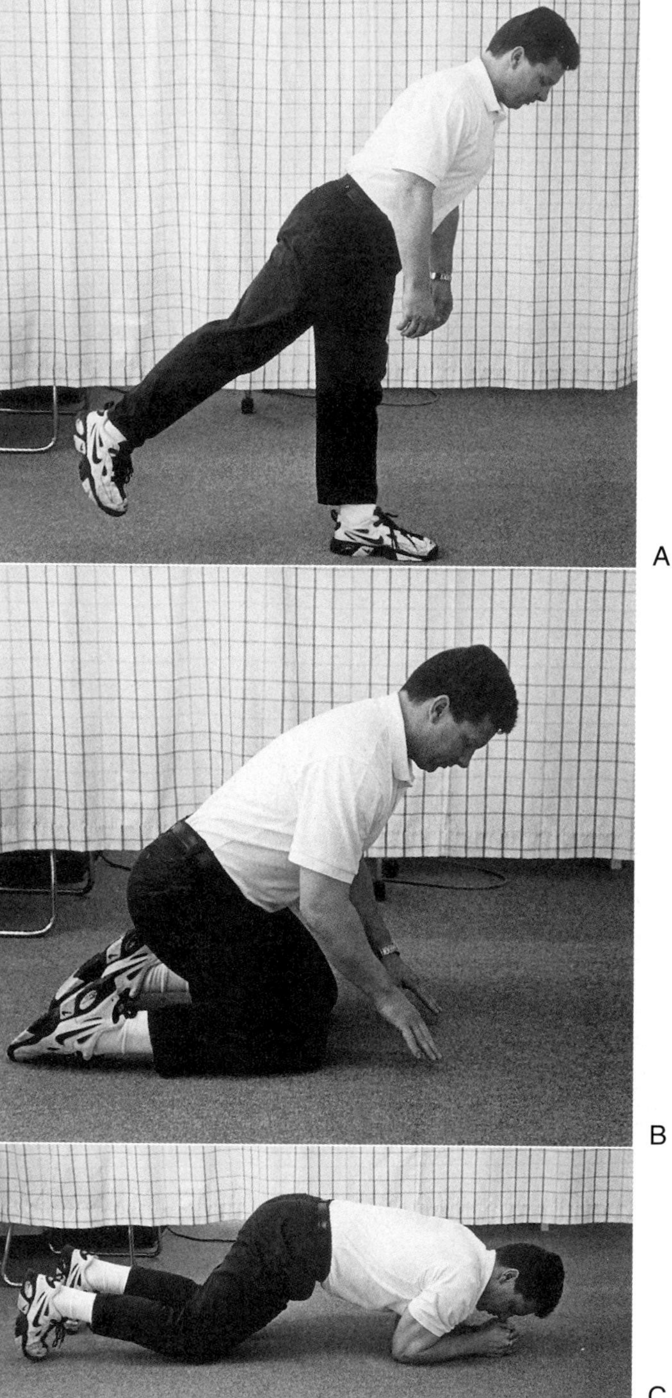

Fig. 14-6 When getting up and down from the floor, the patient moves from a single leg hip hinge (**A**) through a reverse lunge position to double kneeling (**B**). Next, the patient hinges the hips from double kneeling to about 45 degrees. Another balance point occurs here (**C**). From this balance point, the patient rocks forward onto the elbows and rolls as a unit onto the side. To avoid uncontrolled extension, the stomach should never touch the ground. The process is reversed to rise from the ground.

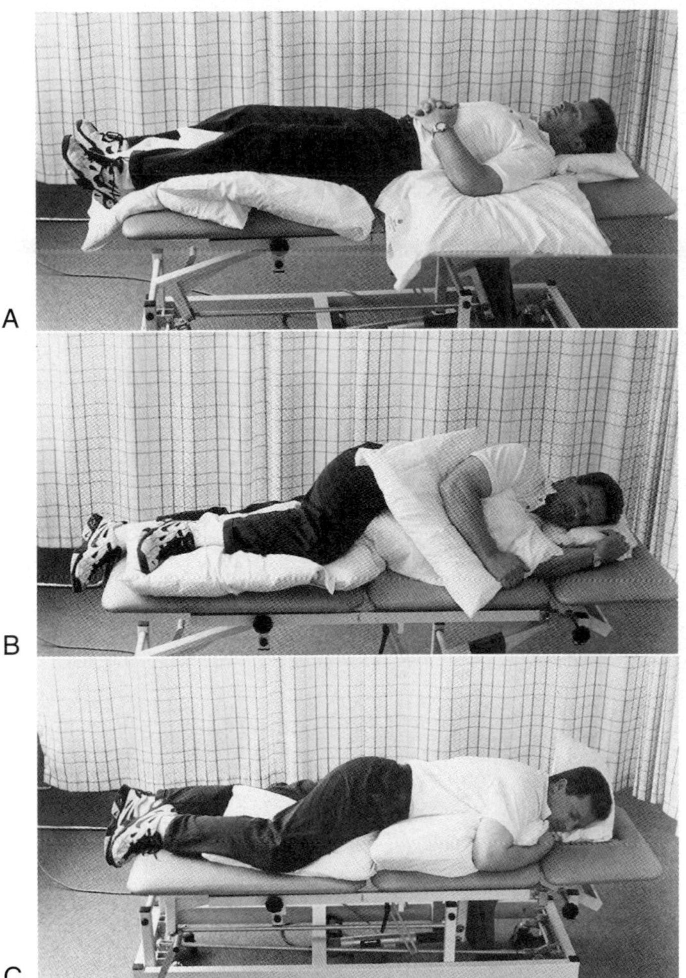

Fig. 14-7 **A**, Supported supine lying. Patients generally prefer to have the whole leg supported rather than just the knees. Any unsupported area becomes uncomfortable and causes the patient to shift and wake. The shoulders also should be supported in whatever degree of protraction exists. Any soft tissue subjected to prolonged stretch eventually becomes uncomfortable. **B**, Supported side lying. The patient needs enough pillows to support the upper extremities (UEs). A body pillow frequently works well. The patient should pull the support directly into the upper thigh and chest and then roll slightly onto it; he or she should not lie on the same side all night. **C**, Three-quarter prone lying is the most popular position. It is similar to supported side lying, except that the patient rolls one-quarter turn more. A wedge-shaped pillow minimizes cervical strain in this position.

these tasks without lumbar motion if they move their hips rather than the spine.

Instead of flexing the lumbar spine, they can "hip hinge" (see Fig. 14-9). Rather than twist in the lumbar spine, they can pivot on another body part (e.g., knees, elbows, hips). When teaching a hip hinge, the PT should point out that the hips should move *back* rather than *down*. After surgery, patients tend to guard and move cautiously. Showing them the way to use their momentum safely in many maneuvers makes the postoperative transition easier. For example, getting out of bed requires less bracing if the legs are moved quickly to the floor, transferring the momentum to the torso (see Fig. 14-4). Outpatient physical therapy begins at this point.

> **Q** Lindsey is 38 years old. She had a lumbar fusion at L4-L5 about 7 weeks ago. She tells her PT that her back pain has been increasing over the past 7 to 10 days. Lindsey has complied with all instructions and restrictions. The PT reviews her chart and exercise program. Over the past 2 weeks, Lindsey has begun doing squats and using the treadmill and the UBE for cardiovascular exercise. She has been stretching her hamstrings, hip flexors, quadriceps, and calf muscles. She also has been doing trunk stabilization exercises in the prone, supine, and quadruped positions. Lindsey also has been strengthening her upper body with biceps curls, seated military presses, and push-ups. Which of these exercises may be aggravating her condition and why?

Nerve root gliding. Patients should extend the knee while lying supine with the spine in a neutral position and the hip flexed to a 90-degree angle. When tension is encountered, the therapist helps the patient work the knee gently back and forth, gradually increasing the ROM. This stretch may cause increased symptoms during the stretch, which should resolve immediately on relaxing. Education should be provided to the patient regarding expected and adverse reactions to neural gliding. **Any lingering symptom is reason to halt the stretch until the therapist can reassess the problem.** Butler[5] describes an excellent approach to evaluation and treatment of neural mobility.

Local inflammation occurs after lumbar spine surgery. Because the body forms scar tissue in response to inflammation, the nerve root can become adherent to the neural foramen or lose elasticity. It is theorized that a nerve root that is kept moving within its sheath cannot develop adhesions.[5,9,29,33] Patients with nonirritable chronic leg symptoms tend to respond well to neural mobilization. However, the patient must keep the spine stabilized while moving the leg.

Decreasing pain and inflammation. Patients should use ice packs for about 20 minutes three or four times per day to help control pain and swelling. Patients can be taught to alternate rest periods with periods of light activity, because sustained postures increase pain and swelling. The therapist may apply modalities in the clinic to control pain after therapy.

Ultrasound should *not* be applied over a healing bony fusion. Patients with severe pain problems can try using a home transcutaneous electrical nerve stimulation (TENS) unit or interferential unit.

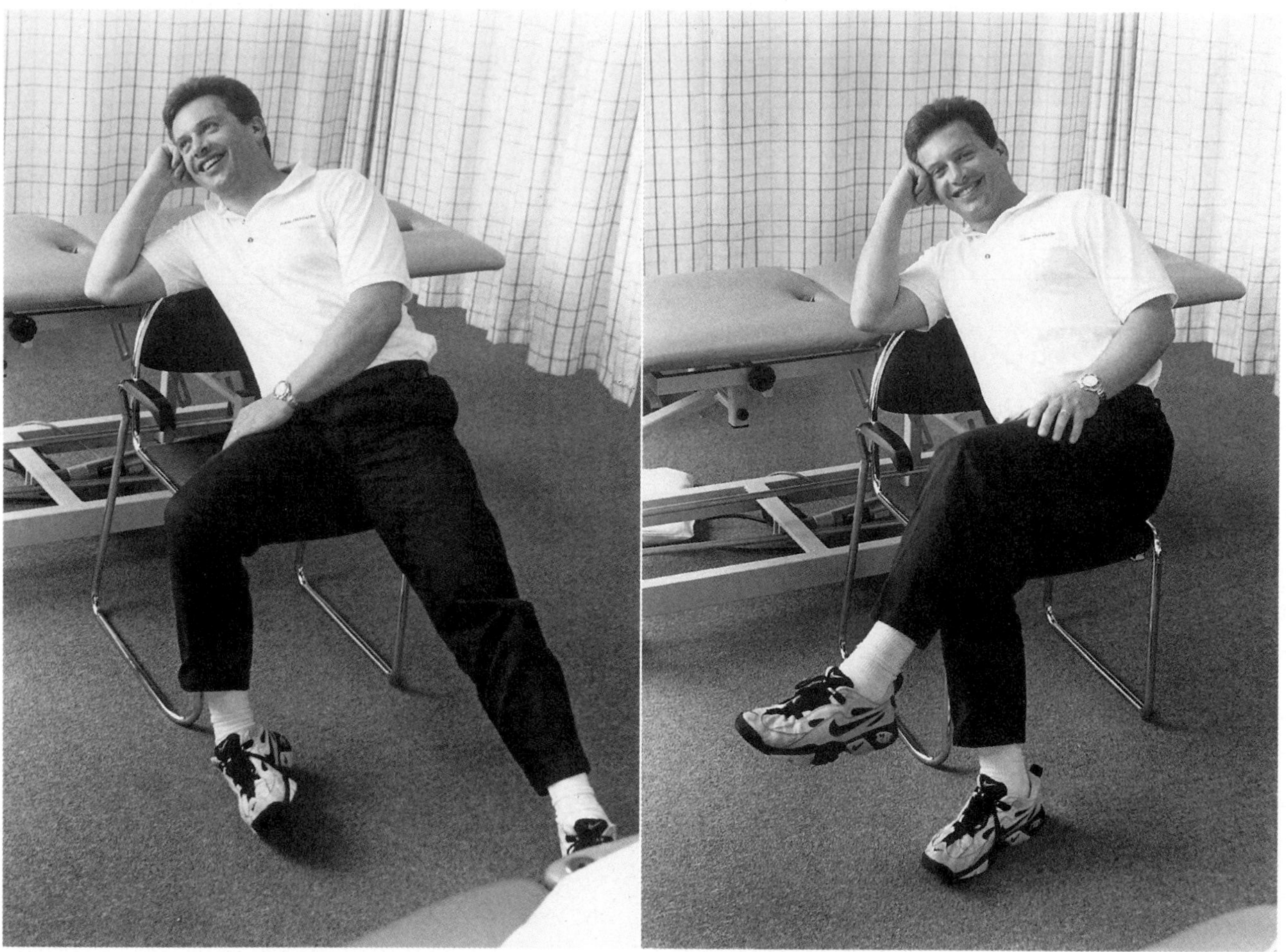

Fig. 14-8 A and B, Alternate sitting postures are important to teach, because patients will want to change sitting postures frequently. As long as a neutral spine position is maintained, the variations are limitless. These positions successfully take the weight off the left pelvis, thereby relieving pressure on the piriformis and sensitive sciatic notch.

If patients know they can control their pain level, they are less fearful of trying activities that may cause a pain flare-up or those that have been painful in the past. They will rely less on inactivity and medication to control pain. Keeping the inflammation to a minimum is important to minimize scarring. The therapist should spend some time initially discovering the patient's fears and alleviating those that are groundless. Not everything has to be accomplished during the first visit. Greater progress will occur in the long run if the therapist initially allays patient fears and teaches the patient ways to control pain. Patients who are sensitive to load bearing through the spine should take frequent short unloading rests throughout the day. Those who cannot tolerate any one position for a length of time can learn to make a circuit of their activities, frequently changing tasks **(avoiding prolonged sustained postures).** Patients with specific position intolerance can benefit from learning ways to avoid that position while doing daily activities. Lumbar rolls are not recommended during this phase, because most patients cannot tolerate pressure on the incision site after surgery.

> **A** Hip flexor stretches should not be initiated until later, when sufficient healing has occurred at the surgical repair area. The iliopsoas originates at the T12-L5 vertebra and intervertebral discs. In addition, exercises such as the military press that load the lumbar spine should be avoided. Finally, all exercises should be executed correctly.

Patient education. Patients should understand the expected postoperative course of events, particularly concerning postoperative pain. Increasing leg pain is not a good sign, even if low back pain diminishes; conversely, decreasing leg symptoms is a good sign, even if low back pain is increasing. Less leg pain is consistent with less neurologic involvement, whereas the low back is expected to be sore because of the incision and altered facet

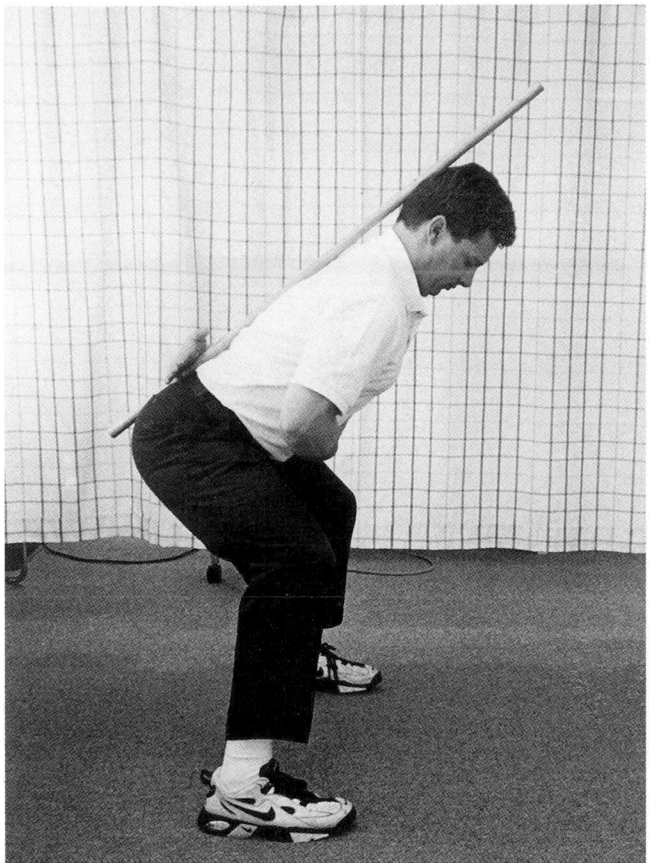

Fig. 14-9 Hip hinging is flexing the hips and knees while maintaining a neutral spine. A dowel can be helpful for patients with difficulty perceiving spinal motion. The spine should *not* be kept vertical but merely straight. This is one of the essential motions patients use to perform functional activities. Hip hinging also can be done on one leg (as in Fig. 14-6, A). This is especially useful when getting up and down from the ground. The position shown is a balance point that patients should learn because it requires little or no effort to maintain. Patients should attempt to move from one balance point to another.

mechanics.[23] Incisional pain can be expected to decrease gradually over 6 to 8 weeks. As patients begin to return to normal activities, an associated increase in muscle soreness frequently occurs. The sooner they recondition themselves, the better they will feel. Patients should be aware that their bodies will be adapting to and remodeling from the surgery for as long as 1 to 2 years. Symptoms often shift and change during that time. The therapist should teach patients to manage flare-ups using ice, rest, and resumption of previous activities within 1 or 2 days.

Patients are generally very fearful after lumbar spine surgery. Anxiety causes increased muscular tension and therefore discomfort. Patients also may be afraid to move, thinking they will somehow disrupt the surgery. Patients can better tolerate flare-ups and variations in their symptoms if they expect them and have been instructed in self-management of these flare-ups. Patients are generally less apprehensive if the therapist is not apprehensive. Most people recover well and should start with that expectation. If the patient appears to be developing neuropathic pain, nerve root signs, symptoms from a new level, or any other complications, then the therapist should note the symptoms calmly and convey the information to the treating surgeon for advice without conveying anxiety to the patient.

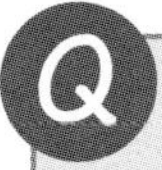

During the initial outpatient treatment, what should be the main focus of the treatment?

Stabilization and reconditioning. The PT should teach patients the following stabilization and reconditioning exercises:

- Bracing
- Squats (see Fig. 13-21)
- Walking

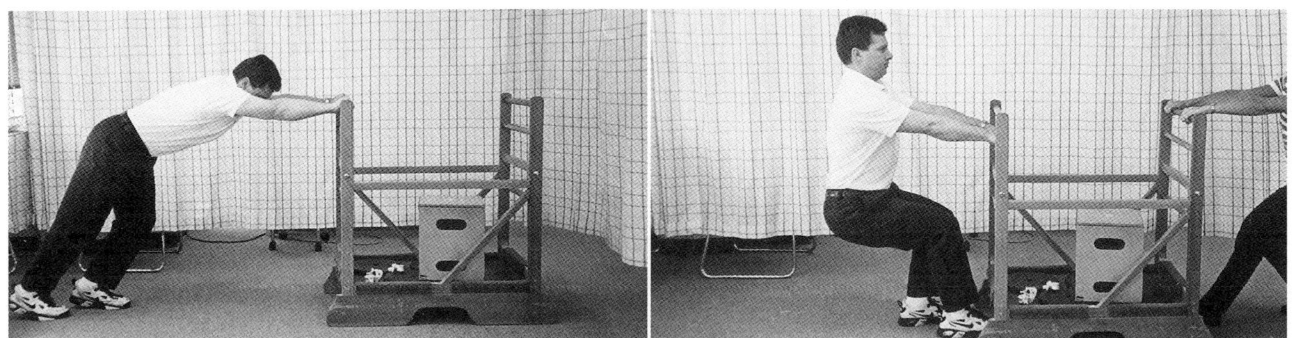

Fig. 14-10 A, To push an object, the patient leans into it with a hip hinge until the body weight begins to move it forward. The heavier the object, the more the patient needs to line the shoulders up behind the hands. Arms can be bent or straight. The patient should take tiny steps, because if the feet move anterior to the hips, then a lumbar flexion moment will occur. B, To pull an object, the patient leans back, maintaining neutral position, until the body weight begins to move the object. The heavier the object, the more the patient needs to flex at the hips and knees. The patient should take tiny steps and hold the upper body erect, because the weight tends to pull the body into flexion.

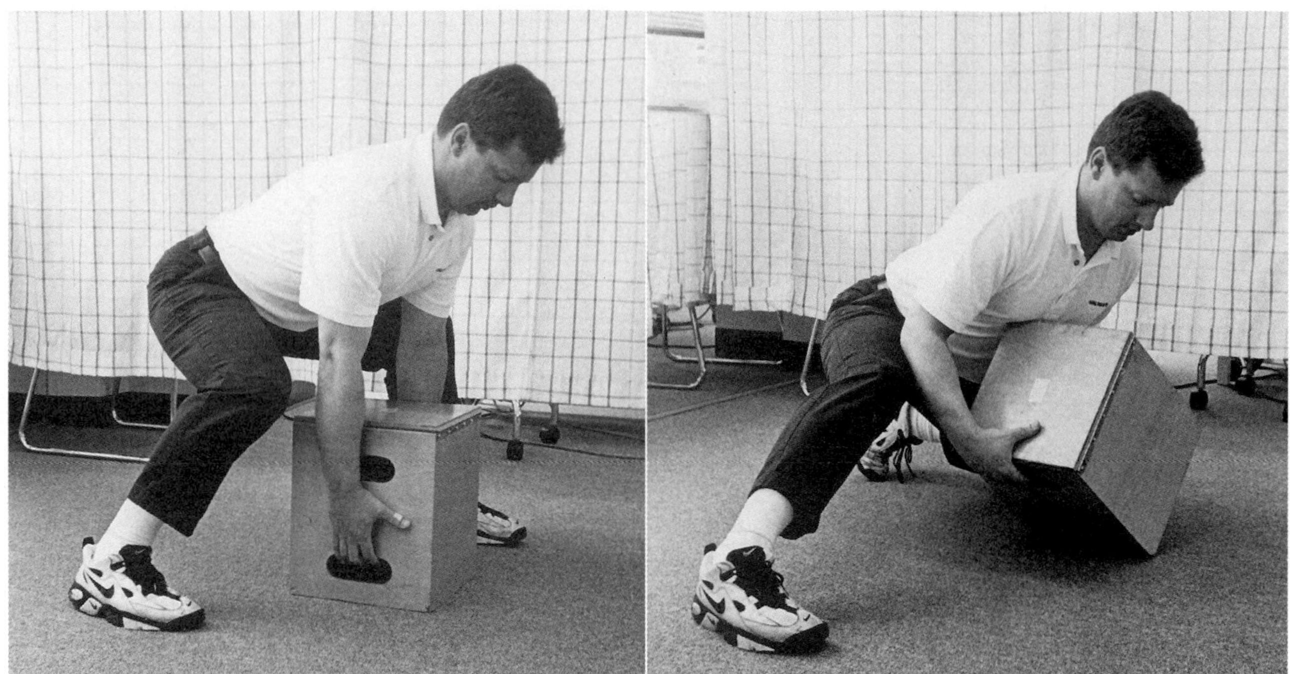

A B

Fig. 14-11 **A,** Lifting from a hip hinge position. The spine remains straight but not vertical. This method works for conveniently placed objects. **B,** To lift a less conveniently placed object safely, the patient goes down onto one knee, then hinges the hips and tilts the object to its maximal height. The patient then locks the object to the chest, reverses the hip hinge, and places the object on the thigh. As the patient stands up, the thigh lifts the majority of the weight.

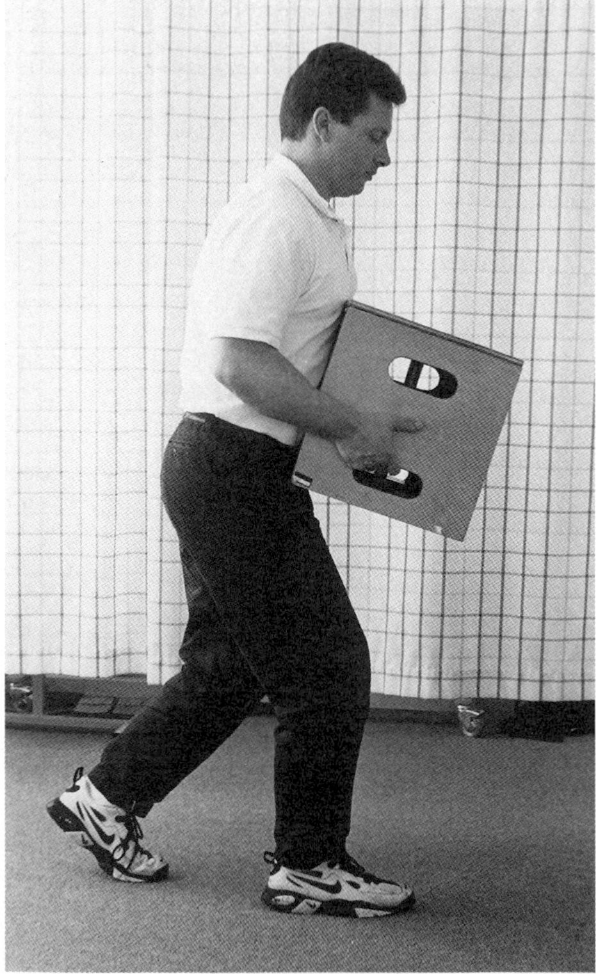

Fig. 14-12 Slight knee flexion reduces the tendency toward lumbar extension while the patient carries objects. It may feel "funny" at first, but with continued practice this flexion becomes simple.

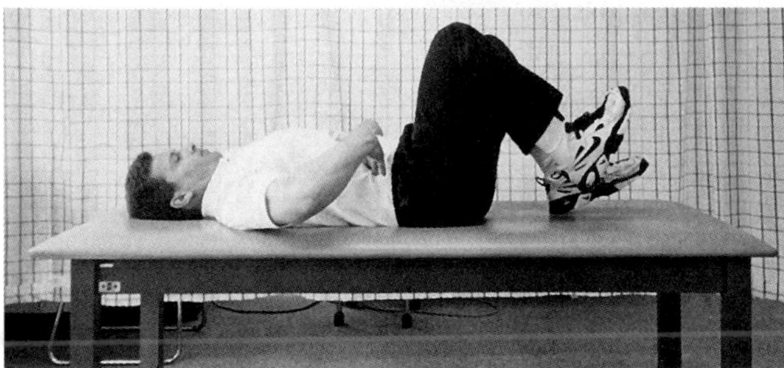

Fig. 14-13 Bracing with tiny steps. The patient creates an abdominal brace by contracting the transverse abdominus, multifidi, and pelvic floor. It is important to remember to move the abdominals without moving the spine. While maintaining the brace, the patient slowly takes the weight off one foot (removing only as much weight from the foot as possible without allowing the hips to rotate or the spine to extend). Eventually the patient should be able to lift the foot an inch off the ground. The patient then alternates feet.

- "Tiny steps," or lower abdominal biased, supported stabilization (initiated after 8 weeks, with physician approval) (Fig. 14-13)
- Cardiovascular reconditioning (using stair climber, brisk walking, and pool exercises when the incision is closed)

Bracing and tiny steps are good exercises to begin strengthening the trunk. Bracing should be taught to include the transverse abdominus, the multifidi, and the pelvic floor muscles.[14,25,32] Patients should perform squats and walking for leg strengthening and conditioning, cardiovascular exercises for cardiovascular conditioning, and overall endurance training for good health.

Maintaining scar and soft tissue mobility. The therapist should use soft tissue techniques to maintain good scar and soft tissue mobility without disrupting the healing of these tissues. Scar tissue tends to contract while healing. This can create a "tight" scar that restricts mobility.[7]

Assessment and treatment for restrictions of thoracic and hip mobility. The following steps will help ease restrictions of the thoracic spine and hip:

- Manual therapy for thoracic motion restrictions
- LE stretches for soft tissue restrictions
- Hamstring stretches (see Fig. 13-19)
- Hip flexor stretches (Fig. 14-14)
- Quadriceps stretches (begin with prone knee flexion before progressing to Fig. 13-20)
- Lumbar flexion stretch (Fig. 14-15)

When initiating this stretch the therapist must not be overly aggressive, obtaining ROM at the expense of compromising the fusion site. Fig. 14-15 demonstrates an ideal ending position for this stretch, which may take several months to obtain.

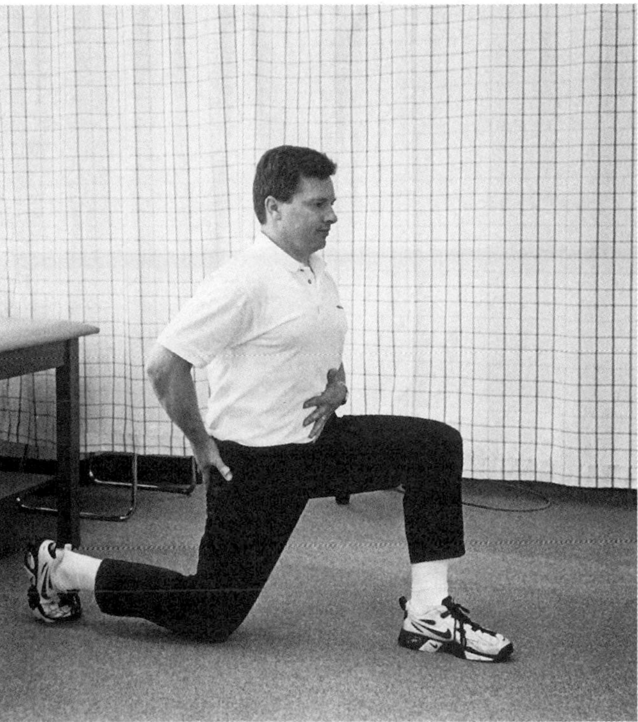

Fig. 14-14 Hip flexor stretch. The patient kneels on one leg with the other leg in front, braces the spine, and gradually begins to shift weight forward to the front foot. The patient should feel a stretch in the groin area of the kneeling leg. The spine should not be extended.

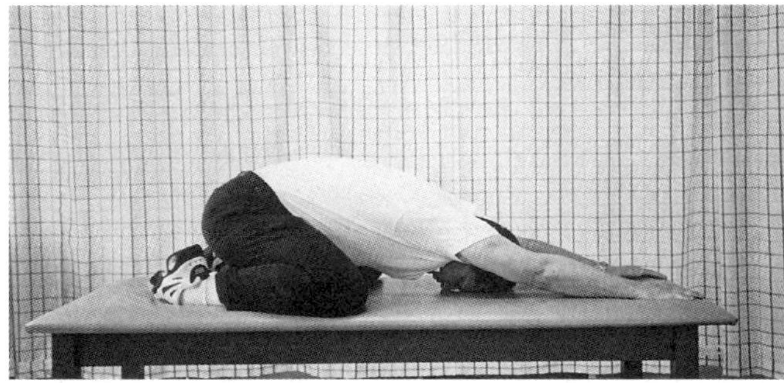

Fig. 14-15 Lumbar flexion stretch. Occasionally when the patient has been working the spinal extensor muscles hard, these muscles may get sore and tight. From an all-fours position, the patient can gradually spread the knees and sit back on the heels, allowing the spine to relax and stretch.

- Up and down from the floor (Fig. 14-16)
- Hip rotator stretches (Fig. 14-17)

The loss of motion caused by the spinal fusion places additional demands for motion on the adjacent segments. One of the most stressful motions in the lumbar spine is rotation, which causes a shearing effect across the disc. The thoracic spine is designed to rotate. Free and easy rotation of the thoracic spine allows this motion to take place in a spinal region better designed to perform this motion. The PT can use manual mobilization techniques

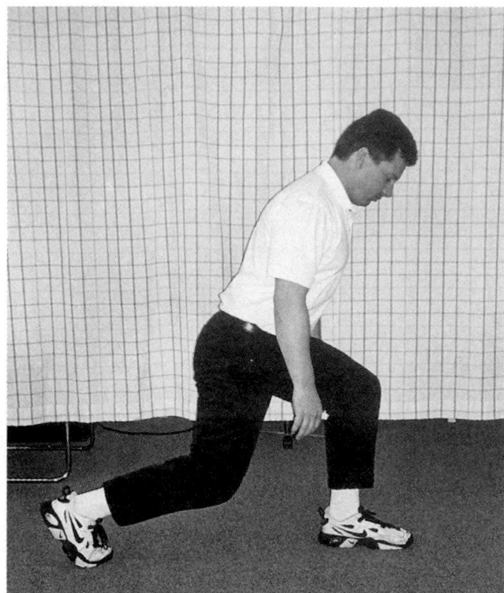

Fig. 14-16 Up and down from the floor. This photo shows the midpoint of getting up or down from the floor.

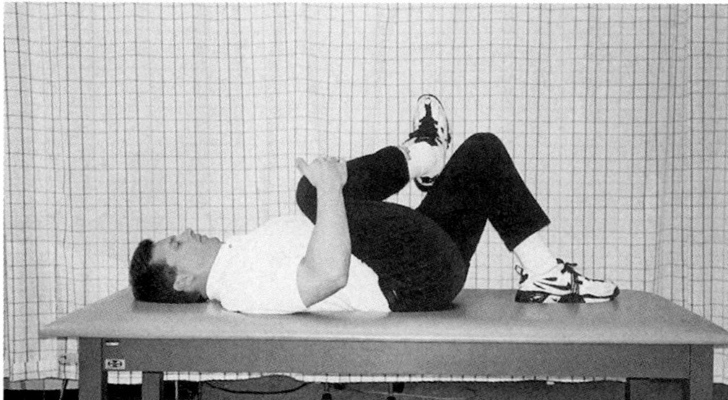

Fig. 14-17 Hip rotator stretch. While lying on the back, the patient crosses the ankle of one leg over the knee of the other leg. The patient performs the stretch by pulling the knee and ankle toward the chest. The patient should feel a stretch deep in the back of the hip.

to increase thoracic spine mobility. Many different approaches to spinal mobilization exist. One can reference Maitland,[22] Mulligan,[24] and Paris[28] for some examples. PTs can teach patients to use two tennis balls taped together to form a fulcrum that can lie over a segment of the thoracic spine and localize motion to the segment above, thus maintaining good segmental mobility of the thoracic spine at home. This can be done in a standing, or later (when appropriate), in a semireclined position for the upper and midthoracic spine.

The hip joint is a large ball-and-socket joint with free motion in all planes. This joint can compensate for the lack of motion in the lumbar spine and should remain as flexible as possible. This can be achieved with stretching of the hip musculature. *Stretching throughout phase II should be very gentle and only pushed to the point the patient can brace to prevent lumbar motion.* Because these muscles attach directly to the lumbar spine or pelvis, the patient should review the principles of stretching. To stretch a muscle, one end must be fixed by something while the other end is pulled away from the fixed end. If patients are not stabilizing the spine while stretching the hips, then they will invariably pull on the lumbar spine, jeopardizing the fusion. All stretching should involve stabilizing one area while pulling against it with another. Iliopsoas stretching is initiated in a later phase. The aggressiveness of any hip stretching is dictated by the patient's ability to control the spine while stretching. **In addition, any stretches that pull on the lumbar spine or healing soft tissues should be avoided until adequate healing has occurred.**

Examples of exercises (performed while bracing) initiated in the later stages of phase II include the following:

- Bridging (see Fig. 13-17)
- Dying bug (see Fig. 13-15)
- Squats (see Fig. 13-21)
- Quadruped with arm and leg raise (see Fig. 13-18)
- Heel lifts
- Superman (avoiding lumbar extension)
- Lateral pulls (light resistance)
- Seated upright rowing machine
- Scapular depression (avoid resisting more than 40% of body weight)
- Push-ups standing and leaning into the wall
- Stair climber
- Upper body ergometer (UBE)
- Brisk walking

A callus is forming at this stage, and patients are expected to tolerate slowly increasing their activity level and returning to normal activities. What the therapist is attempting to develop at this stage is not so much muscle power as kinesthetic sense for the muscles and their role in protecting the spine. Therefore the proper form of each exercise should be emphasized. Muscles learn to do what they are taught. The PT should ensure that the patient is bracing *inward* with the abdominals. If the patient has trouble moving the abdominals without moving the spine, then he or she should get on all fours, find a neutral position for the spine, keep it there, and practice dropping and lifting the stomach without moving the spine. The lifted contractions felt in this position form the brace that is needed to stabilize the spine. The patient can then return to a supine position and practice. When the patient can do this properly, he or she should be able to palpate a contraction of the transverse abdominus and the pelvic floor. Patients generally find they have much less endurance with this brace and need to concentrate to maintain it. This brace is used to stabilize the spine throughout all activities, so patients must learn to grade the contraction. Often they will attempt to give an "all-or-nothing" brace, but they should attempt to brace only as strongly as needed to stabilize the spine during activity. Some activities are easy and some are difficult. For example, the amount of strength required to hold up a feather differs significantly from that used to hold a 5-lb weight, and the body automatically adjusts the degree of contraction of the hand muscles to fit the load.

A

The patient needs to be educated to protect the surgery site and allow for a better recovery with less discomfort. The patient is vulnerable to irritation; good body mechanics and proper posture will help protect the surgery site and allow for a quicker recovery. The therapist must take care to avoid any testing that may irritate the condition. Lumbar spine ROM testing and strength testing of the hip flexors are some examples of testing that must be avoided.

Q

Because anxiety is a key factor in pain perception, how can the therapist decrease the patient's pain levels?

Phase III

TIME: 11 to 19 weeks after surgery
GOALS: Return to work, advance of exercise program, specific skills program, weight program (Table 14-4)

During phase III, patients whose jobs are sedentary or light often begin to return to work, although often on a modified schedule or to modified duties. They begin to establish a routine home maintenance program. Body mechanics are becoming a habit. The exercise program is advancing and approaching its final version. Pain is minimal. Partial and diagonal sit-ups should be added. **Patients should do these without any lumbar rotation or flexion.** The early development of these muscles in their role as spinal stabilizers rather than spinal movers is a crucial component of this phase. After 12 weeks, dips can be added as appropriate. Trunk stabilization exercises begun in phase II are progressed to include more repetitions or to increase in difficulty. Isotonic exercises using weights also may be increased with repetitions or resistance.

At this phase the PT is helping to recondition the patient to the expected level of function, while protecting the spine. The body adapts to the stresses placed on it. The therapist applies stress carefully to the body, in doses that the spine can tolerate, to increase the body's ability to withstand stress. While putting the patient through a conditioning program, he or she should monitor closely for the ability to make a brace that prevents rather than creates motion and modify the program to the patient's sensitivities. **Load-sensitive patients need to avoid overhead lifting for a longer time and should be taught ways to unload the spine while exercising; they may do better in a pool.** Patients with a poor tolerance for any one position do better on a circuit-training program. Exercises should simulate as closely as possible the tasks the patient expects to do.

A

Besides patient education in body mechanics and postures, the therapist needs to increase the patient's awareness of pain expectations. The patient needs to allow 6 to 8 weeks for the incision area to decrease in pain. Increased activity levels at home or in the clinic are associated with an increase in muscle soreness, which can be expected. The therapist should reassure patients that their bodies will be adapting to and remodeling for 1 to 2 years, and symptoms often change during that time. Patients also need to know how to self-manage flare-ups and that most people recover well (they should have that expectation).

Why are stabilization exercises so important for rehabilitating these patients?

Phase IV

TIME: 20 weeks to 1 year after surgery
GOALS: Restore preinjury status, continue home program of conditioning and stabilization (Table 14-5)

During phase IV the body finishes remodeling and adapting to the changes induced during and after surgery. Patients should be fully restored to their preinjury level of function and be independent in caring for the spine. The same programs they have been following in therapy now become home programs of cardiovascular conditioning, stabilization exercises, and hip and thoracic spine stretching. They have a good grasp of body mechanics for everything they need to do. The exercise program has been well outlined in earlier phases. Patients should be able to problem solve unusual situations to determine correct mechanics and manage mild flare-ups independently, knowing which symptoms require professional help.

The bone continues to remodel and adapt to the fusion for as long as 1 year. Patients with fusions frequently develop problems at the level above or below the fusion. For both of these reasons, the patient should learn that spinal care is now a lifetime habit and must be maintained with regular exercise and good mechanics during all daily

Table 14-4 Lumbar Fusion and Laminectomy

Rehabilitation Phase	Criteria to Progress to this Phase	Anticipated Impairments and Functional Limitations	Intervention	Goal	Rationale
Phase III Postoperative 11-19 weeks	No increase in pain Improved tolerance to upright postures	◆ Mild pain ◆ Limited tolerance to upright positions (sit/stand) ◆ Limited trunk, lower extremity, and upper extremity strength	Continue intervention from phase II as indicated ◆ Partial sit-ups (no diagonal movement) ◆ Isometrics with active range of motion— Abdominal bracing with the following: Bridging Dying bug Quadruped with arm and leg raise Heel lifts Superman (avoiding lumbar spine extension) Scapular depressions Push-ups ◆ Progressive resistance exercises— Lateral pull-downs Seated upright/Rows Triceps dips ◆ Cardiovascular conditioning Stair stepper UBE Brisk walking	◆ Independent with most ADLs ◆ Increased trunk and extremity strength ◆ Maintenance of neutral spine while performing strengthening exercises ◆ Performance of 20 minutes of cardiovascular exercise daily	◆ Promote return to independent lifestyle ◆ Develop kinesthetic sense for the muscles and their role in protecting the spine ◆ Improve the ability to brace the spine and maintain a neutral position ◆ Increase strength of trunk and extremities to avoid excess stress on the spine ◆ Start weight training to begin hypertrophy of associate musculature ◆ Promote good cardiovascular fitness

activities (not just those the patient perceives as stressful). Some patients who enjoy exercise prefer extensive exercise programs, but many patients like to keep a minimal program for maintenance. The best home program is one the patient actually does. A realistic home program provides the best chance of consistent follow-through.

Patients returning to a more strenuous job or sports are developing the extra degree of strength and skill to do so. They begin agility drills specific to their sport or job, such as running, cutting, and jumping (see Figs. 13-23 to 13-26). A more comprehensive weight program is established, again geared to the specific activity faced by the patient. The program may require a greater focus on power, endurance, or skill, depending on the activity. Patients should work on maintaining control of a neutral spine during job- or sport-specific challenges during this phase, and the PT should obtain the clearance of the surgeon to begin working on these higher-level activities. The patient must demonstrate good trunk strength and control and good LE strength and flexibility before initiating agility drills.

A certain number of patients can be expected to stop progressing at any stage of rehabilitation. The PT should notify the physician if a patient stops making measurable progress at any stage and, if possible, provide a reason for the lack of progress. Is the patient pain inhibited? Is he or she not making a consistent effort? If the physician determines that no further medical treatment is indicated, then possible recommendations include a functional capacity evaluation, work conditioning or work hardening,

Table 14-5 Lumbar Fusion and Laminectomy

Rehabilitation Phase	Criteria to Progress to this Phase	Anticipated Impairments and Functional Limitations	Intervention	Goal	Rationale
Phase IV Postoperative 20 weeks-1 year	No increase in pain No loss in functional status Patient has decreased reliance on formal therapy Clearance from physician for progression to phase IV	◆ Limited trunk and extremity strength ◆ Limited tolerance to sustained postures ◆ Mild pain associated with activities ◆ Limited with lifting and carrying	Continue exercises from previous phases as indicated ◆ Advance exercises with regard to repetitions and weight ◆ For appropriate patients, initiate running, cutting, and jumping progression. This would not be indicated in a majority of lumbar fusion patients. ◆ Specific activity drills related to home, work, or sport environment ◆ Functional capacity evaluation ◆ Continue progression of interventions in phases II through IV ◆ Progress home exercises ◆ Continue patient education with regard to activity modification and performance with assistive device	◆ Return to work ◆ Increase trunk and extremity strength ◆ Increase muscular endurance ◆ Prepare to return to more strenuous activities ◆ Return to previous level of activity as appropriate ◆ Discharge patient to self-management of flare-ups ◆ Improve trunk strength to previous levels of functioning	◆ Patients with sedentary jobs should be able to resume their schedule ◆ Continue reconditioning to an expected level of function while protecting the spine ◆ Carefully apply stress to the body in tolerable doses to increase the spine's ability to withstand stress ◆ Evaluate the ability to return to previous function ◆ Because patients with lumbar spine fusion may continue to have problems with joints above and below the fusion site, continuation of some level of maintenance must be emphasized ◆ Fusion patients must also maintain constant body awareness, always using proper body mechanics

or a pain management program. Although all therapists would like to relieve pain, some suffering is beyond the ability of current medical science to remove. This is a difficult concept, and patients can be unwilling to accept it. Therapists should make every effort to help patients accept this reality and learn to care for themselves without seeking constant medical intervention. Most people can manage chronic pain and maintain a high functional level despite the pain.

A The most common lumbar spine fusion involves a posterolateral fusion. The paraspinal muscles including the multifidi are stripped off the posterior elements (i.e., spinous process, lamina, transverse processes). This allows for partial tears of the dorsal division of the spinal nerves, therefore having partial denervation of the multifidi. Multifidi are the primary segmental stabilizers, and they do not spontaneously

Continued

recover after low back pain or back surgery. The transverse abdominus is another important muscle that may be cut during a fusion surgery. Trunk stabilization exercises are important for re-educating the multifidi muscles and the other trunk- stabilizing musculature.

SUGGESTED HOME MAINTENANCE FOR THE POSTSURGICAL PATIENT

An exercise program has been outlined at the various phases. The home maintenance on page 289 outlines the rehabilitation the patient may follow. The PT can use it in customizing a patient-specific program.

SUGGESTED HOME MAINTENANCE FOR THE POSTSURGICAL PATIENT

Days 1-5

GOALS FOR THE PERIOD: Educate patient about simple movements, teach nerve mobilization and home care principles

1. Gentle nerve gliding
2. Walking daily as tolerated (should slowly increase in time and speed)
3. Consistent use of proper body mechanics
4. Icing as needed
5. Protection of incision

Weeks 6-10

GOALS FOR THE PERIOD: Educate patient about simple movements, teach neural mobilization and home care principles

1. Progress walking tolerance to 20 to 30 minutes
2. Begin low-level, isometric stabilization
   a. Bracing
   b. Gluteal squeezes
   c. Heel lifts
   d. Ankle pumps to heel lifts
   e. Wall slides (to approximately 135 degrees of knee flexion)
3. Reinforce body mechanics
4. Continue neural mobilization
5. Begin stretching hips and legs, bracing spine in neutral
   a. Hamstrings
   b. Quadriceps
   c. Gluteals
   d. Calves (gastrocnemius and soleus)
   e. Adductors
   f. Piriformis
   g. Hip flexors (initiate after 8 weeks, with physician approval)

Weeks 11-19

GOALS FOR THE PERIOD: Increase activity, emphasize tissue modeling, stabilization, reconditioning, weight programs, and return to work

1. Progress walking tolerance to 30 to 60 minutes daily
2. Increase aggressiveness of stabilization program slowly and to patient's tolerance
   a. Partial sit-ups (no lumbar motion)
   b. Bridging
   c. Dying bug
   d. Squats (to 90 degrees of knee flexion)
   e. Quadruped
   f. Heel lifts
   g. Superman (no lumbar extension)
   h. Push-ups
3. Continue to maintain nerve root mobility
4. After 11 weeks patient can use seated upright rowing machine
5. After 12 weeks patient may add the following exercises:
   a. Latissimus pulls
   b. Scapular depressions
   c. Dips
6. Continue cardiovascular training using the following:
   a. Stair climber
   b. Brisk walking

Week 20 and beyond

GOALS FOR THE PERIOD: Restore preinjury status, continue home program of conditioning and stabilization

1. Progress stabilization program to level required by patient's activity level
2. Continue to work on hip and leg flexibility
3. Develop gym program for independent maintenance of strength, using the following:
   a. Cardiovascular exercise
   b. Stabilization exercises
   c. Latissimus pulls
   d. Seated rowing
   e. Scapular depression
   f. Inclined leg press
   g. Stretches for hips and legs
4. Begin sport- or work-specific activity

References

1. Akuthota V, Nadler SF: Core strengthening, *Arch Phys Med Rehabil* 85(3 suppl 1):S86-92, 2004.
2. Albee FH: A report of bone transplantation and osteoplasty in the treatment of Pott's disease of the spine, *N Y J Med* 95:469, 1912.
3. Biemborn D, Morrissey M: A review of the literature related to trunk muscle performance, *Spine* 13(6):655, 1988.
4. Bourcher HH: A method of spinal fusion, *J Bone Joint Surg* 41B:248, 1959.
5. Butler SD: *Mobilization of the nervous system,* ed 4, Melbourne, 1994, Churchill Livingstone.
6. Crock HV: Anterior lumbar interbody fusion: Indications for its use and notes on surgical technique, *Clin Orthop* 165:157, 1982.
7. Cyriax J: *Textbook of orthopedic medicine: Diagnosis of soft tissue lesions,* vol 1, ed 6, Baltimore, 1975, Williams and Wilkins.
8. Gibson A: A modified technique for spinal fusion, *Surg Gynecol Obstet* 53:365, 1931.
9. Grabiner M, Koh T, Ghazawi AF: Decoupling of bilateral paraspinal excitation in subjects with low back pain, *Spine* 17(10):1219, 1992.
10. Hasue M: Pain and the nerve root, *Spine* 18(14):2053, 1993.
11. Hibbs RA: An operation for Pott's disease of the spine, *JAMA* 59:133, 1912.
12. Hides JA, Richardson CA, Jull GA: Multifidus muscle recovery is not automatic after resolution of acute, first-episode low back pain, *Spine* 21(23):2763-2769, 1996.
13. Hodges PW: Core stability exercise in chronic low back pain, *Orthop Clin North Am* 34(2):245-254, 2003.
14. Hodges PW, Richardson CA: Contraction of the abdominal muscles associated with movement of the lower limb, *Phys Ther* 77:132, 1997.
15. Hodges PW et al: Intervertebral stiffness of the spine is increased by evoked contraction of transverse abdominis and the diaphragm: In vivo porcine studies, *Spine* 28(23)2594-2601, 2003.
16. Kawaguchi Y, Matsui H, Tsuji H: Back muscle injury after posterior lumbar spine surgery, *Spine* 19:2598, 1994.
17. Kirkaldy-Willis WH, Burton CV: *Managing low back pain,* ed 3, New York, 1992, Churchill Livingstone.
18. Knapp DR, Jones ET: Use of cortical cancellous allograft for posterior fusion, *Clin Orthop* 229:99, 1988.
19. Lee D: *The pelvic girdle,* ed 2, Edinburgh, UK, 1999, Churchill Livingstone.
20. Lonstein JE: Use of bank bone for spinal fusions, *Proc Scoliosis Res Soc,* 1984.
21. Lorenz M et al: A comparison of single level fusions with and without hardware, *Spine* 16(8)(suppl):455, 1991.
22. Maitland GD: *Vertebral manipulation,* ed 5, London, 1986, Butterworths.
23. McKenzie RA: *The lumbar spine, mechanical diagnosis and therapy,* Upper Hutt, New Zealand, 1990, Wright and Carman Limited.
24. Mulligan BR: *Manual therapy "NAGS", "SNAGS", "MWMS" etc,* ed 3, Wellington, New Zealand, 1995, Plane View Services.
25. Neumann P, Gill V: Pelvic floor and abdominal muscle interaction: EMG activity and intra-abdominal pressure, *Int Urogynecol J Pelvic Floor Dysfunct* 13(2):125-132, 2002.
26. O'Sullivan P, Twomey L, Allison G: Dysfunction of the neuromuscular system in the presence of low back pain-implications for physical therapy management, *J Man Manip Ther* 5(1):20, 1997.
27. Panjabi M: The stabilizing system of the spine. II. Neutral zone and instability hypothesis, *J Spinal Disord* 5:390, 1992.
28. Paris SV: Mobilization of the spine, *Phys Ther* 49:988, 1979.
29. Rantanen J et al: The stabilizing system of the spine. II. Neutral zone and instability hypothesis, *J Spinal Disord* 5(4):390, 1992.
30. Richardson CA, Jull GA: Concepts of assessment and rehabilitation for active lumbar stability. In Boyling, Palastanga N, editors: *Grieves modern manual therapy: The vertebral column,* ed 2, Edinburgh, 1994, Churchill Livingstone.
31. Richardson C et al: Therapeutic exercise for spinal segmental stabilization in low back pain: Scientific basis and clinical approach, 2000.
32. Sapsford RR, et al: Co-activation of the abdominal and pelvic floor muscles during voluntary exercises. Neurourol Urodyn 2001;20(1):31-42.
33. Shacklock M: Neurodynamics, *Physiother* 81(1):9, 1995.
34. Sihvonen T et al: Local denervation atrophy of paraspinal muscles in postoperative failed back syndrome, *Spine* 18:575, 1993.
35. Smith SA et al: Straight leg raising: Anatomical effects on the spinal nerve root with and without fusion, *Spine* 18(8):992, 1993.
36. Steffee A et al: Segmental spine plates with pedicle screw fixation: A new internal fixation device for disorders of the lumbar and thoracolumbar spine, *Clin Orthop* 203:203, 1986.
37. Trammell TR et al: Luque interpeduncular segmental fixation of the lumbosacral spine, *Orthop Rev* 20:57, 1991.
38. Waddell G: A new clinical model for the treatment of low back pain, *Spine* 12(7):633, 1987.
39. Watkins MB: Posterolateral bone-grafting for fusion of the lumbar and lumbosacral spine, *J Bone Joint Surg* 41A:388, 1959.
40. Weatherly CR, Prickett CF, O'Brien JP: Discogenic pain persisting despite solid posterior fusion, *J Bone Joint Surg Br* 68(1):142, 1986.
41. West JL, Bradford DS, Ogilvie JW: Results of spinal arthrodesis with pedicle screw-plate fixation, *J Bone Joint Surg* 73A:1179, 1991.
42. White A:*Spine* 18:575, 1994.
43. White AH, Schofferman JA: *Spine care: Diagnosis and conservative treatment,* vol 1, St Louis, 1995, Mosby.
44. Wiltse LL et al: The paraspinalis splitting approach to the lumbar spine, *J Bone Joint Surg* 50A:919, 1968.

PART 4

LOWER EXTREMITY

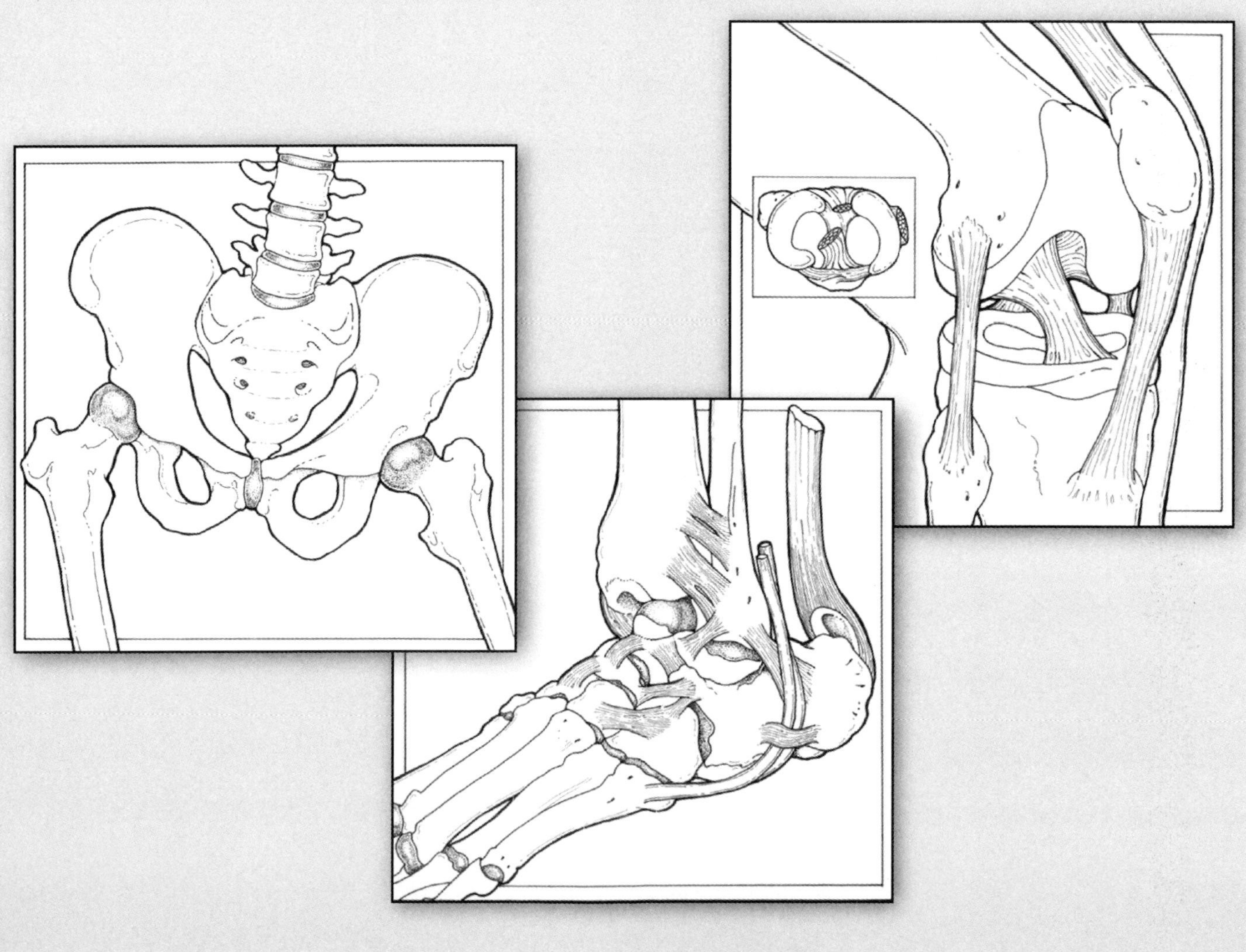

CHAPTER 15

Total Hip Arthroplasty

Edward Pratt
Patricia A. Gray

Each year in the United States approximately 80,000 to 130,000 patients undergo a total hip replacement (THR)[16] procedure hoping to eradicate persistent pain and improve their functional status. The majority of these people have failed to find relief from their symptoms with conservative medical intervention.

SURGICAL INDICATIONS AND CONSIDERATIONS

THR is used to correct intractable damage resulting from osteoarthritis (OA), rheumatoid arthritis, avascular necrosis, and the abnormal muscle tone caused by cerebral palsy.[12] Nonelective THR procedures are performed for fractures in which open reduction internal fixation (ORIF) is deemed inappropriate.

Contraindications for THR surgery include inadequate bone mass, inadequate periarticular support, serious medical risk factors, signs of infection, and lack of patient motivation to observe precautions and follow through with rehabilitation. Surgery also is contraindicated if it is unlikely to increase the patient's functional level.[12]

The prostheses used currently have a projected life span of less than 20 years. Therefore candidates for THR are usually more than 60 years old. Younger patients elect this surgery when their functional status is severely compromised and their pain becomes intolerable. In the case of a fracture, younger patients are treated with an ORIF whenever practical. Given the projected lifespan of current prostheses, younger THR candidates may require a revision surgery later in life.

THR predictably improves function and reduces pain in virtually all patients with disabling disease. Patient satisfaction (with a rating of *very good* or *excellent*) regarding pain relief and improvement of function has been measured as high as 98% at 2 years after THR. The long-term survivability rate has been reported as high as 87.3% to 96.5% at 15 years.[15,34,35]

SURGICAL PROCEDURES

In its essence, THR consists of two parts. First, the remaining arthritic bone and articular cartilage is reamed from the acetabular cup, and a new metal cup with a polyethylene plastic inner liner is press fit into place. Second, the arthritic femoral head is removed and replaced by a femoral head and stem component that is secured into the medullary canal of the proximal femur (Figs. 15-1 through 15-3).

Q Monica had a minimally invasive THR. How will the rehabilitation process change because her procedure was less invasive?

Several aspects of the procedure greatly affect the course of postoperative rehabilitation. First, two approaches are commonly used, each with its own risks and advantages. Second, controversy still exists as to whether it is better to cement or press fit the femoral stem into position.[22] Noncemented implants tend to be more expensive and technically demanding to implant; however, they are easier to revise when they fail. It is not yet clear which technique produces the most durable hip replacement. However, it is generally accepted that noncemented implants are best suited for younger, more active patients and more complicated revisions.[1] Recently, resurfacing arthroplasty has been recommended for young patients with avascular necrosis, because it preserves bone for later conversion to THR if necessary because of implant failure or pain. Many surgeons believe that noncemented femoral components should not have weight borne on them for 6 weeks, whereas cemented femoral components can support weight immediately after surgery. This has been contested recently, and many surgeons now allow patients with noncemented hips to bear weight from the outset.[33] Both approaches have in common the creation of instability around the hip during the early postoperative period. The release of muscle, bone, and joint capsule during accessing of the joint renders the hip vulnerable to dislocation at its extreme ranges of motion (ROM). Patient education of

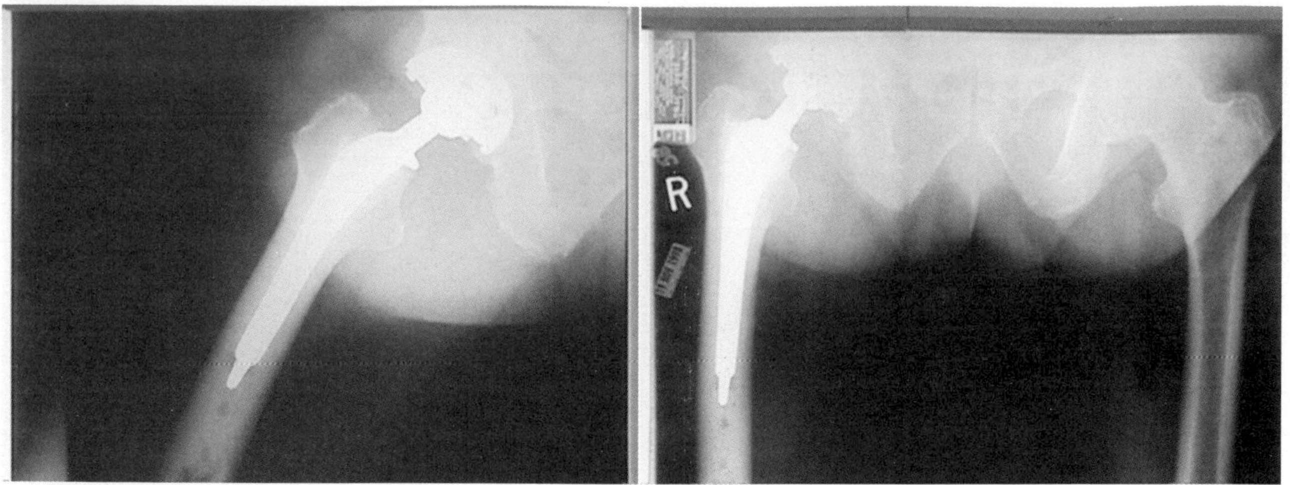

Fig. 15-1 Hybrid cemented total hip arthroplasty.
(Biomet Integral Design, Warsaw, IN.)

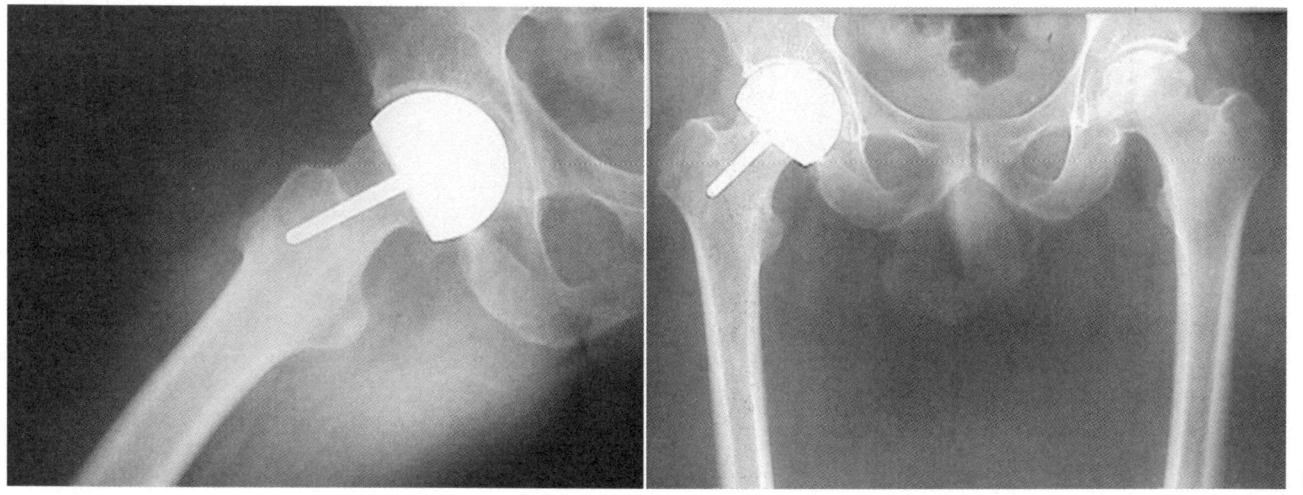

Fig. 15-2 Resurfacing arthroplasty for avascular necrosis.
(Wright Medical Design, Memphis, TN.)

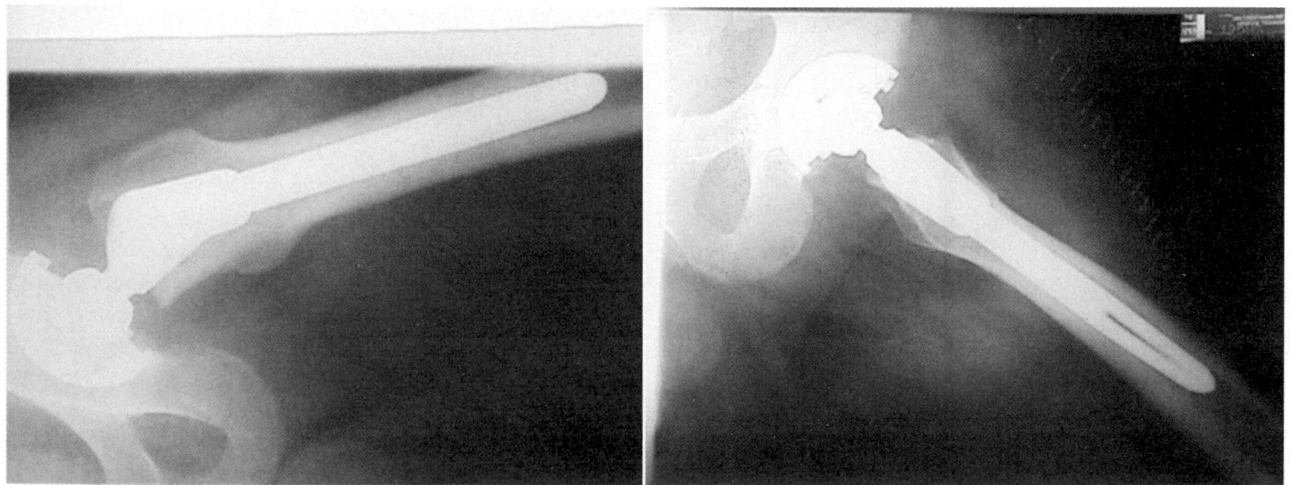

Fig. 15-3 Noncemented modular total hip arthroplasty.
(Biomet Impact Design, Warsaw, IN.)

"hip precautions" becomes extremely important during early convalescence and is alluded to later in this chapter. Controversy remains as to which approach provides the lowest postoperative dislocation rate, the shortest operative time, and the least blood loss.[2] Because of problems with trochanteric nonunion and long-term abductor weakness, the original transtrochanteric approach (in which the greater trochanter or the gluteus medius is completely released) is used most often today in revision surgery. Its main advantage lies in an excellent view of the proximal femoral shaft. The two exposures discussed in the following paragraphs are the posterolateral approach (Gibson) and the anterolateral approach (Watson-Jones).

A Pain and swelling will be less because the trauma to soft tissue is less. The procedure is performed using a smaller opening. This may allow the patient to progress with bed mobility and transfers more quickly and with greater ease and comfort. The surgeon will determine weight-bearing status and rehabilitation progression. However, the hip precautions remain and the rehabilitation is usually similar (because the procedure is similar but performed with a smaller opening and in a smaller area). New materials such as metal-on-metal implants or ceramic implants are starting to be used. It is hoped that these prosthetic hips will have a longer life span.

Posterolateral Approach

The posterolateral approach accesses the hip in the interval between the gluteus maximus and medius. The capsule and short external rotators are released, and the hip is dislocated posteriorly. In extremely large or contracted patients, the surgeon must occasionally release the gluteus maximus and even the adductor magnus at their femoral insertions to translate the proximal femur anteriorly, gaining acetabular exposure. This exposure places traction on the gluteus maximus, medius, and tensor fascia lata. Care must be taken not to place traction on the sciatic nerve or the superior gluteal nerve and artery, which may cause nerve palsy. Repair of the posterior capsule and short external rotators remains controversial, although several recent reports suggest decreased rates of posterior dislocation and heterotopic bone formation when this is done. The posterolateral approach is the author's personal preference for THR, because it preserves the gluteus medius and minimus, as well as the vastus lateralis, making rehabilitation of these muscle groups easier. It also provides for a quicker normalization of gait in the postoperative period, although this is personal surgeon preference and may be disputed by surgeons who prefer the anterolateral approach.

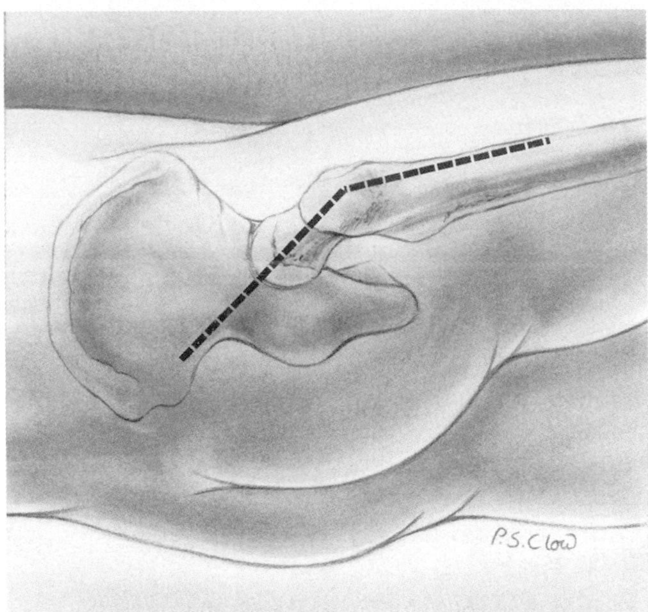

Fig. 15-4 The incision for a posterior approach is centered over the greater trochanter, the distal limb being straight and the proximal limb curved posteriorly.
(From Cameron HU: *The technique of total hip arthroplasty,* St Louis, 1992, Mosby.)

The patient is placed in the lateral decubitus position with the affected hip up; the entire limb is washed, prepared, and surgically draped. The incision is begun 4 to 5 inches superior and medial to the top of the greater trochanter (Fig. 15-4). The line of incision runs down to the greater trochanter, then 3 or 4 inches along the course of the posterior femur. The skin and subcutaneous tissues are incised, and the deep fascia is exposed and divided in line with the skin incision (Fig. 15-5). After mobilizing the fascia, the surgeon inserts a large, self-retaining retractor to hold the fascia apart. The sciatic nerve is then either exposed or palpated to ensure that it is not being stretched or traumatized (Fig. 15-6). The posterior border of the gluteus medius is identified, as well as the interval between the gluteus minimus and piriformis as they pass into the posterior greater trochanter. This interval is developed and a retractor placed around the medius and minimus as they are pulled anteriorly. The remainder of the posterior structures is released from the posterior femoral neck and intertrochanteric line, including the piriformis, obturator internus, superior and inferior gemelli, and the superior half of the quadratus femoris (Fig. 15-7). The surgeon releases the posterior hip capsule with the short external rotators, allowing them to retract together (Fig. 15-8). This decreased dissection around the crucial nervous plane under the inferior border of the piriformis leaves a stronger posterior cuff of tissue to repair at the end of the procedure. The limb is next measured for its length between the ilium and greater trochanter, and the hip is

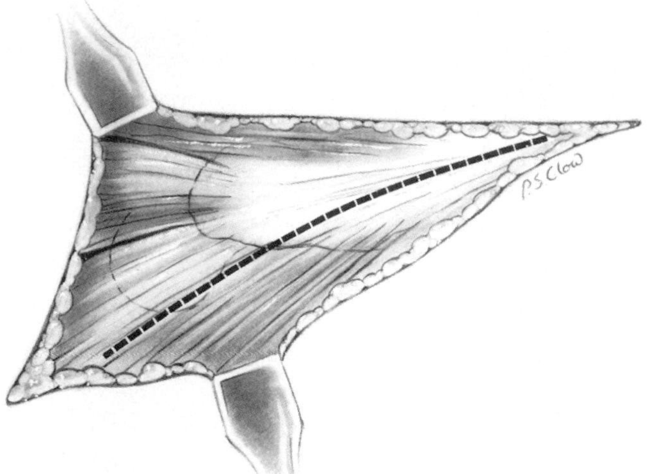

Fig. 15-5 The fascia lata is split in line with the skin incision, and the gluteus maximus is split proximally.
(From Cameron HU: *The technique of total hip arthroplasty,* St Louis, 1992, Mosby.)

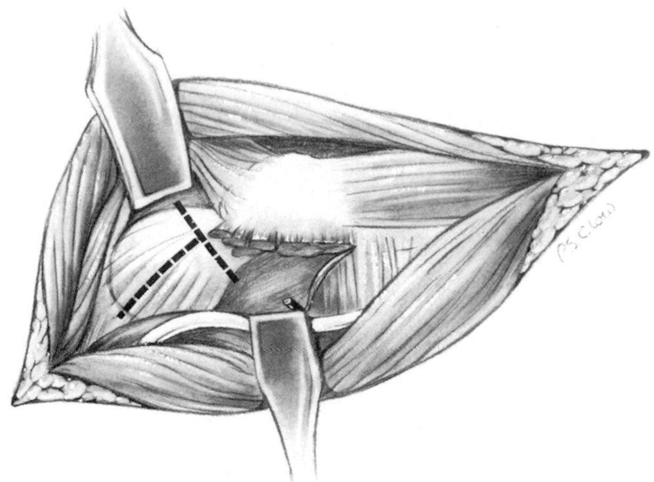

Fig. 15-7 The short external rotators are divided. When the upper part of the quadratus is released, brisk bleeding usually ensues from the medial circumflex femoral artery.
(From Cameron HU: *The technique of total hip arthroplasty,* St Louis, 1992, Mosby.)

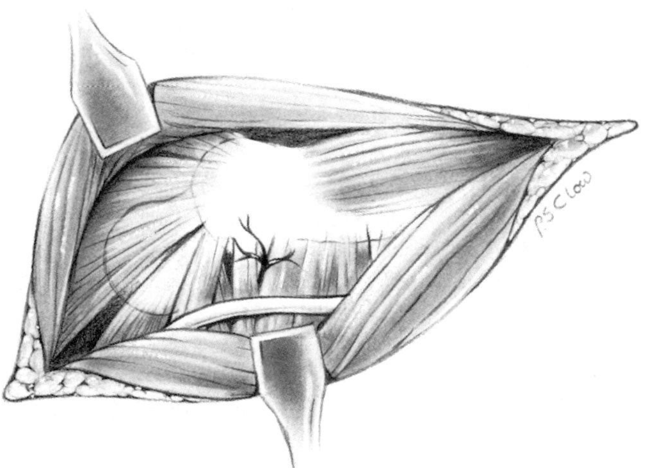

Fig. 15-6 The short external rotators are exposed by blunt dissection. The sciatic nerve lies superficial to the external rotators.
(From Cameron HU: *The technique of total hip arthroplasty,* St Louis, 1992, Mosby.)

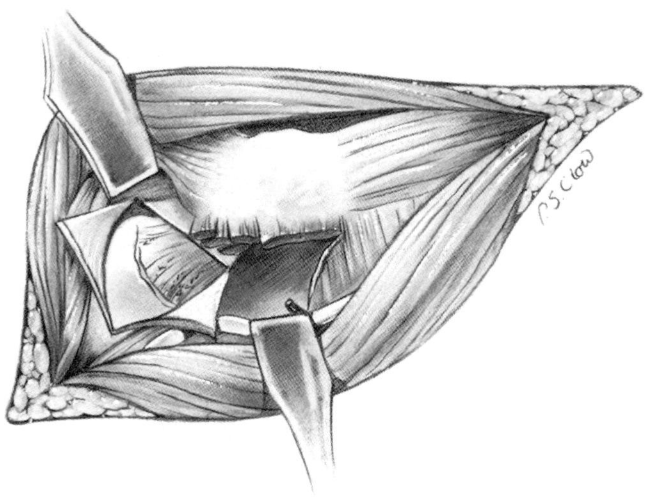

Fig. 15-8 Retraction now exposes the hip joint capsule.
(From Cameron HU: *The technique of total hip arthroplasty,* St Louis, 1992, Mosby.)

posteriorly dislocated. A reciprocating saw is used to cut through the femoral neck, and the arthritic femoral head is delivered from the field. The hip annulus is débrided sharply, and a minimal anterior capsulotomy is performed to help mobilize the proximal femur. As mentioned previously, the surgeon must sometimes go back and release the gluteus maximus, adductor longus, and occasionally even the adductor magnus from the proximal femur so that it can be translated anteriorly. A cobra retractor is placed under the femur and over the front edge of the acetabulum, allowing the femur to be levered anteriorly out of the way of the acetabulum. The acetabulum is then reamed and the acetabular component inserted.

The clinician begins femoral preparation by placing a large retractor under the femur and levering it out of the wound. The surgeon then reams the femoral shaft, increasing the reamer size by 2 mm each pass until good bony contact is made. The intertrochanteric area is then broached or rasped in the same manner until good proximal fill of the femur is obtained. A provisional head is applied, and the joint is placed back together and ranged to check for stability and length. At this stage a stable hip should allow 80 to 90 degrees of flexion, 60 to 80 degrees of internal rotation (IR), and 20 to 30 degrees of external rotation (ER) while being held in neutral abduction. After this the surgeon press fits or cements the implant in place and begins closure. Many surgeons prefer repair of the capsule and short external rotators as a single cuff of tissue held by large No. 2 nonabsorbable sutures through drill holes in the bone. The gluteus maximus and hip adductors are repaired if they were released, and the deep fascia is repaired again with nonabsorbable suture. After closure of subcutaneous tissue and skin, the patient is placed in a triangular-shaped pillow that holds the hip in approximately 30 degrees of abduction. The pillow straps should not be tightened to the point that they compress the common peroneal nerve.

Rehabilitation begins as soon as the patient is coherent. Ankle pumps, quadriceps sets, and leg lifts help reestablish the distal venous circulation, minimizing the risk of thromboembolic disease (TED) and helping with postoperative edema. Standing, sitting, and walking can be started on the first day after surgery if hip precautions are followed carefully.

Anterolateral Approach

The anterolateral approach has been popularized by Smith-Peterson[29] as providing better visibility without the risk of posterior dislocation associated with the posterolateral approach. It avoids the need for postoperative abduction pillows and can allow the patient greater freedom of movement during the initial postoperative period, because hip precautions become less crucial. Because of the reported decreased incidence of posterior dislocation, the anterolateral approach is sometimes preferred in patients who have suffered strokes or those who have cerebral palsy and therefore have a significant muscle imbalance or spasticity that induces flexion and IR of the hip. This approach has been associated with a greater incidence of heterotopic bone formation, greater blood loss, and longer operative times. However, individual surgical expertise seems to have a greater influence on these variables than the exposure chosen.[26,32]

The anterolateral approach uses the interval between the gluteus medius and tensor fascia lata. The superior gluteal nerve near the ilium innervates both of these muscles. Injury to this nerve can result in a partial or complete abductor paralysis that can vary from a temporary neurapraxia to complete and permanent paralysis. In addition, the femoral nerve can be injured through over-retraction of soft tissues in the front of the hip, leaving significant quadriceps weakness. This approach preserves the short external rotators of the hip and prevents direct exposure of the sciatic nerve. The tissues violated include the gluteus medius and minimus, the tensor fascia lata, the vastus lateralis, the referred head of the rectus femoris, the anterior hip capsule, and the iliopsoas tendon.

The patient is placed in the lateral decubitus position with the affected hip up (Fig. 15-9, A); a lateral incision is made with a slight anterior curvature in its proximal aspect. After dividing the subcutaneous tissue, the surgeon incises the lateral fascia and finds and develops the interval between the gluteus medius and the tensor fascia lata (Figs. 15-9, B, and 15-10). The surgeon must be careful not to extend the incision too far proximally, or the investing nerve of both muscles (the superior gluteal nerve) can be injured, resulting in paralysis of the tensor. The vastus lateralis origin is often dissected off its vastus ridge origin to access the anterior hip capsule fully. The capsule is then bluntly released from the front of the femoral neck to gain access to the hip joint itself (Fig. 15-11). The last deep layer of exposure requires the release of the anterior aspect of the gluteus medius off the greater trochanter and the reflection of the rectus femoris off the anterior acetabulum (Fig. 15-12). The gluteus release can be done either through the tendon or through trochanteric

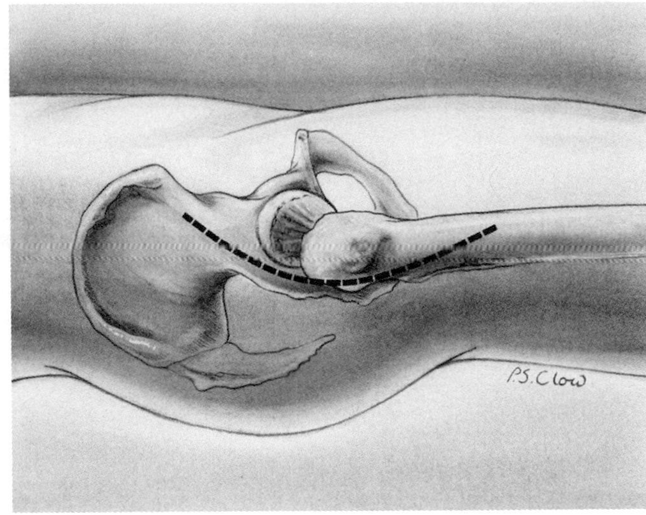

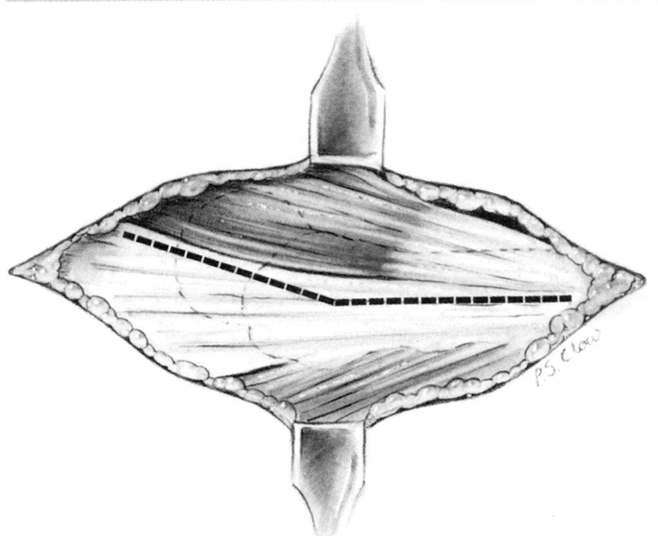

Fig. 15-9 **A**, The skin incision is roughly *C*-shaped and centered over the back of the greater trochanter. **B**, The fascia lata is divided over the summit of the greater trochanter.
(From Cameron HU: *The technique of total hip arthroplasty,* St Louis, 1992, Mosby.)

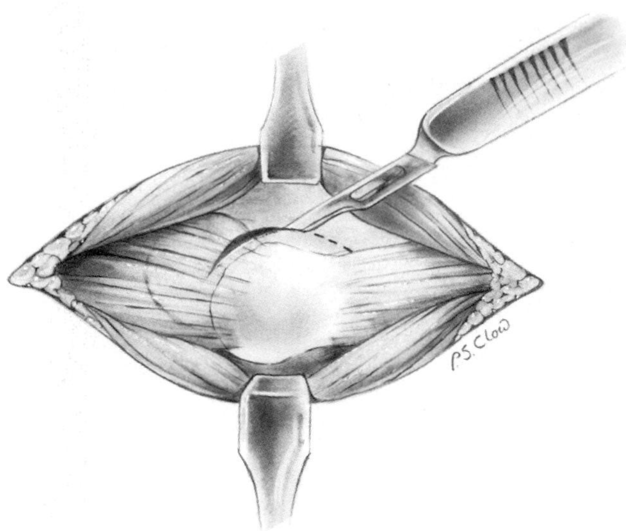

Fig. 15-10 The anterior fibers of the gluteus medius are released from the greater trochanter. The muscle incision is not extended proximally.
(From Cameron HU: *The technique of total hip arthroplasty,* St Louis, 1992, Mosby.)

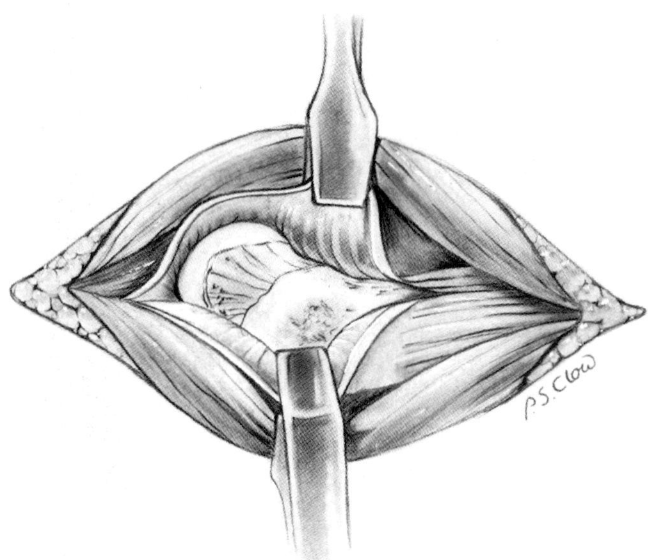

Fig. 15-11 An anterior capsulectomy is carried out with a blunt Homan retractor above and below the femoral neck and a medium Homan retractor placed on the pelvic brim.
(From Cameron HU: *The technique of total hip arthroplasty,* St Louis, 1992, Mosby.)

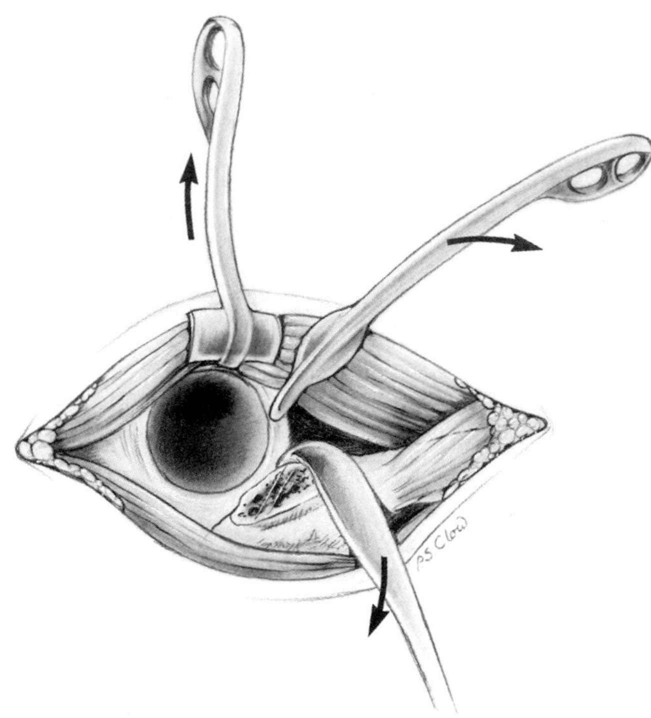

Fig. 15-12 The acetabulum is exposed with a medium Homan retractor on the pelvic brim, a long sharp Homan retractor inferiorly, and a bent Homan retractor posteriorly levering down on the stump of the femoral neck.
(From Cameron HU: *The technique of total hip arthroplasty,* St Louis, 1992, Mosby.)

osteotomy (although trochanteric osteotomy has fallen out of favor to some extent because of the incidence of nonunion). After the gluteus release the hip can be dislocated anteriorly and joint replacement begun much as in the posterolateral approach.

ER and flexion must be avoided postoperatively to prevent dislocation. Hip range of motion (ROM) precautions remain important, especially during the first 6 weeks. Normalization of gait via abductor and quadriceps strengthening remains the focus during early rehabilitation. Pool exercise appears to be extremely helpful in this regard.

Generally a walker or crutches is required for 3 weeks after THR. A cane is used for an additional 3 weeks before unassisted walking is allowed. This varies depending on the age and preoperative condition of the patient. Driving and a return to sedentary activities may be allowed at 3 weeks, and some of the hip precautions can be relaxed at 6 weeks. Improvement in strength and ROM can be expected for as long as 6 months with a motivated patient.

THERAPY GUIDELINES FOR REHABILITATION

The following text can be used as a guideline of rehabilitation after a THR. Flexibility on the part of the therapist is essential, because individual surgeons may impose their own protocols.

The therapist's role is crucial at the postsurgical stage. Santavista's study[27] showed that the majority of patients recovering from a THR report receiving most of their information regarding the recovery phase from physical therapists. Patients depend on their therapists for encouragement and advice. The therapist should set the patients' expectations toward independence and wellness early in this process and prepare them to anticipate a unique recovery progression. Comparisons with other patients should be avoided.

Phase I (Preoperative Training Session)

TIME: a few days before surgery

GOALS: To educate the patient regarding THR precautions with transfers and movements and help patient become independent in exercises for the postoperative phases of recovery

Many institutions have initiated preoperative THR training sessions with the intention of increasing patients' confidence and reducing the length of their hospital stays. These sessions may take place in the physical therapy department or in the patient's home through a home care agency's physical therapist. Educational videos are becoming popular as an adjunct tool.

The preoperative session generally includes an assessment of the patient's strength (including upper-extremity [UE] potential), ROM, neurologic status, vital signs, endurance, functional level, and safety awareness. Any existing edema, contractures, and leg length discrepancies should be noted at this time, as well as knowledge of the patient's scar healing ability.[25] If the evaluation takes place in the patient's home, then the status of stairways and the need for equipment and safety adaptations (e.g., moving furniture and electrical cords) should be evaluated.

Instruction in THR precautions should begin during the preoperative session and be repeated throughout the rehabilitation process.

The precautions after a posterolateral approach to THR prohibit flexion of the hip past 90 degrees, adduction past the body's midline, and IR of the hip. After an anterolateral THR, the patient should observe these precautions and avoid ER (especially with flexion). A review of proper body mechanics for safe functional mobility at home, along with appropriate postoperative sleeping and sitting positions, should accompany the precautions training.

The therapist must teach transitional movements for safe transfer techniques. The proper use of assistive devices such as walkers and crutches according to the patient's projected weight-bearing status follows. **A nonweight-bearing order may be given if the prosthesis is noncemented. Strict adherence to ROM and weight-bearing precautions should be emphasized throughout the entire rehabilitation process.**

Postoperative exercises can be taught at this time. These exercises may include the following:

- Ankle pumps (Fig. 15-13)
- Quadriceps sets
- Gluteal sets
- Active hip and knee flexion (heel slides) while maintaining hip ROM within the physician's recommended guidelines for the surgical technique performed
- Isometric hip abduction
- Active hip abduction

The patient should not perform hip abduction if a trochanteric osteotomy was performed. Dislocation of the THR prosthesis is possible if inappropriate stresses are placed on the new joint. Because the surgical cement is dry and attains its greatest strength within 10 to 20 minutes of its application, it is not a factor in dislocation although many patients worry about it. The integrity of the hip's joint capsule is disrupted by surgery. Movement beyond the limitations of the THR precautions places too much strain on the compromised joint capsule. This is the most frequent cause of postsurgical dislocation. This knowledge may assist in motivating the patient to adhere to his or her precautions and the strengthening program.

Traditional THR exercise programs have become controversial in recent years. The contact pressures on the hip joint during specific activities have been measured and compared with pressures on the hip during gait.

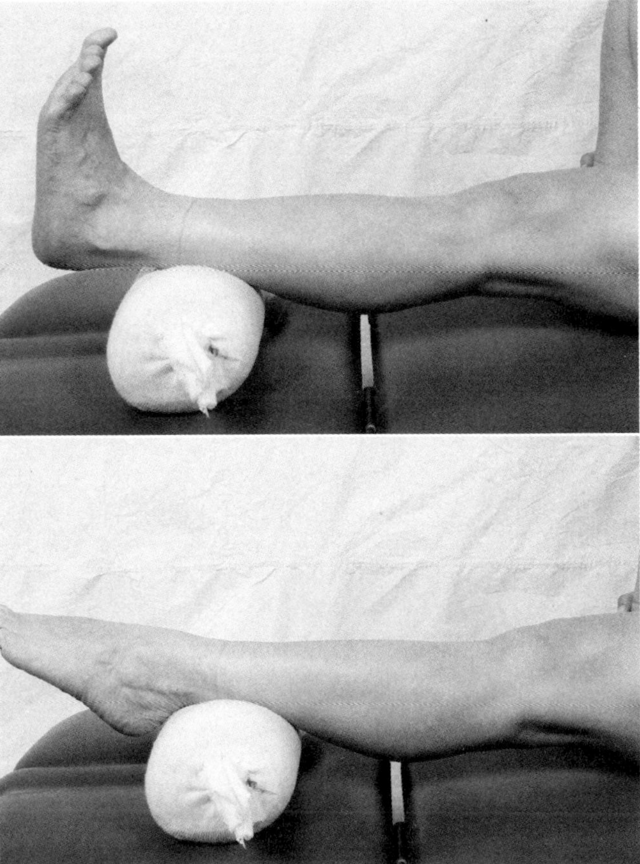

Fig. 15-13 Ankle pumps. The patient lies supine with both knees straight and pumps the feet up and down as far as possible.

Although some practitioners dispute the methodology used, the results of these studies have caused many to question the prescription of some of the standard THR exercises.

Enloe's consensus group[8] eliminated the straight leg raise (SLR) from their "ideal" THR rehabilitation plan, because Strickland and colleagues[31] found that it created greater stresses than the amount incurred at the hip during normal unsupported gait. Lewis and Knortz[19] found that SLRs should be initiated when the patient has regained partial +/or full weight bearing. Gilbert believes that SLRs are unnecessary and may cause dislocation; he warns therapists against using them.[9]

Strickland found that active hip flexion and isometric hip extension produced the greatest stresses on the joint. Based on these findings, Lewis and the consensus group recommend performing gluteal sets at submaximal levels of contraction to avoid the possibility of dislocation.

Givens-Heiss and colleagues[10] found that a maximal isometric hip abduction contraction generated greater peak pressures than both the SLR and unsupported gait.

The Krebs study[19] also found that maximal contraction during exercise generated greater pressures at the hip than did gait. Lewis and Knortz[19] recommend that isometric hip abduction be done at submaximal levels based on the results of these studies and suggests slow, supine hip abduction as an alternative.

Phase IIa (Hospital Phase)

TIME: 1 to 2 days after surgery
GOALS: To prevent complications, increase muscle contraction and control of involved leg, help patient sit for 30 minutes, continuously reinforce THR precautions

Day of Surgery

Postoperative physical therapy (Table 15-1) may begin on the day of surgery when the patient regains consciousness. The patient will be resting in the supine position and wearing TED hose with the legs abducted and strapped to a triangular foam cushion. To avoid damage

Table 15-1 Total Hip Replacement

Rehabilitation Phase	Criteria to Progress to this Phase	Anticipated Impairments and Functional Limitations	Intervention	Goal	Rationale
Phase IIa Postoperative 1-2 days	◆ Postoperative (inpatient) ◆ No signs of infection ◆ Medically stable	◆ Pain ◆ Immobilized postoperatively in bed with abduction pillow ◆ Limited respiratory exchange	◆ Adjust abduction pillow ankle straps ◆ Order foot cradle ◆ Provide patient education regarding total hip precautions ◆ Isometrics—Quadriceps sets, gluteal sets ◆ AROM—Ankle pumps ◆ Encourage use of cough and incentive spirometer On the second postoperative day, begin the following: ◆ Bed mobility training ◆ Transfer training ◆ Gait training (weight bearing per physician's orders) as appropriate	Avoid the following: ◆ Peripheral nerve damage ◆ Heel ulcers ◆ Dislocations of prosthesis ◆ Pooling of fluid in legs ◆ Fluid build-up in lungs ◆ Improve volitional control of involved leg ◆ Initiate mobility training ◆ Sit up in chair 30 minutes ◆ Maintain precautions while performing mobility activities	◆ Decrease strap pressure on legs ◆ Decrease prolonged, unchecked pressure against heels ◆ Prevent excessive stresses on hip ◆ Promote distal venous circulation ◆ Initiate muscle contractions ◆ Prevent respiratory complications ◆ Reinforce precautions to avoid complications ◆ Prepare patient to perform transfers independently ◆ Use assistive device during ambulation for safety and protection of hip

AROM, Active range of motion.

to the peripheral nerves, the therapist is expected to check the tightness of the cushions around the patient's legs.

Pulmonary hygiene exercises typically begin immediately after awakening. The patient's lower-extremity (LE) exercise program also may be initiated at this point with ankle pumps, quadriceps sets, and gluteal sets. Heel booties used to prevent bedsores can be removed for these exercises.

Patients may be groggy and unable to remember the THR precautions at this point; therefore a review is in order. Some may benefit from a sign placed by the bed that lists the ROM precautions or from a knee immobilizer placed on the affected leg to reduce the possibility of making dangerous movements.

Repositioning of the patient every 2 hours (with the abductor pillow in place) is essential at this stage to avoid pressure ulcers. Foot cradles are often attached to the foot of the bed to avoid IR of the operated hip and prevent the heel sores that may develop as a result of pressure from the blankets. Most protocols assign these functions to the nursing staff and begin physical therapy intervention on the first day after surgery. All personnel rendering care to the patient should monitor changes in the limb's vascular and neurologic status closely.

Postoperative Day 1

Acute care physical therapy sessions vary in frequency from one to three times per day and from 5 to 7 days per week, depending on the medical center's protocol.[10] The therapist proceeds after being informed as to the surgical approach used, special precautions, and the patient's weight-bearing status. Assessment and treatment are conducted at the patient's bedside. The patient is situated as described previously.

The THR precautions should be repeated at this time. The patient must observe these precautions until the scheduled follow-up visit with the orthopedist 6 weeks later. The surgeon may relax the precautions or continue them for another 6 weeks. The physical therapist can initiate ankle pumps (see Fig. 15-13), quadriceps sets, and gluteal sets if the patient did not begin them on the day of surgery. **Ankle circles are not indicated, because the patient may inadvertently rotate the affected extremity while performing the exercise. As stated previously, submaximal contraction of the muscles is recommended.** Bilateral UE exercises also begin at this time. Ideally these LE exercises should be repeated ten times every hour.[10] Be aware that some patients may not meet this expectation.

Transfer training begins by assisting the patient in moving safely from a supine to a sitting position and then from sitting to a standing position while observing precautions. Frequently patients are struggling with pain and anxiety and therefore require encouragement. The physical therapist should allot a considerable amount of time for this task and emphasize the use of the UEs when shifting weight. **The patient must avoid pivoting on the operative leg.**

Surgeons usually allow patients to transfer to an appropriate bedside chair and sit up as tolerated, **rarely more than 30 to 60 minutes.** The therapist then supervises their return to bed.

If a patient is not complaining of excessive pain, fatigue, or dizziness, then gait training may begin on the first postoperative day. More frequently, gait training begins on day 2.

> **Q** Sabrina had a noncemented THR surgery 3 days ago. She is TDWB with a walker but continues to place a moderate amount of weight on her affected LE. Because she has difficulty maintaining TDWB during gait, what can be done to help her?

Postoperative Day 2

Treatment on the second postoperative day includes a review of the previous day's activities. The patient should be able to maintain hip ROM within the physician's recommended guidelines for the surgical technique performed.

The physical therapist expands the exercise program to include heel slides and isometric or active assistive hip abduction. Short arc quadriceps sets may require active assistance at this time. Again, submaximal force is recommended for isometric hip abduction. Assistance from the therapist may be necessary for some exercises at first. The use of verbal cues such as "point the moving knee or big toe toward the ceiling" to avoid rotation of the leg also may be helpful.

Gait training usually begins during this session. The patient's assistive device is adjusted to its correct height before instruction and practice in its use is given. Older patients are typically issued a front-wheeled walker. Younger patients may be issued crutches and instructed in the three-point crutch pattern. Patients who have undergone bilateral THR are instructed in the four-point crutch pattern.

The weight-bearing status after a noncemented THR depends on the surgeon's discretion. The patient may be ordered not to bear weight on the affected extremity for several weeks. Most patients with cemented prostheses are instructed to bear weight as tolerated.

Some complex surgeries may require more caution. Concepts such as touchdown weight bearing (TDWB) or partial weight bearing (PWB) are difficult for the patient to grasp at first. If the postoperative order calls for only TDWB, then taping a "cracker" to the sole of the patient's affected forefoot may be helpful in illustrating the concept. Stepping onto a bathroom scale with the affected extremity helps the PWB patient to determine the appropriate amount of pressure (usually 50% of body weight or less) to be put on that leg. Patients who still experience difficulty may benefit from practicing weight shifting on the parallel bars before using a walker.

Patients who have undergone THR frequently walk with the affected leg in abduction. They should be encouraged to normalize their gait pattern early in the recovery phase. Although no maximal distance has been dictated, some facilities encourage the patient to walk a specific minimum distance. The patient's short-term goal is to meet the discharge criteria, which typically demand walking on a level surface for 100 feet.

> **A** A cracker can be taped to the sole of the patient's forefoot. If the patient still has difficulty maintaining TDWB, then she should try using a thick-soled shoe only on the affected leg. If the patient is PWB, say 50%, then a scale can be used to give feedback regarding how it feels to bear 50% of the weight on the LE.

Phase IIb

TIME: 3 to 7 days after surgery
GOALS: To promote transfers and gait independence (using assistive devices as indicated), continuously reinforce THR precautions, discharge to home

Postoperative Day 3 (Until Discharge)

Patients are often moved from the acute care section to a rehabilitation center or skilled nursing facility on day 3 (Table 15-2). Some patients (usually those who are younger and more fit) may be discharged to home care at this time. Treatment at the rehabilitation center is conducted in the physical therapy gym.

Stair training generally begins on day 3. A step-to gait pattern (involved leg not to pass ahead or in front of the uninvolved leg) with minimal weight bearing on the affected leg is taught for ambulation on even surfaces; on steps or stairs, the patient leads up the stairs with the unaffected leg and down the stairs with the affected leg.

Table 15-2 Total Hip Replacement

Rehabilitation Phase	Criteria to Progress to this Phase	Anticipated Impairments and Functional Limitations	Intervention	Goal	Rationale
Phase IIb Postoperative 3-7 days	◆ Good tolerance to Phase IIa ◆ No signs of infection ◆ No significant increase in pain ◆ Medically stable ◆ Gradual improvement in tolerance to inpatient program	◆ Limited bed mobility ◆ Limited transfers ◆ Limited gait ◆ Limited understanding of postoperative precautions	◆ Continue interventions from Phase IIa with progression of activity as tolerated ◆ AROM—Heel slides, hip abduction (if able—otherwise do active assisted hip abduction), terminal knee extension, UE exercises ◆ Bed mobility training ◆ Transfer training; initiate car transfers when appropriate ◆ Gait training; initiate stair training when indicated ("up with good, down with bad") ◆ Evaluation of equipment needs at home ◆ Caregiver training	◆ Maintain postoperative precautions ◆ Improve involved LE AROM within boundaries of precautions ◆ Improve arm strength ◆ Become independent with transfers ◆ Become independent with gait using appropriate assistive device ◆ Promote carryover of precautions at home	◆ Prevent prosthesis dislocation ◆ Restore volitional control of involved LE ◆ Prepare arms to assist during transfer and gait ◆ Emphasize restoration of independence with self-care activities (bed mobility, transfers) ◆ Promote independence with ADLs ◆ Ambulate safely and decrease stress on the involved LE ◆ Ensure patient and caregiver safety (reinforce precautions) and prevent falls

AROM, Active range of motion; *UE*, upper extremity; *LE*, lower extremity; *ADLs*, activities of daily living.

Patients should become comfortable climbing the number of stairs demanded by the home situation. When the patient is not competent with stair climbing, arrangements are sometimes made for the patient to live on the ground floor.

Refinement of these skills continues daily at the rehabilitation center until the time of discharge. By the discharge date, family members or other caregivers must be trained to assist the patient safely whenever necessary.

Common discharge criteria for THR are as follows:

- The patient is able to demonstrate and state the THR precautions.
- The patient is able to demonstrate independence with transfers.
- The patient is able to demonstrate independence with the exercise program.
- The patient is able to demonstrate independence with gait on level surfaces to 100 feet.
- The patient is able to demonstrate independence on stairs.

Written instructions with illustrations pertaining to these criteria are included in a discharge packet for home use. Patients are typically discharged between the fifth and tenth days after surgery. Zavadak and colleagues[36] found that independence in functional activities required the following number of physical therapy sessions:

Supine to sit: 8.1
Sit to stand: 5.5
Ambulate to 100 feet: 8.1
Independent on stairs: 9.5

However, the therapist's expectations should not be unduly influenced by statistics. Munin and colleagues[24] found that fewer than 40% of patients who undergo THR are independent in performing basic tasks at the time of discharge from the rehabilitation center. Approximately 80% of patients were at the supervision level of performance. Advanced age, solitary living conditions, and an increased number of comorbid conditions were the factors that predicted the duration of a patient's treatment stay.[23]

Phase III (Return to Home)

TIME: 1 to 6 weeks after surgery
GOALS: To evaluate the safety of the home, patient independence with transfers and ambulation, plan return of patient to work or previous community activities as appropriate (Table 15-3)

Home Care Phase

Physical therapy home assessment usually occurs within 24 hours after hospital discharge. The elements to be assessed are those listed in the preoperative section, with the addition of the status of the surgical incision. The number of visits authorized by the patient's insurance company may limit the goals set by the therapist. Medicare coverage at this stage is restricted to patients who are homebound or severely limited in their ability to go out. Most patients are no longer homebound after 3 to 4 weeks.

Because managed care insurance has placed constraints on the number of nursing visits allowed, physical therapists are now being trained to remove staples, traditionally a nursing function. Staple removal normally occurs on the twelfth to fourteenth day after surgery.

After hospital discharge, expect to advise the patient regarding appropriate sitting and sleeping positions, furniture adjustments and other safety issues such as slippery rugs or strung-out electrical cords. A review of the home exercise program and precautions is also in order.

Closed kinetic chain exercises (with involved leg firmly planted on the ground or on exercise equipment) such as heel raises and mini-squats can be incorporated into the home program. Cautious stretching may be appropriate for tight Achilles tendons in the standing position. Exercise equipment already in the patient's home may be added to the existing program if it can be used safely.

Shoes often adapt in shape to the stresses imposed by an abnormal gait pattern and may encourage a return to the old pattern if worn after THR surgery. The patient's old misshaped shoes should be replaced if possible.

The patient progresses from the use of a front-wheeled walker or crutches to a single-point cane. This transition usually occurs 3 to 4 weeks after surgery. Occasionally a four-point cane is used as an interim device. Use of the cane is usually discontinued 3 to 4 weeks later. The patient should progress to walking safely with a normalized gait on level and sloped surfaces, jagged sidewalks, curbs, and stairs before discharge.

Enough strength may have been recovered to allow step-over-step stair climbing during the home phase. At first, the patient should practice stepping up onto books or other household items that provide a stable, shallow rise. A modified lunge with the affected extremity placed on the step is another helpful prestep exercise.

Patients may be allowed to drive at 3 to 6 weeks after surgery at the orthopedist's discretion. Permission may be given sooner, depending on the patient's lifestyle requirements and rate of progress. The therapist may need to supervise the patient in getting on and off a bus or in and out of a car safely. A clean plastic trash bag placed over the seat of a car provides a surface that allows the patient to glide-pivot around on the seat to assume the rider's position more easily.

Outpatient Clinic

Physical therapy intervention often ends with the home care phase. Some patients with physically demanding lifestyles may require additional strength and endurance training. Some patients are referred to the clinic because

Table 15-3 Total Hip Replacement

Rehabilitation Phase	Criteria to Progress to this Phase	Anticipated Impairments and Functional Limitations	Intervention	Goal	Rationale
Phase III Postoperative 1-6 weeks	◆ Discharged from hospital or other care center ◆ No loss of ROM ◆ No increase in pain ◆ Need to restore further independence	◆ Limited tolerance to transfers ◆ Limited tolerance to gait ◆ Limited cardiovascular endurance and strength of involved LE	◆ Continuation and progression of phase II interventions ◆ Home evaluation for safety ◆ Patient education review of precautions with performance of bed mobility transfers ◆ Gait training on level surfaces, uneven surfaces, and stairs ◆ Closed-chain exercises (mini-squats, step-up, heel raises) ◆ Pool therapy ◆ Cross-country ski machine (with physician approval) ◆ Treadmill ◆ SLRs ◆ Hip abduction	◆ Improve patient independence ◆ Prevent falls ◆ Prevent complications ◆ Promote safety and independence with community ambulation ◆ Improve LE strength ◆ Return to former employment or previous hobbies as indicated	◆ Promote restoration of independent function ◆ Avoid potential for falls ◆ Avoid prosthesis dislocation ◆ Promote safety with ambulation on all types of surfaces ◆ Improve tolerance of involved LE to single-limb balance activities ◆ Regain cardiovascular conditioning ◆ Resume all ADLs and community activities

ROM, Range of motion; *LE*, lower extremity; *ADLs*, activities of daily living; *SLRs*, straight leg raises.

of lingering gait problems. Others may be referred because they did not meet home care status requirements at the time of hospital discharge. The outpatient therapist should check with the surgeon for the status of precautions and activity level before designing an aggressive exercise program.

Exercises begun in the home or hospital can be expanded on in the clinic. Pool exercise is recommended after THR, **as is simulated cross-country skiing with permission from the surgeon.** As in home care, the goals at this stage depend on the number of visits authorized by the patient's insurance company. Quick independence with a home exercise program should be encouraged.

After Rehabilitation Intervention

The surgeon will determine the patient's return-to-work date. Some patients may require job modification, whereas others may not be allowed to return to their previous jobs. Heavy manual labor is not permitted after THR surgery, and vocational counseling may be necessary.[24] High-impact sports such as running, waterskiing, football, basketball, handball, karate, soccer, and racquetball are contraindicated after THR.[9] The sports most recommended are sailing, swimming, scuba, cycling, and golf. Tennis is not recommended, but doubles tennis is considered less stressful than singles.[21]

Sexual activity after an uncomplicated THR may resume in approximately 1 to 2 months with the surgeon's approval. Studies have shown that most patients feel uncomfortable asking for this type of information. Women tend to prefer the supine position or side lying on the nonoperated side. Men prefer the supine position. The patient is advised to take the more passive role for the first few weeks. The prone position may be resumed in 2 to 3 months after surgery.[30]

Q Before having severe hip pain, Tracy was biking 20 to 30 miles a day, 4 days a week. She also competed in bicycle races and worked out in the gym with light weights three times a week. Should Tracy participate in a long-term exercise program after having a THR if it does not contradict the surgeon's orders? Why?

Patient compliance with home exercise programs is often questionable after the first few weeks and especially after discharge from therapy services. No agreement seems to exist among surgeons as to how long exercise programs should be continued. The surgeon may release the patient from the home exercise program at his or her discretion.

Sheh and colleagues[28] state that flexion showed the slowest rate of recovery in diseased hips. Persistence of weakness was noted in all patients for at least 2 years after hip surgery despite the return of normal stride and phasic activity of muscles. Gluteus maximus or minimus weakness can result in aching near the hip during endurance activities. Sheh states that muscular weakness reduces the protection of the implant fixation surfaces during endurance activities. This may contribute to higher loosening rates reported in active patients.[28] Therefore therapists may want to encourage long-term continuation of exercise programs if this does not contradict the surgeon's orders.

A Sheh et al[28] state that muscular weakness reduces the protection of the implant fixation surfaces during endurance activities. This may contribute to higher loosening rates reported in active patients. Therefore Tracy and other active patients should continue on a long-term exercise program to maintain good muscular strength around the hip.

TROUBLESHOOTING

The THR procedure has been refined to the point that patient progress is now fairly certain and predictable. However, most complications call for a referral back to the surgeon. Examples include the following:

- Thigh pain with walking that clears quickly with sitting down, possibly indicating intermittent claudication
- A positive Trendelenburg sign that does not resolve with treatment, possibly caused by damage to gluteal innervation
- Severe rubor and swelling at the surgical site with accompanying fever, possibly indicating a wound infection
- Unexplained swelling of the limb that does not dissipate with elevation, possibly indicating TED
- General systemic effects, possibly indicating an allergy to the implant materials (rare), postoperative anemia, pulmonary embolus, or other medical complications
- Persistent, severe pain (even referred medial knee pain, unexplained limb shortening or extreme rotation, or pain with rotation of the limb), possibly resulting from dislocation of the prosthesis, heterotopic ossification, or a fracture of the adjacent bone or reflex sympathetic dystrophy

Q Karen is a 75-year-old female who had a THR 3 weeks ago. She is receiving physical therapy at home and has two treatments. Today is her third treatment. Her main complaint is the swelling in her foot. Her last treatments emphasized mobility training. She lives with her daughter. She demonstrates stand by assist (SBA) for most transfers; however, she requires minimal assist to her affected LE when getting in and out of bed. What should be addressed during today's treatment?

Many times the therapist is the first to see a developing complication; therefore good communication with the surgeon is extremely important. Leg length discrepancy is an example. The patient can continue gait training with a temporary shoe insert or with shoes of different heel heights. The surgeon may later prescribe a permanent orthotic. Persistent edema may be treated with medication. Patients should be advised to elevate their legs, rest more often, wear TED hose, pump their ankles, and apply ice to swollen areas. Pain flare-ups in unaffected areas of the body are usually managed with medication. Possible side effects of the medication include nausea, constipation, and hypertension. The therapist can assist in pain reduction with modalities, exercises, and positioning. Significant abnormalities should always be reported to the surgeon.

A The patient was sitting upon arrival of the therapist. Physical therapy performed transfer training back to bed. When the patient was supine, the therapist massaged her foot and lower leg, milking the fluid up towards the heart. The therapist followed up with active/assistive (A/A) ROM for SLR with eccentric lowering of the LE using minimal assistance for guidance. In addition, active assistive hip abduction and adduction (before reaching midline and within the area of hip precautions) were done. Heel cord stretching was also addressed. A discussion regarding using a TED hose and maintaining LE elevation while sitting and in bed followed. In addition, the therapist encouraged the patient to do ankle pumps every hour throughout the day.

CONCLUSION

A rapid, substantial improvement in quality of life can be expected after THR surgery. Better physical function, sleep, emotional behavior, social interaction, and recreation are usually experienced in the first few months. At 2 years after surgery, patients who had undergone THR have reported greater satisfaction with their results than they had predicted in their best preoperative hypothetical scenario.[18]

SUGGESTED HOME MAINTENANCE FOR THE POSTSURGICAL PATIENT

Days 1-2 (in hospital)

GOALS FOR THE PERIOD: Protect healing tissues, prevent postoperative complications, improve volitional control of involved lower extremity (LE)

Isometric Exercises
1. Gluteal sets
2. Quadriceps sets

Active Range of Motion (AROM) Exercises
3. Ankle pumps

Resistive Exercises
4. Resisted shoulder internal rotation (IR) and external rotation (ER) with Theraband
5. Shoulder depressions and triceps dips while seated

Days 3-7 (in hospital)

GOALS FOR THE PERIOD: Improve lower-extremity (LE) and upper-extremity (UE) strength

AROM Exercises
1. Heel slides
2. Hip abduction
3. Terminal knee extension

Weeks 1-6 (after discharge to home setting or as appropriate in interim setting)

GOALS FOR THE PERIOD: Improve strength and balance of lower extremities, promote return to activities and hobbies as indicated

1. Closed-chain exercises (progression to gym equipment and inclined sled): step-ups, mini-squats, heel raises, SLRs, and hip abduction
2. Pool therapy
3. Treadmill (as part of gym program)
4. Heel cord stretches

References

1. American Academy of Orthopaedic Surgeons: *Orthopedic knowledge update 3,* Rosemont, IL, 1987, the Academy.
2. American Academy of Orthopaedic Surgeons: *Orthopedic knowledge update 4: home study syllabus,* Rosemont, IL, 1992, the Academy.
3. Bal BS et al: Early complication of primary total hip replacement performed with a two-incision minimally invasive technique, *J Bone Joint Surg [Am]* 87(11): 2432-2438, 2005.
4. Cameron HU: *The technique of total hip arthroplasty,* St Louis, 1992, Mosby.
5. Chandler HP et al: Total hip replacement in patients under thirty years old, *J Bone Joint Surg* 63A:1426, 1981.
6. Delaunay C, Migaud H: Primary total hip in active patients younger than 50 years of age, *Rev Chir Orthop Reparatrice Appar Mot* 91(4): 351-374, 2005.
7. Engh CA, Glassman AH, Suthers KE: The case for porous-coated hip implants: the femoral side, *Clin Orthop* 261:63, 1990.
8. Enloe LJ et al: Total hip and knee replacement programs: a report using consensus, *J Orthop Sports Phys Ther* 23(1):3, 1996.
9. Gilbert R: Personal communication, June 10, 1998.
10. Givens-Heiss DL et al: In vivo acetabular contact pressures during rehabilitation. II. Postacute phase, *Phys Ther* 72(10):700, 1992.
11. Hoppenfeld S, deBoer P, Thomas HA: *Exposures in orthopedics: the anatomic approach,* Philadelphia, 1984, JB Lippincott.
12. Hicks JE, Gerber LH: Rehabilitation of the patient with arthritis and connective tissue disease. In DeLisa JA, editor: *Rehabilitation medicine: principles and practices,* Philadelphia, 1988, JB Lippincott.
13. Jan MH et al: Effects of a home program on strength, walking speed, and function after total hip replacement, *Arch Phys Med Rehabil* 85(12):1943-1951, 2004.
14. Katti KS: Biomaterials in total joint replacement, *Colloids Surf B Biointerfaces* 39(3):133-142, 2004.
15. Kavanagh BF et al: Charnley total hip arthroplasty with cement: fifteen year results, *J Bone Joint Surg* 71A:1496, 1989.
16. Katz JM et al: Differences between men and women undergoing major orthopedic surgery for degenerative arthritis, *Arthritis Rheum* 37:687, 1994.
17. Krebs D et al: Exercise and gait effects on in vivo hip contact pressures, *Phys Ther* 71(4):301, 1991.
18. Laupacis A et al: The effect of elective total hip replacement on health-related quality of life, *J Bone Joint Surg* 75A(11): 1719, 1993.
19. Lewis C, Knortz K: Total hip replacements, *Phys Ther Forum* May 20, 1994.
20. MacDonald SJ: Metal on metal total hip arthroplasty: the concerns, *Clin Ortho Relat Res* (429):86-93, 2004.
21. McGrorey BJ, Stewart MJ, Sim FH: Participation in sports after hip and knee arthroplasty: a review of the literature and survey of surgical preferences, *Mayo Clin Proc* 70B:202, 1995.
22. Mulroy RD, Jr, Harris WH: The effect of improved cementing techniques on component loosening in total

hip replacement: an 11-year radiographic review, *J Bone Joint Surg* 72B:757, 1990.
23. Munin MC et al: Predicting discharge outcome after elective hip and knee arthroplasty, *Am J Phys Med Rehabil* 74:294, 1995.
24. Munin M et al: Rehabilitation. In Callaghan J, Rosenberg A, Rubash H, editors: *The adult hip,* Philadelphia, 1998, Lippincott-Raven.
25. Petty W: *Total joint replacement,* Philadelphia, 1991, WB Saunders.
26. Roberts JM et al: A comparison of the posterolateral and anterolateral approaches to total hip arthroplasty, *Clin* Orthop 187:205, 1984.
27. Santavista N et al: Teaching of patients undergoing total hip replacement surgery, *Int J Nurs Stud* 31(2):135, 1994.
28. Sheh C et al: Muscle recovery and the hip joint after total hip replacement, *Clin Orthop* 302:115, 1994.
29. Smith-Peterson MN: A new supra acetabular subperiosteal approach to the hip, *Am J Orthop Surg* 15:592, 1917.
30. Stern FH et al: Sexual function after total hip arthroplasty, *Clin Orthop* 269:228, 1991.
31. Strickland EM et al: In vivo acetabular contact pressures during rehabilitation. I. Acute phase, *Phys Ther* 72(10):691, 1992.
32. Vicar AJ, Coleman CR: A comparison of the anterolateral, transtrochanteric, and posterior surgical approaches in primary total hip arthroplasty, *Clin Orthop* 188:152, 1994.
33. Whitesides L: Personal communication (Total Hip Conference), St Louis, 1993.
34. Wickland I, Romanus B: A comparison of quality of life before and after arthroplasty in patients who had arthrosis of the hip joint, *J Bone Joint Surg* 73A:765, 1991.
35. Wroblewski BM: Fifteen twenty-one year results of Charnley low friction arthroplasty, *Clin Orthop* 261:63, 1990.
36. Zavadak KH et al: Variability in attainment of functional milestones during the acute care admission after total hip replacement, *J Rheumatol* 22:482, 1995.

CHAPTER 16

Open Reduction and Internal Fixation of the Hip

Edward Pratt
Patricia A. Gray
Mayra Saborio Amiran

Hip fractures are the bony injuries that require surgical intervention in the United States most frequently. The annual expense for the treatment of these patients has been estimated as high as $7.3 billion. Because the incidence of osteoporosis in our steadily aging population is increasing, the number of hip fractures is expected to increase from 275,000 per year in the late 1980s to more than 500,000 by the year 2040.[1]

SURGICAL INDICATIONS AND CONSIDERATIONS

Numerous classification systems have been devised to describe hip fractures. However, in the context of surgical exposure, soft tissue injury, and rehabilitation potential, they can be simplified into five main categories:

1. Nondisplaced or minimally displaced femoral neck fractures
2. Displaced femoral neck fractures
3. Stable intertrochanteric fractures
4. Unstable intertrochanteric fractures
5. Subtrochanteric fractures

All categories of these fractures can demonstrate good outcomes with surgical intervention and early mobilization.[2] This is true regardless of age, gender, or comorbidities. The rare exception is an incomplete or impacted femoral neck fracture in a nonambulatory or extremely ill individual. The expected postoperative stability of the hip is directly proportional to the severity of the injury, the quality or density of the bone to be repaired, and the technical expertise of the surgeon.

The patient's overall preinjury physical and mental condition is also a predictor of postoperative success. Patients with major cardiopulmonary afflictions, obesity, poor upper body strength, osteoporosis, or dementia in its various forms have increased risk for complications in the treatment of hip fractures. Overall mortality rates of 20% after 1 year, 50% at 3 years, 60% at 6 years, and 77% after 10 years have been reported.[11] This is not surprising, because most hip fractures occur in the older adult population.

The traditional goal of rehabilitation has been to restore patients to the level of function that they had before the injury. In many cases this may not be realistic. Only 20% to 35% of patients regain their preinjury level of independence. Some 15% to 40% require institutionalized care for more than 1 year after surgery. Many—50% to 83%—require devices to assist with ambulation.[17]

Rehabilitation goals must be individualized, with the therapist taking into account all comorbidities, fracture severity, and motivational level of the patient.

SURGICAL PROCEDURES

Nondisplaced or Minimally Displaced Femoral Neck Fractures

Nondisplaced or minimally displaced femoral neck fractures represent the least severe injuries in the spectrum of hip fractures. They are stable and can bear the full weight of the patient immediately after surgery. Moreover, they require no limitations on range of motion (ROM) or exertion in the immediate postoperative period. The preferred surgical procedure is a fluoroscopically aided placement of cannulated 6.5 mm screws through a limited or percutaneous lateral approach. This approach violates the skin, subcutaneous fat, deep fascia of the fascia lata, and fascia and muscle fibers of the vastus lateralis. Typically blood distends the joint capsule, creating some limitation in hip ROM and pain. No major nerves or vessels are at risk in this approach.

The patient is brought to the operating room, and anesthesia is induced. The patient is positioned supine on a fracture table capable of distracting and manipulating the affected limb. After satisfactory position of the

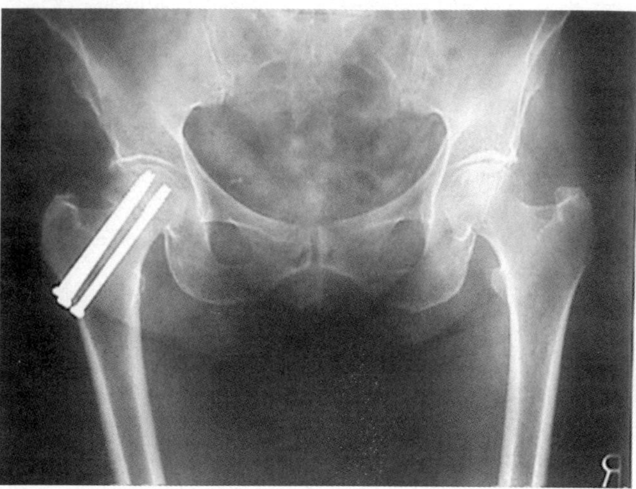

Fig. 16-1 Anteroposterior (AP) radiograph of the pelvis showing proper placement of three cannulated screws across a minimally displaced subcapital femoral neck fracture.

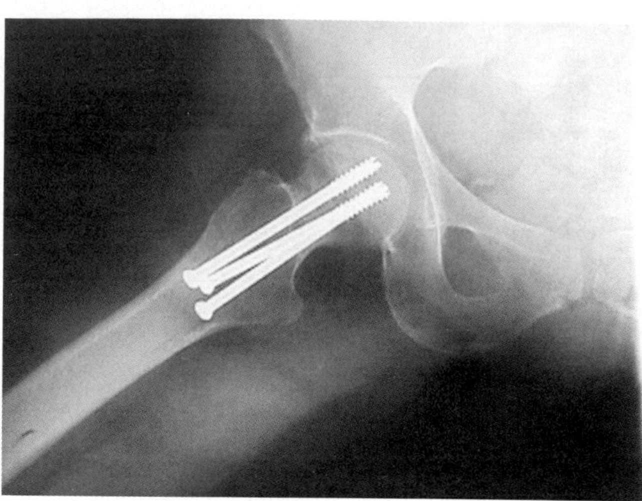

Fig. 16-2 Lateral view of the case illustrated in Fig. 16-1.

fracture fragments is verified with an image intensifier, surgery is begun.

A 2-cm incision is made along the lateral femur in line with the fractured femoral neck. A guide pin is then placed percutaneously through the lateral musculature at or about the level of the lesser trochanter. The pin is introduced up the femoral neck and across the fracture into the subchondral bone of the femoral head. After two to four guide pins have been placed, the outer cortex is drilled with a cannulated drill and cannulated screws are introduced over the guide pins (Figs. 16-1 and 16-2). The soft tissues are repaired, and a dressing is applied. Femoral neck fractures that occur more toward the base of the femoral neck require fixation that is able to resist the bending movement between femoral neck and shaft. These are treated much like intertrochanteric fractures, and the operative procedure is described in that section.

Displaced Femoral Neck Fractures

Femoral neck fractures in which the femoral head has been separated widely from the neck do not heal if reduced and fixed by screws or pins. In these fractures the vascular supply to the femoral head (specifically the medial and lateral femoral circumflex arteries) are often severed. In younger patients it is still desirable to attempt fixation despite the high rate of nonunion and osteonecrosis. When open reduction is attempted, the anterolateral exposure of Watson-Jones is preferred because it preserves the blood supply to the femoral head, which enters through the posteroinferior femoral neck.[23] This approach is discussed in the section on total hip replacement (THR). Older adult patients are often best treated by bipolar, endoprosthetic, or THR procedures using a posterolateral approach.

The posterolateral approach involves violation of the skin; subcutaneous tissue; fascia lata; gluteus maximus; and short external rotators of the hip, including the piriformis, obturator internus, gemelli, and quadratus femoris. The capsule is incised posteriorly and often released anteriorly. Traction is applied on the gluteus maximus, gluteus medius, and gluteus minimus throughout the procedure. Nerves and vessels at risk include the sciatic nerve, the superior gluteal nerve, the inferior gluteal nerve, and their accompanying vessels. Although the psoas is left alone, it is often inflamed and can scar down and across the anterior hip capsule if adequate postoperative mobilization is not encouraged. Generally incisions are healed by 2 weeks, deep soft tissue healing is well advanced by 6 weeks, and full bony healing is expected at 12 weeks.

The patient is anesthetized and placed in the lateral decubitus position with the injured hip up (see Fig. 15-4); the torso is stabilized, and the hip and affected leg are draped to move freely. The initial incision is centered over the greater trochanter and taken distally 3 inches along the femoral shaft, then proximally and medially 4 inches along the course of the fibers of the gluteus maximus. The deep fascia is incised over the greater trochanter and carried distally along the same line as the skin incision, exposing the origin of the vastus lateralis without violating it. The surgeon digitally palpates the interval between the gluteus maximus and tensor fascia lata proximally, then extends the deep incision in this interval. A large, self-retaining retractor is then positioned to hold the deep fascia apart. The greater trochanteric bursa is incised to expose the short external rotators. The interval between the piriformis, gluteus medius, and gluteus minimus is identified, and the glutei are retracted anteriorly. Carefully the short external rotators are taken off the posterior femoral neck along the posterior hip capsule as a single cuff of tissue for later repair. Alternatively the capsule can be released separately with a *T* incision. Generally the surgeon must release the piriformis, gemelli, obturator internus, and half of the quadratus to expose the femoral neck to the level of the lesser trochanter. The hip is then flexed and internally rotated to bring the fracture into view. A saw is used to cut the femoral neck smoothly at the proper level, and the femoral head is retrieved from the acetabulum. The acetabulum is examined, and bone fragments are removed along with the ligamentum teres. After exposure is completed, the prosthesis is installed. It is often inserted in 15 to 20 degrees more anteversion than was present with the biologic hip to minimize the risk of dislocation. This occasionally limits external rotation (ER) after surgery but usually not enough to create a functional impairment.

Closure is somewhat more controversial. The author prefers to repair the capsule and short external rotators with large No. 2 nonabsorbable suture through drill holes in the greater trochanter and intertrochanteric line. This limits the formation of heterotopic bone, decreases the incidence of postoperative dislocation, and improves proprioception during rehabilitation. The deep fascia is then repaired, followed by the subcutaneous tissue and skin.

The initial postoperative rehabilitation is predicated on early mobilization to prevent morbidities associated with recumbency such as deep venous thrombosis (DVT), atelectasis, pneumonia, decubiti, and loss of muscle strength and joint mobility. Full weight bearing is encouraged. After arthrotomy each patient must be educated and drilled regarding potentially dangerous hip positions that can lead to dislocation. The risk inherent in the posterolateral approach is greatest with hip flexion greater than 90 degrees and internal rotation (IR), adduction, or both across the midline. **Patients with prosthetic hips should be instructed to follow their hip precautions religiously for the first 6 weeks after surgery, at which time the soft tissue has regained most of its tensile strength.** Even then they are at greater risk of dislocation than they were before surgery. The next major emphasis of rehabilitation is the regaining of abductor strength. The combination of traction on the abductor tendons, occasional traction neurapraxia on the superior gluteal nerve, and an often-shortened abductor lever arm leads to a Trendelenburg gait. Until abductor strength returns, secondary joint pain can often develop on the spine, knees, and contralateral hip because of the added stresses of shifting the center of gravity to and fro during ambulation.

Intertrochanteric Hip Fractures

Intertrochanteric hip fractures tend to be the most technically challenging. The intertrochanteric region joins the femoral shaft and neck at an angle of about 130 degrees. **The angular movement created by weight bearing is greatest here, and often weight bearing in the initial postoperative period is not feasible.** Morbidity tends to be higher after these fractures, owing to significant comminution of bone and the resultant inadequate stabilization provided by the internal fixation. **These patients often must remain at touch down weight bearing (TDWB) or nonweight bearing until fracture healing is demonstrated.** The most important prognosticator in this subset of patients is the evaluation of fracture stability (i.e., the tendency of the fracture to collapse or angulate under physiologic loads after surgery). Fractures with an intact posteromedial cortex and those at the base of the femoral neck are stable. These fractures tolerate limited weight bearing in the initial postoperative period without shifting. Surgeons best treat patients with these fractures by placing a sliding compression hip screw device in an anatomically aligned fracture.

The best surgical approach for the unstable fracture is controversial. Suggested approaches include hip screw devices with or without medial displacement, third-generation intermedullary reconstruction nail fixation, and calcar replacement endoprostheses. The surgical exposure for placement of a calcar replacement prosthesis is as described under the use of endoprostheses for displaced femoral neck fractures. The exposure and morbidity involved in the placement of an intermedullary nail are discussed in the section on subtrochanteric fractures. The exposure for placement of a dynamic compression hip screw is the same regardless of whether a stable or unstable fracture is being addressed. Typically a long lateral approach is used. This approach violates the skin, subcutaneous tissue, fascia lata, vastus lateralis fascia, and muscle belly. Generally in unstable fractures the lesser trochanter and inserting psoas tendon are left free, limiting hip flexion strength in the initial postoperative period.

Controversy exists as to whether it is better to align unstable fractures anatomically with a highly angled 145- to 150-degree compression plate and allow it to collapse into stability under physiologic loads or to perform a "medical displacement" osteotomy to obtain good posteromedial cortical abutment and stability during surgery (Fig. 16-3).

Both methods can lead to stability or instability; therefore each case must be discussed with the surgeon to ascertain the degree of stability obtained and the amount of weight bearing permitted. In addition, both methods shorten the distance between the insertion of the hip abductors in the greater trochanter and the center of rotation of the hip, creating a mechanical disadvantage for the abductors. This can lead to Trendelenburg gait, which must be overcome during the postoperative rehabilitation period.

The patient is placed supine on a fracture table with the afflicted limb in the traction boot. Care is taken to place

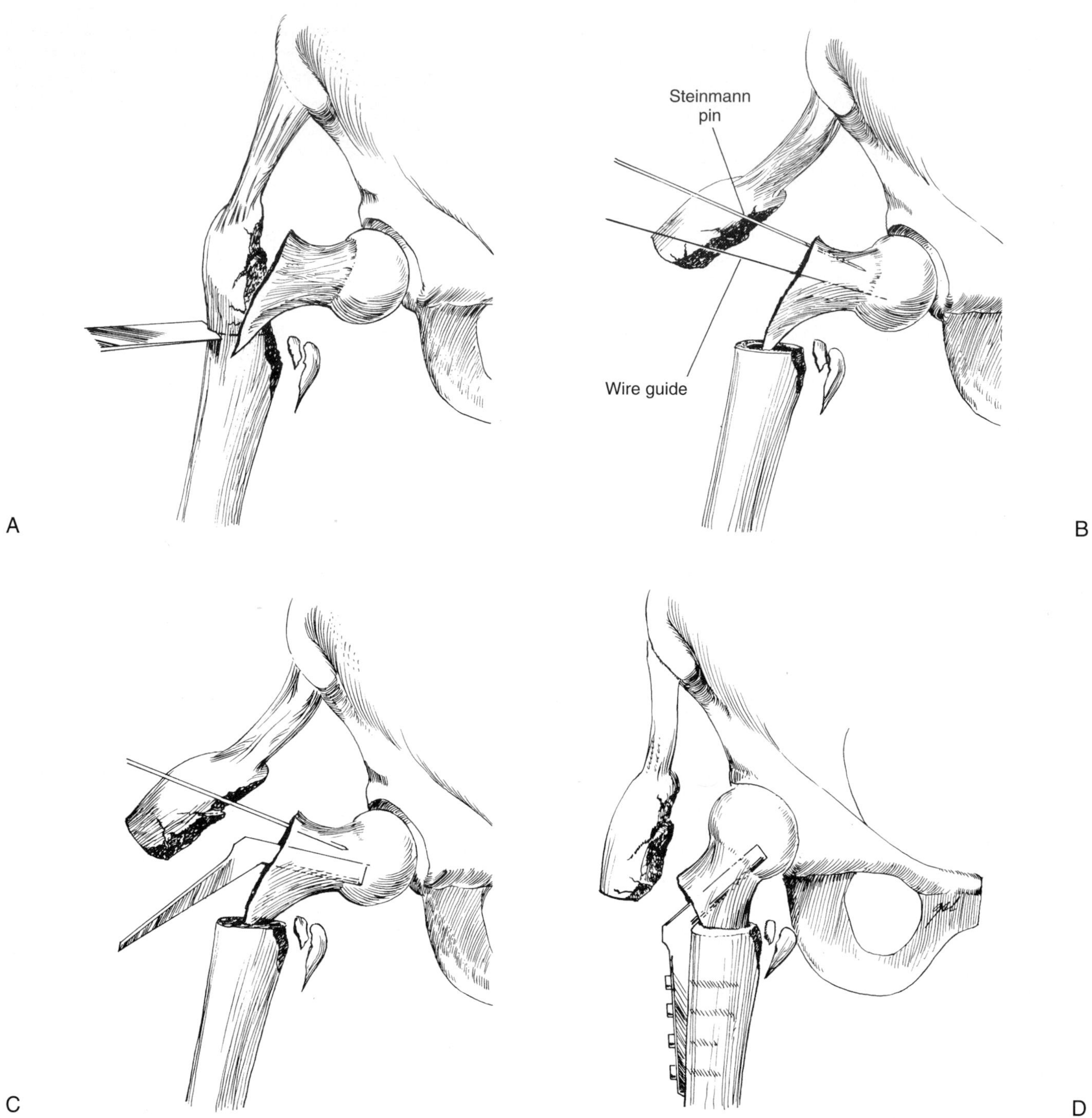

Fig. 16-3 Dimon-Hughston method of internal fixation of unstable trochanteric fractures. **A,** Transverse osteotomy of the lateral shaft. **B,** Insertion of a guide pin with a Steinmann pin for control of fragment. **C,** Insertion of nail in the proximal fragment. **D,** Fixation of the side plate to the shaft.

(From Hughston JC: Intertrochanteric fractures of the hip, *Orthop Clin North Am* 5(3):585, 1974.)

the correct rotation on the distal limb to prevent malalignment. Reduction is carried out under an image intensifier until satisfactory reduction is achieved. Occasionally a satisfactory preoperative reduction is not possible because of posterior sag of the bony fragments, and further reduction must be done manually. After the limb has been prepared and draped, a lateral incision is made from the level of the greater trochanter distally approximately 7 inches, depending on the length of plate to be used. The incision is developed in the same line through skin, subcutaneous fat, and fascia lata. At this point the fascia of the vastus lateralis is followed posteriorly to its origin in the linea aspera. By incising it here the surgeon limits the amount of muscle denervated by the exposure and protects

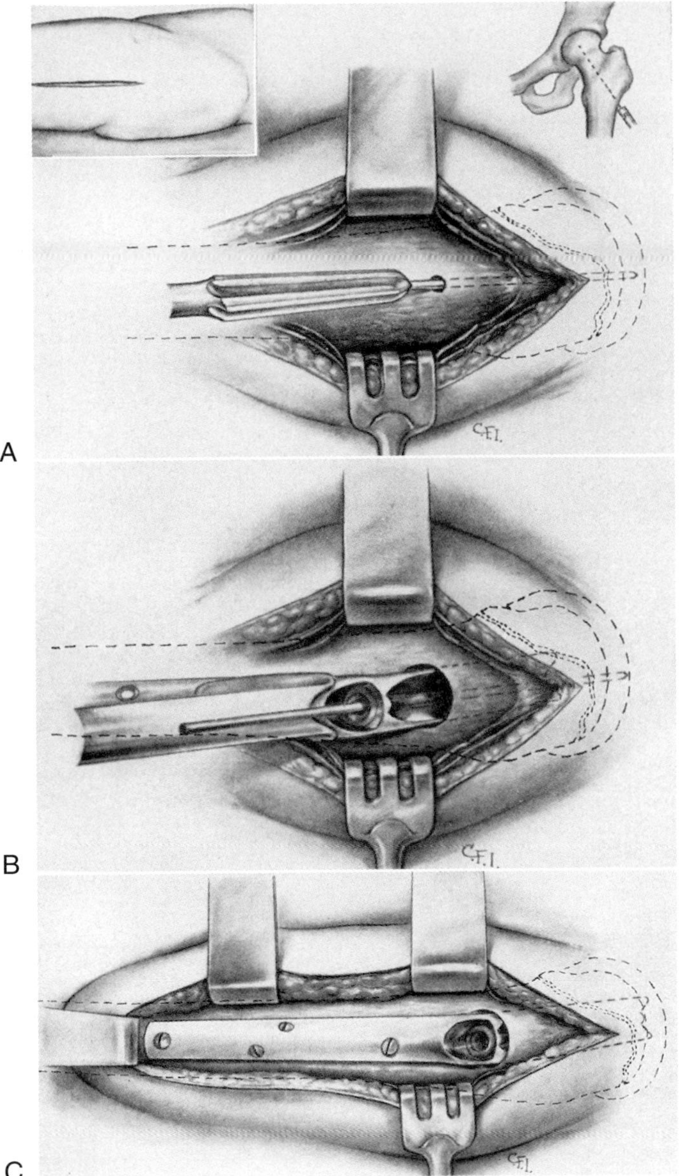

Fig. 16-4 Internal fixation of a trochanteric fracture. A, A guide pin is inserted and its position and that of the fracture are checked by roentgenograms. A cannulated Henderson reamer, placed over the guide pin, is used to make a hole through the lateral cortex. *Left insert,* skin incision; *right insert,* proper position of guide pin in anteroposterior view. B, A Jewett nail is inserted over the guide pin. C, The plate part of the Jewett nail has been fixed to the femoral shaft with screws.

the main muscle mass from damage. The surgeon accesses the lateral cortex of the femoral shaft and places a retractor to maintain anterior retraction of the vastus lateralis, exposing the lateral femoral shaft. After exposure is completed, placement of the fixation device is begun (Fig. 16-4). Closure involves interrupted repair of the fascia of the vastus lateralis, fascia lata, subcutaneous tissue, and skin.

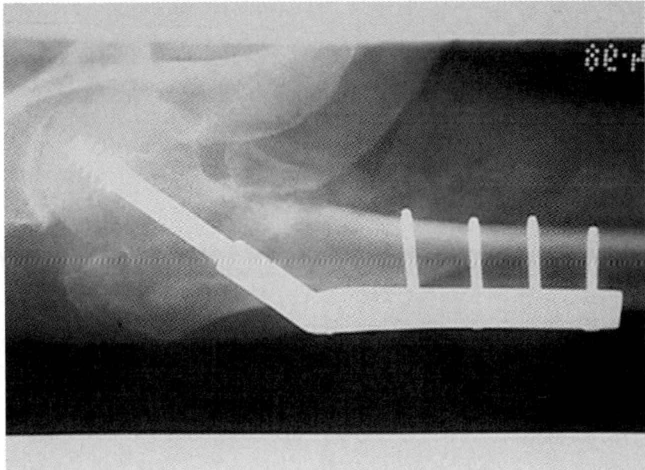

Fig. 16-5 Unstable intertrochanteric fracture of the hip treated with a four-hole compression screw device. The lesser trochanter is often left floating, which can lead to weakness.

The dynamic-compression screw device was not designed to hold the head and neck segment firmly (Fig. 16-5). Rather it allows the ambient muscle forces across the hip joint to pull the fracture fragments together until good bony resistance is encountered. In many comminuted osteoporotic fractures, the ability of the screw device to contract is exceeded before good cortical abutment is obtained between the fracture fragments. **In such cases weight bearing must be curtailed until bony healing ensues, or the screw will "cut out" and all stabilization will be lost.** Again, the skin is healed by 2 weeks, the deep fascia and soft tissues are healed by 6 weeks, and good bony healing is expected by 12 weeks. In older adult osteoporotic patients with severely comminuted fractures, bony healing can sometimes be delayed for as long as 4 to 6 months. In patients with obviously unstable fractures, weight bearing should be delayed until good bony healing is demonstrated on radiographs. The resultant collapse can often leave a limb significantly shorter. Leg length should be checked after healing and a lift provided if appropriate.

Subtrochanteric Hip Fractures

The use of advanced intermedullary nailing techniques has revolutionized the treatment of subtrochanteric fractures. Traditionally, these fractures have been difficult to fix because of the extreme angular force centered in this region, as well as the muscular deforming forces and minimal bony interface between the two fragments available for healing (Fig. 16-6).

Moreover, the bone in this region is more cortical in character, with a poorer blood supply and less osteogenic activity than in the intertrochanteric region. The use of a sliding compression screw device has yielded a higher

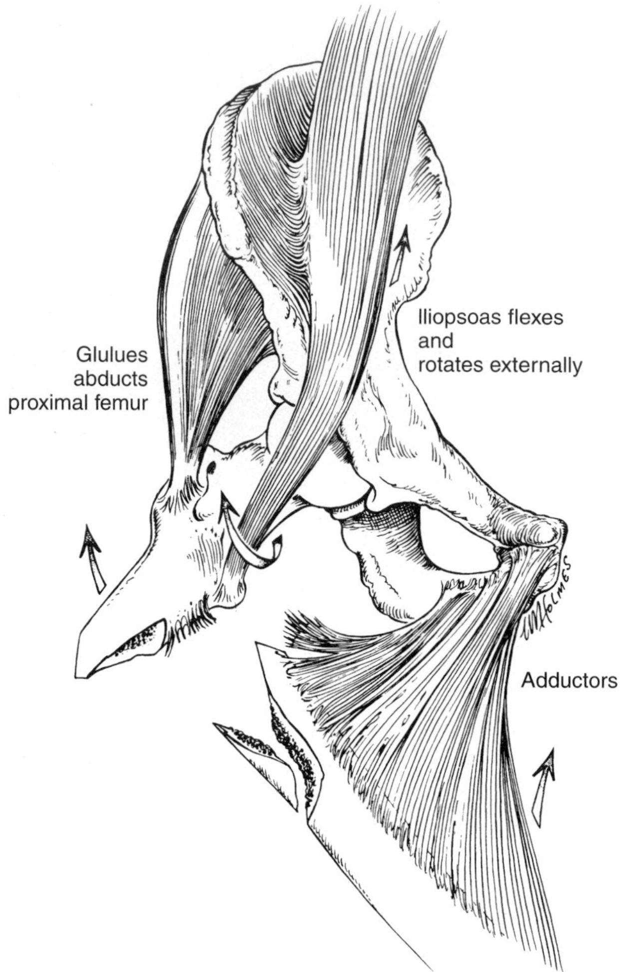

Fig. 16-6 Diagram of pathologic anatomy of subtrochanteric fracture. The proximal fragment is flexed, abducted, and externally rotated, whereas the femoral shaft is shortened and adducted.
(From Froimson AI: Treatment of comminuted subtrochanteric fractures of the femur, *Surg Gynecol Obstet* 131(3):465, 1970.)

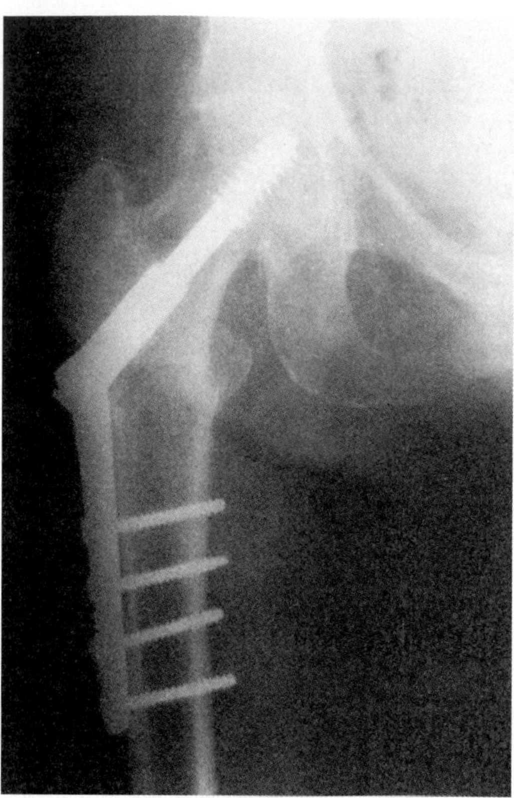

Fig. 16-7 A subtrochanteric fracture of the femur fixed with Richards compression screw-plate device.
(From Crenshaw AH: *Campbell's operative orthopaedics*, vol 3, ed 7, St Louis, 1987, Mosby.)

implant failure and nonunion rate than in other regions. The femur can be stabilized with a static locked intermedullary nail without exposing the fracture or disturbing its periosteal blood supply. The two preferred methods of fixation for patients with these fractures are a routine lateral approach for the placement of an extended compression screw device and the placement of a static locked intermedullary nail. The exposure for the lateral compression plate is discussed in the section on intertrochanteric fractures and deviates only in that the exposure must be taken more distally, causing more damage to the fascia lata and the vastus lateralis. **Although this design stabilizes the fracture, weight bearing usually must be delayed, soft tissue exposure is extensive, and healing is often delayed because of destruction of periosteal blood supply around the fracture.**

The more limited exposure for a static locked or reconstruction nail runs more proximally through the abductors, with a second stab incision for the interlocking screws at the level of the greater or lesser trochanter and a third stab incision laterally along the supracondylar femur. The newer reconstruction nails run the more proximal interlocking screws from the lateral femoral cortex (at the level of the lesser trochanter), across and through the prefabricated holes in the nail in the intermedullary canal. The nails then run up the femoral neck, ending in the hard bone of the subarticular femoral head. The distal interlocking screws pass lateral to medial through the lateral cortex of the femur, nail, and finally through the medial femoral cortex. This design effectively neutralizes deforming forces across the subtrochanteric femur, allowing full weight bearing from the outset (Fig. 16-7).

The patient is placed supine on a fracture table with both legs inserted into traction boots. Traction is applied over a perineal post. The legs are positioned with the involved leg adducted across the midline and slightly flexed at the hip. The uninvolved leg is abducted and extended at the hip, lying adjacent to the operative leg (Fig. 16-8). An incision is started at a point 1 inch proximal to the

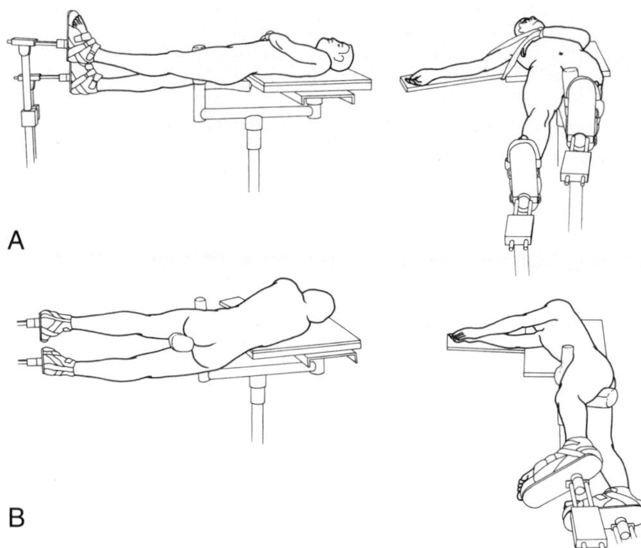

Fig. 16-8 Russell-Taylor interlocking nail technique. **A,** Patient in supine position. **B,** Patient in lateral decubitus position.
(From Crenshaw AH: *Campbell's operative orthopaedics,* vol 3, ed 7, St Louis, 1987, Mosby.)

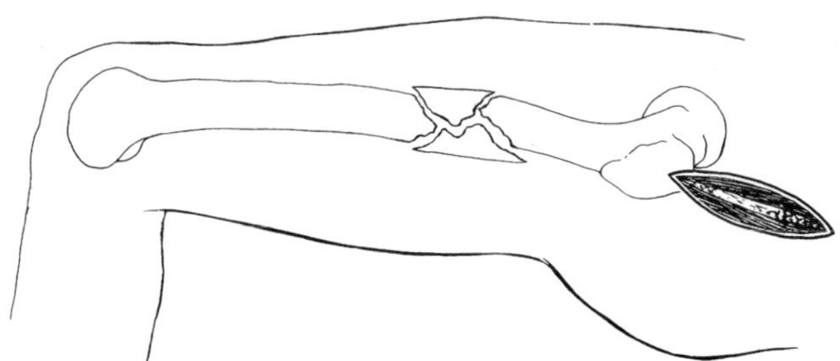

Fig. 16-9 Skin incision at the greater trochanter.
(From Crenshaw AH: *Campbell's operative orthopaedics,* vol 3, ed 7, St Louis, 1987, Mosby.)

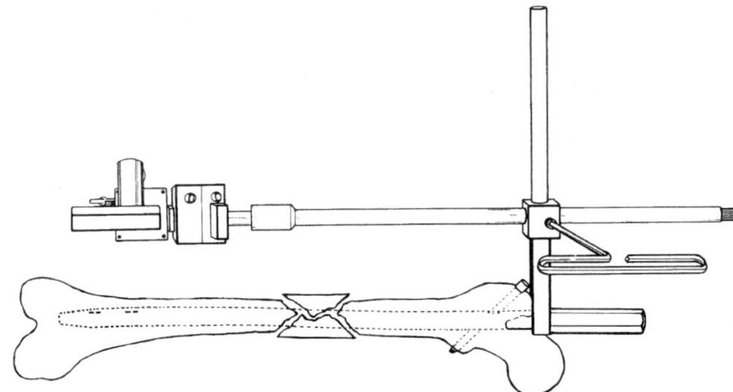

Fig. 16-10 Distal-locking block assembly is attached to the handle of the proximal drill guide.
(From Crenshaw AH: *Campbell's operative orthopaedics,* vol 3, ed 7, St Louis, 1987, Mosby.)

greater trochanter (Fig. 16-9). It is developed proximally and slightly medially 3 inches. The surgeon then extends the incision through the skin and subcutaneous tissue to the fascia of the gluteus medius, which is divided for about 2 inches in line with the skin incision and the fibers of the gluteus medius. Using a small guide pin and fluoroscopy the surgeon makes a small entry point at the base of the superior posterior femoral area, the *piriformis fossa.* The guide pin is passed down the femoral shaft approximately 6 inches, and a cannulated reamer is placed over the guide pin to enlarge the entry hole and begin the reaming process. A larger ball-tip guide that is run down across the fracture and down the intermedullary canal to the intercondylar notch replaces the initial guide pin. After this the canal is reamed with flexible reamers in progressively larger sizes until good cortical fit is obtained. After over-reaming a millimeter or two the surgeon carefully inserts the nail across the fracture under fluoroscopic guidance and then inserts the interlocking screws. The screws at the proximal end of the nail are aimed with the use of a special jig that attaches to the proximal end of the nail (Fig. 16-10). They are inserted percutaneously through the deep fascia and vastus lateralis. The distal screws are usually placed freehand, again percutaneously, using the image to visualize the holes in the nail passing through the iliotibial band and vastus lateralis. Closure consists of repairing the deep fascia, subcutaneous tissue, and skin.

Rehabilitation efforts during the initial postoperative period should consist of regaining control of the proximal hip musculature. Good functional quadriceps contraction and the ability to lift and maneuver the hip against gravity are prerequisites to adequate ambulation. Because of the strength of the fixation, patients can begin full weight bearing immediately after intermedullary reconstruction nailing. Healing normally requires 3 months (Fig. 16-11); nail removal should not be considered before 18 to 24 months.

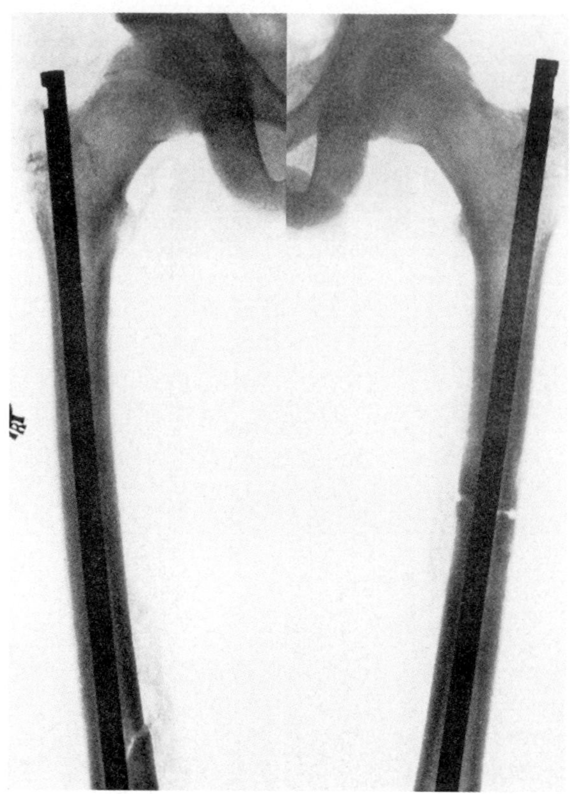

Fig. 16-11 Appearance 2 months after closed reduction of dislocations and medullary nailing of fractures.
(From Crenshaw AH: *Campbell's operative orthopaedics,* vol 3, ed 7, St Louis, 1987, Mosby.)

THERAPY GUIDELINES FOR REHABILITATION

Physical therapy after an open reduction internal fixation (ORIF) procedure for the hip is individualized depending on the health status of the patient before the fracture, the type of ORIF procedure used and the precautions ordered by the surgeon. This chapter provides some general guidelines for the rehabilitation process. The physical therapist (PT) must manage the patient's progress, keeping in mind the patient's ability to heal and the constraints of the patient's insurance carrier. The rehabilitation process can be described in three phases: (1) hospital, (2) home care, and (3) outpatient. In many cases, depending on lifestyle demands, the patient may only go through one or two of these phases.

Q Why are ORIF patients emotionally unique?

Phase I (Hospital Phase)

TIME: 1 to 7 days after surgery
GOALS: Help patient become independent with transfers and gait using appropriate assistive devices, discharge from acute care (Table 16-1)

Table 16-1 Hip Open Reduction Internal Fixation

Rehabilitation Phase	Criteria to Progress to this Phase	Anticipated Impairments and Functional Limitations	Intervention	Goal	Rationale
Phase I Postoperative 1-7 days	◆ Postoperative (inpatient)	◆ Pain ◆ Limited bed mobility ◆ Limited transfers ◆ Limited gait ◆ Limited strength of involved LE	◆ Inpatient on pain medication ◆ Bed mobility training ◆ Transfer training ◆ Gait training ◆ Isometrics—Quadriceps sets, gluteal sets ◆ A/AROM—Hip (flexion, extension, abduction, adduction) ◆ AROM—Heel slides, ankle pumps ◆ Patient education emphasizing safety with all mobility training	◆ Independent or SBA with bed mobility transfers and gait 200 feet using FWW ◆ Independent with home exercise program ◆ Caregiver trained to assist with basic skills ◆ Discharge to home	◆ Emphasize restoration of independence with self care activities (bed mobility, transfers) ◆ Ambulate safely to return to home environment with some degree of independence ◆ Provide exercises to help patient regain muscular control of involved LE ◆ Provide assistance to patient to perform hip ROM ◆ Ensure patient and caregiver safety and prevent falls

LE, Lower extremity; *A/AROM,* active assistive range of motion; *SBA,* stand by assist; *FWW,* front-wheeled walker; *AROM,* active range of motion; *ROM,* range of motion.

Treatments performed on the day of surgery such as incentive spirometry exercises, management of air compression equipment, and donning thromboembolic disease (TED) hose are generally assigned to the nursing staff. When a good recovery from surgical trauma is demonstrated, hospital phase physical therapy usually begins on the first day after surgery.

Postoperative day 1 treatment consists of an evaluation, bed mobility, transfer training, gait training, and a beginning exercise program. The patient's initial goal is to transfer out of bed safely and walk to the bathroom independently using a front-wheeled walker (FWW). Some confusion or an emotional reaction to the event that precipitated the surgery may be encountered on the first postoperative day, and the patient may be groggy or in a great deal of pain. Because ORIF is normally an emergency surgery, the patient does not have the advantage of a preoperative training session. However, bed mobility and transfer training may be easier here than with a patient who has undergone THR, because usually no ROM precautions are in place.

Patients who received sacral anesthesia may show a faster initial rate of progress than those who are administered general anesthesia. The patient's pain medications should be timed to reach peak effectiveness during therapy sessions.

The PT should be informed of the patient's weight-bearing status and any special ROM restrictions. On the first postoperative day, the patient will attempt to walk to a chair and then sit up for approximately 1 hour before returning to bed. This may be repeated two to three times on the first day. The PT will encourage the patient to sit up longer each day.

The PT checks the patient's skin daily for pressure sores, especially at the heels. The patient should be placed properly in bed to preclude the tendency to lie in a frog-legged position with the hips in extreme ER and flexion.

Ankle pumps are the first exercises assigned to a patient. They help to prevent blood clots and to decrease edema in the legs. The patient should perform 10 to 20 repetitions every 30 minutes. Quadriceps sets with and without adductor squeezes (Fig. 16-12), gluteal sets, hamstring sets, and hip abduction sets should be performed three times per day with 10 repetitions of each exercise to begin restoration of proximal hip strength. This program may be expanded to include active assistive and then active hip abduction, adduction, and hip-knee flexion. Repeated encouragement may be necessary.

Ankle proprioceptive neuromuscular facilitation (PNF) patterns done in both diagonal planes may help prepare the patient for weight bearing. Lower extremity (LE) stretching may be done to avoid contractures and to prepare the patient for a normal gait pattern.

The patient can strengthen the upper extremities (UEs) using a Theraband or the hospital bed's triangle as a pull-up bar. Pelvic tilts and single knee-to-chest stretches of the uninvolved extremity can help decrease lumbar soreness and stiffness.

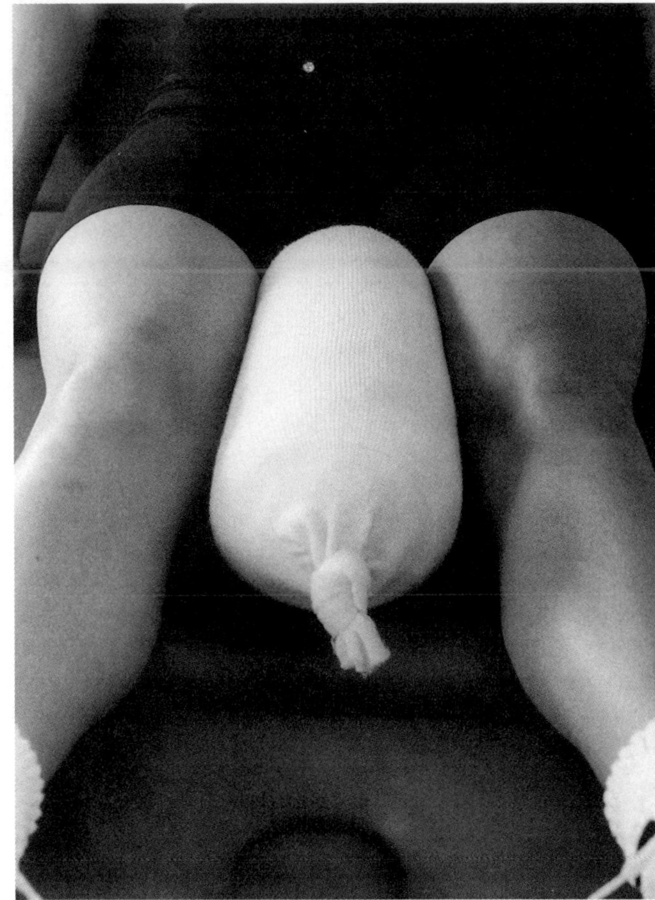

Fig. 16-12 Quadriceps set with the adductor squeezed. The patient sits with the legs stretched out in front. With a pillow between the knees and thighs, the patient squeezes the knees together and tightens the top of the thighs at the same time, holding for a count of 10 seconds.

The patient's weight-bearing status, assigned by the surgeon, can vary depending on the type of procedure performed. A FWW is recommended for patients with weight-bearing restrictions. However, patients who are assigned nonweight bearing may feel more secure using a pick-up walker. A platform walker may be appropriate if UE injuries are present. Agile patients are issued axillary crutches immediately regardless of weight-bearing status.

Patients having difficulty with touchdown weight bearing (TDWB), defined as less than 10 lbs of pressure through the affected leg,[12] or with partial weight bearing (PWB), around 40% of normal weight bearing on the involved extremity, may benefit from weight shift training in the parallel bars. The therapist should wear a very thick-soled shoe worn on the uninvolved leg to help lift the patient (to facilitate TDWB with the involved leg). With PWB status, stepping onto a bathroom scale helps the patient appreciate the appropriate amount of pressure to place on the involved extremity.

Electrical galvanic stimulation is sometimes used to manage edema and electrical stimulation (ES) in the muscle re-education mode can help facilitate quadriceps (especially the vastus medialis oblique) contraction. **However, electrical modalities tend to be very uncomfortable for most patients, especially those with metal implants.** These treatments may be more appropriate at the outpatient stage. The surgeon, as always, should be consulted before the application of these modalities.

Transfer to the skilled nursing facility from acute care is expected on the third day after surgery. Patients are discharged from the hospital when they are medically stable and demonstrate independence with bed mobility, transfers, and ambulation (using an appropriate assistive device). Home caregivers should be trained to assist with these tasks safely before the patient leaves the hospital. Discharge goals are usually attained within 1 or 2 weeks after surgery. Patients may be kept in an extended-care wing longer if no home caregiver is available and assistance is still required for basic mobility. A written exercise program for home use is presented at the time of discharge. The visiting PT in the home will reinforce the skills learned in the hospital.

A They cannot prepare for their surgery because it is an emergency surgery. Some have also been involved in motor vehicle accidents where other loved ones have been injured. Their situation needs to be appreciated and respected.

Q During gait training Julie has difficulty maintaining TDWB on the affected LE. She tends to place approximately 20% of her weight onto her affected leg. She attempts to respond to verbal cues but is unsuccessful. A scale was placed under the affected leg so that Julie could see and feel how much weight she was transferring onto her leg. Although she improved after using the scale, she still could not maintain a safe level of TDWB through the affected leg. What is another way to assist her in maintaining TDWB status?

Phase II (Home Phase)

TIME: 2 to 4 weeks after surgery

GOALS: Improve hip active range of motion (AROM) to 90 degrees, educate patient regarding a home maintenance program, help patient become independent with transfers and to ambulate around the home with appropriate assistive devices, encourage limited community ambulation (Table 16-2)

Home care physical therapy is normally authorized for patients who are homebound or would incur undue hardship by leaving home for treatment. Homebound status is a requirement for reimbursement through Medicare and most other insurance plans. PTs usually schedule visits two to three times per week until the patient is no longer homebound or until goals have been met. This is usually achieved within 2 to 4 weeks of the patient's returning home from the hospital.

Typically the goal of the home care therapist is to ensure the patient's safety at home and to enable a return to previous community activities with the use of an appropriate walking device. However, these goals may be unrealistic, depending on the patient's overall health status, motivation level, or previous level of function. In such a case, the patient is discharged when the PT determines that no more progress can be made.

During the initial home care visit, the PT evaluates the patient's ROM, strength, bed mobility, transfer ability, gait pattern, stair-climbing ability, performance of the home exercise program, endurance, pain level, leg length, overall safety awareness, and skin status. The ability of caregivers to assist the patient must also be assessed.

Equipment needs can include a bedside commode, a raised toilet seat (if the patient has not attained 90 degrees of hip flexion), a shower chair, grab bars installed in the bathroom, railings installed by stairways, and appropriate assistive devices for the progression of gait. Moving furniture and electrical cords to ensure a clear pathway may be necessary.

The patient's understanding of the weight-bearing restrictions and ROM precautions as prescribed by the physician should be demonstrated and recited. Caregivers should be present during this review.

PTs are now being trained to remove staples because of constraints imposed on nursing visits by insurance carriers. Staples are usually removed at about the fourteenth postoperative day. Proper sanitary technique protocols must be followed. The PT should consult the physician if any irregularity in scar healing is noted.

The patient will advance from isometric to active ROM exercises during the home phase. Patients who require an active assist should soon be performing their exercises independently. Bilateral tiptoes (plantarflexion) (Fig. 16-13) and heel cord stretches (Fig. 16-14) while standing can be performed while using a walker or countertop for support. Other closed-chain exercises such as modified lunges and wall slides (Fig. 16-15) are added as appropriate.

Hip flexion, extension, and abduction performed while standing are beneficial for the involved leg. They may be alternated bilaterally, depending on the patient's weight-bearing restrictions. With weight bearing as tolerated (WBAT) status, the patient may attempt balancing exercises on the involved leg. The PT should address chronic deficits in flexibility, strength, and balance that may have precipitated the patient's injury. A balance retraining program may benefit patients who have vestibular or

Table 16-2 Hip Open Reduction Internal Fixation

Rehabilitation Phase	Criteria to Progress to this Phase	Anticipated Impairments and Functional Limitations	Intervention	Goal	Rationale
Phase II Postoperative 2-4 weeks	◆ No signs of infection ◆ No increase in pain ◆ Usually home health status but may be transitioned to outpatient when appropriate	◆ Limited hip ROM ◆ Limited LE strength ◆ Limited with transfers in and out of car ◆ Limited gait	◆ Continuation of exercises as in Phase I ◆ PROM—Stretches as indicated (calf, hamstring, quadriceps, single knee to chest) ◆ AROM—Standing (hip flexion, extension, abduction, adduction); mini-squats, lunges, heel raises, wall slides; sitting (long arc quadriceps, pelvic tilt) ◆ Elastic tubing exercises for UEs ◆ Gait/stair training ◆ Standing balance training (balance boards) with assistance as needed ◆ Car transfers	◆ Increase AROM to hip flexion 90 degrees, abduction 20 degrees, knee flexion 90 degrees ◆ Independent with home exercises ◆ Increase strength in hip to 60%, knee to 70% ◆ Initiate UE strengthening program ◆ Gait—Independent with cane at home; SBA with cane in community (1000 feet) ◆ Improve balance ◆ Perform independent transfers	◆ Develop flexibility to improve sitting posture and tolerance ◆ Improve strength to ensure safety with ambulation and transfers, decreasing dependence on uninvolved LE ◆ Restore presurgical UE strength ◆ Promote independence with community ambulation ◆ Improve balance to prevent falls ◆ Encourage return to previous ADLs and community activities

ROM, Range of motion; *LE,* lower extremity; *PROM,* passive range of motion; *AROM,* active range of motion; *UE,* upper extremity; *SBA,* stand by assist; *ADLs,* activities of daily living.

neurologic involvement. Vision problems should be referred to the physician.

Hamstring and calf stretches may be done in supine using a towel (Fig. 16-16). The quadriceps can be stretched using a towel, with the patient lying prone with knees bent. Pelvic tilt, knee-to-chest, hip rotator stretches, and trunk rotation exercises benefit the low back and the hip.

The patient progresses from using a FWW or two crutches to a cane during this phase. The ability to ambulate safely without an assistive device is sometimes attainable within the time period authorized. Special care should be taken to correct uneven stride length (leading with the involved extremity and stepping-to with the uninvolved extremity), knee flexion in late stance phase, forward flexion at the waist, and overstriding with crutches.[12]

Gait training includes stair climbing. Initially the patient should walk up the stairs leading with the strong leg and descend the stairs leading with the operative leg in a step-to pattern. The patient with WBAT status can practice step-ups onto a book or a step with a very narrow rise using the operative leg (Fig. 16-17). An initial isometric contraction can precede the step-up onto progressively taller rises until the patient is able to walk up and down stairs in a normal step-over-step pattern. Training to step up and down safely from curbs, to walk on uneven surfaces and to transfer in and out of cars also is provided in the home phase.

Home health physical therapy is usually finished within 2 to 4 weeks. The patient should have 90 degrees of hip flexion and 20 degrees of hip abduction at this point. The quadriceps and hip abductor strength should be fair to fair plus (3/5 to 3+/5 with a manual muscle test [MMT]) and the patient should be able to perform all exercises actively.

The majority of ORIF patients are older people with fairly sedentary lifestyles. They may refuse further rehabilitation past the home care phase. Walking programs should be strongly encouraged with these patients.

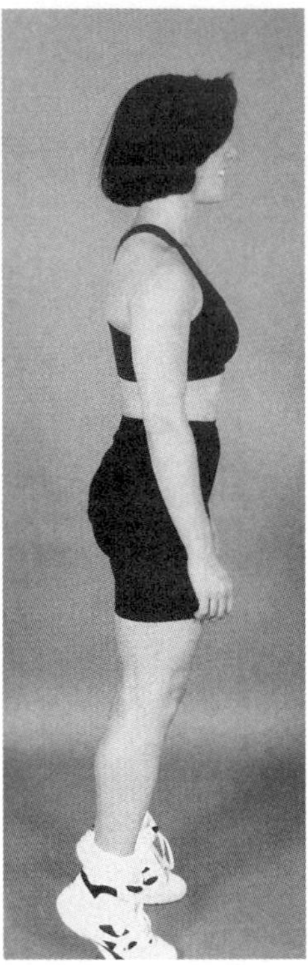

Fig. 16-13 Bilateral tiptoes. The patient stands on the floor with the knees straight and then lifts onto the toes, holds for 5 seconds, and slowly releases downward.

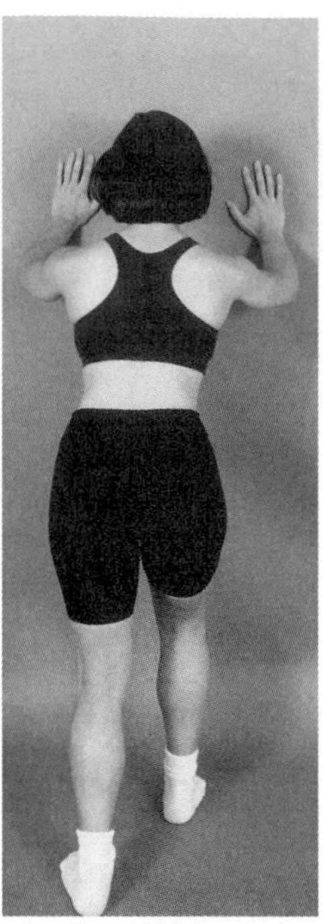

Fig. 16-14 Heel cord stretch. The patient stands with the involved leg and foot back and the toes turned in slightly. He or she then places the hands against a wall and leans forward until a stretch is felt. The patient keeps the heel down, holds for 15 seconds, and slowly releases.

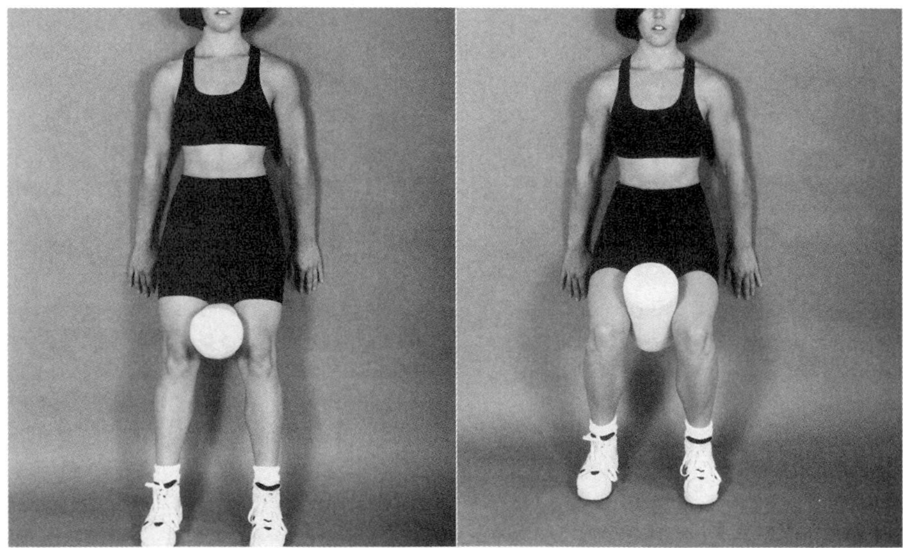

Fig. 16-15 Wall slides using an adductor pillow. **A,** The patient stands with the back against a wall, feet shoulder-width apart, with a pillow between the thighs. **B,** He or she then bends the knees to a 45-degree angle, tightens the thighs, and squeezes the pillow. The patient holds for 10 seconds, then extends the knees and slides up the wall.

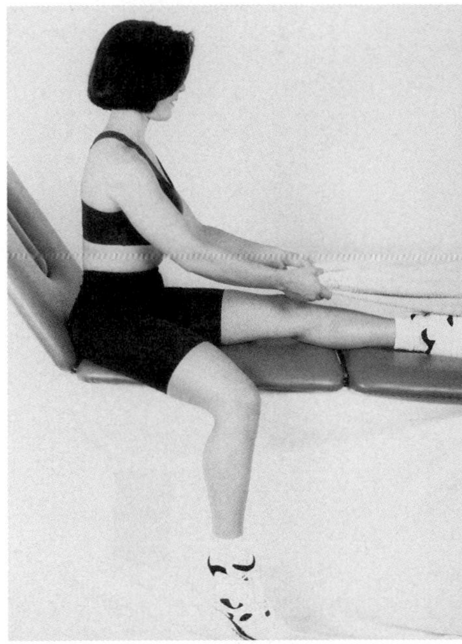

Fig. 16-16 Sitting hamstring stretch. The patient sits with the involved leg straight and the other leg bent off the edge of a table or bed. He or she then hooks a towel around the foot, keeps the back straight, and leans forward until a stretch is felt. The patient holds this position for 15 seconds and slowly releases. Older patients with less flexibility may simply lean back on their hands, initially.

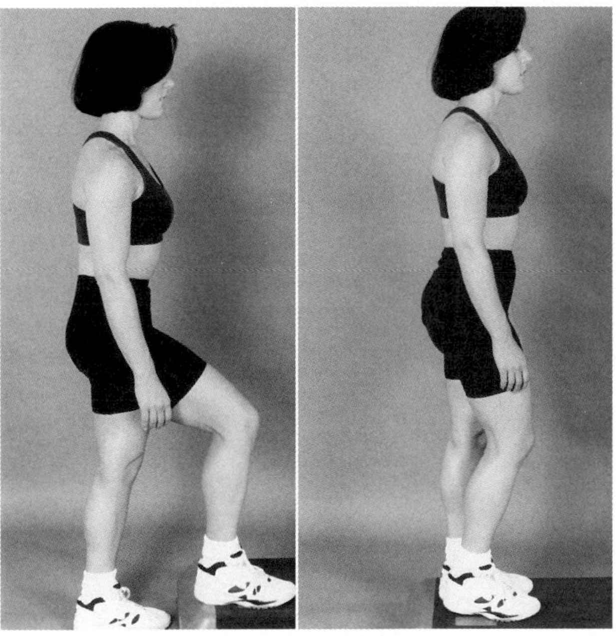

Fig. 16-17 Step-ups. A, The patient slowly steps onto a step with the involved extremity while tightening the muscles of the thigh. B, The patient must control the knee while stepping up.

Swimming and bicycle riding are recommended, when realistic, for long-term exercise programs; tai chi has been shown to decrease the risk of falls in older adults.[9] Active patients with more rigorous lifestyle requirements should go on to outpatient therapy for further strengthening.

With osteoporosis so prevalent in this population, the patient may be advised to consult the primary care physician regarding the propriety of a calcium replacement program or hormone replacement therapy.

A A very thick-soled shoe worn on the uninvolved foot helps lift the patient and facilitates TDWB status.

Q Ruth is 70 years old. She sustained a hip fracture at home when she tripped and fell. She had an ORIF on her left hip 3 months ago. Before her fall, she could walk without an assistive device. Presently she walks at home without an assistive device but needs a cane to ambulate around the community. She rarely goes out because she is so fearful of falling. She has maintained a strengthening home exercise program. Ruth feels that her leg remains weak despite all her exercising. Her LE flexibility is generally restricted throughout. The left leg is more restricted than the right. Ruth's balance and coordination also are impaired. Movements other than forward gait appear labored and slow. Left hip strength is generally 4–/5. Should strengthening, stretching, ROM, balance training, or coordination training be emphasized initially during treatment?

Phase III (Outpatient Phase)

TIME: 5 to 8 weeks after surgery

GOALS: Encourage patient self-management of exercises, help patient become independent in community ambulation, increase strength of LE (Table 16-3)

Outpatient physical therapy is intended to increase the involved extremity's flexibility to full ROM and increase its strength to at least the good minus level (−4/5 MMT). Gait pattern irregularities are to be normalized. Cardiovascular capacity also may be improved. These treatments should be conducted two to three times per week. The duration of outpatient rehabilitation depends on the patient's ability to make objective progress and on whether the intervention or treatment requires the skill of a PT.

All exercises should be done actively by this time. Exercises previously performed in gravity-eliminated positions, such as supine hip abduction (Fig. 16-18) and adduction (Fig. 16-19), are progressed to side-lying gravity-resisted positions. Ankle weights can be added if appropriate. The closed-chain exercises mentioned previously also are performed in the outpatient clinic.

Table 16-3 Hip Open Reduction Internal Fixation

Rehabilitation Phase	Criteria to Progress to this Phase	Anticipated Impairments and Functional Limitations	Intervention	Goal	Rationale
Phase III Postoperative 5-8 weeks	◆ Independence with transfers in and out of car ◆ No loss of hip ROM	◆ Limited AROM and strength of involved LE ◆ Limited tolerance to community ambulation ◆ Limited tolerance to cardiovascular exercises ◆ Limited with resuming more advanced activities	◆ Progression of exercises in Phase I and II, adding resistance where appropriate ◆ Modalities as necessary: heat, ice, ES ◆ Trunk stabilization exercises ◆ UBE ◆ Stationary bicycle ◆ Treadmill ◆ Gait training for uneven surfaces and stairs	◆ Control pain ◆ Regain full AROM of involved LE ◆ Increase LE strength to 75% ◆ Become independent with community ambulation	◆ Progress strength and ROM of involved LE ◆ Use modalities to control any residual activity or prepare tissue for stretching ◆ Promote safety with ambulation on all types of surfaces ◆ Regain cardiovascular conditioning ◆ Resume all ADLs and community activities

ROM, Range of motion; *AROM,* active range of motion; *LE,* lower extremity; *ES,* electrical stimulation; *UBE,* upper body ergometer; *ADLs,* activities of daily living.

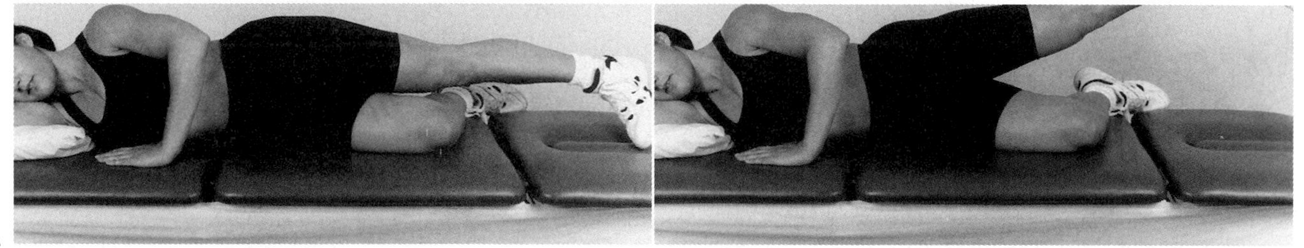

Fig. 16-18 Active hip abduction. **A,** The patient lies on the uninvolved side with the bottom knee bent. **B,** Keeping the top leg straight, he or she lifts upward, holds for 5 seconds, then slowly returns to the starting position.

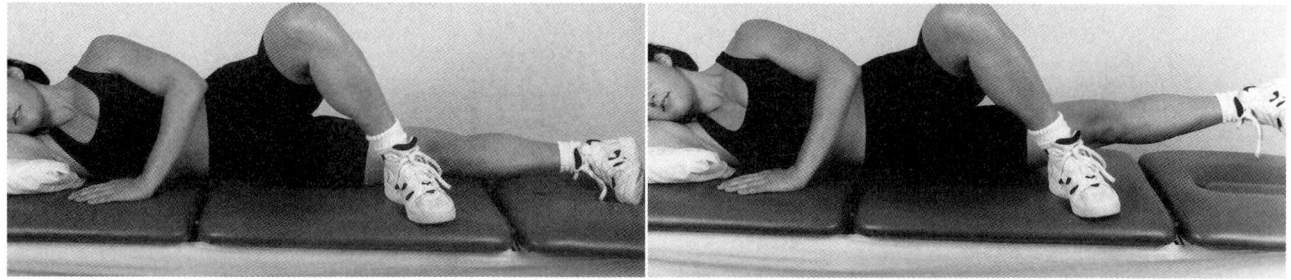

Fig. 16-19 Active hip adduction. **A,** The patient lies on the involved side with the bottom leg straight. **B,** He or she then bends the top knee and places the foot in front of the bottom leg. The patient lifts the bottom leg up approximately 6 to 8 inches and holds for 5 to 10 seconds before slowly returning the leg to the starting position.

Mini-squats and wall squats can emphasize a vastus medialis oblique contraction with the addition of an isometric hip adductor squeeze using a pillow or small ball. Lunges with the involved leg on a small step can progress to stair climbing on larger, more normal-sized steps. Standing balance exercises on the affected leg are appropriate with WBAT status.

Cardiovascular exercise is important during this phase to increase circulation throughout the body and endurance for ambulation. An upper body ergometer (UBE) or a

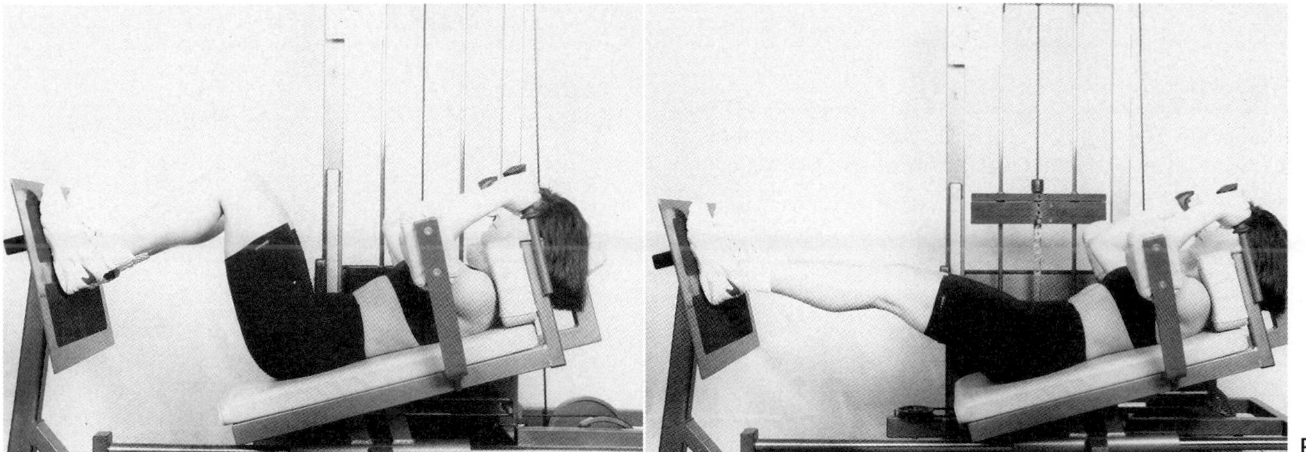

Fig. 16-20 Leg press machine. **A,** The patient should adjust the machine so that the knees are bent approximately 90 degrees while the back is flat. **B,** The patient straightens the legs while exhaling without locking the knees, then slowly releases.

stationary bicycle can be introduced at this phase. The patient's tolerance should be built up to a combined 15 to 30 minutes, if possible.

The modalities mentioned in the hospital phase may be performed here with the approval of the surgeon. Balance retraining programs may be expanded to include various balance boards. Spine stabilization exercises can include those done in the prone and quadruped positions. Inclusion of the leg press (Fig. 16-20) and other weight-training equipment may be appropriate in the clinic phase. At the PT's discretion, a treadmill also may be used to contribute to balance and gait retraining. Placement of a mirror in front of the treadmill can help the patient to observe and correct gait pattern irregularities.

By the end of the outpatient phase, the patient should have a well-rounded program that can be continued at home or at a fitness center. Bicycling, recreational walking, tai chi, and swimming are excellent long-term options for the patient recovering from hip ORIF.

A The therapist ascertained the conditions that were hampering progress with strength, balance, and ease of movement during gait. LE flexibility exercises with the guidance and careful assistance of the therapist were emphasized during the first four visits. Balance, coordination, gait, and strength issues also were addressed. As the flexibility of the LEs increased, advances with strength could be obtained more easily. In addition, the patient was able to move her LEs more freely during lateral or backward movements. Therefore balance and coordination also progressed. Ruth's confidence grew, and in a few weeks she was safely walking and maneuvering around the community without an assistive device.

TROUBLESHOOTING

Complications may arise in the course of rehabilitation. Examples that should be referred to the surgeon include the following:

- Thigh pain with walking that clears with sitting (may represent intermittent claudication)
- A positive Trendelenburg sign that does not resolve with treatment (may result from damage to the gluteal innervation)
- Severe rubor and swelling at the surgical site with accompanying fever (may indicate a septic infection)
- Persistent, severe pain (may result from an expansion of the fracture or loosening of the fixation devices)

Other problems that may arise are the responsibility of the surgeon, but the PT can use palliative measures to assist the patient. Leg length discrepancy is an example. The patient can continue gait training with a temporary shoe insert or with shoes of different heel heights. The surgeon may later prescribe a permanent orthotic.

Persistent edema is treated with medication. Patients should be advised to elevate their legs, rest more often, wear TED hose, pump their ankles, and apply ice to swollen areas.

Pain exacerbations are usually treated with medication. Possible side effects of the medication include nausea, constipation, and hypertension. The therapist can assist in pain reduction with modalities, exercise, and positioning.

SUGGESTED HOME MAINTENANCE FOR THE POSTSURGICAL PATIENT

Days 1-7 (in hospital)

GOALS FOR THE PERIOD: Increase volitional control of involved lower extremity (LE), improve and maintain range of motion (ROM)

Isometric Exercises

1. Quadriceps sets
2. Gluteal sets

Active Range of Motion (AROM) Exercises

3. Heel slides
4. Ankle pumps

Weeks 2-4

GOALS FOR THE PERIOD: Increase LE strength and functional ROM, initiate upper-extremity (UE) strengthening program

1. Stretching as indicated by evaluation

AROM Exercises

2. Standing hip flexion, extension, abduction, and adduction
3. Mini-squats
4. Lunges
5. Wall slides
6. Pelvic tilt
7. Long-arc quadriceps
8. Upper body exercises as indicated

Weeks 5-8

GOALS FOR THE PERIOD: Promote return to previous level of function (as cleared by physician)

1. Continue exercises from weeks 2 to 4
2. Progress to gym activities as indicated and prepare for discharge to community or home gym (treadmill, stationary bicycle)

References

1. American Academy of Orthopaedic Surgeons: *Orthopedic knowledge update 3: home study syllabus,* Rosemont, IL, 1990, the Academy.
2. American Academy of Orthopaedic Surgeons: *Orthopedic knowledge update 4: home study syllabus,* Rosemont, IL, 1992, the Academy.
3. Bray TJ et al: The displaced femoral neck fracture: internal fixation versus bipolar endoprosthesis. Results of a prospective randomized comparison, *Clin Orthop* 230:127, 1988.
4. Brumbeck RJ et al: Design concepts and early utilization of a new femoral interlocking nail, *Am J Orthop* 32(suppl):5-9, 2003.
5. Brumback RJ et al: Intramedullary nailing of femoral shaft fractures. I. Decision making errors with interlocking fixation, *J Bone Joint Surg* 70A:1441, 1988.
6. Brumback RJ et al: Intramedullary nailing of femoral shaft fractures. II. Fracture healing with static interlocking, *J Bone Joint Surg* 70A:1453, 1988.
7. Brumback RJ et al: Intramedullary nailing of femoral shaft fractures. III. Long-term effects of static interlocking fixation, *J Bone Joint Surg* 74A:106, 1992.
8. Brumbeck RJ et al: Immediate weight-bearing after treatment of a comminuted fracture of the femoral shaft with a statically locked intramedullary nail, *J Bone Joint Surg Am* 81(11):1538-1544, 1999.
9. Clark GS, Siebens HC: Geriatric rehabilitation. In DeLisa JA, editor: *Rehabilitation medicine: principles and practice,* ed 3, Philadelphia, 1988, JB Lippincott.
10. Crenshaw AH et al: *Campbell's operative orthopaedics,* ed 9, St Louis, 1998, Mosby.
11. Elmerson S, Zetterberg C, Andersson G: Ten-year survival after fractures of the proximal end of the femur, *Gerontology* 34:186, 1988.
12. Fagerson TL: *The hip handbook,* Newton, MA, 1998, Butterworth-Heinemann.
13. Hoppenfeld S, deBoer P, Thomas HA: *Surgical exposures in orthopedics: the anatomic approach,* Philadelphia, 1984, JB Lippincott.
14. Ions GK, Stevens J: Prediction of survival in patients with femoral neck fractures, *J Bone Joint Surg* 69B:384, 1987.
15. Jensen TT, Juncker Y: Pressure sores common after hip operations, *Acta Orthop Scand* 58:209, 1987.
16. Jette AM: Without scientific integrity, there can be no evidence base, *Phys Ther* 85(11):1122-1123, 2005.
17. Jette AM et al: Functional recovery after hip fractures, *Arch Phys Med Rehabil* 68:735, 1987.
18. Rehnberg L, Olerud C: The stability of femoral neck fractures and its influence on healing, *J Bone Joint Surg* 71B:173, 1989.
19. Ruff ME, Lubbers LM: Treatment of subtrochanteric fractures with a sliding screw-plate device, *J Trauma* 26:75, 1986.
20. Sexson S, Lehner J: Factors affecting hip fractures mortality, *J Orthop Trauma* 1:298, 1988.
21. Weise K, Schwab E: Stabilization in treatment of per- and subtrochanteric fractures of the proximal femur, *Chirurg* 72(11): 1277-1282, 2001.
22. White BL, Fisher WD, Laurin CA: Rate of mortality of elderly patients after fracture of the hip in the 1980's, *J Bone Joint Surg* 69A:1335, 1987.
23. Bertin KC, Rottinger H. Anterolateral mini-incision hip replacement surgery: a modified Watson-Jones approach, *Clin Orthop Relat Res* 429:248-255, 2004.

CHAPTER 17

Anterior Cruciate Ligament Reconstruction

Jim Magnusson
Luga Podesta
Terry Gillette

Anterior cruciate ligament (ACL) injuries can occur at any stage of life from 5 to 85 years old.[120,149] However, most often they occur in the relatively young active (athletic) population. The age group more commonly associated with ACL ruptures is between 15 and 25 years old.[48,51,116,126,147] The extent of the injury and desired level of activity usually dictate when surgical intervention is required. This chapter describes the current surgical considerations, techniques, and rehabilitative guidelines with supportive rationale. The individual clinician must determine the speed and intensity appropriate for each patient.

SURGICAL INDICATIONS AND CONSIDERATIONS

Cause and Epidemiologic Factors

ACL injury has been well documented and classically involves a noncontact mechanism involving rapid deceleration in anticipation to a change of direction (i.e., pivoting motion) or landing motion.[23,26,32,58] Boden and colleagues[23] reported that 72% of ACL tears occurred as a result of noncontact. Most injuries are sustained at foot strike, with the knee close to full extension and with the ground reaction forces lateral to the knee joint causing a "valgus collapse"[23,76]; sagittal plane motion seems to have less influence on the ACL during injury.[23] The incidence of individuals sustaining a ruptured ACL has been reported at 1 in 3000.[58]

Patients describe feeling and sometimes hearing a "pop"[66] and are 1000 times more likely to be participating in a sporting event.[48] Swelling is immediate, which implicates a ligamentous injury because of its associated vascularity. Patients exhibiting instability of the knee that affects pivot shift, demonstrate a positive Lachman's test; positive magnetic resonance imaging (MRI) for ACL rupture should be thoroughly evaluated for surgical considerations. Functionally they have difficulty performing pivoting and deceleration activities related to activities of daily living (ADLs) or sports. Although individuals who have sustained isolated rupture of the ACL may continue to be functional, their level of function is compromised and may require future surgical intervention because of secondary restraint pathology.[19,87,105] The surgeon should thoroughly evaluate the patients desired level of activity to ensure a successful outcome. Multiple studies have made reference to the sequelae of degenerative arthritis and potential for meniscal tears in the ACL-deficient knee.[57,105,152]

Both anatomic and physiologic risk factors have been researched. Some of the anatomic risk factors that may predispose an individual to ACL injury include the following: hypermobility (laxity of joints), hormonal influences on hypermobility, a narrow intercondylar notch, ligament width, tibial rotation, pronated feet, and increased width of the pelvis in the female athlete.[114] Although some causes exist to suggest certain anatomic features, conclusive evidence has not been established between ligament failure and the anatomic risk factors. Physiologic risk factors include poor core strength, lower extremity (LE) deficits in muscular strength and coordination, and foot wear–ground interface. It may be a combination of the previously listed factors that leads to ACL injury, but women are two to eight times more likely to sustain injury than males.[7,85,145] Hormonal influences that affect ligament laxity have been explored, with evidence leaning toward this as a nonfactor. However, menstrual hormones may indirectly contribute to injury by influencing neuromuscular performance and muscle function.[74,145] Although there may be some influence on laxity, more compelling arguments point to strength and coordination differences. Many researchers have further studied the relationship of neuromuscular performance as a potential risk factor. They have identified significant differences in neuromuscular control after the onset of maturation. This deficit was observed in females landing after a jump.

The neuromuscular deficit allowed migration of the knee into a *valgus collapse position*, placing the ACL at risk.[23,74,75,77] Hewett, Myer, and Ford[74] also noted that after maturation (i.e., neuromuscular spurt) males regained their control; however, females did not make similar adaptations. The "drop jump" screening test is a useful exam to help prevent and further understand the mechanisms of an ACL injury.[129]

Leetun and associates[99] looked at lumbopelvic (core) stability as a risk factor for LE injury in female athletes. They concluded that athletes who did not sustain an injury demonstrated better hip abduction and external rotation (ER) strength, and that hip ER strength was the only useful predictor of injury status. **Overall, the therapist must be aware of the potential risk factors that were present leading up to the ACL injury. In this way the rehabilitation program can safely return the patient to the sport and prevent future injury.**

Treatment Options

The timing of when to perform reconstruction (acute versus chronic) has been a source of debate. It has been accepted that a higher risk for complications exists if surgery is performed (1) before obtaining a homeostatic environment, (2) if range of motion (ROM) is limited (especially extension), and (3) when quadriceps and hamstring contraction is inadequate (i.e., unable to perform a straight leg raise [SLR]).[122,152] It is also apparent that with postponing reconstruction in an active population, the risk is higher for meniscal and chondral surface damage.[6,57,92,157]

Researchers have speculated about the age at which reconstruction is not recommended; however, to date no literature has noted any detrimental outcomes based on the age of the patient. In fact, studies have shown no significant difference in outcomes in comparing individuals at the age breaks of 35 and 40 years.[15,96,126,168] Reconstruction of the skeletally immature (SI) patient remains controversial, but the current literature appears to be leaning toward performing reconstruction. Younger populations are sustaining ACL tears; although it has been generally advisable to await physeal closure before reconstruction, some surgeons are having successful outcomes.[154] Appropriateness for reconstruction should be evaluated based on chronologic age, Tanner stage, radiologic findings in the knee, and developmental-psychologic factors.[27,131] Drilling across the physes has not been advocated because of the risks of arresting bone growth. However, Shelbourne and colleagues[154] presented information on a small group of SI patients (Tanner stage 3 or 4 and had clearly open growth plates) who underwent intra-articular patella tendon graft. Surgery emphasized the importance of not overtensioning the graft and meticulous placement of the bone plugs proximal to the physes. They had no growth disturbances on follow-up; when confronted with the potential of new meniscal tears, recurrent instability, effusion, and pain, ACL reconstruction in the SI patient appears to be a viable option.[114,121]

The anticipated functional limitations (modification of activities involving pivoting and deceleration) must be explored and explained to the patient who chooses not to have an ACL-deficient knee reconstructed. Ciccotti and associates[35] reported on nonoperative management of patients from 40 to 60 years. They found that 83% of the patients had a satisfactory result with guided rehabilitation. However, they also mentioned that surgery might be an option for individuals wishing to continue sporting and pivoting activities.

Surgical techniques to replace the deficient ACL continue to evolve. Advances in arthroscopic surgery provide surgeons with the ability to perform these reconstructive procedures using a one-incision endoscopic technique. Research continues in the search for the optimal graft, fixation technique, and surgical reconstructive procedure. In 1920, Hey-Groves[78] and Campbell[30] (in 1939) first described the use of the patella tendon as an ACL graft. Because of these original surgical descriptions, numerous procedures to repair or reconstruct the ACL have been advocated. Attempts at primary repair of the ACL with and without augmentation[29,111,112] were of limited success.[157] Extra-articular ACL reconstruction also was suggested as a technique to reconstruct the ACL-deficient knee.[52,104] However, long-term results were disappointing.[61,163] Intra-articular ACL reconstruction using various tissues, including the patellar tendon, iliotibial band, and combinations of hamstring tendons (semitendinosus, semitendinosus-gracilis), has been extensively described in the literature.[3,34,87,91,125]

The biologic grafts most widely used today are the central third patellar tendon (i.e., bone-patella tendon-bone complex [BPTB]) or multistrand hamstring tendon grafts. Although the hamstring graft has some advantages,[62,86] both procedures are equally successful (surgeon preference dictates choice if problems such as patella dysfunction are not present).[49,72] The endoscopic patellar tendon autograft reconstruction remains the most popular for use in high-level athletes.[26,63]

Graft Selection

The selection of the appropriate graft to replace the ACL is crucial to the ultimate success of the reconstruction. Primary concerns in the selection of an autogenous graft to replace the incompetent ACL include the biomechanical properties of the graft (e.g., initial graft strength and stiffness relative to the normal ACL), ease of graft harvest and fixation, potential for donor-site morbidity, and individual patient concerns. Other factors that ultimately influence graft performance include biologic changes in graft materials over time and their ability to withstand the effects of repetitive loading and stress.[40] Noyes and colleagues[128] studied the biomechanical properties of a number of autograft tissues and showed that an isolated 14 mm wide BPTB graft has 168% the strength of an intact ACL. A graft 10 mm wide is about 120% as strong. The study also determined that a single-strand semitendinosus graft displayed only 70% of the normal ACL strength. The data show that BPTB grafts have comparable tensile strength but increased stiffness in relation to the normal ACL, whereas single-strand semitendinosus grafts have decreased tensile strength but comparable stiffness. Other researchers have shown that multiple strands of semitendinosus or semitendinosus-gracilis composite grafts are stronger relative to the normal ACL.

The graft of choice varies among surgeons. They currently include BPTB autografts and allografts; single-, double-, and quadruple-stranded semitendinosus autografts; and composite grafts using semitendinosus-gracilis autografts. The enthusiasm surrounding the use of allograft replacement of the ACL has recently declined because of the small but tangible risk of infectious disease transmission. The risk of human immunodeficiency virus (HIV) transmission has been estimated to be 1 in 1.6 million using currently available bone- and tissue-banking techniques.[22] Sterilization by means of fresh freezing of allograft tissue may have an advantage over gamma radiation and ethylene oxide. Fielder and associates[54] have determined that 3 mrads or more of gamma radiation are required to sterilize HIV. Furthermore, sterilization procedures have been associated with alterations in graft properties and shown to cause a significant average decrease in stiffness (12%) and maximal load (26%),[137] and a marked inflammatory response with ethylene oxide use. Further studies must be conducted regarding poststerilization ACL allograft performance. Although the use of allografts as ACL replacements can diminish operative time and prevent graft harvest site morbidity, they are not recommended for routine use in primary ACL deficiency. Currently, either BPTB or multistrand semitendinosus autografts are the most widely used ACL substitutes to reconstruct the ACL-deficient knee.

Graft Fixation

Adequate fixation of the biologic ACL graft is crucial during the early postoperative period after ACL reconstruction. Fixation devices must transfer forces from the fixation device to the graft and provide stability under repetitive loads and sudden traumatic loads. Various techniques are now available for fixation, including interference screws, staples, sutures through buttons, sutures tied over screw posts, and ligament and plate washers. Kurosaka, Yoshiyas, and Andrish[97] determined the interference screw to be the strongest method of fixation of BPTB grafts. Interference screw strength depends on compression of the bone plug,[40] bone quality,[40,97] length of screw thread-bone contact,[25] and direction of ligament forces.[40] Robertson, Daniel, and Biden[142] studied soft tissue fixation to bone and determined the screw with washer and the barbed staple to be the strongest methods of fixation.

Graft Maturation

Graft maturation has an influence on the patient whose goals include a return to sports, most of which require pivoting and cutting. The healing properties of autografts have been discussed in the literature.[9,10,38,60,103] Although a majority of the studies the authors of this chapter have reviewed describe maturity of the graft at 100% 12 to 16 months postoperatively, return to sports participation in some protocols occurs at 6 months (if functional tests and isokinetics meet criteria).[45,151]

The graft maturation process begins at implantation and progresses over the next 1 to 2 years. Autografts are strongest at the time of implantation. The implanted graft undergoes a process of functional adaptation (ligamentization), with gradual biologic transformation. The tendon graft undergoes four distinct stages of maturation[9,10,60]:

1. Necrosis
2. Revascularization
3. Cellular proliferation
4. Collagen formation, remodeling, and maturation

Within the first 3 weeks after implantation, cell necrosis of the patella tendon intrinsic graft cells occurs. The graft consists of a collagen network that to this point has relied on a blood supply. As this blood supply is interrupted, the graft undergoes a necrotizing process. Necrosis commences immediately and generally lasts 2 weeks.[38,60,103] Native patella tendon (graft) cells diminish, and replacement cells can be present as early as the first week. Cellular repopulation occurs before revascularization. These cells are thought to arise from both extrinsic sources (i.e., synovial cells, mesenchymal stem cells, bone marrow, blood, ACL stump) and intrinsic sources (i.e., surviving graft cells). Early full ROM is desirable, because as new collagen is formed, its formation and strength are dictated by the stresses placed on it.

As the new cells find their way to this frame and add stability to this weak structure, rehabilitation must be careful not to disrupt or stretch them. Necrosis of the graft allows the metamorphosis of the graft from tendon to ligamentous process. Necrosis of the graft is highlighted by the formation of granulation tissue and inflammation. The bone blood supply and synovial fluid nourish the graft by synovial diffusion.[5] Revascularization occurs within the first 6 to 8 weeks after implantation. By this time the graft is revascularized via the fat pads, synovium, and endosteum,[38,60,103] and the inflammatory response should be under control. Further inflammatory problems signify a delayed healing process and potential graft problems; the physician and therapist should be alert for them.[108,165]

Amiel and colleagues[5] in 1986 described ligamentization of the rabbit patella tendon ACL graft. However, the graft never obtained all the cellular features of normal ACL tissue. Although the graft takes on many of the physical properties of the normal ACL, the cellular microgeometry of the remodeling graft does not closely resemble that of a normal ACL. The revascularization process progresses from peripheral to central.

Bone plugs incorporate into their respective bone tunnels over a 12-week period but are felt to near completion by approximately the sixth postoperative week. The comparative strength of the healed tendon-to-bone attachment versus the healed bone-plug attachment is unknown. Tendon-bone healing begins as a fibrovascular interface develops between the bone and tendon. Bony ingrowth occurs into these interfaces, which extends into the outer tendon tissue. A gradual re-establishment of collagen fiber continuity between bone and tendon occurs, and the attachment strength increases as collagen fiber continuity increases. These ACL autografts approximate 30% to 50% of the normal ACL strength 1 to 2 years postoperatively.[60]

Cellular proliferation and collagen formation take place as a continuing process throughout the maturation process. The function of collagen in the ligament is to withstand tension, and certain types of catalysts are present during the healing process. Transforming growth hormone factor β1 has been isolated during the healing of the medial collateral ligament (MCL) in rats. Administration of this growth hormone during the first 2 weeks after injury was found to increase strength, stiffness, and braking energy of the ligament.[103] Other catalysts of collagen formation (platelet-derived growth factor 1 [basic fibroblast growth factor]) have had equally good results in improving the tensile strength of healing ligaments. Future studies should be performed to validate this intervention.

During the rehabilitation program, pain and edema should dictate the speed at which the patient may progress. In clinics in which it is available, an assessment using the KT-1000 (Medmetric, San Diego, CA) is helpful as well.[2,46,48,152,153,159,161]

SURGICAL PROCEDURE

Endoscopic Bone-Patella Tendon-Bone Complex Anterior Cruciate Ligament Reconstruction

The procedure begins with a complete examination of the knee under anesthesia followed by a thorough diagnostic arthroscopic evaluation. The menisci, joint surfaces, and ligamentous structures are evaluated and additional injuries assessed arthroscopically. The leg is then exsanguinated, and a tourniquet is inflated with 350 mm of pressure. A medial parapatellar incision is made from the inferior pole of the patella to the tibial tuberosity. The skin is dissected down to the peritenon, and skin flaps are made superiorly, inferiorly, medially, and laterally. The peritenon is incised and the patella tendon is exposed. The width of the patellar tendon is noted (Fig. 17-1), and a 10 mm graft is measured from the midpatellar tendon. Two small incisions 10 mm apart are made in the patellar tendon and then extended superiorly and inferiorly with a hemostat. The patellar and tibial bone plugs are measured to provide graft lengths of 20 to 25 mm of patella and 25 to 30 mm of tibial bone. To facilitate bone graft harvest, the corners of the bone plugs are predrilled with a 2 mm drill to decrease stress risers. The perimeters of the bone plugs are then sawed out with a reciprocating saw to a depth of 10 to 11 mm, depending on the size of the patella and tibial tubercle. The graft (Fig. 17-2, A and B) is then taken to the back table, where it is prepared and fashioned to allow passage through the appropriate guides. The surgeon completes the graft by placing one No. 5 Tycron suture in the femoral and three No. 5 Tycron sutures into the tibial bone plugs to facilitate graft passage through the knee. The graft is preserved in a saline-moistened gauze sponge for later use.

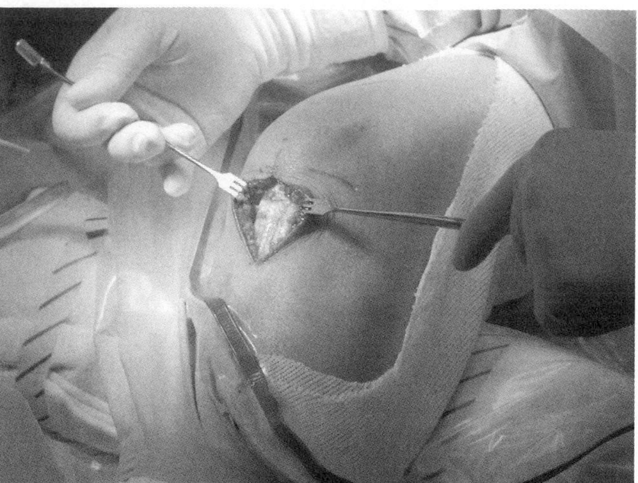

Fig. 17-1 Exposure of the patella tendon in preparation for harvesting.

The remnant of the ACL is resected, along with any hypertrophic tissue. Arthroscopically, the intercondylar notch is then prepared with the aid of a burr to prevent graft impingement. A site is chosen for placement of the tibial tunnel. Through the midline incision, a small area medial to the tibial tubercle is prepared with subperiosteal elevation. Using a tibial guide and under direct visualization, the surgeon drills a guide pin into the knee from the outside in, exiting within the knee at a site chosen anteromedial to the ACL insertion. The tibial tunnel is reamed to the size of the harvested graft. A curette placed over the

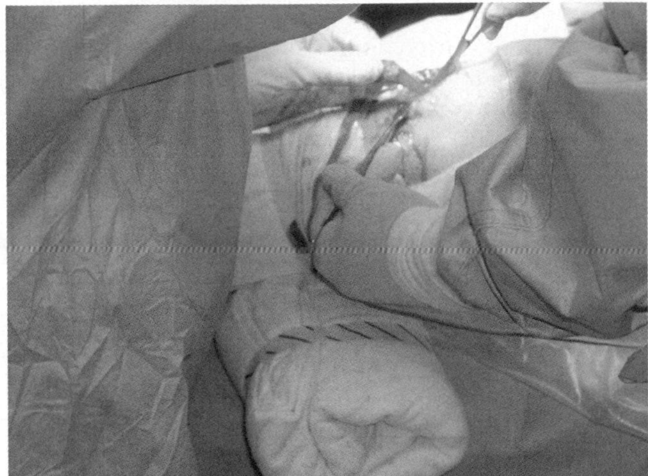

A

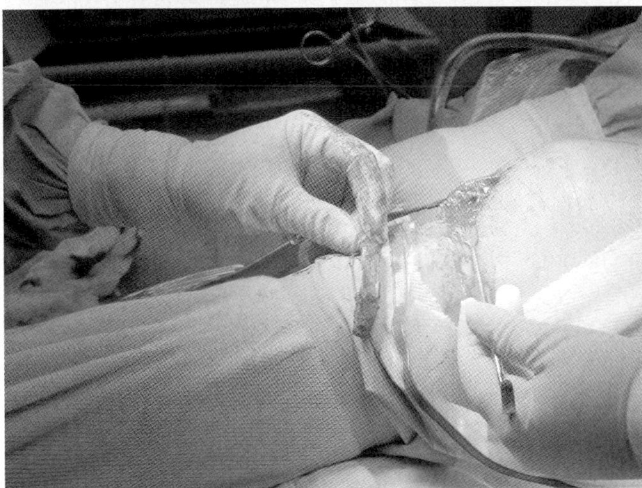

B

Fig. 17-2 Removal of the bone-tendon-bone (BTB) graft from the patella. A, Graft removed from the distal patella. B, Graft completely removed.

guide pin during reaming helps protect the articular cartilage and posterior cruciate ligament from damage. The tibial tunnel must be larger than the femoral tunnel to allow passage of the graft into the knee. The tibial tunnel edges are smoothed with a rasp to prevent graft abrasion after implantation. A fenestrated plug is then placed into the tibial tunnel to prevent fluid extravasation yet allow passage of instruments.

The femoral isometric point is determined on the medial aspect of the lateral femoral condyle, usually 3 to 5 mm anterior to the posterior cortex near the superior intercondylar notch margin (over-the-top position); it is marked with a curette or burr. With the knee flexed past 90 degrees, a fenestrated guide pin is inserted into the knee through the tibial tunnel and drilled through the femoral isometric point and out through the skin with the aid of an over-the-top guide. The femoral tunnel is then reamed to the size of the femoral bone plug to a depth of 30 mm.

The sutures from the femoral bone plug are inserted into the femoral pin and pulled out through the skin. The graft is delivered into the knee, through the tibial tunnel, and into the femoral tunnel under direct visualization. A cannulated interference screw is then inserted into the knee over a nidal guide pin and screwed into the femoral tunnel, compressing the femoral bone plug within the tunnel. Graft isometry is evaluated. The tibial bone plug within the tibial tunnel is secured with interference screw fixation. ROM and stability testing are then performed. The graft is evaluated arthroscopically to assess graft excursion and placement within the intercondylar notch.

The tourniquet is released, hemostasis is obtained, and the knee is irrigated. Loose closure of the patellar tendon is performed with the peritenon approximated to close the anterior defect. The subcutaneous tissue is approximated, and a continuous subcuticular skin closure is performed. The wounds are dressed sterilely. A light compressive wrap and continuous ice water cryotherapy system are applied, and the patient is taken to the recovery room with the knee in a knee immobilizer in full extension.

THERAPY GUIDELINES FOR REHABILITATION

Rehabilitation of the ACL depends on a number of factors. This chapter does not give a precise time frame during which to progress from double-leg squats to single-leg squats; however, the physical therapist should respond as further data emerge and make modifications as indicated. Interpretation of response is usually performed via observation, palpation, and measurement.

Much has been written regarding the rehabilitation of the patient who has undergone ACL reconstructive surgery. A body of literature has addressed the BPTB graft, because this has been the gold standard. Many protocols have been presented to manage such patients.* This chapter focuses on effective guidelines for autograft rehabilitation because it is currently the most common graft selection. The guidelines in this chapter are tailored for an isolated ACL reconstruction, but it is important to be able to modify these guidelines if any additional pathology is present such as meniscal repair or additional ligamentous injury. The rationale behind each component of rehabilitation is discussed.

The factors in developing a program should include the following:

1. Understanding fully the mechanics causing the injury (potential risk factors)

*References 45, 47, 48, 60, 70, 90, 108-110, 127, 132, 146, 148, 150, 151, 155, 156, 158, 161, 170, 172.

2. Respecting the healing constraints of the graft when making a clinical decision regarding modification or progression of the patient's program
3. Designing a program that uses functional training that avoids excessive stress on the graft
4. Emphasizing early ROM (especially full extension)

Preoperative Management

Although the initial visit may be postoperative, it is evident that preoperative care is both physiologically and psychologically beneficial. A 1- to 4-week program of rehabilitation can be used after acute ACL rupture to control edema, improve gait (education), and improve LE strength and ROM.[48,104] The length of the program depends on the degree of swelling and ROM present. During the preoperative examination, the physical therapist should assess the patient's gait, LE ROM, patellofemoral (PF) alignment, degree of edema, and weight-bearing capacity. Passive accessory and functional tests also should be performed as appropriate. The therapist may wish to seek out educational sources (e.g., continuing education programs) for a thorough understanding of rationales and applied techniques.

Gait evaluation focuses on tolerance of weight bearing on the involved leg, stride length, and step length. LE alignment should be assessed from the ground up. After surgery the patient's safety regarding gait must be ensured. Ambulation with crutches in varying degrees of weight bearing on the involved leg on level surfaces (and stairs) is performed to make the patient familiar with one of the first postoperative demands. Evaluation of preoperative knee ROM and PF alignment is helpful in beginning the postoperative planning process. The physical therapist must evaluate both the ankle and the hip (in addition to the knee) to identify any ROM limitations and strength deficits. *Knee ROM limitations greater than -10 degrees of extension have been associated with an increased incidence of arthrofibrosis (which is discussed in the section on complications).*[39,153] Passive accessory testing includes assessing the secondary restraints of the knee, the superior and inferior tibial-fibular articulations, PF complex, and a brief appraisal of the hip and ankle as appropriate.[106] Midpatellar girth measurements are effective in comparing edema of the uninvolved with the involved knee and monitoring progress. PF alignment and mobility are important to assess because of their influence on the pace of the rehabilitation process. *Preoperative PF crepitus is a factor in determining postoperative complications.*[2] Therefore treatment of this dysfunction should be initiated early to avoid setbacks in functional progression (see Chapters 18 and 20 for PF rehabilitation). Weight-bearing tolerance measurement can be as easy as using a weight scale and having the patient perform weight shifting until pain or instability is noted. Other assessments of weight acceptance on the involved leg can include sit-to-stand simulation (90-degree squat) using an inclined sled (calculating the percentage body weight based on the degree of incline) or shuttle (using resistive bands). Treatment for the preoperative phase is listed in Table 17-1. It is useful to initiate a progressive program to increase ROM, decrease edema and pain, and ultimately improve function.

Edema and Pain Management

The control of edema and pain is important both preoperatively and postoperatively. The modalities of choice are ice, electrical stimulation (ES), passive motion with progression to active motion, and elevation. After surgery an inflammatory response occurs as a necessary part of the healing process. However, edema management and pain control should be balanced. Swelling in the knee joint and its surrounding soft tissues is a painful side effect. Joint effusion can inhibit muscle function[159] and limit motion. The percentage of patients with persistent hemarthrosis after reconstruction has been reported to be as high as 12%.[110] Therefore it is important to manage edema and pain from the outset. A good healing environment must be provided to allow the graft to mature. Cryotherapy and ES are commonly used to manage edema and pain.[81,95] However, no studies have shown cryotherapy to be effective in reducing swelling. Nevertheless, cryotherapy can be used to manage and decrease secondary hypoxia, a side effect of swelling.[116] Although the literature has been a forum for debating the effectiveness of cryotherapy,[41,84] the clinical experiences of the authors of this chapter are similar to those of Cohn, Draeger, and Jackson[36] and Lessard and associates,[101] who found that patients receiving cryotherapy were more compliant, had less pain, and took less pain medication. Cryotherapy is effective in pain management.[14,138] Elevation and intermittent compression are used in conjunction with cold to manage postoperative pain and edema.[45,48,110,134]

A continuous flow cold therapy device appears to be more effective than crushed ice in the first week after surgery.[13] Aircast Cryo/Cuff is used immediately postoperatively and at home over the first couple of weeks. The temperatures commonly used are 10° to 20° C.[95] The use of a Cryo/Cuff accomplishes intermittent compression and cooling to maximize efficiency. Ice and exercise are used in an active combination to battle continued edema and pain. Cryotherapy in the form of cold packs or crushed ice can be used for as long as 20 or 30 minutes in conjunction with limb elevation[24,98,118] (above heart level) and exercise (i.e., ankle pumps, quadriceps sets, quadriceps-hamstring cocontraction). Elevation and muscle pumping help the lymph system remove tissue debris and inflammatory byproducts (free-floating proteins too large to filter through the capillaries).[95] The use of cold may be effective in the pain-dominant patient, allowing the therapist to progress ROM exercises. ES also is an effective

Table 17-1 Anterior Cruciate Ligament Reconstruction

Rehabilitation Phase	Criteria to Progress to this Phase	Intervention	Goal	Rationale
Phase Ia Preoperative 1-4 weeks	◆ Preoperative	◆ Cryotherapy 20-30 minutes ◆ Elevation with ankle pumps (10 repetitions per minute) 20-30 minutes ◆ Gait training (emphasizing normal gait pattern-weight shift) ◆ PROM stretches—Supine knee extension, prone hangs, supine wall slides, seated knee flexion ◆ Isometric exercise—Quadriceps/hamstring sets (cocontraction) ◆ A/AROM—Seated knee flexion ◆ AROM-PREs—Heel raises, hip abduction/adduction, ER ◆ Joint and soft tissue mobilization	By the end of 4 weeks: ◆ Self-manage pain ◆ Decrease edema ◆ ROM 0-degree extension to 130-degrees flexion ◆ Independent SLR ◆ Full weight bearing (brace as appropriate) ◆ Good isometric quadriceps contraction ◆ Maintain hip and ankle strength	◆ Pain control ◆ Edema management ◆ Gait training for safety and ease with transition postoperatively ◆ ROM stretches to prevent complications going into surgery ◆ Muscle pump to assist lymph drainage ◆ Graduated exercise to improve neuromuscular coordination ◆ Emphasize self-management of ROM program ◆ Prepare for transfers (supine-sit) ◆ ROM and muscle contraction to assist with edema management and improve ROM ◆ Decrease pain through soft tissue and joint mobilization techniques

PROM, Passive range of motion; *ROM*, range of motion; *SLR*, straight leg raise; *A/AROM*, active assistive range of motion; *ER*, external rotation; *AROM*, active range of motion; *PREs*, progressive resistance exercises.

tool used in the management of pain through the intermittent use of transcutaneous electrical nerve stimulation (TENS) or interferential electrical stimulation (IFC).[89,134]

The types of cold packs used affect the efficiency of cooling. Frostbite is a common concern, as is nerve palsy.[51,136,160] The optimal delivery mechanism is crushed ice in a plastic bag secured in place by an elastic wrap. **Care should be taken to avoid compression or ice over the proximal fibular head (because of the risk of affecting the peroneal nerve).** If the use of a gel pack is considered, compression wrap should not be used and precautions should be taken to avoid frostbite. A cryotherapy application of 20 to 30 minutes (which includes exercises as noted previously) is reinforced as part of the home exercise program, and the patient is instructed to perform it as often as four times daily, depending on the level of edema and pain. Although little consensus exists on this issue, in the management of edema and pain, cryotherapy is the authors' modality of choice for patients who tolerate cold temperatures.

Initial Postoperative Examination

Subjective information is reviewed with the patient regarding medication needs, edema and pain management program compliance, and other pertinent history (if not obtained preoperatively).[106] Baseline measurements of ROM (i.e., knee flexion-extension), girth, and PF mobility are included in the objective examination, along with palpation and observational findings (e.g., gait, transfers).

Many subjective measurements can be obtained using questionnaires. Some of the tests cited in studies are the International Knee Documentation Committee (IKDC), Gillquist, Lysholm, Noyes, Patient-Specific Functional Scale (PSFS), and Tegner.[12,33,35,69,73,124,141,162] Although these tests strive to objectify outcome studies, no consensus has been reached concerning which test is appropriate to use for all ACL reconstructions. Neeb and colleagues[124] attempted to identify a "package" of tests (subjective, functional, and clinical) and found that the clinician must use a comprehensive package to identify impairment and disability. More common is the use of a few questionnaires each yielding different outcome measures: the IKDC (objective assessment), Tegner (ADL assessment), and Lysolm (preoperative versus postoperative assessment).

ROM measurements are essential to monitor each treatment until full motion and function are restored. Patients seen during the first couple of days after surgery should have close to full extension (0 to −10 degrees) and limited flexion (80 to 100 degrees). Full extension must be given the utmost emphasis early in therapy.[48,110,127,151,156,170,172]

Full ROM is expected anywhere from 3 to 10 weeks after surgery.[45,165] Lack of early progress with motion is a red flag for complications and delay in progression through rehabilitation (see the discussion of complications).

Edema can be observed about the knee, leg, and at times the ankle and foot. Girth measurements are typically taken at the midpatella and 10 cm proximally and distally. The authors use the midpatellar measurement to monitor edema. Proximal and distal assessments are continued to monitor progress; they also objectively monitor quadriceps inhibition.[123,159] Girth measurements have long been taken in an effort to relate to muscle strength. Clinically there seems to be no significant relationship between muscle girth and function or strength during the initial rehabilitation period. Measurements of PF alignment should be undertaken in the first postoperative visit and continued during rehabilitation to avoid additional surgeries, slow progression of rehabilitation, and early plateau of exercises.

Palpation assessment of the PF articulation helps confirm any static malalignment problems (glides, tilts, patella alta or baja). Physical therapists can further their evaluation skills with continuing education that emphasizes PF assessment and treatment (see Chapter 18).

Skin temperature should be assessed on a continuing basis to monitor the inflammatory response phase. The physical therapist should assess the incision wound regularly to monitor healing; healing should be complete by 2 weeks after surgery. When appropriate, scar mobilization can be performed in a multidirectional pattern to prevent adhesions.

ROM, edema, pain, and stability testing ultimately determine the progression of exercises throughout rehabilitation. The authors feel that although the KT-1000 assessment of the anterior drawer is the hallmark measurement of how rapidly to progress rehabilitation, the reality is that not every clinic has access to this type of device. *Therefore the clinician must rely on assessment skills, observing closely for any increase in edema or decrease in muscle function (quadriceps, hamstring), and relating those to any subjective complaints.* Increases in laxity of 2 mm or more indicate imminent graft failure[110] and require highly conservative treatment that avoids any stress on the graft for a period of 2 weeks, until signs and symptoms subside. The rehabilitation program should be adjusted to avoid or minimize the stress that caused the setback, and further exercises should then be progressed conservatively.

In addition to the use of positioning and modalities, the authors feel that joint mobilization effectively decreases pain.[106] The continuous passive motion (CPM) device can be used to assist in managing postoperative pain (in addition to restoring ROM). Although CPM may produce no long-term benefits,[109,110,140] it appears helpful for patients with preoperative ROM difficulties.[47]

Although measurement of proprioception is not performed at this initial visit, the clinician must remember that proprioceptive deficits are present because of loss of mechanoreceptor input.[1,37,80] Although proprioception is affected without the ACL, it can improve with proprioceptive exercises and neuromuscular training. Thus exercises that develop neuromuscular control and stress proprioception should be a mainstay of the evolving ACL rehabilitation program.

Postoperative Guidelines and Rationales

The general guidelines listed here are for ACL reconstruction using the BPTB graft. On initial assessment, physical therapists must set treatment goals with patient input to avoid any potential misunderstandings. They also should provide education about graft maturation and the need to progress the rehabilitation program gradually and systematically. The treating therapist can modify the program based on the patient's response to treatment and the healing time frame of the graft.

The use of *closed-chain* versus *open-chain* exercises should be explored when planning rehabilitation of the LE. Closed-chain rehabilitation makes sense for a variety of reasons. Closed-chain activities are less stressful on the graft, have a functional relationship, and are easy for patients to perform at home.[20]

Open-chain exercises place the graft at risk in certain ROMs, appear to be nonactivity specific (except for kicking), and require equipment to progress resistance.

In strengthening the muscles affecting the knee, activation of the quadriceps has the most potential to place increased stress on the graft.[71,139] Grood and associates[68] and Palos and colleagues[132] noted increased anterior tibial translation during the last 30 degrees of extension in an open-chain environment. A number of other researchers and clinicians also support the idea of avoiding open-chain terminal knee extension.[8,55,79,82,128,133,146,148,168]

Performing closed-chain exercises with the foot in a fixed load-bearing position places less stress on the graft.[71,150,156,173] Closed-chain exercises make the exercise more specific to function, thus enhancing functional skills and transitional movements (e.g., weight shifting, sit-stand) in a safe manner.[167] Although open-chain exercises have a place in rehabilitation, the range of these exercises must be limited until graft maturation is adequate to support the stress. Ranges commonly found in the literature are 90 to 30 degrees, again avoiding the last 30 degrees of extension in an open-chain environment.[50,127]

The most common brace used initially is the immobilizer or locked hinged brace. It is used 24 hours a day and is taken off or unlocked only for bathing and appropriate exercises. As the patient gains muscular (quadriceps, hamstrings) control in a weight-bearing position, the brace is unlocked (hinged brace) or discarded (immobilizer). The physical therapist should caution the patient to avoid ambulation on uneven surfaces until adequate dynamic stability is apparent (usually 4 to 6 weeks).

Functional bracing that uses custom or prefabricated (off the shelf) braces is controversial.[21] Malone and Friedhoff[107] found the custom-fitted double upright brace to be the most effective, allowing less slippage or migration. Debate continues regarding the necessity and type of brace that is most appropriate. The authors' preference during phases II and III is to use braces sparingly and determine individually whether bracing is indicated for a specific activity.

> **Q** Tracy is 32 years old and had ACL reconstruction 1 week ago. She arrives at her first outpatient visit with moderate edema about the knee and ankle. She states that she has been compliant with weight bearing and uses her crutches and brace as instructed. What further questions can help the therapist provide a successful edema management program?

Phase I

TIME: 1 to 4 weeks after surgery

GOALS: Patient education and reinforcement of goals, quadriceps contraction, full knee extension, increase active range of motion (AROM) and passive range of motion (PROM), ambulation without an assistive device, initiate joint mobilization (Table 17-2)

The first postoperative visit takes place between 1 and 7 days after surgery. Pain levels, at their most intense at postoperative days 1 and 2, should decline by the seventh day.[18] Measurements are taken as appropriate (the reader should refer to the section on preoperative evaluation). This is the time to re-educate the patient about treatment goals and mechanisms to obtain those goals (including the edema and pain management program) and to initiate mild cardiovascular exercises (e.g., stationary bicycling using the uninvolved leg, upper body ergometer [UBE]). Education at this point regarding graft maturation and expectations regarding home exercise follow through is essential and saves time in future sessions. If patients have difficulty with the supine sleeping posture, the temporary use of a towel under the knee may be helpful in providing enough comfort to sleep if extension is too uncomfortable. However, extra care must be taken by the therapist and patient to not feed in to a potential flexion contracture or extension lag.

DeCarlo and Sell[43] retrospectively examined the number of treatments used in two groups of patients who had undergone ACL reconstruction. One group averaged a mere seven treatments (range of 3 to 18) over a 6-month program that emphasized patient education concerning ROM. Patients "followed written instructions prescribed by a physical therapist for increasing muscle strength." Although this underscores the importance of patient education, these authors cautioned that limited visits for therapy should be considered on an individual basis and should reflect sound clinical rationale. The authors of this chapter suggest a range of 12 to 24 visits over a 6-month period. Most of these visits take place during the first 6 weeks and taper off as clinically indicated; the program should place greater emphasis on patient self-management. *The majority of the literature emphasizes early full extension, progressive weight bearing, and early ROM and mobility.*[45,127,150,151,156,170]

After collecting all data, the physical therapist begins treatment. The patient may be brace free during PROM exercises, but the brace must be used when ambulating, when performing squatting activity, and locked at 0 degrees (extension) with hip AROM exercises until muscle contraction is adequate.

Initially ES is used to assist in obtaining quadriceps contraction. This can be done in conjunction with ES to the hamstrings to facilitate cocontraction. Cocontraction helps stabilize the knee and control tibial translation.[17] Isometrics (i.e., quadriceps and hamstring sets) are initiated along with AROM (i.e., ankle pumps) and cryotherapy in an elevated position (as mentioned in the edema and pain management program). One effective exercise is a quadriceps and hamstring isometric contraction using a closed-chain environment (Fig. 17-3). These are called *spider killers,* because the patient performs the isometric exercise while applying pressure to the ground via the heel (pretending that a spider is under the heel). Passive stretches are used to obtain early full knee extension. With prone hangs (Fig. 17-4) and supine passive knee extension (Fig. 17-5) (towel roll propped under the heel), patients should be well on their way to obtaining full extension. Flexion ROM is emphasized to a lesser extent than extension, but it is still important. Supine wall slides are also included in a home exercise program. The goal by 4 weeks is for the knee to be at 125 degrees of flexion. However, edema, pain, and overall tolerance of the knee to rehabilitation may limit flexion ROM progress.

> **A** Upon further questioning she has not been elevating her leg (above heart level) regularly or performing ROM or isometric exercises. A program was initiated consisting of elevation (20 minutes four times a day) with ankle pumps (10 repetitions every minute).

AROM exercises are performed for the hip and ankle initially to improve strength and endurance. Hip ER and abduction are targeted because of their role in positioning the knee in line with the foot. Supine heel slides and standing hamstring curls assist in gaining flexion ROM and strength. The patient should use a brace with exercises that place stress about the knee to give a sense of security

Table 17-2 Anterior Cruciate Ligament Reconstruction

Rehabilitation Phase	Criteria to Progress to this Phase	Intervention	Goal	Rationale
Phase I Postoperative 1-4 weeks	◆ Postoperative	◆ Brace should be worn for all exercises in **bold** type ◆ Edema and pain management program ◆ PROM—Supine knee extension, prone heel hangs, supine wall slides ◆ Isometrics—Quadriceps/ hamstring sets, cocontraction, towel squeeze ◆ AROM—Heel slides, **SLR (brace locked at 0 degrees)**; hip (flexion, extension, abduction, adduction); standing hamstring curls ◆ PREs—**Supine leg press (0-90 degrees as indicated)**, heel raises; bicycle, step-up exercises (initiate on a 2-inch step) ◆ Gait training using crutches: weight bearing as tolerated, normalize gait (use small obstacle [foam cup] to emphasize hip and knee flexion in conjunction with ankle dorsiflexion) ◆ Weight shifting Joint mobilization as indicated: ◆ Patella glides, tibia-femoral (posterior) glides	Achieve the following by the end of week 4: ◆ ROM 0-125 degrees ◆ Transfers (supine-sit) without assisting involved leg (SLR independent) ◆ Good quality thigh and calf muscle contraction ◆ Full weight bearing ◆ Walk without crutches or cane (household and limited community distances) ◆ Self-manage edema/pain	◆ Provide support and proprioceptive feedback ◆ Prevent complications ◆ Control pain ◆ Manage edema ◆ Provide PROM to improve joint mobility and decrease pain ◆ Initiate home exercise program ◆ Teach isometrics to improve muscle recruitment in preparation for functional activities ◆ Provide AROM to improve neuromuscular coordination, strength, transfers, and gait ◆ Promote self-management of pain ◆ Educate on positions/ movements that will stress the graft ◆ Provide gait training to progress independent ambulation without assistive device ◆ Increase strength and tolerance to weight bearing ◆ Joint mobilization to restore ROM and improve arthrokinematics

PROM, Passive range of motion; *ROM,* range of motion; *SLR,* straight leg raise; *AROM,* active range of motion; *PREs,* progressive resistance exercises.

initially. Exercises that require brace support (locked at 0 degrees) initially include the following:

- ◆ Proprioceptive neuromuscular facilitation (PNF) patterns of the hip[53]
- ◆ Hip flexion, extension, abduction, ER, and adduction

The brace may be unlocked to perform bilateral and, when appropriate, unilateral:

- ◆ Inclined sled (Fig. 17-6)
- ◆ Leg presses

Step-up activities (Fig. 17-7) are performed (when appropriate) with the brace unlocked and motion limited. An inclined sled or leg press can be used for ankle plantar flexion strengthening and initial bilateral squatting and activity within pain-free ranges (usually 20 to 70 degrees, but progressing to 0 to 90 degrees as able). Standing bilateral heel raises can also be initiated limiting weight bearing as appropriate and with the brace locked at 0-degree extension. Stationary bicycling is performed with both legs after a ROM of 110-degrees flexion is obtained; it is initiated not for cardiovascular but for neurophysiologic purposes. The brace should be locked during ambulation until adequate quadriceps contraction is available to control the knee during the stance phase. Exercise repetitions should be carried out to the point of fatigue or 30 repetitions per set. Resistance may be added as appropriate above the knee for hip exercises and at the ankle for standing hamstring curls. The Delorme method[46] is used to guide exercise progression through-

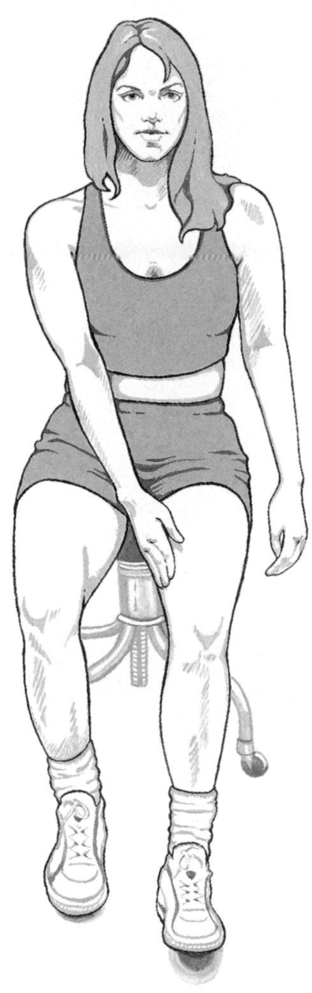

Fig. 17-3 Spider killers. Patient is seated with the involved knee (in this case the left) flexed to a comfortable position (70 to 90 degrees). The patient is instructed to palpate over the vastus medialis oblique while applying pressure down through the heel (ankle dorsiflexed) eliciting a quadriceps and hamstring cocontraction.

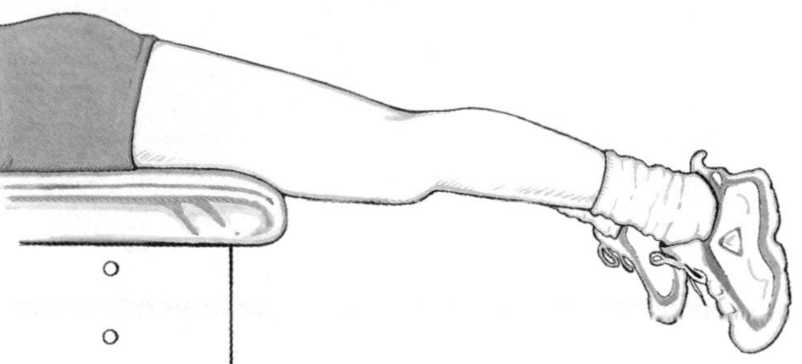

Fig. 17-4 Prone heel hangs. Patient is in the prone position with the involved leg hanging over the edge of the table or bed. Care is taken to avoid pressure on the patella.

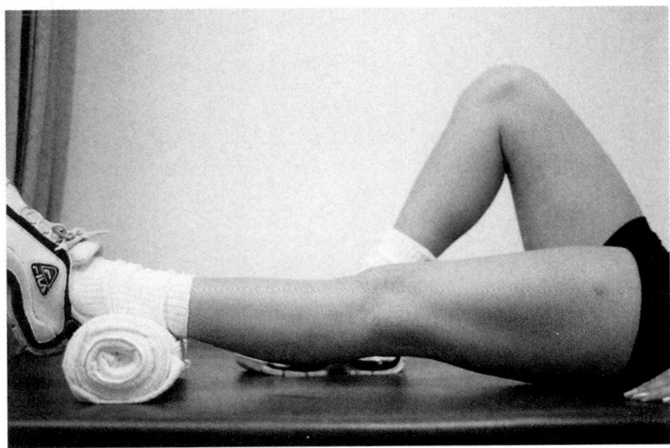

Fig. 17-5 Passive knee extension. Patient is supine or sitting with involved leg straight, into full extension. A towel is placed under the heel, allowing the knee to hang. Care is taken to avoid rotating the hip.

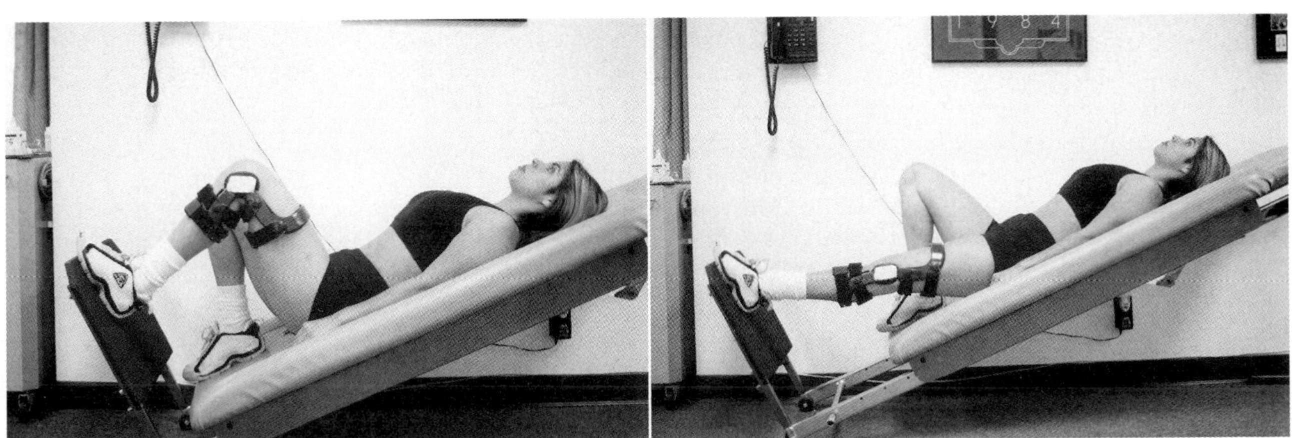

Fig. 17-6 Inclined sled. The use of an inclined sled can be initiated early to recruit volitional muscle contraction in a limited weight-bearing (resistance) environment.

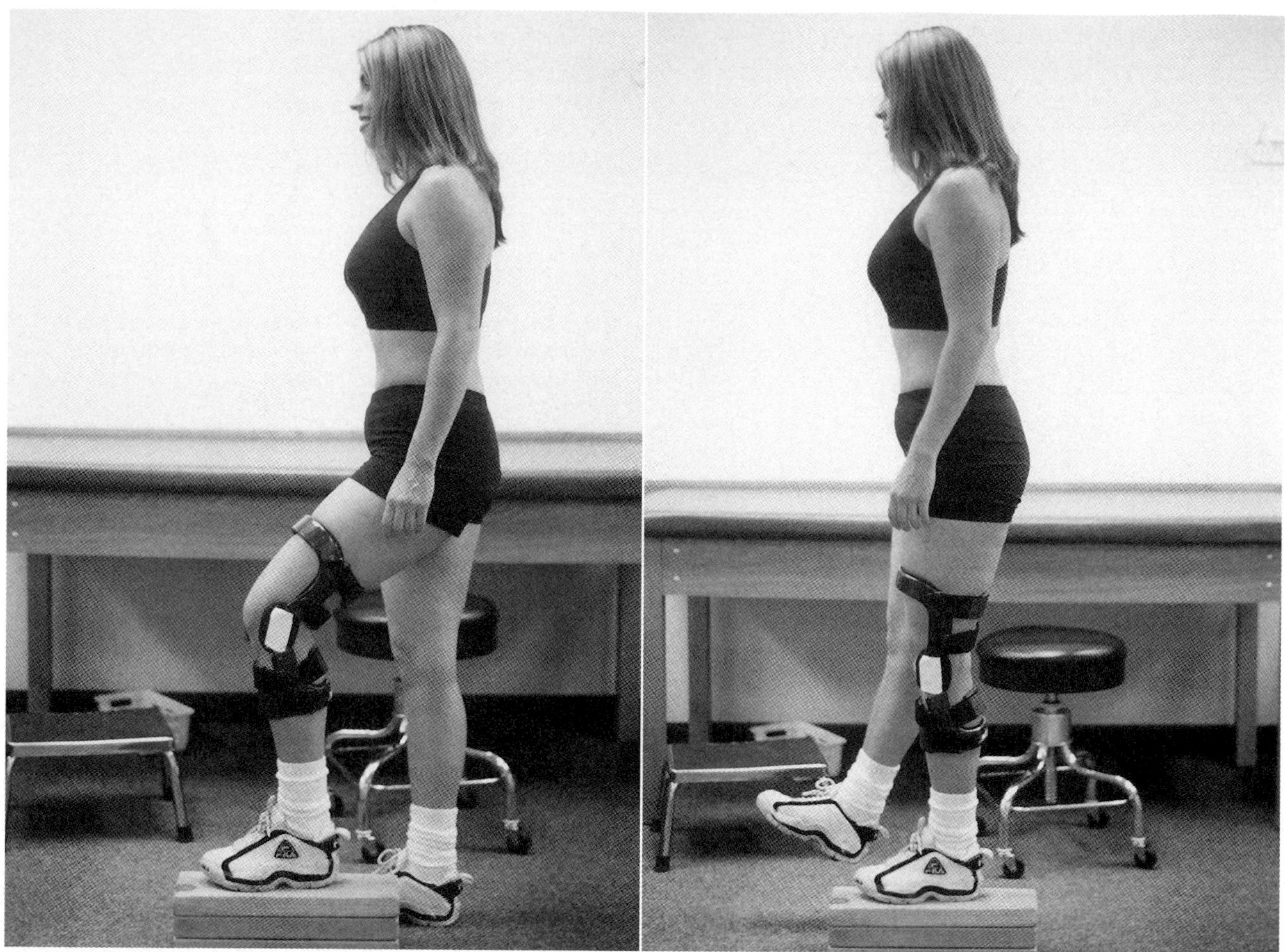

Fig. 17-7 A and B, Step up and down. Patients progress from 2-inch to 6-inch high steps. Care is taken to avoid increased stress on the graft and patella (knee is kept in line with the foot and not allowed to migrate anterior to the toes during the exercise).

out rehabilitation. Upper body and core strengthening exercises can be initiated by the end of the third week using a routine that minimizes stress on the involved leg. Depending on the duration of therapy, the therapist should vary the exercises to keep the treatments from becoming prosaic.[164]

Gait training with weight bearing initially at 25% during the first week should progress to 100% body weight by week 4. Exercises in the form of weight shifting (using crutches as necessary) simulating a normal "step-through" pattern is emphasized. Because of ROM limitations it is important to work on limb advancement during the swing phase of gait. The therapist should facilitate knee flexion during the swing phase by having the patient step over a small obstacle (e.g., towel roll, paper cup), emphasizing the full compliment of hip, knee, and ankle flexion. The physical therapist can wean the patient from crutches as tolerance to weight bearing dictates.

Joint mobilization is initiated in the form of early PF and tibiofemoral (TF) mobilization. To avoid complications, all PF glides are initiated after consideration of incision integrity. The physical therapist instructs patients in self-mobilization techniques as part of the home exercise program. Mobilization of the TF joint also improves extension. Techniques described by Maitland[106] have proven successful in this regard. Posterior gliding of the tibia on the femur also is helpful in gaining flexion ROM (Fig. 17-8). Gentle soft tissue mobilization can be initiated once the incision has healed and no evidence of infection is present.

> **Q** Elizabeth is a 45-year-old woman. She tore her ACL while horseback riding. She had surgery 3 weeks ago to reconstruct her ligament. Knee flexion ROM is progressing nicely. Knee extension is limited, with a PROM of −10 degrees. Inflammation is decreasing. She has pain while performing quadriceps sets and SLRs. What treatment techniques did the therapist use to gain knee extension?

A

Anteroposterior mobilization movements into resistance at end range (using grades III and IV) were applied to the tibia while the knee was in extension. PROM for knee extension increased immediately, and pain with quadriceps sets was alleviated. Anterior-posterior mobilization was applied to the tibia while the knee was at the end range of extension, taking care not to elicit any increased tension on the graft. Mobilizations were performed into resistance (grades III and IV). Extension PROM was increased and pain with quadriceps sets and SLR was alleviated. Full extension appeared to decrease stress on the patello-femoral and tibio-femoral articulations.

Q

Doug is a 45-year-old fireman. He had an ACL reconstruction 9 weeks ago on his left knee. Because of mishaps and personal reasons, physical therapy was not initiated until 5 weeks ago. Presently (9 weeks after surgery) PROM for knee flexion is 110 degrees. The end range is beginning to feel leathery. Soft tissue restrictions appear to be present in the quadriceps. Swelling and complaints of pain are usually minimal. Strength is gradually progressing. What treatment techniques could be used to promote increased knee flexion?

Phase II

TIME: 5 to 8 weeks after surgery
GOALS: Increased ROM, increased independence in performing transfers and in gait performance, full weight bearing (initiate single leg balance and proprioception activities), good management of pain and edema (Table 17-3)

By the end of the fourth week after surgery the physical therapist should be concerned with lingering ROM deficits, edema, and increases in the intensity of pain, because these could signal potential complications (e.g., arthrofibrosis, PF dysfunction, patient noncompliance). At the beginning of the second phase of rehabilitation, the patient should have the following:

- Good self-management of pain and edema
- Zero- to 110-degrees ROM (ideally 125-degrees flexion)
- Independence in lifting the involved leg when performing transfers
- Full weight bearing
- Independence with gait (no crutches or cane) in walking household and limited community distances
- No increase in KT-1000 readings

The hallmark of this phase is the progression to an independent functional status for ADLs. In weeks 5 through 8, joint and soft tissue mobilization is continued on an as-needed basis to maintain extension and improve flexion. If extension is still problematic, then

Table 17-3 Anterior Cruciate Ligament Reconstruction

Rehabilitation Phase	Criteria to Progress to this Phase	Intervention	Goal	Rationale
Phase II Postoperative 5-8 weeks	◆ Postoperative	◆ Braces should be worn (if indicated) for all exercises in **bold** type ◆ Continue Phase I exercises (patient may have functional brace by 6 weeks, depending on physician) ◆ Exercise intensity progressed from AROM to PREs ◆ **PREs—Step up/down, progress to 6-inch step** ◆ **Isokinetics—Limited range (90-30 degrees)** ◆ **Walking program inclusive of boxes and figure eights** ◆ **Balance exercises** ◆ Patient education ◆ Continue joint mobilization	Achieve the following by the end of week 8: ◆ ROM 0-135 degrees ◆ 100% single leg squat 90-0 degrees ◆ Gait with functional brace 1 mile ◆ Transfer sit-stand (equal weight bearing) ◆ Self-manage pain ◆ Stand for 1 hour	◆ Wear brace for additional proprioceptive input to the knee and to increase stability ◆ Increase muscle strength to progress functional activities ◆ Use limited range on open-chain exercises to protect graft ◆ Prepare for return to sport or activity ◆ Increase patient self-reliance for exercise and self-management ◆ Improve joint mechanics and normalize arthrokinematics

ROM, Range of motion; *AROM,* active range of motion; *PREs,* progressive resistance exercises.

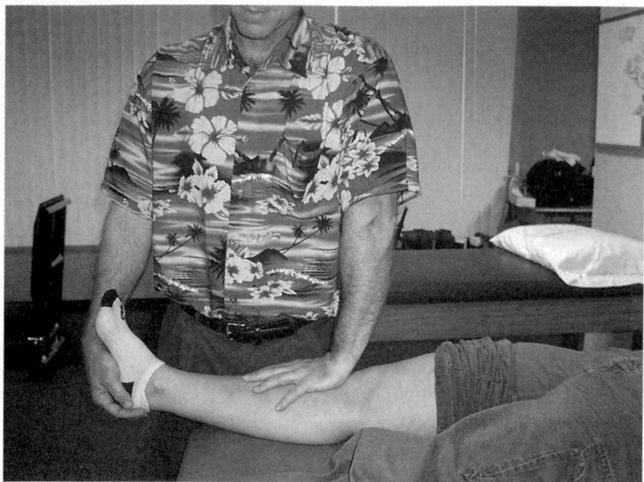

Fig. 17-8 Mobilization for extension range of motion. A posterior glide of the tibia on the femur can be accomplished, avoiding stress to the graft and donor site. Care must be taken to avoid unprotected hyperextension of the knee.

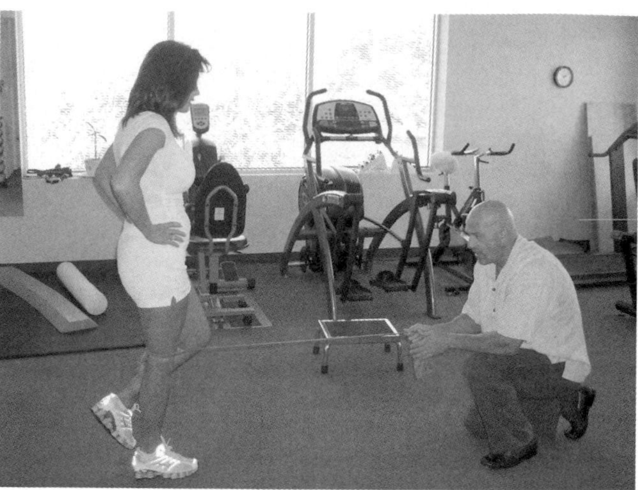

Fig. 17-9 Single-limb balance into terminal extension. This exercise can be initiated with both feet on the floor and resistance band around the distal femur pulling into flexion. The patient should maintain terminal knee extension while avoiding any pain. This exercise can be progressed to allow the patient to perform terminal knee extension movements maintaining their balance.

joint mobilization vigor can be increased (Fig. 17-8). During this mobilization it is imperative that the patient relax the quadriceps muscle so as not to create any anterior shear force on the tibia. By this time patients should continue performing home exercises without much cueing. The brace is worn for the exercises already listed, as well as for gait activities. The therapist increases the exercise intensity from AROM to progressive resistance exercises (PREs). Lateral step-ups are added and forward step-ups are progressed in height (2 to 6 inches) to prepare the patient for community ambulation. Isokinetic exercises are performed in a limited ROM (90 to 30 degrees). The patient continues gait training, shifting the focus from increasing weight-bearing tolerance to normalizing the gait pattern. Resistive tubing can be added to increase resistance emphasizing proprioception and balance during the stance phase (Figs. 17-9 and 17-10). By the end of the eighth week, patients should be walking through figure-eight and box patterns. Another efficient exercise to improve balance and coordination is "the skater" (Fig. 17-11). The patient performs this exercise by maintaining single leg balance with a slight degree of knee flexion. The patient is then instructed to maintain good alignment of the knee (avoiding valgus or varus deviations and not allowing the knee to migrate forward ahead of the toes) and flex at the hip (maintaining a neutral spine with slight extension bias) until the torso is parallel to the ground. This position is maintained initially for 15 seconds and gradually progressed adding time, other balance activities (upper extremity [UE] movements and weights), or both. This will take a lot of control to perform and the therapist *must* guide the patient through the process on a graded basis (i.e., hip flexion to 30, 45, 60, and ultimately 90 degrees), monitoring any symptoms or lack of stability. It will be rare for patients to perform this exercise correctly at the 90-degrees hip flexion position during the first 2 to 3 weeks after initial instruction.

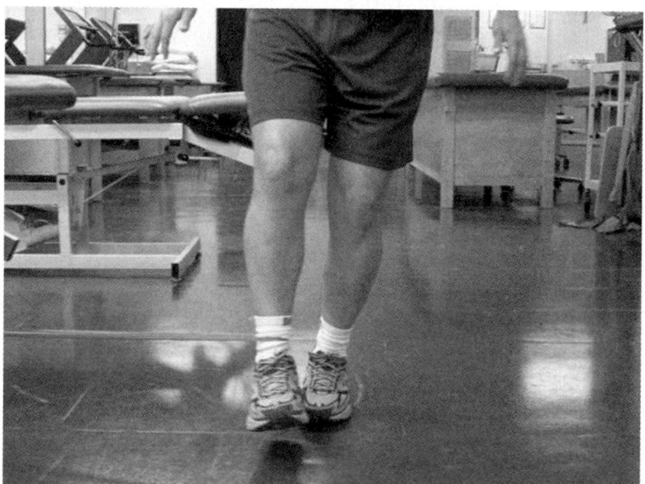

Fig. 17-10 Single-limb balance using elastic band. Standing on the involved leg (in good alignment) the patient performs hip movements (i.e., flexion, extension, abduction, abduction) with the uninvolved leg. Resisted hip adduction is pictured here.

Phase III

TIME: 9 to 16 weeks after surgery

GOALS: Independence in ADLs and readiness for sports participation (Table 17-4)

By the ninth week postoperatively, patients should have close to full ROM, be able to perform a unilateral squat

A Doug assumed a prone position, and the therapist performed gentle contraction and relaxation stretches to the quadriceps. Doug then moved into the supine position with his left knee flexed to its end range. Tibial posterior glides were performed with the knee in flexion (into resistance, grade IV), followed by PROM into flexion with over pressure. Also, soft tissue mobilization to the lateral retinaculum was performed to address patello-femoral restrictions. Next, Doug rode the stationary bicycle. Massage and cryotherapy were used during treatments to decrease swelling. After two or three of these treatments, Doug's knee flexion increased to 0 to 125 degrees.

with 100% body weight (0 to 90 degrees), walk up to 1 mile, tolerate standing for up to 1 hour, and demonstrate independence in self-management of exercises. The hallmark of this phase is progression from being a functionally independent person with ADLs to resumption of the previous level of physical activity (e.g., running, hiking, sports).

The physical therapist should progress the exercises as in prior phases and continue with PREs in the form of open- and closed-chain exercises. Resistance may be progressed further with gait training exercises, thus improving multidirectional (forward, backward, side-to-side, diagonally) weight acceptance of the involved leg.

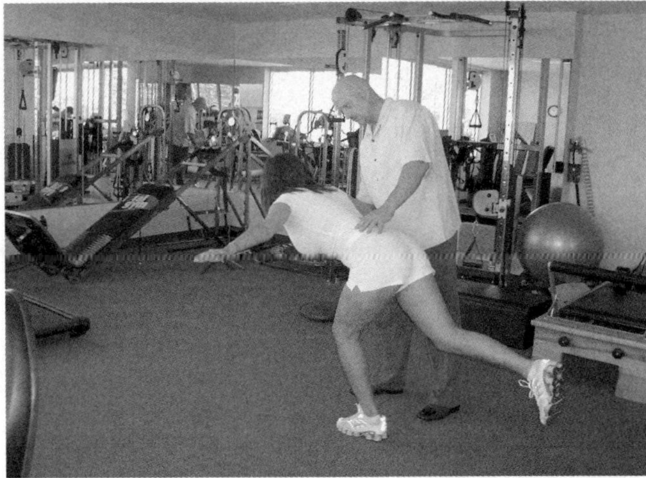

Fig. 17-11 The skater—single-limb balance on the involved leg with partial knee flexion. Slowly (maintaining a neutral spine with slight extension bias) have the patient flex at the hip, maintaining alignment of the knee in both the coronal and sagittal planes. Progress the degree of difficulty by increasing hip flexion so that the torso is parallel to the floor.

The patient may use a variety of equipment to improve strength, balance, proprioception (Fig. 17-12), and cardiovascular conditioning. Dot drills and hopping activities (initially bilateral, then progressing to unilateral) are initiated around week 12 (once weight acceptance on the involved leg is stable and pain free and usually in conjunction with a return to running program).

Table 17-4 Anterior Cruciate Ligament Reconstruction

Rehabilitation Phase	Criteria to Progress to this Phase	Intervention	Goal	Rationale
Phase III Postoperative 9-16 weeks	◆ Same as in Phase II ◆ No loss in ROM ◆ No increase in edema or pain	◆ Brace should be worn if any quadriceps insufficiency is present ◆ Phase I and II exercises as indicated ◆ PREs using closed and open chain (isokinetic) (open chain 90-30 degrees) ◆ Trampoline jogging progressing to single leg balance/hopping, initially bilateral, progressing to unilateral in later phase ◆ Initiate running when cleared by physician (usually by third month) ◆ Sport- and activity-specific drills as appropriate	Achieve the following by the end of week 16: ◆ Come within 10% of full range flexion ◆ Isokinetic test within 25% of uninvolved knee ◆ Run 1+ miles without pain (patient dependent) ◆ Initiate sport- or activity-specific training, modifying appropriately	◆ Increase stability of the knee while limiting stress on the graft ◆ Prepare for functional activities such as jumping and hopping ◆ Prepare to return to sports

ROM, Range of motion; *PREs*, progressive resistance exercises.

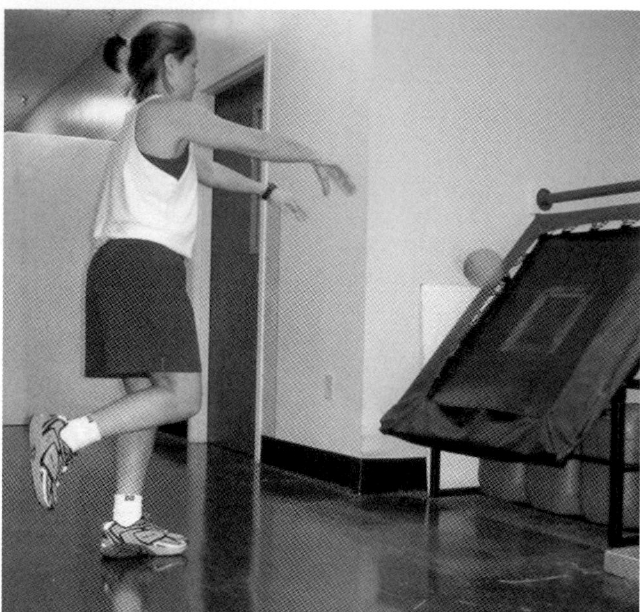

Fig. 17-12 Single-limb balance using medicine ball. Toss and catch activity maintaining good alignment and slight knee flexion.

Box 17-1 Running Program

Week 1
Walk ¼ mile; then run ¼ mile (50% effort) for four repetitions, three times a week.

Week 2
Walk ¼ mile; then run ½ mile (50% effort) for two repetitions, three times a week.

Week 3
Walk ¼ mile, run 1 mile (50% effort); then walk ¼ mile for one repetition, three times a week.

Week 4
Walk ¼ mile, run ¼ mile (50% effort), walk ¼ mile , run ½ mile (75% effort); then walk ¼ mile for two repetitions, three times a week.

Week 5
Walk ¼ mile, run 1 mile (75% effort); then walk ¼ mile for two repetitions, three times a week.

Week 6
Walk ¼ mile walk, run ¼ mile (75% effort), walk ¼ mile, run ½ mile (100% effort); then walk ¼ mile for 2 repetitions, 3 times a week.

Week 7
Walk ¼ mile, run 1 mile (100% effort); then walk ¼ mile for 2 repetitions, 3 times a week.

After the patient tolerates prolonged walking on a level surface (45 minutes to 1 hour) without any pain or edema and has been cleared by the physician, he or she can initiate a running program under the direction of the physical therapist. This usually takes place around the third month. This return to activity depends on the patient's status and must be initiated as appropriate to the patient's previous level of function. A trampoline can be used initially to increase tolerance to landing on the involved side with some cushioning. At this time the therapist must emphasize the posture of the LE upon landing (weight acceptance). Based on the earlier discussion of potential risk factors and the valgus collapse, it is imperative that the patient continues proprioceptive neuromuscular training exercises. The authors of this chapter suggest a simple progression for the return to running based on activity or sport need and allowing a rest day between runs (as shown in Box 17-1).

The program is modified to fit the individual's needs and abilities. The patient should run on level surfaces, using a school track if possible. Along with the running program, the physical therapist should incorporate conditioning for other parts of the body (e.g., abdominals, UEs) as applicable to the sport or activity the patient wishes to resume.

Phase IV

TIME: 4 to 6 months after surgery

GOALS: Return to activity or sport (Table 17-5)

The last phase of rehabilitation focuses on the actual return to the activity or sport. The correct timing of when to release an athlete back to sport participation has been controversial. Graft maturation must be taken into account when making the decision. One graft strength study on sheep noted that the graft at 3 months had only 30% of the tensile strength of the native ACL.[119] Another animal study found that at 52 weeks tensile stress of the graft was only at 47%.[65] It is important to note that these were animal studies; however, they do provide some valuable insight to the physiologic maturation of the graft tissue. Athletes continue to push the limits of the healing process in an effort to resume performing in elite venues. Two case studies cited the return of a professional soccer player just 77 days and a collegiate basketball player just 42 days after ACL reconstruction.[44,144] Although criteria for return to sport may be fulfilled before the desired time frame, the clinician must discuss and weigh short-term and long-term risks and rewards with the athlete, should he or she desire to participate. Although the time frame varies with the demands of the activity, Malone and Garrett[108] note that it is possible to return to the sport at 6 months if the patient has successfully completed "controlled physiologic rehabilitation." Thus initiating the training at the 4-month point allows 2 months of functional training and progression. Isokinetic testing is another piece of the puzzle used to determine whether the patient is ready to return to sport.[67] Shelbourne and associates[156] described criteria for return as follows:

Table 17-5 Anterior Cruciate Ligament Reconstruction

Rehabilitation Phase	Criteria to Progress to this Phase	Intervention	Goal	Rationale
Phase IV Postoperative 17+ weeks	◆ Same as in Phase III	◆ Continuation of exercises from Phases I-III as indicated ◆ Neuromuscular training ◆ Plyometrics—Hopping and jumping activities ◆ Sport-specific activities	Achieve the following before return to sport or activity: ◆ Isokinetic test within 10% ◆ Functional tests within criteria to return to sport ◆ Return to sport by 8-12 months	◆ Improve LE neuromuscular response to sports-related activity ◆ Improve the muscular stability of the knee ◆ Return to sport/activity safely and confidently

LE, Lower extremity.

- Full ROM
- Strength at 65%
- Completion of prescribed running and agility drills

The factors that most rehabilitation programs use to evaluate readiness for return to sport are KT-1000 stability, isokinetic equivalence, and functional tests.[45,47,48,93,109,127,151] **The most useful of these, without denying the importance of others, is functional testing. By using a complement of functional and isokinetic tests, the therapist and physician can determine when return to sport is appropriate.**

The hop and stop,[92] vertical jump, single-leg hop (6 meters for time and distance),[25] triple jump,[25,141] and stair hopping[141] are the most common functional tests referenced in the literature to assess stability and strength after ACL reconstruction. To evaluate readiness to return to previous activities, the authors of this chapter follow an eclectic approach similar to that of Lephart and colleagues[100] who use a combination of functional tests and self-assessment of ability. Two tests are used regularly:

1. Single-leg hop (for distance)—The patient stands on involved leg and performs a long jump type movement. Distance is measured from take-off (toe) to landing (heel). The physical therapist compares the distance with the uninvolved side (three trials each, take best effort of the three).
2. Single-leg hop (for time)—The physical therapist measures off 6 meters, and the patient performs single-leg hops over the measured distance. Time is measured with a stopwatch or other device. The physical therapist compares the distance with the uninvolved side (three trials each, take the best effort of the three).

TROUBLESHOOTING

Carson and associates[31] reviewed 90 failed ACL reconstruction surgeries. Based on their findings a majority of the failures were the result of surgical technical errors. *The most common complications from ACL recon struction are joint stiffness, flexion contractures, patellar irritability (as high as 34%), and quadriceps weakness.*[94,115,165,171] Less frequently, complications include reflex sympathetic dystrophy (less than 1%), neurovascular injury (less than 1%), deep venous thrombosis (DVT), infection and possible fluid extravasation, and compartment syndromes (especially with endoscopic techniques).

The incidence of stiffness is reduced after ACL reconstruction by using proper surgical technique combined with an aggressive rehabilitation program. Improper graft placement with the tibial tunnel too far anterior or inadequate notchplasty can cause graft impingement, blocking terminal knee extension. Intraoperative inspection of the graft throughout a full ROM should always be conducted to ensure that the graft is not impinging within the intercondylar notch.[83]

> **Q** Anne is making excellent progress in therapy. However, at 10 weeks after surgery the therapist notices a palpable "clunk" with her AROM, and extension has become quite painful. What is the therapist's clinical impression?

Arthrofibrosis

One of the most devastating complications after ACL reconstruction is the development of arthrofibrosis. The knee synovium and fat pad become inflamed, leading to a thickened joint capsule. This in turn begins to obliterate the medial and lateral gutters and suprapatellar pouch. The patellar tendon can shorten, produce patella baja, and eventually cause articular damage. Paulos and colleagues[133] have defined three stages in the arthrofibrotic knee:

1. In the early stage, stage 1 (2 to 6 weeks), decreased extension is noted, in addition to quadriceps lag, diminished patellar mobility, joint swelling, and failure to progress in rehabilitation.
2. The active stage, stage 2 (6 to 30 weeks), is defined by a marked decrease in ROM, decreased patellar mobility, quadriceps atrophy, skin changes, and osteopenia. These patients walk with a significant limp.
3. The residual stage, stage 3 (beyond 8 months), is defined by a marked decrease in ROM, patellar rigidity, quadriceps atrophy, patella baja, osteopenia, and possibly arthrosis.

The physical therapist should manage arthrofibrosis early to attempt restoration of full mobility. *A knee with a significant flexion contracture can cause greater impairment than an ACL-deficient knee.* Anti-inflammatory agents, aggressive physical therapy, and patellar mobilization are the initial treatments for all stages of arthrofibrosis. Arthroscopic débridement, open débridement, and dynamic splinting are usually required in the later stages.

Another potential complication in obtaining and maintaining full-extension ROM is the presence of a cyclops lesion.[130,166] This lesion is usually the result of the proliferation of fibrous tissue surrounding the graft and has been shown to be a cause of failure to regain or to lose full extension in the early postoperative period. Some patients who have achieved full extension will develop a gradual loss of full extension and joint line pain with terminal extension. MRI can verify the presence of this nodule that ultimately must be surgically removed. The patient responds quite well once the lesion is débrided. The therapist must be alert for the patient with delayed onset of ROM loss, especially in extension. They should undergo careful evaluation, including radiographs and MRI. If a cyclops lesion is confirmed, then arthroscopic resection should be performed.[130]

A Limitations with extension usually are the result of posterior capsule or notch problems. The presence of *crepitation* or a *palpable clunk* in addition to pain with extension could signify an ACL "nodule." Anne was referred back to her surgeon and an MRI confirmed the presence of a cyclops lesion (nodule). Surgery was scheduled to remove the fibroproliferative tissue.

Anterior Knee Pain

PF pain commonly occurs after ACL reconstruction, although it occurs more frequently after BPTB autograft reconstructions than with hamstring autograft reconstructions. Bach and colleagues[11] reported an 18% incidence of mild PF symptoms in a 2- to 4-year follow-up study, whereas Kartus and associates[94] reported a 33.6% incidence.

Patellar fractures have been reported in the literature as a late complication of BPTB graft harvest. These are believed to be stress fractures that develop because of the decreased vascularity of the patella. Patellar fracture also can occur intraoperatively during graft harvest and has been reported postoperatively. Brownstein and Bronner[28] reported the incidence of patellar fractures at 0.5% and noted that it usually occurs as a result of a fall. They put the patella at highest risk for fracture during rehabilitation at 10 to 14 weeks postoperatively. Pain over the tibial tubercle is less frequently encountered but may occur in those with prominent tibial tubercles. If the patient has limited joint motion preoperatively, especially in extension, then a CPM device should be used immediately postoperatively.[47]

During the first postoperative phase, ROM complications, if present, usually occur in extension. If mobilization and home exercises are not effective, then the patient should try adding weight to the ankle during the prone hanging exercises. Duration and intensity are determined individually, but the authors of this chapter generally start with 3 to 5 lbs for a 5-minute increment and have the patient follow through at home three to five times a day. In addition, the patient can add weights to the knee while performing supine knee extension (towel propped under the heel) and progress in a similar manner.

Treatment for Complications and Troubleshooting

Phases I and II

Strength complications are addressed using ES over the muscles in conjunction with exercise. The physical therapist also can initiate biofeedback on the vasti to assist with balanced muscle contraction. Anterior knee pain related to PF dysfunction can be treated with modalities (i.e., cryotherapy and ultrasound), soft tissue mobilization, patella taping (after the incision has healed), emphasis on proper LE alignment during the offending activity and hip strengthening; assessment of foot biomechanics (the need for orthotics) can also be useful in addressing PF issues.

Persistent swelling may indicate hemarthrosis, synovitis, reinjury, or infection.[31] *If by 4 to 6 weeks the patient has not gained full extension, then the cause may be patellar entrapment.* Use of patellar mobilization to a greater extent and with more vigor and serial casting may be considered. Arthroscopy is usually considered if full extension is not obtained by the eighth week.[104] If reflex sympathetic dystrophy occurs, then it is usually seen by the fifth week postoperatively.

Motion limitations are of primary concern and require aggressive management, as mentioned earlier. Some patients may need to be manipulated or evaluated for surgery during phase II. As the patient progresses with strengthening exercises, the physical therapist should pay careful attention to any residual pain or edema. The PF mechanism must be continually evaluated as the resistance of the exercises is progressed.

Phases III and IV

Complications 9 weeks or more after surgery are usually the result of edema or pain after activity. This can result from the addition of new stressors (e.g., exercises) on the knee joint and soft tissue. If not already initiated, then pool exercises may be a helpful adjunct in continuing to developing strength, maintain ROM, and improve mechanics of the LE in a less than full weight-bearing posture. Exercises in the form of deep-water running and activity-specific drills are a good adjunct to land-based rehabilitation.

SUMMARY

Clinical management after ACL reconstruction can follow many directions. The most efficient management is one in which the patient is an educated and active participant in rehabilitation. If ROM or strength deficits exist preoperatively, then physical therapy must be initiated to ensure a successful surgical outcome. Early restoration of full extension (1 to 4 weeks) is imperative, as is awareness of potential complications that may limit progress. The number of visits depends on the patient's involvement, functional goals, and complications. Return to sports depends on strength, skill acquisition, and response of the knee to the activity.

SUGGESTED HOME MAINTENANCE FOR THE POSTSURGICAL PATIENT

Home exercises are progressed through the four phases of rehabilitation based on the patient's tolerance to activity. Any increase in edema, pain, or laxity should be addressed early, and exercises should be modified to eliminate complications.

Weeks 1-4

GOALS FOR THE PERIOD: Manage pain and edema, improve quadriceps/hamstring contractions, improve range of motion (ROM)

Pain and Edema

1. Cryotherapy with elevation 20 to 30 minutes with ankle pumps (10 repetitions every minute)
2. Use of home electrical stimulation (ES) unit

Strength

1. Isometrics: quadriceps and hamstring sets isolation and cocontraction, 10 to 30 repetitions (can also be done with elevation)

ROM Exercises

1. Supine knee extension
2. Prone heel hangs
3. Heel slides
4. Supine wall slides (supine with involved foot against the wall, gravity assisted into flexion)

Active Range of Motion Exercises (Brace Locked)

1. Hip: flexion, extension, abduction, adduction, abduction with external rotation (ER)
2. Standing hamstring curls

Gait Training

1. Gait training using crutches: weight bearing as tolerated, weaning as appropriate
2. Use small obstacles to work on swing phase of gait clearing involved leg (hip flexion, knee flexion, and ankle dorsiflexion)
3. Once full weight bearing obtained, work on single-limb balance activities.

(Perform exercises three times a day with repetitions and sets determined by strength—usually two sets of as many as 30 repetitions.)

Weeks 5-8

GOALS FOR THE PERIOD: Progress ROM, increase functional strength of hip, knee, and ankle

ROM Exercises

1. Continue passive range of motion (PROM) exercises on an as-needed basis (ROM as needed, progress to prescribed duration with weight on top of knee if full extension is not reached at this time).
2. Add seated passive flexion.

Strength

1. Add step up and down with appropriate-height object (local phone book versus county phone book) and single-limb balance activities.
2. Follow a walking program (as much as 45 minutes of continuous walking on level surfaces daily).
3. Progress back into therapy or community gym environment for cardiovascular exercises: bike, elliptical, treadmill (forward and reverse). Progress upper extremity (UE) exercise program to weight-bearing position gym activities (progressed to include cardiovascular and proprioceptive and neuromuscular training techniques).

Gait Training

1. Work on single-limb balance and walking figure-eight and box patterns.
2. Try walking box and figure-eight patterns.

Weeks 9-16

GOALS FOR THE PERIOD: Progress functional activities, prepare to return to sport or activity

ROM Exercises

1. Should be close to full ROM by this time. Maintenance program should be initiated.

Strength

1. Periodize gym program; initiate running program when appropriate (usually about 3 months).
2. Progress neuromuscular (balance and coordination) training emphasizing proper lower extremity (LE) alignment with activities.
3. Progress balance and coordination activities and continue education on injury prevention with return to specific sport or activity.
4. Add one-legged hopping and jumping activities once cleared for running (usually about week 12).
5. Begin foundational exercises for return to sport emphasizing LE control and neuromuscular training principles.

Week 17 and beyond

GOALS FOR THE PERIOD: Progress back to sport or activity

ROM Exercises:

1. Maintenance

Strength:

1. Gym-based workouts continuing to emphasize proprioceptive and neuromuscular training techniques
2. Perform exercises specific to sport
3. Reassess and progress the periodization program for athlete to adequately prepare for return to sport

References

1. Adachi N et al: Mechanoreceptors in the anterior cruciate ligament contribute to the joint position sense, *Acta Orthop Scand* 73(3):330-334, 2002.
2. Aglietti P et al: Patellofemoral problems after intraarticular anterior cruciate ligament reconstruction, *Clin Orthop Relat Res* 288:195, 1993.
3. Alm A, Lijedahlso SO, Stromberg B: Clinical and experimental experience in reconstruction of the anterior cruciate ligament, *Orthop Clin North Am* 7:181, 1976.
4. Al-Othman AA: Clinical measurement of proprioceptive function after anterior cruciate ligament reconstruction, *Saudi Med J* 25(2):195-197, 2004.
5. Amiel D et al: The phenomenon of "ligamentization": anterior cruciate ligament reconstruction with autogenous patellar tendon, *J Orthop Res* 4:162, 1986.
6. Andriacchi TP, Dyrby CO: Interactions between kinematics and loading during walking for the normal and ACL deficient knee, *J Biomech* 38(2):293-298, 2005.
7. Arendt E, Dick R: Knee injury patterns among men and women in collegiate basketball and soccer. NCAA data and review of literature, *Am J Sports Med* 23(6):694-701, 1995.
8. Arms SW et al: The biomechanics of anterior cruciate ligament rehabilitation and reconstruction, *Am J Sports Med* 12(1):8, 1984.
9. Arnoczky SP: The vascularity of the anterior cruciate ligament and associated structures. Its role in repair and reconstruction. In Jackson DW, Drez D, editors: *The anterior cruciate deficient knee: new concepts in ligament repair*, St Louis, 1987, Mosby.
10. Arnoczky SP, Tarvin GB, Marshall JL: Anterior cruciate ligament replacement using patellar tendon, *Am J Bone Joint Surg* 643:217, 1982.
11. Bach BR Jr et al: Arthroscopy-assisted anterior cruciate ligament reconstruction using patellar tendon substitution. Two-to-four-year follow-up results, *Am J Sports Med* 22(6):758, 1994.
12. Bach BR et al: Arthroscopically assisted anterior cruciate ligament reconstruction using patellar tendon autograft. Five- to nine-year follow-up evaluation, *Am J Sports Med* 26(1):20, 1998.
13. Barber FA: A comparison of crushed ice and continuous flow cold therapy, *Am J Knee Surg* 13(2):97-101, 2000.
14. Barber FA, McGuire DA, Click S: Continuous-flow cold therapy for outpatient anterior cruciate ligament reconstruction, *Arthroscopy* 14(2):130-135, 1998.
15. Barber FA et al: Is an anterior cruciate ligament reconstruction outcome age dependent? *Arthroscopy* 12(6):720, 1996.
16. Barnes L: Cryotherapy: putting injury on ice, *Phys Sports Med* 7130, 1979.
17. Barrata R et al: Muscular coactivation: The role of the antagonist musculature in maintaining knee stability, *Am J Sports Med* 16(2):113, 1988.
18. Beck PR et al: Postoperative pain management after anterior cruciate ligament reconstruction, *J Knee Surg* 17(1):18-23, 2004.
19. Bellabarba C, Bush-Joseph CA, Bach BR Jr: Patterns of meniscal injury in the anterior cruciate-deficient knee: a review of the literature, *Am J Orthop* 26(1):18-23, 1997.
20. Beutler AI et al: Electromyographic analysis of single-leg, closed chain exercises: implications for rehabilitation after anterior cruciate ligament reconstruction, *J Athl Train* 37(1):13-18, 2002.
21. Birmingham TB et al: Knee bracing after ACL reconstruction: effects on postural control and proprioception, *Med Sci Sports Exerc* 33(8):1253-1258, 2001.
22. Bock B, Malinin T, Brown M: Bone transplantation and human immunodeficiency virus: an estimate of the risk of acquired immunodeficiency syndrome (AIDS), *Clin Orthop* 240:129, 1989.
23. Boden BP et al: Mechanisms of anterior cruciate ligament injury, *Orthopedics* 23(6):573-578, 2000.
24. Boland AL: Rehabilitation of the injured athlete. In Strauss RH, editor: *Sports medicine and physiology*, Philadelphia, 1979, WB Saunders.
25. Bolga LA, Keskula DR: Reliability of lower extremity functional performance tests, *J Orthop Sports Phys Ther* 26(3):138, 1997.
26. Bradley JP et al: Anterior cruciate ligament injuries in the National Football League: epidemiology and current treatment trends among team physicians, *Arthroscopy* 18(5):502-509, 2002.
27. Brewer BW et al: Age-related differences in predictors of adherence to rehabilitation after anterior cruciate ligament reconstruction, *J Athl Train* 38(2):158-162, 2003.
28. Brownstein B, Bronner S: Patella fractures associated with accelerated ACL rehabilitation in patients with autogenous patella tendon reconstructions, *J Orthop Sports Phys Ther* 26(3):168, 1997.
29. Cabaud ME, Rodkey WG, Feagin JA: Experimental studies of acute anterior cruciate ligament injury and repair, *Am J Sports Med* 7:18, 1979.
30. Campbell WC: Reconstruction of the ligaments of the knee, *Am J Surg* 43:473, 1939.
31. Carson EW et al: Revision anterior cruciate ligament reconstruction: etiology of failures and clinical results, *J Knee Surg* 17(3):127-132, 2004.
32. Cerulli G et al: In vivo anterior cruciate ligament strain behaviour during a rapid deceleration movement: case report, *Knee Surg Sports Traumatol Arthrosc* 11(5):307-311, 2003.
33. Chatman AB et al: The patient-specific functional scale: measurement properties in patients with knee dysfunction, *Phys Ther* 77(8):820, 1997.
34. Cho KO: Reconstruction of the ACL by semitendinosus, *J Bone Joint Surg* 68B:739, 1986.
35. Ciccotti MG et al: Non-operative treatment of ruptures of the anterior cruciate ligament in middle-aged patients. Results after long term follow-up, *J Bone Joint Surg Br* 76A(9):1315, 1994.
36. Cohn BT, Draeger RI, Jackson DW: The effects of cold therapy in the postoperative management of pain in patients undergoing anterior cruciate ligament reconstruction, *Am J Sports Med* 17(3):344, 1989.

37. Corrigan JP, Cashman WF, Brady MP: Proprioception in the cruciate deficient knee, *J Bone Joint Surg Br* 74(2):247-250, 1992.
38. Corsetti JR, Jackson DW: Failure of anterior cruciate ligament reconstruction: the biologic basis, *Clin Orthop Reatl Res* 323:42, 1996.
39. Cosgarea AJ, Sebastianelli WJ, DeHaven KE: Prevention of arthrofibrosis after anterior cruciate ligament reconstruction using the central third patellar tendon autograft, *Am J Sports Med* 23(1):87, 1995.
40. Daniel DM: Principles of knee ligament surgery. In Daniel DM, Akeson WH, O'Connor J, editors: *Knee ligaments: structure, function and repair*, New York, 1990, Raven.
41. Daniel DM, Stone ML, Arendt DL: The effect of cold therapy on pain, swelling, and range of motion after anterior cruciate ligament reconstructive surgery, *Arthroscopy* 10(5):530, 1994.
42. Daniel DM et al: Fate of the ACL-injured patient. A prospective outcome study, *Am J Sports Med* 22(5):632, 1994.
43. DeCarlo MS, Sell KE: The effects of the number and frequency of physical therapy treatments on selected outcomes of treatment in patients with anterior cruciate ligament reconstruction, *J Orthop Sports Phys Ther* 26(6):332, 1997.
44. DeCarlo M, Shelbourne KD, Oneacre K: Rehabilitation program for both knees when the contralateral autogenous patellar tendon graft is used for primary anterior cruciate ligament reconstruction: a case study, *J Orthop Sports Phys Ther* 29(3):144-153, 1999.
45. DeCarlo MS et al: Traditional versus accelerated rehabilitation following ACL reconstruction: a one-year follow-up, *J Orthop Sports Phys Ther* 15(6):309, 1992.
46. DeLorme TL, Watkins A: *Progressive resistance exercise*, New York, 1951, Appleton-Century.
47. DeMaio M, Noyes FR, Mangine RE: Principles for aggressive rehabilitation after reconstruction of the anterior cruciate ligament. Sports medicine rehabilitation series, *Orthopedics* 15(3):385, 1992.
48. Dietrichson J, Souryal TO: Physical therapy after arthroscopic surgery, "preoperative and post operative rehabilitation after anterior cruciate ligament tears," *Orthop Phys Ther Clin North Am* 3(4):, 1994.
49. Dopirak RM, Adamany DC, Steensen RN: A comparison of autogenous patellar tendon and hamstring tendon grafts for anterior cruciate ligament reconstruction, *Orthopedics* 27(8):837-842, 2004.
50. Doucette SA, Child DD: The effects of open and closed chain exercise and knee joint position on patellar tracking in lateral patellar compression syndrome, *J Orthop Sports Phys Ther* 23(2):104, 1996.
51. Drez D, Faust DC, Evans IP: Cryotherapy and nerve palsy, *Am J Sports Med* 9:256, 1981.
52. Ellison AE: Distal iliotibial-band transfer for anterolateral rotatory instability of the knee, *J Bone Joint Surg Br* 61:330, 1979.
53. Engle RP, Canner GC: Proprioceptive neuromuscular facilitation (PNF) and modified procedures for anterior cruciate ligament (ACL) instability, *J Orthop Sports Phys Ther* 11(4):230, 1989.
54. Fielder B et al: Effect of gamma irradiation on the human immunodeficiency virus, *J Bone Joint Surg Br* 76A:1032, 1994.
55. Fitzgerald GK: Open versus closed kinetic chain exercises: issues in rehabilitation after anterior cruciate ligament reconstructive surgery, *Phys Ther* 77(12):1747, 1997.
56. Fitzgerald GK et al: Hop tests as predictors of dynamic knee stability, *J Orthop Sports Phys Ther* 31(10):588-597, 2001.
57. Foster A, Butcher C, Turner PG: Changes in arthroscopic findings in the anterior cruciate ligament deficient knee prior to reconstructive surgery, *Knee* 12(1):33-35, 2005.
58. Frank CB, Jackson DW: The science of reconstruction of the anterior cruciate ligament, *J Bone Joint Surg Br* 79A(10):1556, 1997.
59. Fu FH, Schulte KR: Anterior cruciate ligament surgery 1996 state of the art? *Clin Orthop Relat Res* 325:19, 1996.
60. Fu FH, Woo SL-Y, Irrgang JJ: Current concepts for rehabilitation following anterior cruciate ligament reconstruction, *J Orthop Sports Phys Ther* 15(6):270, 1992.
61. Garcia R Jr et al: Lateral extra-articular knee reconstruction: long-term patient outcome and satisfaction, *J South Orthop Assoc* 9(1):19-23, 2000.
62. Giron F et al: Anterior cruciate ligament reconstruction with double-looped semitendinosus and gracilis tendon graft directly fixed to cortical bone: 5-year results, *Knee Surg Sports Traumatol Arthrosc* 13(2):81-91, 2005.
63. Gladstone JN, Andrews JR: Endoscopic anterior cruciate ligament reconstruction with patella tendon autograft, *Orthop Clin North Am* 33(4):701-715, 2002.
64. Gobbi A et al: Quadrupled bone-semitendinosus anterior cruciate ligament reconstruction: a clinical investigation in a group of athletes, *Arthroscopy* 19(7):691-699, 2003.
65. Goradia VK et al: Tendon-to-bone healing of a semitendinosus tendon autograft used for ACL reconstruction in a sheep model, *Am J Knee Surg* 13(3):143-151, 2000.
66. Gould JA, Davies GJ: *Orthopedic and sports physical therapy*, vol 2, St Louis, 1985, Mosby.
67. Grace TG et al: Isokinetic muscle imbalance and knee-joint injuries, *Am J Bone Joint Surg* 66:734, 1984.
68. Grood ES et al: Biomechanics of the knee-extension exercise. Effect of cutting the anterior cruciate ligament, *Am J Bone Joint Surg* 66:725, 1984.
69. Grossman MG et al: Revision anterior cruciate ligament reconstruction: three- to nine-year follow-up, *Arthroscopy* 21(4):418-423, 2005.
70. Hardin JA et al: The effects of "decelerated" rehabilitation following anterior cruciate ligament reconstruction on a hyperelastic female adolescent: a case study, *J Orthop Sports Phys Ther* 26(1):29, 1997.
71. Henning C, Lych M, Glick J: An in vivo strain gauge study of the elongation of the anterior cruciate ligament, *Am J Sports Med* 13(1):22, 1985.
72. Herrington L et al: Anterior cruciate ligament reconstruction, hamstring versus bone-patella tendon-bone grafts: a systematic literature review of outcome from surgery, *Knee* 12(1):41-50, 2005.
73. Hertel P et al: ACL reconstruction using bone-patellar tendon-bone press-fit fixation: 10-year clinical results,

Knee Surg Sports Traumatol Arthrosc 13(4):248-255, 2005.

74. Hewett TE, Myer GD, Ford KR: Decrease in neuromuscular control about the knee with maturation in female athletes, *J Bone Joint Surg Am* 86-A(8): 1601-1608, 2004.
75. Hewett TE, Myer GD, Ford KR: Reducing knee and anterior cruciate ligament injuries among female athletes: a systematic review of neuromuscular training interventions, *J Knee Surg* 18(1):82-88, 2005.
76. Hewett TE et al: Biomechanical measures of neuromuscular control and valgus loading of the knee predict anterior cruciate ligament injury risk in female athletes: a prospective study, *Am J Sports Med* 33(4): 492-501, 2005.
77. Hewett TE et al: A review of electromyographic activation levels, timing differences, and increased anterior cruciate ligament injury incidence in female athletes, *Br J Sports Med* 39(6):347-350, 2005.
78. Hey-Groves EW: The crucial ligaments of the knee joint. Their function, rupture, and operative treatment of the same, *Br J Surg* 7:505, 1920.
79. Hirokawa S et al: Anterior-posterior and rotational displacement of the tibia elicited by quadriceps contraction, *Am J Sports Med* 20(3):299, 1992.
80. Hogervorst T, Brand RA: Mechanoreceptors in joint function, *J Bone Joint Surg Am* 80(9):1365-1378, 1998.
81. Hopkins J et al: Cryotherapy and transcutaneous electric neuromuscular stimulation decrease arthrogenic muscle inhibition of the vastus medialis after knee joint effusion, *J Athl Train* 37(1):25-31, 2002.
82. Howell SM: Anterior tibial translation during a maximum quadriceps contraction: is it clinically significant? *Am J Sports Med* 18(6):573, 1990.
83. Howell SM, Taylor MA: Failure of reconstruction of the anterior cruciate ligament due to impingement by the intercondylar roof, *J Bone Joint Surg* 75A:1044, 1993.
84. Hubbard TJ, Denegar CR: Does cryotherapy improve outcomes with soft tissue injury? *J Athl Train* 39(3): 278-279, 2004.
85. Huston LJ, Greenfield ML, Wojtys EM: Anterior cruciate ligament injuries in the female athlete. Potential risk factors, *Clin Orthop Relat Res* (372):50-63, 2000.
86. Ibrahim SA et al: Clinical evaluation of arthroscopically assisted anterior cruciate ligament reconstruction: patellar tendon versus gracilis and semitendinosus autograft, *Arthroscopy* 21(4):412-417, 2005.
87. Insall JJ et al: Bone block iliotibial-band transfer for ACL insufficiency, *J Bone Joint Surg Br* 63:560, 1981.
88. Jacobsen K: Osteoarthritis following insufficiency of the cruciate ligaments in man. A clinical study, *Acta Orthop Scan* 48:520, 1977.
89. Jarit GJ et al: The effects of home interferential therapy on post-operative pain, edema, and range of motion of the knee, *Clin J Sport Med* 13(1):16-20, 2003.
90. Johnson RJ et al: Five to ten year follow-up evaluation after reconstruction of the anterior cruciate ligament, *Clin Orthop* 83:122, 1984.
91. Jones KG: Reconstruction of the anterior cruciate ligament using the central one-third of the patella ligaments, a follow-up report, *J Bone Joint Surg Br* 63A:1302, 1970.
92. Jones HP et al: Meniscal and chondral loss in the anterior cruciate ligament injured knee, *Sports Med* 33(14):1075-1089, 2003.
93. Juris PM et al: A dynamic test of lower extremity function following anterior cruciate ligament reconstruction and rehabilitation, *J Orthop Sports Phys Ther* 26(4):184, 1997.
94. Kartus J et al: Complications following arthroscopic anterior cruciate ligament reconstruction. A 2-5-year follow-up of 604 patients with special emphasis on anterior knee pain, *Knee Surg Sports Traumatol Arthrosc* 7(1):2-8, 1999.
95. Knight KL: *Cryotherapy in sport injury management*, Champaign, IL, 1995, Human Kinetics.
96. Kuechle DK et al: Allograft anterior cruciate ligament reconstruction in patients over 40 years of age, *Arthroscopy* 18(8):845-853, 2002.
97. Kurosaka M, Yoshiyas S, Andrish JT: Biomechanical comparison of different surgical techniques of graft fixation in anterior cruciate ligament reconstruction, *Am J Sports Med* 15:225, 1987.
98. Lange GW et al: Electromyographic and kinematic analysis of graded treadmill walking and the implications for knee rehabilitation, *J Orthop Sports Phys Ther* 23(5):294, 1996.
99. Leetun DT et al: Core stability measures as risk factors for lower extremity injury in athletes, *Med Sci Sports Exerc* 36(6):926-934, 2004.
100. Lephart SM et al: Relationship between selected physical characteristics and functional capacity in the anterior cruciate ligament insufficient athlete, *J Orthop Sports Phys Ther* 16(4):174, 1992.
101. Lessard LA et al: The efficacy of cryotherapy following arthroscopic knee surgery, *J Orthop Sports Phys Ther* 26(1):14, 1997.
102. Liu-Ambrose T et al: The effects of proprioceptive or strength training on the neuromuscular function of the ACL reconstructed knee: a randomized clinical trial, *Scand J Med Sci Sports* 13(2):115-123, 2003.
103. Liu SH et al: Collagen in tendon, ligament, and bone healing: a current review, *Clin Orthop Relat Res* 318:265, 1995.
104. MacIntosh DL, Tregonning RJA: A follow-up and evaluation of the over-the-top repair of acute tears of the anterior cruciate ligament, *J Bone Joint Surg* 59B:511, 1977.
105. Maffulli N, Binfield PM, King JB: Articular cartilage lesions in the symptomatic anterior cruciate ligament-deficient knee, *Arthroscopy* 19(7):685-690, 2003.
106. Maitland GD: *Peripheral manipulation*, ed 3, London, 1991, Butterworth-Heinemann.
107. Malone T, Friedhoff GC: Knee bracing—the prophylactic knee bracing debate, *Biomechanics* (special report) p. 23, May 1997.
108. Malone TR, Garrett WE Jr: Commentary and historical perspective of anterior cruciate ligament rehabilitation, *J Orthop Sports Phys Ther* 15(6):265, 1992.
109. Mangine RE, Noyes FR: Rehabilitation of the allograft reconstruction, *J Orthop Sports Phys Ther* 15(6):294, 1992.
110. Mangine RE, Noyes FR, DeMaio M: Minimal protection program: advanced weight bearing and range of motion

after ACL reconstruction—weeks 1-5, *Orthopedics* 15(4):504, 1992.
111. Marshall JL, Warren RJ, Wickiewicz TL: The anterior cruciate ligament. A technique of repair and reconstruction, *Clin Orthop* 143:97, 1979.
112. Marshall JL, Warren RJ, Wickiewicz TL: Primary surgical treatment of anterior cruciate ligament lesions, *Am J Sports Med* 10:103, 1982.
113. Mayr HO, Weig TG, Plitz W: Arthrofibrosis following ACL reconstruction—reasons and outcome, *Arch Orthop Trauma Surg* 124(8):518-522, 2004.
114. McCarroll JR, Shelbourne KD, Patel DV: Anterior cruciate ligament injuries in young athletes. Recommendations for treatment and rehabilitation, *Sports Med* 20(2):117-127, 1995.
115. McHugh MP et al: Preoperative indicators of motion loss and weakness following anterior cruciate ligament reconstruction, *J Orthop Sports Phys Ther* 27(6):407-411, 1998.
116. McLean DA: The use of cold and superficial heat in the treatment of soft tissue injuries, *Br J Sports Med* 23:53, 1989.
117. McLean SG et al: Sagittal plane biomechanics cannot injure the ACL during sidestep cutting, *Clin Biomech (Bristol, Avon)* 19(8):828-838, 2004.
118. McMaster WC: A literary review on ice therapy in injuries, *Am J Sports Med* 5:124, 1977.
119. Milano G et al: Evaluation of bone plug and soft tissue anterior cruciate ligament graft fixation over time using transverse femoral fixation in a sheep model, *Arthroscopy* 21(5):532-539, 2005.
120. Miller MD, Sullivan RT: Anterior cruciate ligament reconstruction in an 84-year-old man, *Arthroscopy* 17(1):70-72, 2001.
121. Millett PJ, Willis AA, Warren RF: Associated injuries in pediatric and adolescent anterior cruciate ligament tears: does a delay in treatment increase the risk of meniscal tear? *Arthroscopy* 18(9):955-959, 2002.
122. Millett PJ et al: Early ACL reconstruction in combined ACL-MCL injuries, *J Knee Surg* 17(2):94-98, 2004.
123. Morrissey MC: Reflex inhibition of thigh muscles in knee injury, *Sports Med* 7:263, 1989.
124. Neeb TB et al: Assessing anterior cruciate ligament injuries: the association and differential value of questionnaires, clinical tests, and functional tests, *J Orthop Sports Phys Ther* 26(6):324, 1997.
125. Nicholas JA, Minkoff J: Iliotibial band transfer through the intercondylar notch for combined anterior instability, *Am J Sports Med* 6:341, 1978.
126. Novak PJ, Bach BR, Jr, Hager CA: Clinical and functional outcome of anterior cruciate ligament reconstruction in the recreational athlete over the age of 35, *Am J Knee Surg* 9(3):111, 1996.
127. Noyes FR, Barber-Westin SD: Revision anterior cruciate ligament surgery: experience from Cincinnati, *Clin Orthop Relat Res* 325:116, 1996.
128. Noyes FR et al: Biomechanical analysis of human ligament grafts used in knee ligament repairs and reconstructions, *J Bone Joint Surg* 66A:344, 1984.
129. Noyes FR et al: The drop-jump screening test: difference in lower limb control by gender and effect of neuromuscular training in female athletes, *Am J Sports Med* 33(2):197-207, 2005.
130. Nuccion SL, Hame SL: A symptomatic cyclops lesion 4 years after anterior cruciate ligament reconstruction, *Arthroscopy* 17(2):E8, 2001.
131. Paletta GA Jr: Special considerations. Anterior cruciate ligament reconstruction in the skeletally immature, *Orthop Clin North Am* 34(1):65-77, 2003.
132. Paulos L et al: Knee rehabilitation after anterior cruciate ligament reconstruction and repair, *Am J Sports Med* 9(3):140, 1981.
133. Paulos LE et al: Infrapatellar contracture syndrome: an unrecognized cause of knee stiffness with patella entrapment and patella infera, *Am J Sports Med* 15:331, 1987.
134. Podesta L et al: Rationale and protocol for postoperative anterior cruciate ligament rehabilitation, *Clin Orthop* 257:262, 1990.
135. Prodromos CC et al: Stability results of hamstring anterior cruciate ligament reconstruction at 2- to 8-year follow-up, *Arthroscopy* 21(2):138-146, 2005.
136. Proulx RP: Southern California frostbite, *J Am Coll Emerg Phys* 5:618, 1976.
137. Rasmussen T et al: The effects of 4 mrad of gamma irradiation on the internal mechanical properties of bone-patella tendon-bone grafts, *Arthroscopy* 10:188, 1994.
138. Raynor MC et al: Cryotherapy after ACL reconstruction: a meta-analysis, *J Knee Surg* 18(2):123-129, 2005.
139. Renstrom P et al: Strain within the anterior cruciate ligament during a hamstring and quadriceps activity, *Am J Sports Med* 14(1):83, 1986.
140. Richmond JC, Gladstone J, MacGillivray J: Continuous passive motion after arthroscopically assisted anterior cruciate ligament reconstruction: comparison of short versus long-term use, *Arthroscopy* 7(1):39, 1991.
141. Risberg MA, Ekeland A: Assessment of functional tests after anterior cruciate ligament surgery, *J Orthop Sports Phys Ther* 19(4):212, 1994.
142. Robertson DB, Daniel DM, Biden E: Soft tissue fixation to bone, *Am J Sports Med* 14:398, 1983.
143. Rochman S: Accelerating ACL rehab, *Training and Conditioning* 7(2):33, 1997.
144. Roi GS et al: Return to official Italian First Division soccer games within 90 days after anterior cruciate ligament reconstruction: a case report, *J Orthop Sports Phys Ther* 35(2):52-61, 2005.
145. Rozzi SL et al: Knee joint laxity and neuromuscular characteristics of male and female soccer and basketball players, *Am J Sports Med* 27(3):312-319, 1999.
146. Rubenstein RA et al: Effect on knee stability if full hyperextension is restored immediately after autogenous bone-patellar tendon-bone anterior cruciate ligament reconstruction, *Am J Sports Med* 23(3):365, 1995.
147. Sandberg R, Balkfors B: Reconstruction of the anterior cruciate ligament: a 5-year follow-up of 89 patients, *Acta Orthop Scand* 59(3):288, 1988.
148. Seto JL et al: Rehabilitation of the knee after anterior cruciate ligament reconstruction, *J Orthop Sports Phys Ther* 11(1):8, 1989.
149. Shea KG et al: Anterior cruciate ligament injury in pediatric and adolescent soccer players: an analysis of

insurance data, *J Pediatr Orthop* 24(6):623-628, 2004.
150. Shelbourne KD, Klootwyk TE, DeCarlo MS: Update on accelerated rehabilitation after anterior cruciate ligament reconstruction, *J Orthop Sports Phys Ther* 15(6):303, 1992.
151. Shelbourne KD, Nitz P: Accelerated rehabilitation after anterior cruciate ligament reconstruction, *J Orthop Sports Phys Ther* 15(6):256, 1992.
152. Shelbourne KD, Patel DV: Timing of surgery in anterior cruciate ligament-injured knees, *Knee Surg Sports Traumatol Arthrosc* 3(3):148-156, 1995.
153. Shelbourne KD, Patel DV: Treatment of limited motion after anterior cruciate ligament reconstruction, *Knee Surg Sports Traumatol Arthrosc* 7(2):85-92, 1999.
154. Shelbourne KD, Patel DV, McCarroll JR: Management of anterior cruciate ligament injuries in skeletally immature adolescents, *Knee Surg Sports Traumatol Arthrosc* 4(2): 68-74, 1996.
155. Shelbourne KD et al: Correlation of remaining patellar tendon width with quadriceps strength after autogenous bone-patellar tendon-bone anterior cruciate ligament reconstruction, *Am J Sports Med* 22(6):774, 1994.
156. Shelbourne KD et al: Ligament stability two to six years after anterior cruciate ligament reconstruction with autogenous patellar tendon graft and participation in accelerated rehabilitation program, *Am J Sports Med* 23(5):575, 1995.
157. Sherman MF et al: The long-term follow up of primary anterior cruciate ligament repair. Defining a rationale for augmentation, *Am J Sports Med* 19:243, 1991.
158. Silverskiold JP et al: Rehabilitation of the anterior cruciate ligament in the athlete, *Sports Med* 6:308, 1988.
159. Spencer JD, Hayes KC, Alexander IJ: Knee joint effusion and quadriceps reflex inhibition in man, *Arch Phys Med Rehabil* 65:171, 1984.
160. Swenson C, Sward L, Karlsson J.: Cryotherapy in sports medicine, *Scand J Med Sci Sports* 6(4):193-200, 1996.
161. Tegner Y: Strength training in the rehabilitation of cruciate ligament tears, *Sports Med* 9(2):129, 1990.
162. Tegner Y, Lysholm J: Rating systems in the evaluation of knee ligament injuries, *Clin Orthop* 198:43, 1985.
163. Teitge RA, Indelicato PA, Kerlan RK: Iliotibial band transfer for anterolateral rotatory instability of the knee: summary of 54 cases, *Am J Sports Med* 8:223, 1980.
164. Tippett SR, Voight ML: *Functional progressions for sport rehabilitation*, Champaign, IL, 1995, Human Kinetics.
165. Tomaro JE: Prevention and treatment of patellar entrapment following intra-articular ACL reconstruction, athletic training, *JNATA* 26:11, 1991.
166. Tonin M et al: Progressive loss of knee extension after injury. Cyclops syndrome due to a lesion of the anterior cruciate ligament, *Am J Sports Med* 29(5):545-549, 2001.
167. Tovin BJ, Tovin TS, Tovin M: Surgical and biomechanical considerations in rehabilitation of patients with intra-articular ACL reconstructions, *J Orthop Sports Phys Ther* 15(6):317, 1992.
168. Viola R, Vianello R.: Intra-articular ACL reconstruction in the over-40-year-old patient, *Knee Surg Sports Traumatol Arthrosc* 7(1):25-28, 1999.
169. von Eisenhart-Rothe R et al: Femoro-tibial and menisco-tibial translation patterns in patients with unilateral anterior cruciate ligament deficiency—a potential cause of secondary meniscal tears, *J Orthop Res* 22(2):275-282, 2004.
170. Wilk KE, Andrews JR: Current concepts in the treatment of anterior cruciate ligament disruption, *J Orthop Sports Phys Ther* 15(6):279, 1992.
171. Wilk KE, Andrews JR, Clancy WG: Quadriceps muscular strength after removal of the central third patellar tendon for contralateral anterior cruciate ligament reconstruction surgery: a case study, *J Orthop Sports Phys Ther* 18(6):692, 1993.
172. Wilk KE, Reinold MM, Hooks TR: Recent advances in the rehabilitation of isolated and combined anterior cruciate ligament injuries, *Orthop Clin North Am* 34(1):107-137, 2003.
173. Yack HJ, Riley LM, Whieldon TR: Anterior tibial translation during progressive loading of the ACL-deficient knee during weight-bearing and nonweight-bearing isometric exercise, *J Orthop Sports Phys Ther* 20(5):247, 1994.

CHAPTER 18

Arthroscopic Lateral Retinaculum Release

Daniel A. Farwell
Andrew A. Brooks

SURGICAL INDICATIONS AND CONSIDERATIONS

Adaptation resulting from chronic compression in the patellofemoral joint can lead to significant arthrosis in a wide variety of patients, both young and old. Pain, attributed to increased patellofemoral compression, occurs in different aspects of the joint, but the most common site is along the lateral aspect. This patellofemoral pain can originate from mechanical malalignment, the static or dynamic soft tissue stabilizers, or increased load placed across the joint as a result of various activities.[43] Symptoms may include diffuse aches and pains that are exacerbated by stair climbing or prolonged sitting (i.e., flexion of the knees). Crepitus and mild effusion are often associated with patellofemoral arthralgia. Although complaints of "giving way" or collapse are more often linked with ligamentous instability, these symptoms also can be associated with patellofemoral pain. Patients may even complain of joint pain and "locking" when they are experiencing poor patella stabilization during flexion of the knee.

In examining the way lateral retinacular release procedures may affect the arthrokinematics of the patellofemoral joint, the focus should be on the relationship between patella tilt compression and associated tightness in the lateral retinaculum. The function of the patella is to increase the lever of the quadriceps muscle, thus increasing its mechanical advantage. For functional and efficient knee motion, the patella must be aligned so that it can travel in the trochlear groove of the femur. The ability of the patella to track properly depends on the bony configuration of the trochlear groove and the balance of forces of the connective tissue surrounding the joint.

Weakness and stiffness from the hip are factors that appear to influence poor patella alignment (gluteus medius weakness and iliotibial band [ITB] tension). Tensor fascia latae and gluteus maximus fibers combine to form a very thick, fibrous structure that attaches distally into the lateral tibial tubercle (Gerdy's tubercle).[23] The ITB slips into the lateral border of the patella, which interdigitates with the superficial and deep fibers of the lateral retinaculum. This design often leads to excessive compression over the lateral condyle and lateral border of the patella during dynamic activity.

Tilt compression is a clinical radiographic condition of the patellofemoral joint that can lead to retinacular strain (i.e., peripatellar effect) and excessive lateral pressure syndrome (ELPS; i.e., articular effect).[14] A case can definitely be made for a cause-and-effect relationship between tilt compression and retinacular strain. Chronic patella tilting and associated retinacular shortening cannot only produce significant lateral facet overload but also a resultant deficiency in medial contact pressure. This tilt compression syndrome may present as simple soft tissue pain related to the shortening of the lateral retinacular tissue. If left untreated, then histologic studies of painful retinacular biopsies may reveal degenerative fibroneuromas within the lateral retinaculum of patients with chronic patellofemoral malalignment.[15] ELPS results from chronic lateral patella tilt, adaptive lateral retinacular shortening, and resultant chronic imbalance of facet loads. It is prevalent in active, middle-aged adults. In younger patient populations, excessive lateral pressure during growth and development can alter the shape and formation of both the patella and trochlea.[15]

Nonoperative treatment of patella tilt should focus on mobilization of tight quadriceps muscles and the lateral retinaculum. Patellofemoral taping, bracing, and anti-inflammatory medications also are quite helpful. Gait deviation and excessive foot pronation should be corrected to eliminate possible secondary influences on patellofemoral malalignment.[43] The use of resistant weight training or isokinetic exercise (in conjunction with patella taping) can be beneficial in building quadriceps muscle strength.[45]

Patellofemoral Taping

McConnell patellofemoral taping has become a useful technique in the conservative (nonsurgical) rehabilitation

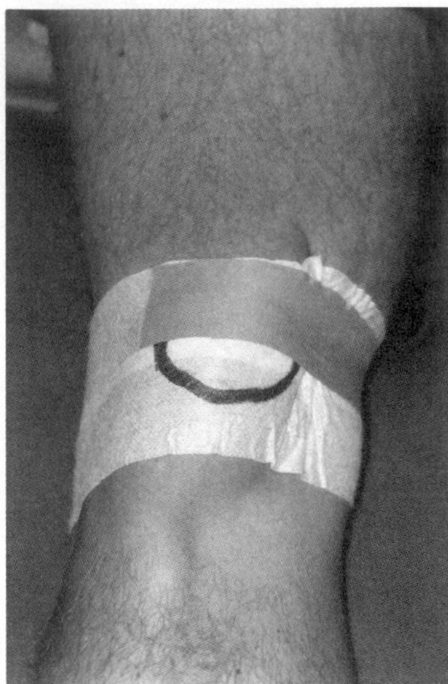

Fig. 18-1 Patella glide. Place a piece of tape on the superior half of the lateral border of the patella and pull the tape medially. Lift the soft tissue over the medial femoral condyle toward the patella to ensure a more secure fixation and less tape slippage.

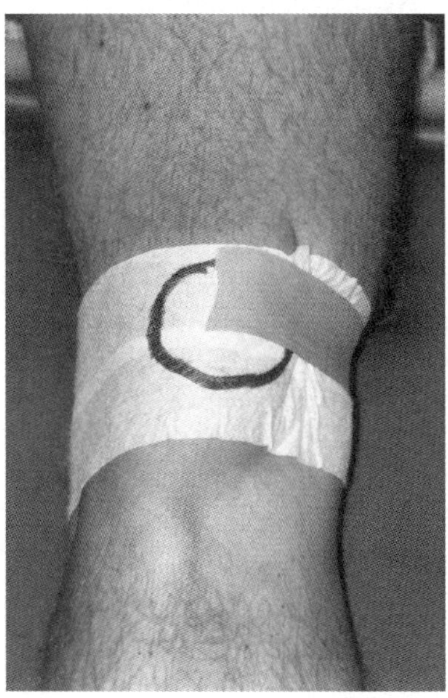

Fig. 18-2 Patella tilt. Place the tape on the medial superior half of the patella. Pull the tape medially to lift the lateral border. Lift the soft tissue over the medial femoral condyle toward the patella to ensure a more secure fixation.

of patellofemoral pain; it can also benefit patients after surgical lateral release as well. Patellar taping has recently been shown to increase vasti muscle activity[6,28] and may enhance knee joint proprioception after surgery.[4] The McConnell patellofemoral program emphasizes closed-chain exercises to correct patella glide (Fig. 18-1), tilt (Fig. 18-2), and rotation (Fig. 18-3) and allow for pain-free rehabilitation. The patient is evaluated dynamically

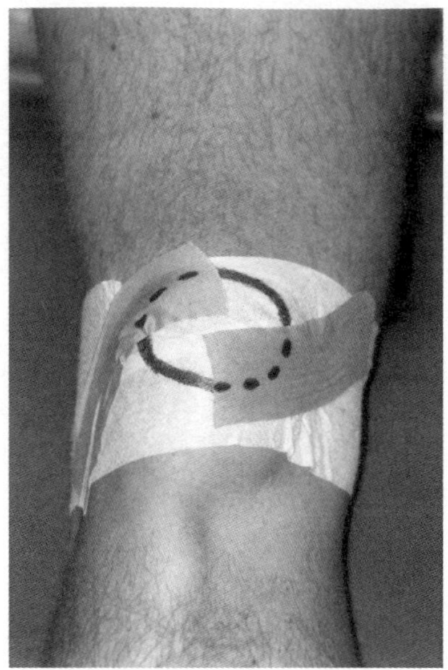

Fig. 18-3 Patella rotation. Place a piece of tape on the inferior-medial quarter of the patella and perform an upward rotation movement of the patella. Place another piece of tape on the superior-lateral half of the patella and perform a downward rotation movement of the patella.

during a functional activity such as walking, stepping down, or squatting. According to Maitland,[29] "The aim of examining movements is to find one or more comparable signs in an appropriate joint or joints." These comparable signs, or reassessment signs, are re-evaluated after each patella correction to determine the effectiveness of the treatment. After an assessment of patella orientation, a specifically designed tape is used to correct for each patella orientation. The patellofemoral joint is principally a soft tissue joint, which suggests that it can be adjusted through appropriate mechanical means (i.e., physical therapy). Two primary components (glide and tilt) may be present either statically or dynamically. Patella orientation varies among patients and even from left to right extremities.

Glide Component

The amount of glide correction depends on the tightness of the structures and the relative amount of activity in the entire quadriceps musculature. The corrective procedure involves securing the edge of the tape over the lateral border of the patella and pulling or gliding the patella more medially. Although this technique is useful for most patellofemoral pain, it is not often used in the post-operative care of patients recovering from lateral retinacular release (see Fig. 18-1).

Tilt Component

Tilt correction is quite often used to stretch the deep retinacular fibers along the lateral borders of the knee.

Increased tension in the lateral retinaculum along with a tight ITB (which inserts into the lateral retinaculum) can produce a lateral "dipping," or tilt, of the lateral border of the patella (see Fig. 18-2).

When focusing on patients recovering from lateral retinacular release, the physical therapist (PT) should remember that the very tissues these taping techniques address have been surgically released. Although patella orientations have most definitely been altered in patients after surgical release, muscle recruitment patterns and joint loading characteristics that may have contributed to the symptoms are still present. McConnell taping procedures produce improved joint loading and allow the patient to return to a more active, pain-free lifestyle when used in conjunction with closed-chain functional exercises.[42]

Although conservative management remains the cornerstone of treatment for patients with anterior knee pain, some patients will not respond and continue to have pain and functional disability. If conservative (nonsurgical) treatment is unsuccessful in providing the patient with appropriate pain relief and function, then surgical intervention should be considered.[36]

In addition to subjective complaints and functional limitations, other indications for surgery include dislocation, subluxation, and failure of previous surgery with or without medial patella position.

Operative procedures that modify patella mechanics are most successful in treating patients with patella articular cartilage lesions. Lateral release procedures should ultimately produce a mechanical benefit to the patient, such as relieving documented tilt.[44]

SURGICAL PROCEDURE

Review of the literature suggests strict indications for lateral release[14]:

1. Chronic anterior knee pain despite a trial of a nonoperative program for at least 3 months
2. Minimal or no chondrosis (Outerbridge grade 2 or less)
3. A normal Q angle
4. A tight or tender lateral retinaculum with clinically and radiographically documented lateral patella tilt

Results may be disappointing for lateral release in the presence of the following conditions:

1. Patellofemoral pain syndrome (anterior knee pain)
2. Advanced patellofemoral arthritis
3. A Q angle greater than 20 degrees

Patients with instability may require medial retinacular imbrication or a distal realignment in addition to an isolated lateral release.

The Southern California Orthopedic Institute (SCOI) technique of arthroscopic lateral release is performed in the supine position without the use of a leg holder; the tourniquet is inflated only when necessary. The procedure is performed with the arthroscope in the anteromedial portal. Routine arthroscopic fluid is used. An 18-gauge spinal needle is inserted at the superior pole of the patella and is used as a marker for the proximal extent of the release. The needle must be withdrawn as the electrosurgical electrode approaches it. With experience, the surgeon can omit the needle marker. The electrosurgical lateral release electrode is inserted through the inferior anterolateral portal using a plastic cannula to protect the skin. The procedure is performed with the generator setting at approximately 10 to 12 watts of power. With the patient's knee extended, the surgeon performs the release approximately 1 cm from the patella edge, progressing from distal to proximal using the cutting mode. The deep and superficial retinaculum, as well as the lateral patellotibial ligament, are released under direct visualization until subcutaneous fat is exposed. The extent of the proximal release is only to the deforming tight structures and should never extend beyond the superior pole of the patella.

An incomplete release is often secondary to inadequate release of the patellotibial ligament. Again, the tourniquet is not inflated during the procedure, and vessels are coagulated as they are encountered. An adequate release is confirmed by the ability to evert the patella 60 degrees. After the release the knee is passively moved through a range of motion (ROM) and correction of lateral overhang during knee flexion is confirmed. The arthroscope should be switched back to the accessory superolateral portal for this assessment. Usual postoperative dressings are applied after the arthroscopic procedure—sterile dressings and an absorbent pad held in place by an elastic toe-to-groin support stocking previously measured for the patient.

Postoperative rehabilitation includes muscle strengthening and ROM exercises the day of surgery, including quadriceps sets and straight leg raising (SLR). The patient continues to do these exercises at home the night of surgery and is given weight bearing as tolerated status with crutches immediately. Crutches are discontinued when adequate quadriceps muscle control has been obtained and patients can walk safely. The vast majority of patients use their crutches for less than 7 days, although some may need them for 2 to 3 weeks depending on quadriceps control.

The SCOI experience with arthroscopic lateral retinaculum release (ALRR) has been reported previously.[37] The researchers monitored 39 patients with a history of recurrent patella subluxation or dislocation in 45 knees for an average of 28 months and noted good to excellent results in 76% of patients. Similar experiences with ALRR have been reported in the literature, with favorable results in 60% to 85% of cases.[1] Arthroscopic treatment compares favorably with open realignment and has a lower complication rate. No postoperative hemarthrosis occurred in

Table 18-1 Lateral Retinaculum Release

Rehabilitation Phase	Criteria to Progress to this Phase	Anticipated Impairments and Functional Limitations	Intervention	Goal	Rationale
Phase I Postoperative 1-2 weeks	◆ Postoperative	◆ Postoperative pain ◆ Postoperative edema ◆ Gait deviations ◆ Limited tolerance to weight-bearing activities ◆ Limited ROM ◆ Limited strength	◆ Ice ◆ Vasopneumatic compression ◆ Grade II patella mobilization ◆ Neuromuscular stimulation ◆ Patellar taping ◆ Knee AROM—Ankle pumps ◆ Knee PROM—Hamstring and ITB stretches ◆ Isometrics—Quadriceps/hamstring sets, quadriceps sets at 20-30 degrees ◆ Home exercises (refer to Suggested Home Maintenance Box)	◆ Decrease pain ◆ Manage edema ◆ Decrease gait deviations ◆ Increase tolerance to weight-bearing activities ◆ ROM 0-135 degrees ◆ Quality contraction of the quadriceps	◆ Decrease edema and pain ◆ Increase neuromuscular coordination with muscle contraction ◆ Restore joint mechanics ◆ Improve joint mobility and stability ◆ Prevent adhesions ◆ Initiate volitional muscle control and increase strength ◆ Increase patient self-management

ROM, Range of motion; *AROM,* active range of motion; *PROM,* passive range of motion; *ITB,* iliotibial band.

the SCOI series; hemarthrosis is the main complication reported in the literature, occurring in 2% to 42% of cases. Small's review[40] of 194 cases of ALRR performed by 21 arthroscopic surgeons found hemarthrosis associated with 89% of the 4.6% total complication rate. Careful coagulation of vessels without an inflated tourniquet can reduce hemarthrosis. If strict criteria are met and proper surgical techniques used, then a consistent result can be obtained with these patients.

The complexity of the patellofemoral articulation and its associated disorders are evident by the significant body of literature on the subject and the abundant surgical procedures involving the joint. A thorough clinical evaluation, including history and physical and radiographic examination, helps to clarify the diagnosis of patellofemoral disorder. Use of the arthroscope for the electrosurgical lateral release is an effective component in the armament of knee surgeons for patients with persistently symptomatic patellofemoral disorders who meet the surgical indications described.

THERAPY GUIDELINES FOR REHABILITATION

Phase I (Acute Phase)

TIME: 1 to 2 weeks after surgery
GOALS: Decrease pain, manage edema, increase weight-bearing activities, facilitate quality quadriceps contraction (Table 18-1)

After knee surgery the goal of rehabilitation is to prevent loss of muscle strength, endurance, flexibility, and proprioception. These issues often are difficult to address immediately after lateral release. The procedure is often associated with significant hemarthrosis resulting from sacrifice of the lateral geniculate artery.[2] Therefore the acute phase of treatment should focus on managing edema and decreasing pain. The use of vasopneumatic compression, electrical stimulation (ES), ice, and intermittent elevation of the limb can assist in decreasing the patient's swelling.

Q Rebecca is 24 years old. She had ALRR done on her right knee 18 days ago. Treatment has focused on decreasing joint effusion, pain, and discomfort. Over the past 2 days her pain has increased, with redness around the knee. What should be done?

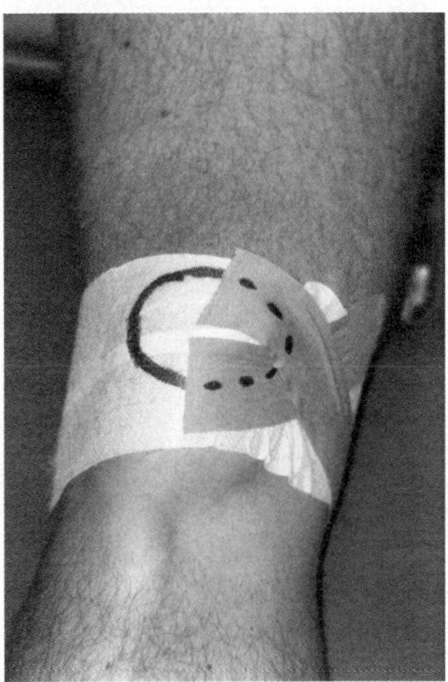

Fig. 18-4 Stabilization taping. After surgery the lateral tissue is often hypersensitive to any type of stretching or pulling. The application of a taping correction for both internal rotation (IR) and external rotation (ER) results in a low-level patella stabilization that the patient finds much easier to tolerate. Taping enables the patient to perform normal knee flexion-extension activity without pain or with less pain. It also decreases effusion.

Other strategies to both decrease joint effusion and begin restoring joint mobility include grade II (mobilizations performed shy of resistance in an effort to decrease pain)[27] patella mobilizations, active calf pumping exercises, and the application of McConnell taping[30] specific to acute lateral release rehabilitation (Fig. 18-4). This procedure places a very mild tilt on the patella, providing a small amount of length to the repair site or lateral retinacular tissue. The tape maintains the new alignment, preventing adhesions that may bind down the released retinaculum during tissue healing. Other taping procedures such as unloading the lateral soft tissue may assist in decreasing pain and discomfort during exercise (Fig. 18-5). This procedure is beneficial in decreasing joint effusion and adds joint stability. It is often used in combination with a patella tilt correction.

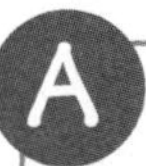

These are signs of infection. The PT should notify the physician immediately.

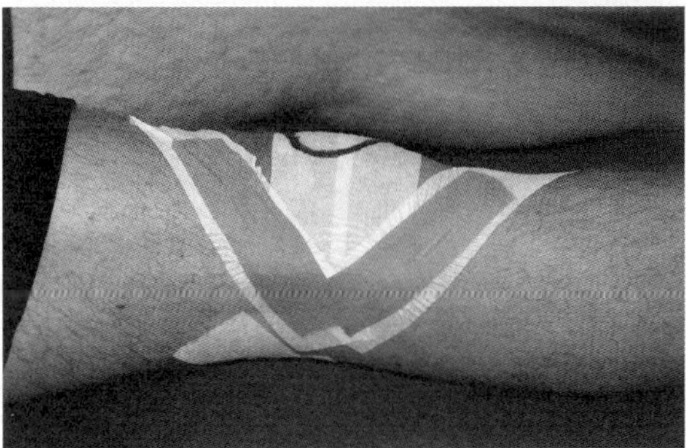

Fig. 18-5 Unloading of lateral soft tissue structures. Taping allows for a decrease in the tension produced over the surgical repair site by inhibiting the effective pull from the iliotibial band (ITB) and vastus lateralis. Unloading the lateral retinaculum may significantly reduce the patient's symptoms. Tape from the posterior aspect of the lateral joint line down to the tibial tubercle and from the posterior lateral joint line to the distal midthigh (approximately 2 to 3 inches above the patella). The tissue inside the tape should be pulled toward the joint line as you pull and secure the tape. The tape should look like a wide *V* lateral to the knee and should not inhibit active motion.

Q Sarah is a 17-year-old basketball player who had ALRR 3 weeks ago. She is complaining of her knee "giving out" during walking. She notes minimal pain, but continues to note pronounced swelling about the knee, especially laterally.

Phase II (Subacute Phase)

TIME: 3 to 4 weeks after surgery
GOALS: Continue to manage edema and pain, improve sit-stand transfer activities, improve strength and stability of the patellofemoral joint, progress functional training to return activity to previous levels (Table 18-2)

As the patient's swelling and pain subside (1 to 2 weeks), the patient moves into a subacute phase. During this phase a more direct and aggressive type of treatment to the knee is implemented. Heat modalities (i.e., moist heat, ultrasound) are used to assist in the absorption and removal of waste products within the joint. Their influence on the cardiovascular system produces increased capillary permeability and vasodilation. The vasodilation brings increased oxygen and nutrients to the knee, which assist in the healing and repairing of the surgically altered tissue.[24] Increased blood flow produces increased capillary hydrostatic pressure. Therefore heat modalities can be very beneficial at this stage of rehabilitation, *but only if the patient's effusion is under control.* If the patient's effusion is displacing the patella from the trochlear groove or the patient cannot perform active isometric quadriceps

Table 18-2 Lateral Retinaculum Release

Rehabilitation Phase	Criteria to Progress to this Phase	Anticipated Impairments and Functional Limitations	Intervention	Goal	Rationale
Phase II Postoperative 3-4 weeks	◆ Incision healed ◆ Edema controlled ◆ Full weight bearing although full ROM and strength may be deficient	◆ Pain with squatting and sit-stand ◆ Gait deviations ◆ Limited stability of patellofemoral joint ◆ Limited tolerance (if any) to prolonged walking, standing, running, or jumping	Continuation of interventions from Phase I, progressed as indicated: ◆ Moist heat and ultrasound (if edema is under control) ◆ Soft tissue mobilization when pain is significantly diminished on palpation ◆ Neuromuscular stimulation ◆ Closed-chain exercises, lunges, standing wall slides, and step-downs (see Figs. 18-6 to 18-8) ◆ Biofeedback in conjunction with exercises ◆ Patellofemoral taping (refer to weaning protocol) ◆ Home exercises	◆ Achieve full ROM ◆ Decrease pain ◆ Increase mobility ◆ Increase strength ◆ Sit-stand without pain ◆ Decrease gait deviations ◆ Increase stability of patellofemoral joint ◆ Tape only for skill-specific activity	◆ Decrease swelling and pain ◆ Increase neuromuscular coordination with muscle contraction ◆ Restore joint mechanics ◆ Functional strengthening using closed-chain exercises ◆ Biofeedback with exercise to improve VMO tonic activity ◆ Improve joint mobility and stability ◆ Increase patient self-management

ROM, Range of motion; *VMO,* vastus medalis oblique.

contractions, then the joint effusion is significant. **Heat applications may be contraindicated until edema is no longer a concern.**

Soft tissue mobilization can be beneficial at this stage to increase circulation, decrease swelling, mobilize healing tissue, and decrease hypersensitivity in the knee joint.[15] Deep massage can assist in the reabsorption of fluid within the knee, yet manipulation of soft tissue structures over the lateral aspect of the knee should be avoided to prevent aggravation of the trauma from surgery.

Soft tissue mobilization should not be initiated in the area of lateral structures before the tissues have begun to heal (1 to 2 weeks) and pain is significantly diminished on palpation of the entire patellofemoral joint.

ES is used to assist in activation of the quadriceps muscle. Specific benefits include decreasing joint edema, increasing local blood flow to the muscle, promoting increased muscle tone, and controlling postoperative pain.[25,32] Electricity also can be used to retard quadriceps atrophy, which results from immobilization or inhibition of the muscle.[17] When used in combination with active isometric and isotonic exercises, ES retrains transposed muscles and promotes muscle awareness in regaining volitional muscle control postoperatively.[24]

Experiments conducted by scientists in the USSR in the 1970s examined the possibility of producing greater intensity of muscle contraction with electrical current. Some studies have found the use of ES during immobilization produces a significant increase in muscle strength.[30,40] By using ES early in the rehabilitative process, PTs can prevent the loss of oxidative capacity, thus shortening postoperative rehabilitation and conditioning time and allowing a more rapid return to functional activities.[8] Although ES can be of great benefit, it should not be used as a replacement for postoperative rehabilitation and strengthening exercise programs.[7]

In summary the use of modalities is beneficial in aiding healing by decreasing acute reactions and altering blood flow, which may provide low-level analgesic effects.[25,33] Understanding the action of these modalities and the way they influence healing is important in predicting their usefulness and appropriateness in the rehabilitation of patients after lateral retinacular release.

> **A** In exploring her situation further it was noted that she was not able to perform an adequate quadriceps contraction. Quadriceps inhibition is a result of the continued edema. A more aggressive edema management program (i.e., elevation, compression, ES three times a day) was initiated along with therapy treatment consisting of ES in conjunction with quadriceps isometrics. A single-point cane was used in the interim until she could demonstrate adequate quadriceps control with walking.

Strengthening

Strengthening of the entire lower kinetic chain is the goal in most patients suffering from anterior knee pain. This goal is no different for patients after lateral retinacular release. Although special attention is paid to the quadriceps muscle, particularly the vastus medialis oblique (VMO), it is the balanced contraction in the vasti group as a whole that is the ultimate goal. Richardson[36] examined the activity level of the quadriceps, specifically the VMO, to better understand the activation patterns of the quadriceps during dynamic motion. The quadriceps were monitored with surface electromyography (EMG) through a full arc of motion in both patients suffering from patellofemoral pain and normal patients. The VMO produced a tonic (constant) pattern of activation throughout a full (0 to 135 degrees) arc of motion in pain-free patients; a phasic (intermittent) activity pattern was observed in patients with patellofemoral pain. *A consistent activation of the entire quadriceps is the goal in quadriceps strengthening. Quality of motion should be emphasized over relative quantity. Exercise beyond 20-degrees flexion (20 to 135 degrees) increases the surface area of contact and gives better stability within the trochlear groove.* Although the development of muscle strength is important, it is not the only goal of rehabilitation. Muscle endurance, flexibility, and the development of correct proprioceptive loading through the entire lower extremity (LE) must be addressed as well. These goals can be accomplished in patients recovering from surgical lateral release by protecting the surgical repair through modalities that speed the tissue repair process and protective taping that adds stability and promotes early functional rehabilitation. Wittingham, Palmer, and Macmillan[47] recently concluded that a combination of patellar taping and exercise was superior to the use of exercise alone. Early quadriceps activation includes isometric quadriceps sets in varying degrees of flexion produced by a proximal load-bearing shift with increased knee flexion.[38] This allows for early muscle strengthening even while joint effusion may still be causing pain in a closed-chain (joint loaded) position. **When effusion and pain have been eliminated for 7 to 14 days, a gradual increase in activity may begin, with cryotherapy being used after activity.** During LE rehabilitation, after the patient can stand or load the joint, the emphasis should be on closed-chain activity because of its relevance to function. The goal is to advance the patient toward functional activities and then slowly introduce a patient-specific exercise program. Specific closed-chain exercises allow for the selection and stimulation of the appropriate muscles at the proper time.[26] These factors, combined with gradual muscle inhibition of the antagonist, produce smooth, coordinated loading of the entire LE.

Although McConnell patellofemoral taping is the modality of choice used by the authors of this chapter to bolster stability at the onset of exercise, a variety of braces may be beneficial in supporting the patellofemoral joint after surgery. Almost any elastic, compressive support around the patellofemoral joint produces an improved ability to exercise. The concept of proprioceptive feedback, together with comfort and affordability, makes post-operative McConnell patellofemoral taping or nonspecific bracing of the knee desirable in patients who do not respond to exercise alone.

> **Q** Diane is 33 years old. She has a history of anterior knee pain for 2 years. Before having ALRR, she used orthotics because she overpronated during gait. She had surgery 6 weeks ago. Complaints of pain are minimal to nonexistent if she avoids all aggravating factors. However, she generally has some soreness from activities of daily living (ADLs) around the home and from taking care of two young children. Diane is performing all the exercises mentioned in phase I and most exercises in phase II without pain. However, she has pain during functional double-leg squats with knee flexion exceeding 60 degrees and knee pain with step-downs from a 4-inch step. What may help Diane progress with her exercise program?

Phase III (Advanced Phase)

TIME: 5 to 6 weeks after surgery
GOALS: Patient self-manages edema and pain, performs gait without deviations, and has unlimited ambulation (Table 18-3)

By phase III patients should have their pain under control using little if any external support (brace or tape). They may continue to benefit from stretching, patella mobilization, and taping in addition to ice after exercise. However, this phase is designed to take the patient back to the preinjury level of function. Exercises are progressed through specificity of training principles. By breaking

Table 18-3 Lateral Retinaculum Release

Rehabilitation Phase	Criteria to Progress to this Phase	Anticipated Impairments and Functional Limitations	Intervention	Goal	Rationale
Phase III Postoperative 4-6 weeks	◆ Pain-free during functional activity (sit-stand, squat 0-90 degrees) ◆ Limited tolerance to walking, running, and standing	◆ Limited endurance with prolonged functional activities ◆ Mild instability of patellofemoral joint during skill-specific exercises ◆ Continued reliance on patellofemoral taping	◆ Closed-chain and stretching exercises as listed in Tables 18-1 and 18-2 ◆ Patella taping ◆ Patella mobilization ◆ Lunges with weights, increased repetitions and speed with exercises ◆ PREs on leg press ◆ Functional specific activity isokinetic training ◆ Knee flexion and extension 270-300 degrees/sec, 10 repetitions at each speed is one set (2-10 sets) ◆ Home exercises	◆ No gait deviations ◆ Good patella stability without taping ◆ Unlimited community ambulation ◆ Leg press body weight ◆ Pain-free with specific activity ◆ Increase strength and velocity of muscle contraction ◆ Patient can self-manage symptoms	◆ Functional strengthening ◆ Decrease pain with functional activities ◆ Improve joint mechanics ◆ Improve joint mobility and stability ◆ Improve endurance of VMO ◆ Increase strength ◆ Specificity of training and progression to community-based gym program (if appropriate) ◆ Use isokinetic principles of strength training ◆ Discharge patient

PREs, Progressive resistance exercises; *VMO,* vastus medalis oblique.

down the activity into its core components, the PT can assess patellofemoral and LE function for any deviations or barriers to performance.

Again, any exercise that increases knee pain and/or swelling needs to be modified or discontinued. After further progress has been gained, the therapist can reassess the patient and attempt the exercise again.

Closed kinetic chain progression consists of the following:

1. Lunges with 5 lb weights in a long-stride position (Fig. 18-6)—Patients must activate the quadriceps and hold the contraction from 0 to 30 degrees eccentrically and back to 0 degrees concentrically without stopping, while moving slowly and maintaining proper alignment.
2. Wall slides at various degrees of flexion with 1-minute holds to promote fatigue (Fig. 18-7)—The patient should progress from 0 to 45 degrees; if a certain angle in the arc of motion appears weaker, then the patient can perform isometric holds at the angle of weakness.
3. Functional single-limb squats from 0 to 30 degrees—Deep flexion squats can be performed by two different methods. In the first, both LEs are aligned directly below the hips, and bilateral knee flexion is initiated. The patient should maintain proper patella alignment directly over the midfoot. The second method is a shortened stride position with the involved LE forward. The patient initiates the squat until the knee is flexed 90 degrees and then rises back to full extension.
4. Functional double-limb squats with elastic tubing
5. Sit-to-stand at increased speed and repetition—The patient initiates sit-to-stand activity (and stand-to-sit activity) without upper extremity (UE) assistance. This exercise can be adjusted from easier to more difficult by lowering the height of the chair.
6. Step-down exercises with an increase in height of step and speed of movement—Proper alignment is crucial, along with slow, controlled movement. The patient must activate the quadriceps before motion is initiated and hold the contraction until heel contact of the opposite leg (Fig. 18-8).
7. Resistive leg press using progressive resistance exercise (PRE) protocols for weight[11,48]
8. Standing (four-wall) elastic tubing exercises for hip flexion, extension, abduction, and adduction (the involved knee acts as the stabilizing leg)—The LE that anchors the body is the "working" leg. The patient should activate the quadriceps and hold throughout the entire active motion of the opposite leg. This may be performed in terminal extension or 10 to 20 degrees of knee flexion of the involved (stabilizing) leg.

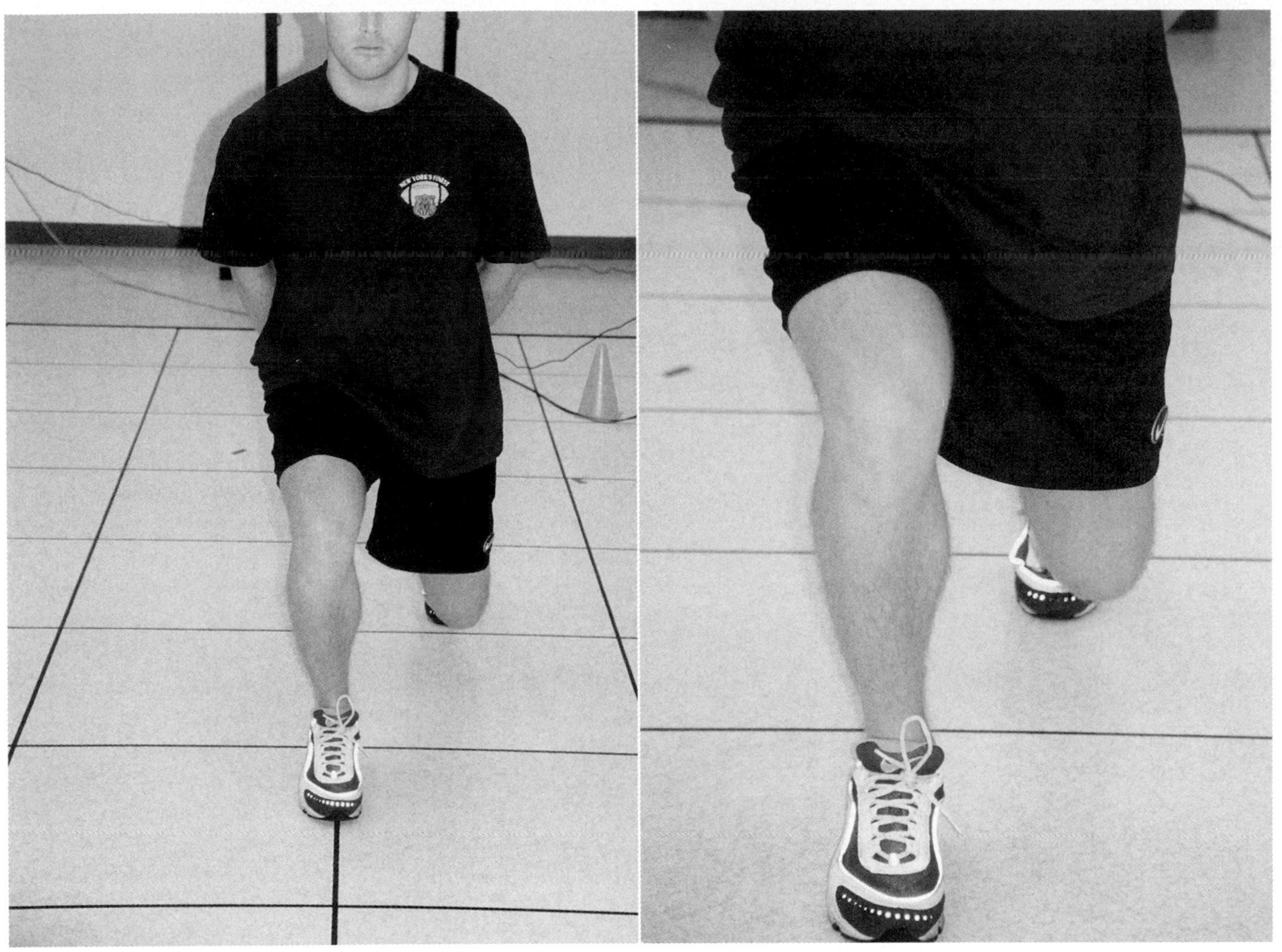

A B

Fig. 18-6 Closed-chain lunge. Instruct the patient to take a "normal" step forward. Have the patient slowly flex the knee to 30-degrees flexion, hold for 3 seconds, and return to 0-degree extension while maintaining proper postural alignment (i.e., anterosuperior iliac spine [ASIS] over midpatella and second toe). The patient should be able to activate the quadriceps tonically (constantly) during the entire motion.

Activity-specific exercises (Fig. 18-9) may include the following: stationary cycle, stair-climbing machine, slide board, and treadmill. The authors of this chapter recommend a 6-week progression to presurgery activity level. Isokinetic exercise is introduced in this phase at a training velocity spectrum protocol between 270 and 300 degree/seconds.[9] The patient performs 10 repetitions at each speed in a ladder progression (50 repetitions equal one set). Patient tolerance for exercise determines the number of sets performed (2 to 10 sets).

After patients can perform the exercises with good control of the patellofemoral joint, they are weaned from formal physical therapy and encouraged to continue their home exercise program as appropriate.

Once you have arrived at the decision to move the patient into a home program, it is important to understand how variable the long-term results can be following this procedure. Recent studies describe favorable results (73% to 86%) after 1 year.[34] This same study indicates that the results are far less favorable (29% to 30%) if the follow-up period is extended to 4 or 5 years. Questions exist concerning the appropriateness of an isolated lateral release procedure improving the biomechanical symptoms it is designed to address.[13] This evidence underscores the importance in identifying muscle strength and muscle length imbalances in the entire lower limb. Any abnormal LE alignment needs to be addressed in advance of discharge to a self-guided program.

A Diane was evaluated for patellofemoral symptoms and treated with the McConnell method of taping. She was able to progress with the closed-chain exercises when the appropriate McConnell taping procedure was used. She was able to perform double-limb squats to 80 degrees of knee flexion without pain. She also could perform two sets of 10 repetitions of step-downs on the 4-inch step without pain. Pain with the single-limb squat persisted but lessened. Therefore single-limb squats were not performed until they could be done without pain.

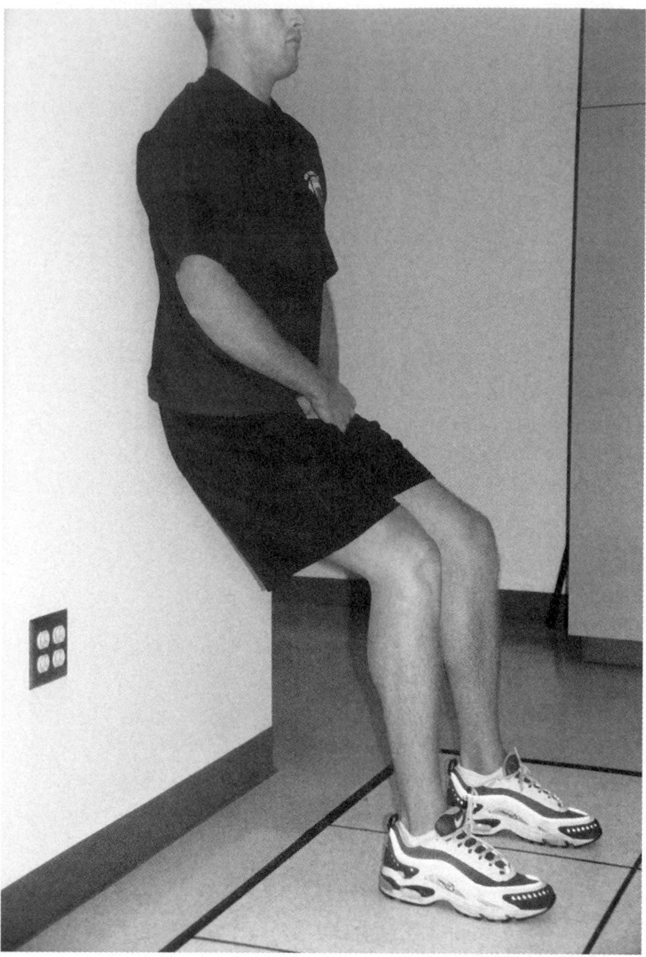

Fig. 18-7 Closed-chain wall slide. This exercise allows the patient to maintain better alignment simply by locking in pelvic tilt. The patient can then move through a particular range of motion (ROM) or the physical therapist (PT) can have the patient perform isometric contractions at various ranges of weakness.

Q Kathy is a 17-year-old soccer player that underwent ALRR because of chronic anterior knee pain. What should be the main focus of her postoperative rehabilitation?

TROUBLESHOOTING

Postural Alignment

A lateral retinacular release procedure produces immediate effects on the patella orientation of the knee, yet the entire lower kinetic chain may still have alignment issues that need to be addressed. When assessing a patient's functional status, the PT should consider equalizing leg lengths, balancing foot posture, restoring normal gait, and regaining appropriate muscle flexibility and strength, which will lead to a restoration of normal posture and balance.[15] By observing static alignment issues, PTs can gather valuable information regarding the way the patient will function dynamically. The interaction of poor alignment measures and quadriceps contraction has been examined.[18] This study compared static and dynamic patellofemoral malalignment measures in subjects with anterior knee pain. Quadriceps contraction altered the malalignment in both type and severity in more than 50% of the cases.

The literature suggests that excessive pronation at the foot is a primary problem because of its association with patellofemoral pain, which inhibits the balance of the entire lower kinetic chain.[43] Increased pronation may lead to increased valgus, compensatory external rotation (ER) of the foot and tibia, and a resultant predisposition to lateral patella tracking with dynamic activity.[19] In such cases, orthotic correction may be indicated even after a

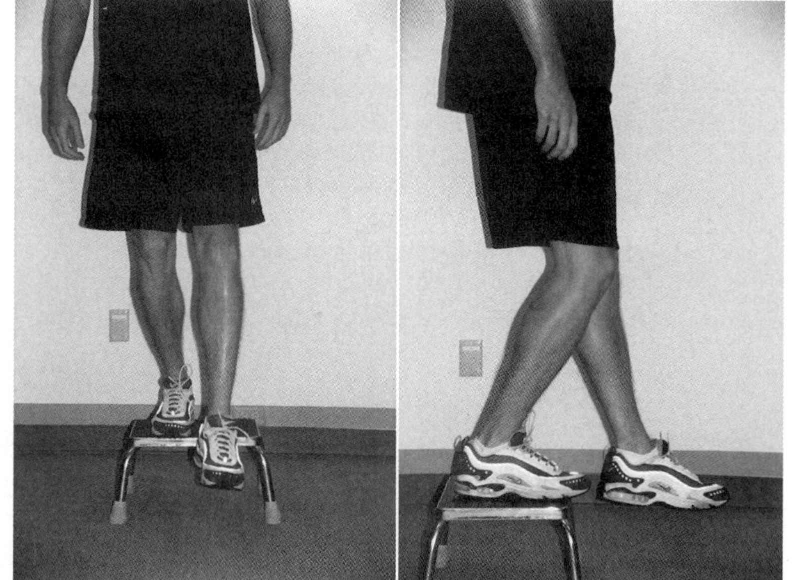

Fig. 18-8 Closed-chain step-down. Patients need to begin on a low-level step (3 to 4 inches) and work up to a standard step (8 inches). Patients must focus on improved alignment. Because the patient is now performing single-limb support activity, he or she should focus on gluteal muscle activation to better stabilize the femur during dynamic activity.

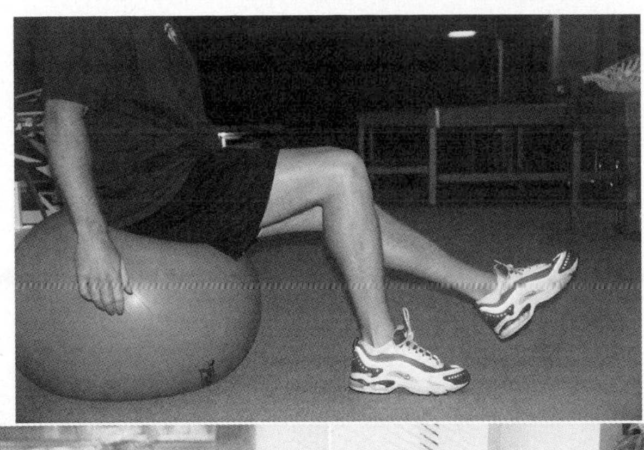

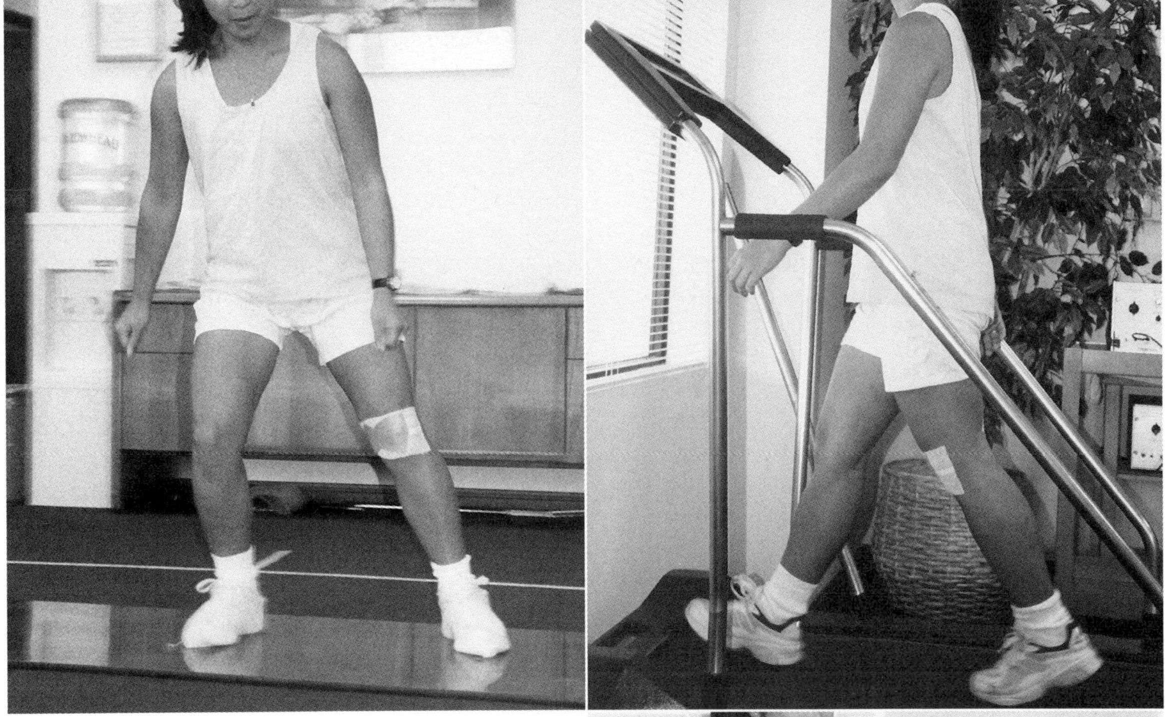

D

Fig. 18-9 Skill-specific training. After the patient is without pain and has developed a quality contraction that is consistent throughout full knee range of motion (ROM), a sport- or activity-specific exercise program is needed to aid in the development of an improved loading pattern and promote coordinated balance in patellofemoral mechanics.

lateral retinacular release procedure to restore proper loading mechanics through the knee.

A Given the chronicity of her symptoms, the therapist should evaluate LE mechanics during gait and with dynamic activities when appropriate. The clinician should focus initially on hip strength and ankle mechanics (pronation dysfunction). Hip weakness can cause a valgus position of the knee, creating increased patellofemoral stress. The hip external rotators and abductors (especially the gluteus medius) are a major component in positioning the knee in proper alignment. Ankle mechanics should also be fully explored and orthotics initiated if appropriate.

Quadriceps Inhibition

Many clinicians tend to use the term *quadriceps inhibition* as though it were synonymous with *quadriceps weakness,* which is not an accurate description. *Reflex quadriceps inhibition* is defined as the inability to perform a quadriceps contraction voluntarily because of direct neurologic suppression.[20,32]

Does true quadriceps inhibition exist? Numerous research articles on the subject describe several mechanisms that could produce a neurogenic influence on voluntary control of the quadriceps.[5,31] The effect of pain on the overall activation of the quadriceps has been examined as a possible cause.[3,46] Effusion also can impair activation of the quadriceps muscle.[10,41] Mechanic receptors within the patellofemoral joint may influence quadriceps function through proprioceptive input.[21,22] Other factors may include training methods, joint position, aging, and even the possible effects of medication.

Any problem resulting in decreased activation of the quadriceps is detrimental to the rehabilitation process. With full activation of the quadriceps femoris muscle, proper strengthening exercises should produce excellent results. However, if voluntary control is absent or compromised, then atrophy and weakness may result. If this situation persists, then volitional exercise protocols may be ineffective and thus temporarily inappropriate for these patients.

Because of the nature of a lateral retinacular release procedure, pain and especially effusion are quite common after surgery. Therefore any treatment techniques that address pain and swelling will ultimately assist in improved recruitment of the quadriceps femoris muscle.

Patellofemoral Tape-Weaning Protocol

Patients using McConnell taping need to learn how to tape themselves. The tape loosens according to the aggressiveness of the patient's activity. The patient should therefore be taught to tighten the tape when necessary.

The patient only needs to wear tape while training the quadriceps to maintain the newly acquired length in the lateral structures. The tape should be removed at night and the skin should be cleaned. This gives the skin a resting period from the pull and friction produced by the tape.

The patient begins closed-chain exercises when pain and effusion are under control. Early home exercises stress "little bits often," meaning multiple VMO sets or quadriceps contractions are performed throughout the day and are linked with a patient's lifestyle. For example, the PT may instruct a patient to perform a quadriceps contraction every time he or she sits down in a chair, palpating the VMO for feedback. When driving a car the patient may perform a quadriceps set at every stoplight, taking care to leave the foot firmly on the brake. As the patient begins to recruit a quality quadriceps contraction successfully, goal setting enters into the program and the patient is asked to attempt repetitions of closed-chain exercises (i.e., lunges, wall slides, squats, step-downs). The more the patient practices, the faster the skill to activate a quality quadriceps muscle contraction is learned.

The patient is ready to be weaned off the taping protocol and continue the program with specific sports-related activity and training when he or she can do the following:

1. Sustain a quarter squat for 1 minute against the wall without pain.
2. Sustain a half squat for 1 minute against the wall without pain.
3. Perform 10 step-downs (off an 8-inch step) for at least 5 seconds per step with good control and alignment and without pain.

If functional activity produces pain and the patient is using patella taping, the PT should first assess the taping procedure to ensure it is correct. The clinician may need to make small adjustments in tension and direction. At the time of discharge from the clinical facility, the patient needs to remember how to self-mobilize the patella, as well as proper alignment and postural issues with closed-chain exercises; the patient should be reminded that exercise should be painless.

SUGGESTED HOME MAINTENANCE FOR THE POSTSURGICAL PATIENT

Weeks 1-2

GOALS FOR THE PERIOD: Decrease pain, manage edema, increase weight-bearing activities, facilitate quality quadriceps contraction

1. Elevate and ice at home two to three times per day (preferably after exercises).
2. Perform ankle pumping and hamstring stretch while elevated on ice (20 to 30 minutes).
3. Perform gentle patella self-mobilizations (Fig. 18-10).
4. Perform active heel slides: one set of 10 repetitions performed three to four times per day.
5. Perform quadriceps sets: two sets of 10 repetitions performed three to four times per day. The physical therapist (PT) should always remember that even though general protocols such as this one may prescribe a number of sets and repetitions, if the patient fatigues and cannot continue to recruit a quality quadriceps contraction, then the exercise is over. Patients are only to count repetitions with quality quadriceps contractions. Quadriceps sets are performed in the sitting or long-sitting position with the knee positioned at 20- to 30-degrees flexion. The heel stays on the floor. Quadriceps sets also may be performed standing if patient finds it is easier to activate the quadriceps in this position. The key to early strengthening is to find which position gives the patient the most success in recruiting a quality quadriceps contraction.

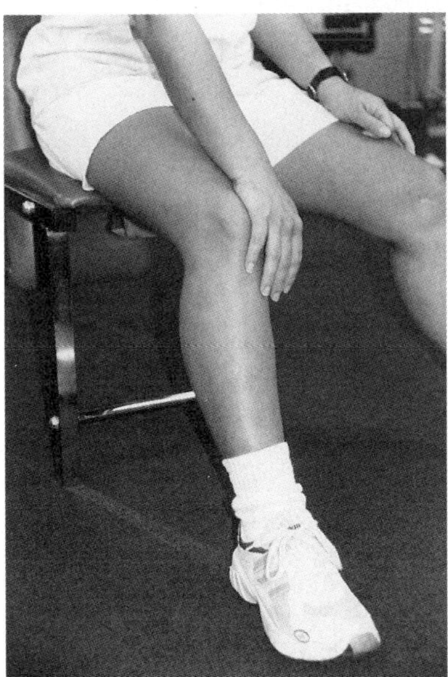

Fig. 18-10 Self-mobilization. The patient should be able to perform active self-stretching to the lateral retinacular tissues. The patient is instructed to place the heel of the hand over the medial half of the patella and push the medial border of the patella down into the trochlear groove. If the exercise is done properly, then the lateral border tilts anteriorly, stretching the lateral retinacular tissue. The knee should be placed in at least 30 degrees of flexion to ensure stability in the trochlear groove and guard against lateral gliding of the patella. The patient progresses into deeper ranges of flexion as pain and lateral tissue tension subside. Each stretch should be held for 5 seconds for two to three repetitions, three to four times a day.

Weeks 3-4

GOALS FOR THE PERIOD: Continue to manage edema and pain, improve sit-stand transfer activities, improve strength and stability of the patellofemoral joint, progress functional training to return activity to previous levels

1. Perform the same exercises as in weeks 1 to 2, but increase the number of repetitions. Generally the patient should perform two sets of 10 to 20 repetitions per day (more or less depending on fatigue).
2. Perform closed-chain exercises (see Figs. 18-6 to 18-9) at home depending on quadriceps and lower extremity (LE) control.
3. Perform self-taping as deemed appropriate by the therapist. Taping should be tailored to the activity.
4. Continue using ice after exercises.

Weeks 5-6

GOALS FOR THE PERIOD: Patient self-manages edema and pain, performs gait without deviations, and has unlimited ambulation

1. Depending on remaining deficits, exercises from weeks 1 to 4 are continued. The need for taping should be minimal; however, if continued taping is required, then patients should be instructed in self-taping techniques.
2. Patient should gradually return to functional activities, with both patient and therapist monitoring for pain and joint effusion.

References

1. Aglietti P et al: Arthroscopic lateral release for patellar pain or instability, *Arthroscopy* 5:176, 1989.
2. Armato DP, Czamecki D: Geniculate artery pseudoaneurysm: a rare complication of arthroscopic surgery, *ATR Am J Roentgenol* 155(3):659, 1990.
3. Arvidsson I et al: Reduction of pain inhibition on voluntary muscle activation by epidural analgesia, *Orthopedics* 9:1415, 1986.
4. Callaghan MJ et al: The effects of patellar taping on knee joint proprioception, *J Athl Train* 37(1):19-24, 2002.
5. Chaix Y et al: Further evidence for non-monosynoptic group I excitation of motoneurons in the human lower limb, *Exp Brain Res* 115(1):35, 1997.
6. Christou EA: Patellar taping increases vastus medialis oblique activity in the presence of patellofemoral pain, *J Electromyogr Kinesiol* 14(4):495-504, 2004.
7. Currier DP, Lehmon J, Lightfoot P: Electrical stimulation in exercise of the quadriceps femoris muscle, *Phys Ther* 59(12):1508, 1979.
8. Currier DP, Petrilli CR, Threlkeld AJ: Effect of graded electrical stimulation on blood flow to healthy muscle, *Phys Ther* 66(6):937, 1986.
9. Davies GJ: *A compendium of isokinetics in clinical usage and rehabilitation techniques,* ed 2, 1984, S&S Publishers.
10. DeAndrade JR, Grant C, Dixon ASJ: Joint distension and reflex muscle inhibition in the knee, *J Bone Joint Surg* 47A:313, 1965.
11. DeLorme TL: Restoration of muscle power by heavy resistance exercise, *J Bone Joint Surg* 27:645, 1945.
12. Ficat P, Hungerford D: *Disorders of the patellofemoral joint,* Baltimore, 1977, Williams and Wilkins.
13. Fithian DC et al: International Patellofemoral Study Group. Lateral retinacular release: a survey of the International Patellofemoral Study Group, *Arthroscopy* 20(5):463-468, 2004.
14. Fu F, Maday M: Arthroscopic lateral release and the patellar compression syndrome, *Orthop Clin North Am* 23:601, 1992.
15. Fulkerson JP: *Disorders of the patellofemoral joint,* ed 3, Baltimore, 1997, Williams and Wilkins.
16. Fulkerson J et al: Histological evidence of retinacular nerve injury associated with patellofemoral malalignment, *Clin Orthop* 197:196, 1985.
17. Gould N et al: Transcutaneous muscle stimulation to retard disuse atrophy after open meniscectomy, *Clin Orthop* 178:190, 1983.
18. Guzzanti V et al: Patellofemoral malalignment in adolescents: computerized tomographic assessment with or without quadriceps contraction, *Am J Sports Med* 22(1):55, 1994.
19. Heckman TP: Conservative vs. postsurgical patellar rehabilitation. In Margine R, editor: *Physical therapy of the knee,* New York, 1988, Churchill Livingstone.
20. Hensyl WR: *Steadman's pocket medical dictionary,* Baltimore, 1987, Williams and Wilkins.
21. Hurley MV et al: Rehabilitation of the quadriceps inhibited due to isolated rupture of the anterior cruciate ligament, *J Ortho Rheum* 5:145, 1992.
22. Johansson J: Role of knee ligaments in proprioception and regulation of muscle stiffness, *Electromyography* 1:158, 1991.
23. Krivickes LS: Anatomical factors associated with overuse sports injuries, *Sports Med* 24(2):132, 1997.
24. Kues JM, Mayhew TP: Concentric and eccentric force-velocity relationships during electrically induced submaximal contractions, *Physiother Res Int* 1(3):195, 1996.
25. Lehmann JF et al: Effect of therapeutic temperatures on tendon extensibility, *Arth Phys Med Rehabil* 51:481, 1970.
26. Lui HI, Corrier DP, Threlkeld AJ: Circulatory response of digital arteries associated with electrical stimulation of calf muscles in healthy subjects, *Phys Ther* 67(3):340, 1987.
27. Lutz GE et al: Rehabilitative techniques for athletes after reconstruction of the anterior cruciate ligament, *Mayo Clin Proc* 65(10):1322, 1990.
28. Macgregor K et al: Cutaneous stimulation from patella tape causes a differential increase in vasti muscle activity in people with patellofemoral pain, *J Orthop Res* 23(2): 351-358, 2005.
29. Maitland GD: *Peripheral manipulation,* ed 5, Newton, MA, 1986, Butterworth-Heinemann.
30. McConnell: Patellofemoral Program course notes, 1997.
31. McMiken DF, Todd-Smith M, Thompson C: Strengthening of human quadriceps muscles by cutaneous electrical stimulation, *Scand J Rehab Med* 15(1):25, 1983.
32. Meunier S, Pierrot-Deseilligny E, Simonetta-Moreau M: Pattern of heteronymous recurrent inhibition in the human lower limb, *Exp Brain Res* 102(1):149, 1994.
33. Morrissey MC: Reflex inhibition of thigh muscles in knee injury. Cases and treatment, *Sports Med* 7:263, 1989.
34. Panni AS et al: Long-term results of lateral retinacular release, *Arthroscopy* 21(5):526-531, 2005.
35. Randall, Iming, Hines: Effect of electronic stimulation flow and temperature of skeletal muscle, *Am J Phys Med* 1953.
36. Richardson C: *The role of the knee musculature in high speed oscillative movements of the knee.* Proceedings of the MTAA 4th Biennial Conference, Brisbane, Australia, 1985, p 59.
37. Shelton GL: Conservative management of patellofemoral dysfunction, *Prim Care* 19(2):331, 1992.
38. Sherman OH et al: Patellar instability: treatment by arthroscopic electrosurgical lateral release, *Arthroscopy* 3:152, 1987.
39. Singerman R, Berilla J, Davy DT: Direct in vitro determination of the patellofemoral contact force for normal knees, *J Biomech Eng* 117:8, 1995.
40. Small NC: An analysis of complications in lateral retinacular release procedures, *Arthroscopy* 5:282, 1989.
41. Soo CL, Currier DP, Threlkeld AJ: Augmenting voluntary torque of healthy muscle by optimization of electrical stimulation, *Phys Ther* 68(3):333, 1988.
42. Spencer JDC, Hayes KC, Alexander IJ: Knee joint effusion and quadriceps reflex inhibition in man, *Arch Phys Med Rehabil* 65:171, 1984.
43. Steine HA et al: A comparison of closed kinetic chain and isokinetic joint isolation exercise in patients with patello-femoral dysfunction, *J Orthop Sports Phys Ther* 24(3):136, 1996.

44. Tiberio D: The effect of excessive subtalar joint pronation on patellofemoral mechanics: a theoretical model, *J Orthop Sports Phys Ther* 9:160, 1987.
45. Vuorinen OP et al: Chondromalacia patellae: results of operative treatment, *Arch Orthop Trauma Surg* 104(3):175, 1985.
46. Werner S, Knutsson E, Ericksson E: Effect of taping the patella and concentric and eccentric torque and EMG of knee extensor and flexor muscles in patients with patello-femoral pain syndrome, *Knee Surg Sports Traumatol Arthrosc* 1(3-4):169, 1993.
47. Whittingham M, Palmer S, Macmillan F: Effects of taping on pain and function in patellofemoral pain syndrome: a randomized controlled trial, *J Orthop Sports Phys Ther* 34(9):504-510, 2004.
48. Wild JJ, Franklin TD, Woods GW: Patellar pain and quadriceps rehabilitation: an EMG study, *Am J Sports Med* 10:12, 1982.
49. Zinovieff AN: Heavy resistance exercises: the Oxford techniques, *Br J Phys Med* 14:29, 1951.

CHAPTER 19

Meniscectomy and Meniscal Repair

Terry Gillette
Andrew A. Brooks

Although meniscal repair was introduced more than 100 years ago,[1] only within the past 10 to 20 years has the meniscus successfully outlived its characterization as a "functionless remains of leg muscle."[25] Only a few years ago it was standard practice to excise the meniscus with impunity because of the perception that it played little role in the function of the knee. Fairbanks[11] called attention to the frequency of degenerative changes after removal of the meniscus and stimulated a new era of research into the anatomy and function of this poorly understood structure. Researchers eagerly investigated the role of the meniscus in load transmission and joint nutrition, and soon the pendulum of orthopedic popular opinion swung in the direction of determining new ways to preserve the injured meniscus.

With the advent of arthroscopic surgery, partial meniscectomy rapidly supplanted total meniscectomy, and research continued to determine the healing capacity of the torn meniscus. From these efforts, meniscal repair has evolved as a successful technique. Ultimately, recognition of the intact meniscus as a crucial factor in normal knee function has led to widespread acceptance of preservation of torn menisci through partial meniscectomy or repair.

SURGICAL INDICATIONS AND CONSIDERATIONS

When assessing the suitability of a meniscal tear for repair, the surgeon must consider several factors: patient age; chronicity of the injury; type, location, and length of the tears (the blood supply of the meniscus exists primarily at the peripheral 10% to 25%); and associated ligamentous injuries.[2] The perfect candidate for a meniscal repair is a young individual with an acute longitudinal peripheral tear of the meniscus that is 1 to 2 cm long, to be repaired in conjunction with an anterior cruciate ligament (ACL) reconstruction. Success rates for meniscal repairs in conjunction with ACL reconstruction has been as high as 90% compared with 75% for isolated meniscus repairs.[26] It appears that the medial meniscus is more suitable for repair than the lateral meniscus. Shelbourne and Dersam[33] performed a repair or partially excised lateral meniscus tears. The surgery was performed in conjunction with ACL reconstruction and the repair was performed using an inside-outside technique. They noted that although no significant statistical difference existed between the two groups (International Knee Documentation Committee [IKDC] grade), the partial meniscectomy group had more pain.[33] Shelbourne and Heinrich[34] also noted that certain types of lateral meniscus tears could be successfully treated with abrasion and trephination or just left in situ.[34] Noyes and Barber-Westin[26,27] studied two different age groups and their response to meniscus repair. They used an inside-outside technique with a majority of the patients undergoing concomitant ACL reconstruction. In looking at the outcomes, 87% of the older (over 40 years old) group, and 75% of the younger (under 20 years old) group were asymptomatic for medial compartment symptoms. They also noted significant improvement in outcomes when the repair was done in conjunction with an ACL reconstruction. Age may not be as significant a factor as the type of tear (degenerative or nondegenerative).[32] The current trend appears to lean toward the preservation of the meniscus whenever possible based on the patient's current and future activity levels. More research is being performed looking at the long-term results and categorizing further the indications for meniscus repair.[20] Outside of these parameters, little consensus exists regarding the relative indications for meniscal repair.

The arthroscopic surgeon should be prepared to perform meniscal repair at the time of any knee arthroscopy. The identification of reparable menisci is usually not possible preoperatively, but often magnetic resonance imaging (MRI) can help demonstrate the location of tears.

Four techniques for repair currently exist:

1. Open meniscal repair
2. Arthroscopic inside-out repair

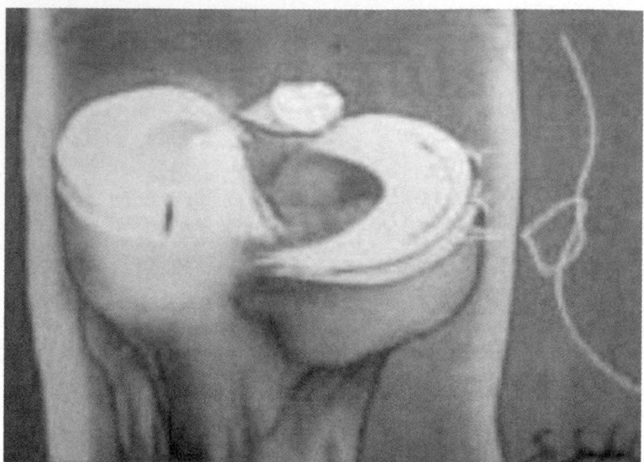

Fig. 19-1 Illustration of meniscus repair.

3. Arthroscopic outside-in repair
4. All-inside arthroscopic repair

Each of these techniques has advantages and disadvantages; application of individual techniques is largely a matter of individual preference.

SURGICAL PROCEDURE

Open Meniscal Repair

Open meniscal repair (Fig. 19-1) is the oldest technique of meniscal repair and has been popularized by Dr. Ken DeHaven.[6] It has a good record of success, even at 1-year follow-up.[8] Open meniscal repairs are best suited for extremely peripheral tears. DeHaven still advocates routine arthroscopic evaluation before considering open repair. The arthroscope is removed from the joint and the knee is prepared. After exposing the capsule through a longitudinal incision, the surgeon prepares the meniscal rim and capsular attachment and places vertically oriented sutures at 3 to 4 mm intervals. The incision is closed in a layered fashion. Long-term follow-up has shown success rates of 70% to 79%.[7,29,30]

Inside-Out Meniscal Repair

The inside-out meniscal repair technique was popularized by Henning[13] in the early 1980s and is the most popular technique for meniscus repair. The surgeon uses long, thin cannulas to allow placement of vertical or horizontal sutures. After identifying the tear arthroscopically, he or she prepares the tear by using a meniscal rasp to create a better biologic environment for healing. A small posterior incision is carried down to the capsule, and sutures are placed arthroscopically using specially designed long Keith needles to pass the suture. The assistant protects the popliteal structures with a retractor while grasping the suture needles. After placing all sutures, the surgeon ties them over the capsule. Success rates have been noted to be 75% to 88%.[30,36]

Outside-In Meniscal Repair

The outside-in meniscal repair technique allows suture placement using an 18-gauge spinal needle placed across the tear from outside the joint to inside. Absorbable polydioxanone suture[14] is passed through the needle into the joint; it is secured with a mulberry knot tied to the end of the sutures. These sutures are tied to adjacent sutures at the end of the procedure over the joint capsule; separate small incisions are made for each pair of sutures. Morgan and colleagues[24] noted an 84% success rate and found the primary reason for failure was an associated ACL deficiency.

All-Inside Meniscal Repair

All-inside meniscal repair allows the meniscus to be repaired without any additional incisions outside the knee. This is truly an all-arthroscopic technique. It is popular because it avoids additional incisions and therefore diminishes neurovascular risk and decreases operative time.[30] Success rates have been noted as high as 90%.[12,30]

All-inside meniscal repair can be accomplished with either suture or biodegradable "darts."[23] The suture technique is accomplished using a specially designed cannulated suture hook to pass suture through both sides of the tear. The sutures are then tied arthroscopically using a knot pusher.

The biodegradable darts are passed across the tear using specially designed cannulas. After preparing the torn meniscal surface, the surgeon reduces the tear and holds it in place with a cannula. A thin cutting instrument is used to make a pathway across the meniscal tear, and the biodegradable dart is passed through the same cannula, fixing the tear. The darts generally completely resorb by 8 to 12 weeks.

THERAPY GUIDELINES FOR REHABILITATION

Limited research is available regarding physical therapy protocols after meniscus repair and long-term outcomes. Clinic protocols vary with the degree of weight bearing, duration of immobilization, control of range of motion (ROM), and return to sports or work. Recent studies have shown the success rates after accelerated rehabilitation programs to be similar to those in conservative rehabilitation programs. These studies found no statistically significant difference in success and repair failure rates between groups using conservative or accelerated programs. The hallmarks of accelerated programs are early full weight-bearing tolerance, unrestricted ROM, and return to pivoting sports.[3,31,35]

An understanding of the clinical implications of knee and meniscus biomechanics helps guide the therapist through the rehabilitation process. Communication among all rehabilitation team members—the physician, therapist, patient, family, and coach—is crucial to a successful rehabilitation outcome. The rehabilitation program must be acceptable to the patient, with goals designed to meet the patient's needs.

Several crucial factors must be considered before initiating a rehabilitation program. These factors influence the speed and aggressiveness of the rehabilitation program. The size of the tear, repair stabilization technique, suture material, number of sutures, and location of the meniscal repair influence initial postoperative weight-bearing tolerance, ROM, and exercise restrictions. *Other factors to consider before initiating a rehabilitation program include degenerative pathology in the weight-bearing articulations or patellofemoral joint, previous patella dysfunction, and concomitant injuries and possible joint laxity (i.e., ACL deficiency or reconstruction, medial collateral ligament injury).* These injuries do not necessarily indicate a potentially unsatisfactory result. The rehabilitation protocol may require modifications to accommodate the effects of these pathologies. Barber and Click[3] evaluated the results of 65 meniscal repairs in patients who underwent an accelerated rehabilitation program. Successful meniscal healing occurred in 92% of patients with a concomitant ACL reconstruction, compared with 67% of patients with ACL-deficient knees and 67% of patients with meniscal pathology alone.

The meniscal repair rehabilitation protocol must be individually tailored to the patient's needs. The rehabilitation process can be broken down into three phases: initial, intermediate, and advanced. These phases may overlap and should be based on objective and functional findings rather than time.

The early phase of the rehabilitation program should emphasize decreasing postoperative inflammatory reaction, restoring controlled ROM, and encouraging early weight bearing as tolerated. Exercise intensity is increased in the later phases of rehabilitation. Closed kinetic chain exercises are progressed through a variety of positions, from simple linear movements to complex multidirectional motions. The final phase of treatment is directed toward return to normal activity (sport or work).

The length of rehabilitation varies among patients. Treatments may be equally distributed among each of the phases of rehabilitation if the number of patient visits must be managed. Fewer treatments are required in the initial phases of rehabilitation if swelling and pain are adequately controlled and ROM is progressing without complications.

Preoperative Care

Ideally the patient should be seen at a preoperative visit, which includes a brief clinical evaluation to record baseline physical data and identify potential latent biomechanical deficits. The evaluation format encompasses a subjective history as outlined in Maitland[18], and objective data are gathered primarily to record baseline measurements. The lower extremity (LE) is evaluated as a functional unit. Strength and ROM are recorded for the hip, knee, ankle, and foot. Foot mechanics also are evaluated and addressed as indicated. Reassessment continues postoperatively with each progression of weight bearing. Girth measurements also are taken about the knee. The remainder of the preoperative visit should include instruction in proper use of crutches, education regarding ROM (heel slides with a 30-second hold for 10 repetitions), instruction in antiembolic exercises (ankle pumps with a 30-second hold for 10 repetitions), and prescription of LE strengthening exercises in the form of isometrics (quadriceps sets, hamstring sets, and cocontraction of quadriceps and hamstrings; all three exercises should be held for 10 seconds for 10 to 20 repetitions) and active range of motion (AROM) of the hip (working the adductors, abductors, and external rotators for 10 to 20 repetitions). Cryotherapy and elevation (for 15 to 30 minutes) and compression wrapping should be reviewed for postoperative pain and swelling management. Depending on individual clinic and physician preference, the patient may be instructed in the use of electrical stimulation (ES). The patient should be instructed in activities of daily living (ADLs), such as bathing and dressing, as appropriate. The physician must clear any preoperative instruction pertaining to exercise and weight-bearing status postoperatively, based on the extent and nature of the surgical repair performed. Home exercises are to be performed three times a day until return for the initial postoperative physical therapy evaluation.

Phase I (Initial Phase)

TIME: 1 to 4 weeks after surgery
GOALS: Manage pain and swelling, increase ROM and strength, increase weight-bearing activities (Table 19-1)

The patient is typically seen for physical therapy 4 to 7 days after surgery. He or she may complain of mild to moderate pain, swelling, and decreased weight-bearing tolerance. The patient may or may not be using pain medication.

Objectively, the patient is nonweight bearing or partial weight bearing to tolerance with crutches for a period of 2 to 6 weeks. Minimal to moderate effusion may be evident. Based on physician preference, the patient may have a postoperative protective brace. Meniscal repairs in the "red zone" (meniscus area that has a blood supply)

Table 19-1 Meniscus Repair

Rehabilitation Phase	Criteria to Progress to this Phase	Anticipated Impairments and Functional Limitations	Intervention	Goal	Rationale
Phase I Postoperative 1-4 weeks	◆ Postoperative	◆ Mild to moderate pain ◆ Nonweight bearing to partial weight bearing to tolerance ◆ Decreased strength ◆ Minimal to moderate effusion ◆ Decreased ROM	◆ Cryotherapy, heat and ice contrast, ES ◆ PROM—Hamstring stretches, gastrocnemius-soleus stretches ◆ Wall slides or passive heel slides (see Fig. 19-2) ◆ Isometrics—Cocontraction quadriceps and hamstring (depending on the repair site), quadriceps sets, hip adductor sets, hamstring sets, resistive exercises ◆ Four-quad program, weight added distally as tolerated ◆ Elastic tubing exercises ◆ Gait training ◆ Low-resistance, moderate-speed stationary cycling ◆ Aquatic therapy; closed kinetic chain activities (initiate near end of phase) ◆ Leg press machine ◆ Partial squats ◆ Heel raises ◆ Standing terminal knee extension with tubing	◆ Manage pain and swelling ◆ Knee ROM 0-120 degrees ◆ Increased muscle strength and endurance ◆ Normalization of gait within healing and weight-bearing limitations	◆ Decrease pain and minimize swelling ◆ Prevent ROM complications ◆ Assist in restoration of joint mechanics ◆ Facilitate return of neuromuscular control ◆ Minimize disuse atrophy ◆ Strengthen knee musculature while protecting the repair site ◆ Increase muscle endurance ◆ Use the properties of water during exercise performance ◆ Functional strengthening

ES, Electrical stimulation; *PROM*, passive range of motion; *ROM*, range of motion.

and larger peripheral repairs may be braced 0 to 90 degrees for up to 14 days. "White zone" (meniscus area that lacks a blood supply) repairs may be braced at 20 to 70 degrees. Extension is increased to 0 degrees, and flexion is increased to 90 degrees after 7 to 10 days. ROM is typically limited within constraints of bracing. Strength of the quadriceps and hamstring may be limited.

On the first visit a comprehensive evaluation is performed, with the physical therapist collecting the new objective data and reviewing and updating the previous

Q Stephen is an active 42-year-old man. He wants to return to skiing as soon as possible. Stephen had a lateral meniscal repair for the posterior horn 2½ weeks ago. The therapist is having Stephen perform cocontraction isometrics of the quadriceps and hamstrings. Stephen wants to know why he cannot start using weights on the seated knee flexion machine (isotonics) for resisted hamstring strengthening. What should the therapist tell him?

subjective data.[18] Subjective data that need to be reviewed postoperatively include medication usage, sleep pattern, pain levels at rest and during activity, and aggravating and easing factors. In addition, the therapist should review the postoperative report that describes the extent and nature of the repair. Goals and rehabilitation expectations are established and reviewed with the patient during the initial visit.

The new and updated objective and clinical data should include visual examination, gait assessment, ROM measurement, strength assessment, palpation, and girth measurement (as described in the section on the preoperative initial visit). Visual observation should focus on areas of atrophy, in particular the vastus medialis oblique (VMO); healing status of incision sites; and swelling about the knee joint and distal LE. Depending on the patient's weight-bearing status or tolerance, gait assessment is either brief or detailed. The primary focus of the brief assessment is safety, correct mechanics, and weight bearing in patients with restricted tolerance. If the patient does not have weight-bearing restrictions and has good gait tolerance, then a more detailed assessment of gait can be made. Gait assessment should focus on proper mechanics and weight-bearing tolerance. The patient's ability to ambulate with normal mechanics throughout each phase of gait should be assessed. Remedial corrective actions are required to decrease potentially harmful loading onto healing structures. Typically patients require cueing to avoid hip external rotation (ER) during the stance phase, because this puts abnormal stresses through the knee, ankle, and foot. Crutches should be used throughout the initial phase of treatment until adequate strength, ROM, and normal gait mechanics are achieved. Static and dynamic foot function (as related to normal gait mechanics) continues to be assessed during this phase of rehabilitation. Dysfunctions must be addressed to decrease abnormal tensile or compressive force affecting healing of the meniscus repair.

Typically on initial evaluation, the patient exhibits a loss of extension of 5 to 10 degrees; flexion ROM is 70 to 90 degrees. The patient exhibits a guarded end feel with motion improving with repetition. Flexibility of the hip musculature, hamstring, and gastrocnemius-soleus complex should be assessed. Appropriate remedial flexibility exercises can be implemented as tolerated in this phase, with the patient avoiding forced knee flexion and rotation about the knee joint. Patients should perform slow static stretches, avoiding ballistic movements, to maintain control of the lower limb and minimize the chance of affecting the healing meniscus repair.[10,15]

The patellofemoral joint should be assessed, especially if the patient reports previous or present patella symptoms. Patella tracking and glides are part of this assessment. Joint mobilization or patellofemoral taping may be helpful in mitigating these symptoms[21] (see Figs. 18-1 to 18-3 and 18-10). All major muscle groups in the LE should be assessed bilaterally. In addition, visible observation and palpation of the VMO during a muscle contraction of the quadriceps indicates VMO function and potential patellofemoral complications. The remaining LE musculature should be assessed, with the therapist identifying any potential weakness that may alter normal closed kinetic biomechanics and therefore increase tensile or compressive forces across the meniscus repair site.

No standard method has been established for assessing girth about the knee joint. Consistency among the team members providing patient care is important when reassessing the patient's condition. Atrophy as measured by girth measurements is not diagnostic of weakness or atrophy in a specific muscle group. Circumference measurement assesses girth of all muscle and joint structures underlying the measurement area. Typical measurement sites for a bilateral comparison include the midpatella, 5 and 10 cm above the knee joint and 5 and 10 cm below the knee joint.

Treatment is initiated after the clinical evaluation is completed (see Table 19-1). Initial phase treatment goals are to decrease pain and manage swelling, restore ROM, increase muscle strength and endurance, and normalize gait within healing and weight-bearing limitations.

A Active knee flexion pulls the medial and lateral meniscus posterior. The lateral meniscus migrates 1 cm posterior, because the popliteus muscle pulls it during knee flexion. This activity places increased stress on the repaired and healing tissues.

Q Nancy underwent a meniscus repair (of a complex tear) 1 month ago. She has noted progressive episodes of clicking in her knee. Especially with sit to stand transitions. Her swelling has increased, and she has had increased difficulty with walking and standing. What course of action should be taken?

Modalities such as heat and ice contrast, ES, and cryotherapy can be used to decrease pain and swelling.[5,17,39]

Instructions in home use of cryotherapy, compression wrapping, and elevation as discussed in the section on preoperative management is initiated for postoperative pain and swelling. The importance of home cryotherapy cannot be overemphasized. The study of Lessard and colleagues[17] on the use of cryotherapy after meniscectomy found statistically significant differences between groups with and without postoperative cryotherapy. Patients reported decreased pain ratings per the McGill Pain Questionnaire, decreased medication consumption, improved exercise compliance, and improved weight-bearing status.

Restoration of ROM is important. The time parameter to achieve full ROM is longer than it is in partial arthroscopic meniscectomies. Although early restoration of ROM is important to normalize joint function, the healing process of the meniscus repair dictates caution, especially with full circumferential peripheral repairs. **Any exercises used to increase ROM should not be forced because of the risk of stressing healing repair sites.** Wall slides or passive heel slides (Fig. 19-2) may be used to increase knee flexion. ROM exercises are to be performed within pain tolerance, held at least 30 seconds, and repeated as tolerated (generally 5 to 10 times). As part of the home exercise program, ROM activity can be repeated two to three times per day.

A She was reinstructed in an edema management program (i.e., elevation, compression, ice). The physician was called and an MRI was ordered (which revealed that the repair had torn). Complex tears have a higher incidence of failures than simple tears.

Q John is a 44-year-old recreational tennis player who underwent repair of his medial meniscus 8 weeks ago. He has progressed rapidly through his exercise program without any significant obstacles. He notes a sudden onset of swelling in his knee, which he relates to performing yard work (i.e., raking leaves, squatting down). Although his knee is swollen, no crepitation or locking is seen. His mild pain symptoms appear localized to the medial joint line. What changes should be made in his program?

Hamstring and gastrocnemius-soleus flexibility exercises can be initiated to the patient's tolerance. Stretches should be held at least 30 seconds and repeated 5 to 10 times, three times a day. Stretches should be sustained and passive in nature, allowing the patient or therapist to control knee joint motions, avoiding potential complications from ballistic-type stretching.[40] The hamstring group can be stretched passively using a long-sit position (with legs straight out in front of the body). A towel can be used to assist with passive ankle dorsiflexion to intensify the stretch. The physical therapist should instruct the patient to maintain a "neutral spine" while performing the stretch (Fig. 19-3). The gastrocnemius-soleus can be stretched using a towel or strap in the early phases of rehabilitation. Progression to stretching of the hip musculature and quadriceps can be performed as the patient's increase in knee ROM dictates. The knee needs to be kept in a relative neutral position to avoid any rotational or compressive forces on the repaired meniscus site. Standing gastrocnemius-soleus stretching can be initiated as weight-bearing tolerance increases.

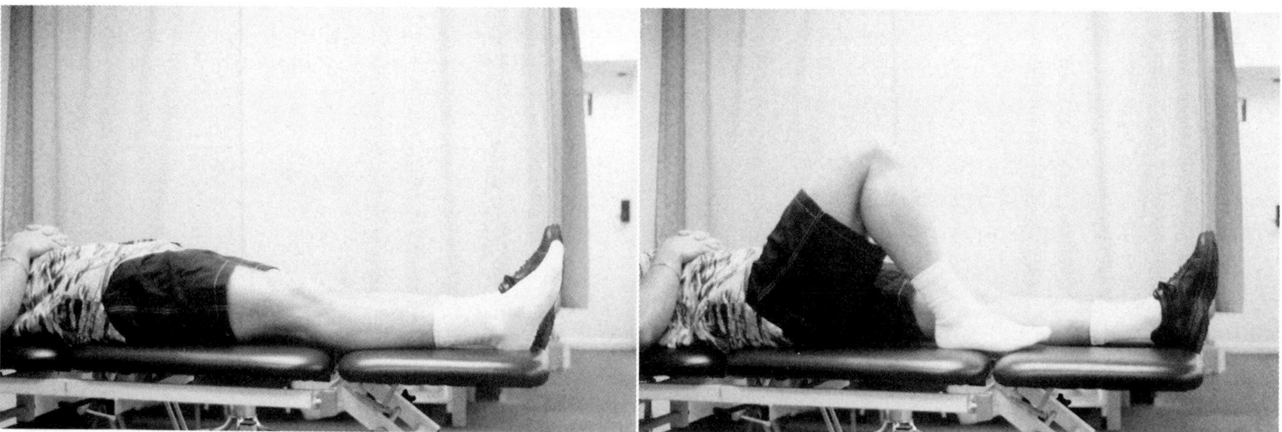

Fig. 19-2 Heel slides. While lying supine the patient slides the involved heel toward the buttock, maintaining the knee in a straight plane and avoiding any hip or tibial rotation.

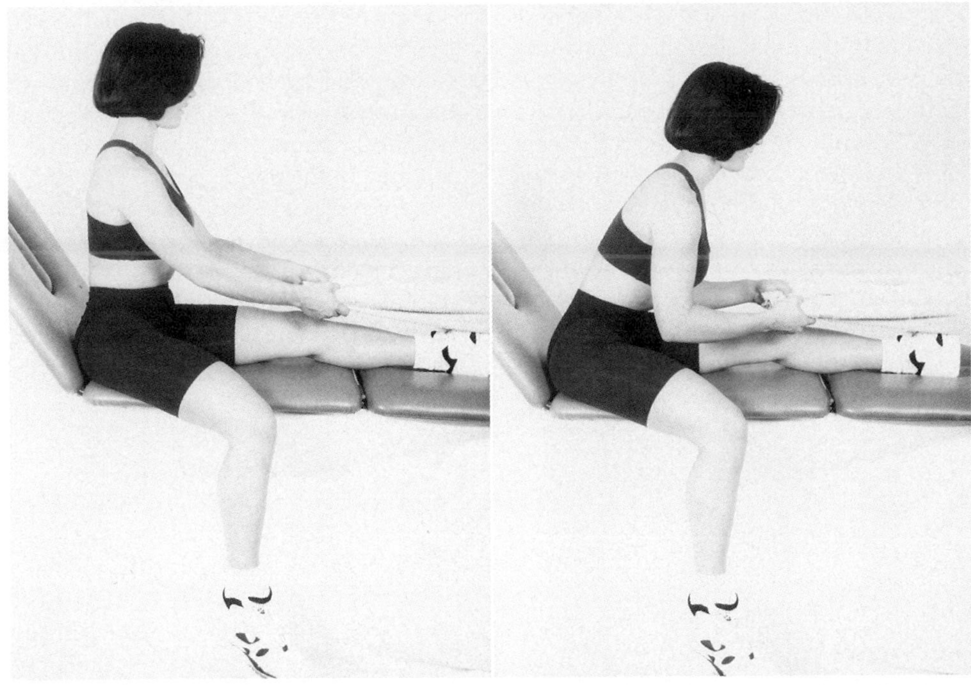

Fig. 19-3 Hamstring stretching. In a long-sit position, the patient leans forward from the hip, avoiding lumbar flexion.

The foot is kept in a neutral position to avoid any tibia rotation caused by supination or pronation, which may increase knee joint compression and tensile forces across the repaired meniscal site.

> **A** It appears that he aggravated his repair site with squatting and pivoting activities. This activity should be avoided until he can clinically demonstrate tolerance to this stress. Use of mini-squats or an inclined sled allows for the careful control of how much compression is delivered to the knee. Pivoting should be avoided for 6 months. John was cautioned about the risk of retearing his meniscus and his swelling was managed with relative rest, ES, ice, and elevation.

Initial strengthening is performed as tolerated in open-chain positions. Closed kinetic strengthening (as discussed in Chapter 17 and shown in Figs. 17-6 and 17-7) can be initiated, depending on the weight-bearing status and tolerance of the patient. All strengthening exercises should be closely monitored for potential adverse reactions and increased pain or swelling.

Strengthening exercises for all LE musculature are initiated with an emphasis on restoration of quadriceps muscle function to minimize potential patellofemoral dysfunction. Isometric exercises should be held for 10 seconds and performed for 10 to 20 repetitions. Quadriceps sets can be performed within the patient's tolerance. A small towel may be required under the posterior aspect of the knee if the patient lacks full extension or if muscle setting in full extension is painful to the knee joint area. The patient is instructed to extend at the hip while tightening the quadriceps muscle, straightening the knee as tolerated. This exercise also may help restore knee extension. The towel should be removed as knee extension increases or becomes less painful. Adductor isometric contractions can be performed, isolated or in conjunction with quadriceps sets (see Chapter 16 exercises). The role of the VMO in patella dysfunction is debatable.[28] Adductor contractions theoretically may facilitate VMO contraction based on the anatomic origin of the horizontal fibers of the VMO to the intermuscular septum of the hip adductor group and the distal adductor tendon insertion into the suprapatellar tendon.[4]

Hamstring isometrics can be performed; they should initially be performed at a submaximal level, with vigor increased based on patient tolerance and response. **Caution should be exhibited when performing hamstring exercises early in rehabilitation, especially with larger peripheral rim or posterior horn meniscus repairs.** Active knee flexion pulls the medial and lateral meniscus posterior. Because the lateral meniscus is more loosely attached, it can migrate posteriorly as much as 1 cm as a result of pull from the popliteus muscle. The medial meniscus may move a few millimeters via the posterior attachment to the joint capsule and influence from the nearby semimembranosus attachment.[2] Cocontraction isometrics of the quadriceps and hamstrings may be used in the first 2 to 4 weeks in patients with the aforementioned repairs to allow adequate meniscal healing.[19]

An open-chain straight leg raise (SLR) "4 quad" program (i.e., four quadrants: hip flexion, abduction, adduction, and extension) can be initiated with the knee fully extended if the patient has adequate LE and quadriceps control. Short arc quadriceps exercises can be added if the patient tolerates end-range extension movement. *Resistance should be added carefully, with the therapist remaining mindful of the role of the quadriceps in pulling the meniscus anteriorly by way of the menisco-patellar ligament, as well as the anterior posterior compressive force exerted by the femoral condyle during knee extension.*[21] The "4 quad" program is a series of SLR exercises held for 10 seconds and 10 to 20 repetitions:

1. Supine SLR
2. Side-lying hip abduction (see Fig. 16-18)
3. Side-lying hip adduction (see Fig. 16-19)
4. Prone hip extension

Progression of this program is based on patient signs and symptoms. Resistance can be added distally as tolerated. The DeLorme strength progression protocol[9] can be used, with gradual increases in resistance based on patient signs and symptoms.

Weight-bearing status and patient tolerance may limit the ability to strengthen the distal musculature. Strengthening of the ankle can be aided by exercises using elastic tubing; the patient should perform three sets of 10 to 20 repetitions. Ankle movements of dorsiflexion, plantar flexion, inversion and eversion, and hip proprioceptive neuromuscular facilitation (PNF) patterns (with the knee extended) can be performed to the patient's tolerance. As with other healing collagen structures, controlled tensile and compressive loading may assist in scar conformation, revascularization, and improvement in the tensile properties of the meniscal repair through the maturation process.[16] Gradual progression and reassessment of activity is crucial.

When initiating any of the closed kinetic chain exercises, the patient must keep the knee and LE in a neutral position. In normal gait the compressive forces on the knee joint may be two to three times normal body weight. The meniscus assumes 40% to 60% of the weight-bearing load. Variations in knee joint angulation or rotation can increase the force across the meniscus 25% to 50%.[25] Variations in foot mechanics that cause rotation or angulation of the knee into varus or valgus can have potentially significant effects on meniscal compressive and tensile forces that may affect the repair site.

Partial weight–bearing, closed kinetic chain activities using leg press (see Fig. 16-20) or inclined squat machines (double leg progressed to single leg [see Fig. 17-6]), partial squats, and heel raises (see Fig. 16-13) can be initiated later in the initial phase. Standing terminal knee extension with tubing can be added to increase quadriceps strength and control with full weight bearing.

Aquatic therapy is an additional treatment option during the initial phase, especially if the patient has limited weight bearing and cannot tolerate traditional therapy because of pain.[38] ROM, LE strengthening, progressive weight bearing, and cardiovascular training can be initiated in the pool.

Low-resistance, moderate-speed stationary cycling can be initiated when knee flexion ROM is around 110 degrees. Toe clips may be optional if hamstring activity is to be minimized because of the location of the repair. Progression is determined by the patient's tolerance to stationary cycling. The goal of initial phase cycling is to increase muscle endurance.

> **Q** Silvia is 40 years old. Before tearing her meniscus, she had two episodes of anterior knee pain over the past 3 years. Silvia had a medial meniscal repair 5 weeks ago. She has been progressing nicely with exercises, and the exercises have been advanced. After treatment she reports pain in the anterior inferior patella region with most of the exercises. Silvia is concerned because she almost slipped and fell after her last physical therapy visit. She denies any episode of her knee locking or becoming stuck. What might be the source of her pain?

Complications in the initial phase of treatment include persistent pain and swelling, arthrofibrosis, adhesions at the porthole sites, patella tendonitis, and patellofemoral pain. Activity modification, use of modalities, heat and cold contrast, cryotherapy, and ES may be helpful in decreasing pain and swelling. *Adhesion of the porthole sites within the distal fat pads may cause painful limitation of knee flexion and active knee extension.* Ultrasound or phonophoresis, along with soft tissue mobilization of incision sites, may be helpful in mitigating distal patella symptoms. Assessment of patellofemoral mechanics (active and passive) is an ongoing process. Patellofemoral taping should be used to control pain and dysfunction.[22]

ROM gradually increases during the initial phase of treatment, approaching full ROM by the end of this phase. Passive and dynamic splints may be helpful in gaining ROM if the joint does not respond to conservative treatment. **Initiation of vigorous stretching or knee joint mobilization should be discussed with the patient and physician.** The therapist should be aware of knee joint symptoms, pain, and swelling as attempts to increase ROM (especially knee flexion) continue.

In addition, the therapist should be cognizant of and recognize meniscus lesion signs and symptoms. These include persistent joint effusion, joint line pain, and locking or giving way of the knee (as opposed to buckling or weakness from decreased LE or quadriceps strength).

If activity modification and use of modalities does not improve the patient's symptoms and objective findings, or if the patient exhibits classic signs of a meniscus tear, then referral to the physician is indicated.

A

Silvia's history, along with the pain distribution pattern, indicates a patellofemoral joint problem that may have become irritated. Meniscal pain often produces complaints of pain near the joint line. Of course, a detailed assessment should be made and the physician notified. In this case the patellofemoral joint was the source of the anterior inferior knee pain. Therefore the patient should be treated for both the patellofemoral symptoms and the meniscal repair. Necessary restrictions should be maintained for each condition. After the patellofemoral symptoms have been significantly reduced or eliminated, the exercise program for the meniscal repair can again be the focus, with consideration of the patellofemoral joint.

Phase II (Intermediate Phase)

TIME: 5 to 11 weeks after surgery

GOALS: Gain full ROM and 90% to 100% strength, progress functional activities, progress to gym program (Table 19-2)

Objective findings rather than time ranges give an indication of progression into the intermediate phase of rehabilitation. In general this phase occurs around 4 to 6 weeks, in part based on improved patient signs and symptoms but also because enough time has elapsed to allow sufficient healing of the meniscal repair. This phase lasts until the patient is ready to enter a return-to-sport program (usually by the week 12). Pain and swelling should be minimal and easily controlled before initiation of this phase. ROM should be full. However, the patient may have a slight restriction of knee flexion, with discomfort at end ROM. Full weight bearing should be tolerated without pain or swelling. The patient should exhibit normal gait mechanics. Good control of the LE musculature should be evident before activity is progressed. The goals of the intermediate phase are to normalize strength, ROM, gait, and endurance, as well as progress the patient into functional activities. Muscle flexibility exercises are continued as needed during this phase. Quadriceps and iliopsoas stretching to improve knee flexion and hip extension can be initiated. Strength exercises are continued and advanced as tolerated. Hamstring strengthening (with isotonic exercise) can be advanced during this phase. Progression is based on DeLorme's principles.[9] *Resistance can be applied to the hamstring group gradually, based on patient tolerance.*

Closed-chain activity can be advanced during this phase of rehabilitation. Progression of activity should be from simple linear movements to complex multidirectional movements. Patients are instructed to perform three sets of 10 to 30 repetitions as indicated. The patient must demonstrate adequate control of LE mechanics and not have adverse reactions (pain and swelling) from the simple linear movements before progressing to complex multidirectional movements. Variables of time, repetitions, ROM, and resistance are used in functionally progressing the rehabilitation program. Full weight–bearing heel raises, lateral step-ups, wall squats, mini-squats with tubing, and partial lunges can be performed. ROM should be limited initially, with most activity being from 0 to 90 degrees. **Constant reassessment should occur, and patient tolerance to the particular activity must be demonstrated before any exercise progression.**

Balance and coordination exercises can be added to the rehabilitation program during the intermediate phase. Initial training is done bilaterally and progressed as tolerated to unilateral activities. Balance boards, trampoline, and elastic cords can be used. Single-limb balance and control can be performed with exercise tubing "T kicks" (Fig. 19-4). The uninvolved extremity has a cord attached distally; the involved extremity remains stationary with the knee in about 10 degrees of flexion. The patient moves the uninvolved extremity into flexion, extension, abduction, adduction, and diagonal planes. Initially the patient performs 10 to 15 repetitions for two sets in each plane of movement. The patient may require support for balance. The exercise can be progressed by altering the tubing resistance, increasing the repetition or time (up to 30 seconds in each plane), and altering the speed of movement.

Cycling can be continued, with the patient modifying the workload parameters of speed, resistance, and duration based on response to the activity. Additional cardiovascular activity (e.g., stair-stepping machine, cross-country ski machine, treadmill) can be added based on patient response and tolerance.

A gradual walking-to-running program can be established toward the end of this phase based on weight-bearing tolerance and adequate closed-chain control and LE strength. (Refer to Chapter 17 for a detailed progressive running program.) Assessment of foot function with appropriate modifications may be helpful in minimizing abnormal joint and meniscus stress before initiating a running program. The running program can start with jogging in place on a trampoline and be progressed to treadmill running. Continued progression is based on patient tolerance and absence of pain and swelling.

Isokinetics strength and endurance training can be initiated during this phase. Tolerance to resisted quadriceps and hamstring strengthening must be demonstrated before an isokinetic program is initiated. A submaximal multispectrum program with a lower velocity speed of 180 degrees/second (three sets of 15 to 20 seconds) and higher velocity speed of 300 degrees per second (three sets up to 30 seconds) can be initiated. Progression is based on patient tolerance and adequate response to training.

Table 19-2 Meniscus Repair

Rehabilitation Phase	Criteria to Progress to this Phase	Anticipated Impairments and Functional Limitations	Intervention	Goal	Rationale
Phase II Postoperative 5-11 weeks	◆ Minimal pain and swelling 4 to 6 weeks to allow sufficient healing ◆ Full weight bearing, normal gait mechanics ◆ Good control of the LE musculature	◆ Decreased strength ◆ Minimal effusion ◆ Decreased ROM (flexion)	◆ Continue exercises as outlined in Phase I Resistive exercise: ◆ Isotonics—Hamstrings ◆ Isokinetics—A submaximal multispectrum isokinetic program ◆ Closed-chain exercise, heel raises, lateral step-up, forward step up/down, wall squats, knee flexion at 45-60 degrees, mini-squats, partial lunges, progression in knee flexion ROM ◆ Balance activities, balance board, trampoline ◆ Elastic tubing activity, T kicks (see Fig. 19-4) ◆ Stationary cycling, modifying the workload parameters of speed, resistance, and duration ◆ Stair-stepping machine later in the phase, cross-country ski machine, or treadmill	◆ Full ROM ◆ 90%-100% LE strength ◆ Normal gait and standing tolerance ◆ Progression to functional activities ◆ Prepare patient for discharge	◆ Restore knee and LE function ◆ Increase muscle strength ◆ Use specificity of training principles to return the patient to previous level of functional activity ◆ Enhance response of joint proprioceptors and neuromuscular coordination ◆ Emphasize stability/ strengthening of involved leg ◆ Improve cardiovascular fitness

LE, Lower extremity; *ROM,* range of motion.

Phase III (Advanced Phase)

TIME: 12 18 weeks after surgery

GOALS: Return to sport or preinjury activities, establish an ongoing training program (Table 19-3)

Progression to the advanced phase of rehabilitation is based on tolerance to intermediate phase treatment. Typically this phase is initiated around 12 to 18 weeks. ROM should be complete without pain. **Caution should be exhibited with full squat or lunge activity. These activities should be avoided early in the advanced phase and gradually introduced with progressive loading toward the end of the phase.** Normal strength in all major muscle groups should be exhibited.

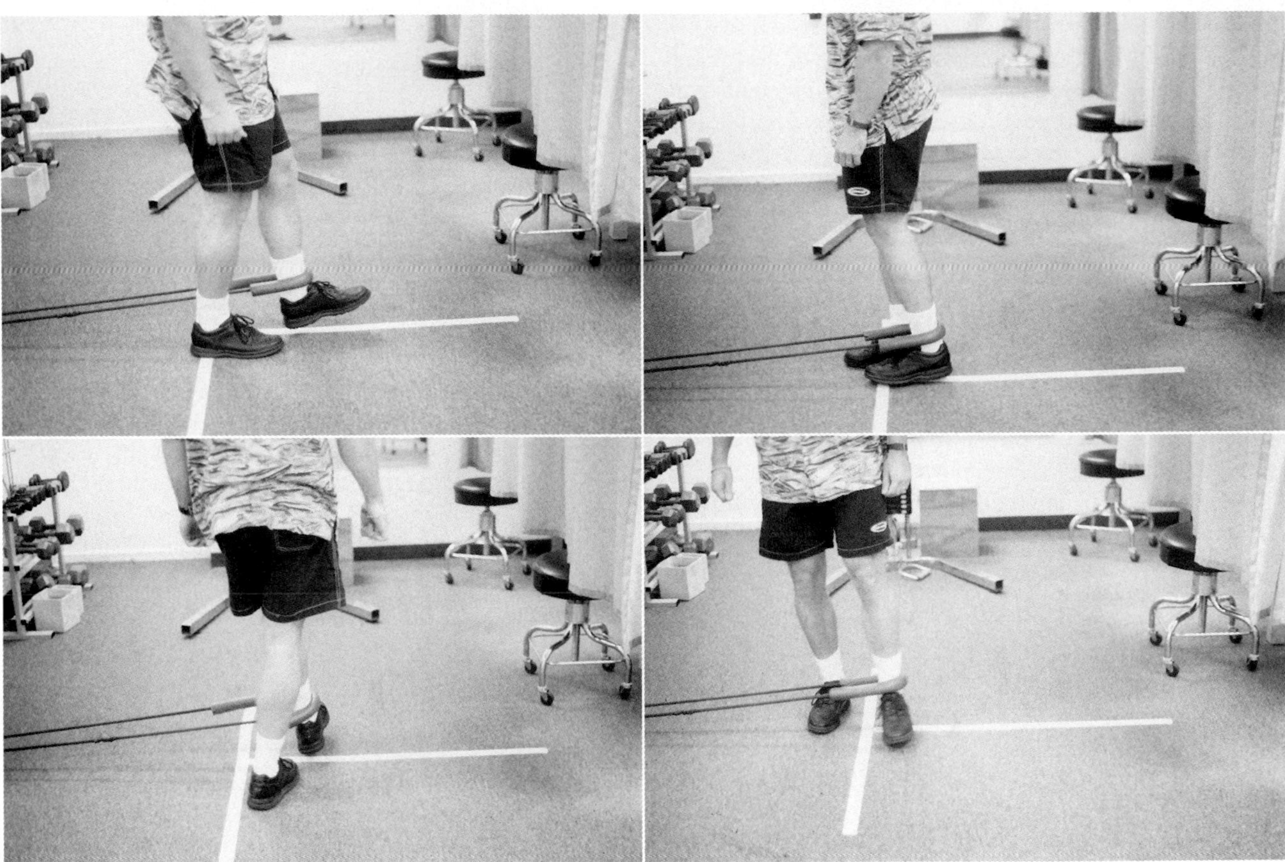

Fig. 19-4 T kicks. This exercise is performed in a standing position, with elastic tubing around the ankle of the uninvolved lower extremity (LE) (foot off ground). The uninvolved LE moves into flexion (A), extension (B), adduction (C), and abduction (D). The emphasis is on maintaining proper LE alignment and avoiding tibial rotation.

Table 19-3 Meniscus Repair

Rehabilitation Phase	Criteria to Progress to this Phase	Anticipated Impairments and Functional Limitations	Intervention	Goal	Rationale
Phase III Postoperative 12-18 weeks	◆ Tolerance to intermediate phase treatment ◆ Full ROM ◆ MMT normal ◆ Good closed-chain control in linear and multidirectional activity ◆ Treadmill 10 to 15 minutes at a pace of 7 to 8 miles per hour without adverse signs and symptoms ◆ Isokinetic strength 70% of the uninvolved extremity	◆ Isokinetic strength and endurance deficit ◆ Decreased ability to perform full squat or lunge ◆ Fair balance and control with higher-level activity	◆ Progression and continuation of exercises as listed in Phases I and II ◆ Depending on previous activity level and functional requirements, agility, sprinting, and track running ◆ Isokinetics—Strength and endurance training	◆ Establish an ongoing training program ◆ Return to preinjury activity or sport ◆ Appropriate performance on functional and isokinetic tests as indicated for return to sport or activity	◆ Continued progression of endurance and strength training ◆ Safe return to functional activity

ROM, Range of motion; *MMT,* manual muscle test.

The patient should exhibit good closed-chain control in linear and multidirectional activity. The goals of this phase are to establish a training program and return to sports or preinjury activity levels. Progression of strength and endurance training continues. Depending on previous activity level and functional requirements, agility, sprinting, and track running can be initiated. An indicator of patient progress in these activities is the ability to jog on a treadmill 10 to 15 minutes at a pace of 7 to 8 miles per hour without adverse signs and symptoms. As with other knee disorders, adequate isokinetic strength (70% of the uninvolved extremity) can be used as an indication for progression to a running and agility program. A deficit of 10% or less is a reliable indicator of return to sport or activity participation.[35] However, other functional tests (as mentioned in Chapter 17) need to be assessed to ensure safe return.

SUGGESTED HOME MAINTENANCE FOR THE POSTSURGICAL PATIENT

An exercise program has been outlined at the various phases. The physical therapist can use it in customizing a patient-specific program.

CONCLUSION

Meniscal repair is an effective technique for preserving certain torn menisci. Although long-term results are still unknown, the meniscus should be preserved whenever possible to avoid the late sequelae of meniscectomy. Numerous techniques are available to achieve this goal and are primarily a matter of surgeon preference. A rehabilitation program must be individually tailored based on scientific evidence, clinical signs and symptoms, and patient needs.

SUGGESTED HOME MAINTENANCE FOR THE POSTSURGICAL PATIENT

Weeks 1-2

GOALS FOR THE PERIOD: Manage pain and swelling, increase range of motion (ROM) and strength, increase weight-bearing activities

1. Heel slides—10 repetitions to be held 30 seconds; pressure within patient's tolerance
2. Ankle pumps—20 to 30 repetitions
3. Isometric muscle contractions—quadriceps, hamstring (if appropriate), adductor, and gluteal isometric contractions (10 to 20 repetitions to be held 10 seconds)
4. Cryotherapy with elevation to be performed as needed throughout the day for 10 to 15 minutes
5. Additional compression garment or wrapping may be helpful

Weeks 3-4

GOALS FOR THE PERIOD: Manage pain and swelling, increase ROM and strength, increase weight-bearing activities

1. Supine wall slides or passive heel slides, 10 repetitions to be held 30 seconds; pressure within patient's tolerance
2. Cocontraction isometrics of the quadriceps and hamstrings, 10 to 20 repetitions to be held 10 seconds (depending on the repair site)
3. Isometric quadriceps, adductor, and hamstring contractions, 10 to 20 repetitions to be held 10 seconds
4. Flexibility exercises for the hamstring and gastrocnemius-soleus; stretches should be held at least 30 seconds and repeated five to 10 times
5. Four-quad program, two to three sets of 10 repetitions, weight added distally as tolerated
6. Elastic tubing exercises (dorsiflexion, plantar flexion, inversion and eversion, and hip proprioceptive neuromuscular facilitation [PNF] patterns), two to three sets of 10 repetitions
7. Low-resistance, moderate-speed stationary cycling
8. Home aquatic therapy (performing active range of motion (AROM) exercises of the hip, knee, and ankle in chest-high water)
9. Continued cryotherapy with elevation to be performed as needed throughout the day for 10 to 15 minutes

Weeks 5-11

GOALS FOR THE PERIOD: Gain full ROM and 90% to 100% strength, progress functional activities, progress to gym program

1. Continued open-chain exercise program, four-quads, short arc quadriceps (SAQs), and PNF patterns with tubing
2. Hamstring, gastrocnemius-soleus, quadriceps, and iliopsoas stretching, 5 to 10 repetitions to be held at least 30 seconds
3. Heel raises, two to three sets of 10 repetitions; lateral step-ups and forward step up and down (using 2-inch height progressions), two to three sets of 10 repetitions; wall squats, knee flexion at 45 degrees advanced to 60 degrees, two sets of 10 repetitions to be held 10 seconds; mini-squats, partial lunges, and progression in knee flexion ROM (add tubing or weight to progress resistance as tolerated), two to three sets of 10 repetitions to be held 5 to 10 seconds
4. Balance activities (bilateral progressed as tolerated to unilateral)—balance board, trampoline (side-to-side and forward-to-back steps)—two sets of 1 minute each
5. Exercise cords activity, T kicks, two to three sets of 10 repetitions
6. Stationary cycling, modifying the workload parameters of speed, resistance, and duration based on the response to the activity
7. Stair-stepping machine, cross-country ski machine, or treadmill, with workload progression based on patient response and tolerance

Weeks 12-18

GOALS FOR THE PERIOD: Return to sport or preinjury activities, establish an ongoing training program

1. Progression of strength and endurance training
2. Functional or sport-specific drills
3. Agility, sprinting, and track running

References

1. Annandale T: An operation for displaced semilunar cartilage, *Clin Orthop Relat Res* 1:779, 1885.
2. Arnoczky SP, Warren RF: Microvasculature of the human meniscus, *Am J Sports Med* 10:90, 1982.
3. Barber FA, Click SD: Meniscus repair rehabilitation with concurrent anterior cruciate reconstruction, *Arthroscopy* 13:433, 1997.
4. Bose K, Kanagasuntheram R, Osman MBH: Vastus medialis oblique: an anatomic and physiologic study, *Orthopedics* 3:880, 1980.
5. Cohn BT, Draeger RI, Jackson DW: The effects of cold therapy on postoperative management of pain in patients undergoing anterior cruciate ligament reconstruction, *Am J Sports Med* 17(3):344, 1989.
6. DeHaven KE: Peripheral meniscal repair: an alternative to meniscectomy, *J Bone Joint Surg* BR63:463, 1981.
7. DeHaven KE, Lohrer WA, Lovelock JE: Long-term results of open meniscal repair, *Am J Sports Med* 23(5):524-530, 1995.
8. DeHaven KE, Stone RC: Meniscal repair. In Sahiaree H, editor: *O'Connor's textbook of arthroscopic surgery*, Philadelphia, 1992, JB Lippincott.
9. DeLorme TL, Watkins A: *Progressive resistance exercise*, New York, 1951, Appleton-Century.
10. DeVries HA: Evaluation of static stretching, procedures for improvement of flexibility, *Res Q* 3:222, 1962.
11. Fairbanks TJ: Knee joint changes after meniscectomy, *J Bone Joint Surg* 30B:664, 1948.
12. Gill SS, Diduch DR: Outcomes after meniscal repair using the meniscus arrow in knees undergoing concurrent anterior cruciate ligament reconstruction, *Arthroscopy* 18(6):569-577, 2002.
13. Henning CE: Arthroscopic repair of meniscus tears, *Orthopedics* 6:1130, 1983.
14. Johnson LL: *Diagnostic and surgical arthroscopy. The knee and other joints*, ed 2, St Louis, 1981, Mosby.
15. Kottke FJ, Pavley DJ, Ptakda DA: The rationale for prolonged stretching for corrections of shortening of connective tissue, *Arch Phys Med Rehabil* 47:345, 1966.
16. Kvist M, Jarvinen M: Clinical, histological and biomechanical features in repair of muscle and tendon injuries, *Int J Sports Med* 3:12, 1982.
17. Lessard LA et al: The efficacy of cryotherapy following arthroscopic knee surgery, *J Orthop Sports Phys Ther* 26(1):14, 1997.
18. Maitland GD: *Peripheral manipulation*, ed 3, London, 1991, Butterworth-Heinemann.
19. Mangine R, Heckman T: The knee. In Saunders B, editor: *Sports physical therapy*, Norwalk, CT, 1990, Appleton & Lange.
20. McCarty EC, Marx RG, DeHaven KE: Meniscus repair: considerations in treatment and update of clinical results, *Clin Orthop Relat Res* Sept:(402):122-134, 2002.
21. McConnell J: The management of chondromalacia patellae: a long term solution, *Aust J Physiother* 32(4):215, 1986.
22. McConnell J, Fulkerson J: The knee: patellofemoral and soft tissue injuries. In Zachazewski JE, Magee DJ, Quillen WS, editors: *Athletic injuries and rehabilitation*, Philadelphia, 1996, WB Saunders.
23. Morgan CD: The all "inside" meniscus repair: technical note, *Arthroscopy* 7:120, 1991.
24. Morgan CD et al: Arthroscopic meniscal repair evaluated by second-look arthroscopy, *Am J Sports Med* 19(6): 632-637, 1991.
25. Norkin CC, Levangie PK: *Joint structure and function: a comprehensive analysis*, Philadelphia, 1992, FA Davis.
26. Noyes FR, Barber-Westin SD: Arthroscopic repair of meniscal tears extending into the avascular zone in patients younger than twenty years of age, *Am J Sports Med* 30(4):589-600, 2002.
27. Noyes FR, Barber-Westin SD: Arthroscopic repair of meniscus tears extending into the avascular zone with or without anterior cruciate ligament reconstruction in patients 40 years of age and older, *Arthroscopy* 16(8): 822-829, 2000.
28. Powers CM: Rehabilitation of patellofemoral joint disorders: a critical review, *J Orthop Sports Phys Ther* 28(5):345, 1998.
29. Rockborn P, Gillquist J: Results of open meniscus repair. Long-term follow-up study with a matched uninjured control group, *J Bone Joint Surg Br* 82(4):494-498, 2000.
30. Rockborn P, Messner K: Long-term results of meniscus repair and meniscectomy: a 13-year functional and radiographic follow-up study, *Knee Surg Sports Traumatol Arthrosc* 8(1):2-10, 2000.
31. Rubman MH, Noyes FR, Barber-Westin SD: Technical considerations in the management of complex meniscus tears, *Clin Sports Med* 15:511, 1996.
32. Shelbourne KD, Carr DR: Meniscal repair compared with meniscectomy for bucket-handle medial meniscal tears in anterior cruciate ligament-reconstructed knees, *Am J Sports Med* 31(5):718-723, 2003.
33. Shelbourne KD, Dersam MD: Comparison of partial meniscectomy versus meniscus repair for bucket-handle lateral meniscus tears in anterior cruciate ligament reconstructed knees, *Arthroscopy* 20(6):581-585, 2004.
34. Shelbourne KD, Heinrich J: The long-term evaluation of lateral meniscus tears left in situ at the time of anterior cruciate ligament reconstruction, *Arthroscopy* 20(4): 346-351, 2004.
35. Shelbourne KD et al: Rehabilitation after meniscal repair, *Clin Sports Med* 15:595, 1996.
36. Spindler KP et al: Prospective comparison of arthroscopic medial meniscal repair technique: inside-out suture versus entirely arthroscopic arrows, *Am J Sports Med* 31(6): 929-934, 2003.
37. Suton JB: *Ligaments: their nature and morphology*, London, 1897, MK Lewis.
38. Tovin BJ et al: Comparison of the effects of exercise in water and on land on the rehabilitation of patients with intra-articular anterior cruciate ligament reconstruction, *Phys Ther* 74(8):710, 1994.
39. Whitelaw GP et al: The use of the Cryo/Cuff versus ice and elastic wrap in the postoperative care of knee arthroscopy patients, *Am J Knee Surg* 8(1):28, 1995.
40. Zachazewski JE: Flexibility for sports. In Saunders B, editor: *Sports physical therapy*, Norwalk, CT, 1990, Appleton & Lange.

CHAPTER 20

Patella Open Reduction and Internal Fixation

Daniel A. Farwell
Craig Zeman

Patella fractures can occur in a wide variety of individuals. Both genders have similar fracture rates. Age-related incidence of patella fractures tends to be shifted to a mature population. Patella fractures are usually caused by direct trauma or a blow to the patella.[4,23,25,35] Depending on the force of the injury, the fracture can be nondisplaced or highly comminuted with significant injury to the extensor mechanism complex. Active extension of the knee is usually preserved with a nondisplaced fracture. However, in a displaced fracture the extensor mechanism is disrupted to the extent that active extension is not possible. Displaced fractures require open reduction internal fixation (ORIF) to maximize active extension of the knee and decrease the incidence of post-traumatic arthritis.

SURGICAL INDICATIONS AND CONSIDERATIONS

Physicians use two main criteria to determine whether surgery is indicated:

1. Fracture displacement of more than 3 or 4 mm
2. Loss of ability to extend the knee actively

Different surgical treatments are based on the type or severity of the fracture. Currently, tension band wiring is the most accepted treatment for displaced patella fractures.[6,15,19] Weber and colleagues[36] noted stability and early range of motion (ROM) is to be performed, there must be a stable repair of the fracture site to avoid displacement of the repair. He noted increased stability by repairing cadaveric patella fractures with a technique in which the wire is anchored directly in bone. He also noted that the retinaculum should be repaired because it added to stability. Bostman and colleagues[5] examined several different approaches and techniques to repair patella fractures and discovered the tension band wiring procedure to be far superior to other methods.

Smith and associates[31] performed a retrospective review of postoperative complications after ORIF of patella fractures. They followed 51 patients treated with the tension band fixation technique until complete healing had occurred at a minimum of 4 months. The authors' objective was to focus on acute, short-term complications after ORIF of patella fracture. Although the study did not specifically assess clinical parameters such as pain or strength, it did point out two important factors to consider during rehabilitation. Approximately 22% of the patella fractures treated with modified tension band wiring and early ROM displaced significantly during the early postoperative period. **Failure of fixation was related to unprotected ambulation and noncompliance. Patient noncompliance in restricting early ROM and weight bearing can cause failure of even technically correct tension band wire fixation.***

Joint congruity must be restored to decrease the development of arthritis, and the extensor mechanism must be restored to regain full extension. Most patients with displaced fractures are candidates for ORIF. If the patient was ambulatory before the injury and can medically tolerate surgery, then surgery should be performed regardless of age. Situations in which non-ambulatory patients with patella fractures lack lower-extremity (LE) function and sensation (neurologic impairment) can be managed conservatively.

Patients with simple two-part fractures have a better chance of a successful outcome than those with highly comminuted fractures. The variability of outcomes relates to the degree of fixation and the ability of the fracture site or sites to consolidate. In some cases of irreducible comminution, the fragments may have to be removed, resulting in a partial or total patellectomy.[1,2,8,11,14,16,26,33,34,35,37] Patellectomy procedures have a lower success rate than stable internal fixation procedures.[9,12,30,32]

---

*References 5, 11, 24, 25, 28.

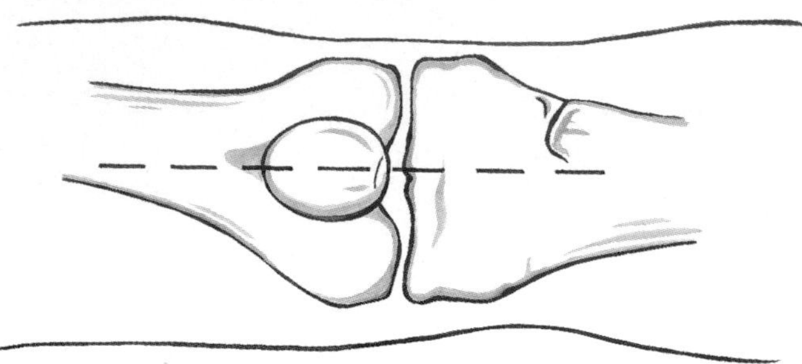

Fig. 20-1 The incision line from which repair of the fracture is initiated.

SURGICAL PROCEDURE

Most methods of ORIF incorporate tension band wiring techniques.[11,22,24,36] The tension band wire is placed around the proximal and distal pole of the patella through the quadriceps and patella tendons. This wire compresses the fracture site. The surgeon maintains rotational control with one or two screws placed across the fracture site from the proximal to the distal pole. The tension band wire is passed under the k-wires or screws to add compressive and rotational stability to the fixation. Another method is to use cannulated screws through which the tension band wire may be passed.

The integrity of the skin over the patella must be evaluated before surgery because of its potential to produce postoperative complications. The therapist should assess this area continually for infection and poor healing, because vascular supply may have been disrupted during the trauma that caused the patella fracture.

Surgery is performed under either general or regional anesthesia. The patient is positioned supine, and a tourniquet is applied to the thigh. It is important that the knee can fully flex and extend so that the surgeon can determine the stable postoperative ROM. The leg is then prepped and draped in sterile fashion. If the skin allows, then a longitudinal midline incision is made over the patella. This incision (Fig. 20-1) is carried down to the peritenon, and full-thickness flaps are developed both medially and laterally to expose the entire patella and extensor mechanism. The peritenon is then incised to expose the fracture and the tendons. The fracture hematoma is débrided from the fracture site, and the raw cancellous bone is delineated to aid in fracture reduction. Two k-wires are then run from the fracture site of the proximal fragment and out the proximal pole of the patella (Fig. 20-2, A to C). The proximal and distal fragments of the patella are brought together to reduce the fracture. The fracture is then held together with bone-holding forceps while the knee is in extension (Fig. 20-2, D). The k-wires are passed back through the middle of the patella and out the distal pole. The bone-holding forceps are then removed (Fig. 20-2, E). Next the tension band wire is placed around the patella and k-wires. It should be positioned as close to the bone and k-wires as possible to minimize complications after ROM is initiated postoperatively (Fig. 20-2, F).

To place the tension wire as close to the bone and k-wire as possible, the surgeon usually passes a hollow needle under the k-wire and over the bone to guide the tension band wire. The tension band wire is then passed through the needle and brought around the patella. The two ends of the tension band wire are then twisted together with pliers to add tension to the system. The surgeon must be careful not to add too much tension to the wire, because this may cause the wire to break early in the rehabilitation process (see Fig. 20-2, G and H).

The surgeon then repairs the extensor mechanism. The medial and lateral retinacula are commonly torn in line with the fracture. These tears are simply repaired using nonabsorbable sutures. After this last repair the surgeon checks the ROM to ensure that the patient can easily obtain full extension and at least 90 degrees of flexion. The surgical site is then closed: first the peritenon, then the subcutaneous tissue, and finally the skin. The wound is dressed with a bulky dressing and placed in an immobilizer. A postoperative water-cooling system or ice pack may be used to assist with pain control immediately.

A partial patellectomy may be performed in patients with comminuted displaced fractures who have at least 50% of the patella remaining.[33] The inferior pole of the patella usually suffers the most trauma, resulting in its removal (Fig. 20-3, A). To do a partial patellectomy the surgeon débrides the bone fragments from the tendon end and then weaves two large 5-0 nonabsorbable sutures into the tendon (5-0 FiberWire is now available that has the strength of 18 gauge wire and the flexibility of suture). The surgeon then drills two holes longitudinally into the remaining piece of the patella. The sutures in the tendon are brought through the holes in the patella and tied over the bone bridge formed by the two holes (Fig. 20-3, B and C).

Most patients require a second operation to remove the hardware placed in the patella.[17] The wires and sutures can become prominent and bother the patient during rehabilitation, slowing progress in gaining ROM.

The fixation of simple fractures is usually the most stable immediately after surgery. If the tension band wire is not placed right next to the screw, then the wire can cut through the tendon until it butts up against the screw, decreasing the compressive effect of the wire and possibly allowing the fracture to displace. Stable fixation of a simple fracture is usually strong enough to allow early passive range of motion (PROM). The amount of ROM is dictated by the surgical procedure and pain tolerance. Time frames to initiate physical therapy vary depending on the degree of comminution. The repair is most vulnerable between 4 to 6 weeks when the bone and tendon have not completely healed and the pins and wires have loosened. After 8 weeks

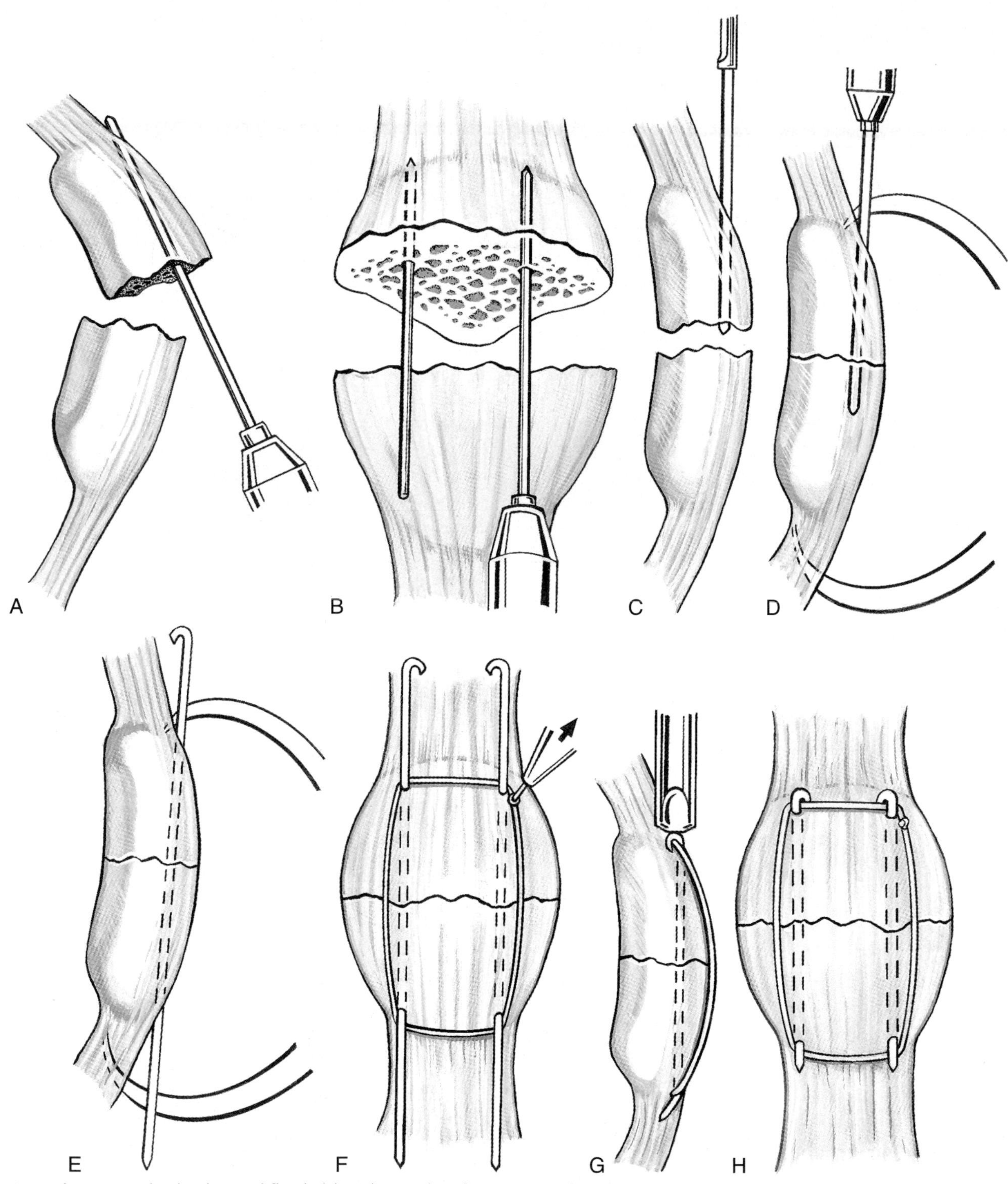

Fig. 20-2 The open reduction internal fixation (ORIF) procedure for transverse fracture of the patella. **A** to **C**, The patella is prepared for the k-wires by drilling congruent holes through both pieces of the fracture. **D** and **E**, Bone forceps are used to approximate the fracture while wires are placed through the drill holes. **F** to **H**, The surgeon finishes the process of tension band wiring, creating stable postoperative fixation.

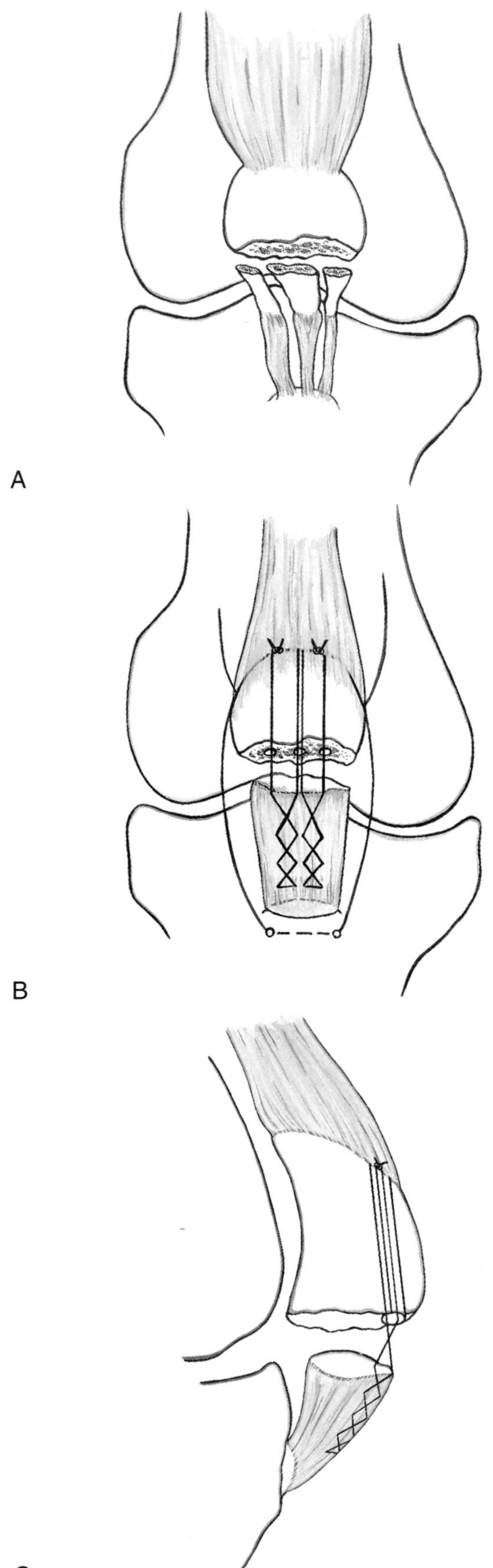

Fig. 20-3 The process of partial patellectomy. A, Comminuted fracture involving the inferior pole of the patella. Front view (B) and side view (C) after débridement of inferior fragments; sutures are woven into the tendon.

the repair should be stable enough to allow aggressive therapy with the goal of regaining full ROM.[7]

The exception to this time frame is the patient who has a comminuted fracture with unstable fixation. This type of situation may require 12 weeks before the initiation of therapy. Most patients return to preinjury activities (sports) by 6 months after surgery.

Outcomes

A successful outcome is a knee with full active extension, full ROM, and without significant pain. The things that can prevent a successful outcome are unstable fixation, incongruous reduction, poor patient compliance, and delays in early PROM exercises. Unstable fixation will decrease the aggression of the rehabilitation program. A poorly reduced joint will make ROM exercises more painful and limit the speed at which the patient will tolerate increases in ROM and strengthening exercises. This procedure is painful. Patients with poor pain tolerance will not regain strength and ROM as easily as patients who are motivated and who can handle an aggressive rehabilitation program. Some early postoperative ROM exercises need to be started to get the best results. If ROM exercises are delayed in the first few weeks for any reason, then it will be more difficult to get back full ROM and strength.

Maximal function after patellar fracture is usually not achieved until 1 year after sugery.[10] Stiffness and anterior knee pain especially with stair climbing or prolonged sitting with the knee flexed are common.[1,12,13,26,32,38] Total patellectomy patients can have an extension lag. Around 70% to 80% of patients with ORIF will end up with a good to excellent result and 20% to 30% with a fair to poor result.[25] A loss of 20% to 49% of extensor mechanism strength can be expected.[13,32,38] About 70% of patients followed long-term will have some complaint about the knee. Long-term results after total patellectomy range from 22% to 85% (good to excellent) and 14% to 64% (fair to poor).[12,13,21,25,26,32,38]

The therapist should call the surgeon with any signs of wound infection. Wound infections after ORIF in patella fractures need to be dealt with quickly, because the hardware is superficial and can easily become infected, which can lead to a deep infection requiring long-term antibiotics.

If in the course of therapy the patient develops an extension lag greater than he or she had earlier in rehabilitation, the surgeon should be called because of the possibility that a loss of fixation has occurred. To help try to confirm this, the fracture site can be palpated for a gap.

THERAPY GUIDELINES FOR REHABILITATION

The treatment of patients who have undergone ORIF for patella fractures requires a cooperative approach from the

Table 20-1 Patella Open Reduction Internal Fixation

Rehabilitation Phase	Criteria to Progress to this Phase	Anticipated Impairments and Functional Limitations	Intervention	Goal	Rationale
Phase I Postoperative 1-4 weeks	◆ Postoperative and cleared by physician to initiate therapy ◆ There may be specific precautions, depending on stability of fixation (communicate with physician)	◆ Edema ◆ Pain ◆ Limited ROM ◆ Limited strength ◆ Limited transfers ◆ Limited gait	◆ Cryotherapy ◆ ES for muscle stimulation ◆ PROM—Knee extension, knee flexion, supine wall slides ◆ Isometrics—Quadriceps/hamstring sets, quadriceps sets at 20 to 30 degrees ◆ AROM—Standing hamstring curls, supine heel slides ◆ Gait training using crutches and weight bearing as tolerated in immobilizer ◆ Weight shifting ◆ Gentle joint mobilization to the patella (resistance free)	◆ Control pain ◆ Manage edema ◆ Improve muscle contraction ◆ PROM—Knee extension 0 degrees, flexion 90 degrees ◆ Initiate volitional muscle contraction ◆ Improve tolerance to flexion ROM ◆ Avoid excessive stress on the extensor mechanism during ambulation ◆ Decrease pain	◆ Initiate self-management of pain ◆ Use ES to improve muscle contraction ◆ Restore joint ROM as indicated by physician ◆ Prepare for independence with transfers (SLR independent) ◆ Begin to prepare extensor mechanism to accept load ◆ Restore independence with ambulation ◆ Improve stability of involved LE ◆ Control pain through resistance-free mobilization to the patella

ROM, Range of motion; *ES,* electrical stimulation; *PROM,* passive range of motion; *AROM,* active range of motion; *SLR,* straight leg raising; *LE,* lower extremity.

orthopedist and the physical therapist (PT). This concept is most evident when considering the challenge in treating patients after surgery. The goal of treatment is to provide a structurally stable patellofemoral joint and allow for full functional recovery of the involved LE. Factors that influence the choice of treatment include the following:

1. The overall health of the patient and the way it may influence wound and fracture healing
2. The location and configuration of the fracture
3. Immobilization after surgery (osteopenia of the entire LE, muscle atrophy, and possible contracture of the knee joint) versus ORIF (which allows for early ROM and patella mobilization)
4. Patient compliance with prescribed treatment plan (home program)

Although rehabilitation after a patella fracture treated with ORIF is crucial, a wide range of protocols may be used depending on the factors listed previously, the physician's chosen fixation technique, and the patient's goals (which differ among athletes, sedentary adults, and children). The information the PT collects from both the physician and the patient aids in determining the design and time parameters of the rehabilitation program.

The remainder of this chapter deals only with the simple transverse fracture. However, the clinician is reminded to respect the previously discussed four factors influencing treatment when planning rehabilitation for all patella fractures.

Phase I

TIME: 1 to 4 weeks after surgery
GOALS: Control pain, manage edema, gain 0 to 90 degrees of PROM, improve quadriceps and hamstring contraction (Table 20-1)

The acute phase of rehabilitation (the first 4 weeks) after ORIF of the patella is the time when reinjury is most likely. Attention to detail and communication with the treating physician are crucial during this period.

Controversy exists over when to initiate ROM. Hung and colleagues[15] initiates knee motion 1 week after surgery, whereas Lotke and Ecker[20] often immobilizes patients for as long as 3 weeks before beginning any type of motion. Bostman and associates[5,6] not only immobilizes his patients an average of 38 days but also states that he sees no correlation between the initial time of immobilization and the final outcome. Biomechanical studies that have demonstrated the appropriateness of tension band wiring and early ROM have generally used a simple transverse fracture pattern as the model.[3] Complications such as poor bone quality and comminuted patella fractures may prevent the desired fixation and thus preclude any early joint ROM.

> **Q** James is 45 years old and had patella ORIF 3 weeks ago. He arrives for his initial evaluation in an immobilizer with his incision well healed. He weighs 250 pounds and is 5-feet 10-inches tall. What modality and procedures would be most appropriate to improve his gait pattern?

The PT performs an evaluation on the first postoperative visit, respecting the surgical procedure and any restrictions noted by the surgeon. Observation of the surgical site is documented and continually assessed to prevent wound complications.

If the surgical site shows any signs of infection, then the PT should notify the surgeon immediately. Crutches are used postoperatively, and weight bearing is as tolerated with the immobilizer in place. Patients may eventually progress to independent ambulation (with the immobilizer still in place) after they tolerate full weight bearing and are cleared by the physician (usually between 3 to 6 weeks). Smith and associates[31] reported four complete failures after ORIF with tension band wiring. No inadequacies were detected during the initial procedures, and all four failures resulted from falls while walking unprotected in the early postoperative period.

ROM measurements of the knee are taken passively, with the PT again observing any restrictions. Quality of muscle contraction in the extensor mechanism is noted, and active knee flexion is assessed. Girth measurements may be taken to assess atrophy of the thigh and calf; however, this has little overall benefit compared with functional assessment.

Early ROM is the goal in any operative treatment of patella fractures, yet the definition of early ROM varies, depending on who performs the procedure.[5,6,15,20] Although the acute phase of rehabilitation tends to focus on knee joint range, gait deviations can produce problems later in rehabilitation if they are not addressed early. Patients often are treated in some type of immobilizer. A hinged brace can be used to allow for motion while stabilizing the fracture.

Initial treatments focus on restoring ROM (0 to 90 degrees), improving quadriceps activation and hamstring muscle control, progressing gait (weight-bearing tolerance), managing edema, and controlling pain. A program of elevation and ice (20 to 30 minutes three times a day) is used as necessary to manage edema and control pain. **Electrical stimulation (ES) for pain control is avoided because of the proximity of the screw and wires.** However, ES can be used to assist in quadriceps contraction when appropriate. Gentle mobilization (grades I and II shy of resistance) of the patella also is used to control pain.

Initial exercises of the knee involve PROM, limited active range of motion (AROM), and isometrics. Passive stretches are performed to restore flexion and extension. The vigor of the stretch should be in concert with the guidelines established by the surgeon. In general, patients are expected to reach 90 degrees of flexion and full extension by 4 weeks. Supine wall slides can be easily performed in the clinic or at home. (Refer to the section on Suggested Home Maintenance for the Postsurgical Patient.) Regaining full extension is usually not a problem; however, limitations of extension can be treated quite successfully (see Figs. 17-4 and 17-5).

Active exercises primarily focus on using the hamstrings to flex the knee. Heel slides and standing hamstring curls are initiated to aid in increasing muscle control and progressing ROM.

Isometric exercises involve quadriceps and hamstring cocontraction and isolated quadriceps contractions at 20 to 30 degrees flexion. Quality is observed and ES is helpful in recruitment.

Gait training focuses on increasing the acceptance of weight on the involved leg. Weight shifting can be given as part of the home program. After the incision is healed and the surgeon allows it, aqua therapy can be initiated with an emphasis on proper weight shifting and gait mechanics.

> **A** Given his size, pool therapy would be the most appropriate tool to improve his gait pattern and limit body weight stress on the patella. Warm water can help decrease pain, improve ROM, and stresses that land based therapy place on the joint.

Phase II

TIME: 5 to 8 weeks after surgery
GOALS: Self-manage pain, increase strength, increase ROM to 90%, initiate quadriceps AROM (6 to 8 weeks), have minimal gait deviations on level surfaces (Table 20-2)

The subacute or midphase of rehabilitation (from weeks 5 to 8) is the transition from limited functional activity to aggressive functional activity. The actual exercise protocol is similar to any other type of patellofemoral rehabilitation. The only real difference with ORIF patella fracture is that a true fixation of the fracture has been obtained. Motion at the fracture site tends to activate secondary callus formation, especially with tension band

Table 20-2 Patella Open Reduction Internal Fixation

Rehabilitation Phase	Criteria to Progress to this Phase	Anticipated Impairments and Functional Limitations	Intervention	Goal	Rationale
Phase II Postoperative 5-8 weeks	◆ No signs of infection ◆ No significant increase in pain ◆ No loss of ROM	◆ Pain ◆ Limited ROM ◆ Limited strength ◆ Limited gait	◆ Continuation and progression of interventions from Phase I ◆ Patellofemoral taping ◆ Gait training; discontinue crutches when indicated ◆ LE exercises continued from Phase I ◆ A/AROM—Stationary bike used as a ROM assist for flexion ◆ AROM—Knee extension (when cleared by physician, usually between 6-8 weeks)	◆ Self-manage pain ◆ Decrease gait deviations ◆ Increase LE strength ◆ PROM of knee to 90% ◆ Independent with home exercises	◆ Prepare patient for discharge ◆ Assist patellofemoral mechanics ◆ Promote return to unassisted gait in the community ◆ Restore LE stability and strength ◆ Promote restoration of normal joint mechanics ◆ Initiate extensor mechanism strengthening and improve tolerance to patellofemoral compression with tracking

ROM, Range of motion; *PROM,* passive range of motion; *LE,* lower extremity; *A/AROM,* active assistive range of motion.

wiring of a patella fracture. The danger in moving a nonfixated fracture (i.e., a fracture with no established callus formation) is that a nonunion may develop. A nonunion of bone is caused by excessive motion directly at the fracture site, which keeps the callus from forming sufficiently. This underlines the importance of maintaining immobility in some patella fractures during the rehabilitative process.[18]

> **Q** Meghan is 25 years old and had patella ORIF 6 weeks ago. She has only 60 degrees of flexion and guards with any attempts at manual therapy (soft tissue mobilization, joint mobilization) to improve ROM. The "end feel" of her flexion is a soft end feel that does not provide much resistance (no catching or hard end feel). She also has been negligent in performing her home exercise program. What changes did the therapist suggest to improve Meghan's outcome?

Another factor to consider is that patella fractures involve joint surfaces. Incongruency of the articular surfaces can lead to articular cartilage degeneration and possible early arthritis if not treated. Incongruity of the patellofemoral joint may alter the joint mechanics, producing areas of noncontact or excessive pressure over the patella.[29] Issues of patellofemoral contact area and joint reaction force must be evaluated during this phase of rehabilitation. The use of patellofemoral taping (see Figs. 18-1 to 18-3) can be useful in limiting imbalances over the fractured surface of the patella. By this phase the patient is demonstrating increased competency in ambulating with the brace and decreased reliance (if any) on the crutches. Exercises are progressed as in phase I, and the patient is instructed to perform two sets per day (repetitions to fatigue). Closed-chain exercises are initiated on a progressive basis based on patient healing and quadriceps and LE control.

Modalities at this stage are primarily ice for pain control. ES of the quadriceps is continued as indicated to progress muscle recruitment. Moist heat can be used to prepare the knee for stretching after edema is controlled.

PROM stretches are progressed as indicated to obtain full flexion. Vigor of grades of mobilization is increased into resistance as indicated.

AROM for the quadriceps is initiated between 6 to 8 weeks (or when the fracture is deemed stable enough to tolerate it). The stationary bike can be used as a ROM assistive device and progressed for strengthening and cardiovascular purposes after flexion allows full revolution without hip hiking. Surgeon approval is required before initiating resistance training on bicycle.

The rehabilitation at this point begins to mimic that prescribed for the patient recovering from lateral release in terms of exercises and progressions. Taping can be initiated in this phase as deemed appropriate by the therapist.

A Meghan was instructed to, when possible, take her pain medication before coming to therapy. The therapist also explained that 20% to 30% of patients have a "poor" outcome. If her case was to be successful (and the surgeon saw no reason why it should not be), then she must gain flexion ROM. At some point she needs to take responsibility for her care. After this intervention, her ROM improved as did her tolerance to manual techniques.

Q Jessica is 40 years old. She fractured her patella when she fell off a footstool and onto her knees. She had a patella ORIF surgery 9 weeks ago. Her knee flexion ROM is limited, and peripatella pain is a factor when performing ROM stretches. ROM exercises for knee flexion have been emphasized during the past few treatments along with modalities for pain control. Little progress has been noted. What treatment techniques may be the most helpful?

Phase III

TIME: 9 to 12 weeks after surgery

GOALS: Return to full function, develop endurance and coordination of the LE, continue to address limitations with steps and running (with physician clearance) (Table 20-3)

The advanced stage of rehabilitation (from weeks 9 to 12) focuses on functional, skill-specific activity. Most of the effort and work is spent on building back the patient's quadriceps, hamstring, and gastrocnemius-soleus muscle strength.

Depending on remaining deficits, exercises from the previous two phases are continued. The therapist should keep in mind that the time frame will vary depending on many factors, including type of fracture, fixation, and the patient's response to rehabilitation. **Furthermore, isokinetics should be avoided until the physician approves them.** The need for taping should be minimal, but if continued taping is needed, patients are instructed in self-taping techniques. Monitoring for pain and joint effusion gives the therapist feedback on the way to progress activities aggressively. Long-term strengthening of the muscles surrounding the patellofemoral joint with the development of endurance and coordination over time are the goals of this phase.

Table 20-3 Patella Open Reduction Internal Fixation

Rehabilitation Phase	Criteria to Progress to this Phase	Anticipated Impairments and Functional Limitations	Intervention	Goal	Rationale
Phase III Postoperative 9-12 weeks	◆ Pain free at rest ROM 0-90 degrees ◆ Good quadriceps control during gait ◆ Minimal gait deviations	◆ Limited endurance with prolonged functional activities ◆ Mild pain of patellofemoral joint during skill-specific exercises ◆ Limited tolerance to stairs and single-limb squat and balance	◆ Closed-chain and stretching exercises as listed in Phases I and II ◆ Patella taping ◆ Patella mobilization ◆ PREs on leg press ◆ Function-specific activity: bicycle, treadmill, isokinetic training (when cleared by physician) ◆ Home exercises (refer to Suggested Home Maintenance section)	◆ Unlimited community ambulation ◆ No gait deviations ◆ Good sitting and standing tolerances ◆ Good patella stability without taping ◆ Patient self-management of symptoms	◆ Decrease pain with functional activities ◆ Improve joint mechanics ◆ Improve joint mobility and stability ◆ Provide functional strengthening ◆ Improve endurance of VMO ◆ Increase reliance on patient self-management

ROM, Range of motion; *PREs*, progressive resistance exercises; *VMO*, vastus medalis oblique.

A The PT should assess the patella for limited mobility. If mobility is limited, which is likely, then patella mobilizations using grades into resistance (grades III and IV) can be helpful. The therapist should receive clearance from the physician before initiating mobilization into resistance. If it is limited, then increasing inferior patella movement may particularly help knee flexion ROM. The patellofemoral contact area and reaction forces also must be evaluated. Patellofemoral taping can be useful in limiting imbalances over the fractured surfaces of the patella. Complaints of pain with flexion may decrease, particularly with closed-chain exercises.

Q Jessica's knee ROM is now full 12 weeks after surgery. She performs a series of exercises for leg strengthening. She begins by stretching her hamstrings and gastrocnemius-soleus muscles. She then performs the following:

- Standing mini-squats against the wall (see Fig. 16-15)
- Leg presses using 100 lbs and keeping knee flexion less than 60 degrees (see Fig. 11-20)
- Lunges with 5 lb weights in a long-stride position (see Fig. 13-6)
- Wall slides between 0 and 45 degrees with a 1-minute hold (see Fig. 13-7)
- Sit-stand (see Fig. 21-15)
- Standing (four-wall) elastic tubing hip flexion, abduction, and adduction on the uninvolved side (see Fig. 19-3, A to D)
- Step-downs on an 8-inch step, holding contraction until the heel of the opposite leg makes contact (see Fig. 18-8)

Although she had minimal discomfort during the exercise regimen, she had increased complaints of pain for 2 days after the exercises. Which of these exercises is most likely to be an aggravating factor?

By this stage patients should be close to discharge because they are fairly functional with sitting, standing, and walking tolerances. Limitations with stairs and squatting activities continue to be present. Prolonged standing and walking should be continually improving, with the focus on a progressive increase in activities. Running and jumping should be initiated on an individual basis as determined by the surgeon (potentially after removal of hardware).

A The 8-inch step-downs are the most aggressive exercises, because they produce the highest patellofemoral compression forces. The knee is most likely flexed beyond 50 degrees while performing an eccentric contraction during full weight bearing on the affected extremity.

SUGGESTED HOME MAINTENANCE FOR THE POSTSURGICAL PATIENT

An exercise program has been outlined at the various phases. The home maintenance section outlines rehabilitation guidelines the patient may follow. The PT can use it in customizing a patient-specific program.

TROUBLESHOOTING

Issues that prevent a successful outcome are unstable fixation, incongruous reduction, poor patient compliance, and delays in early PROM exercises. Patients with poor pain tolerance do not regain strength and ROM as easily and may be left with residual deficits. Maximal function after patella fracture has been noted to take as long as 1 year.[10] Residual problems of anterior knee pain and stiffness are common complications.[1,12,13,26,32,38] An estimated 70% to 80% of patients recovering from patella ORIF have good to excellent results, although 20% to 30% have fair to poor results.[25] Residual loss of extensor strength has been recorded in the 20% to 49% range.

Prolonged immobilization is detrimental to the final result regardless of the treatment.[25] Although it produces a risk of wound infection, the benefits of ROM outweigh the risk of wound complications. However, this situation is especially tenuous in patients who suffer open patella fractures, because they are at a higher risk for infection.

SUGGESTED HOME MAINTENANCE FOR THE POSTSURGICAL PATIENT

Weeks 1-4

GOALS FOR THE PERIOD: Control pain, manage edema, gain 0 to 90 degrees of passive range of motion (PROM), improve quadriceps and hamstring contraction

1. Elevate and ice at home two to three times per day (preferably after exercises).
2. Perform ankle pumping and hamstring stretches with the extremity elevated and on ice (20 to 30 minutes).
3. Perform supine wall slides (when appropriate)—one set of five repetitions three to four times a day.
4. Perform active heel slides—one set of 10 repetitions performed three to four times per day.
5. Perform quadriceps sets (on clearance from the physician)—two sets of 10 repetitions performed three to four times per day. Even though general guidelines such as this may prescribe a number of sets and repetitions, if the patient fatigues and cannot continue to recruit a quality quadriceps contraction, then the exercise is over. Patients are only to count repetitions with quality quadriceps contractions. The heel should stay on the floor. Quadriceps sets also may be performed standing if the patient finds it easier to activate the quadriceps in this position. The key to early strengthening is to find which position the patient is most successful in recruiting a quality quadriceps contraction.

Weeks 5-8

GOALS FOR THE PERIOD: Self-manage pain, increase strength, increase ROM to 90%, initiate quadriceps active range of motion (AROM) (6 to 8 weeks), have minimal gait deviations on level surfaces

1. Perform the same exercises as in weeks 1 to 4, increasing the number of repetitions. Exercises should generally be performed in two sets of 10 to 20 repetitions per day (based on fatigue).
2. Initiate closed-chain exercises based on patient tolerance to resistance. Spider killers (see Fig. 17-3) are initiated in pain-free ranges. In addition, simulated leg press exercises with elastic tubing can be performed. Patients begin with two sets of 10 repetitions and progress based on tolerance.
3. Perform self-taping as deemed appropriate by therapist.
4. Continue use of ice after exercises.

Weeks 9-12

GOALS FOR THE PERIOD: Return to full function, develop endurance and coordination of the LE, continue to address limitations with steps and running (with physician clearance)

1. Depending on remaining deficits, continue exercises from the previous 8 weeks. The need for taping should be minimal; if continued taping is required, then patients are instructed in self-taping techniques.
2. Progress closed-chain exercises to include stepping exercises at home using threshold of doorway for balance.
3. Gradually return to functional activities while monitoring for pain and joint effusion.

References

1. Andrews JR, Hughston JC: Treatment of patellar fractures by partial patellectomy, *South Med J* 70:809, 1977.
2. Anderson LD: In Crenshaw AH, editor: *Campbell's operative orthopaedics*, ed 5, St Louis, 1971, Mosby.
3. Benjamin J et al: Biomechanical evaluation of various forms of fixation of transverse patella fractures, *J Orthop Trauma* 1:219, 1987.
4. Bohler L: *Die technik der knochenbruchandlung*, ed 13, 1957, Wein Wilhelm Maudrich Verlag.
5. Bostman O et al: Comminuted displaced fractures of the patella, *Injury* 13:196, 1981.
6. Bostman O et al: Fractures of the patella treated by operation, *Arth Orthop Trauma Surg* 102:78, 1983.
7. Bray TJ, Marder RA: Patellar fractures. In Chapman MD, Madison M, editors: *Operative orthopaedics*, ed 2, Philadelphia, 1993, JB Lippincott.
8. Brooke R: The treatment of fractured patella by excision: a study of morphology and function, *Br J Surg* 24:733, 1937.
9. Burton VW: Results of excision of the patella, *Surg Gynecol Obstet* 135:753, 1972.
10. Crenshaw AH, Wilson FD: The surgical treatment of fractures of the patella, *South Med J* 47:716, 1954.
11. DePalma AF: *The management of fractures and dislocations*, Philadelphia, 1959, WB Saunders.
12. Duthie HL, Hutchinson JR: The results of partial and total excision of the patella, *J Bone Joint Surg* 40B:75, 1958.
13. Einola S, Aho AJ, Kallio P: Patellectomy after fracture. Long-term follow-up results with special reference to functional disability, *Acta Orthop Scand* 47:441, 1976.
14. Heineck AP: The modern operative treatment of fracture of the patella. I. Based on the study of other pathological states of bone. II. An analytical review of over 1,100 cases treated during the last ten years, by open operative method, *Surg Gynecol Obstet* 9:177, 1909.
15. Hung LK et al: Fractured patella: operative treatment using tension band principle, *Injury* 16:343, 1985.
16. Jakobsen J, Christensen KS, Rassmussen OS: Patellectomy—a 20-year follow-up, *Acta Orthop Scand* 56:430, 1985.
17. Johnson EE: Fractures of the patella. In Rockwood CA, Green DP, Bucholz RW, editors: *Fractures in adults*, ed 3, Philadelphia, 1991, JB Lippincott.
18. Klassen JK, Trousdale RT: Treatment of delayed and non-union of the patella, *J Orthop Trauma* 11(3):188, 1997.
19. Lexack B, Flannagan JP, Hobbs S: Results of surgical treatment of patellar fractures, *J Bone Joint Surg Br* 67:416, 1985.
20. Lotke PA, Ecker ML: Transverse fractures of the patella, *Clin Orthop* 158:1880, 1981.
21. MacAusland WR: Total excision of the patella for fracture: report of fourteen cases, *Am J Surg* 72:510, 1946.
22. Magnusen PB: *Fractures*, ed 2, Philadelphia, 1936, JB Lippincott.
23. McMaster PE: Fractures of the patella, *Clin Orthop* 4:24, 1954.
24. Muller ME, Allgower M, Willinegger H: *Manual of internal fixation: technique recommended by the AO group*, New York, 1979, Springer-Verlag.
25. Nummi J: Fracture of the patella: a clinical study of 707 patellar fractures, *Ann Chir Gynaecol Fenn* 60(suppl):179, 1971.
26. Peeples RE, Margo MK: Function after patellectomy, *Clin Orthop* 132:180, 1978.
27. Mehta A: *Physical medicine and rehabilitation: state of the art reviews*, vol 9, no 1, Philadelphia, 1995, Hanley & Belfus.
28. Rorabeck CH, Bobechko WP: Acute dislocation of the patella with osteochondral fracture: a review of eighteen cases, *J Bone Joint Surg* 58A:237, 1976.
29. Sanders R: Patella fractures and extensor mechanism injuries. In Bronner BD et al, editors: *Skeletal trauma*, Philadelphia, 1992, WB Saunders.
30. Sanderson MC: The fractured patella: a long-term follow-up study, *Aust N Z J Surg* 45:49, 1974.
31. Smith ST et al: Early complications in the operative treatment of patella fractures, *J Orthop Trauma* 11(3):183, 1997.
32. Sutton FS et al: The effect of patellectomy on knee function, *J Bone Joint Surg* 58A:537, 1976.
33. Thompson JEM: Comminuted fractures of the patella: treatment of cases presenting with one large fragment and several small fragments, *J Bone Joint Surg* 58A:537, 1976.
34. Watson-Jones R: Excision of the patella (letter), *Br Med J* 2:195, 1945.
35. Watson-Jones R: *Fractures and other bone and joint injuries*, Edinburgh, 1939, E&S Livingstone.
36. Weber MJ et al: Efficacy of various forms of fixation of transverse fractures of the patella, *J Bone Joint Surg* AM62:215, 1980.
37. West FE: End results of patellectomy, *J Bone Joint Surg* 62A:1089, 1962.
38. Wilkinson J: Fracture of the patella treated by total excision: a long-term follow-up, *J Bone Joint Surg* 59B:352, 1977.

CHAPTER 21

Total Knee Arthroplasty

Nora P. Cacanindin
Julie Wong
Michael D. Ries

INTRODUCTION

Osteoarthritis (OA), more commonly known as *degenerative joint disease*, is one of the leading causes of disability worldwide.[12] In the United States, it is estimated that OA may affect 25 million adults, of which 15 million are limited in their daily activities.[2] When conservative management fails to decrease pain or restore mobility, surgical intervention becomes the treatment of choice. Arthroscopic surgeries may be beneficial in early stages with mechanical symptoms,[2] but when this also fails, a total knee arthroplasty (TKA) is usually recommended.

According to the National Center for Health Statistics, 381,000 TKAs were performed in 2002.[125] Most were performed on people aged 65 and older,[124] reflecting the aging population of Baby Boomers. Understanding the surgical procedure of the TKA and designing appropriate programs for rehabilitation are essential to ensure successful and cost-effective outcomes in anticipation of this future growth.

The scope of this chapter focuses on the primary TKA. It is referred to as TKA, rather than total knee replacement (TKR), to distinguish it from total knee revision (which is also referred to as *TKR*). In addition, minimally invasive surgery (MIS)-TKA is also described. This new surgical approach may become routine for future patients. As more published results become known and compared with the well-established outcomes of traditional TKA, MIS-TKA may be the next generation in joint arthroplasty surgery. Physical therapists should understand, participate in, and advise on the rehabilitation aspects of this new advancement.

SURGICAL INDICATIONS AND CONSIDERATIONS

TKA is an effective treatment for symptomatic OA or inflammatory arthritis of the knee that is not responsive to conservative therapy. Earlier stages of arthritis may be treated with nonsteroidal anti-inflammatory drugs (NSAIDs), activity restrictions, exercise, bracing, orthotics, and weight loss. Other treatments include injections of hyaluronic acid or cortisone. However, when conservative measures fail and arthritic symptoms limit functional activity, surgery is a more appropriate treatment option. If symptoms are mechanical and associated with catching or locking more than weight-bearing pain, they may result from a torn or degenerative meniscus. Magnetic resonance imaging (MRI) is useful to delineate meniscal pathology from degeneration of the articular cartilage. Arthroscopic débridement may be beneficial for treatment of meniscal pathology but does not appear to be as helpful for management of articular cartilage degeneration.[85] If cartilage degeneration occurs primarily in the medial tibiofemoral (TF) compartment with varus deformity, then valgus osteotomy of the tibia can be effective in relieving medial-sided knee pain and delay the need for total joint replacement.[67] Osteotomy is most appropriate for treatment of unicompartmental OA in a young active patient, a knee with adequate range of motion (ROM), and limited varus deformity. Relative contraindications include obesity, flexion contracture, significant lateral compartment or patellofemoral arthritis, TF subluxation, and advanced age. For lateral compartment OA with valgus deformity, distal femoral rather than proximal tibial osteotomy is preferred. However, osteotomy generally requires a longer rehabilitation period, and outcomes are less predictable than for TKA.[111]

Prosthetic options include metallic interposition hemiarthroplasty, as well as unicompartmental and TKA. The McKeever and MacIntosh metallic interposition hemiarthroplasties were used before the development of TKA.[80,84] The implant is a metallic spacer placed between the femoral and tibial surfaces. Favorable results may be achieved most commonly in a patient with arthritic changes in one compartment who is not considered an appropriate candidate for ostoeotomy because of obesity, limited motion, or arthritic involvement of the opposite compartment.[29,65] However, pain may develop from articulation of the joint surface with the metallic implant. More recently surgeons have become interested in use of a mobile metallic Uni spacer (Centerpulse, Austin, TX), which is intended to distract the medial compartment and transfer loads to the lateral compartment.[47] However, results appear less predictable than unicompartmental or TKA.

Unicompartmental and TKA resurface both the femoral and tibial articlar portions of the joint and are effective in relieving arthritic pain. Unicompartmental arthroplasty is indicated for degenerative arthritis limited to either the medial or lateral TF compartment with preservation of the opposite TF and patellofemoral compartments. Unicompartmental arthropasty preserves both cruciate ligaments, the opposite TF compartment, and the patellofemoral joint, which is typically associated with more favorable knee kinematics, ROM, and overall joint function than TKA. However, failure of the unicondlylar arthroplasty may occur from the development of arthritic symptoms in the patellofemoral or opposite TF compartment, requiring conversion to TKA. Mechanical failure or polyethylene wear may also limit the longevity of unicondylar replacement. Although the indications for use of unicondylar replacement as an alternative to TKA are controversial, unicondylar replacement is generally considered less predictable in terms of longevity of the arthroplasty, particularly when used in situations in which some arthritic involvement of the opposite TF or patellofemoral compartment exists.

TKA is an effective treatment for severe arthritic knee pain. Both the medial and lateral TF and usually the patellofemoral compartments, are resurfaced in TKA. After TKA, reliable improvement in pain and function can be expected, and survivorship rates of 90% to 95% after 10 years have frequently been reported.* **Early failures may result from infection, instability, malalignment, stiffness, reflex sympathetic dystrophy, and patellar problems. Relative contraindications include active infection, extensor mechanism disruption, severe loss of bony or ligament support, and uncontrolled cardiac disease or medical comorbidities that substantially increase the risk of perioperative morbidity and mortality.** However, using proper surgical technique, implant selection, appropriate postoperative pain management, and rehabilitation can avoid these problems. Recent developments including computer-assisted surgery (CAS), more kinematic or high-flexion implant designs, and use of MIS may further improve the results of TKA.

TKA performed through a conventional skin incision centered over the rectus tendon proximally and extending distal to the tibial tubercle, with a medial parapatellar arthrotomy, is associated with reliable pain relief, improvement in function, and 90% to 95% 10-year survivorship.* However, many patients experience significant pain and inflammation, which typically occurs to some extent for 6 months after arthroplasty and may limit participation in rehabilitation exercises. Less invasive or MIS permits TKA to be performed with reduced soft tissue trauma. Early reports indicate that MIS is associated with less blood loss, less pain, and earlier return of quadriceps function and ROM.[46,72,116] However, a minimally invasive approach may compromise surgical exposure and result in increased complications. Minimally invasive total hip arthroplasty has been reported to have a higher complication rate than with use of a standard approach.[123] With use of small cutting blocks and avoiding dissection of the suprapatellar pouch, reliable results can be achieved with a complication rate that is not greater than conventional TKA.[45,72,116] Particularly, when combined with a preoperative patient education program and multimodal postoperative pain management, TKA performed through a minimally invasive approach appears to offer significant advantages compared with conventional TKA. However, more muscular patients, those with prior surgery, stiffness, poor skin vascularity, or significant deformity requiring soft tissue releases may not be appropriate candidates for a minimally invasive approach.

*References 5, 10, 25, 70, 78, 122.

*References 5, 10, 25, 70, 78, 122.

SURGICAL PROCEDURES TRADITIONAL

Preoperative Evaluation

Preoperative evaluation always includes a thorough history and physical examination, determination of the type of arthritis, other joint involvement and status, walking distance, current and expected activity level, and sports involvement. Other significant concerns include history of deep venous thrombosis (DVT) or pulmonary embolus (PE) and previous surgery such as joint replacement, corrective osteotomy, and internal fixation of a hip, femur, or tibial fracture. Close attention is paid to joint alignment (varus or valgus), stability, ROM (especially the presence or absence of flexion contracture), muscle tone, and leg lengths.

Preoperative radiographs are crucial. Ideally they should include bilateral and single-leg-stance weight-bearing films from hip to ankle on one cassette. This combination demonstrates any femoral or tibial deformity and aids in determining overall lower extremity (LE) alignment. The angle between the mechanical and anatomic axis is measured on the femur to ensure that the distal femoral osteotomy will be perpendicular to the mechanical axis and parallel to the proximal tibial osteotomy (Fig. 21-1).

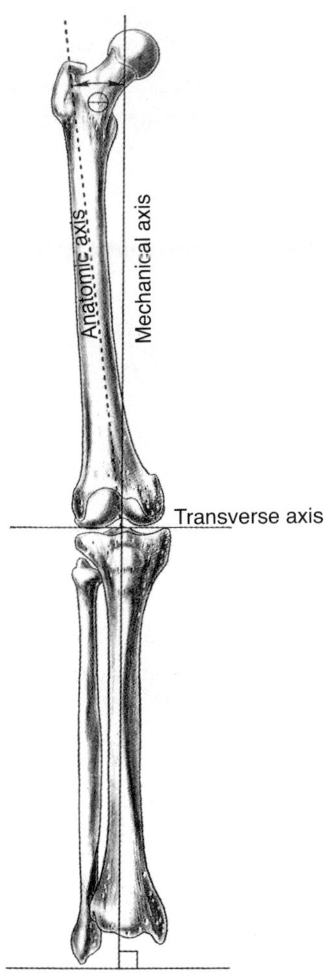

Fig. 21-1 The anatomic axis parallels the femoral shaft, whereas the mechanical axis is a straight line from the center of the femoral head to the center of the knee and the center of the ankle.
(Courtesy Zimmer, Inc., Warsaw, IN.)

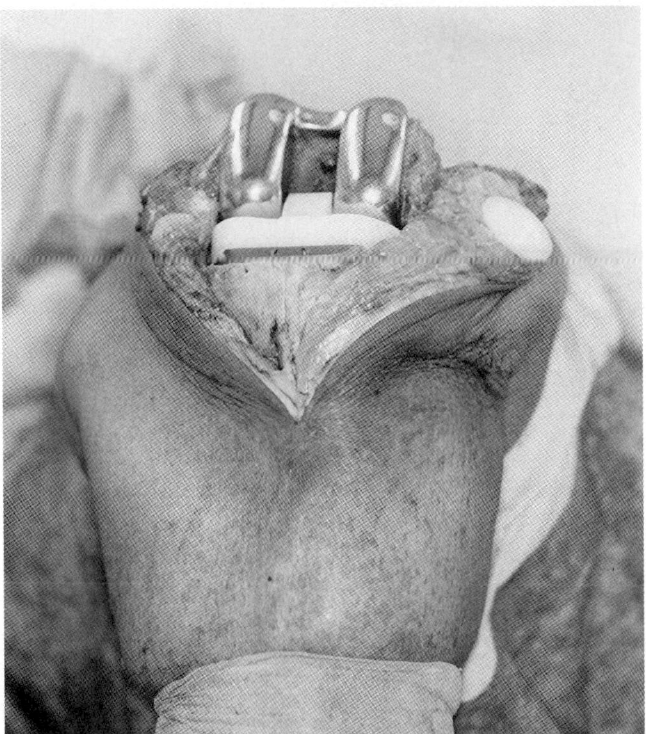

Fig. 21-2 Final result of the author's choice for total knee arthroplasty (TKA). (Note: This is Dr. Vaupel's choice and not Dr. Ries'.)

Routine roentgenograms should also include anteroposterior (AP) standing films, as well as lateral and patellar views.

Procedure

Numerous implant and fixation choices are available for TKA:

1. Cemented, uncemented, or hybrid
2. Metal-backed tibia or all-polyethylene tibia
3. Metal-backed patella or all-polyethylene patella
4. Patella resurfacing or patella retaining
5. Posterior cruciate or bicruciate substituting, posterior cruciate-retaining, or mobile-bearing surfaces

The technique described here is the primary TKA using the cemented implant, metal-backed tibia, all-polyethylene patella with posterior cruciate substitution (Fig. 21-2). Currently this combination is commonly used with consistent long-term results published to date.*

Surgical Technique

An antithrombotic stocking or pump is placed on the uninvolved leg in the preoperative holding area. The patient is questioned as to which knee is to be replaced as a final check to avoid the mistake of operating on the wrong knee. An intravenous antibiotic, usually first-generation cephalosporin, is given before the skin incision is made. The patient is placed supine on the operating room table with a tourniquet about the proximal thigh. A general endotracheal or regional anesthetic is required. A sandbag is taped to the operating room table, or a commercial leg-holding device is often used to help stabilize the leg during the procedure. The entire LE is sterilely prepared and draped. The LE is exsanguinated with an Esmarch bandage, and a tourniquet is inflated to an appropriate pressure.

Exposure

A longitudinal midline skin incision is made extending from proximal to the patella to just distal to the tibial

*References 16, 24, 97, 98, 110.

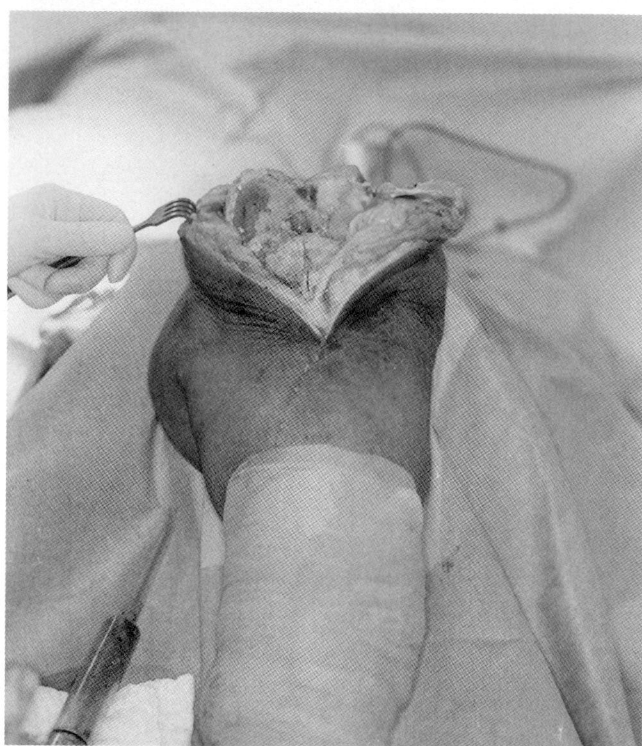

Fig. 21-3 Surgical exposure of the left knee. Note the full-thickness skin flaps, medial arthrotomy, and eversion of the patella. This varus knee demonstrates severe wear of the medial femoral condyle.

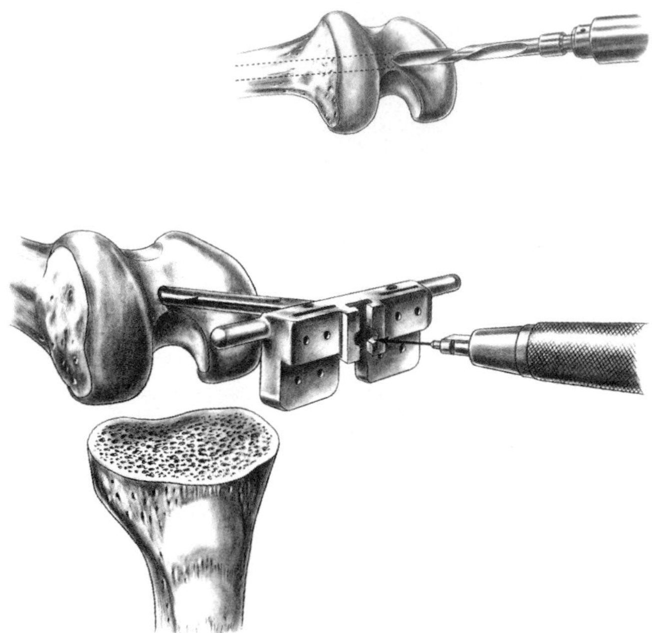

Fig. 21-4 The intramedullary femoral guide ensures placement parallel to the anatomic axis.
(Courtesy Zimmer, Inc., Warsaw, IN.)

tuberosity. Full-thickness skin flaps, including the deep fascia, are developed medially and laterally (Fig. 21-3). Medial arthrotomy is made extending from the quadriceps tendon and ending medial to the tibial tuberosity. The patella is everted laterally. After flexing the knee to 90 degrees, the surgeon trims osteophytes from about the femoral condyles, intercondylar notch, and tibial plateaus. The cruciate ligaments are excised.

Ligament Balancing

Ligamentous balance is then addressed by inserting spreaders in the medial and lateral femoral tibial joints, both in flexion and extension. Equal spacing is then attained by excision of osteophytes and soft tissue releases. The four most common deformities encountered are varus, valgus, flexion, and recurvatum. For deformities with combined varus and flexion contracture, the semi-membranosus insertion is released. Occasionally, in the severe flexed varus deformity, release of the pes anserinus insertion is necessary.

Varus deformity. Osteophytes protruding off the medial tibia are removed and the medial capsule is incised. If necessary, then the medial collateral ligament is subperiosteally stripped off the tibia.

Valgus deformity. A lateral retinacular release is commonly required. The iliotibial band may require Z-lengthening. The popliteus tendon, lateral collateral ligament, and posterolateral capsule may be released, depending on the severity of the deformity. The biceps femoris tendon rarely requires a Z-lengthening. Peroneal nerve neuropraxia may occur, especially with flexion contracture in association with valgus deformity.

Flexion deformity. Excising posterior femoral osteophytes and releasing posterior capsular adhesions usually address a minor contracture. Further correction requires excision of more bone from the distal femur and possible posterior capsular release.

Genu recurvatum. Implanting the components more tightly than usual creates a slight flexion contracture.

Osseous Preparation

The proximal tibia is osteotomized with a power sagittal saw perpendicular to its long axis, approximately 5 mm distal to its articular surface, and angled posteriorly approximately 3 degrees. Either intramedullary or extra-medullary cutting guides are used. Small tibial defects are addressed with cement. Larger defects require either bone grafting or specialized wedge components. Attention is then drawn to the femur. An intramedullary femoral guide is placed through a drill hole in the center of the trochlea (Fig. 21-4). The intramedullary rod must parallel the femoral shaft in both the AP and lateral planes, ensuring placement parallel to the anatomic axis of the femur. Cutting guides are attached to the intramedullary guide to allow precise osteotomies of the anterior and

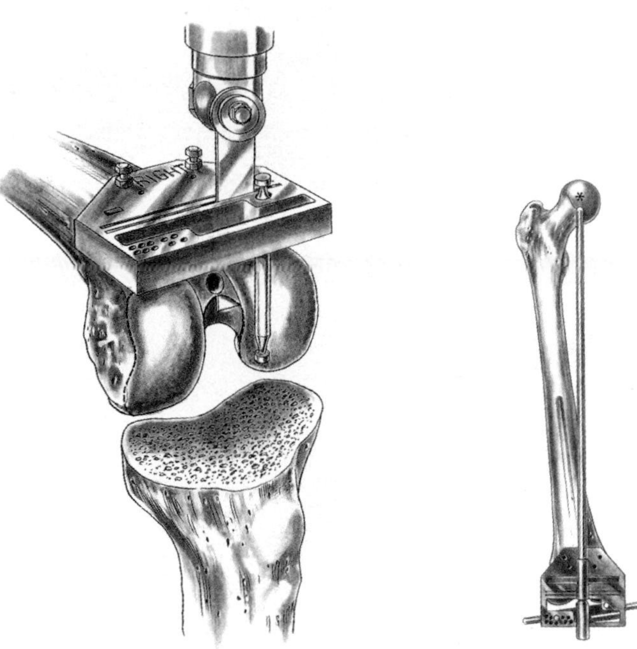

Fig. 21-5 The distal femoral guide attaches to the intramedullary guide with a proper amount of valgus (usually 6 degrees) to ensure the osteotomy is made perpendicular to the mechanical axis.
(Courtesy Zimmer, Inc., Warsaw, IN.)

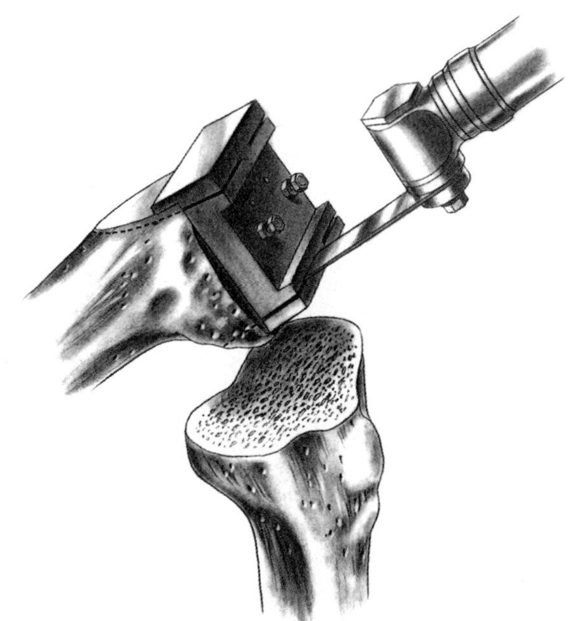

Fig. 21-6 Anterior and posterior femoral osteotomies.
(Courtesy Zimmer, Inc., Warsaw, IN.)

distal femur. The distal femoral osteotomy is usually made 6 degrees to the anatomic axis to produce distal femoral alignment perpendicular to the mechanical axis (Fig. 21-5).

An AP measuring guide is used to determine the appropriate site for the femoral component. An AP cutting

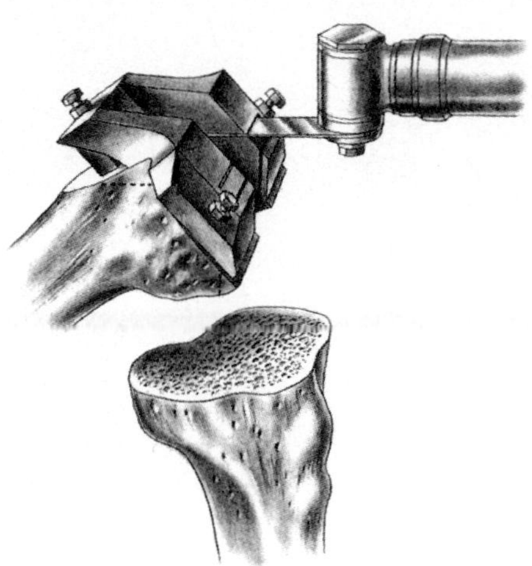

Fig. 21-7 Single guide used to perform anterior and posterior chamfers and remove the intercondylar notch.
(Courtesy Zimmer, Inc., Warsaw, IN.)

guide is placed to remove the anterior and posterior femoral condyles. This affords excellent visibility and access to remove any remaining meniscus, cruciate ligament, and osteophytes (Fig. 21-6).

The flexion and extension gaps are measured with standardized blocks. Ideally, the same gap has been produced between the distal femur and tibia in extension and posterior femur and tibia in flexion. This ensures proper soft tissue tension and ligamentous balance. **If full extension is not attained, then further bone is removed from the distal femur.** For very severe flexion contractures, such as those encountered in some cases of hemophilic arthropathy or juvenile rheumatoid arthritis, resection of the distal femur to the level of the collateral ligament insertions may be required. Further bone resection is a relative contraindication to TKA if the ligament insertions are compromised, and use of a more highly contrained or revision prosthesis is necessary. A guide is then used to chamfer the anterior and posterior femoral condyles and remove the intercondylar notch (Fig. 21-7).

Sizing guides are used to determine the proper-sized tibial component. After orienting the guide in the AP and medial and lateral planes, the surgeon ensures proper rotation with the use of an alignment rod extending to the middle of the ankle joint. A bone punch is then used to compress the soft cancellous bone in the tibial metaphysis to accommodate the keel on the tibial component (Fig. 21-8). Trial tibial and femoral components are placed to ensure proper sizing, soft tissue tensioning, ligamentous balance, and ROM.

The surgeon measures patella thickness with a caliper. The articular surface is removed with a power saw or reamer. A template is used to drill one or more holes in

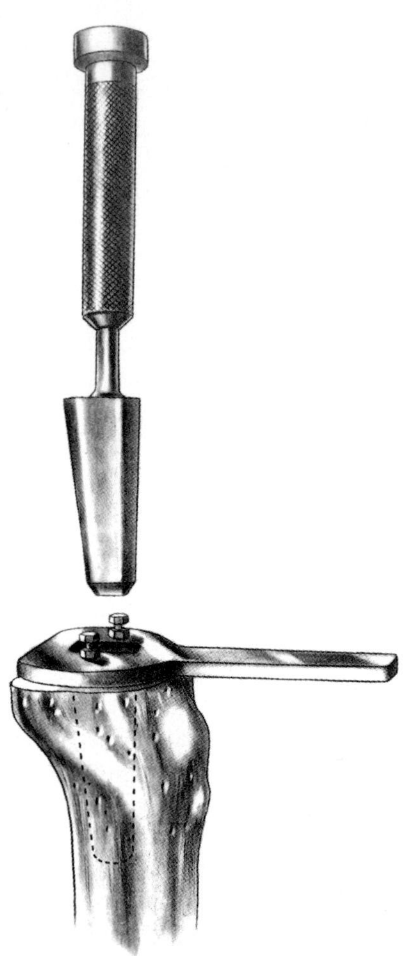

Fig. 21-8 A tibial template is rotationally aligned and sized appropriately to allow proper placement of the tibial stem punch.
(Courtesy Zimmer, Inc., Warsaw, IN.)

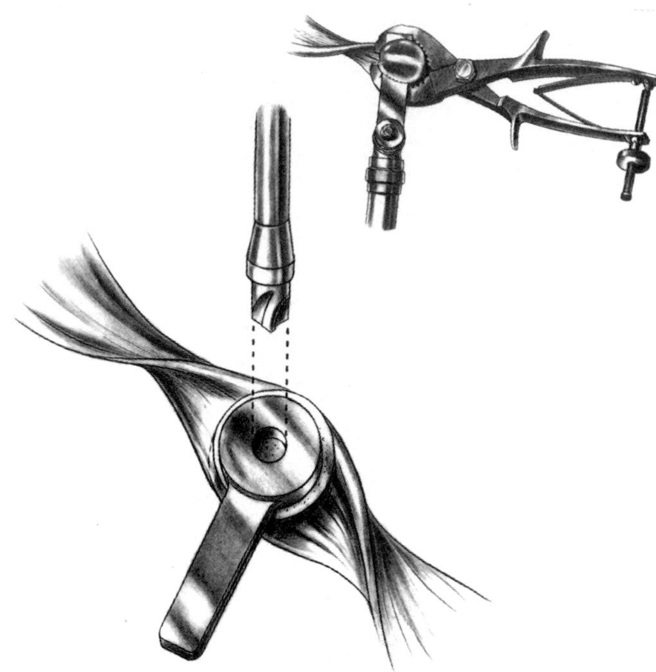

Fig. 21-9 A patella template ensures the proper size and placement of the patella component.
(Courtesy Zimmer, Inc., Warsaw, IN.)

the patella for additional peg fixation (Fig. 21-9). The component is placed slightly medial on the patella to assist in patella tracking. The thickness is again checked with the caliper; if the patella is thicker than before, then more patella is removed to restore normal patella thickness.

Patella tracking is now observed without finger pressure (Fig. 21-10). If the patella tracks laterally, then a lateral retinacular release is performed. Efforts are made to preserve the superior lateral geniculate artery, thereby preserving the blood supply to the patella.

All trial components are removed, the tourniquet is deflated, and bleeding is controlled. The tourniquet is reinflated, all bony surfaces are cleansed with pulse lavage, and bone cement is mixed. All components may be cemented at one time, or a second batch of cement may be prepared to allow sequential implantation of the components. All excess cement is trimmed while soft. After the cement has hardened, the tibial spacer may be exchanged to allow final adjustments with regard to ROM and stability.

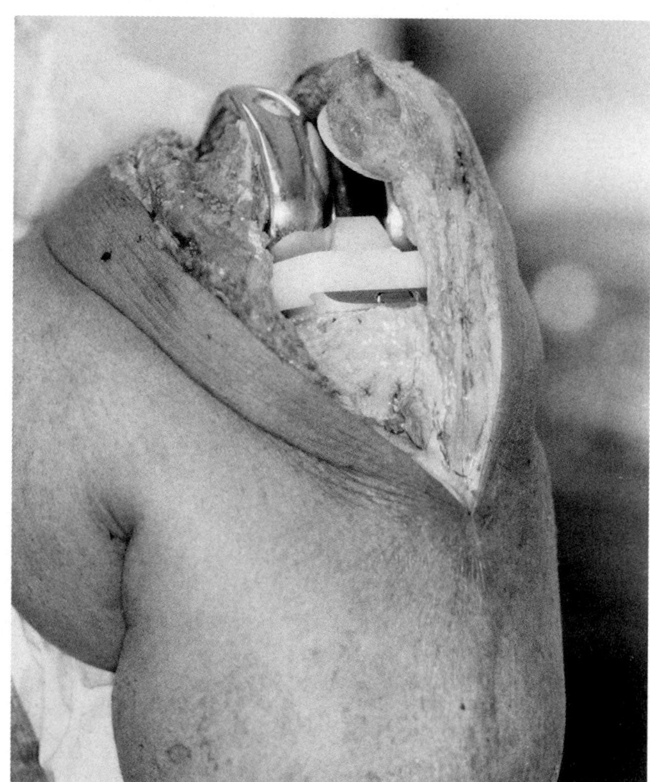

Fig. 21-10 Final component cemented in place. Central tracking of patella without finger pressure should be noted.

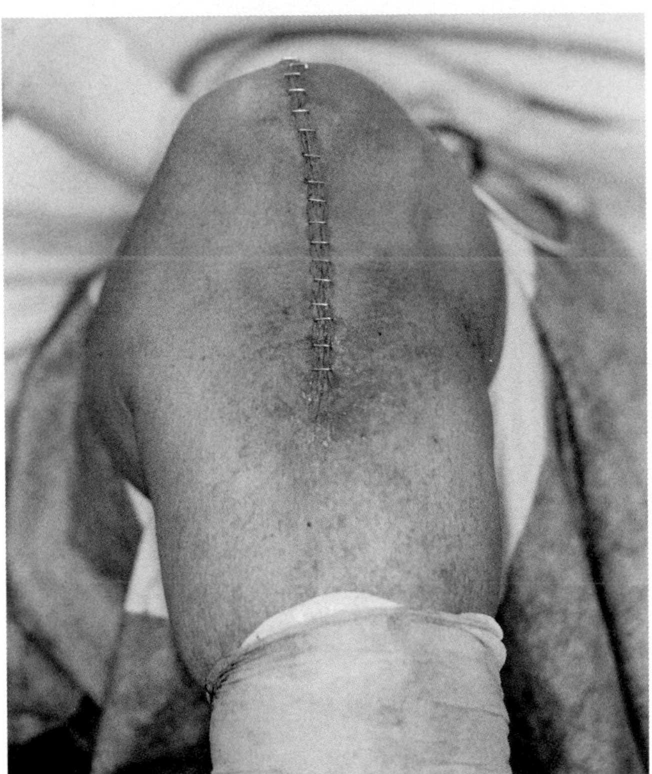

Fig. 21-11 The wound is closed in layers with nonabsorbable sutures in arthrotomy incisions, running absorbable sutures in subcutaneous layer incorporating Scarpa's fascia, and staples in the skin. Suction drainage is performed supralaterally to avoid quadriceps mechanism.

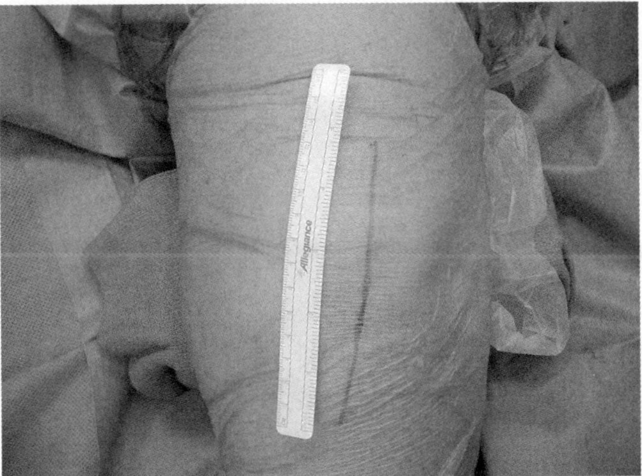

Fig. 21-12 Skin incision extends from the proximal pole of the patella to the tibial tubercle.

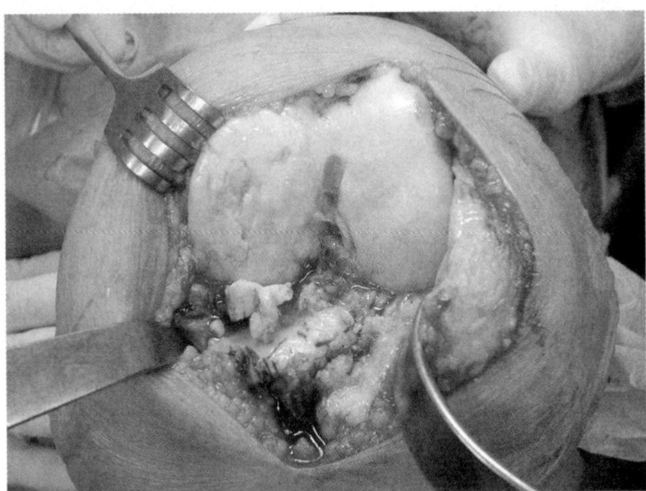

Fig. 21-13 The patella is subluxed laterally but not everted while the knee is flexed.

The wound is irrigated thoroughly and closed over a suction drain. An antithrombotic stocking is applied over a sterile dressing, and the patient is transferred to the recovery room (Fig. 21-11).

MINIMALLY INVASIVE SURGERY

Surgical Technique

The minimally or less invasive skin incision extends from the superior pole of the patella to the tibial tubercle (Fig. 21-12). In most patients the length of the incision is approximately 12 cm, but it may be longer or shorter depending on the size of the patient. Full-thickness skin and subcutaneous tissue flaps are raised to mobilize the superficial skin layer and permit adequate deep exposure.

Either a medial parapatellar, midvastus, or quadriceps-sparing (subvastus) arthrotomy may be used to expose the knee. Excellent results have been reported using the mini-midvastus approach, whereas the quadriceps-sparing approach is more restrictive and may only be appropriate for thin patients with mobile extensor mechanisms and no intra-articular deformity. Typically for muscular male patients, either more proximal dissection of the vastus medialis (in a midvastus approach) or a medial parapatellar arthrotomy is necessary to displace the extensor mechanism laterally. A portion of the fat pad is excised to facilitate exposure. Lateral patellar subluxation is necessary, but eversion of the patella while the knee is flexed does not necessarily increase exposure and may contribute to quadriceps inhibition and postoperative knee pain (Fig. 21-13).

The skin and subcutaneous tissue may be considered as a "mobile window." By extending the knee, the skin incision is moved more proximally and exposure is centered over the distal femur, whereas flexing the knee permits more distal exposure over the proximal tibia (Figs. 21-14, A and B, and 21-15). Cutting guides for minimally invasive TKA are smaller than conventional instruments but permit accurate bone cuts.

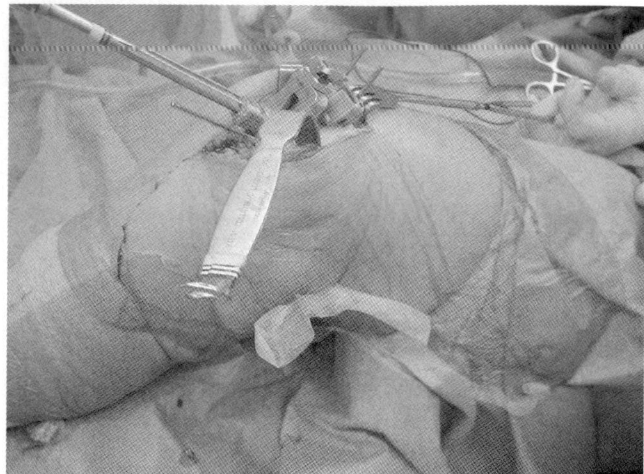

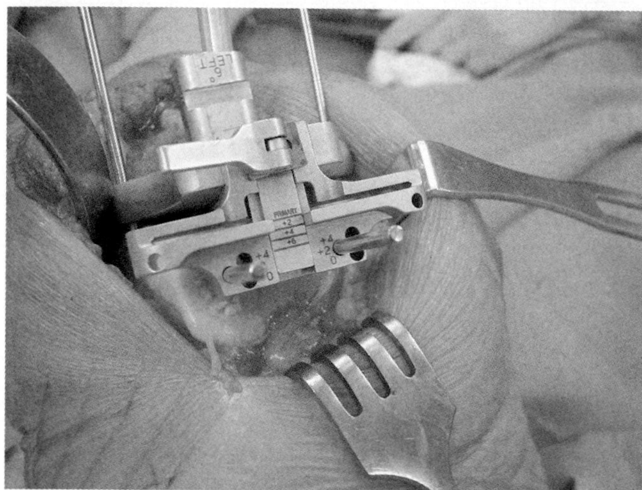

Fig. 21-14 **A,** To expose the distal femur, the knee is partially flexed to 45 to 60 degrees, which moves the center of the skin incision more proximally. **B,** The distal femoral cutting block is positioned, and the distal femoral cut is made with the knee partially flexed.

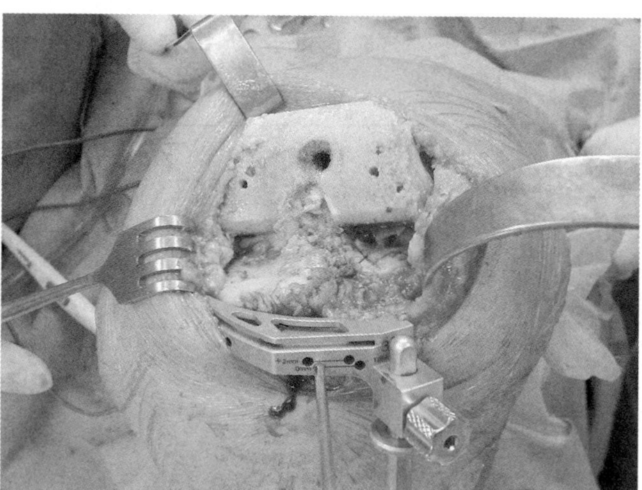

Fig. 21-15 To expose the proximal tibia and resect the tibial surface, the knee is fully flexed.

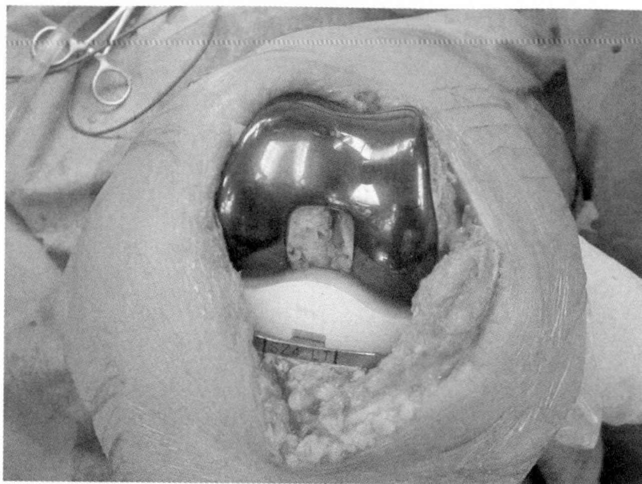

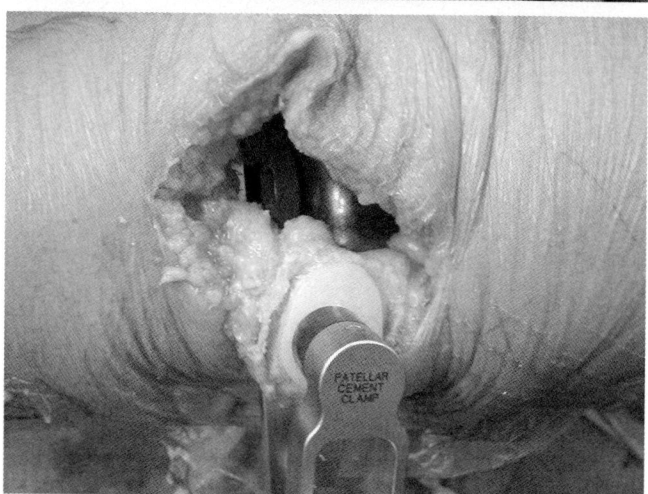

Fig. 21-16 **A,** The femoral and tibial components are implanted. **B,** With the knee fully extended, the patella is everted and resurfaced.

With the knee in extension, tension in the extensor mechanism is reduced and the patella may be everted for resurfacing without traumatizing the suprapatellar pouch (Fig. 21-16, A and B).

THERAPY GUIDELINES FOR REHABILITATION

Successful postoperative management of the patient ideally begins preoperatively. In many cases, the patient has already been seen by a physical therapist (PT) for a conservative course of treatment. Although the goal of rehabilitation at this time may be to avoid surgery, the PT must bear in mind that the treatment plan is similar to those for preoperative care:

1. Patient education regarding the disease process and prognosis

2. Behavioral and health modification for joint protection
3. Cardiovascular conditioning as an adjunct to weight loss
4. An individualized exercise program to address strength and flexibility issues
5. Functional training to maximize the patient's ability

Much can be done for these patients in this phase of the disease process. A successful outcome for postoperative TKA can be predicted by the patient's functional ability and status preoperatively.[69,75,101]

In the event that a TKA is the intervention of choice, then preoperative treatment is modified to include the assembly of a multidisciplinary team. This group includes the orthopedic surgeon, PT, nursing staff, occupational therapist, and social service worker. Although each team member is responsible for his or her area of expertise, all are committed to the common goal of providing the best possible care to get the maximal benefit and outcome.

During this phase the patient should be educated and familiarized with the surgical procedure and the phases of the rehabilitation process. This serves both to identify and anticipate any special problems or needs that the patient should incur. It will also reinforce the active role of the patient in his or her own long-term care. Recommendations may involve home planning, dental hygiene, and social planning.

In the era of managed care, many hospitals have formed preoperative educational classes for this purpose. In a group atmosphere, patients can begin to understand the rehabilitation process and formulate realistic goals and expectations. Informational pamphlets outlining all pertinent information are also helpful. Good preoperative care and communication between the team and the patient can guarantee a smooth transition through the postoperative process.

Phase I (Inpatient Acute Care)

TIME: 1 to 5 days after surgery
GOALS: Prevent complications, reduce pain and swelling, promote ROM, restore safety and independence (Table 21-1)

The goals for this initial period of rehabilitation are standard for any postoperative care. These pertain to the prevention of any possible complications. Medical considerations include (1) the prevention of infection, (2) the prevention of PE, (3) the prevention of DVT, and (4) the reduction of pain and swelling. Functional goals include (1) the promotion of ROM and (2) the restoration of safety and independence in activities of daily living (ADLs) and gait. The treatment plan is formulated with these specific considerations in mind.

Medical Considerations

Intravenous antibiotics are continued for 24 hours. DVT prophylaxis is initiated. This typically consists of antithrombotic pumps, Coumadin, low molecular–weight heparin, or a combination of these treatments.

Monitoring the surgical incision for drainage, erythema, excessive pain, or swelling is continued throughout the patient's stay.

It is vital for the therapist to be aware of the signs and symptoms of wound infection, as well as other complications such as DVT or PE. If signs and symptoms of possible DVT develop, further knee ROM exercises should be restricted until diagnostic testing is completed and DVT is ruled out or an appropriate level of anticoagulation therapy is achieved. Specific signs, symptoms, and tests are discussed in the Trouble Shooting section of this chapter. Any symptom *must* be brought to the immediate attention of the nursing staff and surgeon.

Functional Considerations

Restoration of functional ROM is essential for the success of TKA. Continuous passive motion (CPM) has been used and shown to be beneficial in regaining mobility. CPM may be initiated in the recovery room.

In one study, CPM patients were able to achieve 90 degrees of flexion in 9.1 days versus their non-CPM counterparts, who required 13.8 days to reach the same goal.[14,119] Unfortunately, CPM was found to be ineffective in the enhancement of knee extension.[14,48]

Many surgeons choose to begin immediate postoperative CPM.[87,128] Because of wound concerns, others choose to begin on postoperative day 2.[81] The beneficial effects of CPM include the improvement of wound healing,[103] accelerated clearance of hemarthrosis,[91] reduced muscle atrophy,[4,23] reduced adhesion formation,[18,20,37,92] reduction in the incident of DVT,[79] decreased hospital stay,[41] and decreased need for medication.[12,19] Although excellent function and ROM can be achieved without the use of CPM, many surgeons and patients find that CPM is useful in reducing the frequency of complications after TKA.[42,81,128]

The protocol of CPM application varies in the literature. In general, the initial settings range from zero to 25 to 40 degrees of flexion. The range is then either increased 5 to 10 degrees per day or to patient tolerance. CPM can be used from 4 to 20 hours per day. Its use is discontinued at the end of the acute hospital stay or when maximum knee flexion of the CPM machine is attained.

Another modality that has proven to be useful in improving ROM and quadriceps strength is neuromuscular electrical stimulation (NMES). In conjunction with the CPM, the application of NMES was shown to reduce extensor lag and the length of stay in the acute care setting.[42]

Exercises are taught at bedside beginning on postoperative day 2 or 3.[30,87] Breathing exercises promote full excursion of the rib cage. Ankle ROM exercises (i.e., pumping, circumduction) along with instruction in proper elevation and positioning of the LE is encouraged

Table 21-1 Total Knee Arthroplasty

Rehabilitation Phase	Criteria to Progress to this Phase	Anticipated Impairments and Functional Limitations	Intervention	Goal	Rationale
Phase I Inpatient acute care 1-5 days	Postoperative and cleared by physician to initiate therapy	◆ Edema ◆ Pain ◆ Limited ROM ◆ Limited strength ◆ Limited bed mobility and transfers ◆ Limited gait	◆ CPM setup and patient instruction beginning with 0-40 degrees and progressing 5-10 degrees as tolerated 5-10 hours/day ◆ Inspect wound for drainage, erythema, and excessive pain ◆ Breathing exercises ◆ Patient education to control edema (elevation and pumps) and positioning to prevent knee flexion contracture ◆ PROM—Knee extension and flexion, supine heel slides ◆ Isometrics—Quadriceps, hamstrings, and gluteal sets 10 repetitions three times ◆ AROM—Ankle dorsiflexion, plantar flexion, and circumduction ◆ Transfer and bed mobility training ◆ Gait training with weight bearing as tolerated or as physician orders (using walker or crutches) in immobilizer until adequate quadriceps control is attained After second day, progress to: ◆ Initiation of A/AROM exercises twice daily ◆ AROM—Heel slides (supine and seated) TKEs, SLRs	◆ Independent with the following: (1) Bed mobility; (2) Don/doff clothing, and corset if indicated; (3) transfers; (4) gait using assistive device as appropriate ◆ Demonstrate appropriate body mechanics with self-care and basic ADLs ◆ Independent with gait for 100 feet on level surfaces using appropriate assistive device ◆ Progress self-management of ROM exercises ◆ Decrease pain and edema	◆ Restore ROM of knee ◆ Improve wound healing, reduce adhesion formation, prevent complications ◆ Wound and surgical site protection is important as patient begins to perform exercises and ambulation (Note: Infection and DVT are major postoperative complications of TKA.) ◆ Use gravity feed and muscle pump to minimize edema and prevent DVT ◆ Reduce reflex inhibition of quadriceps resulting from pain and edema ◆ Prepare patient for independence with transfers ◆ Begin to prepare extensor mechanism to accept loads ◆ Restore independence with ambulation ◆ Improve stability of involved LE ◆ Prevent disuse atrophy and reflex inhibition ◆ Prepare for home disposition, facilitate independence

CPM, Continuous passive motion; *ROM*, range of motion; *PROM*, passive range of motion; *ADLs*, activities of daily living; *DVT*, deep venous thrombosis; *TKA*, total knee arthroplasty; *AROM*, active range of motion; *LE*, lower extremity; *A/AROM*, active assistive range of motion; *SLR*, straight leg raises; *TKE*, terminal knee extension.

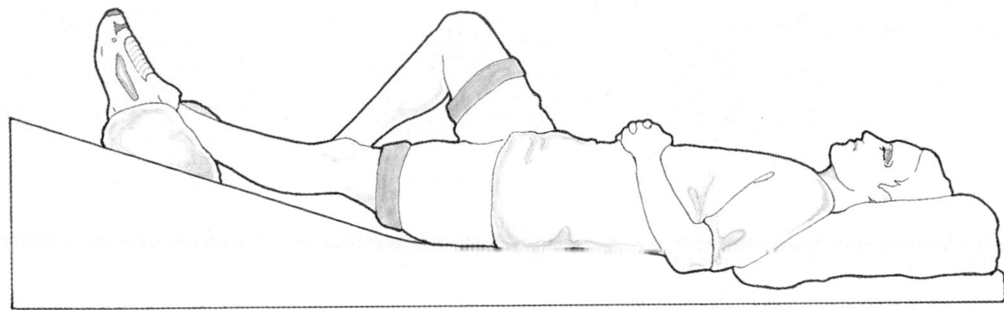

Fig. 21-17 With the leg straight, a pillow is positioned under the ankle to increase end-range extension and venous drainage and decrease compression of the posterior tibial vein.

(Fig. 21-17). The purpose of these exercises are to engage the muscle pump and passive gravity feed to decrease distal edema and avoid DVT.

Isometric gluteal sets, hamstring sets, and quadriceps sets are taught to prevent disuse atrophy and quadriceps reflex inhibition. Patients are encouraged to do these exercises independently, thereby increasing the patient's active participation. It is recommended that this program be initially performed 10 repetitions every hour, and progressed to 20 repetitions, three times daily.[30]

This exercise program is advanced throughout the first week of rehabilitation. Active assistive range of motion (A/AROM) exercises such as seated heel slides or therapist-assisted knee flexion and passive knee extension are performed to improve mobility. Straight leg raises (SLRs) and terminal knee extensions (TKEs) further strengthen the quadriceps muscles, thus improving the dynamic stabilizers of the knee.[30,109] These exercises will become the home program once the patient is discharged.

The patient is also instructed in ADLs such as dressing, bathing, transfers, reaching, and picking up items. Usually this comes under the supervision of the occupational therapist, although in some smaller settings, the PT is responsible. The ADLs should be reviewed and performed until the patient can demonstrate safety and independence. The need for any special assistive devices are assessed and issued.

Progressive gait training begins with a walker or crutches on postoperative day 2 or 3,[30] proceeding throughout the acute care hospitalization. Safety, balance, and patient independence are the primary goals for this intervention. Negotiating level surfaces, ramps, curbs, stairs, or other activities relevant to the patient are practiced.

Current clinical care pathways recommend that the average length of stay in the acute hospital should be approximately 3 to 5 days,[30,86] with physical therapy sessions twice daily. The patient is discharged when deemed medically stable. Specifically, from a rehabilitation standpoint, the patient should be able to demonstrate 80 to 90 degrees of motion,[30] transfer supine to sit and sit to stand independently, ambulate 15 to 100 feet, and ascend and descend three steps[107] or as the home situation dictates.[30] If unable to do these tasks or if any medical postoperative complications occur, then the patient may be transferred to an extended care unit (ECU) or skilled nursing facility (SNF) for further care.

Phase IIa (Inpatient Extended-Care Skilled Nursing Facility)

TIME: 6 to 14 days after surgery

GOALS: Prevent complications, reduce pain and swelling, promote ROM, restore safety and independence (Table 21-2)

The goals of this short-term rehabilitation phase are the same as for in the acute hospital. Treatment efforts continue, with physical therapy scheduled twice a day for a length of stay of approximately 3 to 7 days or until goals are met. Sometimes it becomes necessary to begin training family members or caregivers in assisting the patient during gait and transfers. Social services are often necessary to assist in planning home care needs or placement in long-term care facilities.

Phase IIb (Outpatient Home Health)

TIME: 1 to 3 weeks after surgery

GOALS: Become safe in home environment with transfers, gait, and most ADLs (Table 21-3)

Once discharged home, physical therapy treatments are reduced to 3 times weekly. During this phase of rehabilitation, the goals are expanded to facilitate functional ROM, endure safe and independent ADLs, transfers, and gait in the community. It is important for the therapist to assess the home for safety and make changes as appropriate. Recommendations may include but are not limited to the installation of nonskid rugs, safety rails, ramps, and the elimination of potential obstacles around the house.

The home exercise program initiated in the inpatient setting is reviewed and refined.

If extension mobility is lacking, then more aggressive knee extension exercises are instructed (Fig. 21-18).

Table 21-2 Total Knee Arthroplasty

Rehabilitation Phase	Criteria to Progress to this Phase	Anticipated Impairments and Functional Limitations	Intervention	Goal	Rationale
Phase IIa Extended care or skilled nursing (inpatient) 6-14 days	No signs of infection No significant increase in pain No loss of ROM Discharge from acute care Progressive stiffness, wound drainage, other complications that may preclude home discharge If patient is unsafe for home disposition, transfer to extended care unit (ECU) Discharged to home	• Edema and pain • Limited ROM • Limited strength • Limited gait tolerance	• Continuation and progression of interventions from phase I • Transfer training (car, sit-stand varying seat heights) • Progressive gait training using appropriate assistive device • Aggressive knee extension and flexion exercises • PROM—Flexion (prone and standing) • A/AROM—Flexion (seated, on step, on bicycle) • AROM—SLR, heel raises, leg curls, step-ups, step-downs, one-fourth squats • Joint mobilization • Soft tissue and myofascial release (respecting incision) • Careful ongoing monitoring of edema	• Self-management of pain and edema • Independence with bed mobility and transfers • Independent gait in community distances (300-500 feet) • Knee PROM 0-110 degrees • Advance independence with home exercises • Improve functional LE strength	• CPM may be discontinued if ROM is improving • Prepare for discharge from ECU (transition to home health or outpatient) • Promote return to unassisted gait in the community • Obtain close to if not functional ROM (110 degrees necessary for stair climbing) • Maximize LE strength and stability • Prevent disuse atrophy • Treat hip weaknesses resulting from altered weight-bearing and compensatory postural strategies (Note: Postoperative stiffness is a major complication of TKA. Manipulation criteria varies among surgeons—see text.)

CPM, Continuous passive motion; *ECU*, extended care unit; *PROM*, passive range of motion; *ROM*, range of motion; *A/AROM*, active assistive range of motion; *LE*, lower extremity; *AROM*, active range of motion; *SLR*, straight leg raising; *TKA*, total knee arthroplasty.

Postoperative pain may limit a patient's ability to perform knee ROM exercises. If postoperative pain is not adequately controlled, then more effective pain management strategies should be considered, including inpatient pain management for very severe cases. If knee flexion is limited, then more progressive active and active assistive exercises are given (Fig. 21-19, A to C). Functional strengthening exercises are progressed in both the open and closed-chain positions. Examples of closed-chain exercises are bilateral toe raises, sit-to-stand exercises (Fig. 21-20, A and B), one-quarter squats, and progressive step-ups and step-downs (Fig. 21-21, A and B). Closed-chain exercises have been shown to be highly effective in recruiting the vastus medialis oblique (VMO) and vastus lateralis (VL) as compared with open-chain isometric exercises.[21,44,114] Specific transfers in the home and the car are practiced. Progression in gait includes advancing the patient to crutches or cane as his or her balance dictates. Ambulation on uneven, ramped, and outdoor surfaces are also reviewed. Home physical therapy is discontinued when the patient is not home bound.

Table 21-3 Total Knee Arthroplasty

Rehabilitation Phase	Criteria to Progress to this Phase	Anticipated Impairments and Functional Limitations	Intervention	Goal	Rationale
Phase IIb Home health 2-3 weeks (depending on need for ECU or SNF)	No signs of infection No significant increase in pain No loss of ROM If at home, good family support for assistance with ADLs and safety	Limited ROM Limited strength ◆ Difficulty with gait on uneven surfaces and stairs Unable to attend outpatient rehabilitation (homebound)	◆ Assess home safety and make changes as appropriate ◆ Car transfers and gait training on uneven surfaces ◆ Continuation of exercises as listed previously to increase knee ROM and strength ◆ Progressive weight bearing per physician's orders and patient's ability	◆ Safe and independent in home setting ◆ Independent ambulation using appropriate assistive device ◆ Independent in community distances ◆ ROM 0-110 degrees	◆ Prevent complications such as falling ◆ Return to independent living ◆ Prepare for discharge to outpatient rehabilitation facility ◆ Strengthen lower kinetic chain ◆ Prevent disuse atrophy ◆ 110 degrees of flexion required for stair climbing and use of stationary bicycle ◆ Avoid postoperative contracture and need for manipulation

ECU, Extended care unit; *SNF,* skilled nursing facility; *ROM,* range of motion.

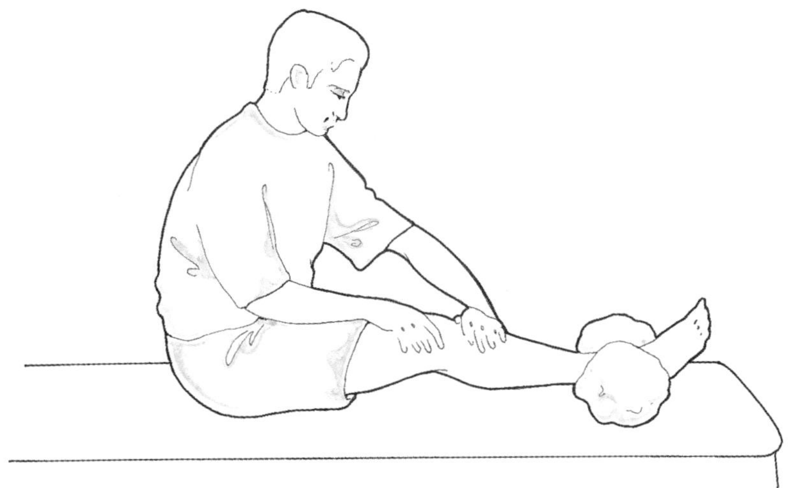

Fig. 21-18 TKE with passive overpressure. With the knee straight, a pillow is positioned under the ankle. Manual overpressure is applied above and below the patellofemoral joint to increase TKE passively.

Q Noreen is a 55-year-old patient who had TKR 7 weeks ago. Her pain levels have prevented ROM gains beyond –8 to 95 degrees. Her preoperative ROM was -5 to 120 degrees. Her ROM in the last week has plateaued and may have even decreased. What should the therapist's next course of care be?

Phase III (Outpatient Care)

TIME: 3 to 8 weeks after surgery
GOALS: Normalize gait; reduce reliance on assistive devices; increase ROM; improve weight bearing, balance, strength, endurance, and proprioception (Table 21-4)

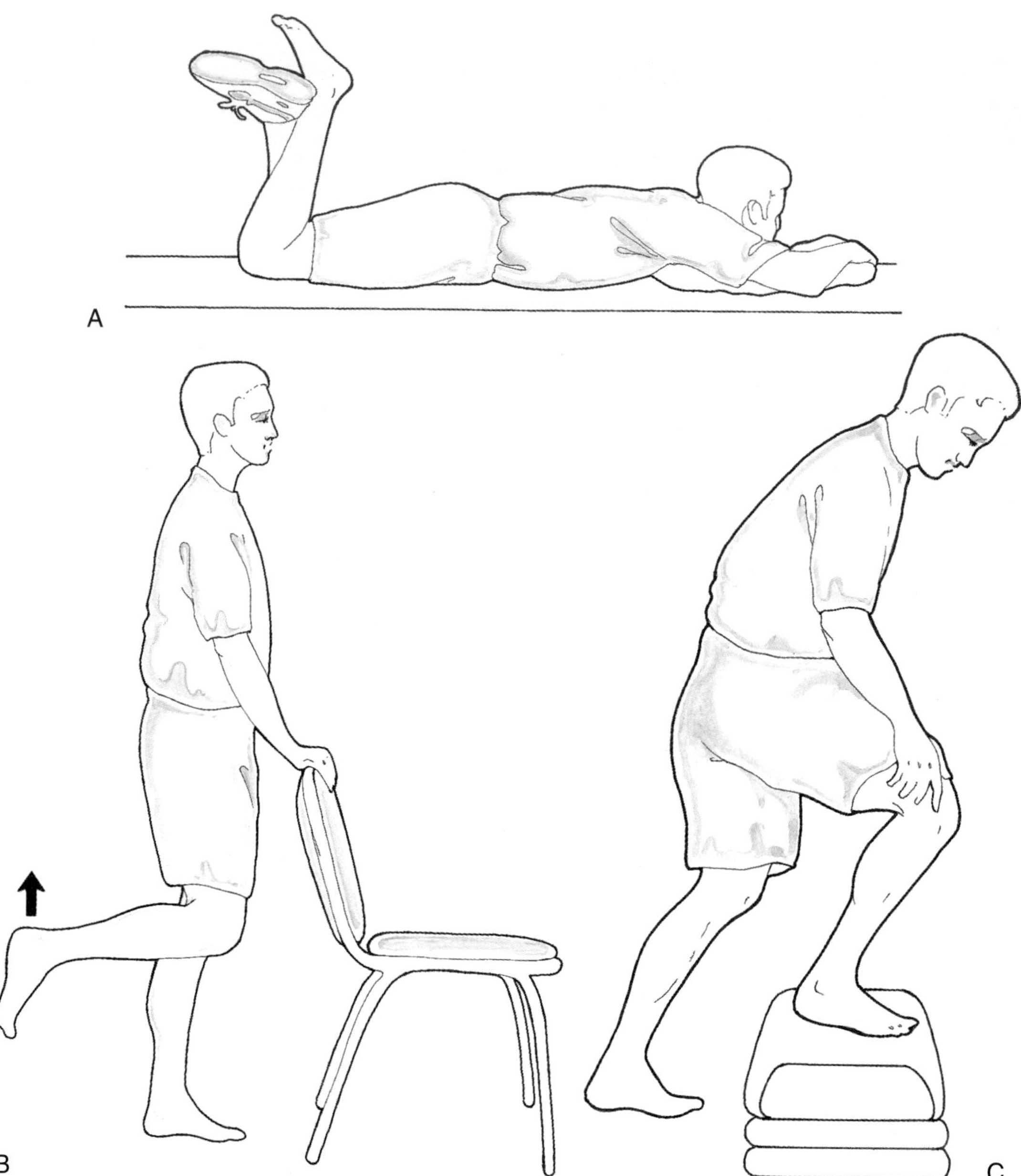

Fig. 21-19 A, Prone knee flexion. In a prone position the patient bends the operated knee as far as possible while using the uninvolved knee to apply passive overpressure to increase knee flexion. B, Standing open-chain knee flexion. In a standing position with upper extremity (UE) support, the patient actively bends the involved knee, bringing the heel to the buttocks while maintaining upright posture. C, Standing closed-chain knee flexion. In a standing position the patient places the foot of the involved leg flat on a step; then the patient places the hands above the knee, slowly leans forward on the involved leg, and guides the knee into more flexion.

This phase of rehabilitation may begin on postoperative week 2 for the highly advanced and active patients or week 3 to 4 for those proceeding slowly. The length of this stage is also dependent on factors such as the patient's goals, and potential functional abilities. It is always recommended that the therapist review the insurance benefits and explain to the patient all options for rehabilitation should there be any insurance limitations.

Common difficulties encountered with TKAs include patellar instability and lack of motion. Routine functional activities usually require ROM from zero to 110 degrees. **Full extension is necessary to normalize the gait cycle[17,52,88] and to facilitate quadriceps strength.[64]** Full normal ROM may not be a realistic goal for all patients. Posoperative ROM may be restricted, particularly if preoperative and intraoperative ROM is restricted. Stair climbing, sitting on a regular toilet seat or chair (17-inch

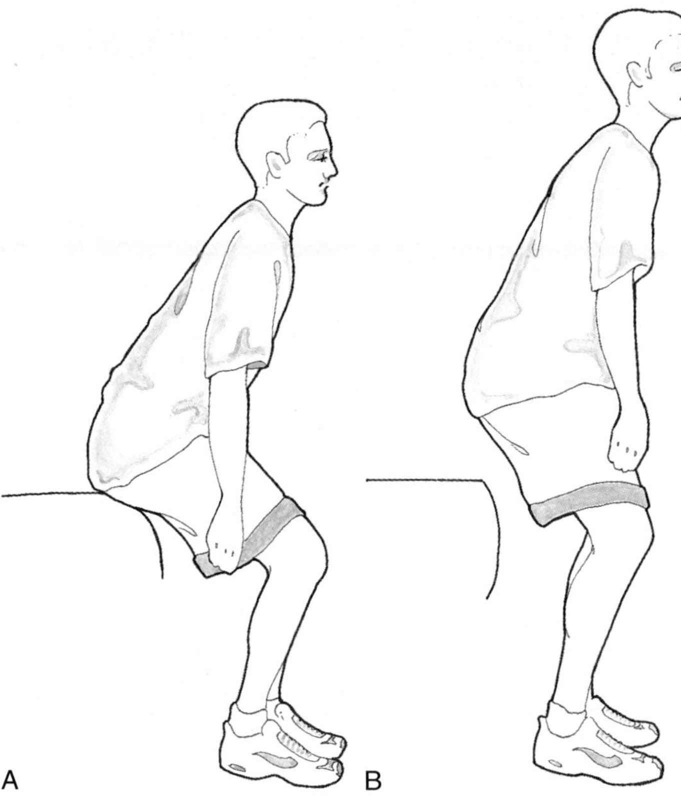

Fig. 21-20 Sit-to-stand exercise. **A,** Start position. **B,** End position. Without using the upper extremities (UEs) for support, the patient practices controlled and balanced sit-to-stand transfers from various heights.

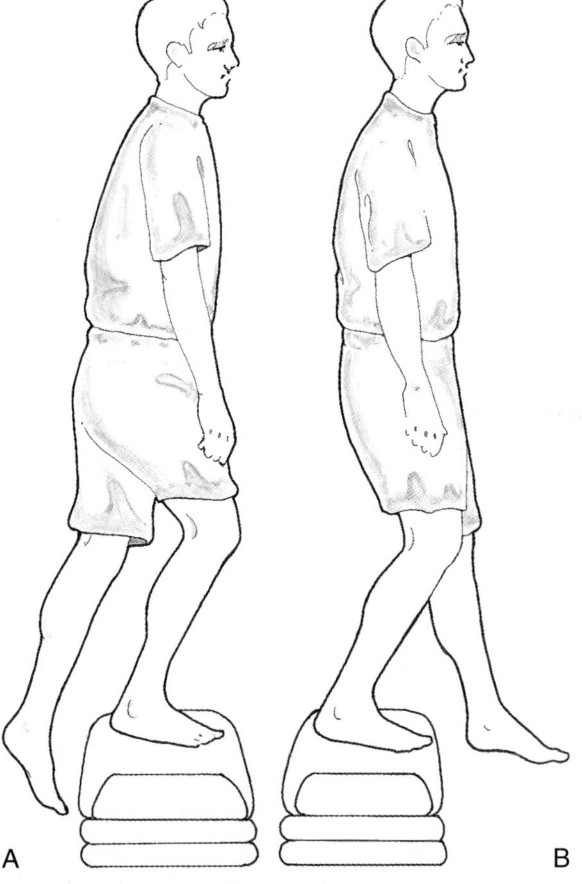

Fig. 21-21 **A,** Step-up progression. Patient practices controlled step-up with the involved leg from progressive heights. **B,** Step-down progression. Patient practices controlled step-downs with the uninvolved leg from progressive heights.

Table 21-4 Total Knee Arthroplasty

Rehabilitation Phase	Criteria to Progress to this Phase	Anticipated Impairments and Functional Limitations	Intervention	Goal	Rationale
Phase III Outpatient care 3-8 weeks	◆ No longer homebound ◆ Safe and independent with ambulation using assistive device ◆ Safe and independent with car transfers ◆ Patients may access outpatient care if caregiver or family member is assisting with transfers and gait	◆ Limited ROM ◆ Limited community ambulation using assistive device ◆ Limited lower extremity strength	◆ Initiate aquatic therapy if available with concurrent land-based treatment ◆ Continuation of ROM stretches and soft tissue procedures ◆ Progression of (repetitions or weight) intensity with previous exercises ◆ Squats, leg press, and bridging ◆ Bicycling, walking, or swimming for cardiovascular conditioning 20 minutes three to five times a week (as indicated per general health issues) ◆ Hip external rotator exercises ◆ BAPs (foam roller) ◆ Return to previous activities (see text)	◆ Normalize gait pattern and reduce reliance on assistive device ◆ Increase ROM to 110-125 degrees or as indicted by comparison with uninvolved knee ◆ Single-leg half-squat to 65% body weight ◆ Full weight bearing with single-leg stance ◆ Improve balance, strength, endurance, and proprioception of LE	◆ Reduce stress on the compensatory muscle and joints to prevent chronic imbalance issues ◆ Aquatic (buoyant) environments allow for increased ease of mobility and load-bearing stresses on joints ◆ Zero-110-125 degrees of flexion required to use bicycle and stairs ◆ Improved extension and flexion reduces compensatory gait patterns such as "hip hiking" ◆ Decrease stress on the uninvolved leg with sit-stand transfers ◆ Increase VMO/VL in closed-chain exercises ◆ Provide aerobic conditioning for weight control ◆ Address hip weakness caused by altered weight-bearing and compensatory postural strategies ◆ Improve tolerance to community ambulation and prevent falls ◆ Resume previous activities to restore quality of life

ROM, Range of motion; *LE,* lower extremity; *BAPs,* balance and proprioception exercises; *VMO,* vastus medalis oblique; *VL,* vastus lateralis.

height), and stationary bike riding requires 110 degrees of knee flexion.[1] If motion is limited, then a manipulation under anesthesia (MUA) may be warranted.

General indications for a manipulation include less than 70 degrees at postoperative week 4[77] or a progressive loss of flexion.[32,77]

Manipulation carries risks of fracture or other complications that may further compromise the outcome of the TKA.[77] Relative contraindications to manipulation include severe osteoporosis and markedly restricted intraoperative ROM. Muscle strength and flexibility imbalances of the hip, knee, ankle, and foot can occur after knee injury or surgery.[27,51,60,64] Reflex inhibition, faulty joint mechanics, altered gait, presurgical disuse atrophy, immobilization, or nerve injury have been shown to cause altered function of the muscles in the lower kinetic chain.[11,93,102,104] Therefore it is essential for the PT to fully assess the entire LE for any loss of ROM or muscle strength and then develop a comprehensive rehabilitation program to address the findings.

A successful plan must include aerobic conditioning for weight reduction.[120] Because obesity (defined as body mass index [BMI]) of more than 30) is often associated with OA, many patients with a TKA are overweight and deconditioned.

Increased forces such as those found in obesity can be the cause of wear to the weight-bearing surfaces.[36,106] One study found that subjects were actually 12 to 13 kg (25 to 30 lbs) heavier and had 4% to 6% more body fat 1 year after TKA.[120] On the other hand, after total joint replacement, many patients have been shown to resume routine walking and recreational activities that improved maximum oxygen consumption 1 year after the surgery.[100] Nonimpact activities such as stationary bicycling, distance walking, and swimming are suggested for cardiovascular conditioning.[106]

Aquatic therapy programs have proven to be effective in rehabilitation of total joint replacements.[15,33,115] The buoyant and warm environment can provide pain relief, increase circulation, and decrease weight bearing for the patient. Many can immediately start to work on ROM, strengthening, and normalizing gait without the assistance of a walker. The therapist can challenge the patient by progressing him or her from shoulder-deep water (approximately 24% weight bearing) to waist-deep water (50% weight bearing).

Changes in equilibrium after LE injuries have been cited in the medical literature.* Balance activities and single-leg exercises should be incorporated to offset any compensatory postural changes that have occurred as a result of decreased weight bearing, altered gait, and pain. The use of rocker boards, half foam rollers, and other balance apparatuses can be helpful to improve the patient's proprioception, balance, and postural control strategies.

In regards to long-term rehabilitation goals, the patient's primary concern should be to maintain a pain-free functional activity level for as long a period as possible. With a TKA, certain restrictions in activities are warranted. Generally those recreational activities and sports that involve high repetitive compression or impact loading are not encouraged because of the possibility of loosening or osteolysis of the joint implant.[3,51,61] Joint forces at the TF interface are 1.5 to 4.0 times body weight when walking,[69] 1.2 times body weight when cycling, and increases to 2.0 to 8.0 times body weight when running.[31] Patellofemoral joint forces show comparable increases. During walking, these are 0.5 times body weight[34] and with running they increase to 3.0 to 4.0 times body weight.[95] Failures of TKAs may occur because of loosening of the implant. Therefore patients with joint replacement are encouraged to participate in those activities that maintain cardiovascular fitness while subjecting the implant to reduce impact-loading stresses.

In the gym, using a treadmill (walking only), ski machine, stair-climbing machine, elliptical machine, or stationary bicycle is acceptable. Outdoor sports that are allowable include golfing, hiking, cycling, cross-country skiing, swimming, fishing, hunting, scuba diving, sailing, and occasional light doubles tennis.[106] Baseball, basketball, rock climbing, downhill skiing, football, martial arts, parachuting, singles tennis, racquetball, running, soccer, sprinting, and volleyball are discouraged.

A A phone call to the orthopedist is warranted to explore if she is appropriate for a MUA. After consultation with the physician, a MUA was scheduled and performed. The patient returned to therapy and gained full extension and 125 degrees of flexion. The patient's post-MUA physical therapy should also include taking medication before her treatments to manage pain and maintain and improve the gains in ROM made from the MUA.

REHABILITATION FOR MINIMALLY OR LESS INVASIVE SURGERY TOTAL KNEE ARTHROPLASTY

Minimally invasive surgery is one of the most recent advancements in primary TKA. Because of the smaller incision, quadriceps muscle and tendon sparing, less intraoperative blood loss, deletion of patella eversion procedure, and reduction of pain, rehabilitation can occur on an accelerated timeline. Shorter hospital stays; less overall use of analgesics; and more rapid return of ROM, strength, and function are the benefits.[8,71,118]

In one observation, hospital length of stay was decreased from 7 days to 2 to 3 days.[89] Physical therapy can begin on postoperative day 1, with ROM, ADLs, and gait training. It has been shown that the average MIS-TKA patient regained 90 degrees of flexion within 3.2 days after surgery.[71]

Depending on the patient's age, motivation, previous function, and fitness level, gait and ADL training is progressed immediately. Early studies after MIS-TKA show that patients used crutches or walkers for 1 to 2 weeks, then advanced to a cane for 1 to 2 weeks thereafter. Many ambulated without the use of an assistive device 4 weeks after surgery. Most were independent with

*References 38, 40, 66, 112, 117.

bed and bath transfers and all other ADLs after 2 weeks. Many were climbing stairs at 1 month and descending stairs at 2 months. Driving is allowed at 3 to 6 weeks.

As with traditional TKAs, light-impact activities such as hiking, swimming, and cycling are permitted when comfortable. High-level activities such as running, skiing, and singles tennis remain unadvised in the long term.[8,89]

MIS-TKA outcomes show that a large percentage of patients were satisfied with the cosmetic benefit as well as the quicker recovery and excellent early function. Patients achieved discharge goals 18% faster than those who had traditional TKA. Good function and knee scores were achieved after 3 to 4 months as compared with the usual 1-year result.[8,71,89]

TROUBLESHOOTING

Although the treatment guidelines given here provide a framework for postoperative rehabilitation of TKA, they should not be used as strict protocols. In fact, modifications are expected, because each patient has individual needs, abilities, and goals. Continual reassessment of the patient's status and subsequent alterations in the treatment plan are necessary to achieve optimal results. The therapist must have the necessary abilities and skills to anticipate any potential complications and implement appropriate changes in the treatment plan. The following section describes additional procedures and modalities that can be used to refine the therapy to meet the patient's individual needs.

Medical Complications

During the initial stage of postoperative care, the most serious complications are wound infection, PE, DVT, persistent joint effusion, and lymphedema. **As previously stated, the therapist must know all symptoms and signs that may indicate any of these medical problems. Any of these complications can severely deter rehabilitation progress in terms of time frame and overall prognosis.**

Wound Infection

Systemic signs of a potential wound infection include patient complaints of feeling cold, shivering, breaking out in goose bumps, feeling cold in the extremities, and exhibiting minimal diaphoresis. Knee flexion can increase skin tension. If skin necrosis develops, then ROM exercises should be limited until adequate soft tissue healing has occurred. Other symptoms of infection include increased warmth and erythema about the surgical site, passive drainage, and an increase in body temperature up to 104° F.[68] Wound dressings should be checked and changed daily until the staples are removed.[1] Although uncommon (less than 1%), infection remains a serious problem, usually requiring additional surgery and intravenous antibiotic therapy.

Methods to reduce infection include proper skin preparation and drape; prophylactic antibiotics, such as cephalosporin or vancomycin before surgery; local antibiotics in cement, particularly for immune-compromised patients (e.g., rheumatoid arthritis, diabetes mellitus, human immunodeficiency virus [HIV], cancer); and minimizing the length of surgery and tissue trauma.[96]

Q John is 69 years old. He had a left TKR 8 days ago. He is now semireclined in his hospital bed. When the therapist helps him out of bed during transfer, John complains of feeling light-headed. He usually requires a few moments for his head to clear, but today he needs a little more time to adjust. Gait training is initiated, and suddenly Marc has difficulty breathing. What do these symptoms indicate?

Pulmonary Embolus

PE is a potentially fatal, but rare, complication. PE can be life threatening and requires prompt diagnostic testing and treatment. Patients at risk for PE are those who may have proximal lower extremity deep vein thrombosis (PDVT). PDVTs are located at or proximal to the trifurcation of the popliteal vein and considered the more dangerous form of LE DVT, because the thrombi are larger than those associated with calf DVT and are more likely to lead to PE.[99]

Clinical signs of PE include tachycardia, distended cervical veins, hypotension, and chest pain. Pulmonary symptoms include tachypnea, rales, wheezing, and pleural effusion.[68] Sudden dyspnea is the most frequent symptom. Pleuritic pain is also common in patients with severe embolization. If any of these signs or symptoms occur, then the PT should immediately notify the nursing staff and physician.

A Rapid heart rate, hypotension, and dyspnea are signs of a possible PE—a potentially fatal complication. Cardiovascular signs may include tachycardia, distended jugular veins, hypotension, and chest pain. Pulmonary symptoms include tachypnea, rales, wheezing, and pleural effusion. Sudden dyspnea is the most common symptom.

Deep Venous Thrombosis

Because of decreasing lengths of hospitalization, patients are seen in outpatient settings with elevated risks of DVT. Significant signs and symptoms of DVT include complaints of pain and swelling in the involved extremity, calf tenderness, and a positive Homans' sign. Specifically, the patient may report a dull ache, tight feeling, or frank pain in the calf or entire leg. The signs and symptoms include slight swelling in the involved calf; distention of the superficial venous collaterals; tenderness, induration, or spasm of the calf muscles, with or without pain, produced by dorsiflexion of the foot (Homans' sign); warmth of the affected leg when both legs are exposed to room temperature; and a slight fever or tachycardia.[66] However, DVTs are also often asymptomatic. When signs and symptoms of possible DVT develop, further ROM exercises should be restricted until definitive diagnostic testing is performed.

Additionally, improved assessment of risk for DVT can be obtained by the use of a clinical decision rule (CDR). A series of studies found that patients could be categorized into low-, moderate-, and high-risk groups based on their CDR scores. The use of the CDR may aid in improving the accuracy of probability estimates of DVT and subsequent referral decisions.[99]

Persistent Joint Effusion

A patient sometimes complains of postoperative stiffness, pain, and swelling. The patient should be reassured that this usually resolves within the first few weeks after surgery. **Persistent joint effusion can forestall the rehabilitation process.** Knee ROM exercises can be continued if an effusion is present, but the effusion may limit motion and should be treated with ice before and after exercise. Soft tissue mobilization is an effective procedure that can enhance muscle recovery and reduce soreness after intense physical activity.[13,73] Increasing blood flow may increase oxygen delivery to the injured tissue, enhance healing, and restore homeostasis.[54] If edema, swelling, and inflammation are significant factors in muscle soreness sensation,[108,113] then massage may be able to reduce soreness in the involved muscles. Persistent effusion may be aspirated, not only to relieve pressure and stiffness but also to rule out an indolent infection.

Lymphedema and Total Knee Arthroplasty

Lymphedema is abnormal swelling caused by the presence of excess lymphatic fluid within the tissues. This swelling occurs when the lymphatic system malfunctions or is damaged from a decrease in developmental transport capacity of the lymph vessels, trauma, surgery, radiation, or infection.

Although lymphedema is a minor complication, persistent swelling can occur.[126]

Lymphedema, which is present before surgery, should be minimized with use of support stockings and, if necessary, diuretic medications. If lymphedema develops after surgery, rehabilitation can be continued, but compressive stockings should be used to limit the amount of swelling. Because abundant lymph vessels are found at the medial aspect of the knee, trauma to this area or surgery can lead to lymphedema. Lymph flow swelling in this area of bottleneck occurs as a result of tissue trauma in this area. A patient who has venous insufficiency and undergoes TKA also has an increased risk of developing lymphedema postoperatively.[90,126]

In treating lymphedema, therapy consists of manual lymph drainage, special compressive bandaging, exercise, and skin care. With proper treatment, edema can be reduced by as much as 60% and in some cases up to 74%. Once the limb is reduced, the patient graduates from the compressive bandages to a proper compression class stocking. Anti-embolism stockings, such as T.E.D.® hose stockings[129] (12 to 20 mm Hg), are worn postsurgery as DVT prophylaxis from bed rest, mild edema, or mild varicosities. Class I (20 to 30 mm Hg) are used for mild lymphedema, mild venous insufficiency, moderate varicose veins, or DVT prevention in individuals with clotting disorders. Higher grades of Class II to IV (30 to 50+ mm Hg) are available for individuals with moderate to severe lymphedema, cardiovascular insufficiency, or prevention of DVT in postthrombotic syndrome.[90,121]

Q Gemma is 55 years old. She had severe degenerative joint disease in her right knee and underwent a TKR 8 weeks ago. She says the pain around the knee has considerably decreased. However, she complains of pain around the area of the fibular neck. The area also is sensitive to palpation. Gemma has intermittent pain radiating down the lateral surface of the lower leg. What is the probable cause of these symptoms?

Functional Complications

A The peroneal nerve travels around the fibular neck. The symptoms described indicate peroneal nerve irritation. On further investigation the PT noted altered sensation over the dorsum of the foot, with the exception of the first web space. In addition, right dorsiflexion and eversion strength both equaled 4/5 – 5/5 (5/5 is "normal" strength on a manual muscle test [MMT]). Normal strength was demonstrated throughout the left LE. Dural nerve root stretches for the sciatic and peroneal nerve were initiated. After the first treatment using nerve tissue mobilization to target these nerves, strength returned to normal for dorsiflexion and eversion. After three treatments using dural mobilization, the pain was decreased by 90% and the sensation tested normal.

Peroneal Nerve Neuropraxia

Peroneal nerve neuropraxia may arise more frequently in patients with (1) flexion contractures associated with valgus deformity, (2) those who had epidural anesthesia for postoperative control of pain or previous laminectomy, and (3) those who had a previous proximal tibial osteotomy.[55]

In peroneal nerve neuropraxia, the common peroneal nerve and its branches are tethered at the fibular neck. Clinical findings of nerve entrapment or injury include local tenderness around the fibular neck with pain, diminished sensation, or paresthesia radiating over the lateral surface of the lower leg and the dorsum of the foot.[65,94] Nerve conduction velocity testing and electromyographic (EMG) studies will be positive for neuropathic dysfunction in the motor distribution of the common peroneal nerve distal to the injury or entrapment site at the fibular neck. Clinically, the patient displays an inability to walk or stand on the heel because of the weakness of the ankle dorsiflexors. Additionally, instability when attempting toe walking results from the muscle imbalance and associated sensory abnormalities at the ankle joint. The muscles affected are those in the anterior and lateral compartments of the leg.

When the superficial peroneal nerve is compressed, a decrease in sensation is noted over the dorsum of the foot, with the exception of the first web space. The involvement of the deep peroneal nerve produces a diminution of sensation in the first web space of the foot and affects the muscles of the anterior compartment, including the extensor hallucis brevis and the extensor digitorum brevis.

Complete common peroneal nerve palsy results in a severely affected gait pattern. Without an ankle-foot orthosis, the patient suffers from a foot drop with associated steppage gait in profoundly affected cases or foot slapping in milder ones. The ankle is unstable and vulnerable to ankle inversion sprains. The functional result of partial peroneal nerve palsy depends on which nerve components are the most affected. Loss of the peroneal muscles in the lateral compartment results in a chronically inverted foot, with weight bearing occurring more laterally than normal and invariably affecting the position and stability of the foot and ankle throughout the stance phase of the gait cycle. Loss of the anterior compartment muscles, especially the tibialis anterior, affects the entire gait cycle. The loss of the dorsal intrinsic muscles of the foot has a relatively minor effect on basic weight-bearing functions.

Physical therapy interventions for nerve entrapment include examination of the joint mechanics of the proximal and distal tibiofibular joints and determination of the specific muscle weakness and sensory loss. Manual techniques include joint mobilization as appropriate, facilitation of the recruitment of the affected muscles, and dural nerve root stretches for the sciatic and peroneal nerves.

Q Sharon is a 60-year-old patient who had TKA 4 weeks ago. She complains that her operative leg is shorter than the other leg. No preoperative leg length difference was noted, and the physician noted that there were no relative changes made that would account for decreased leg length. What possible explanation could there be for this?

Muscle Imbalance

A detailed evaluation of the entire lower kinetic chain is necessary for the successful treatment of patients with TKA. Altered gait, faulty mechanics, and muscle imbalances have more than likely existed before the TKA. These factors contribute greatly to the eventual surgical outcome.

Most of the present understanding regarding muscle imbalances and neuromotor retraining comes from the work of Janda,[58,59] Lewit,[74] and Sahrmann.[104] Muscle imbalance is a multifactorial problem and can be highly complex. In simplistic terms, the result of muscle imbalance is that the tight muscles become tighter, weak muscles become weaker, and motor control becomes asymmetric.[43]

According to Janda,[58,59] muscle balance is continually adapting the body's posture to gravity. When an injury occurs, faulty posture and weight bearing alter the body's center of gravity, which initiates mechanical responses requiring muscle adaptation. Change in the mechanical behavior of a joint causes neuroreflexive alteration of muscle function through aberrant afferent mechanoreceptor stimulation of articular reflexes.[9]

Postural-tonic muscles respond to dysfunction with facilitation, hypertonicity, and shortening. Dynamic-phasic muscles respond with inhibition, hypotonicity, and weakness. In the lower quadrant, Janda[58,59] identified a common pattern of muscle imbalance. Hyperactive muscles include the iliopsoas, rectus femoris, tensor fascia latae, quadratus lumborum, the thigh adductors, piriformis, hamstrings, and the lumbar erector spinae musculature. Muscles that display inhibition or reflexive weakness include the gluteus maximus, medius, and minimus; quadriceps (vasti); rectus abdominis; and external and internal obliques. Sahrmann,[104] Dorman et al,[26] and Bullock-Saxton, Janda, and Bullock,[11] similarly identified weakness in the entire LE in the presence of knee dysfunction.

Quadriceps weakness, especially in the early stages of TKA rehabilitation, must be addressed. A knee immobilizer may be needed for ambulation in the hospital setting if quadriceps strength is not great enough to stabilize the knee. Biofeedback or NMES can be beneficial in "jump starting" the recruitment of the quadriceps. In cases of patella instability, quadriceps strength should be restored as soon as possible. Soft tissue work, friction massage, and assisted stretches to the iliotibial band (ITB) may be beneficial.

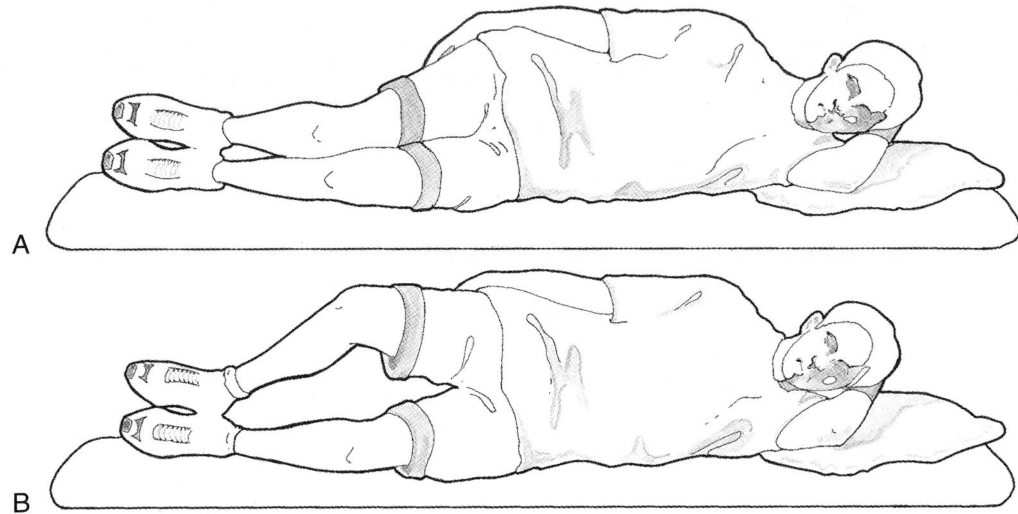

Fig. 21-22 Hip lateral rotation. **A,** Start position. The patient lies on the uninvolved side with the shoulders and hips perpendicular to the table and the knees flexed to 45 degrees. **B,** End position. The patient then lifts the top knee toward the ceiling, keeping the feet in contact. The patient should emphasize movement from the hip and not allow the pelvis to roll backward.

Faulty joint mechanics at the hip, knee, and ankle affect the overall surgical result. A study by Dorman et al[26] found that inhibition or facilitation of the gluteus medius is influenced by the position of the sacroiliac joint. An anterior rotation (an apparent long leg) manifested a significantly weaker muscle than one in posterior rotation (an apparent short leg). Exercises that address gluteus medius weakness include hip abduction and lateral hip rotation (Fig. 21-22).

Altered ankle movements and instability disturb the overall sense of balance and influence gait safety accordingly. Joint mobilization techniques to correct associated dysfunctions in the joints of the LE can be helpful. A stiff knee can be helped with contraction and relaxation techniques to the muscles that may be guarding or fatigued.[15,77]

> **A** Upon further evaluation it was found that the patient had a posteriorly rotated ilium, creating an apparent leg length difference. Faulty joint mechanics at the hip, knee, and ankle affect the overall surgical result. Manual techniques and exercises were used to address the posterior rotation. Exercises that address gluteus medius weakness include hip abduction and lateral hip rotation (see Fig. 21-22).

OUTCOMES

TKA is a method to improve "quality" of life. This is accomplished primarily through pain relief, resulting in increased functional mobility. Results are generally reported using the Hospital for Special Surgery[56] or the Knee Society[57] rating systems. Haas' patients[46] from the Hospital for Special Surgery who had MIS showed favorable outcomes (Table 21-5) compared with the traditional TKA. They were able to do a SLR on postoperative day 1, walk without a cane on postoperative day 8, alternate stair climbing by week 6, and full knee ROM by week 8.

It should be noted that despite extensive rehabilitation efforts, various studies have shown outcomes of diminished functional capacity. Self-report measures of perceived abilities indicate that at 1 year after TKA, most individuals have regained 80% of normal function. However, stiffness and pain occasionally still remained a problem.[35,83,112] Lingard's study[75,76] showed that the most improvement in pain reduction and functional improvement was made in the first 3 months after TKA, with little change after 12 months.[22,62] Walsh et al[120] also showed that at 1 year after TKA, little pain was noted during activities of walking, stair climbing, and concentric muscle testing. Slower walking speeds for both males and females were reported (62% and 25% decrease at normal pace

Table 21-5 Functional Outcomes—Minimally Invasive Surgery Compared with Traditional Total Knee Arthroplasty

Functional Measure	Minimally Invasive Surgery (MIS)	Traditional Total Knee Arthroplasty (TKA)
◆ Straight leg raise (SLR)	◆ Postoperative day 1	◆ Unable to do SLR
◆ Walk without a cane	◆ Postoperative day 8	◆ Days 6-14 with assistive device
◆ Knee flexion at 3 months postoperatively	◆ 122-degrees flexion	◆ 110-degrees flexion
◆ Knee flexion at 1 year postoperatively	◆ 125-degrees flexion	◆ 116 degrees-flexion

and 31% and 6% decrease at fast pace, respectively). Clinical relevance points to the fact that 17% of these individuals were not able to cross safely at a typical city intersection. Other recent studies have shown slower sit-to-stand and up-and-go tests,[50] quadriceps weakness,[81,103] and smaller girth circumference[103] for individuals at greater than 1 year after surgery.

With these studies in mind, the development and implementation of a well-designed, comprehensive treatment plan is paramount. Addressing the entire lower quadrant with an appropriate exercise program will only serve to enhance the course of rehabilitation and ensure a more successful outcome.

References

1. Aliga NA: New venues for joint replacement rehab, *Adv Dir Rehab* 17(4):43, 1998.
2. American Academy of Orthopaedic Surgeons: *Osteoarthritis of the knee—a compendium of evidence-based information and resources,* San Francisco, 2004, the Academy.
3. Amstutz HC et al: Mechanism and clinical significance of wear debris-induced osteolysis, *Clin Orthop* 276:7, 1992.
4. Anderson MA: Continuous passive motion. In Iglarsh ZA, Richardson JK, Timm KE, editors: *Orthopaedic physical therapy clinics of North America,* vol 1, Philadelphia, 1992, WB Saunders.
5. Berger RA et al: Long-term follow-up of the Miller-Galante total knee replacement, *Clin Orthop* 388:58, 2001.
6. Boldt JG et al: *Comparison of isokinetic strength in resurfaced and retained patella in bilateral TKA.* Scientific exhibit presented at the 71st Annual Meeting of the American Academy of Orthopedic Surgeons, San Francisco, March 2004.
7. Bong MR, DiCesare PE: Stiffness after total knee arthroplasty, *J Am Acad Orthop Surg,* 12(3):164, 2004.
8. Bonutti P: *Minimally invasive total knee arthroplasty—two year follow-up.* Paper presented at the 71st Annual Meeting of the American Academy of Orthopedic Surgeons, San Francisco, March 2004.
9. Bookout MR, Geraci M, Greenman PE: *Exercise prescription as an adjunct to manual medicine.* Course notes, Tucson, AZ, March 1997.
10. Buehler KO et al: The press-fit condylar total knee system: 8- to 10-year results with a posterior cruciate-retaining design, *J Arthroplasty* 15:698, 2000.
11. Bullock-Saxton JE, Janda V, Bullock MI: Reflex activation of gluteal muscles in walking, *Spine* 18(6):704, 1993.
12. Burks R, Daniel D, Losse G: The effect of continuous passive motion on anterior cruciate ligament reconstruction stability, *Am J Sports Med* 12:323, 1984.
13. Cafarelli E, Flint F: The role of massage in preparation for and recovery from exercise, *Sports Med* 14:1, 1992.
14. Chiarello CM, Gunderson L, O'Halloran T: The effect of continuous passive motion duration and increment on range of motion in total knee arthroplasty patients, *J Orthop Sports Phys Ther* 25(2):119, 1997.
15. Cocchi R: No pain with gain—aquatic total knee replacement therapy, *Adv Phys Ther* 8(3):7, 1997.
16. Colizza WA, Insall JN, Scuderi GR: The posterior stabilized total knee prosthesis. Assessment of polyethylene damage and osteolysis after a 10 year minimum follow up, *J Bone Joint Surg* 77A:1713, 1995.
17. Corcoran PJ, Peszczynski M: Gait and gait retraining. In Basmajian JV, editor: *Therapeutic exercise,* ed 2, Baltimore, 1978, Williams & Wilkins.
18. Coutts RD: Continuous passive motion in the rehabilitation of the total knee patient, its role and effect, *Orthop Rev* 15(3):126, 1986.
19. Coutts RD et al: The effect of continuous passive motion on total knee rehabilitation (abstract), *Orthop Rev* 7:535, 1983.
20. Coutts RD, Toth C, Kaita JH: The role of continuous passive motion in the rehabilitations of the total knee patient. In Hungerford DS, Krackow DA, Kenna RV, editors: *Total knee arthroplasty: A comprehensive approach,* Baltimore, 1984, Williams & Wilkins.
21. Cuddeford T, Williams AK, Medeiros JM: Electromyographic activity of the vastus medialis oblique and vastus lateralis muscles during selected exercises, *J Man Manip Ther* 4(1):10, 1996.
22. Dalury DF et al: The long term outcome of TKA patients with moderate loss of motion, *J Knee Surg* 16 (4):215, 2003.
23. Dhert WJA et al: Effects of immobilization and continuous passive motion of postoperative muscle atrophy in mature rabbits, *Can J Surg* 31:185, 1988.
24. Diduch DR et al: Total knee replacement in young active patients. Long term follow up and functional outcome, *J Bone Joint Surg* 79A(4):575, 1997.
25. Dixon MC et al: Modular fixed-bearing total knee arthroplasty with retention of the posterior cruciate ligament. A study of patients followed for a minimum of fifteen years, *J Bone Joint Surg* 87A:598, 2005.
26. Dorman TA et al: Muscles and pelvic clutch, *J Man Manip Ther* 3(3):85, 1995.
27. Elmqvist L et al: Does a torn anterior cruciate ligament lead to change in the central nervous system drive of the knee extensors? *Eur J Appl Physiol* 58:203, 1988.
28. Elmqvist L et al: Knee extensor muscle function before and after reconstruction of the anterior cruciate ligament tear, *Scand J Rehabil Med* 21:131, 1989.
29. Emerson R, Potter T: The use of the McKeever metallic hemi-arthroplasty for unicompartmental arthritis, *J Bone Joint Surg* 67A:208, 1985.
30. Enloe LJ et al: Total hip and knee replacement treatment programs: A report using consensus, *J Orthop Sports Phys Ther* 23(1):3, 1996.
31. Ericson MO, Nisell R: Tibiofemoral joint forces during ergometer cycling, *Am J Sports Med* 14(4):285, 1986.
32. Esler CN et al: Manipulation of TKR: Is the flexion gained retained? *J Bone Joint Surg Br* 81(1):27, 1999.

33. Farina EJ: Aquatic vs. conventional land exercises for the rehabilitation of total knee replacement patients (abstract), *VII World FINA Med & Sci Aspects of Aquatic Sports.*
34. Ficat RD, Hungerford DS: *Disorders of the patellofemoral joint,* Baltimore, 1977, Williams & Wilkins.
35. Finch E et al: Functional ability perceived by individuals following total knee arthroplasty compared to age-matched individuals without knee disability, *J Orthop Sports Phys Ther* 27(4):255, 1998.
36. Foran JRH et al: The outcome of total knee arthroplasty in obese patients, *J Bone Joint Surg Am* 86(8):1609, 2004.
37. Frank C et al: Physiology and therapeutic value of passive joint motion, *Clin Orthop* 185:113, 1984.
38. Friden T et al: Disability in anterior cruciate ligament insufficiency—an analysis of 19 untreated patients, *J Orthop Res* 6:833, 1988.
39. Friedhoff G, Davies G, Malone T: Chain links, *Biomechanics* 5(3):59, 1998.
40. Gauffin H et al: Function testing in patients with old rupture of the anterior cruciate ligament, *Int J Sports Med* 11:73, 1990.
41. Gosc JC: Continuous passive motion in the postoperative treatment of patients with total knee replacement: A retrospective study, *Phys Ther* 67(1):39, 1987.
42. Goth RS et al: Electrical stimulation effect on extensor lag and length of hospital stay after total knee arthroplasty, *Arch Phys Med Rehabil* 75(9):957, 1994.
43. Greenman PE: *Principles of manual medicine,* ed 2, Baltimore, 1996, Williams & Wilkins.
44. Gryzlo SM et al: Electromyographic analysis of knee rehabilitation exercises, *J Orthop Sports Phys Ther* 20(1):36, 1994.
45. Haas SB: Minimally invasive total knee arthroplasty: A comparative study, *Clin Orthop* 428:68, 2004.
46. Haas SB: *Minimally invasive knee arthroplasty.* Course notes, Western Orthopedic Association, Seascape, CA, May 2005.
47. Hallock RH, Fell BM: Unicompartmental tibial hemiarthroplasty: Early results of the UniSpacer knee, *Clin Orthop Relat Res* 416:154, 2003.
48. Hansen CH et al: *Meta-analysis of continuous passive motion use in total knee arthroplasty.* Research presented at the APTA Scientific Meeting, Orlando, 1998.
49. Hanssen AD et al: Surgical options for the middle-aged patient with osteoarthritis of the knee joint, *J Bone Joint Surg* 82A:1768, 2000.
50. Hasson S et al: *An evaluation of mobility and self report on individuals with total knee arthroplasty.* Research presented at the APTA Scientific Meeting, Orlando, June 1998.
51. Herlant M et al: The effect of anterior cruciate ligament surgery on the ankle plantar flexors, *Isokinet Exerc Sci* 2(3):140, 1992.
52. Hertling D, Kessler RM: *Management of common musculoskeletal disorders,* ed 2, Philadelphia, 1990, JB Lippincott.
53. Howie DW et al: The response to particulate debris, *Orthop Clin North Am* 24(4):571, 1993.
54. Hunt ME: Physiotherapy in sports medicine. In Torg JS, Welsh RP, Shephard RJ, editors: *Current therapy in sports medicine,* Toronto, 1990, Decker.
55. Idusuyi OB, Morrey BF: Peroneal nerve palsy after total knee arthroplasty, assessment of predisposing and prognostic factors, *J Bone Joint Surg* 78:177, 1996.
56. Insall JN et al: A comparison of four models of total knee-replacement prosthesis, *J Bone Joint Surg* 58A:754, 1976.
57. Insall JN et al: Rational of the knee society clinical rating system, *Clin Orthop* 248:13, 1989.
58. Janda V: Muscles, central nervous motor regulation and back problems. In Korr I, editor: *The neurobiologic mechanisms in manipulative therapy,* New York, 1977, Plenum Press.
59. Janda V: *Muscles as a pathogenic factor in low back pain in the treatment of patients.* Proceedings of the IFOMT 4th Conference, Christchurch, NZ, 1980.
60. Jaramillo J, Worrell TW, Ingersoll CD: Hip isometric strength following knee surgery, *J Orthop Sports Phys Ther* 20(3):160, 1994.
61. Jasty M, Smith E: Wear particles of total joint replacements and their role in periprosthetic osteolysis, *Curr Opin Rheumatol* 4(2):204, 1992.
62. Jones CA et al: Determinants of function after TKA, *Phys Ther* 83(8):696, 2003.
63. Kawamura H, Bourne RB: Factors affecting range of flexion after TKA, *J Orthop Sci* 6(3):248, 2001.
64. Kisner C, Colby LA: *Therapeutic exercise foundations and techniques,* ed 2, Philadelphia, 1990, FA Davis.
65. Kopell HP, Thompson WAL: Peripheral entrapment neuropathies of the lower extremity, *N Engl J Med* 262(2):56, 1960.
66. Koralewicz et al: Comparison of proprioception in arthritic and age-matched normal knees, *J Bone Joint Surg Am* 82:1592, 2000.
67. Koshino T et al: Regeneration of degenerated articular cartilage after high tibial valgus osteotomy for medial compartmental osteoarthritis of the knee, *Knee* 10:229, 2003.
68. Krupp MA, Chatton MJ: *Current medical diagnosis and treatment,* Los Altos, CA, 1979, Lange Medical.
69. Kuster MS et al: Joint load considerations in total knee replacement, *J Bone Joint Surg* 79B(1):109, 1997.
70. Laskin RS: The Genesis total knee prosthesis: A 10-year follow-up study, *Clin Orthop* 388:95, 2001.
71. Laskin RS: *TKR through a mini midvastus MIS approach and comparison of standard approach TKR.* Paper presented at the 71st Annual Meeting of the American Academy of Orthopedic Surgeons, San Francisco, March 2004.
72. Laskin RS et al: Minimally invasive total knee replacement through a mini-midvastus incision: An outcome study, *Clin Orthop* 428:74, 2004.
73. Lehn C, Prentice WE: Massage. In Prentice WE, editor: *Therapeutic modalities in sports medicine,* St Louis, 1995, Mosby.
74. Lewit K: *Manipulative therapy in rehabilitation of the motor system,* London, 1975, Butterworth.
75. Lingard EA: *Five-year patient reported outcomes of TKA.* Poster presented at the 71st Annual Meeting of the American Academy of Orthopedic Surgeons, San Francisco, March 2004.
76. Lingard EA et al: Predicting the outcome of total knee arthroplasty, *J Bone Joint Surg Am* 86:2179, 2004.

77. Lux PS, Hoernschemeyer DG, Whiteside LA: *Manipulation and cortisone injection following total knee replacement (abstract).* Paper presented at the 64th Annual Meeting of the American Academy of Orthopedic Surgeons, San Francisco, February 1997.
78. Lyback CO et al: Survivorship of AGC knee replacement in juvenile chronic arthritis: 13-year follow-up of 77 knees, *J Arthroplasty* 15:166, 2000.
79. Lynch JA et al: Mechanical measures in the prophylaxis of postoperative thromboembolism in total knee arthroplasty, *Clin Orthop* 260:24, 1990.
80. MacIntosh DL: Hemi-arthroplasty of the knee using a space occupying prosthesis for painful varus and valgus deformities. Proceedings of the joint meeting of the Orthopaedic Associations of the English Speaking World, *J Bone Joint Surg* 40A:1431, 1958.
81. Maloney WJ et al: The influence of continuous passive motion on outcome in total knee arthroplasty, *Clin Orthop* 256:162, 1990.
82. Marks R: The effects of 16 months of angle-specific isometric strengthening exercises in midrange on torque of the knee extensor muscles in osteoarthritis of the knee: A case study, *J Orthop Sports Phys Ther* 20(2):103, 1994.
83. McAuley JP et al: Outcome of knee arthroplasty in patients with poor preoperative ROM, *Clin Orthop* (404):203, 2002.
84. McKeever DC: Tibial plateau prosthesis, *Clin Orthop* 18:86, 1960.
85. Moseley JB et al: A controlled trial of arthroscopic surgery for osteoarthritis of the knee, *N Engl J Med* 347(11):81, 2002.
86. Mukand J et al: Critical pathways for TKR—protocol saves time and money, *Adv Dir Rehab* 6(8):31, 1997.
87. Munin MC et al: Early in-patient rehabilitation after elective hip and knee arthroplasty, *JAMA* 279(11):880, 1998.
88. Murray MP: Gait as a total pattern of movement, *Am J Phys Med* 46(1):290, 1967.
89. Nickenig T: Medical marvels, *Adv Dir Rehab* 13(10):40, 2004.
90. Norton School of Lymphatic Therapy. Course notes, Boston, August 2004.
91. O'Driscoll SW, Kumar A, Salter RB: The effects of continuous passive motion in the clearance of hemarthrosis from synovial joint: An experimental investigation in the rabbit, *Clin Orthop* 176:305, 1983.
92. Parisien JS: The role of arthroscopy in the treatment of postoperative fibroarthrosis of the knee joint, *Clin Orthop* 229:185, 1988.
93. Patla-Paris C: Kinetic chain: Dysfunctional and compensatory effects within the lower extremity (manual), *Orthop Phys Ther Home Study Course* 91(1):1, 1992.
94. Piegorsch K: Peripheral nerve entrapment syndromes of the lower extremity (manual), *Orthop Phys Ther Home Study Course* 91(1):1, 1991.
95. Pitman MI, Frankel VH: Biomechanics of the knee in athletes. In Nicholas JA, Hershman EB, editors: *The lower extremity and spine in sports medicine,* St Louis, 1995, Mosby.
96. Ranawat CS: *Optimizing outcomes in orthopedic surgery.* Course notes, 71st Annual Meeting of the American Academy of Orthopedic Surgeons, San Francisco, March 2004.
97. Ranawat CS et al: Long-term results of the total condylar knee arthroplasty, *Clin Orthop* 286:94, 1993.
98. Rand JA, Illstrup DM: Survivorship analysis of total knee arthroplasty. Cumulative rates of survival of 9200 total knee arthroplasties, *J Bone Joint Surg* 73A:397, 1991.
99. Riddle DL et al: Diagnosis of lower-extremity deep vein thrombosis in outpatients with musculoskeletal disorders: A national survey study of physical therapists, *Phy Ther* 84(8):717, 2004.
100. Ries MD et al: Improvement in cardiovascular fitness after total knee arthroplasty, *J Bone Joint Surg* 78:1696, 1996.
101. Ritter MA et al: Predicting range of motion after TKA, *J Bone Joint Surg Am* 85-A(7):1278, 2003.
102. Ross M, Worrell TW: Thigh and calf girth following knee injury and surgery, *J Orthop Sports Phys Ther* 27(1):9, 1998.
103. Ross MD et al: *A comparison of quadriceps strength and girth between involved and uninvolved limbs in individuals with total knee arthroplasty.* Research presented at the APTA Scientific Meeting, Orlando, June 1998.
104. Sahrmann SA: *Diagnosis and treatment of movement impairment syndromes.* Course notes, San Francisco, June 1997.
105. Salter RB: The biological concept of continuous passive motion of synovial joints, *Clin Orthop* 242:12, 1989.
106. Savory CG: Total joint replacement patients should stick to low-impact sports, *Biomechanics* 5(3):71, 1998.
107. Shields RK et al: Reliability, validity, and responsiveness of functional tests in patients with total joint replacement, *Phys Ther* 75(3):169, 1995.
108. Smith LL: Acute inflammation: The underlying mechanism in delayed onset muscle soreness, *Med Sci Sports Exerc* 23:542, 1991.
109. Spencer JD, Hayes KC, Alexander IJ: Knee effusion and quadriceps reflex inhibition in man, *Arch Phys Med Rehabil* 65:171, 1984.
110. Stearn SH, Insall JN: Posterior stabilized prosthesis. Results after follow up of 9 to 12 years, *J Bone Joint Surg* 74A:980, 1992.
111. Stukenborg-Colsman C et al: High tibial osteotomy versus unicompartmental joint replacement in unicompartmental knee joint osteoarthritis: 7-10-year follow-up prospective randomized study, *Knee* 8:187, 2001.
112. Swanik CB et al: Stifness after TKA, *J Bone Joint Surg Am* 86:328, 2004.
113. Tidius PM: Exercise and muscle soreness. In Torg JS, Welsh RP, Shephard RJ, editors: *Current therapy in sports medicine,* Toronto, 1990, Decker.
114. Tippett SR: Closed chain exercise, *Orthop Phys Ther Clin N Am* 1:253, 1992.
115. Toran MW: Pooling resources for sports medicine, *Adv Dir Rehab* 7(3):59, 1998.
116. Tria AJ, Coon TM: Minimal incision total knee arthroplasty, *Clin Orthop* 416:185, 2003.
117. Tropp H, Odenrick P: Postural control in single-limb stance, *J Orthop Res* 6:833, 1988.

118. Vaughan LM: *Minimal incision TKA-5 year follow-up.* Paper presented at the 71st Annual Meeting of the American Academy of Orthopedic Surgeons, Symposia AR Knee, Mar 2004.
119. Vince KG et al: Continuous passive motion after total knee arthroplasty, *J Arthroplasty* 2(4):281, 1987.
120. Walsh M et al: Physical impairments and functional limitations: A comparison of individuals one year after total knee arthroplasty with control subjects, *Phys Ther* 78(3):248, 1998.
121. Weiss JM: Treatment of leg edema and wounds in a patient with severe musculoskeletal injuries, *Phys Ther* 78(10):1104, 1998.
122. Worland RL et al: Ten to fourteen year survival and functional analysis of the AGC total knee replacement system, *Knee* 9:133, 2002.
123. Woolson ST et al: Comparison of primary total hip replacements performed with a standard incision or a mini-incision, *J Bone Joint Surg* 86A:1353, 2004.
124. American Academy of Orthopaedic Surgeons/American Association of Orthopaedic Surgeons: Website home page. Available at: http://www.aaos.org. Accessed 7/19/06.
125. Centers for Disease Control and Prevention, National Center for Health Statistics: Website home page. Available at: http://www.cdc.gov/nchs/index.htm. Accessed 7/19/06.
126. Lymphnotes.com: Total knee replacement and lymphedema. Available at: http://www.lymphnotes.com/article.php/id/207. Accessed 7/19/06.
127. Lymphnotes.com: What is lymphedema? Available at: http://www.lymphnotes.com/cat.php/id/8/. Accessed 7/19/06.
128. Yashar AA et al: Continuous passive motion with accelerated flexion after total knee arthroplasty, *Clin Orthop* 345:38, 1997.
129. Anti-embolism.com. Anti-embolism hosiery (TED). Available at: http://anti-embolism.com/. Accessed 8/28/06.

CHAPTER 22

Lateral Ligament Repair

Robert Donatelli
Will Hall
Brian E. Prell
Richard D. Ferkel

The ankle requires both static and dynamic stability. Mobility is crucial for normal ankle function in the midst of rapidly changing postures of the foot during sporting and everyday weight-bearing activities. Lateral ligament injuries of the ankle account for 13% to 56% of all injuries in sports requiring running or jumping such as soccer, basketball, and volleyball.[12,15] The large majority of these injuries can be successfully treated conservatively with casting, bracing, nonsteroidal anti-inflammatory drugs, and physical therapy. Approximately 85% of all ankle sprains involve the lateral structures of the ankle.[10,25] The majority of ankle sprains heal without any residual functional instability.[10] Despite adequate trials of conservative measures, however, approximately 10% to 30% of all acute ligamentous injuries have recurrent symptoms of chronic pain, swelling, and instability with activities.* Functional instability of the ankle is reported to be as high as 20% after ankle sprains.[8] When conservative measures fail to produce satisfactory proprioceptive performance and mechanical stability, surgical repair or reconstruction of the injured lateral ligament structures should be considered.

SURGICAL INDICATIONS AND CONSIDERATIONS

The etiology of the unstable ankle is usually a plantar flexion inversion injury that tears the anterior talofibular (ATF) ligament and possibly the calcaneofibular (CF) ligament and anterior inferior tibiofibular (AITF) ligament. The unstable ankle is generally caused by a traumatic event such as an ankle sprain. It also can be associated with ankle fractures but virtually never develops insidiously.

A lateral ankle reconstruction is an elective surgery used to treat chronic instability that results from a continuum of ankle injuries. Ankle injuries can result in permanent damage to the ligaments that support the lateral ankle. Various studies have examined the benefits of surgical versus functional treatment in lateral ligament injuries of the ankle. These studies have shown that operative repair was associated with patients' delayed return to work, restricted range of motion (ROM), impaired ankle mobility, and increased complications after surgery, including undefined pain.* This is in contrast to conservative treatment, which includes functional bracing and early mobilization. The surgical option is used when nonoperative treatments have failed, such as physical therapy, bracing, activity modification, and steroid injections. Postoperative physical therapy is a vital link in returning the patient to an active lifestyle.

Indications for reconstruction of the ankle's lateral ligaments include recurrent giving way with activities of daily living (ADLs) and sports that is refractory to conservative treatment, a positive physical examination, abnormal inversion, and/or positive anterior drawer stress x-rays (Fig. 22-1, A and B).

Patients of all ages and types are candidates for this type of surgery, but few patients older than 40 years undergo ankle reconstruction because of decreased activity levels and a decreased ability to adjust functions and lifestyle to avoid recurrent buckling episodes. Surgeons should take care when considering this procedure for patients with generalized ligamentous laxity and collagen disorders that may result in failure. In addition, advanced degenerative joint disease or arthrofibrosis may be relative contraindications to this surgery.

SURGICAL PROCEDURES

More than 50 different surgical procedures for correction of lateral ankle instability have been described.[3] The majority of reconstructive procedures use part, or all, of

*References 1, 2, 10, 13, 23

*References 14, 20, 24, 30

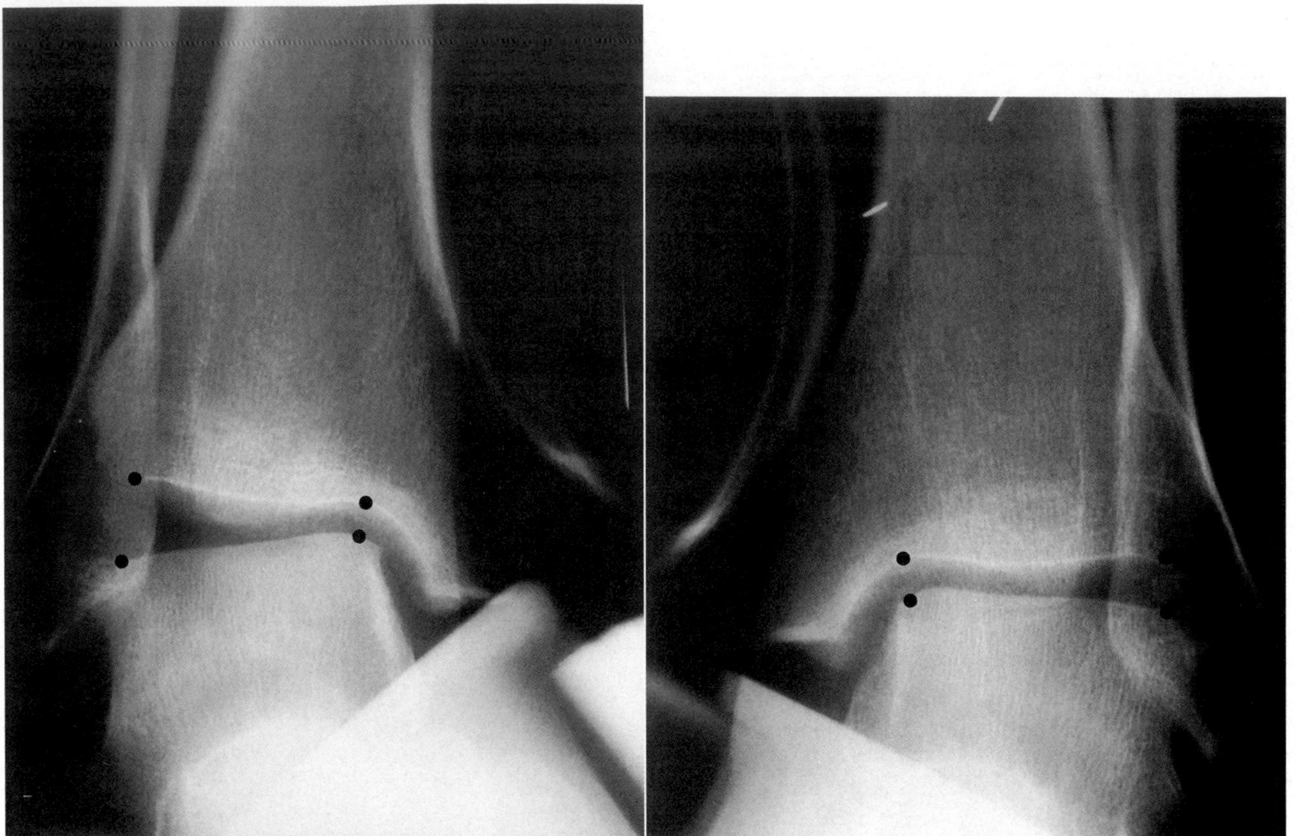

Fig. 22-1 Inversion stress testing on the Telos device. The right ankle (**A**) demonstrates increased talar tilt compared with the left ankle (**B**).

the peroneal brevis tendon. Common procedures include the Watson-Jones, Evans, Chrisman-Snook, and Elmslie procedures and their modifications. Anatomic repair with direct suturing of the torn ligaments, imprecation, reinsertion to the bone, and in some instances augmentation with local tissue have increased recently in popularity.[8,17,21] Direct repair of the ATF and CF ligaments was described by Broström in 1966 and later modified by Gould in 1980.[5,17] Direct repair of torn lateral ligaments has the advantage of being simple and reliable, avoiding the use of normal tendons. It restores the original anatomy, requires less exposure, and maintains full ankle motion.

Procedure

The patient is taken to the operating room and examined under anesthesia. If the surgeon has any questions about the degree of ankle instability, stress x-ray films (stressing the ankle in both inversion and anterior drawer) are taken. The thigh is then secured on a well-padded thigh holder in preparation for ankle arthroscopy, as described in Chapter 24. The lower extremity is prepared and draped in standard fashion. Arthroscopy is performed first; the authors of this chapter have found that 93% of patients have additional intraarticular ankle pathology associated with lateral ankle instability.[25] In addition, a similar report by Taga showed 95% of patients have additional intraarticular pathology at the time of ankle reconstruction.[31]

The intraarticular pathology is identified and addressed through arthroscopic surgery. The scarred anterior talofibular ligament is identified and assessed to make sure it is adequate for the modified Broström repair. After the arthroscopy is completed, the nurse removes the thigh support and places the leg flat on the surgical table. The ankle is re-swabbed with a sterile antibacterial solution. An additional clean surgical drape is placed over the foot and ankle, and gloves are changed. New sterile instruments are used to perform the open portion of the procedure. Arthroscopic methods are available for surgical reconstruction of the lateral ankle ligaments, but at this time open stabilization as described by Broström gives a better, more reproducible result.

After arthroscopy the ankle is prepared and the tourniquet inflated. An incision is made over the lateral aspect of the ankle. This incision may be obliquely shaped in the skin folds or more vertical from the fibula toward the sinus tarsi, depending on the surgeon's preference and the clinical situation. The senior author prefers the vertical incision because it allows better assessment of the peroneal tendons and can be extended distally and proximally if other procedures need to be done. Dissection is carried down through the subcutaneous tissues and the extensor retinaculum is carefully exposed because it is to be used for later reattachment. The surgeon must take care to avoid the intermediate dorsal cutaneous nerve, the lateral branch of the superficial peroneal nerve (which often lies near the end of the ATF ligament), and the sural nerve (which lies over the peroneal tendons). An oblique capsular incision is then made along the anterior border of the fibula from the AITF ligament to the CF ligament, leaving a small 3- or 4-mm cuff of tissue on the fibula for reattachment of the torn ligament complex (Fig. 22-2). The stretched ATF ligament is found as a thickening in the anterior capsule, and the CF ligament is found in the distal portion of the wound under the tip of the fibula, running deep to the peroneal tendons. The CF ligament often is attenuated or avulsed from the fibular tip.

A "pants-over-vest" overlapping suture technique is used to imprecate or shorten the torn ligaments and provide a double layer of reinforcement to the repair. Suturing is done starting from the ligament portion attached to the talus, so that the knots are tied distal and inferior to the fibula. This helps prevent postoperative knot prominence and skin irritation with shoe wear. The sutures are tied with the ankle in neutral position, and a posterior drawer is applied to reduce the talus. The ankle is checked to make sure full ROM has been maintained during the repair. The extensor retinaculum is then pulled proximal over the repair and sutured to the fibular periosteum (Fig. 22-3, A and B). ROM is again checked, as is the stability of the ankle. The tourniquet is released, and bleeding tissues are coagulated. The subcutaneous tissue and skin are then closed in the standard fashion. The patient is placed in a short-leg well-padded cast that is split in the recovery room to allow for swelling.

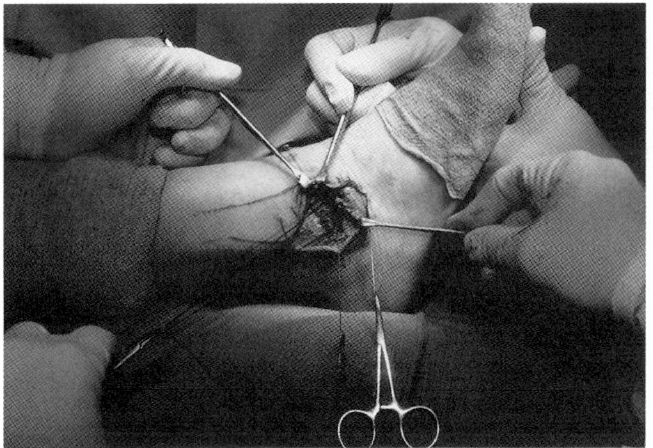

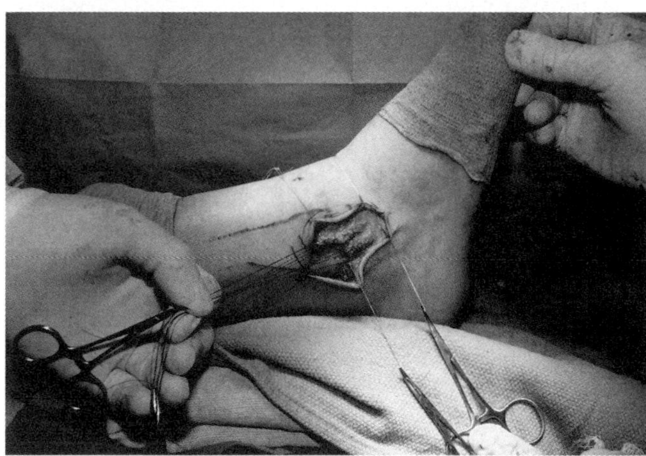

Fig. 22-2 **A,** An oblique incision is made over the fibula, in line with the anterior talofibular ligament and the extensor retinaculum and lateral ligaments are exposed. **B,** An oblique capsular incision is made along the anterior border of the fibula from the AITF ligament to the CF ligament, leaving a small 3- to 4-mm cuff of tissue on the fibula for reattachment of the ligament complex.

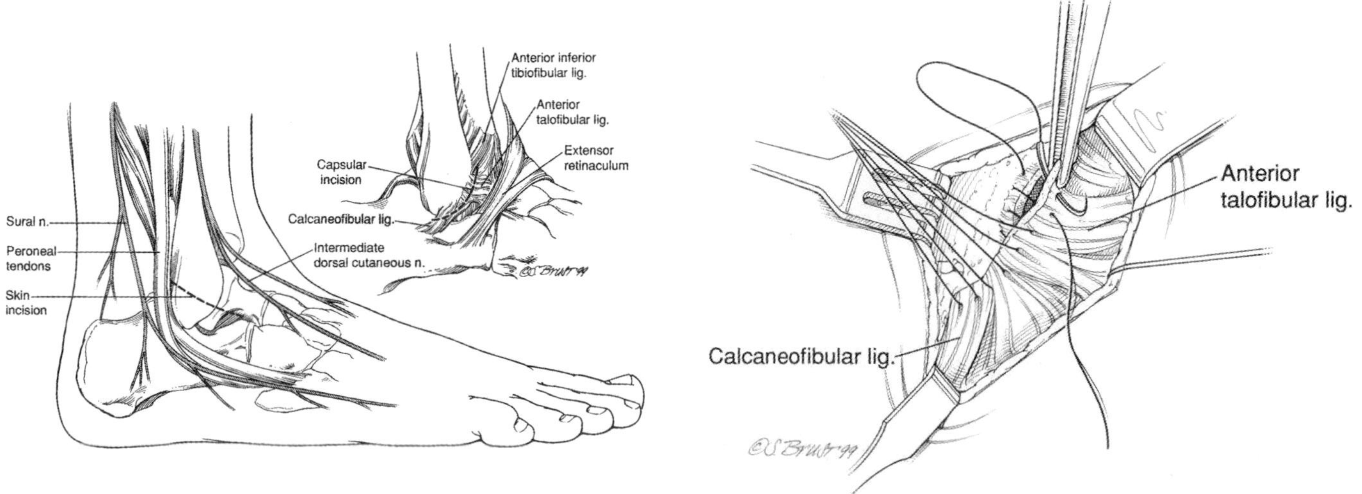

Fig. 22-3 **A,** The anterior talofibular and calcaneofibular ligaments are reefed in a "pants-over-vest" fashion with nonabsorbable suture. **B,** The extensor retinaculum is pulled proximally over the repair and sutured to the fibular periosteum.

The patient's cast is changed at one and two weeks and the stitches are removed. Weight bearing is started at week 3 in a cast or cast boot, at the surgeon's discretion. Physical therapy with mobilization starts usually at week 6 or sometimes sooner.

SURGICAL OUTCOMES

A lateral ankle reconstruction is considered to be successful when the patient has full ROM and a pain-free ankle and can return to all ADLs and sports without restriction. Liu and Baker[26] studied the static restraints of various surgical procedures in 40 cadaveric ankles. They found no significant difference between the Watson-Jones and Chrisman-Snook procedures, but the modified Broström procedure produced the least anteroposterior (AP) displacement and talar tilt at all different forces tested.

Hennrikus[19] prospectively compared the Chrisman-Snook and modified Broström procedure in 40 patients. Although both produced 80% good-to-excellent results, the former procedure had a much greater proportion of complications and the latter procedure had a higher functional score. Hamilton performed the modified Broström procedure on 28 ankles; 54% of the patients were high-level ballet dancers.[18] At 64 months follow-up, he noted 27 of 28 good-to-excellent results. Peters[27] reviewed the literature and found 460 ankles treated with anatomic modified Broström repairs had an average of between 87% and 95% good-to-excellent results.

Recently, Chams and Ferkel[6] reviewed the results of 21 patients who underwent the modified Broström procedure. The average patient age was 27.5 years and the average follow-up occurred at 57 months. They found 95% good-to-excellent results with an American Orthopaedic Foot and Ankle Society's (AOFAS) ankle/hindfoot score of 97.1. When the anterior talofibular ligament is not adequate to use for a Broström repair, we use either an autogenous or allograft hamstring graft with biotenodesis screws through the talus and calcaneus to reconstruct the ATFL and CFL.[9,32]

Challenges

Despite having a stable ankle postoperatively, some patients still complain of pain, aching, swelling, and crepitation.[31] Many of these complaints may be related to preexisting intraarticular pathology such as degenerative joint disease, loose bodies, chronic synovitis, and chronic scarring. Occasionally the ankle can be made too tight at the time of reconstruction; this severely limits the patient's ability to invert. This is the single most serious complication after ankle reconstruction. If a patient does not have full motion after surgery, especially full inversion and eversion, rehabilitation is significantly compromised and the patient tends to develop a painful valgus hindfoot.

Precautions and Contraindications

The physical therapist should increase the level of rehabilitation gradually for the patient after surgery. Too-vigorous exercise and the use of isokinetic machines can lead to increased pain, shear stress, and swelling that can last for weeks to months. If this occurs, the ultimate results can be compromised and the patient, physician, and physical therapist can all become quite frustrated. Every patient progresses at a different rate and the exercise program should be customized to the individual needs of each patient.

Rehabilitation Concerns

The therapist should contact the physician whenever pain appears to be out of proportion to expectations. In addition, any wound drainage, evidence of fever or infection, and increased laxity should alert the therapist to interact with the surgeon. If the patient has an acute episode of pain or feels a "pop" or significant change during rehabilitation or ADLs, the surgeon should be alerted immediately.

Q Will, who is 18 years old, tore his ATF ligament while playing basketball. The tear occurred over a 1-year period after accumulating multiple ankle sprains. He had an ATF ligament repair 8 weeks ago. Since then his physical therapy has consisted of massage, ultrasound, AROM and PROM exercises, cryotherapy with compression, and a home exercise program. His main complaint is stiffness during gait, while ascending stairs, and during attempts to squat partially. Dorsiflexion is limited by 10 degrees with moderate edema noted. What treatment is most likely to improve Will's dorsiflexion ROM and decrease edema?

THERAPY GUIDELINES FOR REHABILITATION

The first 6 weeks after surgery are important for the succes of the surgery. Whether the reconstruction was done with primary ligamentous repair (as in the Broström procedure), with tendon augmentation (as in the Chrisman-Snook procedure), or with hamstring reconstruction, the initial tissue healing stage is important.[19,23] The surgical reconstruction to correct the ligamentous instability is only as good as the stability gained from soft tissue healing. Soft tissue healing is considered the maximal protection stage.

Evaluation

The initial postoperative evaluation gives the therapist a baseline from which to proceed in returning the patient to desired independent function. Initial ROM measurements are taken both for active range of motion (AROM) and passive range of motion (PROM). PROM is measured within a pain-free range, especially while measuring forefoot inversion.

The physical therapist has a responsibility to the surgeon and the patient to protect the lateral ligamentous reconstruction. Forefoot inversion stresses the reconstructed tissues and must be carefully engaged. Manual muscle testing to determine strength of the lower extremity can be part of the initial evaluation. However, muscle testing at the ankle is delayed until the patient has progressed and accommodated to resisted exercises at the ankle.

The therapist should avoid having the patient perform a single-leg heel raise, which is usually advocated to determine normal gastrocnemius-soleus strength, because of decreased proprioception and the significant muscle deficits resulting from the effects of immobilization. The incision is assessed for mobility and hypersensitivity after complete healing has occurred. Operative damage to the sural nerve and the lateral branch of the superficial peroneal nerve has been reported as a cause of decreased sensation in the involved ankle.[8,22] Joint effusion and soft tissue edema can be factors in limited ROM, proprioception deficits, and the inability to strengthen the joint. Joint and soft tissue mobility also are assessed at the limits of ROM.

> **A** The patient was reassessed for associated restrictions. A mobilization technique was performed at the proximal and distal fibula. An AP movement was applied to the proximal fibular head, and a posteroanterior (PA) movement was applied to the lateral malleolus to increase dorsiflexion. This was followed by stretching and ROM exercises to reinforce dorsiflexion. Will's dorsiflexion PROM increased to 18 degrees. Pain with gait, stairs, and squatting was dramatically decreased after the first treatment.

Phase I

TIME: Weeks 4-6 after surgery

GOALS: Decrease pain and swelling, restore joint and soft tissue mobility, increase strength in lower extremity and ankle, increase proprioception, normalize gait, maintain cardiovascular fitness, and provide patient education (Table 22-1)

During this maximal protection phase the patient is casted and allowed to progress from non–weight bearing to weight bearing. The patient remains non–weight bearing and the cast is removed at the first postoperative visit for wound inspection. A second cast is applied for an additional week and the stitches are removed. Weight bearing is initiated during the third week and the cast is removed at the sixth week. At this point the patient is placed in a controlled action motion (CAM) walker brace and compression stocking or in a small brace, depending on the individual patient. At 6 weeks the patient is started on ROM and strengthening exercises in physical therapy, as well as pool exercises. Some authors have advocated a limited ROM of 10 degrees dorsiflexion and 10 degrees of plantar flexion, with partial weight bearing from 2 to 6 weeks after surgery.[28] Formal physical therapy is usually initiated at 6 weeks when the cast is removed. At this time the tissues should be adequately healed and ready to tolerate stresses within a pain-free ROM. Studies have shown that motion is beneficial to nourish cartilage, prevent soft tissue contractures, and restore joint mobility.[16]

After performing the initial evaluation, the physical therapist can implement appropriate treatment. Initially, the therapist performs grade I and II joint mobilization along with PROM, especially inversion, within pain-free ranges. At 6 weeks after surgery the ligaments should have healed sufficiently to allow gentle active movement.[22]

However, at this stage the soft tissue is unable to withstand significant forces into inversion.[10] The patient is able to perform AROM for plantar flexion and dorsiflexion using pain as a guide; submaximal multiangle isometrics for all planes also are used at this stage of the rehabilitation. Soft tissue and joint mobilizations are started to reverse the effects of immobilization and surgical trauma. Effusion, pain, and soft tissue edema are treated with the appropriate modalities. Research has suggested that ice independently is not effective in reducing postoperative edema. Instead, studies have reported an increased effectiveness of reducing post-op edema using cold compression therapy.[4,29,34] Efforts to normalize full weight-bearing gait without assistive devices should include gait training drills. Proper foot mechanics throughout the stance phase of gait can be emphasized if pain is minimal or absent.

A home exercise program emphasizing increased frequency and decreased intensity of exercises should be initiated at this time. The therapist should clearly instruct the patient on precautions to protect healing tissues. The program may be altered as needed by the therapist.

Precautions

The therapist should take a few precautions during this phase.

Careful monitoring of exercise progression and intensity of the workout session is crucial to avoid overstressing healing tissues. The therapist must caution the patient to avoid aggressive stretching and strengthening of lateral ankle tissues early in the rehabilitation program; progress should be cautious and slow. Exercises that cause increased symptoms in the lateral ankle complex must be modified or avoided.

> **Q** Leigh is a 30-year-old woman who tore her left ATF ligament while performing step aerobics. She had an ATF ligament repair 10 weeks ago. She has complained of knee and back pain on the unilateral side. She has asymmetric pelvic imbalance, with left iliac crest higher than the right and the left anterosuperior iliac spine (ASIS)/posterior superior iliac spine (PSIS) higher than the right. Decreased knee extension left versus right. Progress with exercises has decreased because of pain during many of the closed-chain exercises such as single-leg stance, double-heel lifts, mini-squats, and walking more than 8 minutes on the treadmill. What types of activities can be performed for her unilateral imbalances while increasing core stability?

Phase II

TIME: Weeks 6-8 after surgery
GOALS: Return gait within normal range, maintain normal ROM, increase strength, control pain and swelling, increase proprioception (Table 22-2)

Phase II is overlapped with phase I as the patient's ROM begins to progress and therapeutic exercise options are expanded. At this stage rehabilitation is similar to that advocated in the literature for lateral ankle sprains.[10] Multiplane isometrics and AROM against gravity progress to exercises with appropriate grades of submaximal resistance using weights or rubber tubing. Peroneal strengthening is a major focus because repeated trauma resulting from the instability may lead to weakness of these muscles.[10] Activities to increase strength may occur

Table 22-1 Lateral Ligament Repair

Rehabilitation Phase	Criteria to Progress to this Phase	Anticipated Impairments and Functional Limitations	Intervention	Goal	Rationale
Phase I Postoperative 4-6 weeks	Postoperative Cleared by physician to begin rehabilitation	◆ Edema ◆ Pain ◆ Patient casted for 6 weeks ◆ Limited weight bearing (non–weight bearing for 3 weeks, then progressive weight bearing per physician) ◆ Limited ROM ◆ Limited strength	◆ Patients usually begin therapy at about 6 weeks ◆ Modalities as needed ◆ PROM—(stretches within pain-free ranges) Plantar flexion, dorsiflexion, and eversion; take care when gently stretching into inversion ◆ Isometrics—Submaximal multi-angle exercises for all planes ◆ AROM—Ankle—supine and seated plantar flexion and dorsiflexion ◆ Progressive resistance exercises (PREs)—Hip—All ranges ◆ Soft tissue mobilization ◆ Joint mobilization as indicated ◆ Gait training—Progress to full weight bearing using appropriate assistive device ◆ Patient education	◆ Manage edema ◆ Decrease pain ◆ Increase ROM ◆ Increase tolerance of muscle contraction	◆ Provide maximal protection in this phase: patient is casted for 6 weeks; communication with physician is imperative regarding weight-bearing status ◆ Begin restoring joint and soft tissue mobility ◆ Initiate muscle contraction and prepare for strengthening exercises ◆ Improve hip strength to prepare for normal gait ◆ Provide gait training to improve tolerance to accepting weight on involved leg ◆ Avoid overstressing healing tissues; adapt program as symptoms dictate

Table 22-2 Lateral Ligament Repair

Rehabilitation Phase	Criteria to Progress to this Phase	Anticipated Impairments and Functional Limitations	Intervention	Goal	Rationale
Phase II Postoperative 6-8 weeks	No increase in pain No loss of ROM Improved tolerance to weight bearing	◆ Mild edema ◆ Mild pain ◆ Limited strength ◆ Limited ROM ◆ Limited gait	Continuation of Phase I interventions as indicated ◆ Isometrics—Multiplane submaximal inversion and eversion (pain-free) ◆ AROM—Ankle—all ranges against gravity Standing bilateral heel raises Squats and lunges ◆ Treadmill ◆ Stationary bicycle (using low resistance) ◆ Elastic tubing (light resistance) exercises initiated late phase II; dorsiflexion, plantar flexion, inversion, and eversion ◆ Balance board progressed from seated to standing with bilateral, then unilateral, support ◆ Proprioceptive neuromuscular facilitation (PNF) ◆ Pool therapy—Deep water running and light jumping	◆ Control edema and pain ◆ Increase strength ◆ Promote equal weight bearing with sit-stand ◆ Minimize gait deviations on level surfaces ◆ Increase tolerance to single-limb stance ◆ Improve proprioception and stability of ankle ◆ Increase tolerance to advanced activities	◆ Continue modalities to control edema and pain ◆ Improve strength and stability of ankle joint in numerous directions ◆ Improve strength with mild resistance initially ◆ Progress exercises incorporating functional activities ◆ Maintain consistent cadence and work on endurance ◆ Later in phase II, ankle should be able to tolerate increased resistance with inversion and eversion motions ◆ Proprioception exercises with varying degrees of weight bearing and manual resistance aids in return of proprioception ◆ Buoyancy effect of water aids progression of more advanced activities

on land or in a pool. On land, early proprioceptive activity is initiated with the use of a balance board as a means of increasing functional stability.[11] The patient progresses from sitting to standing, with bilateral and then unilateral support. One-leg standing also is initiated. Bilateral heel raises are started and progressed to unilateral as tolerated by the patient and according to the therapist's discretion. Proprioceptive neuromuscular facilitation (PNF) is an excellent strengthening tool for the lower kinetic chain. In the pool, activities may include light jogging and jumping exercises in shallow water. Lunges and squats also are effective. The patient should continue with deep water running exercises for increased cardiovascular fitness. Gait training is an important aspect of the rehabilitation program and should be given priority. An aberrant pattern reinforces itself and leads to continued limitations in ROM and strength. Walking on a treadmill at a moderate speed with a low-to-moderate grade as tolerated aids in gait training.

A The therapist explained to Leigh that any activities causing her to substitute secondary to increased pain must be modified. The patient was reassessed, and associated restrictions at the pelvis were recorded. A long axis distraction was performed to correct pelvic asymmetry. Appropriate hamstring stretches were performed to increase muscle length. As exercise was modified and asymmetries were corrected, Leigh was able to perform the following closed-chain exercises: forward lunges, backward lunges, lateral lunges, heel raises with mini-squat, and single-heel raises performed on a leg press machine using 70 lb. She was also able to perform backward walking, minimal walking on a treadmill, and jogging or running in the pool. As strength and tolerance to exercise increased, Leigh progressed to more challenging exercises, which included core stabilization activities.

Q Karen is 22 years old and plays basketball primarily on the weekends. She tore her ATF during a pick-up game when she stepped abnormally causing her ankle to turn into extreme inversion. She had an ATF ligament repair 11 weeks ago. Progress with exercise has decreased because of pain during many closed-chain activities. What factors could be involved that would cause pain during these activities?

Phase III

TIME: Weeks 8-10 after surgery

GOALS: Focus on training to allow return to work and sports, continue ankle mobilization and passive stretching, prevent pain and swelling (Table 22-3)

When ROM and gait are within normal limits, isokinetic strengthening for inversion and eversion can be initiated. At this time the patient should be able to tolerate a submaximal strengthening program without exacerbation of symptoms. Resistive exercises for plantar flexion and dorsiflexion are initiated at 8 weeks. Inversion and eversion resistive exercises must be performed to the tolerance of the patient. Single-leg stance with opposite leg-resisted flexion, abduction, extension, and adduction can be performed with increasing resistive band tension. All resistive exercises should be performed without pain. Three-way lunge, single-leg stance with three-point reach and three-point step with the opposite leg can be initiated cautiously. The ability to perform pain-free weight training and isokinetic training is a good indication that soft tissue strength is progressing well.

The therapist must monitor the progression of resistive exercises to ensure that symptoms are not exacerbated. The patient may be ready for discharge after phase III or may progress to phase IV depending on the prior level of fitness or activity and goals.

A During an additional assessment, it was found that Karen had restrictions with AP proximal fibular glides and PA distal fibular glides. Calcaneal eversion was also limited. Graded mobilizations were performed at the proximal and distal fibular heads, which released the calcaneal eversion and decreased the patient's pain during activity.

Q Jason is a 30-year-old man who suffered an ATF tear after slipping on wet grass while performing yard work. He had an ATF ligament repair 12 weeks ago. He reports that his ankle pain has started to decrease but that he is noticing progressively increased pain at the third through fifth distal metatarsal heads. The pain is progressing to affect gait. What should the therapist assess?

Phase IV

TIME: Weeks 11-18 after surgery

GOAL: Return to sporting activities (Table 22-4)

The goal of rehabilitation is, in general, for the patient to return to sporting activity 11 to 18 weeks after surgery; an ankle brace is used initially on return to sporting activities.[8,19] Exercise should continue with the therapist monitoring patient progress. Exercises in this phase are more advanced, and chances of re-injury are greater. In this final phase of rehabilitation the patient should be able to perform all exercises safely and correctly, with proper form and technique and with little verbal cueing from the therapist.

After the AROM and PROM are within normal limits and strength has returned to normal, sport-specific and functional training can be implemented. Exercise options include plyometrics, trampoline activities, box drills, figure-eight drills, carioca, slide board, and lateral shuffles (Fig. 22-4 through Fig. 22-7). Many of the initial ankle injuries resulted from sporting activities such as cutting activities and movements requiring quick reflexes and balance. These activities should be incorporated into the rehabilitation program.

Table 22-3 Lateral Ligament Repair

Rehabilitation Phase	Criteria to Progress to this Phase	Anticipated Impairments and Functional Limitations	Intervention	Goal	Rationale
Phase III Postoperative 8-10 weeks	No loss of ROM No increase in pain Continued progress in therapy	◆ Limited gait on uneven surfaces ◆ Limited ROM ◆ Limited strength ◆ Mild edema and pain associated with increased activity	Continue interventions as in phase I and II (joint and soft tissue mobilization performed as indicated) ◆ Elastic tubing (mild to moderate resistance) Ankle—All ranges ◆ Isotonics—Ankle—All ranges ◆ Isokinetics—Performed at pain-free intensities ◆ Joint Mobilization: Grades III and IV to decrease stiffness and increase ROM ◆ Single-leg stance with opposite leg-resisted flexion, abduction, extension, and adduction can be performed with increasing resistive band tension ◆ Three-way lunge, single-leg stance with three-point reach and three-point step with the opposite leg can be initiated cautiously	◆ Full AROM and PROM ◆ 80% ankle strength ◆ Self-management of edema and pain	◆ By the end of this phase the patient should have full ROM and hands-on care can be eliminated ◆ Exercises should use a combination of varying resistance in different positions to acquire proprioceptive strength and stability ◆ Exercises are progressed to include activity-specific drills emphasizing specificity of training principles

A The therapist, when learning of this clinical change, assessed the foot position and compared findings bilaterally. The patient was found to have increased rear foot pronation and forefoot supination on the affected side as compared with the unaffected side. The therapist attempted a temporary orthotic trial and posted the patient using a 3-degree medial rear foot wedge and a 3-degree lateral forefoot wedge on the affected extremity. At the next session, the patient reported decreased ankle and distal metatarsal pain on the affected side. The patient would later be fitted for permanent orthotics.

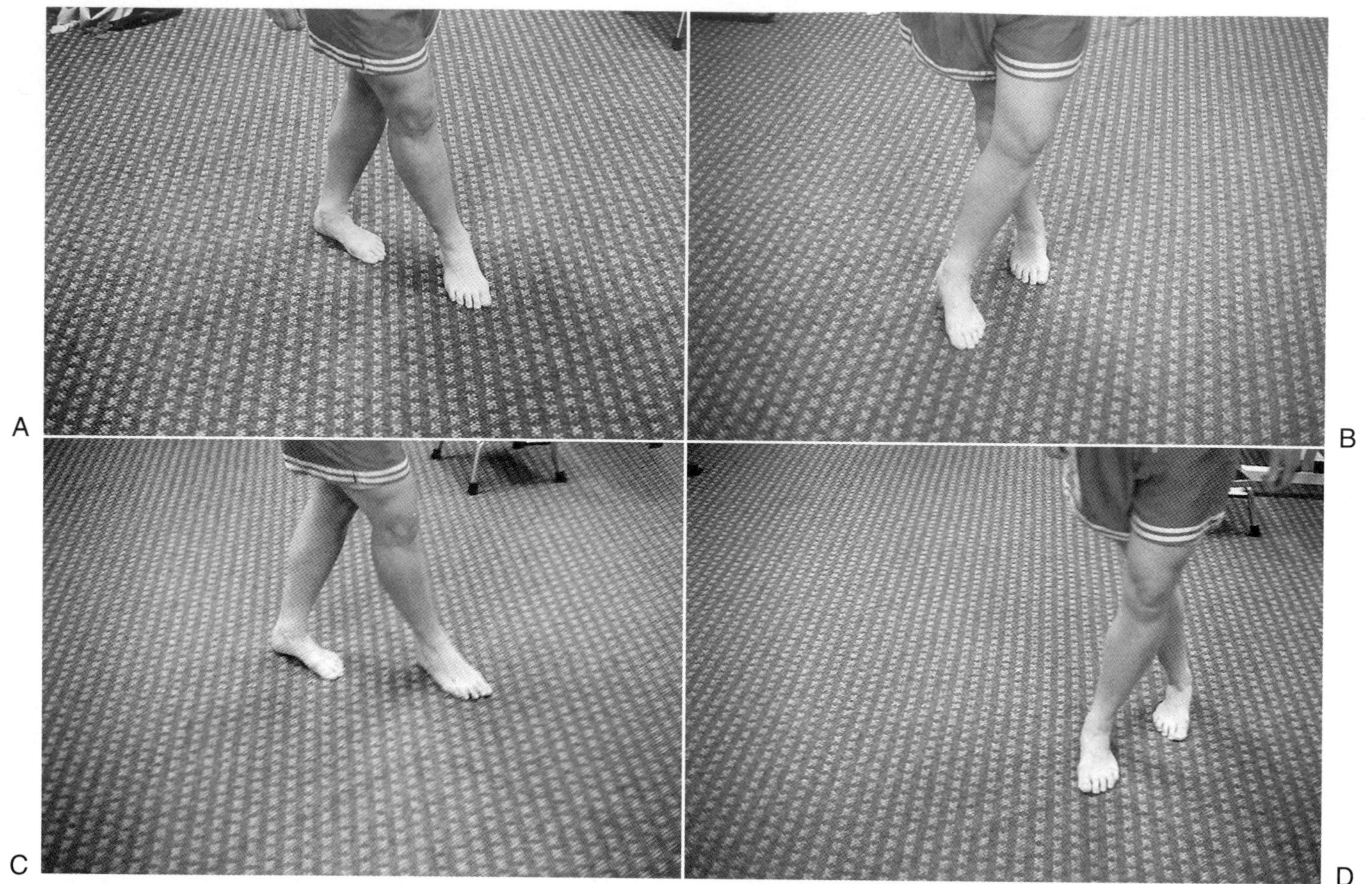

Fig. 22-4 Carioca.

Table 22-4 Lateral Ligament Repair

Rehabilitation Phase	Criteria to Progress to this Phase	Anticipated Impairments and Functional Limitations	Intervention	Goal	Rationale
Phase IV Postoperative 11-18 weeks	Good progression through previous phases with the need to return to higher-level activities and sports Normal ROM Normal strength	◆ Limited strength and tolerance to higher-level activities	Continuation of exercises from phases I through III as indicated ◆ Use ankle brace as appropriate ◆ Plyometrics, trampoline activities, figure-8 drills, carioca, slide board, and lateral shuffle ◆ Increase demand of pivoting and cutting exercises ◆ Four-square hopping ankle rehabilitation (see Fig 24-11) ◆ Progress towards box drills	◆ Prevent reinjury with return to sport ◆ Discharge to gym program ◆ Return to sport	◆ Patient's opportunity for re-injury is highest with the addition of advanced exercises; clinicians should ensure proper performance of drills (plyometrics, pivoting, cutting) ◆ Functional training for sports ◆ After patients can perform drills safely and adequately they are discharged with communication to coaches and trainer

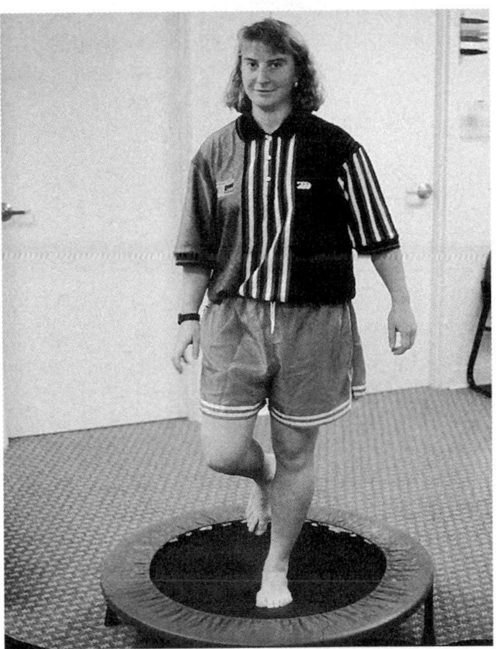

Fig. 22-5 Trampoline stork standing.

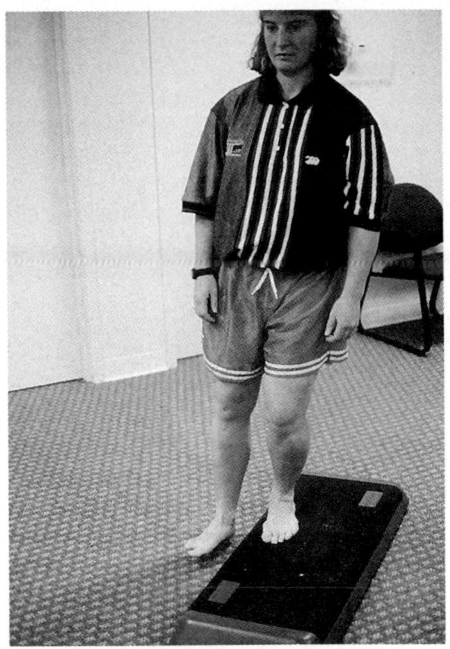

Fig. 22-7 Step-ups.

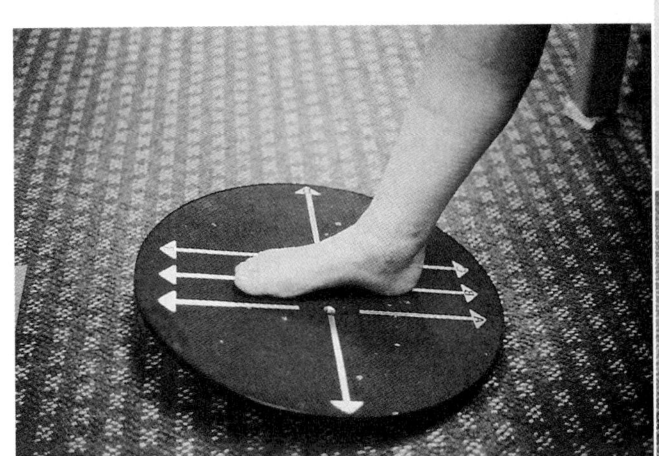

A

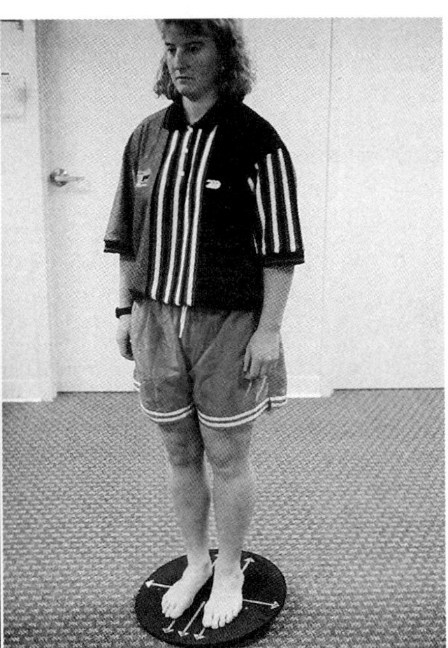

B

Fig. 22-6 Balance board exercise.

Q Jim is 17 years old and tore his ATF while rounding second base during a high school baseball game. He had an ATF ligament repair 16 weeks ago. He has progressed well through rehabilitation but was having difficulty initiating higher-level activities. How did the therapist progress this athlete in order for him to return to baseball for the next season?

SUGGESTED HOME MAINTENANCE FOR THE POSTSURGICAL PATIENT

An exercise program has been outlined at the various phases. The home maintenance box on page 431 outlines rehabilitation suggestions the patient may follow. The physical therapist can use it in customizing a patient-specific program.

TROUBLESHOOTING

Limited dorsiflexion can be a problem with most patients because of limited talar tibia-fibula mobility as a result of joint restrictions and soft tissue tightness. If restrictions exist at the talocrural joint, long-axis distraction thrust techniques are useful (see Fig. 23-6). In addition, mobilization of the talus, tibia, and fibula can be useful. Anterior and posterior glides to these bones help restore dorsiflexion (see Fig. 23-9). The gastrocnemius and soleus muscle group can be the major limiting factor in dorsiflexion ROM. Low-load prolonged stretching techniques can be beneficial in increasing soft tissue extensibility. The load of the stretch is to the patient's tolerance for 20 to 30 minutes, one or two times per day.

Another method to prevent chronic ankle sprains is to use biomechanical foot orthotics. In theory, biomechanical foot orthotics are designed to enhance joint position, increasing the shock-absorbing capabilities of the lower limb and improving muscle function.

A The therapist initiated activities that were sports specific to increase functional stability. The patient performed multidirectional single-leg hopping, including forward, backward, and side to side. The patient began box exercises, including shuffle sprint and box *X* with pivot. He was progressed in proprioceptive activities, including unilateral leg stand with opposite LE resistive-band flexion, extension, and abduction, and biomechanical ankle platform system (BAPS) board activities. The exercises were progressed, increasing the time from 1 to 2 minutes.

Q Steve is an 18-year-old senior track athlete being actively recruited by several Division I universities for pole vaulting. During a track meet, the patient performed his vault and, upon landing, severely inverted his right ankle. He entered the clinic with severe bruising around the ankle with + 2 pitting edema. He was tender over the lateral malleoli and peroneals, as well as the lateral ligaments. He has no significant gait deviations and has reported that he has been jogging. What is the differential diagnosis and course of treatment?

SUMMARY

A successful outcome for lateral ligamentous reconstruction includes no recurrent instability, normal ROM and strength, and no pain with weight-bearing activities. A successful functional outcome is achieved if the patient experiences no instability on returning to daily activities or sporting activities. The first step toward a good outcome is adequate postoperative stabilization. However, the success of the surgical procedure depends on postoperative rehabilitation in which the patient, surgeon, and therapist work closely to achieve a functional ankle.

A The therapist first instructed Steve to cease jogging activities immediately and used the tuning fork and tapping method to rule out possible fracture, which was negative. Radiographs later showed no fracture present. The patient was positive with talar tilt, anterior drawer, and high ankle sprain. The patient demonstrated MMT within normal limits for all ankle motions except ankle eversion, which showed pain and weakness at 3+/5. Grossly, the patient had full ROM with pain at end range. The course of treatment included initial edema reduction and pain management while maintaining full ROM. Because of peroneal involvement, the therapist was able to begin strengthening in all planes except eversion, which was limited to isometrics. The patient later performed proprioception and plyometric exercises and returned to pole-vaulting after 8 weeks, with an ankle-stabilizing orthosis (ASO) ankle brace.

SUGGESTED HOME MAINTENANCE FOR THE POSTSURGICAL PATIENT

Weeks 6-8

GOALS FOR THE PERIOD: Improve gait, increase ROM to normal, gradually increase strength, control pain and swelling, and increase proprioception

1. AROM in plantar flexion, dorsiflexion, and eversion
2. Isometrics for plantar flexion, dorsiflexion, and eversion
3. Towel calf non–weight bearing stretch for gastrocnemius-soleus muscle group
4. Towel-crunching exercise
5. Four-way hip non–weight bearing exercise to initiate total lower extremity strength
6. Seated heel and toe raises

Weeks 8-10

GOALS FOR THE PERIOD: Maintain normal ROM, continue to increase strength and improve proprioception

1. Rubber tubing with appropriate resistance for dorsiflexion and plantar flexion
2. Submaximal isometric exercises of inversion and eversion (performed without pain)
3. Stationary bicycle
4. Heel raises (bilateral)
5. Step-ups, step-downs
6. Single-leg stance

Weeks 11-18

GOALS FOR THE PERIOD: Progress with strengthening, increase endurance, and return to previous level of function (sport activity)

1. Standing gastrocnemius-soleus stretch
2. Increased resistance of rubber tubing
3. Straight-ahead running if gait is normal
4. Heel raises progressing to single-leg raises
5. Sports-specific training
6. Functional training
7. Return to sport as cleared by the therapist and physician with ankle bracing

References

1. Bahr R, Fetal P: Biomechanics of ankle ligament reconstruction: an in vitro comparison of the Broström repair, Watson-Jones reconstruction, and a new anatomic reconstruction technique, *Am J Sports Med* 25:424, 1997.
2. Balduini FC et al: Management and rehabilitation of ligamentous injuries to the ankle, *Sports Med* 4:364, 1987.
3. Berlet GC, Anderson RB, Davis WH: Chronic lateral ankle instability, *Foot Ankle Clin* 4:713, 1999.
4. Bleakley C, McDonough S, MacAuley D: The use of ice in the treatment of acute soft-tissue injury: A systematic review of randomized controlled trials. *Am J Sports Med* 32(1), 2004.
5. Broström L: Sprained ankles VI. Surgical treatment of "chronic" ligament ruptures, *Acta Chir Scand* 132:551, 1966.
6. Chams RN, Ferkel RD: Long term follow-up of the modified Broström procedure after arthroscopic evaluation. Accepted publication, *Foot Ankle Int* 2006.
7. Chrisman OD, Snook GA: Reconstruction of lateral ligament tears of the ankle: An experimental study and clinical evaluation of seven patients treated by a new modification of the Elmslie procedure, *J Bone Joint Surg* 51A:904, 1969.
8. Colville MR, Grondel RJ: Anatomic reconstruction of the lateral ankle ligaments using a split peroneus brevis tendon graft, *Am J Sports Med* 23:210, 1995.
9. Coughlin MJ, Schenck RC, Grebing BR, Treme G: Comprehensive reconstruction of the lateral ankle for chronic instability using a free gracilis graft, *Foot Ankle Int* 25:231-241, 2004.
10. DeMaio M, Paine R, Drez D: Chronic lateral ankle instability-inversion sprains: Part I & II, *Orthopedics* 15:87, 1992.
11. Eils E, Rosenbaum D: A multi-station proprioceptive exercise program in patients with ankle instability. *Med Sci Sports Exerc* 33(12), 2001.
12. Ekstrand J, Trapp II: The incidence of ankle sprains in soccer, *Foot Ankle* 11:41, 1990.
13. Evans DL: Recurrent instability of the ankle: A method of surgical treatment, *Proc R Soc Med* 46:343, 1953.
14. Evans GA, Hardcastle P, Frenyo AD: Acute rupture of the lateral ligament of the ankle. To suture or not to suture? *JBJS* 66(2), 1984.
15. Garrick JG: The frequency of injury, mechanism of injury and epidemiology of ankle sprains, *Am J Sports* 5(6):241, 1977.
16. Gebhard JS et al: Passive motion: The dose effects on joint stiffness, muscle mass, bone density, and regional swelling, *JBJS* 75A:163, 1993.
17. Gould N, Seligson D, Gassman J: Early and late repair of lateral ligament of the ankle, *Foot Ankle* 1:84, 1980.
18. Hamilton WB, Thompson FM, Snow SW: The modified Broström procedure for lateral ankle instability, *Foot Ankle* 13:1, 1993.
19. Hennrikus WL et al: Outcomes of the Chrisman-Snook and modified-Broström procedures for chronic lateral ankle instability. A prospective, randomized comparison, *Am J Sports Med* 24:400, 1996.

20. Kaikkonen A, Kannus P, Jarvinen M: Surgery versus functional treatment in ankle ligament tears. A prospective study, *Clinical Orthopaedics & Related Research* (326), 1996.
21. Karlsson J et al: Reconstruction of the lateral ligaments of the ankle for chronic lateral instability, *J Bone Joint Surg* 70A:581, 1988.
22. Karlsson J et al: Comparisons of two anatomic reconstructions for chronic lateral instability of the ankle joint, *Am J Sports Med* 25:48, 1997.
23. Keller M, Grossman J: Lateral ankle instability and the Broström-Gould procedure, *Foot and Ankle* 35:513, 1996.
24. Kerkoffs GMMJ, Handoll HHG, De Bie R, Rowe BH, Struijs PAA: Surgical versus conservative treatment for acute injuries of the lateral ligament complex of the ankle in adults. *Cochrane Review* 3, 2002.
25. Komenda G, Ferkel RD: Arthroscopic findings associated with the unstable ankle, *Foot Ankle Int* 20(11):708, 1999.
26. Liu SH, Baker CL: Comparison of lateral ankle ligamentous reconstruction procedures, *Am J Sports Med* 22:313, 1994.
27. Peters WJ, Trevino SG, Renstrom PA: Chronic lateral ankle instability, *Foot Ankle* 12:182, 1991.
28. Sammarco GJ, Carrasquillo HA: Surgical revision after failed lateral ankle reconstruction, *Foot Ankle Int* 16:748, 1995.
29. Scheffler NM, Sheitel PL, Lipton MN: Use of Cryo/Cuff for the control of postoperative pain and edema. *J Foot Surg* 31(2), 1992.
30. Specchiulli F, Cofano RE: A comparison of surgical and conservative treatment in ankle ligament tears. *Orthopedics* 24(7), 2001.
31. Taga I et al: Articular cartilage lesions in ankles with lateral ligament injury. An arthroscopic study, *Am J Sports Med* 21:120, 1993.
32. Takao M, Oae K, Uchio Y, Ochi M, Yamamoto H: Anatomical reconstruction of the lateral ligaments of the ankle with a gracilis autograft, *Am J Sports Med* 33:814, 2005.
33. Watson-Jones R: *Fractures and other bone and joint injuries,* Baltimore, 1940, Williams & Wilkins.
34. Wilke B, Weiner RD: Postoperative cryotherapy: Risks versus benefits of continuous-flow cryotherapy units. *Clin Podiatr Med Surg* 20(2), 2003.

CHAPTER 23

Open Reduction and Internal Fixation of the Ankle

Robert Donatelli
Will Hall
Brian E. Prell
Richard D. Ferkel

The treatment of ankle fractures dates back to antiquity. Evidence of healed ankle fractures has been noted in the remains of mummies from ancient Egypt.[11] Hippocrates recommended that closed fractures be reduced by traction of the foot, but few other advances in the understanding and treatment of ankle fractures were made until the middle of the 18th century.[1,16,20] Operative treatment of ankle fractures was popularized by Lambotte and Danis; the AO group began a systematic study of fracture treatment in 1958.[3,8,18,33] Since these original investigators, significant progress has been made in the treatment of ankle fractures.

An ankle fracture is a debilitating injury, especially if the fracture is unstable. The treatment of choice for an unstable ankle fracture is open reduction and internal fixation (ORIF). As technology and surgical techniques have advanced, so have the outcomes for ORIF.[23] Anand and Klenarman[4] report that, in a sample of 80 patients older than 60 years, 88.5% were satisfied with their postoperative outcome.

Much of the current understanding of the mechanism of ankle fractures has developed from the work of Lauge-Hansen.[21] In his system, the position of the foot (pronation or supination) at the time of the injury is described first and the direction of the deforming force is described second. Ankle fractures currently are classified most commonly by two systems: Lauge-Hansen and Danis.[21] The latter system is based on the level of the fracture of the fibula. Fractures also are classified by the number of bones that are affected—that is, a bimalleolar fracture involves injury to two areas of the ankle, whereas a trimalleolar fracture indicates that the medial, lateral, and posterior malleoli have all been fractured.

SURGICAL INDICATIONS AND CONSIDERATIONS

Ankle fractures are treated conservatively if minimal displacement has occurred with little rotation and shortening of the fracture fragments. The ankle mortise must be secure with the medial clear space (the space between the medial malleolus and talus) measuring 3 mm or less. In addition, the lateral clear space (the space between the lateral fibula and the lateral dome of the talus) also must measure 3 mm or less. Moreover, the talus must be reduced beneath the tibial plafond and not subluxated forward or backward. If the fracture is felt to be stable, it can be treated in a cast, usually below the knee, extending to the tips of the toes with the foot in an appropriate position for the type of fracture deformity. In some instances, after swelling resolves, the fracture can displace; in this case ORIF should be performed. In general, ORIF should be performed on all patients, regardless of age, gender, activity level, or vocation, as long as they are healthy enough to undergo the procedure. However, exceptions do exist, including paraplegics and quadriplegics and patients who are nonambulatory and lack sensation to the lower extremities.

Preoperative variables that predict a successful outcome include an otherwise healthy patient who is well motivated to recover after surgery. Systemic diseases such as osteoporosis, diabetes, alcoholism, and tobacco abuse can all affect the ultimate outcome of surgery. These variables affect wound healing as well as the healing of the fracture itself.

SURGICAL PROCEDURE

Surgical Options

The currently accepted method for fracture ORIF is the AO (Association for the Study of Internal Fixation [ASIF]) technique developed in Switzerland. This technique emphasizes the use of plates and screws and wires as needed to achieve rigid fixation. A careful preoperative assessment of not only the patient's health, but also the fracture and the patient's swelling and skin tension, is important to a successful outcome. In some cases surgery may have to be delayed for as long as 14 days to allow swelling to resolve so the skin can be closed at the end of surgery without a wound slough. Recently, a foot and ankle pump device has been used to reduce swelling rapidly to permit earlier surgery and fewer complications.

Initially, patients may be too swollen to wear a cast. In this instance a bulky dressing with cast padding and bias-type compression wrap is applied with a posterior splint. The patient remains non–weight bearing with crutches and elevates the injured ankle above the heart to promote reduction of swelling.

Procedure

Four criteria must be fulfilled to achieve the best possible functional results in the treatment of ankle fractures:

1. Dislocations and fractures should be reduced as soon as possible.
2. All joint surfaces must be precisely reconstituted.
3. Reduction of the fracture must be maintained during the period of healing.
4. Motion of the joint should be instituted as early as possible.

The patient is taken to the operating room and either epidural or general anesthesia is provided. Prophylactic antibiotics are administered and the injured extremity is prepared and draped as described in Chapter 22. Recent research at the Southern California Orthopedic Institute indicates that a high percentage of patients have intra-articular pathology associated with ankle fractures.[23] Almost 75% of patients with displaced ankle fractures have an osteochondral lesion of the talus that is not evident on preoperative x-ray films and can only be seen on arthroscopy before ORIF. On the basis of these results and Lantz's research[19] (which found a 49% incidence of injuries to the talar dome articular cartilage in isolated malleolar fractures), the authors recommend arthroscopy before ORIF of all ankle fractures. This approach is also supported by Hintermann's recent study.[13]

The arthroscopic evaluation is done as described in Chapter 24. All intraarticular pathology is documented and appropriately treated. The surgeon must examine carefully for osteochondral lesions of the talus, tears of the deltoid ligament, and dislocations of the posterior tibial tendon, which may impede fracture reduction. Some fractures can be reduced and internally fixated by arthroscopic means alone.[24] A typical example is a patient with a fracture of the medial malleolus that was debrided arthroscopically and fixated percutaneously with two cannulated screws (Fig 23-1). Recently, we have reported on the long-term results of treating Tillaux fractures in this manner.[14] After the arthroscopic portion of the procedure is completed, if the fracture is not amenable to all-arthroscopic reduction, the ankle is prepared and draped again, gloves are changed, and new sterile instruments are used.

Incisions are made over the lateral, medial, or posterior malleolus, depending on the nature of the fractures. When a fracture apparently involves only the medial malleolus,

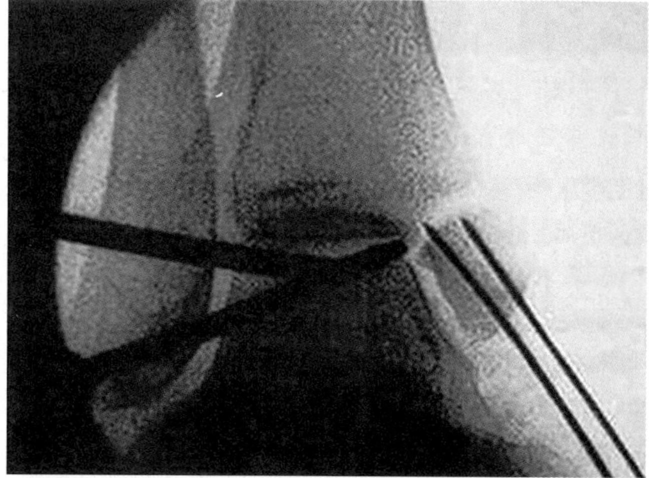

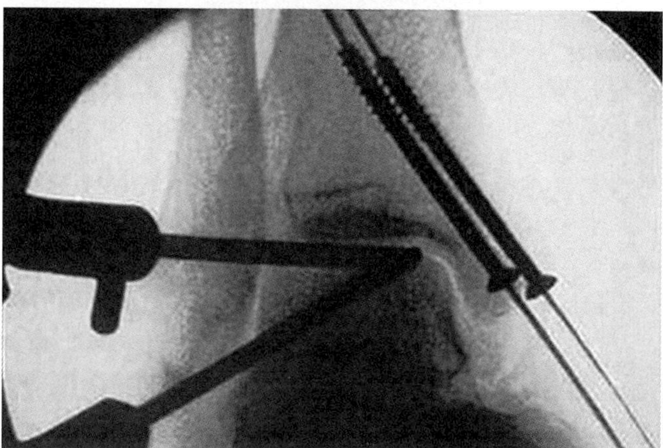

Fig. 23-1 A, Intraoperative fluoroscopy view confirming parallel guide wire insertion used to manipulate the medial malleolus fragment. Fracture reduction is checked arthroscopically as the wires are advanced proximally across the fracture site. **B,** Cannulated screws are subsequently inserted and checked under fluoroscopy and also arthroscopically to verify anatomic reduction.

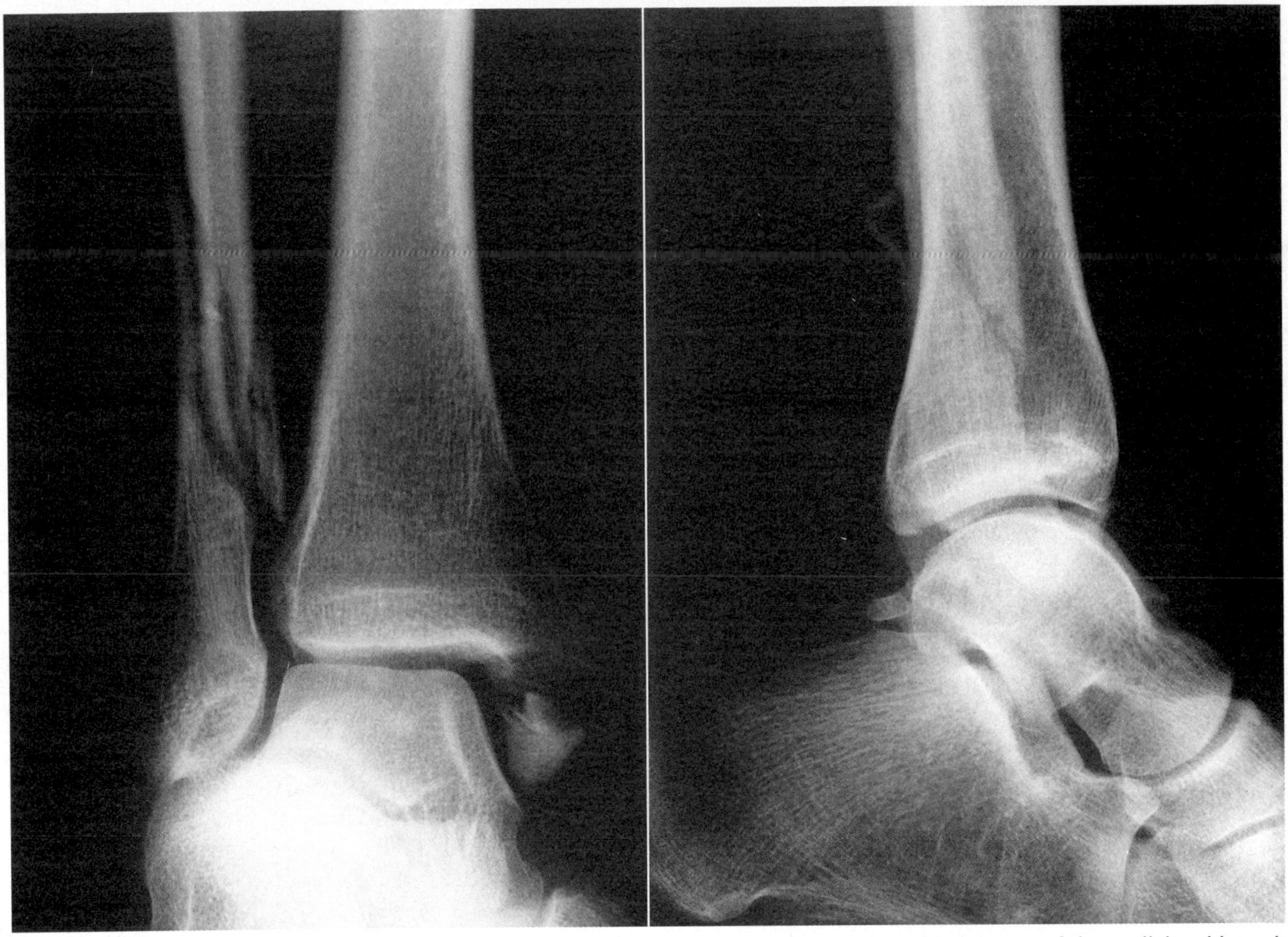

Fig. 23-2 Bimalleolar ankle fracture. Anteroposterior (AP) (A) and lateral (B) radiographs demonstrating fractures of the medial and lateral malleoli.

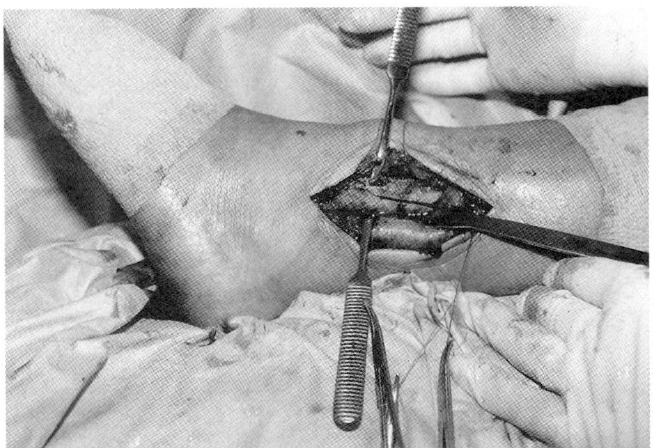

Fig. 23-3 The malleolus fracture of the left ankle is exposed and the periosteum is elevated with sharp dissection.

the surgeon should search for an injury to the syndesmosis with subsequent tearing of the interosseous membrane, which may result in a high fibular fracture. This type of fracture, which also is known as a Maisonneuve type of fracture, could even occur at the fibular head and may be missed if the surgeon is not diligent. In this instance the medial malleolar fracture is reduced anatomically, usually with two screws inserted proximally through a small incision from the tip of the medial malleolus. The deltoid ligament is split in line with its fibers, and the two screws are inserted parallel to each other under fluoroscopic control. If the syndesmosis and interosseous membrane have been torn and are unstable, one or two syndesmotic screw(s) are inserted through the fibula and tibia, exiting the medial border of the tibia with the foot in maximal dorsiflexion. The screw(s) are not placed with compression because compressing the syndesmosis restricts motion postoperatively. When both the medial and lateral malleoli have been fractured, the lateral malleolus is approached first (Fig. 23-2). The surgeon makes an incision over the fracture site and extends it proximally and distally. Dissection is carried down to the periosteum and the fracture site. The fracture is exposed and the periosteum is elevated with sharp dissection (Fig. 23-3). The surgeon uses a curette to remove the hematoma and applies reduction clamps to assist in reducing the fracture. Reduction of the fracture usually also requires traction and rotation of the foot and ankle. When anatomic reduction has been achieved, frequently one or two lag screws are used to provide interfragmentary compression across the fracture site. After this is accomplished, an appropriately sized plate is centered over the fracture site and stabilized with screws (Fig. 23-4). An incision is then made over the medial malleolus as previously described, the fracture site is exposed, the hematoma is removed, and the fracture is reduced. The surgeon inserts one or two screws. Postoperative x-ray films are taken to verify anatomic reduction of the fractures and appropriate positioning of the screws and plate (Fig. 23-5).

In ORIF of a trimalleolar fracture, the lateral and medial malleoli are addressed as previously mentioned. Using the fluoroscope, the surgeon then reduces the posterior malleolar fracture by manipulating the fragment into place and making a small incision along the anterolateral aspect of the distal tibia. Two guide pins are inserted to reduce the fragment and one or two cannulated screws are inserted from anterior to posterior to hold the posterior malleolar fragment in place. In general, posterior malleolar fracture fragments do not require internal fixation if they involve less than 30% of the articular surface.

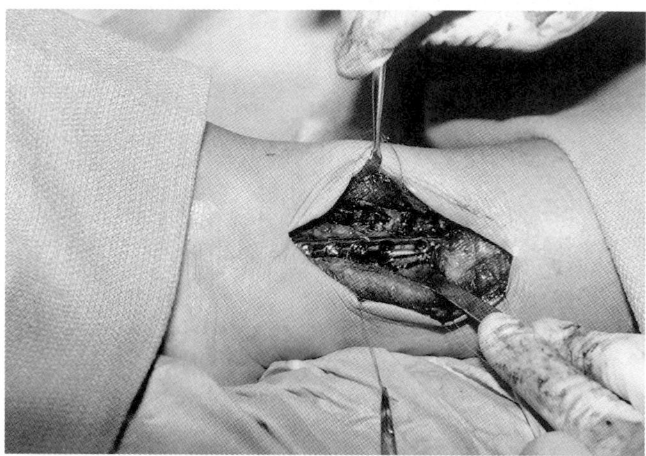

Fig. 23-4 Lag screws are used to provide interfragmentary compression across the fracture site. An appropriately sized plate is then centered over the fracture site, and the fracture is stabilized with screws.

Postoperative Considerations

After surgery the patient is placed in a well-padded short-leg cast; the cast is split in the recovery room to allow for swelling. The procedure can be done on an outpatient basis if the pain level is not too severe, but in some instances the patient may be required to stay 1 or 2 days in the hospital. After discharge the patient is non–weight bearing on crutches. The cast is changed at 1 week after surgery, the wound is inspected, and all new dressings are applied. At 2 weeks after surgery the stitches are removed and a new short-leg cast is applied for 2 additional weeks. At 4 weeks after surgery, another short-leg cast is applied and the patient starts partial weight bearing, gradually increasing to full weight bearing without crutches. After the fracture has healed, the patient can wear a supportive brace and start pool and then land physical therapy. In patients with stable, reliable fixation, sometimes early motion can be initiated after the third or fourth post-operative week to facilitate early return of motion and strength.[12]

When a syndesmosis screw has been inserted, the patient must be non–weight bearing for 6 to 8 weeks; the screw is

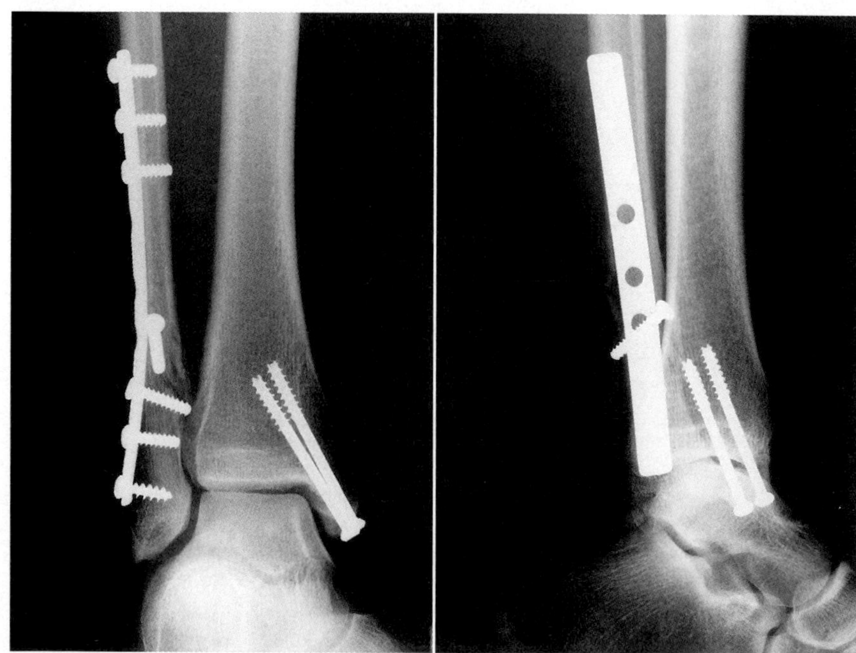

Fig. 23-5 **A** and **B**, Postoperative anteroposterior (AP) and lateral radiographs are taken to verify anatomic reduction of the fractures with appropriate positioning of the screws and plate.

removed at 10 to 12 weeks postoperatively. The screw will break with weight bearing if it is left in place. Physical therapy is started 6 to 8 weeks after surgery. After the screw is removed, the patient can be full weight bearing and initiate physical therapy.

SURGICAL OUTCOMES

A successful outcome is defined as a fully healed fracture, with the patient achieving near full or complete range of motion (ROM) with normal strength and function.[34] Function is defined differently for each patient—an athlete's function is different from that of a sedentary, elderly patient. Several different grading systems, including subjective, objective, and functional data, are used to evaluate ankle fracture results. However, ankle fracture results are difficult to compare because of the multitude of fracture patterns and different circumstances of treatment. Results can be affected by many things, including severity and type of injury, associated intraarticular problems, preexisting arthritis,[17] age and reliability of the patient, quality of the bone, and other site injuries. Finally, it should be noted that there is a potential for superficial nerve injury after surgical repair as well as syndesmosis instability.[26]

THERAPY GUIDELINES FOR REHABILITATION

The physical therapist normally evaluates the patient approximately 6 weeks after surgery. In most cases, the patient has been casted for those 6 weeks and has had partial weight bearing status between 2 and 4 weeks. Studies have reported that clinical outcomes may be improved in patients with trimalleolar fractures who have full weight bearing status in an ankle orthosis between 2 to 4 weeks after surgery.[2] Some authors also suggest early active range of motion (AROM) for plantar flexion and dorsiflexion as soon as the surgical incision has healed.[2,15]

Evaluation

The initial evaluation establishes the baseline deficits from which further goals and treatment are formulated. AROM and passive range of motion (PROM) are assessed within the patient's tolerance. ROM is a primary limitation noted at the initial evaluation. Joint effusion and soft tissue edema are evaluated as well using either a "figure 8" technique with a standard measuring tape or by applying volumetrics. The patient's ambulation is assessed to determine abnormal movement patterns secondary to an antalgic gait. At this stage the patient may have acute pain and be in a fracture boot or other type of orthosis. Often, the patient may experience hardware-related pain, which may have an affect on functional outcomes.[7] The physical therapist inspects and evaluates scar mobility. Joint and soft tissue mobility is assessed with an emphasis on the way restrictions limit ROM and function. After enough mineralization and calcium formation has occurred according to the physician, an assessment of the arthrokinematic movements of the ankle joint can be done. For example, posterior glide of the talus is often markedly restricted and has been correlated to restrictions in dorsiflexion and normal gait. In addition, posterior and anterior glide of the proximal and distal fibular heads have been shown to increase AROM and PROM (Box 23-1).

Box 23-1

- Asses PROM within pain tolerance
- Asses AROM within pain tolerance
- Asses joint effusion and soft tissue edema
- Asses ambulation secondary to antalgic gait
- Asses scar mobility
- Asses soft tissue mobility (including muscle tightness)
- Asses joint mobility after 8-10 weeks (after enough mineralization and calcium formation has occurred per MD)

After evaluation and discussion, the physical therapist and patient formulate a treatment plan and goals. Belcher et al[6] reported impaired function as long as 24 months after an ORIF surgery for a trimalleolar fracture.

Phase I

TIME: Weeks 6-8 after surgery
GOALS: Minimize pain and swelling, normalize ROM, initiate AROM and therapeutic exercises, normalize gait, increase joint and soft tissue mobility, maintain cardiovascular fitness, and provide patient education (Table 23-1)

Treatment goals initially are to decrease pain and swelling, increase ROM and strength, and normalize gait. AROM and PROM are initiated immediately for all planes of movement under the supervision of the physical therapist.

AROM can progress from movement with lessened gravity (e.g., in a pool) to movement using gravity as resistance. Soft tissue mobilization of restricted structures is particularly useful in decreasing pain and increasing ROM. Around 8 weeks, with physician approval, joint mobilization of the ankle is implemented using distraction and glide maneuvers (Figs. 23-6 and 23-7).[9]

Ankle joint mobilizations into resistance are deferred until enough mineralization and calcium formation have occurred (usually 8 weeks).

The rehabilitation program also includes gait training and lower extremity strengthening in shallow and deep

Table 23-1 Ankle Open Reduction Internal Fixation

Rehabilitation Phase	Criteria to Progress to this Phase	Anticipated Impairments and Functional Limitations	Intervention	Goal	Rationale
Phase I Postoperative 6-8 weeks	◆ Cleared by physician to begin rehabilitation postoperatively	◆ Limited weight-bearing per physician ◆ Pain ◆ Edema ◆ Limited ROM ◆ Limited strength	◆ Encourage use of compression stocking ◆ Cryotherapy with compression ◆ ES (with pads carefully placed) ◆ Elevation ◆ PROM (pain free) for ankle dorsiflexion, plantarflexion, inversion, and eversion ◆ Joint mobilization grades II and III (at 8 weeks with physician approval) ◆ Isometrics (submaximal) for ankle dorsiflexion, plantarflexion, inversion, and eversion ◆ AROM (pain free) for ankle dorsiflexion, plantarflexion, inversion, and eversion ◆ PNF patterns ◆ Weight-shifting exercises ◆ Stationary bicycle ◆ Seated balance board activities ◆ Soft tissue mobilization ◆ Gait training as indicated by weight-bearing status ◆ Instruction for locating neutral pelvic position ◆ Initial core stabilization exercises ◆ Home exercise program	◆ Manage edema ◆ Decrease pain ◆ Increase PROM ◆ Increase strength ◆ Decrease gait deviations, improve tolerance to weight bearing ◆ Improve soft tissue mobility ◆ Improve joint mobility	◆ Control edema and decrease pain using ES, rest, ice with compression, and elevation ◆ Improve ROM in pain-free ranges to avoid increase in edema and pain ◆ Movement nourishes articular cartilage and improves tolerance to exercise ◆ Physician must give weight-bearing status to progress gait; weight-shifting exercises and intermittent loading (bicycle) can be useful in progressing tolerance of ankle and foot to compression ◆ Soft tissue and joint mobilization useful in restoring ROM and gating pain ◆ Core stabilization to maintain neutral pelvic position and improve gait biomechanics ◆ Self-manage exercises

ROM, Range of motion; *ES,* electrical stimulation; *PROM,* passive range of motion; *AROM,* active range of motion; *PNF,* proprioceptive neuromuscular facilitation.

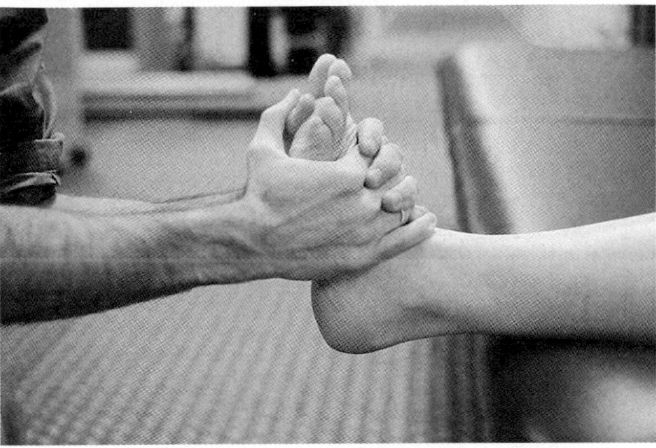

Fig. 23-6 Long-axis distraction of the talus.

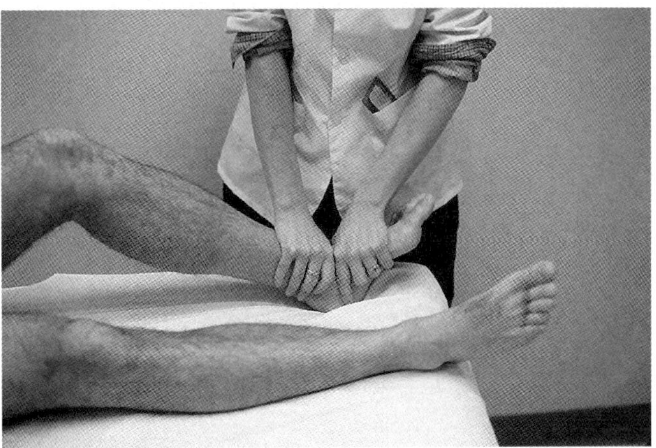

Fig. 23-7 Posteroanterior (PA) glide of the talus.

water in addition to land therapy. Ankle AROM exercises also are initiated in the pool.

The patient should avoid jumping and running exercises in shallow water at this time. However, if lack of ROM and gait are significant problems at the time of the patient's initial physical therapy evaluation, the therapist may decide to begin land therapy in combination with pool therapy to address specific problems and monitor the patient more closely.

A compressive stocking is useful to help control soft tissue edema and joint effusion, especially during initial weight-bearing activities. The patient is instructed in a home exercise program incorporating ice, elevation, compression, and light active exercises such as stationary bicycling or AROM exercises to reduce soft edema and joint effusion. Pain and swelling are managed with appropriate modalities such as pulsed ultrasound or electrical stimulation. **However, these modalities shouldn't be performed over the metal implants.**

> **Q** Amy is a 30-year-old female who suffered a bimalleolar fracture while playing soccer. She underwent an ORIF procedure on her ankle 15 weeks ago. Amy complains of tightness, which progressively increases throughout the day as she performs her functional daily activities. How did the therapist address this issue in her treatment plan?

Phase II

TIME: Weeks 9-12 after surgery

GOALS: Minimize pain and swelling, normalize ROM, normalize gait, decrease soft tissue restrictions, increase strength of intrinsic and extrinsic foot and ankle muscles (Table 23-2)

The second phase is initiated after pain and swelling have subsided, usually 9 to 12 weeks after surgery. The second phase of treatment blends with the first as ROM and gait progress to normal. Progressive resistive exercises (PREs) are used to strengthen the anterior and posterior tibialis, peroneals, and gastrocnemius and soleus muscle groups. A home program, using elastic tubing for resistance, is helpful to augment supervised physical therapy in the office. Treatment options for strengthening exercises include the stationary bicycle, stair-climbing machine, step-ups, step-downs, calf raises, and isokinetic exercises. Specific muscle strengthening for the gastrocnemius and soleus muscles is important to examine because of the likelihood of muscle atrophy. A total lower extremity strengthening program is indicated, as well as a program to maintain cardiovascular fitness. Joint and soft tissue mobilization is continued as indicated. Submaximal isokinetics can be implemented using high speeds such as 120 to 180 degrees per second. The higher velocities prevent excessive resistance that could exacerbate the patient's symptoms. Proprioceptive activities are increased as the patient begins to demonstrate increased balance; use of a balance board is helpful in developing proprioception. The patient progresses heel raises from sitting to standing to single-leg standing. Modalities such as compression wraps and ice packs are used as indicated for postexercise pain and swelling. Electrical stimulation may be used if the pads are appropriately placed away from plates and pins. The intensity of the rehabilitation should be altered if pain or swelling limit the rehabilitation progression. **Weight-bearing exercises and resisted exercises done too aggressively will exacerbate the symptoms and could delay the rehabilitation process for several weeks.**

Table 23-2 Ankle Open Reduction Internal Fixation

Rehabilitation Phase	Criteria to Progress to this Phase	Anticipated Impairments and Functional Limitations	Intervention	Goal	Rationale
Phase II Postoperative 9-12 weeks	◆ No signs of infection ◆ No loss of ROM ◆ No significant increase in pain	◆ Edema and pain present but under control ◆ Limited ROM ◆ Limited strength ◆ Gait deviations	◆ Continue interventions as in Phase I as indicated ◆ Modalities as needed ◆ PROM (stretches)—Gastrocnemius- soleus, tibialis posterior and anterior ◆ AROM—Sitting heel raises (bilateral and progressed to single leg and from sitting to standing) ◆ Isotonic or elastic tubing exercises—Dorsiflexion, plantarflexion, inversion, eversion ◆ Treadmill ◆ Stationary bicycle ◆ Stair-climbing machine ◆ Multihip exercises ◆ Knee flexion/ extension ◆ Closed-chain exercises ◆ Leg press machine ◆ Bilateral heel raises ◆ Step-ups and step-downs ◆ Lateral step-ups and step-downs ◆ Mini-squats ◆ Partial lunges ◆ Isokinetics (submaximal)—120-180 degrees per second ◆ Balance exercises	◆ Self-manage edema ◆ Decrease pain ◆ Increase ROM ◆ Increase strength ◆ Decrease gait deviations ◆ Improve functional strength of gait ◆ Increase endurance ◆ Increase proprioception and prevent reinjury	◆ Progress home exercises and use modalities as indicated ◆ Provide specific LE stretches ◆ Improve tolerance to body weight as resistance for exercises ◆ Use varying resistance to progress strength ◆ Use gym equipment to progress functional strength and endurance; progress to cardiovascular levels when able ◆ Use closed-chain and balance exercises to strengthen foot intrinsic and ankle muscles in a weight-bearing position

ROM, Range of motion; *PROM*, passive range of motion; *AROM*, active range of motion; *LE*, lower extremity.

A

When a patient complains of stiffness, it is always necessary to determine if the problem is joint or soft-tissue in nature. The therapist assessed the patient and found significant restrictions with proximal fibular anteroposterior (AP) glides and distal fibular posteroanterior (PA) glides. These were treated appropriately, and the patient immediately noticed a decrease in her "stiffness."

Q

Lauren is a 23-year-old female who suffered a bimalleolar fracture secondary to a motor vehicle accident. Lauren has progressed well; however, she has noticed increased purulent discharge from her incision at an area that is having difficulty closing. Upon assessment, increased skin temperature and redness around the incision was also noted. What was done?

Phase III

TIME: Weeks 13-18

GOALS: Maintain normal limits of ROM, joint and soft tissue mobility, gait, and muscle strength; increase coordination for higher-level activities; improve balance and proprioception (Table 23-3)

The third phase of rehabilitation begins approximately 13 to 18 weeks from the time of surgery. The fracture is usually healed by this phase of rehabilitation.[15] The patient has progressed to normal ROM and demonstrates a normal gait and increased strength with manual muscle testing. Before progressing to a more aggressive program the patient should be cleared by the surgeon. Therapeutic exercises should progress to include strengthening exercises that are 60% to 70% of maximal effort. This submaximal effort is best determined by the patient's ability to lift a specific amount of weight 10 times. The ninth and tenth repetitions should be difficult for the patient. Isokinetic strengthening programs can be initiated. The use of various speeds during the workout session is referred to as *velocity spectrum.* The authors of this chapter have found velocity spectrum training useful in promoting strength and power of the extrinsic muscles of the foot and ankle.

Functional training should be initiated for the patient wishing to return to sporting activities or vigorous work. Treadmill walking on an incline or retrograde can be an excellent method of training for the endurance athlete. Pool activities can be used initially for running and jumping.

A

The physician was notified, and the patient was sent for a follow-up visit. Tests showed the patient had developed an infection at the incision site, and she was placed on a broad-spectrum antibiotic. Whirlpool treatment was initiated, maintaining the water at 98° F to 100° F for 20 minutes 3 times per week. General wound care was provided, and her rehabilitation schedule continued in a modified fashion.

Q

Brittany is a 30-year-old female who suffered a bimalleolar fracture and had ORIF 16 weeks ago. Brittany has returned to her position as an art teacher, which requires her to stand frequently throughout the day. Since returning, Brittany reports she has had increased lateral ankle pain, which is greater in the afternoon and evening. How did the therapist treat this patient?

Phase IV

TIME: Week 19 and beyond

GOALS: Return to sporting activities or daily activities without restrictions (Table 23-4)

Phase IV is the last phase, starting at 19 weeks after surgery. This phase is used to condition the patient for a return to sports, work, or any activity requiring vigorous movement. Sport-specific activities are carefully implemented with the use of an ankle brace.

Plyometric exercises simulate many sporting activities because of the pre-stretch to the muscle before contraction. Some examples of plyometric exercises include depth jumping, trampoline, hopping, and jumping over obstacles. However, plyometric exercises are stressful to joints and soft tissue structures and should be initiated after normal muscle strength is obtained throughout the lower limb.

A

Brittany was assessed and it was found that her AROM and strength were within normal limits. She had the option of having the hardware removed once healing occurred; however, Brittany refused to have additional surgery. Brittany was issued a home TENS unit and was instructed in its use, as well as the precautions and contraindications. She was also issued an ankle-stabilizing orthosis (ASO) brace to wear during work and with activities requiring prolonged walking and running. Finally, the therapist discussed various options for allowing changes in the length of time she stands during the day (the therapist recommended she use a stool while lecturing).

Table 23-3 Ankle Open Reduction Internal Fixation

Rehabilitation Phase	Criteria to Progress to this Phase	Anticipated Impairments and Functional Limitations	Intervention	Goal	Rationale
Phase III Postoperative 13-18 weeks	◆ Continued progression with Phase II activities ◆ No loss of ROM ◆ No increase in pain	◆ Limited strength ◆ Limited gait ◆ Limited with jumping and running	◆ Continuation of Phase I and II interventions as indicated ◆ Treadmill using incline and retrograde ◆ Isokinetic velocity spectrum ◆ Agility drills—Lateral shuffles, carioca, and initiate low-level plyometrics ◆ Pool therapy—Running and jumping in chest- to waist-deep water as indicated	◆ Full ROM ◆ No gait deviations ◆ Ankle muscle strength 80%-90% ◆ Increase coordination, balance, and proprioception ◆ Prepare for return to sport	◆ Progress Phases from I and II as indicated; discontinue reliance on modalities to control pain ◆ Use uneven surface ambulation and agility drills to improve tolerance of the ankle and foot to the community environment and return to sport ◆ Progress isokinetics to train ankle for endurance activities ◆ Use water to aid in progression of tolerance to advance activities while unweighted ◆ Use FCE to determine work tolerances if activity is in question

ROM, Range of motion; *FCE,* functional capacity evaluation.

Table 23-4 Ankle Open Reduction Internal Fixation

Rehabilitation Phase	Criteria to Progress to this Phase	Anticipated Impairments and Functional Limitations	Intervention	Goal	Rationale
Phase IV Postoperative 19+ weeks	◆ Continued progress in Phases I to III	◆ Limited with higher-level activities	◆ Continuation of exercises from Phases I to III as indicated ◆ Work- and sport-simulated exercises ◆ FCE	◆ Return to work and sport activities	◆ Use specificity of training principles to return to previous activities ◆ Use FCE to determine work tolerances if activity is in question

FCE, Functional capacity evaluation.

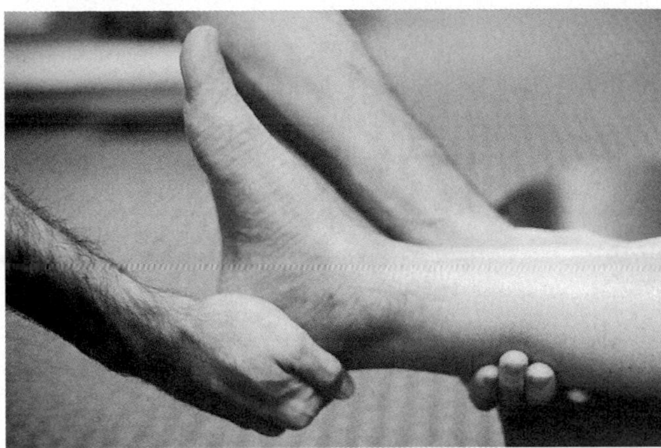

Fig. 23-8 Calcaneal distraction.

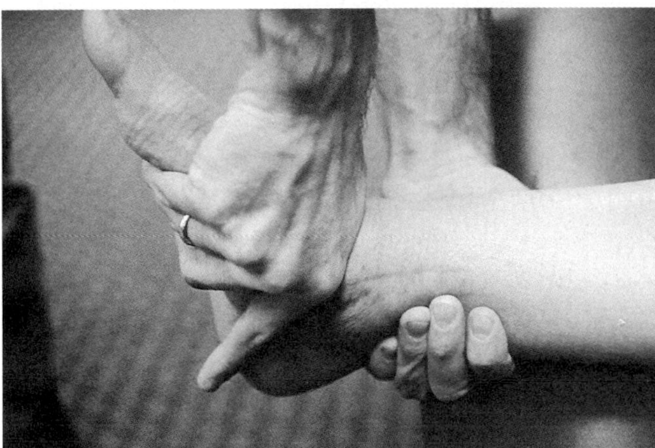

Fig. 23-9 Post-talus glides.

PRECAUTIONS

A trimalleolar fracture is a serious injury. Secondary problems and complications can occur during postoperative rehabilitation. Occasionally low back or sacroiliac pain develop as a result of the antalgic gait with the cast or fracture boot. This is treated symptomatically with emphasis on the need to normalize gait as soon as possible or restrict ambulation activities.

Overuse injuries such as plantar fascitis secondary to a preexisting over-pronation may be treated with modalities and foot orthosis. Because limited dorsiflexion is sometimes an issue, a low-load prolonged stretch for dorsiflexion over 2 to 30 minutes is effective. This can be done in conjunction with moist heat or ultrasound to the gastrocnemius and soleus muscle group. Specific joint mobilizations are shown in Figs. 23-8 and 23-9.

> **Q** Sarah is a 23-year-old college senior who suffered a right ankle bimalleolar fracture and had ORIF 6 weeks ago. On arriving to the clinic for a treatment session, she complained of experiencing increased right calf pain exacerbated with weight bearing. Sarah also reported that she noticed her right calf felt "hot" to touch as compared with the left. She has not slept well the last 2 nights secondary to the previously mentioned symptoms. How did the therapist proceed?

SUGGESTED HOME MAINTENANCE FOR THE POSTSURGICAL PATIENT

An exercise program has been outlined at the various phases. The home maintenance box on page 445 outlines rehabilitation suggestions the patient may follow. The physical therapist can use it in customizing a patient-specific program.

TROUBLESHOOTING

Residual problems after surgical anatomic restoration of the ankle joint include chronic pain, loss of motion, recurrent swelling, and perceived instability. The cause of such poor outcomes is often unclear, but it may be related to missed occult intraarticular injury.[5,27,31,32] Other post-operative problems that can develop include malunion or nonunion, loosening or fracture of the internal fixation devices, infection, and wound problems. These complications are rare. Unless contraindicated, the physical therapist must work on mobilization of the scar or scars as well as general stretching and mobilization of the joint. Care should be taken to increase soft tissue and ankle flexibility gradually and not to stretch or stress the joint excessively to gain more rapid and improved ROM. Pool therapy should be used initially, with some land therapy; as the patient progresses, land therapy increases and pool therapy is diminished. The physical therapist also must take care to avoid pushing the ankle too hard, resulting in increased swelling, pain, and subsequent loss of motion.

The physician should be notified immediately if the patient develops significantly increased pain, swelling, loss of motion, or wound healing problems. In addition, if signs of infection or loosening of the internal fixation develop, the physician should be notified immediately.

A Further assessment by the therapist revealed a positive Homans' sign at the right calf. The physician was notified, and the patient was sent immediately to the hospital for an ultrasound, which showed the patient had developed a deep vein thrombosis (DVT). The patient was admitted to the hospital where anticoagulant therapy was initiated.

Q Braeden is a 19-year-old male who suffered a bimalleolar fracture 20 weeks ago with corresponding ORIF. He received physical therapy at another facility after his surgery for 10 weeks. Braeden has been referred to the therapist's facility with chief complaint of pain inferior to the lateral malleolus and at the Achilles tendon insertion. Pain is minimal in the morning and progressively worsens throughout the day. The patient was noted to have decreased calcaneal abduction and demonstrated increased pronation on the affected side. The patient was also noted to have 5 degrees of dorsiflexion. How did the therapist proceed?

SUMMARY

In the next century, continued advances in surgical techniques and rehabilitation will allow patients to return earlier to their work and sports activities. As additional physicians and physical therapists specialize in foot and ankle problems, more basic and clinical research will be carried out to "push the envelope" of progress to improve foot and ankle care.

A Grade III and IV joint mobilization was performed for AP talar glides and grades III and IV physiologic calcaneal abduction. A contract-relax technique was initiated to increase dorsiflexion. The patient was then taught how to perform the contract-relax technique as a home exercise. Exercises to increase strength in the peroneals and the gastrocnemius and soleus complex were also performed. Additionally, a 3-degree wedge was inserted into the right shoe medially to decrease the angle of pronation. The patient was later casted for custom orthotics.

SUGGESTED HOME MAINTENANCE FOR THE POSTSURGICAL PATIENT

Weeks 6-8

GOALS FOR THE PERIOD: Minimize pain and swelling, improve ROM, initiate AROM and therapeutic exercises, improve gait, and maintain cardiovascular fitness

1. AROM of the ankle (plantar flexion, dorsiflexion, inversion, and eversion)
2. Stretching exercises for the gastrocnemius-soleus muscle groups in a non–weight bearing position (use of a towel or strap to stretch these muscles is recommended)
3. Seated heel and toe raises
4. Ice, elevation, and compression
5. Lower extremity conditioning using the stationary bicycle and/or pool

Weeks 9-12

GOALS FOR THE PERIOD: Normalize ROM and gait, increase strength of the intrinsic and extrinsic foot and ankle musculature, and improve cardiovascular condition

1. Standing heel raises
2. Resistive exercises using elastic bands or tubing for all ankle movements
3. Step-ups and step-downs
4. Single-leg standing progressed to standing on a pillow with eyes open and then with eyes closed (for balance and proprioception)
5. Walking program, including hills as appropriate
6. Lower extremity conditioning using a stationary bicycle, stair-climbing machine, treadmill, pool, leg press, and toe raises
7. Weight-bearing stretching exercises to the posterior calf muscles

Weeks 13-18

GOALS FOR THE PERIOD: Maintain normal ROM, gait, and strength; increase coordination for higher-level activities; improve balance and proprioception; and transition to sporting activities

1. Strengthening exercises with increasing resistance
2. Pool activities such as jumping, running, and cutting drills
3. Agility drills such as side shuffles, backward walking, and carioca
4. Lower extremity conditioning continued from phase II

Week 19 and Beyond

GOALS FOR THE PERIOD: Return to previous level of function (sport- and activity-specific exercises) without restrictions

1. Maximal strengthening of lower extremity muscles
2. Land-based functional activities such as running, jumping, and cutting
3. Sports simulated activities

References

1. Adams F: *The genuine works of Hippocrates*, London, C and J Adlard, 1849.
2. Ahl T et al: Early mobilization of operated on ankle fractures, *Acta Orthop Scand* 64:95, 1993.
3. Allgower M, Muller ME, Willenegger H: *Techniques of internal fixation of fractures*, Berlin, Springer-Verlag, 1965.
4. Anand N, Klenarman L: Ankle fractures in the elderly: MVA versus ORIF, *Injury* 24:116, 1993.
5. Anderson IF et al: Osteochondral fractures of the dome of the talus, *J Bone Joint Surg* 71A:1143, 1989.
6. Belcher GL et al: Functional outcome analysis of operatively treated malleolar fractures, *J Orthop Trauma* 11:106, 1997.
7. Brown OL, Dirschl DR, Obremskey WT: Incidence of hardware related pain and its affect on functional outcomes after open reduction and internal fixation of ankle fractures, *J Orthop Trauma* 15(4):271.
8. Danis R: Le vrai but et les dangers de l'ostesynthese, *Lyon Chirugie* 51:740, 1956.
9. Donatelli R: *Biomechanics of the foot and ankle*, Philadelphia, FA Davis, 1996.
10. Eilis E, Rosenbaum D: A multi-station proprioceptive exercise program in patients with ankle instability, *Med Sci Sports Exerc* 33(12):1991-1998, 2001.
11. Elliot S, Wood J: *The archeology survey of the Nubia report, 1907-1908*, vol 2, Cairo, 1910.
12. Godsiff SP et al: A comparative study of early motion and immediate plaster splintage after internal fixation of unstable fractures of the ankle, *Injury*, 24:116, 1993.
13. Hintermann B, Regazzoni P, Lampert C, Stutz G, Gachter A: Arthroscopic findings in acute fractures of the ankle, *J Bone Joint Surg* 82B:345, 2000.
14. Hommen JP, Ferkel RD: Arthroscopic treatment of the juvenile Tillaux ankle fracture, accepted for publication in *Arthroscopy*, 2006.
15. Hovis WD, Bucholtz RW: Polyglycolide bioabsorbable screws in the treatment of ankle fractures, *Foot Ankle Int* 18(3):128, 1997.
16. Hughes SPF: A historical view of fractures involving the ankle joint, *Mayo Clin Proc* 50: 611, 1975.
17. Jarde O, Vives P, Havet E, Gouron R, Meunier W: Malleolar fractures. Predictive factors for secondary osteoarthritis. Retrospective study of 32 cases, *Acta Orthop Belg* 16(4):382, 2000.
18. Lambotte A: *Chirurgie operatoire des fractures*, Paris, Masson & Cie, 1913.
19. Lantz BA et al: The effect of concomitant chondral injuries accompanying operatively reduced malleolar fractures, *Int Orthop Trauma* 5:125, 1991.
20. Lauge N: Fractures of the ankle. Analytic historic survey as the basis of new, experimental, retrogenologic and clinical investigations, *Arch Surg* 56:259, 1948.
21. Lauge-Hansen N: "Ligamentous" ankle fractures: Diagnosis and treatment, *Acta Chir Scand* 97:544, 1949.
22. Leeds HC, Ehrlich MG: Instability of the distal tibiofibular syndesmosis after bimalleolar and trimalleolar ankle fractures, *J Bone Joint Surg Am* 66(4):490, 1984.
23. Loren GJ, Ferkel RD: Arthroscopic assessment of occult intraarticular injury in acute ankle fractures, *Arthroscopy* 18(4):412-421, 2002.
24. Loren GJ, Ferkel RD: Arthroscopic strategies in fracture management of the ankle. In: Chow JCY (ed): *Advanced Arthroscopy*. New York, Springer, 2001.
25. Michaelson J, Curtis M, Magid D: Controversies in ankle fractures, *Foot Ankle* 14:170, 1993.
26. Redfern DJ, Sauve PS, Sakellariou A: Investigation of incidence of superficial peroneal nerve injury following ankle fracture, *Foot Ankle Int* 24(10):771, 2003.
27. Renström Per AFH: Persistently painful sprained ankle, *J Am Acad Orthop Surg* 2:270, 1994.
28. Rozzi SL, Lephart SM, Sterner R, Kuligowski L: Balance training for persons with functionally unstable ankles, *J Orthop Sports Phys Ther* (8):478-486, 1999.
29. Schmidt R, Benesch S, Bender A, Claes L, Gerngross H: The potential for training of proprioceptive and coordinative parameters in patients with chronic ankle instability, *Z Orthop Ihre Grenzgeb* 143(2):227-232, 2005.
30. Simanski CJ, Maegele MG, Lefering R, Lehnen DM, Kawel N, Reiss P, et al: Functional treatment and early weightbearing after an ankle fracture: A prospective study, *J Orthop Trauma* 20(2):108-114, Feb. 2006.
31. Stone JW: Osteochondral lesions of the talar dome, *J Am Acad Orthop Surg* 4:63, 1996.
32. Taga I et al: Articular cartilage lesions in ankles with lateral ligament injury. An orthoscopic study, *Am J Sports Med* 21:120, 1993.
33. Weber BG: *De verletzungen des oberon Sprunggellenkes, Aktuelle Probleme in der Chirurgie,* Bern, Verlag Hans Huber, 1966.
34. Wiss DA (ed): *Masters Techniques in Orthopaedics: Fractures.* Philadelphia, Lippincott Williams & Wilkins, 2006.

CHAPTER 24

Ankle Arthroscopy

Deborah Mandis Cozen
Richard D. Ferkel
Lisa Maxey

The first arthroscopic inspection of a cadaveric joint was performed by Takagi in Japan in 1918.[20] In 1939 he reported on the arthroscopic examination of an ankle joint in a human patient.[20] With the advent of fiberoptic light transmission, video cameras, instruments for small joints, and distraction devices, arthroscopy has become an important diagnostic and therapeutic modality for disorders of the ankle. Arthroscopic examination of the ankle joint allows direct visualization during stress testing of intraarticular structures and ligaments about the ankle joint. Various arthroscopic procedures have been developed with less attendant morbidity and mortality to patients.[2,5,6,9-11]

SURGICAL INDICATIONS AND CONSIDERATIONS

Diagnostic indications for ankle arthroscopy include unexplained pain, swelling, stiffness, instability, hemarthrosis, locking, and abnormal snapping or popping. Operative indications for ankle arthroscopy include loose body removal, excision of anterior tibiotalar osteophytes, debridement of soft tissue impingement, and treatment of osteochondral lesions, synovectomy, and lateral instability (Fig. 24-1). Other indications include arthrodesis for posttraumatic degenerative arthritis and treatment for ankle fractures and postfracture defects.

Absolute contraindications for ankle arthroscopy include localized soft tissue or systemic infection and severe degenerative joint disease. With end-stage degenerative joint disease, successful distraction may not be possible, precluding visualization of the ankle joint. Relative contraindications include reflex sympathetic dystrophy, moderate degenerative joint disease with restricted range of motion (ROM), severe edema, and tenuous vascular supply.

Methods

Ankle arthroscopy is usually performed in one of three ways: (1) in the supine position, (2) with the knee bent 90 degrees over the end of the table, or (3) in the decubitus position. The method of choice is determined by the surgeon and surgical circumstances. Different types and sizes of arthroscopic equipment can be used depending on surgeon preference and availability.

SURGICAL PROCEDURE

The procedure described is that used most commonly by the author of this chapter; a more detailed description of ankle arthroscopy can be found in his textbook.[7] The patient is taken to the operating room and placed in the supine position. The hip is flexed to 45 degrees, and the leg is placed onto a well-padded thigh support. The thigh support is placed proximal to the popliteal fossa and distal to the tourniquet. The lower extremity is then prepared and draped so that good access is available posteriorly. A tourniquet is applied as needed.

A noninvasive distraction strap is placed over the foot and ankle. Distraction is used to separate the distal tibia from the talus so that at least 4 mm of joint space opening is obtained (Fig. 24-2). Without distraction the surgeon has difficulty positioning the arthroscopic instruments in the ankle without scuffing the articular cartilage; visualizing the central and posterior portions of the ankle also is difficult without adequate joint separation. The distraction device is carefully positioned so as not to injure the neurovascular structures, and approximately 30 lbs of force is placed across the ankle for no more than 60 to 90 minutes.

Before applying the distraction strap, the surgeon should identify and outline the dorsalis pedis artery, the deep peroneal nerve, saphenous vein, tibialis anterior tendon, peroneus tertius tendon, and superficial peroneal nerve and its branches on the skin with a marker. Identification of the superficial peroneal nerve and its branches is facilitated by inverting and plantar flexing the foot and flexing the toes.

The surgeon uses three primary portals or access areas to insert the arthroscope and instrumentation (Fig. 24-3). These include the anteromedial, anterolateral, and posterolateral portals. Accessory portals can be used as needed, but are rarely required. Portals are made by nicking the skin only and then spreading with a clamp through the

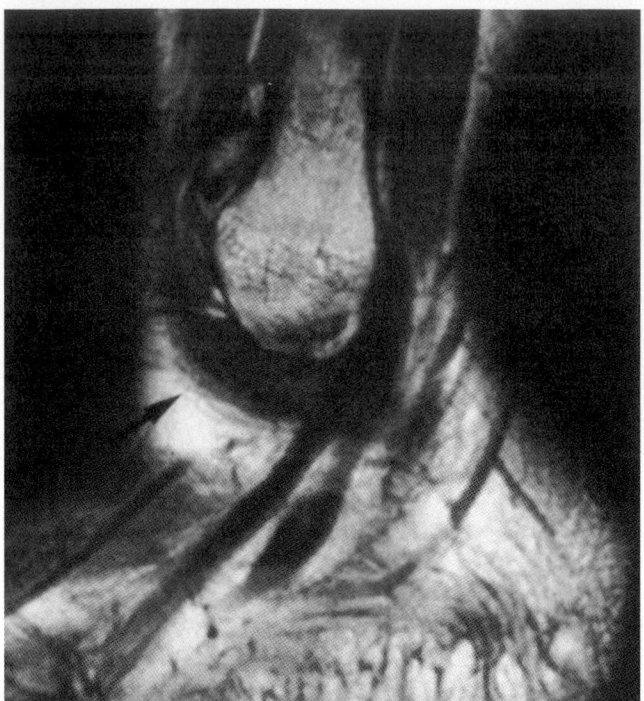

Fig. 24-1 Sagittal T-weighted magnetic resonance image (MRI) showing low-signal intensity consistent with anterolateral soft tissue impingement of the ankle.

subcutaneous tissue and into the ankle joint. The surgeon must take great care to avoid injuring the neurovascular and tendinous structures.

Recently, techniques have been developed for arthroscopy in the prone position, using the posterolateral and posteromedial portals. This allows access for treatment of

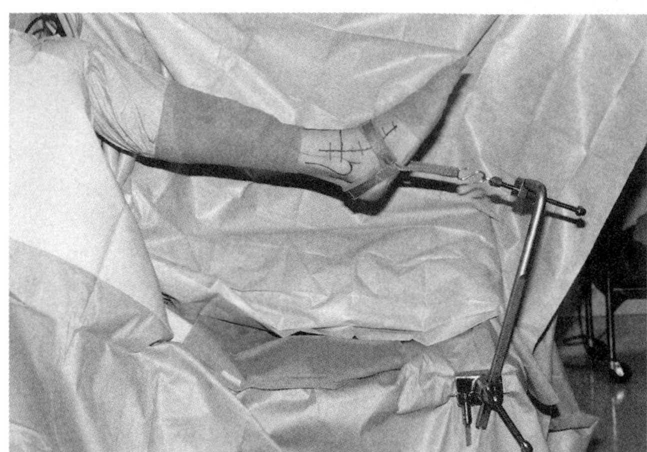

Fig. 24-2 Noninvasive distraction is used to increase the space between the distal tibia and the talus.

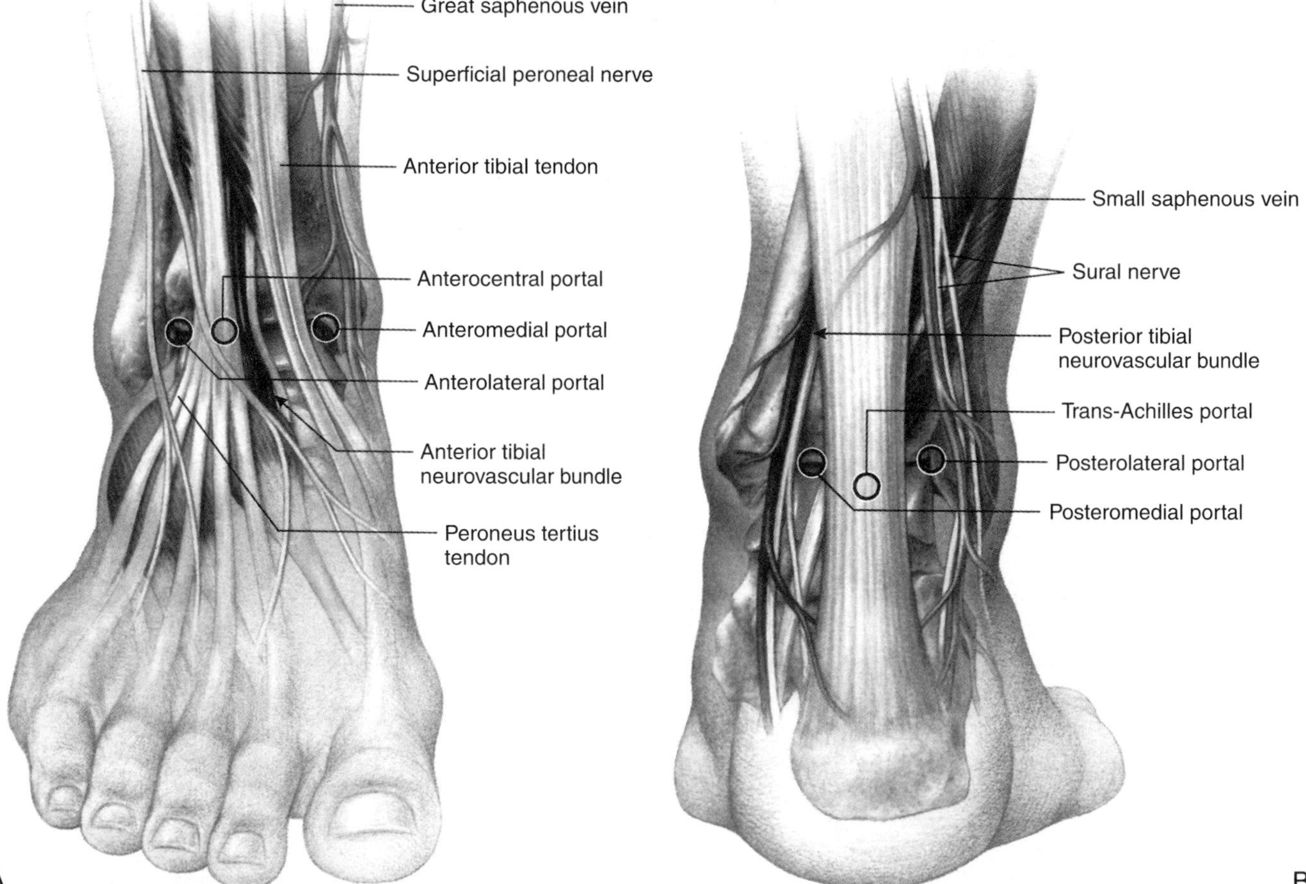

Fig. 24-3 Anteromedial, anterolateral, and posterolateral portals are commonly used for insertion of the arthroscopic instrumentation. (From Ferkel RD, Scranton P: Current concepts review: arthroscopy of the ankle and foot, *J Bone Joint Surg* 75A:1233, 1993.)

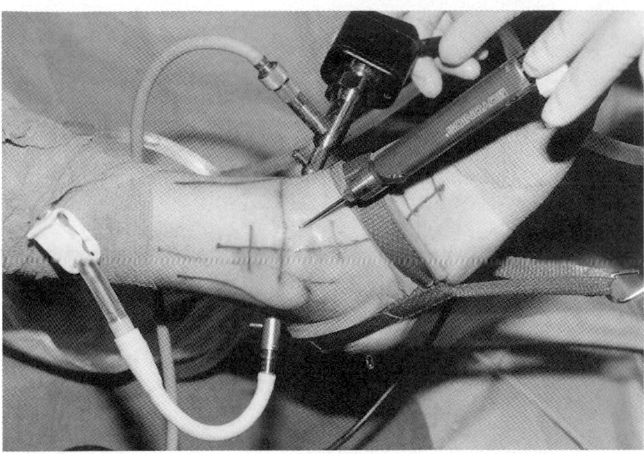

Fig. 24-4 Synovectomy performed with an intra-articular shaver.

osteochondral lesions of the talus, os trigonum, and flexor hallucis longus tendinitis or tears.[1,18]

The anteromedial portal is established first and a 2.7-mm, 30-degree oblique small-joint videoscope is inserted. The surgeon establishes the anterolateral portal under direct vision, using extreme care to avoid injuring the superficial peroneal nerve branches. The arthroscope is then positioned in the posterior portion of the ankle so the posterolateral portal can be made just lateral to the Achilles tendon, entering the ankle beneath the posterior ankle ligaments.

A 21-point arthroscopic examination of the ankle is performed to ensure a systematic evaluation.[7] After completing the arthroscopic evaluation, the surgeon identifies the pathology and treats it accordingly, using small joint instrumentation ranging in size from 1.9 to 3.5 mm. These instruments include baskets, knives, intraarticular shavers, and burrs. Scar tissue is removed using baskets and an intraarticular shaver. Synovectomy is performed with an intraarticular shaver (Fig. 24-4). Osteochondral lesions of the talus are carefully evaluated and, if they are found to be loose, excised with a ring curette and banana knife. The surgeon can use trans-malleolar or transtalar drilling, or microfracture techniques, to promote fibrocartilage formation and new circulation in the avascular area. Acute ankle fractures can be evaluated arthroscopically; the surgeon can perform percutaneous screw insertion while monitoring fracture reduction arthroscopically.

After the procedure is performed, the wounds are closed with a nonabsorbable suture, and a compression dressing and posterior splint are applied. The patient remains non–weight bearing on crutches for 1 week. The splint and the stitches are then removed. *If an osteochondral lesion has been treated with one of the previously mentioned methods, the patient may be required to be non–weight bearing for 4 to 6 weeks.* During this time the patient is initially in a removable splint and is allowed to exercise the ankle actively to promote new fibrocartilage formation. Weight-bearing status and rehabilitation are determined by the type of arthroscopic procedure performed and individual patient goals.

SURGICAL OUTCOMES

Numerous papers have been published regarding the outcome of arthroscopic surgery of the ankle. Results vary depending on the type of procedure and the study that was undertaken.[2,12-14,16,17,19] In general, a large percentage of patients should achieve a successful outcome depending on the nature of the pathology. Expectations after surgery include a full ROM, strength, and full function. Results are heavily influenced by the preoperative ROM, strength, and severity of the pathologic condition surgically addressed.

> **Q** Paul had arthroscopic ankle surgery for an excision of an anterior tibiotalar osteophyte. He had surgery 7 weeks ago and has returned to working as a store manager. He is on his feet most of the day. He is anxious about recovering quickly and doing his usual routine. During his last visit he complained of increased soreness at times. The pain has not been decreasing, and swelling persists. During his home exercises, Paul works hard on the resisted exercises. How can the therapist help Paul to progress?

THERAPY GUIDELINES FOR REHABILITATION

Several factors must be considered in planning a successful rehabilitation. Rehabilitation guidelines may vary greatly for the same injury or surgery depending on patient age, severity of injury, healing rate of tissue, and previous level of activity. The physician, physical therapist, and patient must work together as a team to develop an appropriate treatment plan to achieve the same goals. The phases in each of the following rehabilitation protocols may overlap by 1 to 3 weeks depending on the factors mentioned previously and, therefore, may need to be modified to meet the needs of each patient.

The physical therapist should consider six basic rehabilitation principles when planning an ankle rehabilitation protocol:

1. **Never over-stress healing tissue.**
2. Ankle rehabilitation involves more than just strengthening. *Control of acute symptoms and sufficient increase*

in joint mobility need to be addressed before efficient ankle strengthening can be accomplished. Also, increased proprioception should be emphasized in all ankle rehabilitation programs.
3. The effects of immobilization must be minimized.
4. Neutral position of the subtalar joint during exercise is important for efficient strengthening of the intrinsic and extrinsic muscle groups of the ankle joint.
5. The ultimate goal of rehabilitation is not only to return the patient to the previous level of function safely, but also to prevent re-injury. Therefore, patient education should be addressed from the moment rehabilitation begins until the time of discharge.
6. Avoid isolating treatment to only the joint involved. The entire lower kinetic chain should be assessed to identify dysfunctional links within the chain that may have contributed to the original injury.

The following rehabilitation program is designed for a patient who developed chronic sprain pain after an inversion basketball injury and underwent arthroscopic debridement for anterolateral soft tissue impingement of the ankle.

A Paul was advised to sit at work and at home whenever possible and to elevate his foot when he is sitting. The therapist evaluated his resisted home exercises and cautioned him to use only moderate resistance. The patient was told that exercising too aggressively will only delay his progress and cause increased pain and swelling. In addition, he was told that overstressing his ankle by being on his feet all day would also delay his progress. If he decreases the irritability factors regarding his ankle, then he will recover faster (and the pain and swelling should start to decrease).

Q Christine is a 32-year-old woman who underwent an ankle arthroscopy procedure for débridement of soft tissue impingement 5 weeks ago. Since then her physical therapy has consisted of massage, ultrasound (US), AROM and PROM exercises, resisted exercises, cryotherapy, and a home exercise program. Her main complaint is pain during gait, while descending stairs, and during attempts to squat partially. Dorsiflexion is minimally limited, and minimal swelling persists. What treatment may be particularly helpful to Christine?

Phase I: Acute Phase

TIME: Week 1
GOALS: Provide adequate soft tissue and joint healing after surgery in preparation for the appropriate rehabilitation protocol (Table 24-1)

Patient is placed in a splint and is non–weight bearing.

Phase II: Early Rehabilitation

TIME: Weeks 2-5
GOALS: Decrease inflammation and pain, restore normal gait, increase ankle joint ROM, restore soft tissue flexibility, increase strength and proprioception, maintain cardiovascular fitness, increase patient knowledge and awareness (Table 24-2)

Rehabilitation program. The splint is removed and the patient is progressed to full weight bearing. Exercises are performed on land two to three times per week. Pool exercises are indicated only if the patient has difficulty with full weight bearing, has persistent problems with pain and swelling, or is unable to tolerate land exercise two times per week.

Table 24-1 Ankle Arthroscopy

Rehabilitation Phase	Criteria to Progress to this Phase	Anticipated Impairments and Functional Limitations	Intervention	Goal	Rationale
Phase I Postoperative 1 week	◆ Postoperative and cleared by physician to initiate therapy ◆ Specific precautions if any, depending on the stability of fixation (communicate with physician)	◆ Nonweight bearing	◆ Splint extremity to prevent reinjury	◆ Protect surgical site and promote adequate healing in preparation for physical therapy	◆ Patient is not yet ready for rehabilitation exercises this soon after surgery; sufficient healing time is crucial

Table 24-2 Ankle Arthroscopy

Rehabilitation Phase	Criteria to Progress to this Phase	Anticipated Impairments and Functional Limitations	Intervention	Goal	Rationale
Phase II Postoperative 2-5 weeks	◆ Splint removed ◆ Weight-bearing status progressed to full weight bearing as tolerated ◆ Physician's orders to begin physical therapy	◆ Pain ◆ Swelling ◆ Decreased ROM and flexibility ◆ Decreased proprioception ◆ Decreased weight-bearing ability	◆ Land therapy two times a week (or land therapy two times a week and pool therapy one time a week) ◆ Pain control modalities ◆ Joint mobilization and PROM ◆ AROM ◆ Gait training ◆ PREs using elastic bands or manual resistance ◆ Intrinsic muscle strengthening (e.g., towel curls) ◆ BAPS board and balancing exercises ◆ Cardiovascular conditioning—Stationary bicycle, UBE, deep-water pool running ◆ Closed-chain exercises—Bilateral heel raises, partial squats, leg press machine, lunges ◆ After 4 weeks step-ups, step-downs, slide board, mini-trampoline, treadmill, and stair climber may be added ◆ Home exercise program ◆ Patient education	◆ Decrease pain and swelling ◆ Increase ankle joint ROM ◆ Increase strength and proprioception ◆ Restore normal gait to full weight bearing ◆ Increase soft tissue flexibility ◆ Maintain cardiovascular fitness ◆ Increase patient knowledge and awareness of injury and rehabilitation	◆ Modalities decrease pain and swelling ◆ Joint mobilizations decrease pain and increase ankle ROM ◆ AROM and PREs increase strength ◆ BAPS board and balancing exercises increase proprioception and coordination ◆ Stabilize MTP joints for effective propulsion ◆ Improve cardiovascular fitness ◆ Provide functional strengthening ◆ Home exercise programs and education improve patient follow-through at home

ROM, Range of motion; *PROM,* passive range of motion; *AROM,* active range of motion; *PREs,* progressive resistance exercises; *BAPS,* biomechanical ankle platform system; *UBE,* upper body ergometer.

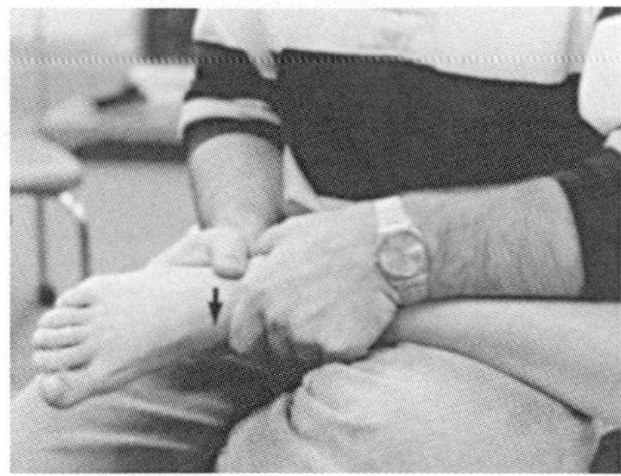

Fig. 24-5 Medial glide of the calcaneus on the talus to increase calcaneal eversion (pronation).
(From Andrews JR, Harrelson GL, Wilk KE: *Physical rehabilitation of the injured athlete,* ed 3, Philadelphia, WB Saunders, 2004.)

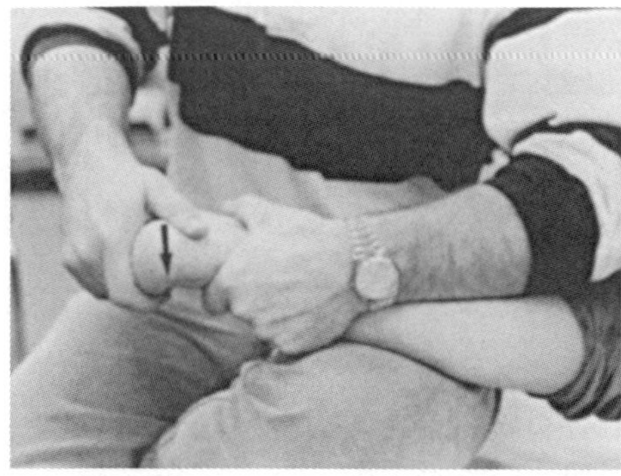

Fig. 24-6 Lateral glide of the calcaneus on the talus to increase calcaneal inversion (supination).
(From Andrews JR, Harrelson GL, Wilk KE: *Physical rehabilitation of the injured athlete*, ed 3, Philadelphia, WB Saunders, 2004.)

Decrease Inflammation and pain. The following modalities are useful in treating and decreasing pain and swelling:

- ◆ Ice and elevation
- ◆ Electrical stimulation
- ◆ Soft tissue massage
- ◆ Phonophoresis
- ◆ Grade I and II ankle and forefoot joint mobilizations
- ◆ Active ankle circles and pumps

Passive accessory movements are performed by the clinician to decrease pain and swelling and increase joint mobility within the anatomic limit of the joint's ROM. After ankle immobilization, sustained stretch techniques can be used as a beginning technique to stretch a tight joint capsule. Sustained stretch uses the gliding component of the joint motion to restore joint play and improve mobility. Gentle oscillatory distraction can be used to reduce swelling and pain (grades I and II). After pain and swelling have been reduced, more specific capsular stretching can be initiated to improve limited joint ROM (grades III and IV).

The following accessory joint mobilizations are performed according to specific joint limitations and individual patient needs:

- ◆ Medial and lateral glides of the subtalar joint to increase ankle inversion and eversion (Figs. 24-5 and 24-6)
- ◆ Posterior glide of the talocrural joint to increase dorsiflexion (see Fig. 23-8)
- ◆ Anterior glide of the talocrural joint to increase plantar flexion
- ◆ Distraction of the subtalar joint (see Fig. 23-8)
- ◆ Distraction of the talocrural joint to increase joint play at the ankle mortise (see Fig. 23-6)
- ◆ Talar rock to increase general calcaneal movement medially and laterally
- ◆ Forefoot metatarsal anterior and posterior glides

Restore normal gait. Full weight bearing emphasizing heel-toe gait and sufficient push-off with gait training drills helps the patient learn a normal gait pattern.

Increase ankle joint ROM and restore soft tissue flexibility. The following exercises can be used to help the patient increase ROM and improve flexibility:

- ◆ Passive range of motion (PROM) to ankle joint and forefoot
- ◆ Active range of motion (AROM) exercises in all directions
- ◆ Grade II to III ankle and forefoot joint mobilizations
- ◆ Hamstring and Achilles tendon stretching (non–weight bearing)

Increase strength. Proceed with caution during the initial part of this phase. When progressing with PREs and adding weight-bearing strengthening exercises, the patient can easily aggravate the ankle. The patient may have a 1- to 2-week setback or delayed recovery secondary to irritability and overstressing tissues. The patient needs to be aware that overactivity with exercises, or weight-bearing activities, can lead to setbacks. The following exercises are useful in helping the patient increase strength in the lower extremity and ankle intrinsic and extrinsic muscle groups:

- ◆ Manual resistance as tolerated (light to moderate) in all planes of motion
- ◆ Active resistive exercises using elastic bands (starting with light-resistance red bands; Fig. 24-7)
- ◆ Intrinsic muscle strengthening (e.g., towel curls)
- ◆ "Windshield wipers"
- ◆ Upper extremity and general hip and knee strengthening on isotonic gym equipment
- ◆ Toe push-ups

Intrinsic muscle strengthening (e.g., towel curls) entail closed-chain exercise to increase strength and endurance in the long and short toe flexors. The function of the intrinsic muscles is to stabilize the metatarsophalangeal

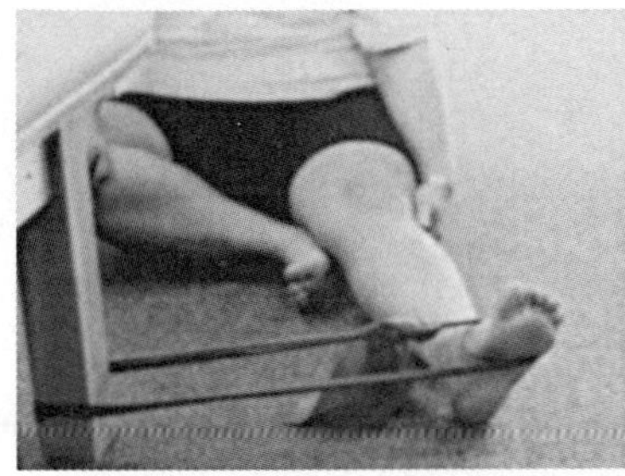
A

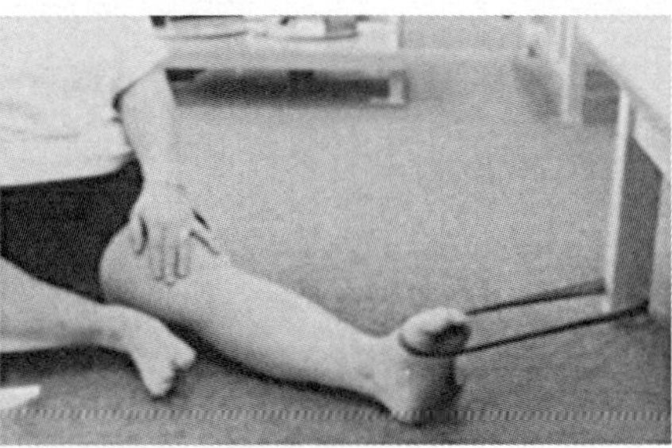
B

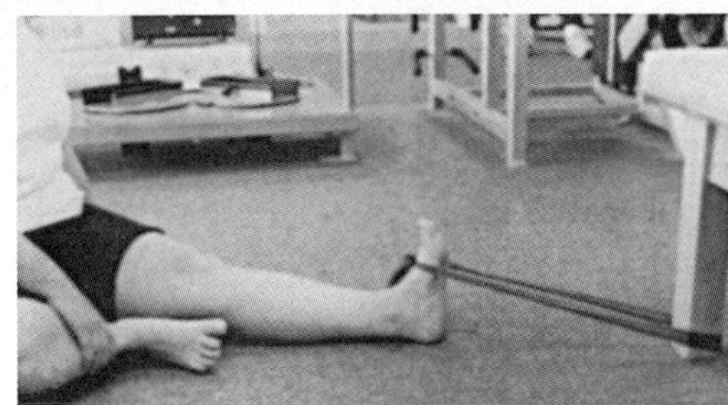
C

Fig. 24-7 Elastic bands or surgical tubing can be used for resisted exercises. **A**, Eversion; **B**, Inversion; **C**, Dorsiflexion.
(From Andrews JR, Harrelson GL, Wilk KE: *Physical rehabilitation of the injured athlete*, ed 3, Philadelphia, WB Saunders, 2004.)

(MTP) joints for effective propulsion, converting the toes into rigid beams to provide stability and terminal stance. The patient sits with both feet on the ground with hips and knees flexed to 90 degrees. The heels are directly under the knees, with the feet placed on a towel spread over a smooth surface. The patient flexes the toes repeatedly to curl the towel up and under the arches and then fully extends the toes. Flexion of the knees to 90 degrees emphasizes the long tow flexors; flexion of less than 90 degrees emphasizes the short toe flexors.

Windshield wipers are a closed-chain exercise to strengthen and increase endurance in the ankle extrinsic stabilizing muscles, the posterior tibialis, and peroneus longus. The patient sits with the hips and knees flexed to 90 degrees. Both feet are flat on the ground, shoulder width apart. The patient places both fists between the knees to stabilize them, then pivots on the heels and moves the feet inward and outward, keeping the feet *completely* flat against the ground.

Upper and lower extremity strengthening and endurance training are done to maintain fitness in other areas of the body while the foot and ankle joint is healing. The physical therapist must address the entire lower kinetic chain (i.e., hip, knee, ankle joints) for successful rehabilitation to occur. Abnormalities and weaknesses in one link of the chain (e.g., the hip) directly affect the mechanism of the foot and ankle, leading to re-injury or insufficient strengthening. Before patients achieve full weight-bearing status, physical therapists can help them build and maintain strength in the hip and knee joints with traditional exercises that do not involve the ankle joint. After the patient has full weight-bearing status, closed kinetic chain exercise should be emphasized for lower extremity strengthening. These exercises provide decelerated training for the large lower extremity muscle groups, as well as enhanced neuromuscular training benefits of speed, balance, and coordination. Closed kinetic chain exercises are performed with the distal segment of the extremity fixed, allowing motion to occur at the proximal segments. In the beginning of phase II, these exercises include partial squats, leg presses, lunges, elastic resistive bands, and heel raises. At the end of phase II (4 weeks), step-ups and step-downs (see Fig. 22-7), stair climbing, treadmill walking, slide boards, and mini-trampoline can be added to the program.

Increase proprioception. The following exercises encourage increased proprioception:

- Biomechanical Ankle Platform System (BAPS) board—start with non–weight bearing in sitting (all planes) and progress to weight bearing as tolerated in standing (Fig. 22-6)
- Balance exercises, including single-limb stance (i.e., stork exercises) (Fig. 22-5)

Maintain cardiovascular fitness. The following exercises can be used by the patient to increase cardiovascular fitness:

- Stationary bicycle
- Upper body ergometer (UBE)
- Deep-water pool running

Increase patient knowledge and awareness. The physical therapist should provide the following to the patient to increase knowledge and awareness:

- Home exercise program
- Specific instructions concerning pathology of injury, precautions and limitations with activities, rate of progression, and specific goals

A mobilization technique was performed at the talocrural joint. An anteroposterior (AP) movement was applied to the talus, while stabilizing the distal tibia, to increase dorsiflexion. This was followed by stretching and ROM exercises to reinforce dorsiflexion. Christine's dorsiflexion PROM increased to 15 degrees. Pain with gait, stairs, and squatting was dramatically decreased after this treatment.

Q Jessica is a 40-year-old woman who had an ankle arthroscopy done with the removal of a loose body from an osteochondral lesion 9 weeks ago. She was nonweight bearing for 5 weeks and has been in therapy; progress with exercise has decreased because of pain during many of the closed-chain exercises such as single-leg stance, double-heel lifts, mini-squats, and walking more than 8 minutes on the treadmill. What types of closed-chain exercises can Jessica do to progress with her strengthening?

Phase III: Advanced Rehabilitation

TIME: Weeks 6-8
GOALS: Alleviate pain and swelling, improve ROM, strength, and proprioception (Table 24-3)

Rehabilitation program

Alleviate pain and swelling. The patient should continue with modalities only as needed for control of pain and swelling. Iontophoresis can be used for specific or localized pain.

Return ROM to within normal limits. The physical therapist should continue with manual ankle joint mobilizations as needed until full ROM has been achieved. General lower extremity stretching should be continued before and after exercise. The patient can add posterior tibialis, anterior tibialis, and peroneal stretching, if indicated.

Improve strength. The following exercises are recommended to help the patient increase in strength:

- ◆ Ankle proprioceptive neuromuscular facilitation (PNF), using moderate to maximal resistance
- ◆ Increased elastic band resistance

Table 24-3 Ankle Arthroscopy

Rehabilitation Phase	Criteria to Progress to this Phase	Anticipated Impairments and Functional Limitations	Intervention	Goal	Rationale
Phase III Postoperative 6-8 weeks	◆ Patient progressing well with decreased pain and minimal swelling ◆ Improved strength from 3/5 to 4/5 and near normal ROM ◆ Full weight bearing with very slight gait deviations	◆ Localized pain ◆ Persistent swelling ◆ Minimal limitations in ROM ◆ Decreased strength and proprioception	◆ Iontophoresis ◆ Ankle joint mobilization grades III and IV ◆ PNF ◆ Resistance exercises ◆ Closed-chain exercises, advancing as able ◆ Mini-trampoline and advanced balancing exercises	◆ Alleviate pain and swelling ◆ Decrease use of modalities except for ice after high-level exercises ◆ Improve ROM to within normal limits ◆ Improve strength and proprioception to within normal limits	◆ Iontophoresis decreased localized pain ◆ Aggressive ankle mobilization decreases end-range tightness in ankle and forefoot ◆ Exercises provide strengthening in functional patterns ◆ Strengthening of extrinsic muscles improves function ◆ Advanced functional strengthening speeds the return to previous level of function ◆ Advanced trampoline and balancing exercises develop functional proprioceptive skills

ROM, Range of motion; *PNF,* proprioceptive neuromuscular facilitation.

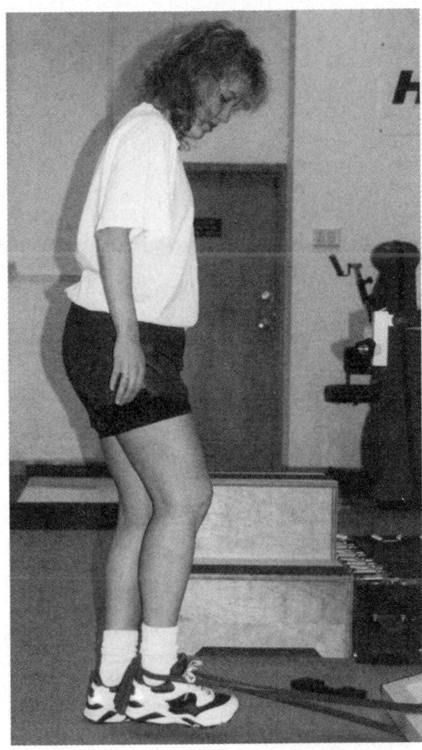

Fig. 24-8 Contralateral kicks to simulate closed-chained pronation and supination. The elastic band goes around the unaffected lower extremity.
(From Andrews JR, Harrelson GL, Wilk KE: *Physical rehabilitation of the injured athlete*, ed 3, Philadelphia, WB Saunders, 2004.)

- Increased resistance in windshield wipers and towel curls
- Concentric and eccentric gastrocnemius and soleus strengthening in weight bearing with resistance
- Step-ups and step-downs (Fig. 22-7)
- Retro stair-climbing machine (Retro rehabilitation is the performance of certain activities in reverse direction. This decreases knee joint loading while increasing quadriceps strength and power. Stability is decreased and, therefore, proprioception is more difficult to control.)
- Treadmill walking
- Closed kinetic chain exercises with sports cord (begin with light resistance)
- Closed kinetic chain exercises with elastic band or surgical tubing (begin with light resistance; Figs. 24-8 and 24-9)
- Slide board
- Front and side lower extremity lunges, with weight if tolerated
- Continued upper-extremity strengthening to maintain strength and endurance for return to sports

Improve proprioception. The following exercises promote improved proprioception:

- BAPS board, weight bearing and with weights
- Trampoline drills that incorporate balance exercises and weight shifting

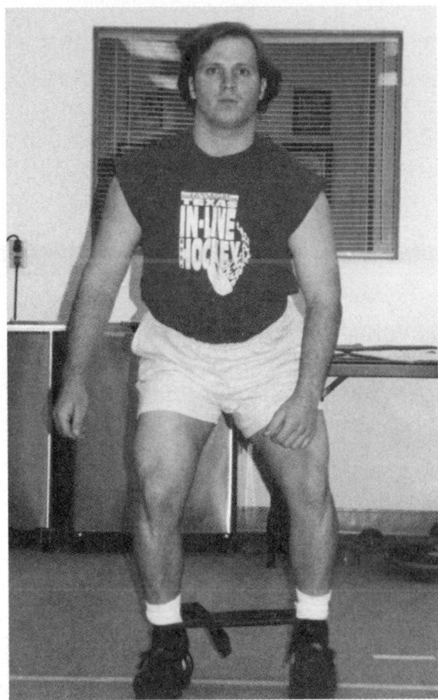

Fig. 24-9 Tubing-resisted side steps.
(From Andrews JR, Harrelson GL, Wilk KE: *Physical rehabilitation of the injured athlete*, ed 3, Philadelphia, WB Saunders, 2004.)

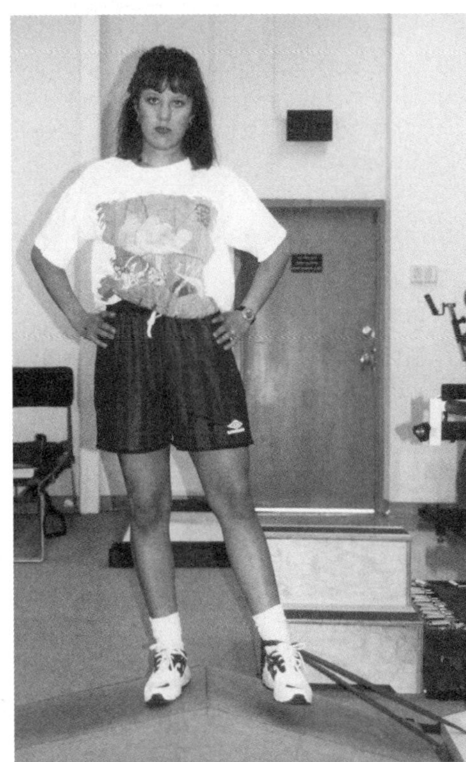

Fig. 24-10 Proprioceptive training on inclined surfaces. The elastic band goes around the unaffected lower extremity.
(From Andrews JR, Harrelson GL, Wilk KE: *Physical rehabilitation of the injured athlete*, ed 3, Philadelphia, WB Saunders, 2004.)

- Stork exercises with dynamic movement of uninvolved side and applied external resistance
- Proprioceptive training on inclined surfaces (Fig. 24-10)

A The therapist explained to Jessica that any activities that cause prolonged pain and swelling must be stopped. Any painful exercises should be eliminated or safely altered until she can perform them correctly without pain. Jessica was able to perform the following closed-chained exercises: forward lunges, backward lunges, lateral lunges, and single-heel raises performed on a leg press machine using 75 lbs. She could also perform backward walking, minimal walking on the treadmill, and jogging or running in the pool. As strength and tolerance to exercise increased, Jessica progressed to more challenging exercises.

Q Rebecca is a 45-year-old mother of young children. She underwent ankle arthroscopy surgery for a synovectomy 5 weeks ago. When she is on her feet for more than a couple hours, she has prolonged soreness. Yesterday she was on her feet for several hours in the afternoon and intermittently for the rest of the day. Today she is in for treatment; she has minimum to moderate swelling and complains of minimum to moderate levels of pain with weight-bearing activities. What type of treatment should Rebecca receive today?

Phase IV: Specificity of Sport

TIME: Weeks 9-12

GOALS: Provide sport-specific training to return to basketball, prepare for discharge from physical therapy to a structured sport-specific home exercise program, have patient demonstrate good knowledge and technique with home exercise program and good awareness of physical limitations to avoid reinjury (Table 24-4)

The time of this final phase of rehabilitation varies greatly depending on the patient's progression through the earlier phases of rehabilitation. As the athlete prepares to be challenged by higher-level activities, a progression needs to be used to recreate the stresses, forces, and movements that will occur in the sporting activities. **In addition, before implementing this advanced phase of rehabilitation, the patient must be free of pain and swelling and have proprioception and ROM within normal limits.**

Rehabilitation program. During this phase the patient works on advanced strengthening and proprioceptive training. Exercises are tailored to the specific sport. Exercises that are useful for a basketball player in phase IV follow:

- Running and side-stepping on a treadmill
- Cross-over stepping on a stair-climbing machine
- Squat jumping on a trampoline
- Lower-extremity plyometric exercises
- Running and agility drills with a sport cord (forward, backward, side to side)

Table 24-4 Ankle Arthroscopy

Rehabilitation Phase	Criteria to Progress to this Phase	Anticipated Impairments and Functional Limitations	Intervention	Goal	Rationale
Phase IV Postoperative 9-12 weeks	◆ No pain or swelling ◆ Normal strength (5/5) ◆ Good proprioception ◆ Full ankle ROM in all planes ◆ Normal gait without deviations	◆ Patient requires sport-specific training to increase functional strength, endurance, and proprioception for a safe return to sport	◆ Sport-specific drills and exercises emphasizing power, agility, and speed ◆ Running ◆ Plyometric ◆ Duplication of sport activities	◆ Full return to sports without limitations ◆ Excellent patient knowledge and performance of home exercises and clear understanding of the pathology of injury	◆ Advanced sport-specific training helps ensure a safe return to sport

ROM, Range of motion.

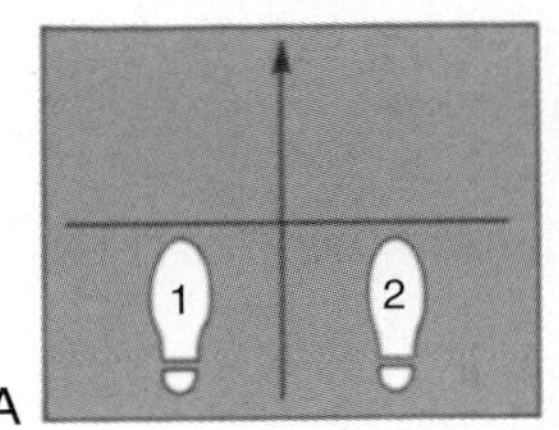

A

Side to side: Hop laterally between two quadrants.

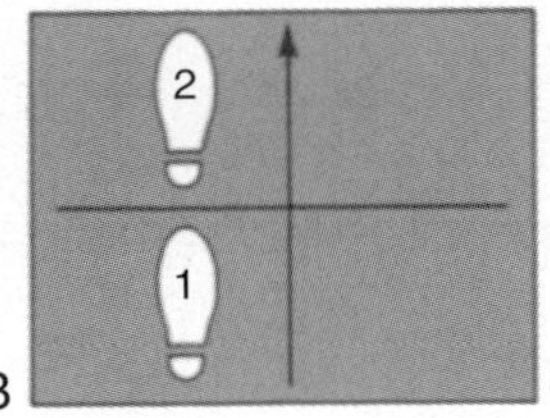

B

Front to back: Hop forward and backward between two quadrants.

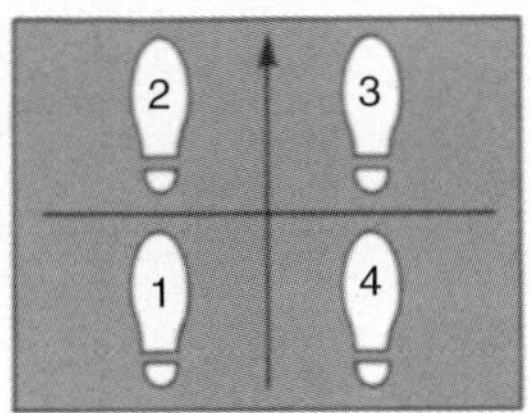

C

Four square: Hop from square to square in a circular pattern. Sets are performed clockwise and counterclockwise.

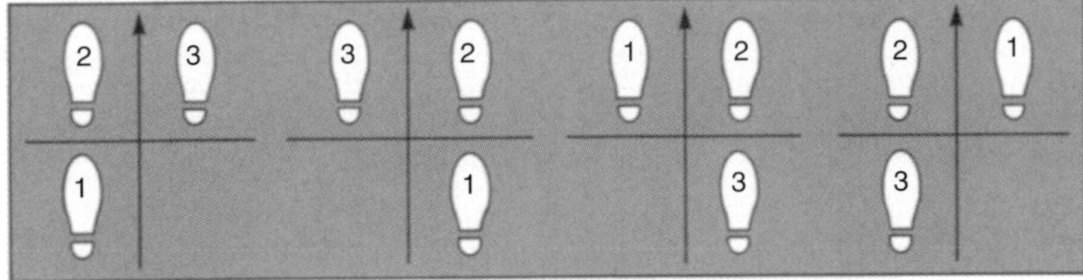

D

Triangles: Hop within three different quadrants. There are four triangles, each requiring a different diagonal hop.

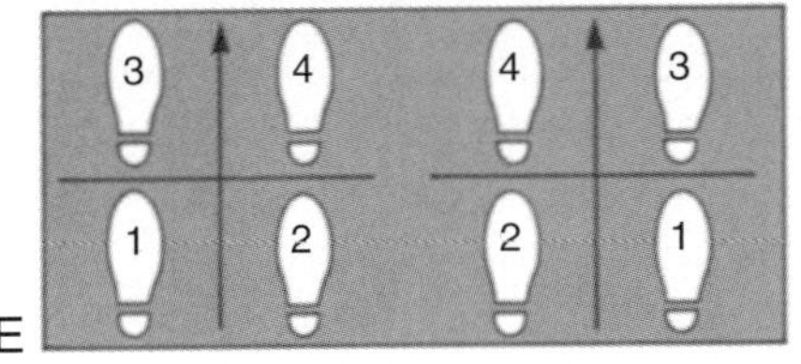

E

Crisscross: Hop in an X pattern.

F

Straight-line hop: Hop forward and then backward along a 15- to 20-ft. line.

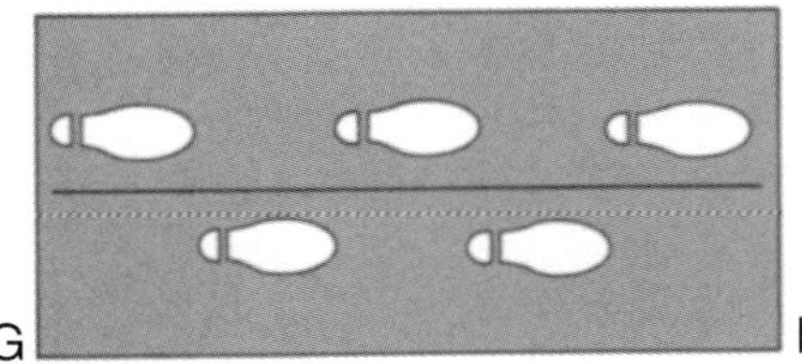

G

Line zigzag: Hop from side to side across a 15- to 20-ft. line while moving forward and then backward.

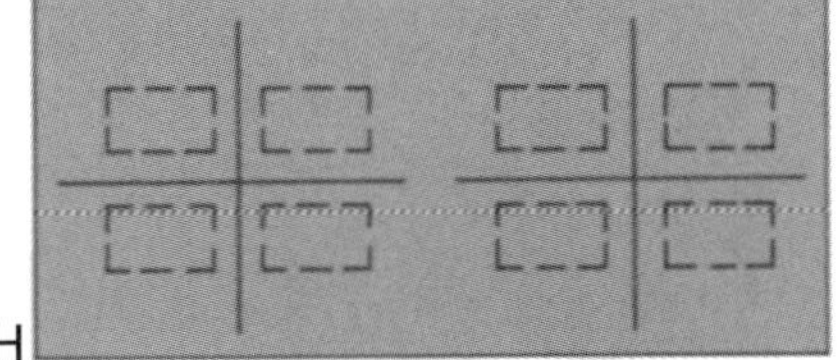

H

Disconnected squares: While performing the first five patterns, hop into squares marked in the quadrants.

Fig. 24-11 A-H, Four-square hopping ankle rehabilitation. The eight basic hopping patterns in the four-square ankle rehabilitation program are arranged in order of increasing difficulty. The arrows denote the direction the athlete is facing. Number 1 is the starting point.
(From Toomey SJ: Four-square ankle rehabilitation exercises, *Phys Sportsmed* 14;281, 1986.)

- Agility drills on basketball court (or a simulated court outside), including figure eights, cutting drills, and cariocas (Fig. 22-4)
- Advanced trampoline exercises with resistance (e.g., throwing plyoball, using body blade)
- Four-square hopping to simulate athletic activity (Fig. 24-11)
- Videotaping patient playing basketball and reviewing tape with patient to assess weaknesses and biomechanical problems with form that may lead to re-injury or other related injuries in the future

Advanced mini-trampoline exercises in single-limb stance with added external resistance are used to incorporate sport-specific activities. The soft surface of the trampoline provides an element of instability, thus requiring more control in the weight-bearing lower extremity. The patient maintains balance using a single-limb stance while performing upper extremity skills such as throwing, batting, and dribbling. He or she can then progress to incorporate walking (swinging leg), specific dance moves, and kicking actions performed by the non–weight-bearing leg.

The athlete can be guided in returning to sports activities with some basic progression principals:

- ◆ non–weight-bearing exercises
- ◆ partial weight-bearing exercises
- ◆ full weight-bearing exercises
- ◆ stable surface balance training
- ◆ walking
- ◆ weight-bearing balance board activities (bilateral then unilateral)
- ◆ stepping sideways, backwards, diagonals, etc.
- ◆ cariocas
- ◆ rebounder jogging
- ◆ jogging
- ◆ running
- ◆ bilateral jumping and hopping
- ◆ backpedaling
- ◆ figure eight running
- ◆ cutting and twisting
- ◆ plyometrics
- ◆ single-leg hopping and jumping

The program must be structured to challenge the athlete according to his physical status and abilities, and then progressed as able. Modifications are made depending on the goals of the athlete.

Before ending the formal rehabilitation program, the physical therapist should review proper training technique and the home exercise program with the patient in detail.

A When pain or swelling limits the progress of rehabilitation, the intensity of rehabilitation needs to be altered. The therapist focused on controlling pain and decreasing swelling. Joint mobilization using glides and distraction maneuvers was performed on the talocrural joints. Gentle PROM was performed. No resisted or AROM exercises were done today because of pain and swelling. Massage was done to promote circulation and decrease swelling. Ice packs were used in conjunction with a compression device. Swelling and pain decreased after treatment. The patient was encouraged to avoid aggravating her symptoms.

SUGGESTED HOME MAINTENANCE FOR THE POSTSURGICAL PATIENT

A home maintenance program for ankle exercises has been outlined in Chapter 22.

TROUBLESHOOTING

After ankle arthroscopy, patients may have soreness or numbness and tingling over the portal sites. In addition, residual swelling and discoloration may occur. Patients begin physical therapy 2 or 3 weeks after surgery. If rehabilitation is begun too soon, significant swelling and pain may develop with loss of motion and strength; these sequelae may be difficult to reverse. If formal physical therapy is delayed for at least 2 to 3 weeks, the author of this chapter has found these problems to be significantly diminished. The rest period allows for gentle ROM and strengthening, promotes soft tissue healing, and gives the residual swelling, edema, and soreness time to abate. Some patients may require additional special precautions depending on the type of procedure that is performed; the physical therapist should consult with the physician after reviewing the operative report for specific cautions and guidelines.

Complications can occur in ankle arthroscopy, and we have previously reported on our complication rate of 9%. The most common complication after ankle arthroscopy is injury to the surrounding nerves. Injury to the superficial peroneal nerve is the most frequent complication seen in ankle arthroscopy, and this can be associated with transient or permanent numbness on the dorsum of the foot, extending into the toes.[8]

CONCLUSION

The therapist should notify the physician immediately if any wound opening, drainage, redness, or increased swelling and pain occur. In addition, if physical therapy has been progressing well and suddenly the patient develops problems with rehabilitation, the therapist should notify the physician. If the patient does not attend physical therapy, is not cooperative, or tries to rush the program, this also should be discussed with the physician.

References

1. Acevedo JI, Busch MT, Ganey TM, Hutton WC, Ogden JA: Coaxial portals for posterior ankle arthroscopy: An anatomic study with clinical correlation on 29 patients, *Arthroscopy* 16:836, 2000.
2. Andrews JR, Previte WJ, Carson WG: Arthroscopy of the ankle: technique and normal anatomy, *Foot Ankle* 6:29, 1985.
3. Baker CL, Andrews JR, Ryan JB: Arthroscopic treatment of transchondral talar dome fractures, *Arthroscopy* 2:82, 1986.
4. Chen Y: Arthroscopy of the ankle joint. In Watanabe M (ed): *Arthroscopy of small joints,* New York, Igaku-Shoin, 1985.
5. Drez D, Jr, Guhl JF, Gollehon DL: Ankle arthroscopy: technique and indications, *Foot Ankle* 2:138, 1981.
6. Ferkel RD, Hommen JP: Arthroscopy of the ankle and foot. In Mann RA, Coughlin M, Saltzman C (eds): *Surgery of the foot and ankle,* ed 7, St Louis, Elsevier, 2006.
7. Ferkel RD: *Arthroscopic surgery: The foot and ankle,* Philadelphia, Lippincott-Raven, 1996.
8. Ferkel RD: Complications in ankle and foot arthroscopy. In Ferkel RD (ed): *Arthroscopic surgery: The foot and ankle,* Philadelphia, Lippincott-Raven, 1996.
9. Ferkel RD, Fischer SP: Progress in ankle arthroscopy, *Clin Orthop* 240:210, 1989.
10. Ferkel RD et al: Arthroscopic treatment of anterolateral impingement of the ankle, *Am J Sports Med* 19:440, 1991.
11. Ferkel RD, Zanotti RM, Komenda GA, et al: Arthroscopic treatment of osteochondral lesions of the talus: Long term results, submitted for publication, *Am J Sports Med*, 2006.
12. Johnson LL: *Diagnostic and surgical arthroscopy,* ed 2, St Louis, 1981, Mosby. Operatively reduced malleolar fractures, *J Orthop Trauma* 5:125, 1991.
13. Liu SH et al: Arthroscopic treatment of anterolateral ankle impingement, *Arthroscopy* 10:215, 1994.
14. Nam EK, Ferkel RD: Ankle and subtalar arthroscopy. In Thordarson DB (ed): *Orthopaedic surgery essentials: Foot and ankle*, Philadelphia, Lippincott Williams & Wilkins, 2004.
15. O'Connor RL: *Arthroscopy*, Kalamazoo, MI, Upjohn, 1977.
16. Parisien JS, Shereff MJ: The role of arthroscopy in the diagnosis and treatment of disorders of the ankle, *Foot Ankle* 2:144, 1981.
17. Parisien JS, Vangsness T: Operative arthroscopy of the ankle: Three years experience, *Clin Orthop* 199:46, 1985.
18. Sitler DF, Amendola A, Bailey CS, Thain LMF, Spouge A: Posterior ankle arthroscopy, *J Bone Joint Surg* 84A:763, 2002.
19. Stetson WB, Ferkel RD: Ankle arthroscopy. Part I: Technique and complications. Part II: Indications and results. *J Am Acad Orthop Surg* 17, 1996.
20. Takagi K: The arthroscope, *J Jpn Orthop Assoc* 14:359, 1939.

CHAPTER 25

Achilles Tendon Repair and Rehabilitation

James E. Zachazewski
Jane Gruber
Eric Giza
Bert R. Mandelbaum

Achilles tendon injuries, whether acute or chronic, occur in many individuals. The severity of these injuries varies from mild, overuse-related inflammatory responses to acute, traumatic tendon rupture. Treatment options are nonoperative immobilization with a cast or functional bracing or else operative repair with open or percutaneous procedures. Postoperative management varies with the length of immobilization and timing of early motion. This chapter describes current trends in surgical intervention, outlines rehabilitative guidelines and techniques, and details the rationales associated with treating Achilles tendon ruptures.

SURGICAL INDICATIONS AND CONSIDERATIONS

Anatomy

The Achilles tendon complex is composed of contributions from the gastrocnemius, soleus, and plantaris (collectively known as the *triceps surae*) and inserts directly into the central third of the posterior calcaneal surface. The tendon is round in cross-section to a level 4 cm proximal to calcaneus, where it flattens and rotates 90 degrees so that its medial fibers insert posteriorly. This biomechanical "winding" of the fibers increases stored energy for higher shortening velocity and muscle power.[101]

During dorsiflexion the tendon articulates with the superior third of the calcaneus. This articulation is cushioned by the retrocalcaneal bursa, which lies between the tendon and the superior third of the calcaneus.

The Achilles tendon does not possess a true synovial sheath. The peritendinous structures of the Achilles are composed of a triple-layered tissue.[104] The superficial layer of tissue is the most durable and is analogous to the deep fascia. This layer comprises the posterior boundary of the superficial posterior compartment. The middle layer, the mesotendon, provides the major blood supply for the central portion of the Achilles tendon. The deepest layer of tissue is quite delicate and thin; however, it can always be isolated from the most superficial layer of the tendon, the epitenon.

The Achilles tendon is supplied with blood and nutrients by three different sources.[104] The most abundant supply is at the proximal and distal portions of the tendon, and the poorest is in the central portion of the tendon. As originally demonstrated by Lagerrgren and Lindholm[69] and corroborated by others,[7,15] a gradual decrease occurs in the number of blood vessels in the central part of the tendon 2 to 6 cm proximal to the calcaneal insertion (Fig. 25-1).

Nutrient branches emanate directly from the muscle to nourish the distal gastrocnemius aponeurosis and proximal portion of the tendon.[102] The insertion of the Achilles tendon is supplied by anastomotic branches between the periosteal vessels and the tendon vessels. As already noted, the major blood supply comes from the mesotendon. Vessels enter the tendon itself via a network of fine connections with the deepest peritendinous layer. These vessels come off the deepest layer radially and enter the tendon perpendicular to its long axis. They then course proximally and distally. Because of the external forces that may be encountered by the posterior aspect of the tendon as a result of friction supplied by the skin, most of these fine vessels are found along the anterior aspect of the tendon, where they are afforded more protection (Fig. 25-2).

Pathogenesis

The theoretic explanation for tendon injuries suggests a continuum of events, including hypovascularity and repetitive microtrauma, that results in localized tendon

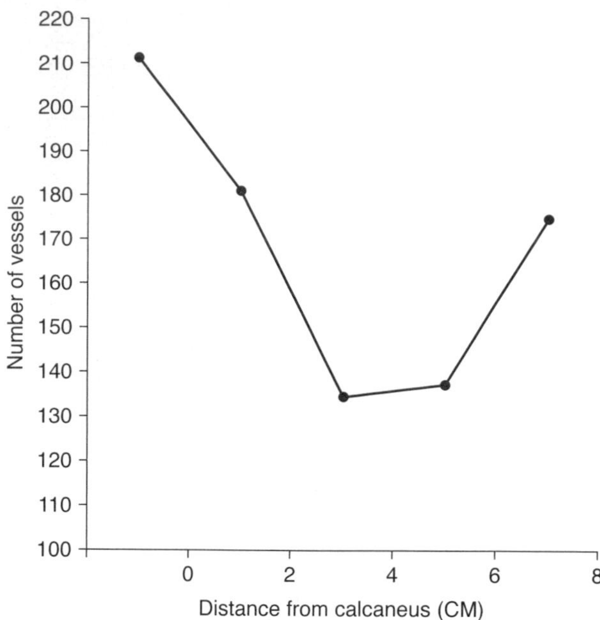

Fig. 25-1 The number of intratendinous vessels of the Achilles tendon varies depending on the distance from the calcaneus.
(From Carr AJ, Norris SH: The blood supply of the calcaneal tendon, *Br J Bone Joint Surg* 71B:100, 1989.)

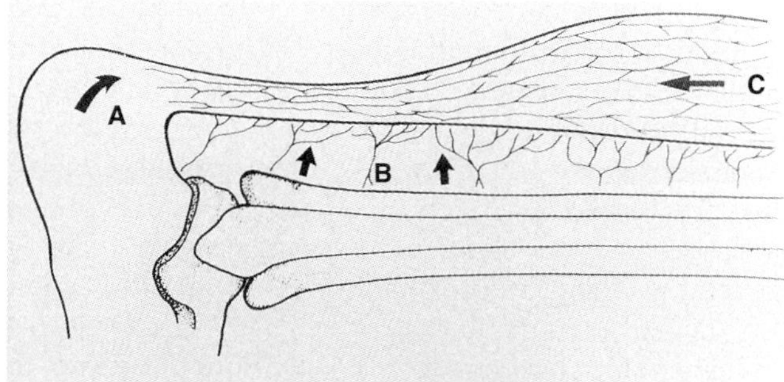

Fig. 25-2 Diagram of the blood vessels of the Achilles paratenon, showing supply for the osseous junction (**A**), the mesotendon (**B**), and the musculotendinous junction (**C**).
(From Carr AJ, Norris SH: The blood supply of the calcaneal tendon, *Br J Bone Joint Surg* 71B:100, 1989.)

degeneration and weakness and ultimately rupture with the application of an otherwise normal load that exceeds the tendon's physiologic capacity. Based on clinical and histologic findings, the traditional description of Achilles tendonitis is not preferred,[2] and Achilles tendon pathology is classified into three different categories: (1) paratendinitis, (2) paratendinitis with tendinosis, and (3) pure tendinosis.[5,10,95]

Paratendinitis involves inflammation only in the paratenon, regardless of whether it is lined by synovium. The paratenon thickens, and adhesions may form between the paratenon and the tendon.[68] However, patients will rarely have isolated paratendinitis, and some authors believe that this process is the predecessor to tendinosis.[2]

Paratendinitis with tendinosis involves not only inflammation of the paratenon but also a degenerative change within the substance of the tendon. Paddu, Ippolito, and Postacchini[95] and Kvist and Kvist[68] have noted thickening, softening, and yellowing of the tendon, as well as cleavage planes and vascular budding at surgery for this condition. As in tendinitis, pain also is commonly noted because of the inflammatory process.

Pure tendinosis often appears as a nodule that is mobile with plantar flexion.[2] It can present as a chronic nodule in the sedentary middle-aged person or as a contribution to the pathology of rupture in the tendons of persons older than 35 years who have suffered spontaneous rupture.[60] Histopathologic changes such as hypoxic and mucoid degeneration, lipomatous infiltration, and calcifying tendinopathy have been noted at the time of surgical repair of acute ruptures.[60,95]

Hippocrates was the first to record an injury to the Achilles tendon. Ambrose Pare was the first to describe Achilles tendon ruptures in 1575, and Gustave Paoaillon was report operative repair of the tendon.[83,101,104] Theories that implicate the degenerative changes that take place in the Achilles tendon with the increased mechanical loads associated with various activities are the most common explanations of the pathogenesis of these ruptures.[82,83] A combination of hypovascularity and repetitive microtrauma results in degenerative changes and inflammation, putting the tendon at risk for rupture. Healing and regeneration are hindered or halted because of poor blood supply to the tendon and recurrent microtrauma. Alfredson, Thorsen, and Lorentzon[3] have shown that microtears in the tendon lead to areas of chronic damage that lack normal levels of prostaglandin E2, which are needed for healing. The combination of these factors may account for the fact that most ruptures occur 2 to 6 cm proximal to the tendon's insertion into the calcaneus. Associated intrinsic factors include age (which leads to decreased vascularity and decreased deoxyribonucleic acid [DNA] synthesis),[4,49,110] endocrine function, and nutrition.[24] Extrinsic factors of compression and friction on the posterior aspect of the tendon (from the skin and inappropriately compressive footwear) further hinder vascularity, healing, and regeneration. Fluroquinolone antibiotics are also associated with Achilles tendon rupture. Their use inhibits transcription of *decorin*, a protein important in collagen architecture, and the odds ratio for tendon rupture in patients taking the medication is 4.2.[114] Acute Achilles ruptures are also often the result of corticosteroid injection for chronic inflammation of the tendon.[2]

Normally, tendons are able to tolerate high forces associated with daily activities and athletics. However, if degenerative changes take place, then the mechanical load usually tolerated may exceed the tendon's physiologic capacity. Mechanically, a tendon may be damaged or ruptured by a sudden application of force. This often involves a forceful lengthening or eccentric muscle

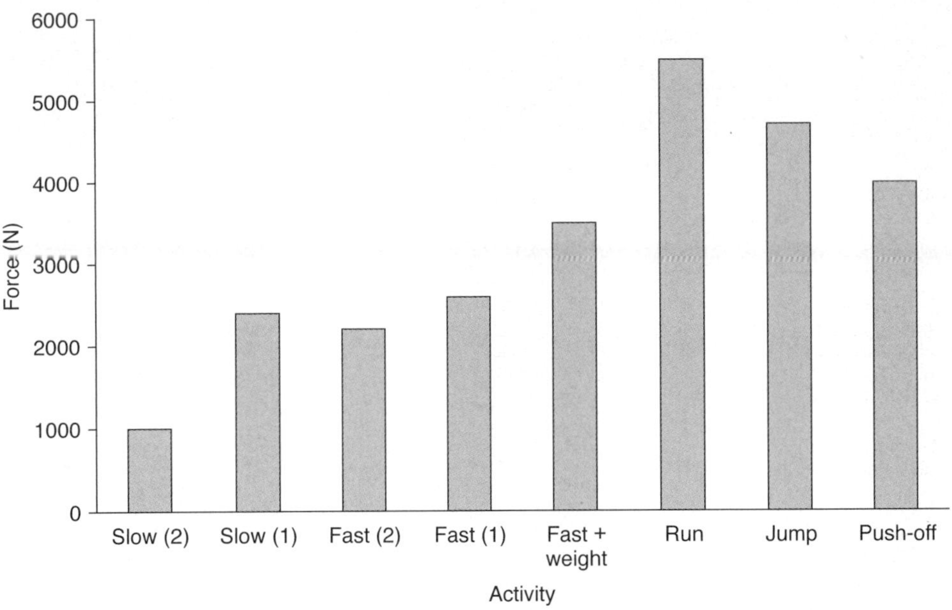

Fig. 25-3 Increasing Achilles tendon forces during toe-raising exercises over the edge of a step and three sports-related activities. Slow (2), weight on both feet, slow speed; slow (1), weight on one foot, slow speed; Fast (2), weight on both feet, fast speed; Fast (1), weight on one foot, fast speed; Fast weight, extra weight added to body; run, spring running; jump, landing from 50 cm; push-off, change in direction from backward to forward running. The slow and fast movements represent progressive steps in the clinical exercise program to treat Achilles tendinitis.

(From Curwin SL: Tendon injuries: pathophysiology and treatment. In Zachazewski JE, Magee DG, Quillen WS, editors: *Athletic injuries and rehabilitation*, Philadelphia, 1996, WB Saunders.)

contraction. Sudden maximal muscle activation results in a larger than normal force that is applied rapidly to the tendon, causing the rupture. The high load forces that cause such rupture are usually associated with vigorous activities such as sports. The forces to which the Achilles tendon is exposed during activities such as running and jumping have been calculated to be between 4000 and 5500 N[25,26,43]; they are summarized in Fig. 25-3.[24] Arner and Lindholm[6] describe three activities that can rupture a tendon:

1. Pushing off with weight bearing on the forefoot while extending the knee (e.g., running, sprinting, jumping)
2. Sudden dorsiflexion with full weight bearing as might occur with a slip, fall, or sudden deceleration
3. Violent dorsiflexion when jumping from a height and landing on a plantar-flexed foot

Curwin[24] best summarized the possible progression of tendon injury (Fig. 25-4).

Epidemiology

Reports regarding the incidence, cause, and conservative, surgical, and postoperative management of Achilles tendon ruptures have increased during the past 50 to 60 years. The number of cases reported may be attributed not only to the observation and diligence of the health care community in publishing their research and thus improving patient care but also to the fact that the general population has increased its level of participation in recreational activity.

Although spontaneous tendon ruptures are rare, the Achilles tendon appears to be the one that is most frequently ruptured. Kannus and Jozsa[60] report that 44.6% (397 out of 891) of tendon ruptures treated surgically between 1968 and 1989 involved the Achilles tendon, whereas the biceps brachii accounted for 33.9%. Achilles tendon ruptures are usually traumatic and occur between the ages of 30 and 40 years,[8,20,58] which is younger than for other tendon ruptures (Fig. 25-5).

Most ruptures are suffered by recreational athletes rather than highly competitive, very active athletes. Of the 105 patients with Achilles ruptures described by Nistor,[94] only 9 participated in competitive sports. Of the remaining patients, 35 exercised twice a week, 41 once a week, 20 took walks and occasionally exercised, and two were physically inactive. Of the 111 patients who ruptured their Achilles tendon while participating in a sports activity in Cetti and colleagues' report,[20] 92 (83%) averaged only 3.6 hours of athletic activity per week. Of the 292 Achilles tendon ruptures documented by Jozsa and associates,[58] 59% occurred during recreational athletic activity—141 of these (83.2%) in men and 29 (16.8%) in women. No patients in this study by Jozsa and colleagues participated in competitive athletics. In their study, more than 625 of the Achilles tendon ruptures occurred in professional or white-collar workers who tended to have generally sedentary lifestyles except when involved in sports. A

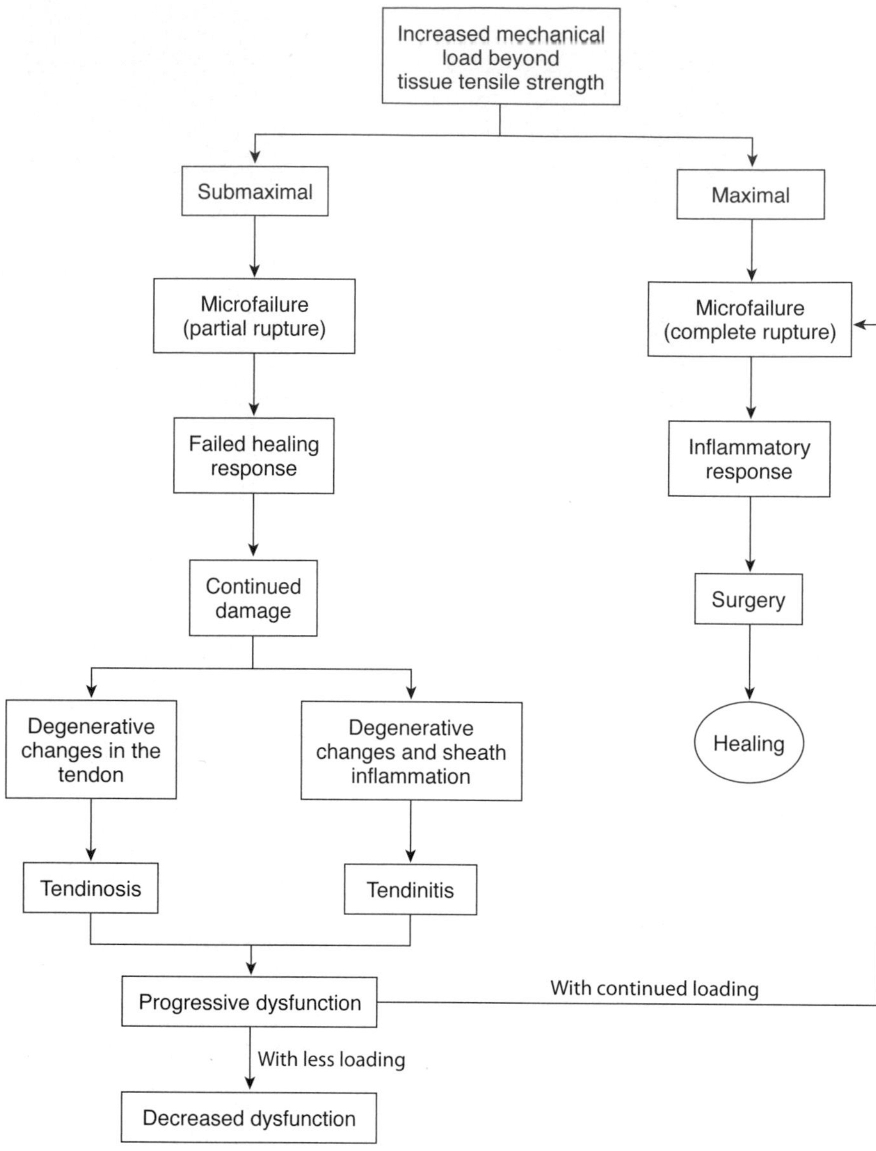

Fig. 25-4 Progression of tendon injury. The inflammatory response may be limited and barely noticed by the athlete, even as degenerative changes continue. As the remaining collagen fibers are overloaded and more are damaged, the inflammatory response recurs, possibly weeks or months after the initial injury. After the tendon is in the inflammatory stage, it can be treated as an acute injury and should heal normally. In rare cases the tendon may rupture because applied forces exceed the tensile strength of the now-weakened tendon.
(Adapted from Curwin SL: Tendon injuries: pathophysiology and treatment. In Zachazewski JE, Magee DG, Quillen WS, editors: *Athletic injuries and rehabilitation,* Philadelphia, 1996, WB Saunders.)

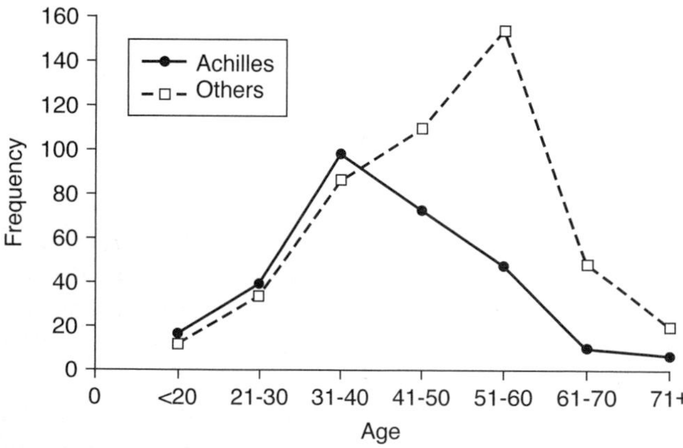

Fig. 25-5 Age distribution of patients with Achilles tendon ruptures.
(From Josza L et al: The role of recreational sport activity in Achilles tendon rupture, *Am J Sports Med* 17:338, 1989.)

review of numerous studies demonstrates that athletic activities that require sudden acceleration or deceleration are most likely to cause a rupture (Table 25-1). Ruptures not attributed to athletic activity are usually caused by falls or stumbles that also produce sudden acceleration and deceleration movements. Overall, Achilles tendon ruptures have been demonstrated to be more common in men than in women. Ratios of 2:1,[14] 4:1,[22] 1.6:1,[53] 8.7:1,[94] 10:1,[8] and 12:1[95] have been reported.

Diagnosis of Acute Achilles Tendon Rupture

In most situations the history is diagnostic. Patients describe hearing a *pop* as though someone had shot them in the back of the ankle. Prodromal symptoms of Achilles aching have been reported in 5% to 30% of cases.[60,80] The

Table 25-1 Distribution of Achilles Tendon Ruptures According to Sport

	Study											
Sport	Frings[37] (1969) Germany	Nillius, Nilsson, & Westin[93] (1976) Sweden	Inglis & Sculco[52] (1981) USA	Cetti & Christenson[18] (1983) Denmark	Holz[50] (1983) Germany	Schedl, Fasol, & Spangler[103] (1983) Austria	Zolinger, Rodriquez, & Genoni[120] (1983) Switzerland	Kellam, Hunter, & McElwain[62] (1985) Canada	Jozsa et al[57] (1987) Hungary	Cetti et al[20] (1983) Denmark	Soldatis, Good-fellows, & Wilber[107] (1997) USA	Karjalainen et al[61] (1997) Finland
Soccer	102	35	18	7	168	13	300	33	58	10	3	2
Handball	32	9	4	19	57	—	—	—	10	7	—	1
Volleyball	—	—	4	—	6	14	—	5	3	3	4	2
Basketball	—	—	29	—	6	—	—	—	23	—	10	1
Badminton	4	38	—	20	—	—	—	—	—	58	—	7
Tennis	5	15	—	—	23	4	—	—	12	3	3	3
Table tennis	4	5	20	—	—	—	—	—	2	—	—	—
Other ball games	9	—	20	—	—	—	230	—	5	—	—	—
Gymnastics	43	19	—	5	47	7	110	—	12	10	—	—
Running	46	6	—	—	42	5	—	—	14	—	—	1
Jumping	31	—	5	—	18	—	—	17	14	—	—	—
Climbing	—	—	—	1	—	—	—	—	—	—	—	—
Rock climbing	—	—	—	—	—	—	—	—	3	—	—	—
Weight lifting	—	—	—	—	—	—	—	—	6	—	—	—
Trampoline	—	—	—	1	—	—	—	—	—	—	—	—
Bicycling	—	—	1	—	39	—	—	—	3	—	—	—
Skiing	6	—	12	—	73	19	570	4	4	—	—	—
Dancing	—	—	10	—	—	—	—	—	7	1	—	1
Jogging	—	—	9	—	—	—	—	—	—	—	—	—
Racquetball	—	—	—	—	—	—	—	—	—	—	2	—
Aerobics	—	—	—	—	—	—	—	—	—	—	—	1
Baseball	—	—	—	—	—	—	—	—	—	—	4	—
Others	30	7	—	—	—	6	30	—	—	19	4	1
Total	317	134	131	53	479	68	1240	59	173	111	30	20

Adapted from Jozsa L et al: The role of recreational sport activity in Achilles tendon rupture. A clinical, pathoanatomical, and sociological study of 292 cases, *Am J Sports Med* 17(3):338, 1989.

rupture commonly occurs in the "watershed area," between 2 and 6 cm proximal to the calcaneus.[69] Avulsion fractures of the calcaneus are relatively uncommon.[7] A careful history and physical exam are important, as it has been shown that 22% of primary care physicians miss the diagnosis of acute Achilles rupture.[20] The physical examination is characterized by palpation of the defect and documentation by Thompson test,[112] which indicates discontinuity and loss of plantar flexion when the calf is squeezed. The therapist best performs a Thompson test by asking the patient to kneel on a chair with the feet hanging over the edge and the calf muscles relaxed. In this prone position, the examiner can usually denote a difference in resting angle from the contralateral side. Radiographic evaluation rules out the presence of a bony injury. Magnetic resonance imaging (MRI) can be helpful in demonstrating the presence, location, and severity of tears of the Achilles tendon. MRI also is helpful in assessing the status of an Achilles tendon repair.[87] Ultrasonography has been used to define Achilles tendon discontinuity[48] in countries where MRI is not routinely used.

After an accurate diagnosis is made, definitive treatment can be implemented by establishing the objectives for management. If any questions remain regarding the diagnosis or severity of the tear, then MRI and ultrasonography can be used to enhance diagnostic accuracy. The physical therapist (PT) should define the patient's functional and athletic goals, personal needs, and temporal priorities before making therapeutic judgments.

Nonoperative Versus Operative Management

Treatment for Achilles tendon ruptures was nonoperative until the twentieth century. It included immobilization with strapping, wrapping, and braces for varying periods of time.[117] In 1929 Quenu and Stoianovitch[97] stated that a rupture of the Achilles tendon should be operated on without delay. Christensen[22] (1953) and Arner, Lindholm, and Orell[7] (1958) compared patients treated surgically and those managed nonoperatively; the surgical group had better results. As the field of sports medicine progressed with new surgical techniques, including rigid internal fixation combined with rehabilitation, the optimal treatment for Achilles tendon rupture became controversial. Some studies supported nonoperative management of Achilles ruptures,[70,94] as shown in the following editorial statement made in 1973: "In view of the excellent results obtainable by conservative treatment, it is doubtful whether surgical repair in closed rupture of the Achilles tendon can be justified."[1] Skin healing complications are lower in nonoperative groups (0.5% nonoperative versus 14.6% operative); however, rerupture rates are much lower with surgery (15.6% nonoperative versus 6.7%).[20,53,55,118] In a meta-analysis of reports on Achilles tendon injury, Khan and associates[65] found that open operative treatment of acute Achilles tendon ruptures significantly reduces the risk of rerupture compared with nonoperative treatment, but it produces a significantly higher risk of other complications, including wound infection.

In 2003, Weber and colleagues[116] compared the results of acute ruptures in 23 patients treated nonoperatively to 24 patients treated operatively. Patients in the nonoperative group were allowed full weight bearing in 20-degrees patellofemoral (PF) cast for 6 weeks and were verified with weekly ultrasonography and cast changes. Patients in the operative group were placed in casts and were non–weight bearing for 6 weeks with variable rehabilitation protocols. The results showed a decreased return to work and crutch time for nonoperative cases, with 4 of 23 rerupture at 7 to 12 weeks. Patients in the operative group had only 1 of 24 rerupture at 3 years. This study demonstrates that nonoperative treatment may be acceptable for some patient populations, but that operative treatment, even with traditional postoperative immobilization, yields a lower rerupture rate. The surgeon must explore the goals and expectations of the patient and decide which treatment is most appropriate. Indications for nonoperative treatment include concomitant illness in the patient, a sedentary lifestyle, or lower functional and athletic goals.

Early nonoperative options were well accepted and tolerated. But in the past 20 years, patient expectations and functional goals have increased so that surgical options have gained acceptance and preference. In contrast, the patient selected for operative repair should be an individual who is extremely interested in optimal functional restoration.

Recently an emphasis has been placed on less invasive operative techniques and the postoperative management of Achilles tendon repair. These postoperative treatment programs, regardless of surgical technique, avoid cast immobilization and are well tolerated, safe, and effective with well-motivated athletes and patients who especially desire the highest functional outcome.*

Acute Care of the Achilles Tendon Rupture

In the last century the literature has proposed numerous approaches to the management of acute Achilles tendon ruptures. The most important design principles of the option selected should include the following:

1. The option and procedure are safe and effective.
2. The method allows the patient to accomplish realistic goals.
3. The surgeon can execute the method successfully.
4. The risks of the method are acceptable to the patient and surgeon.

---

*References 17, 19, 23, 75, 83, 85, 99.

The categorical options for the surgical treatment of acute Achilles tendon rupture include repair, repair with augmentation, and reconstruction.

SURGICAL PROCEDURE

Repair

The rationale for any repair method is to restore continuity of the ruptured tendon end, facilitate healing, and restore muscle function. The technical difficulty is taking relative "mop ends" and opposing them in a stable fashion. Bunnell[13] and Kessler[64] were the first to popularize the end-to-end suture technique for ruptured tendons. Ma and Griffith[79] described a percutaneous repair in 1977; however, a higher rerupture rate also occurred in their series. Beskin[8] introduced the three-bundle suture, and Cetti[17] demonstrated the suture weave in 1988, which was further modified by Mortensen and Saether[88] in 1991 as a six-strand suture technique. Nada[92] described the use of external fixation for Achilles tendon ruptures in 1985. Richardson, Reitman, and Wilson[98] described good results using a pull-out wire, which has the advantage of minimal suture reaction but requires a second procedure for suture removal. Each of these techniques has advantages and disadvantages, hence the wide spectrum of options. The surgeon's selection of a method should be based on technical training, an accurate pathoanatomic diagnosis, and the patient's goals and desires.

Repair with Augmentation

Historically, augmentation procedures evolved to supplement the repair construct of mop ends plus suture. Most augmentation procedures involved the local use of gastrocnemius fascia flaps or the plantaris tendon if available. Christensen[22] described the use of the gastrocnemius aponeurosis flap to augment Achilles tendon repair in 1981. Silfverskiold[106] described a central rotation gastrocnemius flap, and Lindholm[77] devised a method of two turndown flaps. Lynn[78] (1966) used the plantaris tendon, fanning it out to use the membrane to reinforce the repair. Kirschembaum and Kellman[66] modified the technique in 1980 by placing the fascial flaps centrally rather than separating them. Chen and Wertheimer[21] (1992) demonstrated the use of suture anchors distally at the calcaneus to repair the gastrocnemius turndown flap with semirigid fixation. Overall, these methods can facilitate the continuity and strength of the repair construct when doubt persists concerning the repair's integrity. In practice these techniques are applied only in limited situations, but they should still be in the surgeon's armamentarium.

Reconstruction

Acute ruptures are usually managed with the repair techniques already described with or without augmentation. Usually these are appropriate to promote continuity and healing of acute ruptures. Neglected, chronic ruptures, however, require reconstruction with endogenous or exogenous materials. Endogenous materials include fascia lata,[12] peroneus brevis transfer,[111] flexor digitorum longus,[84] and flexor hallucis longus.[115] Exogenous materials include carbon fiber,[56] Marlex mesh,[51] Dacron vascular grafts,[75] polylactic acid (PLA) implant, and a polypropylene braid.[42] Once again, the surgeon must be familiar with these procedures and understand their advantages and disadvantages before applying them in appropriate scenarios.

Concepts of Achilles Tendon Repair

Prolonged cast immobilization has been used with both operative and nonoperative treatment of Achilles tendon ruptures. Although cast immobilization may promote healing, it also promotes one or more of the following manifestations of "cast disease"[44,91]:

- Muscle atrophy
- Joint stiffness
- Cartilage atrophy
- Degenerative arthritis
- Adhesion formation
- Deep venous thrombosis (DVT)

Immobilization after tendon surgery was considered the single factor most responsible for postsurgical complications as long ago as 1954.[6,22,79] Various clinical studies in the literature document residual isokinetic strength deficits between 10% and 16% after cast immobilization of Achilles tendon injuries, regardless of whether they were managed operatively or nonoperatively.*

The AO Group of Switzerland found that stable and rigid internal fixation of bone fractures allows early range of motion (ROM) and maximal rehabilitation, thus minimizing atrophy and the manifestations of cast disease. This principle indicates that early mobilization of tendon ruptures should be promoted as long as stable fixation is ensured. In support of this concept, it has been demonstrated that early motion limits atrophy,[9] promotes fiber polymerization to collagen,[96] and increases the organization of collagen at the repair site, leading to increased strength.[29,30,32,40] Krackow, Thomas, and Jones[67] initially described a suture technique that allows "rigid" internal fixation without tendon necrosis. This technique, coupled with complete repair of the peritenon, should result in progressive and successful healing of the Achilles tendon rupture without postoperative cast immobilization.

*Resources 10, 52, 74, 94, 105.

Mandelbaum, Myerson, and Forster[83] reported on the successful use of the Krackow modified suture technique in a series of 29 athletes with acute Achilles tendon rupture. Postoperatively the patients were not rigidly immobilized and were started on early ROM and conditioning programs. No patients in this series experienced rerupture, persistent pain, frank infection, or skin necrosis as a complication. By 6 weeks postoperatively, 90% of patients had full ROM. By 6 months, 92% had returned to sports participation; strength deficits were less than 3% on isokinetic testing. Rigid internal fixation of Achilles tendon tears allowed a more functional rehabilitation process in this series, including early motion and weight bearing. Maffulli and colleagues,[80] who reported on the operative results of 42 patients who were randomized to a traditional protocol of postoperative immobilization or a full weight–bearing protocol, strengthened these results. In the full weight–bearing group, patients were placed in a full weight–bearing cast for 2 weeks, then a full weight–bearing dorsiflexion splint for 4 weeks. In the traditional protocol, the patients were immobilized in a cast for 4 weeks, then a full weight–bearing cast for 2 more weeks. They found that the full weight–bearing group had no crutch use at 1.5 weeks, a quicker return to work, less calf atrophy, greater patient satisfaction, less patient visits, and equal isometric strength to the traditional group.[80] This method of accelerated but controlled postoperative management has proven to be safe and highly effective at returning the athlete and patient to activities of daily living (ADLs) and sports with the highest level of function.[82,83,109]

Preoperative Treatment

After the diagnosis is made, the patient should be placed in a compressive elastic or cohesive tape wrap to minimize swelling. They should be encouraged to use ice and elevate the extremity. If possible, then the patient should be allowed to ambulate in a cam walker boot or with a cane to promote circulation and prevent venous thrombosis. Surgery should be performed in an outpatient setting 7 to 10 days after the injury. This delay allows consolidation of the tendon ends, making repair technically easier.

Surgical Technique

Surgery is performed with the patient in the prone position under general, regional, or local anesthesia. Care should be taken to note the resting tension of the opposite foot. To be most accurate, both feet can be prepped to allow accurate side-to-side comparison of tendon length. Either a straight midline or an anteromedial incision is made just medial to the gastrocnemius. A direct incision is made through the peritenon, which is split and tagged. Before repair of the tendon, any adhesions between the anterior surface of the muscle and tendon unit and the paratenon are removed. A relaxing incision in the anterior surface of the paratenon is made down to the muscle of the flexor hallucis longus, which will facilitate closure of the paratenon. Each end of the tear is sewn with a No. 2 nonabsorbable suture using the Krackow suture technique (Fig. 25-6). The recently introduced synthetic, polyethylene sutures such as Fiberwire (Arthrex, Naples, FL) or Orthocord (Depuy Mitek, Norwood, MA) are now commonly used for the repair and have been shown to have superior strength to traditional braided sutures.[27] The sutures are tensioned appropriately to achieve the same resting angle as the contralateral extremity. If any doubt exists regarding the amount of tension, then the contralateral side may be used for comparison. The suture knots are passed to the anterior aspect of the tendon and secured. The peritenon is then closed anatomically with 4-0 absorbable suture. The ankle is taken through a ROM to evaluate the stability of the repair construct. The wound is closed with dermal mattress sutures with the knots based on the medial side to protect the tendon, and a posterior splint is applied. On the second day after surgery, the splint is removed and the ankle is taken gently through active range of motion (AROM). Gentle ROM exercises are begun. The sutures are removed by about day 14, and a progressive weight-bearing program is initiated using a walker boot.

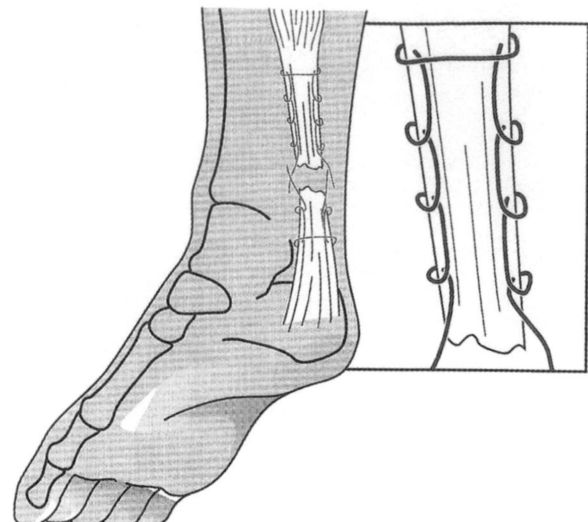

Fig. 25-6 Krackow suture technique.
(Courtesy Santa Monica Orthopaedic and Sports Medicine Group, Santa Monica, CA.)

Percutaneous Repair

Percutaneous repair of the Achilles tendon has become an acceptable alternative method to open repair. Proponents of the technique have cited a lower wound complication rate and similar rerupture rates.* Halasi, Tallay, and

*References 11, 45, 46, 76, 113.

Berkes[46] performed an endoscopically assisted repair on 123 patients and had no wound problems, a return to sport in 4 to 6 months, and no wound complications. Although sural nerve irritation can be a complication of the technique, it has been postulated that endoscopic assistance of the procedure lowered the sural nerve complication rate.

Percutaneous Repair Technique

Buchgraber and Pässler[11] described the following surgical technique. Patients are placed in a prone position and given a short-acting general anesthetic. The tendon defect is identified by palpation, and a transverse or longitudinal incision is made along the skin folds across its center. The associated hematoma is deliberately left in place. Using a 15.3 mm blade, stab incisions are made at the medial and lateral aspects of the tendon approximately10 to 12 cm above the site of the tear. Another two stab incisions of the same length are made above the calcaneus medial and lateral to the insertion of the Achilles tendon. To prevent sural nerve injury, a mosquito clamp is placed in the proximal lateral stab incision to retract the skin and the underlying fascia. With the help of a cutting needle (Aesculap, Tuttlingen, Germany) a 1.2 mm polydioxanone suture (PDS) cord is pulled through proximally from the medial to the lateral stab incision. Then the cutting needle is introduced through the incision overlying the tear, passed through the tendon proximally, and advanced toward the lateral proximal stab incision. Using the cutting needle, the end of the PDS cord at this site is passed out through the central incision. Next the cutting needle is pushed into the tendon tissue from the lateral distal stab incision, brought out centrally to load it with the lateral end of the PDS cord, and pulled out distally. This end of the cord is grasped with the needle and introduced through the medial distal stab incision, brought out through the lateral distal stab incision, and pulled through medially. In the final step, the needle is passed through the proximal tendon end from the central incision and brought out at the medial proximal stab incision. The foot is put repeatedly through the full ROM to ensure that the cord will dig into the tendon tissue. The ends of the cord are tied with the foot in slight plantar flexion. Once the first knot is tied, the foot is dorsiflexed several times to check the tension on the cord. The procedure is concluded with another two knots added in a crisscross pattern.[11]

Potential Complications

The major complication with nonoperative treatment is a higher rerupture rate and an incomplete return of function and performance. Complications associated with the surgical technique include infection, anesthetic problems, rerupture, deep vein thrombosis (DVT), and an incomplete return of function. Infection can be a disastrous complication, because soft tissue coverage is a major problem and can only be resolved with vascularized flaps and a reconstructive tendon procedure.[73]

THERAPY GUIDELINES FOR REHABILITATION

Consideration Toward the Healing Tendon

The use of early motion during postoperative rehabilitation requires the PT to have a working knowledge of the process of tissue healing. With this knowledge, the therapist can apply appropriate amounts of stress at the correct times, progressing the rehabilitation program at an optimal pace and ensuring a good clinical outcome. Extensive summaries by Leadbetter[72] and Curwin[24] and Curwin and Stanish[26] fully describe tendon physiology and healing.

Fig. 25-7 summarizes the stages of the healing process and the implications they have for traditional postoperative management of Achilles tendon repairs and motion in the early postoperative period. Tendon healing occurs in four consecutive, related phases, with somewhat overlapping time frames.

Stages of Healing

Inflammatory Response

Minutes after injury, laceration, or the initiation of surgical repair, a coagulation response occurs, triggering the formation of a fibrin clot. This clot contains fibronectin, which is essential to reparative cell activity. Fibronectin eventually creates a scaffold for cell migration and supports fibroblastic activity. Soon after this clot forms, polymorphonuclear leukocytes and macrophages invade the area to clear cellular and tissue debris. The resulting arachidonic acid cascade is the primary chemical event during this stage. This stage is usually complete in less than 6 days unless infection and wound disturbance occur.

Q Kerry had an Achilles tendon repair 7 weeks ago. She is partial weight bearing and uses a fixed protective splint. At 9 weeks she will initiate non–weight-bearing stretching exercises for all ankle motions. During phases I and II (weeks 1 through 8) of the healing process, fibroblastic proliferation continues, producing a rapid increase in the amount of collagen. Even though collagen amounts are increased, the repaired tissue is weak and requires protection (e.g., restricted weight bearing and nonaggressive ROM stretches). Why do the healing tissues remain weak despite the increase in collagen fibers?

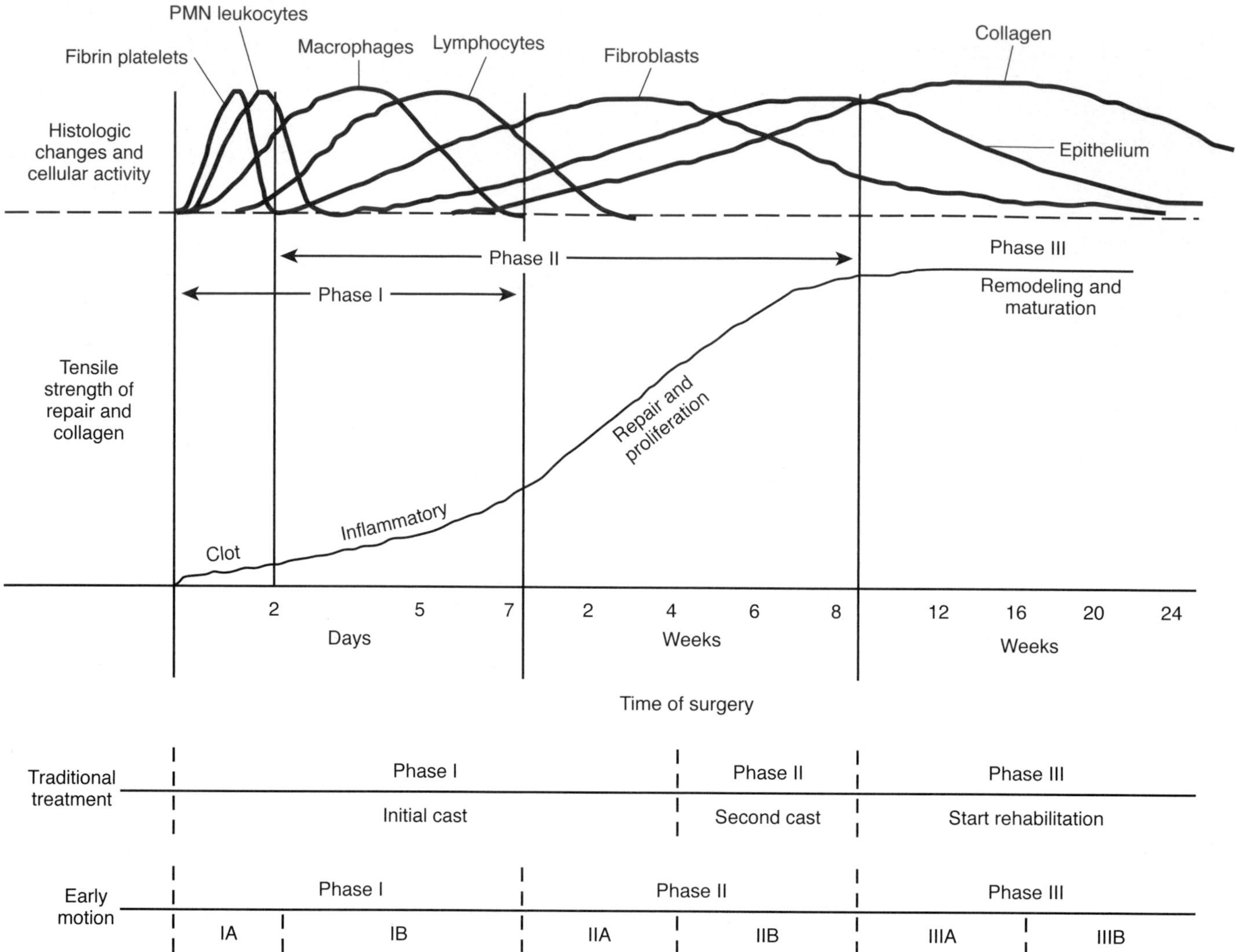

Fig. 25-7 Phases of tissue healing and rehabilitation timelines.

Repair and Proliferation

The repair and proliferation stage may begin as early as 48 hours after injury and may last for 6 to 8 weeks. Tissue macrophages are the key factors early in this stage. The macrophage is mobile and capable of releasing various growth factors, chemotactants, and proteolytic enzymes when necessary or appropriate for the activation of fibroblasts and tendon repair.[72] Fibroblastic proliferation continues and produces increasing amounts of collagen. Type III collagen, which has poor cross-link definition, small fibril size, and poor strength, is initially deposited rapidly. As the repair process continues, collagen deposition shifts to type I collagen, which has greater cross-link definition, fibril size, and strength. The deposition of type I collagen accelerates and continues throughout this stage and well into the remodeling and maturation stage.

Changes in the postoperative internal structure of 21 surgically repaired Achilles tendons have been documented by Karjalainen and colleagues[61] during the healing process using MRI. After surgery, patients were placed in casts in equinus position for 3 weeks without weight bearing and for another 3 weeks in a short walking cast in neutral position, with weight bearing as tolerated. After cast removal, patients began AROM and walking exercises. MRI was repeated at 3 weeks, 6 weeks, 3 months, and 6 months after repair to document changes (Fig. 25-8). During this stage the postoperative cross-sectional area of repaired Achilles tendon increased dramatically, measuring 2.9 and 3.4 times the size of the uninjured contralateral tendon at 3 and 6 weeks, respectively. Diffuse, high-intensity heterogeneous signal was present at the repair site for all 21 tendons at 3 weeks and in 13 of 21 tendons at 6 weeks. In the other eight tendons, early formation of high-intensity intratendinous signal was present in the center of the tendon at the level of repair.

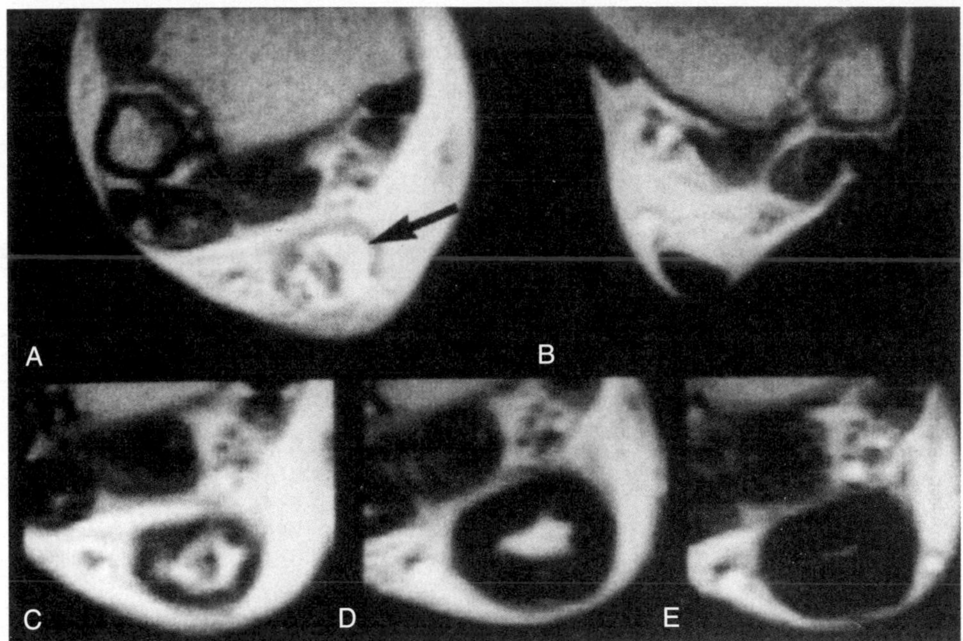

Fig. 25-8 T_2 weighted magnetic resonance imaging (MRI) (TR, 2000 ms; TE, 80 ms) of the normal reunion process of ruptured and surgically repaired Achilles tendon. **A,** The affected tendon shows a high-intensity signal (*arrow*) with a peripheral thin rim of low-intensity signal area and also low-intensity elements centrally. **B,** The unaffected side. **C,** At 6 weeks the intratendinous lesion and the margin of the Achilles tendon are better visualized. **D,** At 3 months the periphery of the healing tendon has returned to its normal low-intensity signal level. The intratendinous lesion inside the tendon is rather small. The cross-sectional area is seven times as large as the unaffected side (**B**). **E,** At 6 months the scar is barely visible and the edema around the tendon has decreased compared with previous images.
(From Karjalainen PT et al: Magnetic resonance imaging during healing of surgically repaired Achilles tendon ruptures, *Am J Sports Med* 25(2):164, 1997.)

> **A** Type III collagen is deposited; it has poor cross-link definition, small fibril size, and poor strength. As the repair process continues, the collagen deposition shifts to type I collagen, which has better cross-link definition, fibril size, and strength.

Remodeling and Maturation

Remodeling and maturation of collagen fibrils and cross-links characterize the third healing stage. Overall a trend toward decreased cellularity and synthetic activity, increased organization of the extracellular matrix, and a more normal biochemical profile is evident.[71] Functional linear alignment of the collagen fibrils is usually present by 2 months.[72] Although maturation appears to be complete a number of months after the injury, biochemical differences in collagen type and arrangement, water content, DNA content, and glycosaminoglycan content persist indefinitely. The material properties of these scars never become identical to those of intact tendon.[5] Biomechanical properties can be reduced by as much as 30% despite the completion of all stages of healing and maturation.[5,26,38,39] Karjalainen and associates[61] found that the cross-sectional area of the tendon continues to increase. The area is 6.1 times the size of the unaffected tendon at 3 months and 5.6 times the size at 6 months. A variably sized, high-intensity signal demonstrating a central intratendinous lesion was detected in 19 of 21 repaired tendons at 3 months. The development of an intratendinous lesion appears to be a normal part of the healing process after surgical repair and casting.

Future Directions

Gene therapy and growth factors have an emerging role in the treatment of bone, cartilage, and tendon healing.[47,100] Tendon callus can be influenced by cartilage derived morphogenic protein-2 (CDMP-2).[100] Using an animal model of rabbit Achilles tendon tears, Forslund and Aspenberg[35] showed that failure load and stiffness in a CDMP-2 group were greater at 14 days compared with controls. Future treatments may include addition of growth factors to the repair site.

Postoperative Management: Traditional Immobilization and Remobilization Versus Early Motion

Since surgical repair of Achilles tendon ruptures began almost 50 years ago,[117] the most common method of postoperative management has traditionally been to immobilize the repair in a plaster cast or other type of restrictive device until healing is considered complete, then begin ROM and strengthening exercises.* Based on an understanding of connective tissue physiology and the success achieved with other types of surgical repairs, such as anterior cruciate ligament (ACL) reconstruction, several authors have begun using early postoperative motion to minimize the deleterious effects of immobilization on joints (e.g., stiffness and loss of muscle strength, endurance, and flexibility)[9,39,81,119] and facilitate an earlier return to preoperative functional levels.† Numerous studies have compared cast immobilization to early postoperative motion. The *Cochrane Database of Systematic Reviews* considered five appropriately designed studies to find that functional bracing appeared to reduce hospital stay, time off work, and sports, as well as possibly lowering overall complication rates.‡ However, no studies have compared different rehabilitation regimens. The guidelines presented are a compilation of various approaches considering appropriate tendon healing.

Q Doug is 43 years old and underwent an Achilles tendon repair 9 weeks ago. The physician has chosen the traditional immobilization approach for rehabilitation. He presented today 1 week after cast removal and is still quite painful with ambulation (stance phase). What can the therapist do to help control his symptoms.

Guidelines for Traditional Immobilization and Remobilization

Phases I and II

TIME: 1 to 8 weeks after surgery
GOALS: Minimize deconditioning, control edema and pain, encourage independent gait (non–weight bearing until cleared by the physician to progressive weight bearing, usually at 4 weeks) with assistive device as appropriate

During traditional postoperative rehabilitation of surgically repaired Achilles tendon ruptures, a cast is in place throughout phases I and II of the healing process (Table 25-2). The PT can do little to influence healing and affect the outcome of the surgical repair. Casting, usually for 6 to 9 weeks, incorporates varying degrees of plantar flexion to protect the repair from stress. Casts that were initially applied with the foot in plantar flexion are usually changed to neutral (zero-degrees dorsiflexion) for the final 3 to 4 weeks of immobilization. During this period a conditioning program is designed to maintain the patient's general strength and cardiovascular conditioning. After the cast is removed, the PT can further protect the tendon from full stress by using a heel lift of varying heights for as long as 8 weeks, if needed. Crutches with progressive weight bearing also may be used to control mechanical stress.

A The PT can assist in protecting the tendon from full stress by using a heel lift of varying heights, and wean the height as able. In addition, by using crutches, progressive weight bearing may be used to control mechanical stress. Modalities can also be used to help manage any residual pain and inflammation.

Phase III

TIME: 9 to 16 weeks after surgery
GOALS: Normalize gait, increase ROM and strength, improve scar mobility

With the traditional approach, the rehabilitation program does not truly begin until phase III. The scar and tissue have begun to mature and therefore ROM, joint mobilization, stretching, strengthening, gait training, and return to function may progress as tolerated (Table 25-3). The sequence of treatment depends more on resolving the patient's physical impairments and functional limitations than on the timeline of healing. Impairments are resolved to re-establish function, develop skills, and return the patient to full activity and sports participation.

The initial goal is to restore ROM. Restoration of mobility must occur before the patient can begin to work on strength. Active exercises in the sagittal (dorsiflexion and plantar flexion) and transverse (inversion and eversion) planes are initiated and progressed with the knee flexed and extended. The therapist should use joint mobilization techniques to assist in gaining joint ROM and stretching exercises to gain muscle flexibility and improve joint ROM (see figures in Chapter 23 describing mobilization of the ankle).

Any symptoms of pain and swelling that occur must be controlled during this phase through the use of appropriate modalities and adjustments in the intensity of the treatment plan and home program. Soft tissue mobilization can be used to reduce scar adhesion. These adjuncts for restoring ROM, muscle and tendon flexibility, and strength are continued throughout the program as appropriate (see Table 25-3).

Phase IV

TIME: 17 to 20 weeks after surgery
GOALS: Demonstrate normal gait on level surfaces, initiate running program, have full ROM, increase strength, improve balance and coordination

The therapist can initiate strengthening as ROM progresses. Initially, isometric techniques are used for all

*References 20, 34, 41, 53, 62, 107.
†References 16, 33, 75, 82, 83, 108.
‡References 19, 59, 63, 65, 80, 86, 89, 118.

Table 25-2 Achilles Tendon Repair (Traditional Rehabilitation)

Rehabilitation Phase	Criteria to Progress to this Phase	Anticipated Impairments and Functional Limitations	Intervention	Goal	Rationale
Phase I Postoperative 1-4 weeks	◆ Postoperative	◆ Edema ◆ Pain ◆ Non–weight bearing ◆ Cardiovascular and muscular deconditioning	◆ Cast in equinus ◆ Provide elevation and ice ◆ Instruct and monitor non–weight-bearing crutch gait on all surfaces ◆ Design and implement cardiovascular- and muscular-conditioning program	◆ Control edema and pain ◆ Protect repair ◆ Minimize deconditioning	◆ Immobilization in equinus minimizes stress on surgical repair during healing process ◆ Elevation and ice assist in minimizing pain and swelling ◆ Non–weight-bearing status protects repair ◆ Maintenance of cardiovascular and muscular conditioning crucial to general health and return to preoperative level of function when out of cast
Phase II Postoperative 5-8 weeks	◆ Stable edema and pain ◆ Well-healed incision present at cast change	◆ Abolished or diminishing postoperative pain and swelling ◆ Atrophy of lower leg and foot muscles ◆ Progressive weight-bearing status allowed ◆ Cardiovascular and muscular deconditioning	◆ Recasted in neutral dorsiflexion ◆ Elevation and ice as needed ◆ Instruct in progressive weight bearing to full weight bearing using appropriate assistive devices ◆ Modify cardiovascular and muscular conditioning program as appropriate	◆ Control symptoms of edema and pain if they occur ◆ Continue to protect repair ◆ Encourage full weight bearing during gait cycle ◆ Minimize deconditioning	◆ Decreased rate of atrophy occurs when muscles are immobilized in lengthened position[39] ◆ Progressive weight bearing to full weight bearing allows loading and proprioceptive input ◆ Conditioning program should be progressed as patient's condition allows

motions. Strength training then progresses to the use of elastic tubing and manual resistive techniques, such as proprioceptive neuromuscular facilitation (PNF). Isokinetic exercise and body weight resistance can be added if symptoms do not arise from the other techniques. The patient should begin double-heel raises before single-heel raises to reduce tensile stress and the potential for symptoms such as pain and swelling. The heel raises should initially be performed on a level, flat surface, after which the patient can progress to doing them over the edge of a stair to use the full ROM available. Proprioceptive and balance activities should be initiated concurrently with strengthening. The PT can begin a running progression, sport-specific skill development, and functional activities after the patient has a normal gait and full ROM and can rapidly perform heel raises. Isokinetic measurement of strength, power, and endurance at 4 to 6 months may *assist* in the determination of return to sport activity, but it is not the determining factor.

The success of Achilles tendon repair using traditional immobilization and rehabilitation has been favorably measured, primarily by rerupture rates, strength, calf circumference, tendon width, and return to previous activity levels. Rerupture rates have been reported at an average of less than 2%.[117] Strength measurements include the ability to perform single-toe raises, manual muscle

Table 25-3 Achilles Tendon Repair (Traditional Rehabilitation)

Rehabilitation Phase	Criteria to Progress to this Phase	Anticipated Impairments and Functional Limitations	Intervention	Goal	Rationale
Phase III Postoperative 9-16 weeks	◆ Out of cast ◆ No increase in pain ◆ No increased loss of ROM ◆ Incision healed	◆ Altered gait cycle (preswing phase of gait) ◆ Limited joint ROM and muscle flexibility ◆ Atrophy and limited strength ◆ Soft tissue edema and joint swelling ◆ Tendon hypertrophy ◆ Scar tissue adhesion ◆ Limited cardiovascular fitness	◆ Ice, elevation, and NSAIDs ◆ Therapeutic ultrasound and/or whirlpool ◆ PROM (stretches)—Gastrocnemius-soleus, peroneals, tibialis anterior, tibialis posterior ◆ Exercises, pool therapy, and joint mobilization as listed under the early motion program ◆ AROM and isometrics in all directions, progressing to resisted exercises using tubing or manual resistance (PNF) ◆ Gait training—Heel lift if required; return to progressive weight bearing with appropriate assistive devices (crutches or cane) to obtain normal gait cycle if necessary to avoid secondary overuse/tendonitis syndrome; progress as indicated based on symptoms of gait cycle	◆ Control edema and pain if occur ◆ Initiate normalization of gait cycle ◆ Obtain full ROM ◆ Improve strength of all foot and ankle musculature ◆ Reduce scar tissue adhesion ◆ Promote cardiovascular and muscular conditioning	◆ Modalities have been demonstrated to improve ease of tissue deformation when used in conjunction with mobilization and stretching ◆ Restore normal ROM ◆ Initiate strength through ROM to improve overall function ◆ Increase strength and endurance ◆ Gait deficits in the preswing phase may result from limited dorsiflexion and decreased plantar flexion strength; heel lifts assist in reducing stress on musculotendinous structures in foot and ankle during the early gait cycle out of cast; heel lift can be decreased or eliminated as indicated ◆ Overuse symptoms should be addressed as appropriate to minimize severity and longevity
Phase IV Postoperative 17-20 weeks	◆ No symptoms from ROM, flexibility, and strengthening exercises initiated during weeks 9-16 ◆ Able to sustain isometric single-leg toe raise and lower body	◆ Mild or minimal alteration in gait cycle without assistive devices ◆ Restricted joint ROM and muscle flexibility ◆ Unable to do repeated single-leg heel raise ◆ Limited strength	◆ Continue intervention from Phase III as indicated ◆ Continue joint mobilization techniques as appropriate ◆ Continue stretching exercises;	◆ Normal gait cycle on level surfaces; initiate running program when normal gait cycle is evident ◆ Full symmetrical ankle joint ROM and	◆ Progress intensity of rehabilitation program as indicated ◆ Restore arthrokinematics ◆ Promote patient self-management and stretching program ◆ Prepare for

Table 25-3 Achilles Tendon Repair (Traditional Rehabilitation)—cont'd

Rehabilitation Phase	Criteria to Progress to this Phase	Anticipated Impairments and Functional Limitations	Intervention	Goal	Rationale
	weight eccentrically under control ◆ AROM dorsiflexion 5 degrees ◆ PROM dorsiflexion 10 degrees ◆ Symmetrical plantar flexion, inversion, and eversion ◆ No assistive devices required for ambulation	◆ Limited proprioception ◆ Soft tissue edema ◆ Tendon hypertrophy ◆ Minimal scar tissue adhesion ◆ Cardiovascular and muscular deconditioning	initiate body weight stretching over edge of step ◆ Continue strength program for foot and ankle musculature as listed in early motion program ◆ Modify cardiovascular and muscular conditioning program as needed ◆ Isokinetics and body weight resistance exercises such as heel raises (if no increase in symptoms occurs with previous exercises) ◆ Balance and proprioceptive activities (e.g., BAPS board, single-leg balance activities) ◆ Near end of the phase (see criteria on page 472-473), begin running progression and sport-specific skill development	muscle flexibility ◆ Continue to improve foot and ankle strength; repeated single-leg heel raise ◆ Symmetrical single-limb balance ◆ Reduce scar tissue adhesion ◆ Promote cardiovascular and muscular conditioning	discharge ◆ Promote symmetrical strength of foot and ankle via single-limb balance, isokinetic testing, and progressive plyometric program initiated in water and progressed to land ◆ Continue and progress based on each patient's response to intervention ◆ Provide good cardiovascular maintenance program based on patient's needs ◆ Increase strength and improve function ◆ Improve balance and coordination on uneven surfaces ◆ Transition into high-level occupational activities or sports

ROM, Range of motion; *NSAIDs,* nonsteroidal anti-inflammatory drugs; *PROM,* passive range of motion; *AROM,* active range of motion; *PNF,* proprioceptive neuromuscular facilitation; *BAPS,* biomechanical ankle platform system.

tests, and isokinetic strength measurements. Authors using peak torque measurements of isokinetic plantar flexion strength have reported that the gastrocnemius and soleus strength of the repaired Achilles tendon ranges from 83% to 101% of the uninvolved extremity.[117] Outcome measures in studies that have been reported in the literature are difficult to use in comparing various studies.[117] These studies used different operational definitions, set forth different methodologies, and collected data at different times, making meaningful comparison difficult.

Guidelines for Early Motion

As early as 1984, in an effort to reduce the effects of immobilization, various authors began to present methods of repair that would allow early motion and rehabilitation.* Orthoses or specialized splinting were developed to protect the repair postoperatively.[16,59,89,108] Regardless of the type of repair, rehabilitation programs that emphasize

*References 33, 59, 63, 65, 75, 76, 83, 89, 90.

early motion must consider the strength and integrity of the repaired Achilles tendon as it changes during the various stages of healing.

> **Q** Scott is 35 years old and is undergoing his initial evaluation 7 days after surgery. What part of his history will help the therapist avoid being too aggressive and putting the repair at risk?

Phase Ia

TIME: 1 to 2 days after surgery
GOALS: Prevent infection, control edema and pain, increase AROM, prevent complications, promote independent gait using assistive device as appropriate

Phase Ib

TIME: 3 to 7 days after surgery
GOALS: Demonstrate AROM dorsiflexion to 5 degrees and plantar flexion 50% of uninvolved side, control edema and pain

When using an early motion program for postoperative rehabilitation, the therapist must keep in mind the phases of tissue healing and the degree to which tissues can tolerate tensile stress. During phases Ia and Ib of the early motion program, the primary concerns are evaluating wound status, decreasing swelling, and initiating ROM exercises (Table 25-4). However, ROM should not be pushed aggressively. The patient should work through PROM within the limits of pain and swelling intermittently throughout the day. The PT may prescribe ice, compression, and elevation to decrease swelling.

> **A** His general health, family, and past medical history are keys to determining if any factors may delay the healing process. Diabetes, peripheral vascular disease, medications (corticosteroids/NSAIDs), anticoagulants, smoking, past responses to healing (surgical, nonsurgical, or both), pain tolerance, nutrition, and high body mass index (BMI) all influence soft tissue healing response.

Phase IIa

TIME: 2 to 4 weeks after surgery
GOALS: Increase AROM and PROM, strength, and weight-bearing tolerance (on day 14) to partial weight bearing and full weight bearing as early as 3 weeks[59]

During phase IIa (Table 25-5) of the early motion program, emphasis is placed on gaining active dorsiflexion past neutral, following a full weight-bearing program in a protective splint or boot with a fixed hinge (Fig. 25-9), and initiating a gentle strength-training program of all the muscle groups in a range that minimizes tensile stress on the repair.

During phases Ia and IIa, therapeutic ultrasound can be used to assist in the healing response. In some instances therapeutic ultrasound has been shown to increase collagen synthesis and tensile strength in experimentally repaired rabbit Achilles tendon.[28,31,40,54] Enwemeka[28] and Enwemeka, Rodriguez, and Mendosa[31] reported favorable results that enhanced the healing response using 1 MHz at doses of 0.5 W/cm^2 and 1 W/cm^2 for 5 minutes during nine consecutive treatments. Jackson, Schwane, and Starcher[54] noted changes in collagen synthesis and breaking strength as early as 5 days after injury when giving continuous therapeutic ultrasound at 1.5 W/cm^2 for 4 minutes over 8 consecutive days and then every other day for up to 21 days. Freider and associates[36] reported similar results in partially ruptured, nonsurgically repaired Achilles tendons of Marland rats that received continuous therapeutic ultrasound at 1.5 W/cm^2 three times a week for either a 2- or a 3-week period. Although the results of studies using animal models may not be directly applicable to the human response, the therapeutic use of therapeutic ultrasound in the inflammatory and proliferative stages could prove beneficial. Using therapeutic ultrasound during these stages is a common clinical intervention.

Phase IIb

TIME: 5 to 8 weeks after surgery
GOALS: Demonstrate normal gait on level surfaces, encourage full ROM (symmetrical), increase strength and proprioception

During phase IIb (Table 25-6) the patient should strive to obtain full symmetrical ROM, achieve a normal gait cycle on level surfaces and in controlled environments without the protective boot, progress the strength program, and initiate proprioceptive training.

> **Q** Kim is 40 years old and ruptured her Achilles tendon playing tennis. She had surgery 7 weeks ago and is eager resume her prior activity level. What exercises can she safely perform, laying the foundation for her return to the court?

Phase IIIa

TIME: 9 to 16 weeks after surgery
GOALS: Demonstrate normal gait for all activities, have full weight bearing, increase strength and endurance; initiate walking or jogging program, isokinetics, and pool therapy plyometrics as appropriate (toward end of phase)

Table 25-4 Achilles Tendon Repair (Early Motion)

Rehabilitation Phase	Criteria to Progress to this Phase	Anticipated Impairments and Functional Limitations	Intervention	Goal	Rationale
Phase Ia Postoperative 1-2 days	◆ Postoperative	◆ Pain ◆ Soft tissue and joint edema ◆ Altered weight bearing, non–weight bearing with crutches	◆ Instruct in surgical site protection ◆ Provide ice, compression, and elevation ◆ Teach toe curls and pumps ◆ AROM (out of splint)—Ankle dorsiflexion, plantar flexion within pain limits two times a day ◆ Patient education—Instruction and monitoring of non–weight-bearing crutch gait	◆ Monitor wound status for drainage ◆ Prevent wound infection ◆ Control pain and swelling ◆ Increase AROM ◆ Prevent complications	◆ Surgical site inspection and cleanliness is crucial when patient is out of splint for ROM ◆ Ice, compression, and elevation with a Cryocuff over sterile wound dressing minimizes swelling ◆ Toe curls and AROM dorsiflexion and plantar flexion provide muscle pump to minimize edema
Phase Ib Postoperative 3-7 days	◆ No signs of infection	◆ Pain ◆ Soft tissue and joint edema ◆ Altered weight bearing, non–weight bearing with crutches until day 14	◆ Monitor wound for infection ◆ Provide ice, compression, and elevation ◆ AROM—Increase frequency to three times a day for dorsiflexion and plantar flexion ◆ Therapeutic ultrasound ◆ Instruction and monitoring of non–weight bearing crutch gait	◆ Minimize joint stiffness ◆ Facilitate healing ◆ Reduce soft tissue and joint swelling ◆ Active dorsiflexion to −5 degrees ◆ 50% active plantar flexion ROM compared with opposite side	◆ As in Phase Ia ◆ Therapeutic ultrasound has been demonstrated to assist in fibroblastic proliferation and facilitate collagen development along lines of stress[28,31,36]

AROM, Active range of motion; *PROM,* passive range of motion.

Phase IIIb

TIME: 17 to 20 weeks after surgery

GOALS: Return to preoperative level of activity or sport

During phase IIIa (Table 25-7) emphasis is on increasing the velocity of activity, increasing the patient's strength to perform a repeated single-leg heel raise, and improving the endurance of the gastrocnemius and soleus group to tolerate a functional progression. During phase IIIb (Table 25-8) a full functional progression is initiated to return the patient to the desired level of function.

All authors using the early motion program, regardless of the type of augmentation used during surgery, have reported excellent results. Success was measured by the same methods as for traditional rehabilitation. Limitation of ROM for dorsiflexion and plantar flexion are rare; patients are able to walk heel-toe and do single-leg raises at the time of follow-up examination. In addition, isokinetic peak torque levels are within 5% of the uninvolved side.[16,83]

Table 25-5 Achilles Tendon Repair (Early Motion)

Rehabilitation Phase	Criteria to Progress to this Phase	Anticipated Impairments and Functional Limitations	Intervention	Goal	Rationale
Phase IIa Postoperative 2-4 weeks	◆ Absence of wound drainage and infection ◆ Stable edema and pain levels ◆ Diminishing postoperative pain ◆ No increase in pain with touchdown weight bearing using crutches ◆ A well-healed incision should be present by week 3 to progress to the more active interventions (pool therapy) outlined in this phase	◆ Diminishing postoperative pain ◆ Diminishing soft tissue and joint swelling ◆ Scar adhesion ◆ Touchdown and progressive weight-bearing status ◆ Restricted ROM ◆ Decreased strength ◆ Altered cardiovascular endurance and conditioning	◆ Continue interventions as noted in Phase I ◆ Joint mobilization progress techniques for distraction—Anteroposterior and medial-lateral glides ◆ Progressive soft tissue mobilization and scar massage ◆ Progressive weight-bearing exercises and gait training in walking splint ◆ Start touchdown weight bearing on day 8; progress from partial to full weight bearing as pain and symptoms allow beginning on day 14 ◆ Isometrics—Out of splint ◆ Ankle in neutral —Inversion and eversion ◆ Start plantar flexion isometrics in late Phase IIa ◆ Pool therapy—Walk or run under full buoyancy conditions (non–weight bearing only!) ◆ AROM (out of splint)—Ankle (early Phase IIa, all directions, knee flexed and extended; late Phase IIa, gentle dorsiflexion stretching with towel or strap, knee flexed and	◆ Minimize joint stiffness ◆ Facilitate healing ◆ Decrease edema ◆ Minimize scar adhesion ◆ Increase weight-bearing tolerance to full weight bearing, beginning on day 14 ◆ Initiate isometric strength program ◆ Improve general muscular strength and endurance ◆ Early Phase IIa —Active dorsiflexion to 0 degrees with knee extended, 5 degrees with knee flexed ◆ Late Phase IIa —Active dorsiflexion to 0-5 degrees with knee extended, 5-10 degrees with knee flexed ◆ Minimize cardiovascular deconditioning	◆ Therapeutic ultrasound is most effective in first 3 weeks and less effective thereafter; discontinued by late Phase IIa ◆ Repair is strong enough and symptoms are stable enough to initiate full weight bearing in protective brace; reduce weight-bearing status as necessary based on symptom fluctuation and patient activity pattern ◆ Isometrics to facilitate strengthening and diminish edema and atrophy are performed in neutral position to reduce stress on repair ◆ Pool exercises facilitate ROM and strength in non–weight-bearing environment ◆ Ice, compression, and elevation with a Cryocuff over sterile wound dressing minimizes swelling ◆ Toe curls and AROM dorsiflexion and plantar flexion provide muscle pump to minimize edema ◆ Sufficient strength present at repair site based on healing and surgical technique to allow AROM to zero-degrees

Table 25-5 Achilles Tendon Repair (Early Motion)—cont'd

Rehabilitation Phase	Criteria to Progress to this Phase	Anticipated Impairments and Functional Limitations	Intervention	Goal	Rationale
Phase IIa Postoperative 2-4 weeks (continued)			extended towel curls with toes) ◆ Gait training wearing protective splint, with weight bearing to tolerance ◆ Elastic tubing or band exercises—Inversion, eversion, and plantar flexion and dorsiflexion; progress as tolerated if pain and symptoms allow ◆ Isotonics—Weight training program for all unaffected muscle groups ◆ Cardiovascular exercise using stationary bicycle to tolerance in walking sprint		dorsiflexion and all other motions to symptom tolerance with knee flexed and extended ◆ Towel curls facilitate muscle pump action to diminish edema and atrophy ◆ By 4 weeks, sufficient strength to allow start of plantar flexion isometrics and isotonics within symptom limits, using light resistance; performed in non–weight bearing ◆ Maintenance of general muscular strength and cardiovascular endurance necessary to resume full ADLs and recreational activities when feasible; walking splint protects repair during activity

ROM, Range of motion; *AROM,* active range of motion; *ADLs,* activities of daily living.

Reruptures are rare and are usually attributed to lack of retraining before a return to sports.[90] However, these outcomes are also difficult to compare for the same reasons as cited for traditional rehabilitation programs.

The success of early motion rehabilitation challenges the traditional use of cast immobilization after surgical repair. The *Cochrane Database of Systematic Reviews* concludes that functional bracing either produces better or no worse outcomes than cast immobilization.

The various postoperative protocols have not yet been compared. Patients are generally immobilized in equines for 6 weeks, then rehabilitation is progressed per impairments. Protected AROM begins as early as day 1. In some cases AROM begins at 2 weeks.[89] Mobility and strength progress. The walker boot is removed most frequently at 6 weeks, sometimes with use of a heel lift for several weeks.

The superiority of early motion for Achilles tendon repairs compared with traditional postoperative casting cannot yet be fully determined. Although studies reported to date state that the results are excellent, the different rehabilitation philosophies cannot be compared critically because of differences in operational definitions, criteria monitored, postoperative time when the data are collected, and surgical technique. Although the ultimate level of function achieved appears to be the same regardless of the rehabilitative program, the authors of this chapter believe that using early motion after Achilles tendon repair enables the patient to obtain a more independent and active quality of life sooner than that seen with traditional postoperative casting. However, patient compliance and

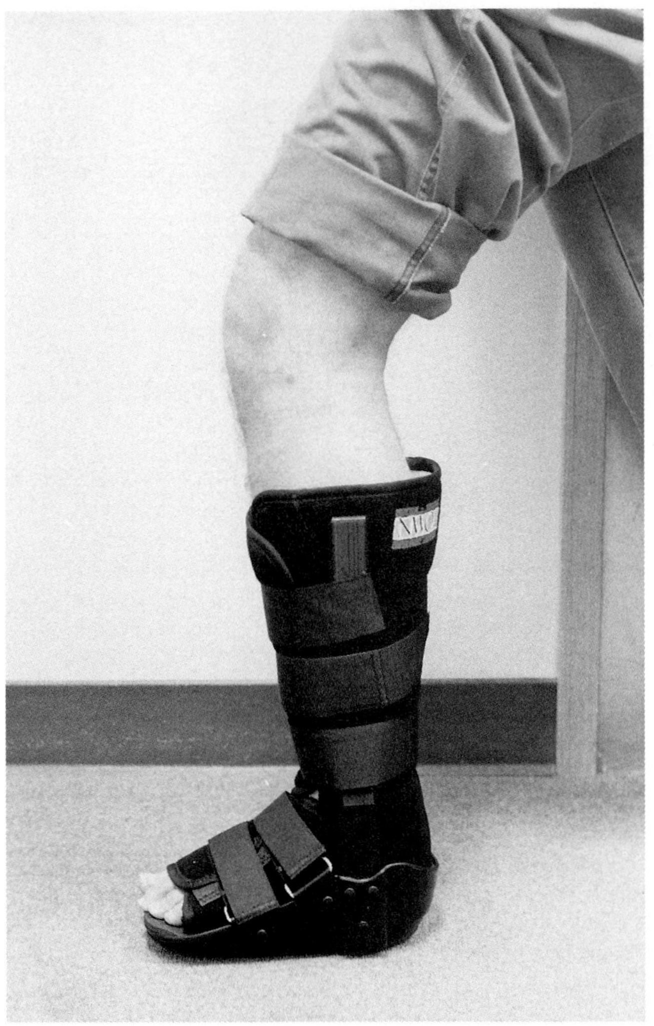

Fig. 25-9 Protective splint and boot for initiating progressive and full weight bearing. A fixed hinge should be used.

ongoing oversight of the rehabilitation program are crucial factors that must always be considered.

> **A** At this stage of Kim's rehabilitation, she can safely perform deep-water running (in a floatation vest without feet touching the bottom), core training exercises that avoid straining the repair (sitting or supine using a medicine ball), and upper extremity (UE) exercises (scapula stabilization and rotator cuff program).

SUGGESTED HOME MAINTENANCE FOR THE POSTSURGICAL PATIENT

Adherence to a home exercise program is crucial for a successful return to full ADLs and recreational function after Achilles tendon repair. The suggestions provided in this chapter do not constitute a fixed protocol. The home program for any patient must be individually determined based on the patient's postoperative condition, anticipated follow-through, and individual needs. Frequency, sets, and repetitions are determined similarly based on the therapist's professional opinion of what is needed in a particular situation.

Table 25-6 Achilles Tendon Repair (Early Motion)

Rehabilitation Phase	Criteria to Progress to this Phase	Anticipated Impairments and Functional Limitations	Intervention	Goal	Rationale
Phase IIb Postoperative 5-8 weeks	◆ No loss of ROM ◆ No increase in symptoms ◆ Full weight bearing in walking splint ◆ Incision healed ◆ Mild edema ◆ Pain controlled ◆ AROM ◆ Dorsiflexion to neutral or better ◆ Plantar flexion, inversion/ eversion symmetrical	◆ Minimal postoperative pain ◆ Limited ROM ◆ Limited strength ◆ Tendon hypertrophy and continued soft tissue swelling ◆ Altered gait cycle out of walking splint ◆ Unable to do a single-leg heel raise ◆ Altered proprioception and joint reaction time	◆ Continue interventions as noted in Phases I and II ◆ PROM—Initiate weight-bearing dorsiflexion stretch with knee extended and flexed ◆ AROM (out of splint) ◆ Gait training out of walking splint to tolerance ◆ Strength training	◆ Full symmetrical ROM in all motions ◆ Normal gait cycle on level surfaces and controlled environments out of walking splint ◆ Initiate isokinetic and isotonic strength-training	◆ Continue mobilizations to increase soft tissue strength and mobility and restore joint ROM sufficient to initiate gait training out of splint; gait should be practiced in controlled environment out of splint for safety as appropriate; discontinue use of splint at physician's

Table 25-6 Achilles Tendon Repair (Early Motion)—cont'd

Rehabilitation Phase	Criteria to Progress to this Phase	Anticipated Impairments and Functional Limitations	Intervention	Goal	Rationale
Phase IIb Postoperative 5-8 weeks (continued)			—Initiate double-leg heel raises ◆ Isokinetics—Submaximal velocity spectrum ◆ Plantar flexion and dorsiflexion, emphasizing endurance ◆ Weight training program for all unaffected muscle groups ◆ Stationary bicycle to tolerance without walking splint ◆ Pool therapy for ROM (walking or running under total buoyant conditions); heel raises in waist- to chest-deep water	program for gastrocnemius-soleus complex ◆ Improve cardiovascular conditioning ◆ Improve muscular strength and endurance ◆ Improve proprioception and joint reaction time	and therapist's discretion ◆ Weight-bearing dorsiflexion required for normal ADLs; repair should be sufficiently strong; discontinue if symptoms occur ◆ Gastrocnemius-soleus/repair initially conditioned with isometrics; repair now strong enough to tolerate increased strength training on a progressive weight and force basis

ROM, Range of motion; *AROM,* active range of motion; *PROM,* passive range of motion; *ADLs,* activities of daily living.

Table 25-7 Achilles Tendon Repair (Early Motion)

Rehabilitation Phase	Criteria to Progress to this Phase	Anticipated Impairments and Functional Limitations	Intervention	Goal	Rationale
Phase IIIa Postoperative 9-16 weeks	◆ No longer requires walking splint for ADLs; may require use of splint for extended ambulatory periods in early parts of phase ◆ Pain-free gait during ADLs walking out of splint ◆ Minimal difference in dorsiflexion ROM versus uninvolved side	◆ Gait deviations in preswing phase of gait resulting from limited plantar flexion, strength, and endurance, not insufficient dorsiflexion ◆ Unable to perform single-leg heel raise ◆ Unable to jump and run ◆ Mild pain and muscle and tendon fatigue at end of day if walking for a significant period	◆ Continue interventions from Phases I and II as indicated, especially weight-bearing dorsiflexion stretch ◆ AROM—Progress towards single-leg heel raises, add resistance up to 1.5 times body weight as symptoms dictate ◆ Gait training—Treadmill walking on level surfaces and	◆ Discontinue use of walking splint ◆ Repeated single-leg heel raise from level surface ◆ Normal gait cycle for all ADLs ◆ Full symmetrical weight-bearing dorsiflexion ◆ Initiate fast-walking or jogging program ◆ Decrease complaints of	◆ Plantar flexion weakness will compromise gait; emphasis placed on improving functional plantar flexion strength and endurance (single-leg heel raise); higher gait velocities affected until late in this phase or into Phase IIIb ◆ Incline treadmill use will develop strength and endurance of gastrocnemius-soleus muscles

Continued

Table 25-7 Achilles Tendon Repair (Early Motion)—cont'd

Rehabilitation Phase	Criteria to Progress to this Phase	Anticipated Impairments and Functional Limitations	Intervention	Goal	Rationale
	◆ Full plantar flexion, inversion, and eversion	◆ Limited tolerance to tendon-loading activities (concentric and eccentric)	slight incline, uneven surface walking, stair climbing; progress to jogging toward end of phase if symptom free (no sprinting, cutting, or jumping activities); jogging on mini-trampoline ◆ Isokinetics—Submaximal effort velocity spectrum plantar flexion and dorsiflexion ◆ Pool therapy (waist deep)—Plyometrics (hopping, bounding, and jumping in waist-deep water) ◆ Cardiovascular exercises	mild pain or muscle and tendon fatigue at end of day with walking activities ◆ Increase plantar flexion strength and endurance ◆ Improve plantar flexion strength and endurance at maximal velocities ◆ Prepare for land-based agility drills ◆ Improve cardiovascular fitness level	◆ Uneven surface and stair training improves proprioception and community ambulation ◆ Jogging and running must be initiated only if patient is symptom free, has a normal gait, and is able to perform multiple single-leg heel raises at moderate to high velocities to avoid overloading tendon and initiating an inflammatory cycle ◆ Use of mini-trampoline will facilitate achievement of dorsiflexion at varying velocities, simulate higher-level function, and develop higher-velocity eccentric load tolerance ◆ Continued development of strength and endurance required throughout this phase to achieve full ADLs and recreational function ◆ Plyometric activities in the pool facilitate functional use without full weight-bearing stress ◆ Use gait training activities and stair machine to provide aerobic training

ADLs, Activities of daily living; *AROM,* active range of motion; *ROM,* range of motion.

Table 25-8 Achilles Tendon Repair (Early Motion)

Rehabilitation Phase	Criteria to Progress to this Phase	Anticipated Impairments and Functional Limitations	Intervention	Goal	Rationale
Phase IIIb Postoperative 17-20 weeks	◆ Normal gait on all surfaces and inclines ◆ Able to fast walk or jog without gait deficits ◆ Able to do repeated single-leg heel raises with moderate to high velocities ◆ Asymptomatic with all ADLs, treadmill walking, and jogging	◆ Unable to hop or jump on single leg without performance deficit or compensatory movement ◆ Difficulty with sprinting or cutting during higher-level recreational activities	◆ Review of past rehabilitation program to address areas that may not have been appropriately addressed ◆ Development of individualized strength, flexibility, ROM, and functional progression program to alleviate impairments and functional limitations	◆ Resolve all impairments and functional limitations that limit full return to preoperative level of function	◆ Most patients and athletes have only minor performance deficits by this time; deficits (which may continue to exist) require individualized attention based on their presentation and the way they affect athlete or patient in question; these areas may not have been appropriately addressed earlier or athlete or patient might have tried to progress too fast; any impairments or functional limitations are usually resolved within this phase and time period

ADLs, Activities of daily living; *ROM,* range of motion.

SUGGESTED HOME MAINTENANCE FOR THE POSTSURGICAL PATIENT: TRADITIONAL REHABILITATION PROGRAM

Weeks 1-4

GOALS FOR THE PERIOD: Manage edema, improve function

1. For edema: Use ice and elevation; perform toe curls and pumps.
2. For function: Use non–weight-bearing crutch gait.

Weeks 5-8

GOALS FOR THE PERIOD: Manage edema, improve function

1. For edema: Use ice, compression, and elevation as needed; perform toe curls and pumps as needed.
2. For function: Progress to full weight bearing to tolerance with appropriate assistive devices if needed.

Weeks 9-16

GOALS FOR THE PERIOD: Improve range of motion (ROM), continue strength training, and achieve functional improvement

1. For ROM:
   a. Initiate non–weight-bearing stretching exercises for all ankle motions (dorsiflexion, plantar flexion, inversion, and eversion).
   b. Initiate weight-bearing dorsiflexion stretch with knee flexed and extended.
2. For strength training:
   a. Initiate isometric and elastic band strengthening exercises for all muscle groups.
   b. Progress to double-leg heel raises as tolerated.
3. For function:
   a. Begin ambulation out of cast to symptom tolerance.
   b. Use heel lift and cane or crutches as appropriate to limit symptoms.

Weeks 17-20

GOALS FOR THE PERIOD: Improve ROM, continue strength training, and achieve functional improvement

1. For ROM: Continue all stretching exercises.
2. For strength training:
   a. Initiate single-leg heel raises.
   b. Progress to additional weight heel raises with up to 1.5 times body weight provided no symptoms of pain, swelling, or inflammation develop.
3. For function:
   a. Initiate walking on all types of surfaces and inclines and declines.
   b. Progress to fast walking and jogging toward the end of this phase if no symptoms have occurred and patient is able to do single-leg toe raises repeatedly.
   c. **NO sprinting, cutting, or jumping allowed.**

Week 20 and beyond

GOALS FOR THE PERIOD: Continue strength training, achieve functional improvement

1. For strength training:
   a. Do single-leg heel raises over the edge of a step.
   b. Do weight lifting to tolerance.
2. For function:
   a. Initiate jogging when able.
   b. Initiate hopping, skipping, and jumping activities.
   c. Return to all recreational and sports activities.

SUGGESTED HOME MAINTENANCE FOR THE POSTSURGICAL PATIENT: EARLY MOTION PROGRAM

Week 1

GOALS FOR THE WEEK: Manage edema, improve ROM, and begin work on function

1. For edema: Use ice, compression, and elevation; perform toe curls and pumps.
2. For ROM: Perform active range of motion (AROM) three times daily; perform plantar flexion and dorsiflexion out of the splint within pain limits with the knee flexed and extended.
3. For function: Use non–weight-bearing crutch gait.

Weeks 2-4

GOALS FOR THE PERIOD: Manage edema, improve ROM, continue strength training, work on function

1. For edema: Use ice, compression, and elevation as needed; perform toe curls and pumps as needed.
2. For ROM in early phase IIa (days 7-21): Perform AROM three times daily in all directions out of the splint (plantar flexion, dorsiflexion, inversion, and eversion) with the knee flexed and extended.
3. For ROM in late phase IIa (days 21-28): Perform *gentle* dorsiflexion stretching with a towel or strap with the knee flexed and extended three times daily.
4. For strength training in early phase IIa (days 7-21): Perform isometric inversion and eversion in neutral dorsiflexion.
5. For strength training in late phase IIa (days 21-28): Perform isometric plantar flexion and dorsiflexion; progress to light elastic band exercises if free of pain and swelling.
6. For function (note: use walking boot at all times): Start touchdown weight bearing on day 8; perform progressive weight bearing at day 14 if no increase in pain and symptoms is noted.

Weeks 5-8

GOALS FOR THE PERIOD: Improve ROM, continue strength training, and improve function

1. For ROM:
   a. Continue phase IIa activities as appropriate.
   b. Initiate weight-bearing dorsiflexion stretch with knee flexed and extended.
2. For strength training:
   a. Continue phase IIa activities as appropriate.
   b. Initiate double-leg heel raises.
3. For function:
   a. Begin ambulation out of the walking splint to symptom tolerance.
   b. Use heel lift and cane as appropriate to limit symptoms.

Weeks 9-16

GOALS FOR THE PERIOD: Improve ROM, continue strength training, and improve function

1. For ROM: Continue phase IIb activities as appropriate to gain full ROM
2. For strength training:
   a. Progress towards single-leg heel raises.
   b. Progress to additional weight heel raises with up to 1.5 times body weight if no symptoms of pain, swelling, or inflammation occur.
3. For function:
   a. Initiate walking on all types of surfaces and inclines and declines.
   b. Progress to jogging toward end of phase if no symptoms have occurred.
   c. **NO sprinting, cutting, or jumping allowed.**

Weeks 17-20

GOALS FOR THE PERIOD: Continue strength training and achieve functional improvement

1. For strength training:
   a. Do single-leg heel raises over the edge of a step.
   b. Perform weight lifting to tolerance.
2. For function:
   a. Initiate hopping, skipping, and jumping activities.
   b. Return to all recreational and sports activities.

References

1. Achilles tendon rupture (editorial), *Lancet* 1:189, 1973.
2. Alfredson H, Lorentzon R: Chronic Achilles tendinosis: recommendations for treatment and prevention, *Sports Med* 29:135, 2000.
3. Alfredson H, Thorsen K, Lorentzon R: In situ microdialysis in tendon tissue: high levels of glutamate, but not prostaglandin E2 in chronic Achilles tendon pain [see comment], *Knee Surg Sports Traumatol Arthrosc* 7:378, 1999.
4. Almekinders LC, Deol G: The effects of aging, antiinflammatory drugs, and ultrasound on the in vitro response of tendon tissue, *Am J Sports Med* 27:417, 1999.
5. Amadio PC: Tendon and ligament. In Cohen IK, Diegelmann RF, Lindblad WJ, editors: *Wound healing: biochemical and clinical aspects*, Philadelphia, 1992, WB Saunders.
6. Arner O, Lindholm A: Avulsion fracture of the os calcaneus, *Acta Chir Scand* 117:258, 1959.
7. Arner O, Lindholm A, Orell SR: Histologic changes in subcutaneous rupture of the Achilles tendon, *Acta Chir Scand* 116:484, 1959.
8. Beskin JL et al: Surgical repair of Achilles tendon ruptures, *Am J Sports Med* 15:1, 1987.
9. Booth FW: Physiologic and biochemical effects of immobilization on muscle, *Clin Orthop* 219:15, 1987.
10. Bradley JP, Tibone JE: Percutaneous and open surgical repairs of Achilles tendon ruptures, *Am J Sports Med* 18:188, 1990.
11. Buchgraber A, Pässler HH: Percutaneous repair of Achilles tendon rupture. Immobilization versus functional postoperative treatment, *Clin Orthop Relat Res* 341:113, 1997.
12. Bugg EI Jr, Boyd BM: Repair of neglected rupture or laceration of the Achilles tendon, *Clin Orthop* 56:73, 1968.
13. Bunnell S: Primary repair of severe tendons, *Am J Surg* 47:502, 1940.
14. Carden DG et al: Rupture of the calcaneal tendon. The early and late management, *J Bone Joint Surg* 69B:416, 1987.
15. Carr AJ, Norris SH: The blood supply of the calcaneal tendon, *J Bone Joint Surg* 71B(1):100, 1989.
16. Carter TR, Fowler PJ, Blokker C: Functional postoperative treatment of Achilles tendon repair, *Am J Sports Med* 20:459, 1992.
17. Cetti R: Ruptured Achilles tendon. Preliminary results of a new treatment, *Br J Sports Med* 22:6, 1988.
18. Cetti R, Christenson SE: Surgical treatment under local anesthesia of Achilles rupture, *Clin Orthop* 173:204, 1983.
19. Cetti R, Henriksen LO, Jacobsen KS: A new treatment of ruptured Achilles tendons, *Clin Orthop* 308:155, 1994.
20. Cetti R et al: Operative versus nonoperative treatment of Achilles tendon rupture. A prospective randomized study and review of the literature, *Am J Sports Med* 21(6):791, 1993.
21. Chen DS, Wertheimer SJ: A new method of repair for rupture of the Achilles tendon, *J Foot Surg* 31:440, 1992.
22. Christensen IB: Rupture of the Achilles tendon: analysis of 57 cases, *Acta Chir Scand* 106:50, 1953.
23. Crolla RMPH et al: Acute rupture of the tendo calcaneus, *Acta Orthop Belgica* 53:492, 1987.
24. Curwin S: Tendon injuries: pathology and treatment. In Zachazewski JE, Magee DJ, Quillen WS, editors: *Athletic injuries and rehabilitation*, Philadelphia, 1996, WB Saunders.
25. Curwin SL: *Force and length changes of the gastrocnemius and soleus muscle-tendon units during a therapeutic exercise program and three selected activities*, master's thesis, Halifax, Nova Scotia, Canada, 1984, Dalhousie University.
26. Curwin S, Stanish W: *Tendinitis: its etiology and treatment*, Lexington, MA, 1984, Collamore Press.
27. De Carli A et al: Effect of cyclic loading on new polyblend suture coupled with different anchors, *Am J Sports Med* 33:214, 2005.
28. Enwemeka CS: The effect of therapeutic ultrasound on tendon healing. A biomechanical study, *Am J Phys Med Rehabil* 67:264, 1988.
29. Enwemeka CS: Inflammation, cellularity, and fibrillogenesis in regenerating tendon: implications for tendon rehabilitation, *Phys Ther* 69:816, 1989.
30. Enwemeka CS: Connective tissue plasticity: ultrastructural, biomechanical, and morphometric effects of physical factors on intact and regenerating tendons, *J Orthop Sports Phys Ther* 14(5):198, 1991.
31. Enwemeka CS, Rodriguez O, Mendosa S: The biomechanical effects of low intensity ultrasound on healing tendons, *Ultrasound Med Biol* 16:801, 1990.
32. Enwemeka CS, Spielholz NI, Nelson AJ: The effect of early functional activities on experimentally tenotomized Achilles tendon in rats, *Am J Phys Med Rehabil* 67:264, 1988.
33. Fernandez-Fairen M, Gimeno C: Augmented repair of Achilles tendon ruptures, *Am J Sports Med* 25(2):177, 1997.
34. Fitzgibbons RE, Hefferon J, Hill J: Percutaneous Achilles tendon repair, *Am J Sports Med* 21(5):724, 1993.
35. Forslund C, Aspenberg P: Improved healing of transected rabbit Achilles tendon after a single injection of cartilage-derived morphogenetic protein-2, *Am J Sports Med* 31:555, 2003.
36. Freider S et al: A pilot study: the therapeutic effect of ultrasound following partial rupture of Achilles tendons in male rats, *J Orthop Sports Phys Ther* 10(2):39, 1988.
37. Frings H: Uber 317 falle von operrierten subkutanen Achil-lesrupturen be sportiern und sportlerinnen, *Arch Orthop Unfallchir* 67:64, 1969.
38. Gamble JG: *The musculoskeletal system: pathological basics*, New York, 1988, Raven Press.
39. Gelberman RH et al: Effects of early intermittent passive mobilization on healing canine flexor tendons, *J Hand Surg* 7(2):170, 1982.
40. Gelberman RH et al: Flexor tendon repair in vitro: a comparative histologic study of the rabbit, chicken, dog, and monkey, *J Orthop Res* 2:39, 1984.
41. Gerdes MH et al: A flap augmentation technique for Achilles tendon repair, postoperative strength and functional outcome, *Clin Orthop* 280:241, 1992.
42. Giannini S et al: Surgical repair of Achilles tendon ruptures using polypropylene braid augmentation, *Foot Ankle* 15:372, 1994.

43. Gregor RV, Komi PV, Jarvinen M: Achilles tendon forces during cycling, *Int J Sports Med* 8(suppl):9, 1987.
44. Haggmark T et al: Calf muscle atrophy and muscle function after non-operative vs. operative treatment of Achilles tendon ruptures, *Orthopaedics* 9(2):160, 1986.
45. Haji A et al: Percutaneous versus open tendo achillis repair, *Foot Ankle Int* 25:215, 2004.
46. Halasi T, Tallay A, Berkes I: Percutaneous Achilles tendon repair with and without endoscopic control, *Knee Surg Sports Traumatol Arthrosc* 11:409, 2003.
47. Hannallah D et al: Gene therapy in orthopaedic surgery, *J Bone Joint Surg Am* 84:1046-, 2002.
48. Harcke H, Grisson LE, Finkelstein MS: Evaluation of the musculoskeletal system with sonography, *AJR Am J Roentgenol* 150:1253, 1988.
49. Hastad K, Larsson HG, Lindholm A: Clearance of radiosodium after local deposit in the Achilles tendon, *Acta Chir Scand* 116:251, 1959.
50. Holz U: Die Achilles shenen ruptur–klinische und ultratrukturturelle aspekte. In Chapchal G, editor: *Sportverletzungen und Sportschagen*, Stuttgart, 1983, Georg Tieme.
51. Hosey G et al: Comparison of the mechanical and histologic properties of Achilles tendons in New Zealand white rabbits secondarily repaired with Marlex mesh, *J Foot Surg* 30:214, 1991.
52. Inglis AE, Sculco TP: Surgical repair of ruptures of the tendo Achilles, *Clin Orthop* 156:160, 1981.
53. Inglis AE et al: Ruptures of the tendo Achilles, *J Bone Joint Surg* 58A:990, 1976.
54. Jackson BA, Schwane JA, Starcher BC: Effect of ultrasound on the repair of Achilles tendon injuries in rats, *Med Sci Sports Exerc* 23(2):171, 1991.
55. Jacobs D et al: Comparison of conservative and operative treatment of Achilles tendon rupture, *Am J Sports Med* 6:107, 1978.
56. Jenkins DHR et al: Induction of tendon and ligament formation by carbon implants, *J Bone Joint Surg* 59B:53, 1977.
57. Jozsa L et al: Pathological alterations of human tendons, *Morphol Igazsagugy Orr Sz* 27(2):106, 1987.
58. Jozsa L et al: The role of recreational sport activity in Achilles tendon rupture. A clinical, pathoanatomical, and sociological study of 292 cases, *Am J Sports Med* 17(3):338, 1989.
59. Kangas J et al: Early functional treatment vs early immobilization in tension of the musculotendinous unit after Achilles rupture repair: a prospective, randomized, clinical study, *J Trauma* 54(6):1171, 2003.
60. Kannus P, Jozsa L: Histopathological changes preceding spontaneous rupture of a Achilles tendon, *J Bone Joint Surg* 73A(10):1507, 1991.
61. Karjalainen PT et al: Magnetic resonance imaging during healing of surgically repaired Achilles tendon ruptures, *Am J Sports Med* 25(2):164, 1997.
62. Kellam JF, Hunter GA, McElwain JP: Review of the operative treatment of Achilles tendon rupture, *Clin Orthop* 201:80, 1985.
63. Kerkoffs GM et al: Functional treatment after surgical repair of acute Achilles tendon rupture: wrap vs walking cast, *Arch Orthop Trauma Surg* 122(2):102, 2002.
64. Kessler I: The grasping technique for tendon repair, *Hand* 5:253, 1973.
65. Khan RJ et al: Interventions for treating acute Achilles tendon ruptures, *Cochrane Database Syst Rev* (3), 2004.
66. Kirschembaum SE, Kellman C: Modification of the Lindholm procedure for plastic repair of ruptured Achilles tendon: a case report, *J Foot Surg* 19:4, 1980.
67. Krackow KA, Thomas SC, Jones LC: A new stitch for ligament-tendon fixation. Brief note, *J Bone Joint Surg* 68A:764, 1986.
68. Kvist H, Kvist M: The operative treatment of chronic calcaneal paratendonitis, *J Bone Joint Surg* 62B(3):353, 1980.
69. Lagerrgren C, Lindholm A: Vascular distribution in the Achilles tendon: an arteriographic and microangiographic study, *Acta Chir Scand* 116:491, 1959.
70. Laseter JT, Russell JA: Anabolic steroid-induced tendon pathology: a review of the literature, *Med Sci Sports Exerc* 23:1, 1991.
71. Laurant TC: Structure, function and turnover of the extracellular matrix, *Adv Microcirc* 13:15, 1987.
72. Leadbetter WB: Cell matrix response in tendon injury, *Clin Sports Med* 11(3):533, 1992.
73. Leppilahti J et al: Free tissue coverage of wound complications following Achilles tendon rupture surgery, *Clin Orthop* 328:171, 1996.
74. Leppilahti J et al: Isokinetic evaluation of calf muscle performance after Achilles rupture repair, *Int J Sports Med* 17:619, 1996.
75. Levy M et al: A method of repair for Achilles tendon ruptures without cast immobilization, *Clin Orthop* 187:199, 1983.
76. Lim J, Dalal R Wasseem M: Percutaneous vs open repair of the ruptured Achilles tendon—a prospective randomized controlled study, *Foot Ankle Int* 22(7):559, 2001.
77. Lindholm A: A new method of operation in subcutaneous rupture of the Achilles tendon, *Acta Chir Scand* 117:261, 1959.
78. Lynn TA: Repair of the torn Achilles tendon, using the plantaris tendon as a reinforcing membrane, *J Bone Joint Surg* 48A:268, 1966.
79. Ma GW, Griffith TG: Percutaneous repair of acute closed ruptured Achilles tendon: a new technique, *Clin Orthop* 128:247, 1977.
80. Maffulli N et al: Early weightbearing and ankle mobilization after open repair of acute midsubstance tears of the achilles tendon, *Am J Sports Med* 31:692, 2003.
81. Malone TR, Garrett WE, Zachazewski JE: Muscle: deformation, injury, repair. In Zachazewski JE, Magee DJ, Quillen WS, editors: *Athletic injuries and rehabilitation*, Philadelphia, 1996, WB Saunders.
82. Mandelbaum BR, Hayes WM, Knapp TP: Management of Achilles tendon ruptures, *Foot Ankle* 2(3):1, 1997.
83. Mandelbaum BR, Myerson MS, Forster R: Achilles tendon ruptures, a new method of repair, early range of motion, and functional rehabilitation, *Am J Sports Med* 23(4):392, 1995.
84. Mann RA et al: Chronic rupture of the Achilles tendon: a new technique of repair, *J Bone Joint Surg* 73A:214, 1991.
85. Marti RK, Weber BG: Achillessehnenruptur-functionalle Nachbehandlung, *Helv Chir Acta* 4:293, 1974.

86. Mclauchlin GJ, Handoll HHG: Interventions for treating acute and chronic Achilles tendonitis, *Cochrane Database Sys Rev* (3), 2004.
87. Mink JH, Deutsch AL, Kerr R: Tendon injuries of the lower extremity: magnetic resonance assessment, *Top Magn Reson Imaging* 3:23, 1991.
88. Mortensen NHM, Saether J: Achilles tendon repair: a new method of Achilles tendon repair tested on cadaverous materials, *J Trauma* 31:381, 1991.
89. Mortenson NH, Skov O, Jenson PE: Early motion of the ankle after operative treatment of a rupture of the Achilles tendon. A prospective, randomized clinical and radiographic study, *J Bone Joint Surg Am* 81(7):983, 1999.
90. Motta P, Errichiello C, Pontini I: Achilles tendon rupture. A new technique for easy surgical repair and immediate movement of the ankle and foot, *Am J Sports Med* 25(2):172, 1997.
91. Muller ME et al: General considerations. In Muller ME et al, editors: *Manual of internal fixation: techniques recommended by the AO-Group*, Berlin, 1979, Springer-Verlag.
92. Nada A: Rupture of the calcaneal tendon, *J Bone Joint Surg* 67B(3):449, 1985.
93. Nillius SA, Nilsson BE, Westin WE: The incidence of Achilles tendon rupture, *Acta Orthop Scand* 47(1):118, 1976.
94. Nistor L: Surgical and non-surgical treatment of Achilles tendon rupture, *J Bone Joint Surg* 63A(3):395, 1981.
95. Paddu G, Ippolito E, Postacchini F: A classification of Achilles tendon disease, *Am J Sports Med* 4(4):145, 1976.
96. Pepels WRJ, Plasmans CMT, Sloof TJH: The course of healing of tendons and ligaments (abstract), *Acta Orthop Scand* 54:952, 1983.
97. Quenu J, Stoianovitch I: Les ruptures du tendon d'Achilles, *J Chir Paris* 67:647, 1929.
98. Richardson LC, Reitman R,Wilson M: Achilles tendon ruptures: functional outcome of surgical repair with a "pull-out" wire, *Foot Ankle Int* 24: 439, 2003.
99. Rippstein P, Jung M, Assal M: Surgical repair of acute Achilles tendon rupture using "mini-open" technique, *Foot Ankle Clin* 7(3):611, 2002.
100. Rodeo SA: What's new in orthopaedic research, *J Bone Joint Surg Am* 85:2054, 2003.
101. Romanelli D, Almekinders L,Mandelbaum B: Achilles rupture in the athelete: current science and treatment, *Sports Med Arthroscopy Rev* 8:377, 2000.
102. Schatzker J, Branemark PI: Intravital observation of the microvascular anatomy and microcirculation of tendon, *Acta Orthop Scand Suppl* 126:3, 1969.
103. Schedl R, Fasol P, Spangler H: Die Achillessehnen-ruptur als sportverletzung. In Chapchal G, editor: *Sportverletzungen und Sportschagen*, Stuttgart, 1983, Georg Tieme.
104. Schuberth JM: Achilles tendon trauma. In Scurran BL, editor: *Foot and ankle trauma*, ed 2, New York, 1996, Churchill Livingstone.
105. Shields CL et al: The Cybex II evaluation of surgically repaired Achilles tendon ruptures, *Am J Sports Med* 6:369, 1978.
106. Silfverskiold N: Uber die subkutane totale Achillessehn-enruptur und deren Behandlung, *Acta Chir Scand* 84:393, 1941.
107. Soldatis JJ, Goodfellows DB, Wilber JH: End to end operative repair of Achilles tendon rupture, *Am J Sports Med* 25(1):90, 1997.
108. Solveborn S-A, Moberg A: Immediate free ankle motion after surgical repair of acute Achilles tendon ruptures, *Am J Sports Med* 22(5):607, 1994.
109. Soma CA, Mandelbaum BR: Repair of acute Achilles tendon ruptures, *Orthop Clin North Am* 26(2):239, 1995.
110. Strocchi R et al: Human Achilles tendon: morphological and morphometric variations as a function of age, *Foot Ankle* 12:100, 1991.
111. Teuffeur AP: Traumatic rupture of the Achilles tendon. Reconstruction by transplant and graft using the lateral peroneus brevis, *Orthop Clin North Am* 5:89, 1974.
112. Thompson TC, Doherty JH: Spontaneous rupture of tendon of Achilles: a new clinical diagnostic test, *J Trauma* 2:126, 1962.
113. Tomak SL, Fleming LL: Achilles tendon rupture: an alternative treatment, *Am J Orthop* 33:9, 2004.
114. van der Linden PD et al: Increased risk of achilles tendon rupture with quinolone antibacterial use, especially in elderly patients taking oral corticosteroids [see comment], *Arch Int Med* 163:1801, 2003.
115. Wapner KL, Hecht PJ, Mills RH Jr: Reconstruction of neglected Achilles tendon injury, *Orthop Clin North Am* 26:249, 1995.
116. Weber M et al: Nonoperative treatment of acute rupture of the Achilles rendon: results of a new protocol and comparison with operative treatment, *Am J Sports Med* 31:685, 2003.
117. Wills CA et al: Achilles tendon rupture. A review of the literature comparing surgical versus non-surgical treatment, *Clin Orthop* 207:156, 1986.
118. Wong J, Varrass V, Maffulli N: Quantitative review of operative and non-operative management of Achilles tendon ruptures, *Am J Sports Med* 30(4)565, 2002.
119. Zachazewski JE: Muscle flexibility. In Scully R, Barnes ML, editors: *Physical therapy*, Philadelphia, 1989, JB Lippincott.
120. Zolinger H, Rodriquez M, Genoni M: Zur atiopathogeneseund diagnostik der Achillesehnenrupturen im sport. In Chapchal G, editor: *Sportverletzungen und Sportschagen*, Stuttgart, 1983, Georg Tieme.

APPENDIX

A

Transitioning the Throwing Athlete Back to the Field

Luga Podesta

Injuries to athletes happen every day. Some can be easily treated, while others require surgery and/or lengthy rehabilitation. An arm injury to a baseball player is potentially career ending and therefore needs very special attention. Every baseball player knows the demands put on an arm in training and competition, so we also realize the need for very intense and specialized rehabilitation. During my playing career I had three serious shoulder injuries. Much time and energy was spent on the strengthening of my shoulder, but the critical time of rehabilitation was the transition from physical therapy into a throwing program. An aggressive full-body conditioning program, including plyometrics, was essential in assisting my shoulder to function correctly when throwing a baseball. This program paved the way for a smooth transition onto the field and a successful return to competition.

Mike Scioscia
Anaheim Angels

A great deal of literature exists detailing the surgical technique and postoperative rehabilitation of the injured shoulder. However, little has been written on the difficult task of transitioning the throwing athlete from the rehabilitation setting back to throwing sports after surgery. This appendix outlines a program to return the throwing athlete back to his or her sport after surgery.

Numerous surgical procedures can be performed on a throwing athlete's shoulder for a variety of pathologic conditions (e.g., glenohumeral [GH] instability, labral tears, rotor cuff tears, impingement syndrome, acromioclavicular joint injury). Because one short appendix cannot describe each surgical procedure and the postoperative rehabilitation course recommended for it, the program described in this appendix is based on the assumption that the athlete has already been cleared to begin an advanced throwing and conditioning program.

ASSESSMENT

Regardless of the surgical procedure performed, the physical therapist (PT) must assess the athlete's overall physical condition before beginning a more aggressive conditioning and throwing program. Knowledge of the athlete's flexibility, strength, and endurance is essential for the development of a program specific for his or her needs. The athlete's throwing mechanics must be carefully evaluated throughout rehabilitation and the transition back to throwing sports.

STRENGTHENING AND CONDITIONING

In the past a great deal of emphasis was placed on developing mobility in the postoperative shoulder and developing strength in the shoulder-supporting musculature, including the rotator cuff and scapular stabilizers. Very little attention was given to the remainder of the musculature that plays a significant role in permitting the athlete to throw effectively and without injury.

Dynamic stability of the throwing shoulder requires fine, coordinated action of the GH and scapulothoracic stabilizers to facilitate synchronous function of the GH joint. After surgery, proper neuromuscular control must be re-established to prevent asynchronous muscle-firing patterns, which can result in dysfunction.[3,6]

Neuromuscular control is defined as a purposeful act initiated at the cortical level.[24] Payton, Hirt, and Newton[24] stated that motor control is an involuntary associated movement organized subcortically that results in a well-learned skill operating without conscious guidance. The fine coordinated activity necessary for propelling a ball rapidly and accurately requires subcortical control of the muscles responsible for throwing.

Kinesthesia is the ability to discriminate joint position, relative weight of body parts, and joint movement, including speed, direction, and amplitude.[21] Proprioception is the ability to discriminate joint position. The ability to throw requires that joint proprioceptors (muscle and joint afferents present in ligament and synovial tissues) function normally. Joint proprioceptors within the GH joint are responsible for signaling a stretch reflex when the GH capsule is taut to prevent translation at extremes of motion.[9] Many throwers recovering from surgery, especially those who have undergone procedures for instability, complain of stiffness and tightness in their shoulders. Neuromuscular controls may have been arrested by trauma and surgery, resulting in a new subcortical sense of joint tightness during throwing that was not present before the shoulder-stabilization procedure.

The upper extremity (UE) and shoulder represent the last link in the kinetic chain during the overhead-throwing motion, which begins distally as ground reactive forces are transferred caudally. Biomechanical analysis shows that tremendous forces are generated and extreme motion occurs in the shoulder with overhand throwing. Angular velocities in excess of 7000 degrees/second have been recorded during the transition from external rotation (ER) to internal rotation (IR) when throwing.[23,25] Shearing forces on the anterior shoulder are estimated at 400 N.[23] Approximately 500 N of distraction force occurs during the deceleration phase of the throwing motion.[23] These forces are short in duration, develop quickly, occur at extremely high intensity, and must be performed repeatedly. The direction and magnitude of the forces generated when throwing a ball cause anteroposterior (AP) translational and distraction vectors that stress the GH constraints.

However, these forces are not entirely generated in the shoulder. The shoulder-supporting musculature is not capable of generating the forces and motions measured at the shoulder during throwing. Throwing a ball effectively requires the athlete to generate, summate, transfer, and regulate these forces from the legs through the throwing hand. To generate the forces measured with throwing, the shoulder relies on its position at the end of the kinetic chain. It has been reported that 51% to 55% of the kinetic energy created is generated in the lower extremities (LEs).[4,29] Use of ground reaction forces sequentially linked with the activity of the large LE and trunk muscles generate a significant proportion of the forces measured. Biomechanical data show that the shoulder itself contributes relatively little of the overall total energy necessary to the throwing motion. However, it provides a relatively high contribution to the total forces (21%), indicating that the shoulder, because of its position at the end of the kinetic chain, must effectively transfer and concentrate the developed energy. Conditioning of the shoulder and UE musculature is important in returning throwing athletes back to their sports. Moreover, the trunk and LE musculature must be adequately conditioned to provide the foundation to generate the forces required for effective and safe throwing.

When designing a program to return a throwing athlete back to sports, the PT should consider two primary objectives: (1) enhancing current performance levels and (2) preventing injury. Gambetta[18] has outlined ten key principles that are basic to the development of a conditioning program for the throwing athlete (Box A-1). The many components of the program must work together to produce optimal performance. The quality of the effort and the overall intensity should be emphasized first. The clinician should monitor each exercise and eventually scrutinize the throwing technique to ensure optimal training effect and minimize the potential for injury.

The development of muscle balance is essential for coordinated, efficient movement to occur, especially around the shoulder where muscle imbalance can easily develop. Muscles (e.g., rotator cuff) cannot simply be trained solely and in isolation, as in the early phases of most postoperative programs. After base strength has been developed in the postoperative shoulder, functional activities and more sport-specific exercises must be added to mimic the activities the athlete will be performing.

The development of core strength in the abdominals, trunk, and spinal-stabilizing muscles cannot be overemphasized. Without adequate core strength, the throwing athlete becomes vulnerable to improper postural alignment, which can lead to compensatory movements that place even greater stress on the shoulder, further predisposing the athlete to injury. After adequate strength has been achieved in the shoulder-supporting musculature, abdominals, spinal stabilizers, and LEs, endurance training can be added.

Only after sufficient strength and endurance are developed and normal, synchronous muscle-firing patterns are re-established, can a more functional and

Box A-1 Basic Conditioning Principles

- Develop muscle synergy.
- Train for performance, not work capacity.
- Train for muscle balance.
- Train movements, not muscles.
- Develop structural (core) strength before extremity strength.
- Use body weight resistance before external resistance.
- Build strength before strength endurance.
- Develop synergists before prime movers.
- Promote joint integrity before mobility.
- Teach fundamental movement skill before specific sport skill.

sport-specific activity such as throwing be added. The ultimate success of the training program depends on its overall design in introducing a variety of training stimuli to maximize total conditioning. An ideal conditioning program should contain a preparation period, an adaptation period, and an application period.[18] The preparation period should consist of general work, including strength and endurance training. Specialized work incorporating joint dynamics of the sport occurs during the adaptation period. Finally, the application period incorporates the specific joint actions and movements required to perform the sport.

ISOTONIC EXERCISES

A progressive weight- and functional-training program should start with body weight exercise. This allows the athlete to develop the proper exercise techniques and regain the synchronous muscle-firing patterns required to perform the overhand sport. This method of training also is adaptable to the more advanced plyometric exercises that follow after base strength has been gained.

Weight training is one of the most popular methods of training and can be performed with either free weights or machines. Free weight training with dumbbells is preferable, because it allows for unilateral training while permitting a full range of motion (ROM) of the extremity. Machines are better used in training the LEs. The use of rubber tubing or bands is another popular method of early strength training for the overhand-throwing athlete. These exercises can be performed as a warm-up for more strenuous weight resistance exercises or as a cooldown exercise; they can accommodate all muscle actions. Rubber tubing or band exercises also allow for unilateral training of the extremity through a full ROM. They can be performed during the rehabilitation period and should continue when the thrower returns to play. Isotonic strengthening can be tailored to each athlete's needs and can be used to maintain strength in all muscle groups. Jobe's UE exercise program[19] is the most popular group of isotonic exercises performed. They can be initiated early in the rehabilitation period and continued throughout the athlete's career. However, they *must* be performed correctly to maximize their benefit (Table A-1).

Core strength should first be developed using isotonic training. Only after base strength is developed should the intensity of the exercise program be increased (Table A-2).

Table A-1 Jobe's Shoulder Exercises*

Exercise	Weight (lb)	Sets/Repetitions
Shoulder flexion	3-5	3-4/10-15
Shoulder elevation	3-5	3-4/10-15
Shoulder abduction	3-5	3-4/10-15
Shoulder abduction	3-5	3-4/10-15
Military press	3-5	3-4/10-15
Horizontal abduction	3-5	3-4/10-15
Shoulder extension	3-5	3-4/10-15
External rotation (ER) I (side lying)	1-5	3-4/10-15
ER II (prone)	1-5	3-4/10-15
Internal rotation (IR)	1-5	3-4/10-15
Horizontal adduction	3-5	3-4/10-15
Rowing	3-5	3-4/10-1

*All exercises should be performed three times a week.
(Modified from Jobe FW et al: *Shoulder and arm exercises for the athlete who throws,* Inglewood, CA, 1996, Champion Press.)

PLYOMETRIC EXERCISES

Plyometric training was first introduced in the late 1960s by Soviet jump coach Yuri Verkhoshanski.[30] American track coach Fred Wilt[33] first introduced plyometrics in the United States in 1975. The majority of the literature concerning plyometric exercise discusses its use in the LEs. Adapting these principles to the conditioning of throwing athletes is logical, considering the maximal explosive concentric contractions and rapid decelerative eccentric contractions that occur with each throwing cycle. Although agreement regarding the benefits of plyometric exercise in the training program is well documented, controversy exists regarding its optimal use.[7,8,20,26]

Plyometric exercise can be broken down into three phases: (1) the eccentric (or setting) phase, 92) the

Table A-2 Isotonic Core-Strengthening Exercises

Exercise*†	Sets/Repetitions
Chest	
Bench press (close grip)	2-3/8-10
Legs squats	2-3/8-10
Leg press	2-3/8-10
Knee extensions	2-3/8-10
Leg curls	2-3/8-10
Lunges	2-3/8-10
Calf press	2-3/8-10
Toe raises	2-3/8-10
Back	
Latissimus pull-downs	2-3/8-10
Shoulder shrugs	2-3/8-10
Seated rows	2-3/8-10
Bent-over rows	2-3/8-10
Abdominals Crunches (to be performed in sequence)	
Feet flat	3/15, rest 30 seconds
Weight on chest	3/15, rest 60 seconds
Knees bent	1/25, rest 60 seconds
Knees up with weight	1/25

*All exercises should be performed two to three times a week.
†Wide-grip bench press, behind-neck pull-down, deep squats, and behind-neck military press should not be performed.

amortization phase, and (3) the concentric response phase. The setting phase of the exercise is the preloading period; it lasts until the stretch stimulus is initiated. The amortization phase of the exercise is the time that occurs between the eccentric contraction and the initiation of the concentric contraction. During the concentric phase the effect of the exercise (a facilitated contraction) is produced and preparation for the second repetition occurs.

Clinicians believe physiologic muscle performance is enhanced by plyometric exercise in several ways. The faster a muscle is loaded eccentrically, the greater the resultant concentric force produced. Eccentric loading of a muscle places stress on the elastic components, increasing the tension of the resultant force produced.

Neuromuscular coordination is improved through explosive plyometric training. Plyometric exercise may improve neural efficiency, thereby increasing neuromuscular performance.

Finally, the inhibitory effect of the Golgi tendon organs, which serve as a protective mechanism limiting the amount of force produced within muscle, can be desensitized by plyometric exercise, thereby raising the level of inhibition. This desensitization and the resultant raise in the inhibition level ultimately allow increased force production with greater applied loads.

Through neural adaptation the throwing athlete can coordinate the activity of muscle groups and produce greater net force output (in the absence of morphologic change within the muscles themselves). The faster the athlete is able to switch from eccentric or yielding work to concentric overcoming work, the more powerful the resultant response. Effective plyometric training requires that the amortization phase of the exercise be quick, limiting the amount of energy wasted as heat. The rate of stretch rather than the length of stretch provides a greater stimulus for an enhanced training effect. With slower stretch cycles the stretch reflex is not activated.

Before implementing a plyometric training program, the patient must have an adequate level of base strength to maximize the training effect and prevent injury. Remedial shoulder exercises focusing on the rotator cuff and shoulder-supporting musculature are continued to develop and maintain joint stability and muscle strength in the arm decelerators. These exercises also should be used to warm up before the plyometric drill and cool down after it has been concluded.

Plyometric exercise is contraindicated in the immediate postoperative period, in the presence of acute inflammation or pain, in athletes with gross shoulder or elbow instability, or in both. Plyometric training also is contraindicated in athletes who do not have an adequate degree of base strength and who are not participating in a strength-training program. This form of exercise is intended to be an advanced form of strength training. Post-exercise muscle soreness and delayed-onset muscle soreness are common adverse reactions that the clinician should be aware of before beginning an athlete on this type of exercise. **Tremendous amounts of stress occur during plyometric exercises; therefore they should not be performed for an extended period.** A plyometric program should be used during the first and second preparation phases of training.

The plyometric training program for the UE can be divided into four groups of exercise as described by Wilk[32] (Table A-3):

1. Warm-up exercises
2. Throwing movements
3. Trunk extension and flexion exercises
4. Medicine ball wall exercises

Warm-up exercises are performed to provide the shoulder, arms, trunk, and LEs an adequate physiologic warm-up before beginning more intense plyometric exercise. The facilitation of muscular performance through an active warm-up has been ascribed to increased blood flow, oxygen use, nervous system transmission, muscle and core temperature, and speed of contraction.* The athlete should perform two to three sets of 10 repetitions for each warm-up exercise before proceeding to the next group of exercises.

Throwing movement plyometric exercises attempt to isolate and train the muscles required to throw effectively. Movement patterns similar to those found with overhead throwing are performed. These exercises provide an advanced strengthening technique at a higher exercise level than that of more traditional isotonic dumbbell exercises. The exercises in this group are performed for two to four sets of six to eight repetitions two to three times weekly. Adequate rest times should occur between each session for optimal muscle recovery.

Plyometric exercises for trunk strengthening include medicine ball exercises for the abdominals and trunk extensor musculature. The athlete performs two to four sets of eight to ten repetitions two to three times weekly.

The final group of exercises, the Plyoball wall exercises, require the use of 2 lb and 4 lb medicine balls or Plyoballs and a wall or pitchback device to allow the athlete to perform this group of exercises without a partner. This group of drills starts with two-handed throws with a heavier 4 lb ball and concludes with one-handed plyometric throws using the lighter 2 lb ball. All the exercises in this phase of the program should be performed in the standing and kneeling positions to increase demands on the trunk, UE, and shoulder girdle and eliminate the use of the LEs. The same number of repetitions and sets should be performed two to three times weekly (Fig. A-1).

Plyometric training of the LEs is essential in developing the throwing athlete's explosive strength needed for speed,

*References 1, 2, 11, 16, 21.

Table A-3 Plyometric Exercises

Exercise*	Equipment	Sets/Repetitions
Warm-Ups		
Medicine ball rotation	9-lb ball	2-3/10
Medicine ball side bends	9-lb ball	2-3/10
Medicine ball wood chops	9-lb ball	2-3/10
Tubing		
Internal rotation (IR), external rotation (ER), and 90-degree shoulder abduction	Medium tubing	2-3/10
Diagonal patterns (D2)	Medium tubing	2-3/10
Biceps	Medium tubing	2-3/10
Push-ups		2-3/10
Throwing Movements		
Medicine ball soccer throw†	4-lb ball	2-4/6-8
Medicine ball chest pass†	4-lb ball	2-4/6-8
Medicine ball step and pass†	4-lb ball	2-4/6-8
Medicine ball side throw†	4-lb ball	2-4/6-8
Tubing Plyometrics		
IR and ER		6-8 repetitions
Diagonals		6-8 repetitions
Biceps		6-8 repetitions
Push-ups	6- to 8-inch box	10 repetitions
Trunk Extension and Flexion Movements		
Medicine ball sit-ups	4-lb ball	2-3/10
Medicine ball back extension	4-lb ball	2-3/10
Medicine Ball Exercises (Standing and Kneeling)		
Soccer throw	4-lb ball	2-4/6-8
Chest pass	4-lb ball	2-4/6-8
Side-to-side throw	4-lb ball	2-4/6-8
Backward side-to-side throws	4-lb ball	2-4/6-8
Forward two hands through legs	4-lb ball	2-4/6-8
One-handed baseball throw	2-lb ball	2-4/6-8

*All exercises should be performed two to three times a week.
†Throw with partner or pitchback device.
(Modified from Wilk KE, Voight ML: Plyometrics for the shoulder complex. In Andrews JR, Wilk KE, editors: *The athlete's shoulder,* New York, 1994, Churchill Livingstone.)

lateral mobility, and acceleration. LE plyometric training also helps develop the coordination and agility necessary to compete effectively. High demands are placed on the musculature supporting the hips, knees, and ankle joints during plyometric jump exercises. The PT *must* monitor exercise loads performed and allow adequate recovery time between sets. Proper technique in performing these exercises is vital to prevent injury. A variety of jump exercises can be used to train the LEs when preparing the throwing athlete to return to athletic competition (Table A-4).

Rapid box jumps are performed to develop explosive power in the calf and quadriceps musculature. An explosive but controlled jump up onto the box then down off the box is performed; box height can be increased as the exercise is mastered. The athlete should immediately jump back on the box, spending as little time as possible on the ground.

Alternating-height box jumps train the quadriceps, hamstrings, gluteals, and calf muscles and help develop explosive power. Box jumps are performed using three to five plyometric boxes of varying heights (from 12 to 24 inches) placed in a straight line two feet apart from one another. Starting at the smallest box, the athlete performs controlled jumps from the box to the ground to

Table A-4 Lower Extremity (LE) Plyometric Exercises

Exercise*	Equipment	Sets/Repetitions
Rapid box jumps (alternating height)	Boxes of varying heights	2-3/8-10
Box jumps	12- to 24-inch boxes	3-4 sets
Depth jump and sprint†	24-inch box	5-8 repetitions
Depth jump and base steal†	24-inch box	5-8 repetitions

*All exercises should be performed two to three times per week.
†Jump from a 24-inch box followed by an immediate 10-yard sprint.

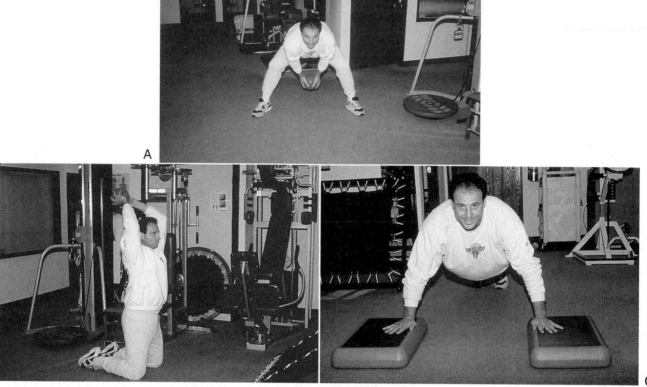

Fig. A-1 A, Medicine ball wood chop warm-up exercises. B, Medicine ball soccer throw exercises from the knees. C, Plyometric push-up. (Photos by Dr. Luga Podesta, Oxnard, CA.)

the next tallest box, spending as little time on the ground as possible; the athlete should rest for 15 to 20 seconds between sets.

The depth jump and sprint and the depth jump with base steal focus on teaching muscles to react forcefully from a negative contraction to an explosive positive contraction. The athlete immediately explodes into a 10-yard sprint or 10-yard base steal after jumping off a 24-inch box.

AEROBIC CONDITIONING

Although the initial postoperative emphasis is on rehabilitation of the shoulder, the transition from formal therapy to return to play requires the throwing athlete to regain the preinjury aerobic condition. Therefore the aerobic conditioning component of the training program must not be neglected. Aerobic fitness can be developed using a variety of exercises (Box A-2).

For any method of aerobic activity to be effective, the exercise should be performed continuously for 20 to 40 minutes four to five times weekly. Because this type of conditioning is long and repetitious, the athlete should enjoy the activity being performed.

Box A-2 Aerobic Conditioning Exercises

- Running
- Bicycling
- Versa-Climber
- Stair-climbing machine
- Elliptical runner
- Cross-country ski machine
- Rowing machine
- Swimming

THROWING

The overhead-throwing motion is not unique to throwing a baseball. Similar muscular activity is required to throw a softball, football, or javelin. However, the majority of research performed on overhead throwing has been conducted on the overhead pitch.

The clinician must appreciate the highly dynamic nature of the throwing motion to be effective in preparing and progressing the rehabilitating athlete through a safe throwing program. A thorough understanding of normal and abnormal throwing mechanics and the biomechanical forces placed on the throwing arm are essential for the therapist wishing to implement a throwing program in the rehabilitation setting.

Baseball

Pitching

Pitching a baseball is the most violent and dynamic of all overhead-throwing activities, producing angular velocities in excess of 7000 degrees/second across the shoulder. Maximal stability of the GH joint occurs at 90 degrees of shoulder elevation.[27] Because muscle weakness can result in abnormal compression and shear forces, muscle balance is necessary to maintain stability of the humeral head in the glenoid fossa. *A favorable balance between compression and shear forces occurs at 90 degrees of shoulder elevation, placing the shoulder in the optimal position for joint stability.*[3,24,27,28] *All throwers therefore should maintain 90 degrees of GH elevation relative to the horizontal surface regardless of technique or pitching style.*

Dynamic control of the GH joint during throwing depends on the rotator cuff and biceps muscle strength.[3,6] An abnormal throwing pattern can result from GH instability and inadequate control of the rotator cuff and biceps tendon. Neuromuscular conditioning and control of the GH joint allows for safer throwing by facilitating the dynamic coordination of the rotator cuff and scapulothoracic stabilizers.

The throwing or pitching motion can be divided into six phases (Fig. A-2):

1. Windup
2. Early cocking
3. Late cocking
4. Acceleration
5. Deceleration
6. Follow-through

Windup is the preparatory phase of the throwing motion. Relatively little muscle activity occurs during this phase. From a standing position the athlete initiates the throw by shifting the weight onto the supporting back leg. The weight shift from the stride leg to the supporting leg sets the rhythm for the delivery. Windup ends when the ball leaves the gloved nondominant hand (Fig. A-3, *A*).

During **early cocking** the shoulder abducts to approximately 104 degrees and externally rotates to 46 degrees.[11] The scapular muscles are active in positioning the glenoid for optimal contact with the humeral head as the arm is abducted. The supraspinatus and deltoid muscles work synergistically to elevate the humerus. The deltoids position the arm in space, and the supraspinatus stabilizes the humeral head within the glenoid[10] (Figs. A-3, B-H, and A-4).

The stride forward is initiated during the early cocking phase of throwing. The athlete should keep the trunk and back closed as long as possible to retain the energy stored, which later results in velocity.

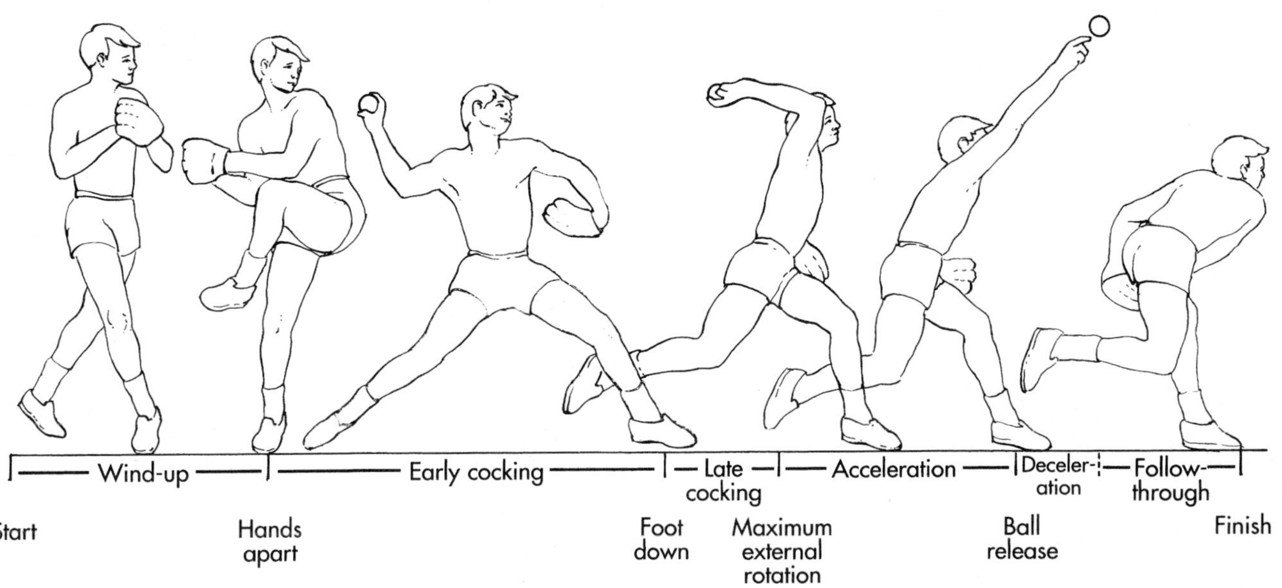

Fig. A-2 Phases of the baseball pitch.
(From Jobe FW: *Operative techniques in upper extremity sports injury*, St Louis, 1996, Mosby.)

Text continued on p. 14

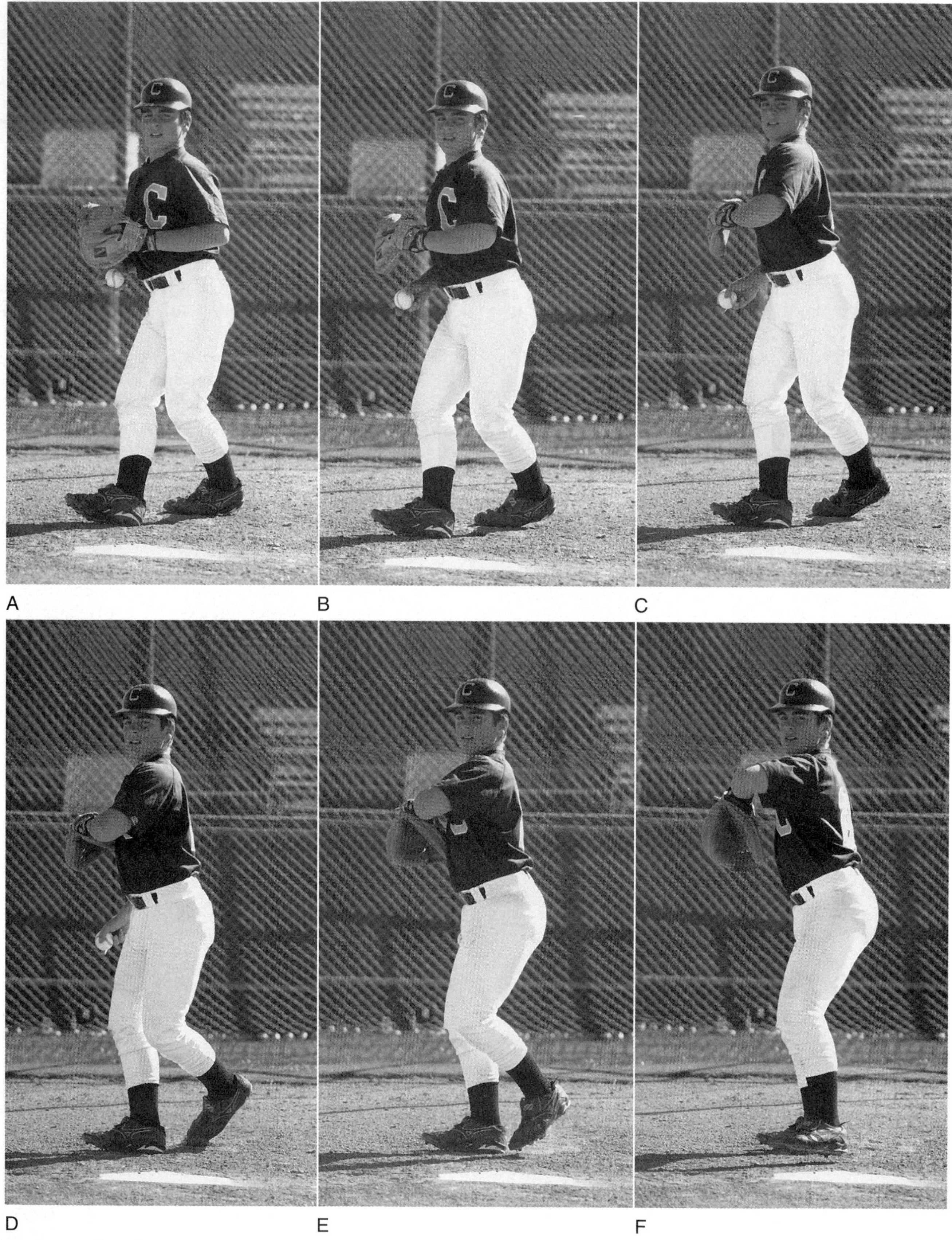

Fig. A-3 Front view of the throwing motion. **A** to **E**, The crow hop step begins the throwing motion. The pelvis and chest are rotated 90 degrees from the target. The hands separate as weight is shifted to the back leg. **F** to **J**, During the cocking phase of throwing, the throwing arm is elevated and externally rotated.

Continued

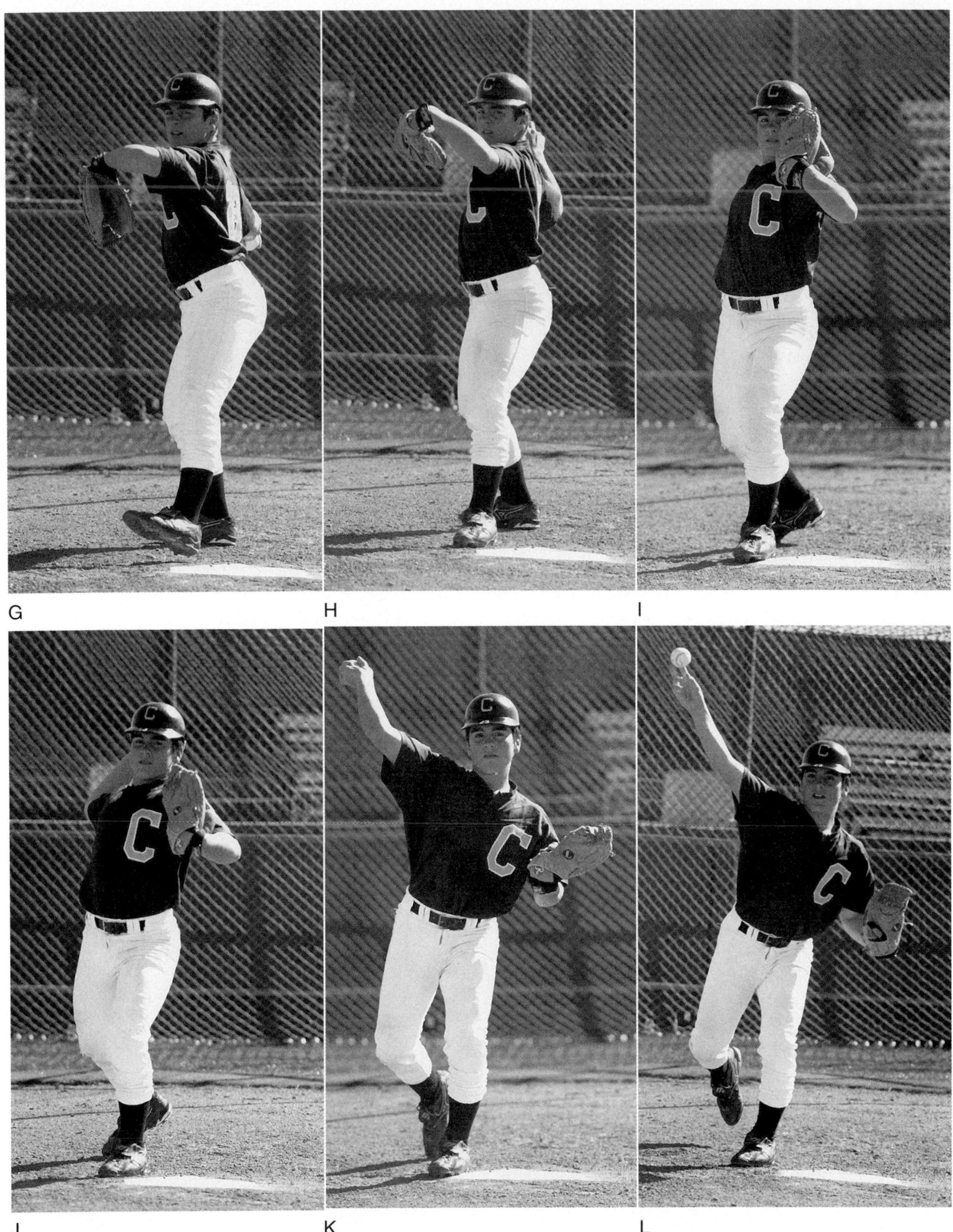

Fig. A-3, cont'd Front view of the throwing motion. The front foot is planted in a slightly closed position as the pelvis begins to rotate. Front view of the throwing motion. K to L. During the acceleration phase, the elbow is above the height of the shoulder and weight is shifted to the front foot as the pelvis rotates.

Continued

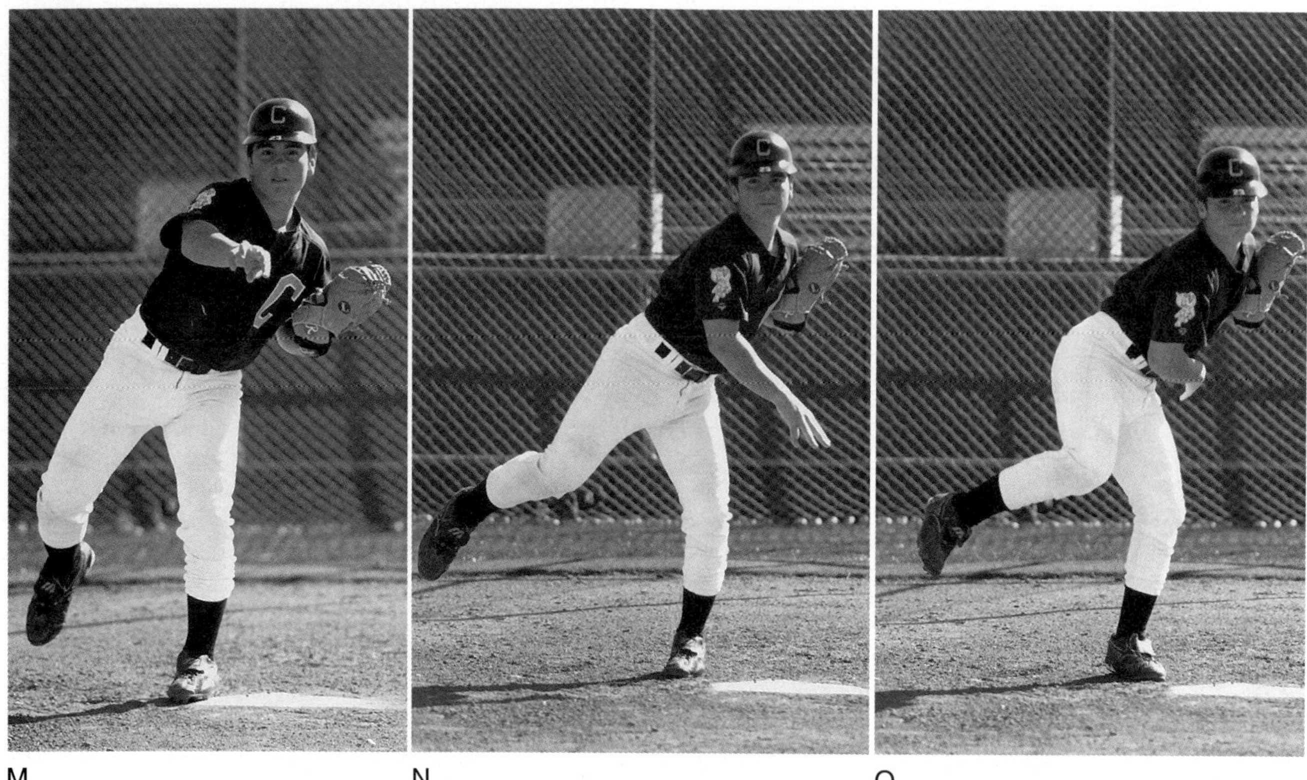

M N O

Fig. A-3, cont'd M to O, The deceleration and follow-through phases.
(Photos by Marsha Gorman, Camarillo, CA.)

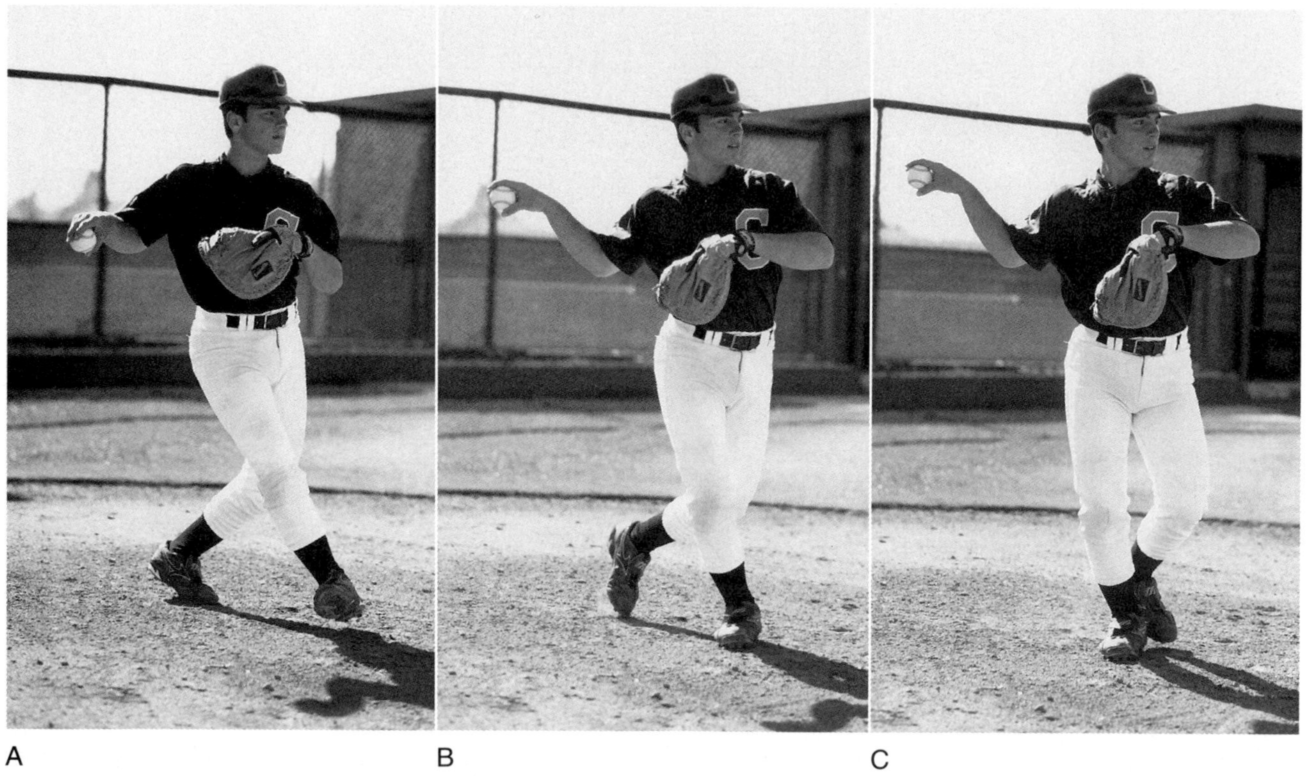

A B C

Fig. A-4 Side view of the throwing motion. **A** to **C**, The windup and cocking phases of throwing.

Continued

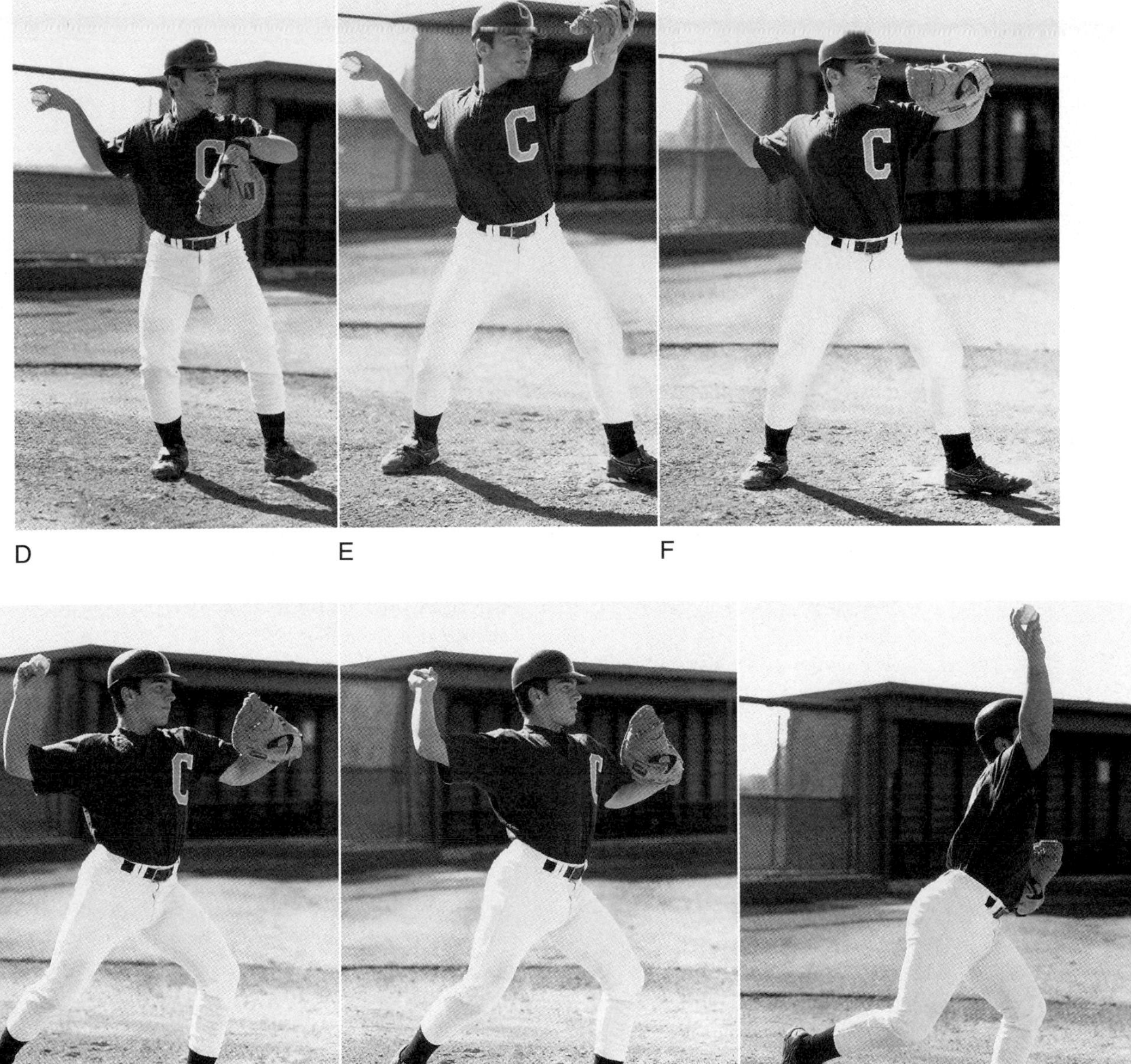

Fig. A-4, cont'd Side view of the throwing motion. **D** to **G**, The windup and cocking phases of throwing. **H** to **I**, The acceleration phases.

Continued

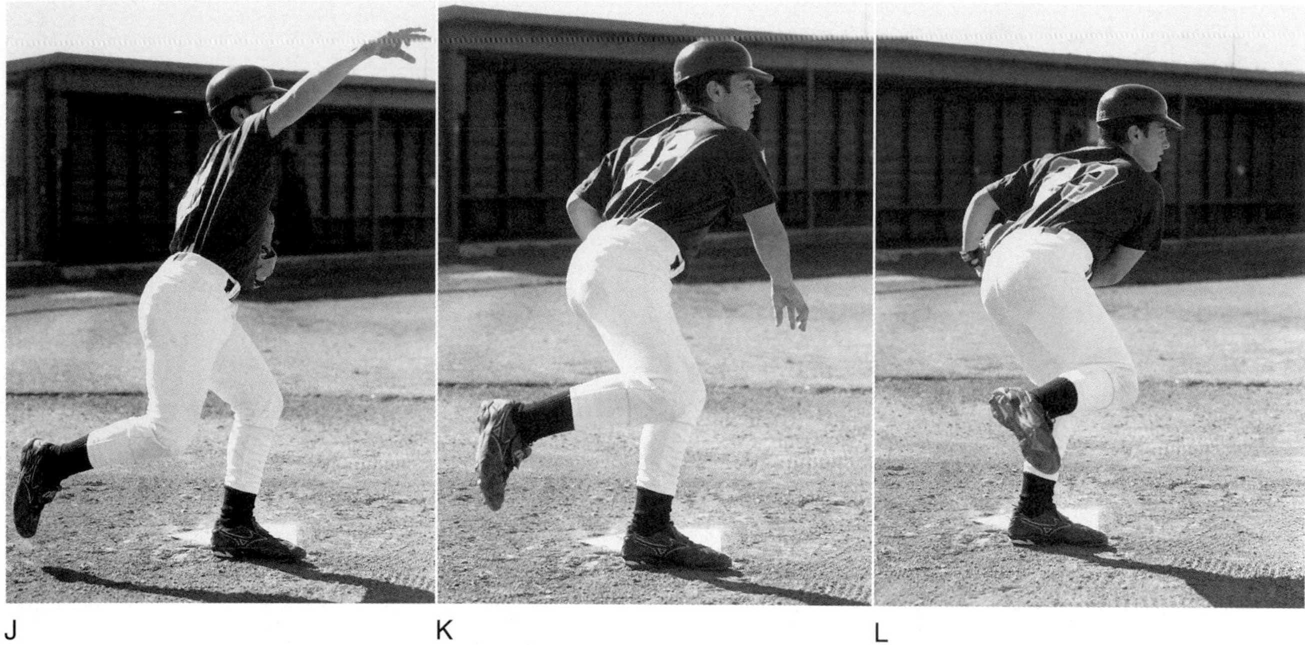

Fig. A-4, cont'd Side view of the throwing motion. **J**, The acceleration phases. **K** to **L**, The deceleration and follow-through phases. (Photos by Marsha Gorman, Camarillo, CA.)

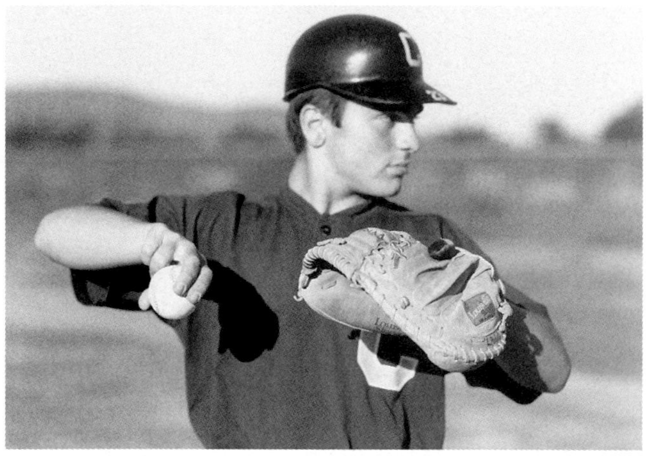

Fig. A-5 The proper technique for gripping the ball and releasing it from the glove. The ball is gripped loosely across four seams in the fingertips of the index and middle fingers. The thumb is placed under the ball, with the index and middle fingers held together. The hands separate with a supinating motion of the forearms forcing the thumbs of both the glove and ball hand downward. (Photo by Marsha Gorman, Camarillo, CA.)

As the stride leg moves toward the target, the ball breaks from the glove and the throwing arm swings upward in rhythm with the body. The positioning of the breaking hands followed by the downward then upward rotation of the throwing arm ensures optimal positioning of the arm (Fig. A-5). Establishing this synchronous muscle-firing pattern is one of the most crucial aspects of the throw. If the throwing arm and striding leg are synchronized properly, then the arm and hand will be in the early cocked position when the stride foot contacts the ground (see Figs. A-3, H, and A-4, D).

The direction of the stride should either be directly toward the target or slightly closed (to the right side of a right-handed thrower) (see Figs. A-3, H, and A-4, E). When the stride is too closed, the hips are unable to rotate and the thrower is forced to throw across the body, losing kinetic energy from the LEs. When the stride is too open (i.e., the stride foot lands too far to the left of a right-handed thrower), the hips rotate too early, forcing the trunk to face the batter too early and dissipating stored kinetic energy. This also places tremendous stress on the anterior shoulder. After the stride leg contacts the ground, the stride is completed and cocking of the throwing arm is initiated.

During the **late cocking phase** of throwing the humerus maintains its level of abduction while moving into the scapular plane. The arm externally rotates from 46 degrees to 170 degrees.[11] In this position the humeral head is positioned to place an anterior-directed force, potentially stretching the anterior ligamentous restraints.

The trunk moves laterally toward the target, and pelvic rotation is initiated. As the trunk undergoes rotation and extension, the elbow is flexed, and the shoulder externally rotates. When the trunk faces the target, the shoulder should have achieved maximal ER. At the end of this phase, only the arm is cocked as the legs, pelvis, and trunk have already accelerated (see Figs. A-3, I and J, and A-4, F and G).

During the **acceleration phase** the humerus internally rotates approximately 100 degrees in 0.005 seconds. Tremendous torque and joint compressive forces and high angular velocities across the GH joint are present at this time.[11,17,23]

The acceleration phase begins when the humerus begins to internally rotate. Just before the beginning of IR, the elbow should begin to extend (see Figs. A-3, K, and A-4, H and I). When ball release occurs, the trunk is flexed, the elbow reaches almost full extension, and the shoulder undergoes IR (see Figs. A-3, L, and A-4, J). At ball release the trunk should be tilted forward with the lead knee extending. Acceleration ends with ball release.

The **deceleration phase** of the throwing motion is the first third of the time from ball release to the completion of arm motion (see Figs. A-3, M and N, and A-4, K). During deceleration excess kinetic energy that was not transferred to the ball is dissipated. High calculated forces and torque also occur during this phase.[5,13]

Follow-through occurs during the final two thirds of the throwing motion, during which time the arm continues to decelerate and eventually stops (see Figs. A-3, O, and A-4, L). After ball release, the throwing arm continues to extend at the elbow and internally rotates at the shoulder. Internal angular velocities drop from their maximal level at ball release to zero. *A proper follow-through is crucial in minimizing injury to the shoulder during this violent stage of throwing. Follow-through is completed when the throwing shoulder is over the opposite knee. This is achieved by allowing the supporting leg to rotate forward, finishing the rotation of the trunk across the body.*

Football

The throwing mechanics necessary to throw a football are very similar to those required to throw a baseball.[15] The most significant differences between the two are the size and weight of the ball and the positioning of the throwing hand during the acceleration and ball release phases of the throwing motion. Although the precise throwing mechanics are not well defined, studies are currently underway to determine and describe the specific mechanics. Similar forces and stresses appear to be applied to the shoulder and elbow. Dynamic control of the entire kinetic chain during the football throw is essential for the quarterback to be effective throwing to the right, left, and on the run. Neuromuscular conditioning and control of the LEs, core, and UEs allows for safer throwing by facilitating the dynamic coordination of the entire kinetic chain.

The football-throwing motion can be divided into six phases:

1. Windup
2. Early cocking
3. Late cocking
4. Acceleration
5. Deceleration
6. Follow-through

Windup is the preparatory phase of the throwing motion. From a squatting position, the quarterback steps backward from behind the center varying distances (i.e., steps) positioning the body to initiate the throw by shifting the weight onto the supporting back leg. The weight shift from the stride leg to the supporting leg sets the rhythm for the delivery. Windup ends when the ball and supporting hand separate (Fig. A-6, A and B).

During **early cocking** the shoulder abducts and externally rotates (Fig. A-7, A and B). The stride forward is initiated during the early cocking phase of throwing. The athlete should keep the trunk and back closed as long as possible to retain the energy stored, which later results in velocity.

As the stride leg moves toward the target, the ball breaks from the hand and the throwing arm swings upward in rhythm with the body. Establishing this synchronous muscle-firing pattern from the feet to the LEs through the pelvis and trunk to the shoulder to the UE and finally the hand is one of the most crucial aspects of the throw. If the throwing arm and striding leg are synchronized properly, then the arm and hand will be in the early cocked position when the stride foot contacts the ground.

The direction of the stride should either be directly toward the target or slightly closed (to the right side of a right-handed thrower) regardless of the direction of the throw—straight, right, or left.

During the **late cocking phase** of throwing (Fig. A-8, A and B) the humerus maintains its level of abduction while moving into the scapular plane. The arm externally rotates, the trunk moves laterally toward the target, and pelvic rotation is initiated. As the trunk undergoes rotation and extension, the elbow is flexed and the shoulder externally rotates. When the trunk faces the target, the shoulder should have achieved maximal ER. At the end of this phase, only the arm is cocked, because the legs, pelvis, and trunk have already accelerated.

During the **acceleration phase** (Fig. A-9, A and B) the humerus internally rotates applying tremendous torque and joint compressive forces and high angular velocities across the GH.

The acceleration phase begins when the humerus begins to internally rotate. Just before the beginning of IR, the elbow should begin to extend. When ball release occurs, the trunk is flexed, the elbow reaches almost full extension, and the shoulder undergoes IR and the forearm maximally pronates (Fig. A-10). At ball release the trunk should be tilted forward with the lead knee extending. Acceleration ends with ball release.

The **deceleration phase** of the throwing motion is the first third of the time from ball release to the com-

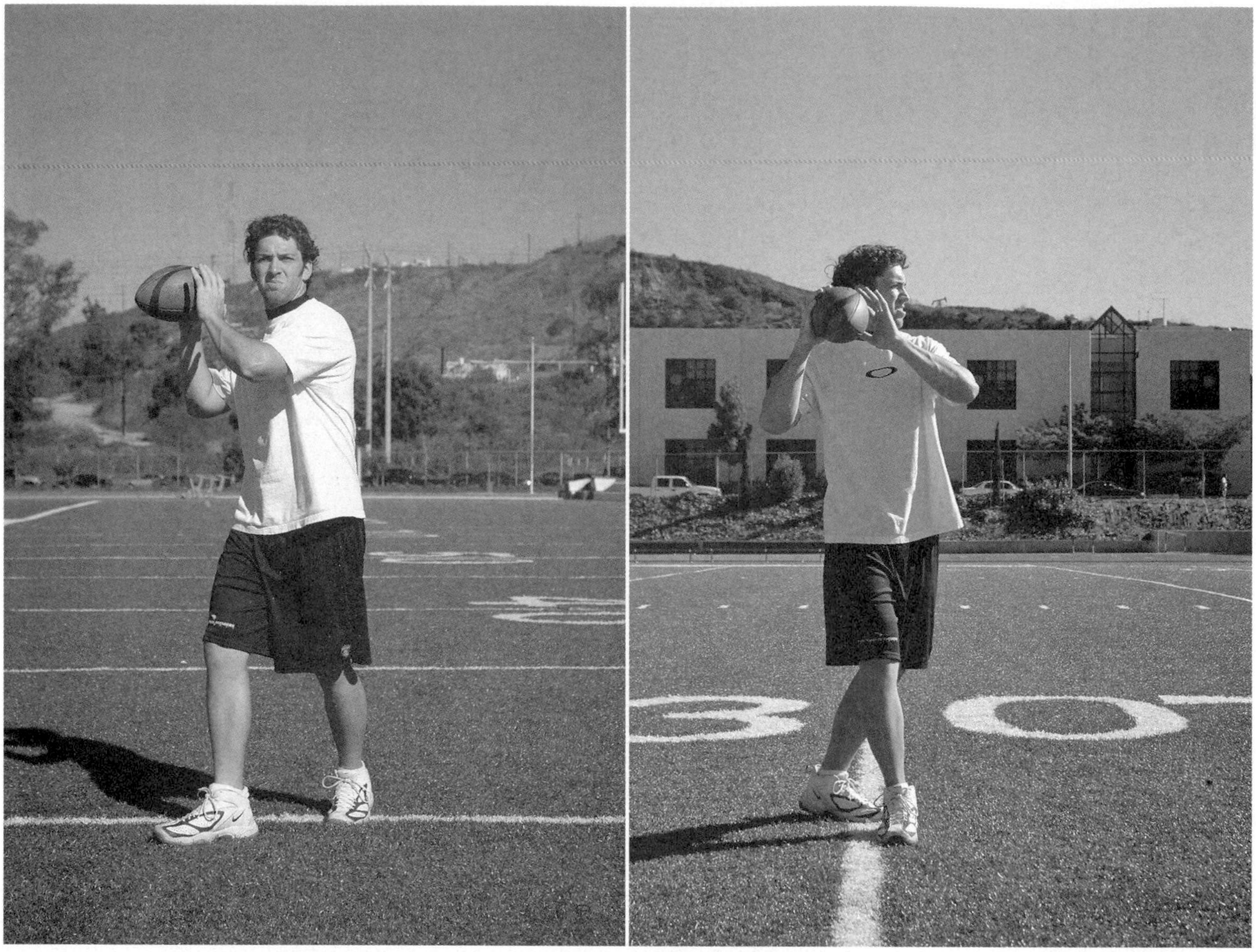

A B

Fig. A-6 A and B, The wind up phase.

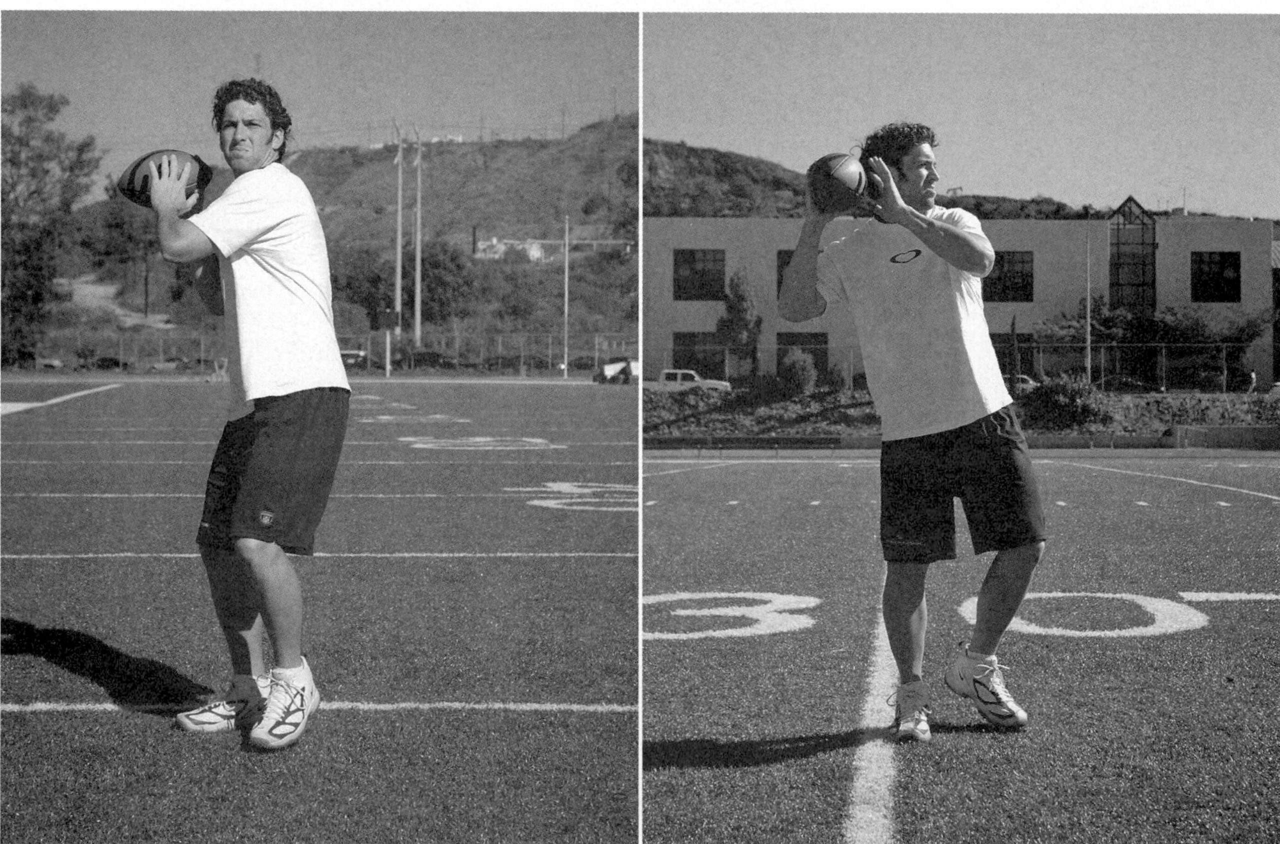

Fig. A-7 A and B, The early cocking phase.

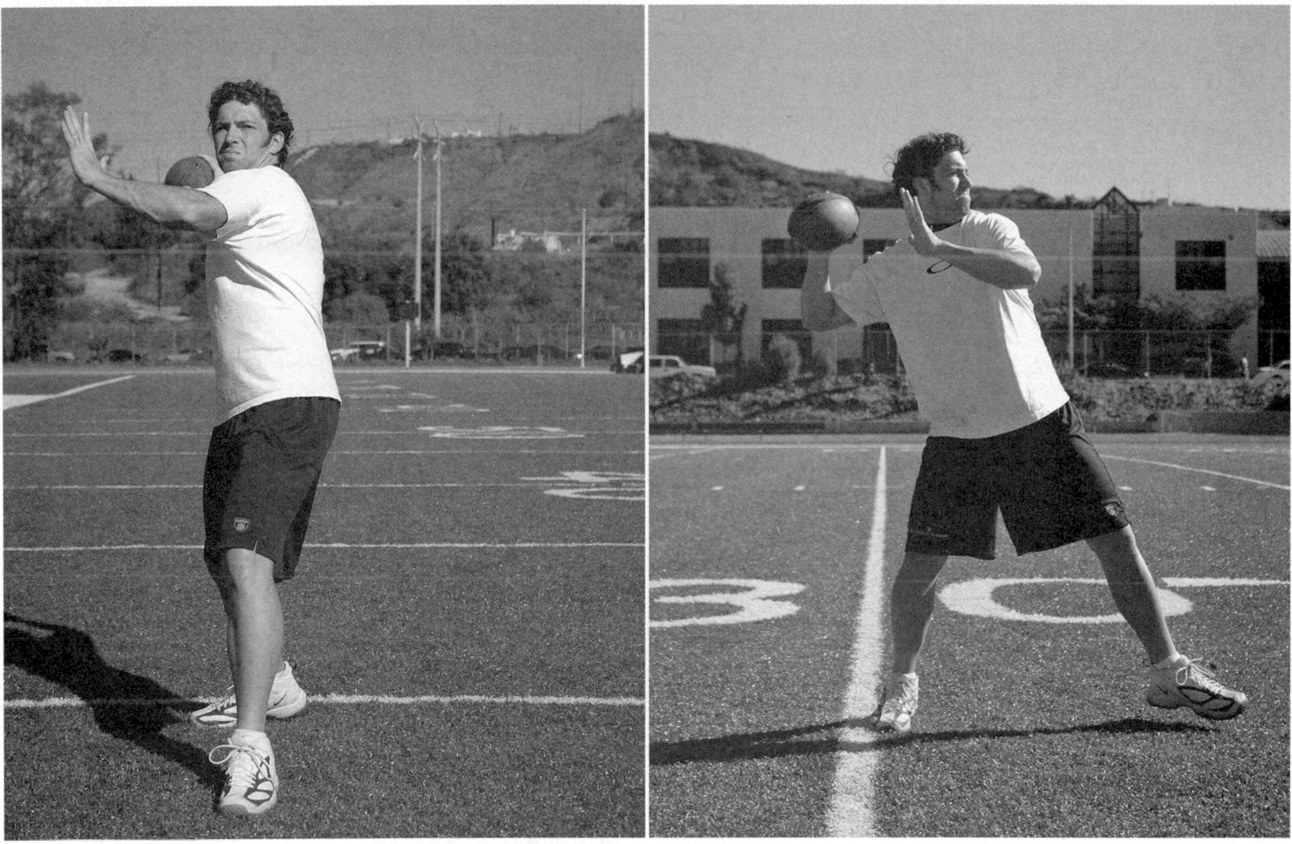

Fig. A-8 **A** and **B**, The late cocking phase.

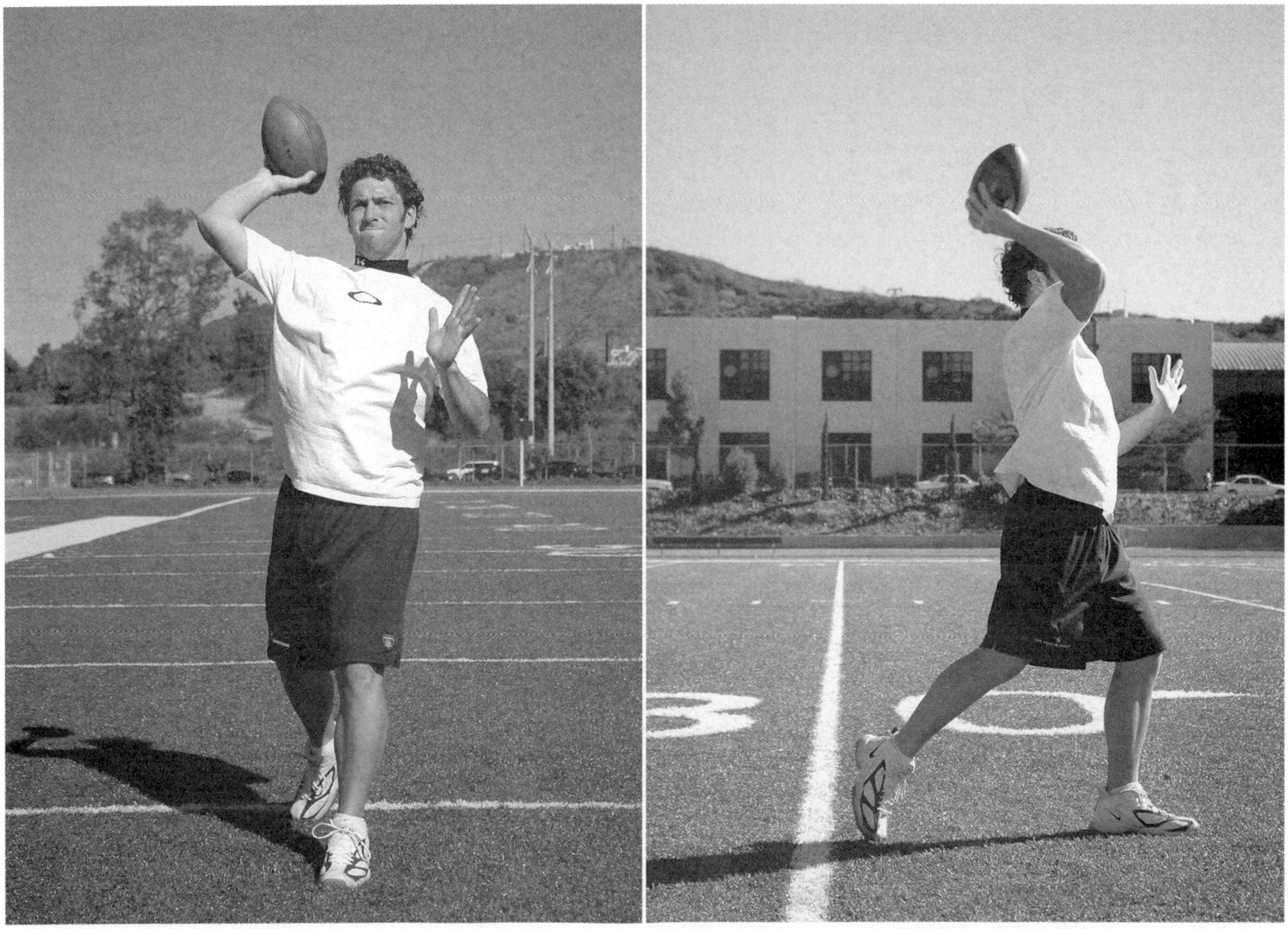

A B

Fig. A-9 **A** and **B**, The acceleration phase.

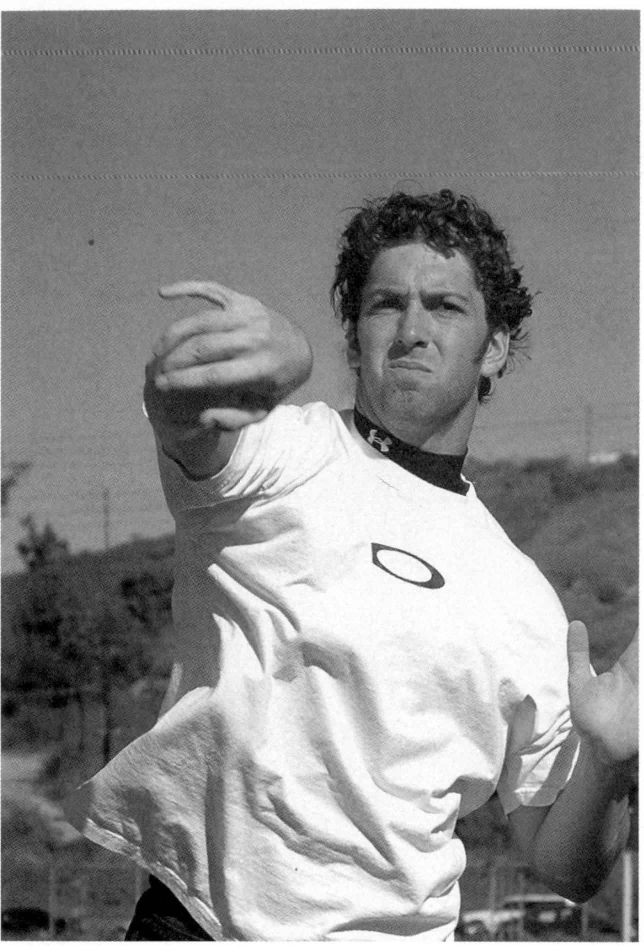

Fig. A-10 Maximal pronation occurs toward the end of the acceleration phase.

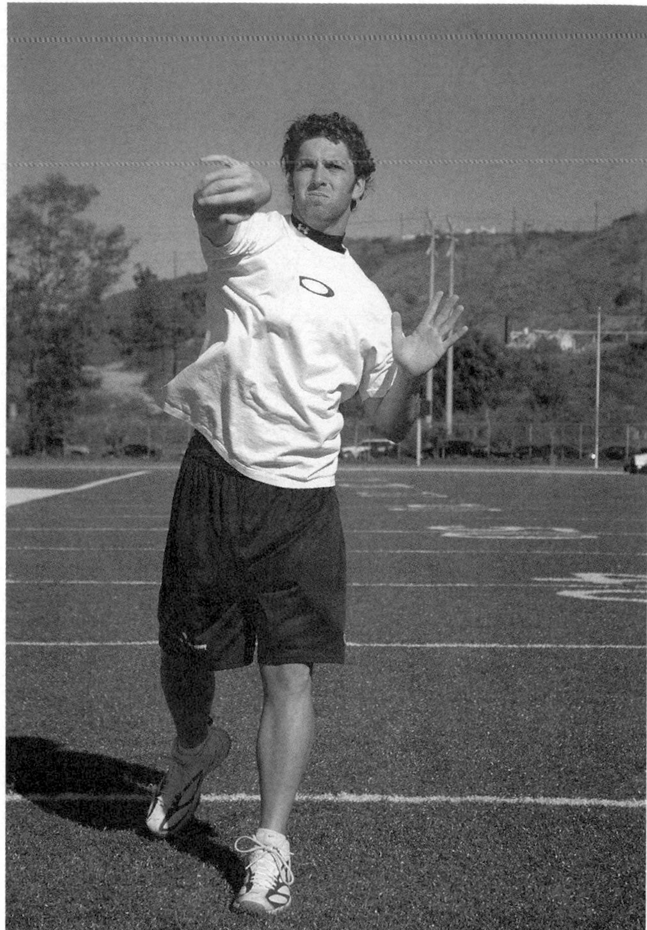

Fig. A-11 The deceleration phase.

pletion of arm motion (Fig. A-11). During deceleration excess kinetic energy that was not transferred to the ball is dissipated.

Follow-through (Fig. A-12) occurs during the final two thirds of the throwing motion, during which time the arm continues to decelerate and eventually stops. After ball release, the throwing arm continues to extend at the elbow and internally rotates at the shoulder. A proper follow-through is crucial in minimizing injury to the shoulder during this violent stage of throwing. Follow-through is completed when the throwing shoulder is over the opposite knee. This is achieved by allowing the supporting leg to rotate forward, finishing the rotation of the trunk across the body.

INTERVAL BASEBALL THROWING PROGRAM

The purpose of the interval throwing program is to return motion, strength, and confidence gradually to the throwing arm after injury or surgery. The interval throwing program allows the throwing patient the opportunity to re-establish timing, movement patterns, coordination, and synchronicity of muscle firing before returning to competition.[30] This is accomplished by slowly increasing the throwing distances and eventually the velocity of the throws. The program should be individualized to each athlete. No set timetable is prescribed for the completion of the program; each patient's time spent completing the program may vary. The throwing program is designed to minimize the chance of injury by emphasizing proper prethrowing warm-up, stretching, and cooldown. It should be performed in the presence of a coach, trainer, or therapist knowledgeable in throwing mechanics. Careful supervision cannot be overstressed.

The participants must resist the temptation to increase the intensity of the throwing program and understand that this may increase the incidence of reinjury, which would greatly retard the rehabilitation process.

Before initiating the interval throwing program the athletic patient must exhibit the following criteria:

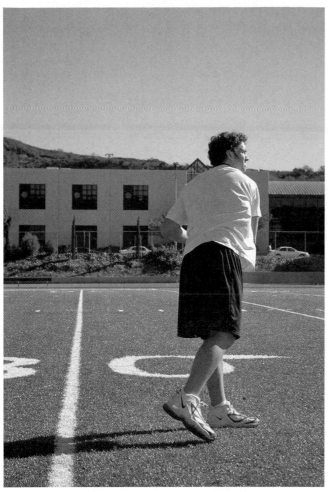

Fig. A-12 The follow-through phase.

1. Full and painless ROM
2. No pain or tenderness
3. Satisfactory muscle strength and conditioning
4. Normal or clinically stable examination

Specific attention throughout the interval throwing program to the maintenance of proper throwing mechanics is crucial (Box A-3). Participants in the rehabilitation program may find videotaping throwing sessions extremely helpful in assisting with the analysis of the athlete's throwing mechanics.

Proper warm-up before beginning to throw cannot be overemphasized.

A common mistake is for the thrower to begin throwing to warm up. Instead, the thrower should increase the blood flow to muscles and joints before throwing. Running or jogging long enough to break a sweat can accomplish this.

The athletic patient must warm up to throw, not throw to warm up.

A "crow hop" throwing technique uses a hop, skip, and throw to accentuate LE and trunk involvement in the throw. The use of the crow hop method simulates the throwing motion and emphasizes proper throwing mechanics (see Figs. A-3, A to F, and A-4, A to D).

Throwing flat-footed encourages improper throwing mechanics and places increased stress on the throwing shoulder.

The throwing athlete progresses through each step of the program, throwing every other day, or three times weekly. **The thrower progresses to the next step after the prescribed number of throws can be completed without pain or residual pain. If pain or difficulty throwing occurs, then the athlete should regress to the previous level or attempt the same level during the next session.** The ultimate goal is for the athlete to throw 75 repetitions at 180 feet without pain for positional players and 150 feet for pitchers. Box A-4 illustrates a progressive interval throwing program.[31]

When progressing through a pitcher-specific interval throwing program, it is extremely important to ensure that the person or target receiving the throws is at the same height as the thrower. When throwing on flat ground, the thrower should be throwing to a standing target. When throwing off the pitching mound, the target can get into a squatting position. Throwing on flat ground to a squatting catcher changes the point of ball release, which may lead to increased stress across the anterior shoulder and elbow. Pattern throwing (Fig. A-13) also can be implemented to develop arm strength:[18]

1. Proper warm-up before throwing (i.e., jogging, running, bicycling)
2. Throwing from a kneeling position, facing the direction of the throw with the arm already in the abducted position for a distance of 20 feet, easy effort, for 10 repetitions, with emphasis on proper grip
3. Kneeling on one knee facing the target with the arm in the abducted position (right-handed thrower on the

Box A-3 **Throwing Evaluation Checklist**

- Foot position—Crow hop, back foot 90 degrees to the target
- Body position—Nondominant hip and shoulder to the target
- Hand break—Ball release from glove, thumbs down
- Ball hand and glove position—Ball facing away from the target, glove side elbow points to target flexed 90 degrees, glove down
- Arm position—Elbow above shoulder level
- Front foot plant—Step toward the target, "toes to target," slightly closed
- Trunk rotation—Hips rotate before shoulders
- Balance—Stand tall, weight back
- Finish—Stride foot posts, back leg and hip rotate through

right knee, left-handed thrower on the left knee) from a distance of 30 feet, easy effort, 10 repetitions, with emphasis on hitting the target and maintaining proper follow-through
4. Standing with the feet in a straddle position facing the target with the shoulders turned and the ball in the glove at a distance of 40 feet, medium effort, with emphasis on follow-through
5. Standing in a regular throwing position at a distance of 40 feet, throwing medium effort for 10 repetitions, with emphasis on staying closed and pointing the front shoulder to the target

SUMMARY

Rehabilitation goals for the shoulder after surgery emphasize pain management, re-establishing ROM, and developing strength in the shoulder-supporting musculature. To return the throwing athlete to sports after surgery requires further intense strengthening and conditioning to regain preinjury form and performance. Progressive strengthening followed by aerobic conditioning helps prepare the thrower recovering from surgery for an eventual return to throwing. After throwing has been introduced into the rehabilitation regimen, careful attention to throwing technique is imperative to prevent reinjury. An interval throwing program is followed to establish a time frame for a safe, gradual, and progressive return to throwing.

The program described in this appendix should only serve as a guide for the progressive return of the thrower to throwing; it is not a specific postoperative protocol applicable to all patient athletes. Each patient's program requires individualization and should progress at its own rate.

Box A-4 Progressive Interval Throwing Program

- Warm-up
- Run to break sweat
- Stretching

45-foot phase (half the distance to first base from home plate)

Step 1:
a. Warm-up throwing—25 feet
b. 45 feet (25 throws)
c. Rest 10-15 minutes
d. Warm-up throwing
e. 45 feet (25 throws)

Step 2:
a. Warm-up throwing
b. 45 feet (25 throws)
c. Rest 10 minutes
d. Warm-up throwing
e. 45 feet (25 throws)
f. Rest 10 minutes
g. Warm-up throwing
h. 45 feet (25 throws)

60-Foot phase (distance from home plate to pitching mound)

Step 3:
a. Warm-up throwing
b. 60 feet (25 throws)
c. Rest 10-15 minutes
d. Warm-up throwing
e. 60 feet (25 throws)

Step 4:
a. Warm-up throwing
b. 60 feet (25 throws)
c. Rest 10 minutes
d. Warm-up throwing
e. 60 feet (25 throws)
f. Rest 10 minutes
g. Warm-up throwing
h. 60 feet (25 throws)

90-Foot phase (distance from home plate to first base)

Step 5:
a. Warm-up throwing
b. 90 feet (25 throws)
c. Rest 10-15 minutes
d. Warm-up throwing
e. 90 feet (25 throws)

Step 6:
a. Warm-up throwing
b. 90 feet (25 throws)
c. Rest 10 minutes
d. Warm-up throwing
e. 90 feet (25 throws)
f. Rest 10 minutes
g. Warm-up throwing
h. 90 feet (25 throws)

120-Foot phase (distance from home plate to second base)

Step 7:
a. Warm-up throwing
b. 120 feet (25 throws)
c. Rest 10-15 minutes
d. Warm-up throwing
e. 120 feet (25 throws)

Step 8:
a. Warm-up throwing
b. 120 feet (25 throws)
c. Rest 10 minutes

Continued

Box A-4 **Progressive Interval Throwing Program—cont'd**

d. Warm-up throwing
e. 120 feet (25 throws)
f. Rest 10 minutes
g. Warm-up throwing
h. 120 feet (25 throws)

150-Foot phase (distance from home plate to grass behind second base)

Step 9:
a. Warm-up throwing
b. 150 feet (25 throws)
c. Rest 10-15 minutes
d. Warm-up throwing
e. 150 feet (25 throws)

Step 10:
a. Warm-up throwing
b. 150 feet (25 throws)
c. Rest 10 minutes
d. Warm-up throwing
e. 150 feet (25 throws)
f. Rest 10 minutes
g. Warm-up throwing
h. 150 feet (25 throws)

180-Foot phase (distance from home plate to the outfield)

Step 11:
a. Warm-up throwing
b. 180 feet (25 throws)
c. Rest 10-15 minutes
d. Warm-up throwing
e. 180 feet (25 throws)

Step 12:
a. Warm-up throwing
b. 180 feet (25 throws)
c. Rest 10 minutes
d. Warm-up throwing
e. 180 feet (25 throws)
f. Rest 10 minutes
g. Warm-up throwing
h. 180 feet (25 throws)

Step 13:
a. Warm-up throwing
b. 180 feet (25 throws)
c. Rest 10 minutes
d. Warm-up throwing
e. 180 feet (25 throws)
f. Rest 10 minutes
g. Warm-up throwing
h. 180 feet (25 throws)

Step 14:
a. Return to position or begin throwing from the mound (see Box 3-1)

(Modified from Wilk KE, Arrigo CA: Interval sport programs for the shoulder. In Andrews JR, Wilk KE, editors: *The athlete's shoulder*, New York, 1994, Churchill Livingstone.)

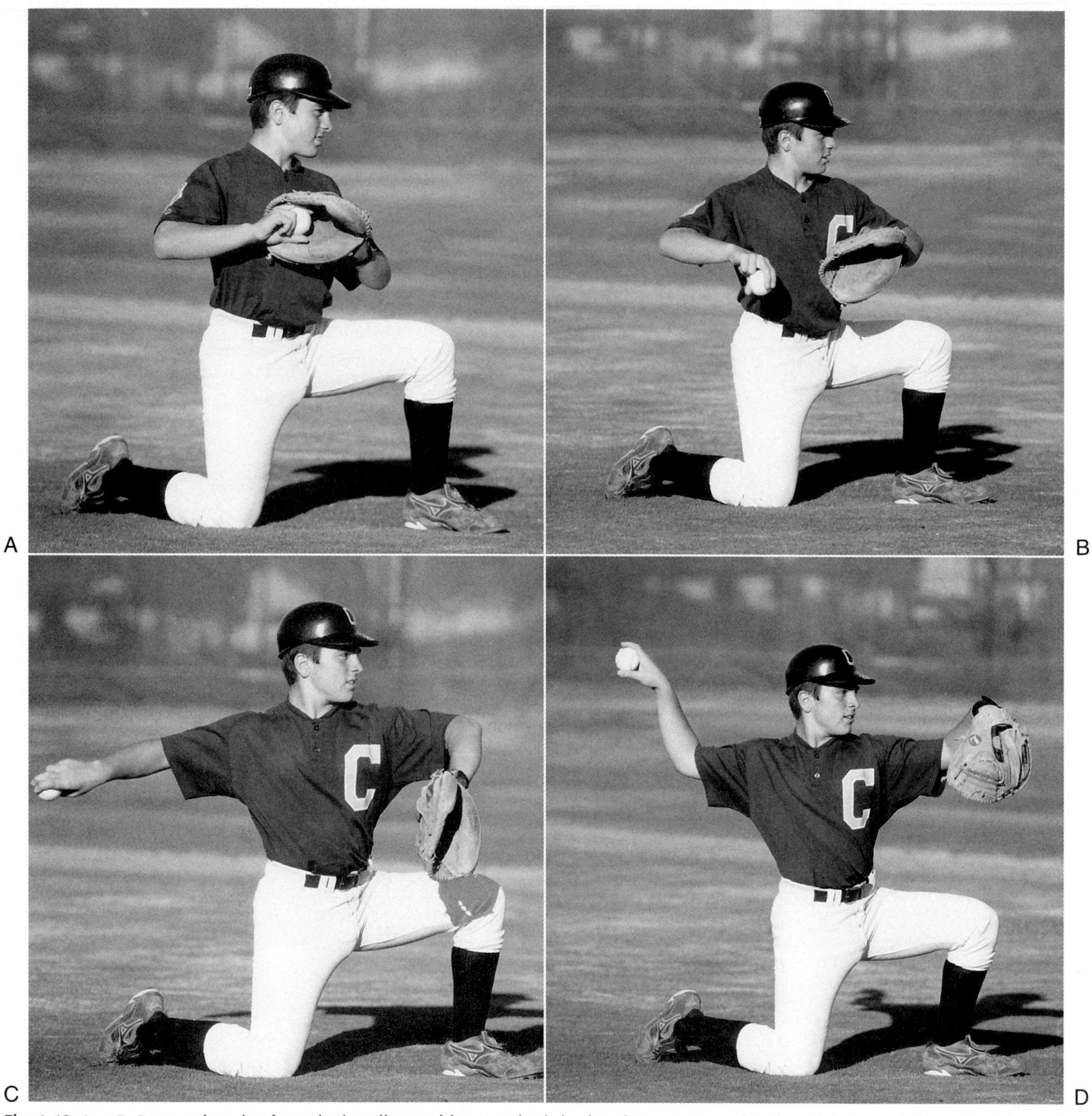

Fig. A-13 A to D, Pattern throwing from the kneeling position. Emphasis is placed on proper positioning of the hand, elbow, shoulder, and trunk throughout the entire throwing motion.
(Photos by Marsha Gorman, Camarillo, CA.)

Continued

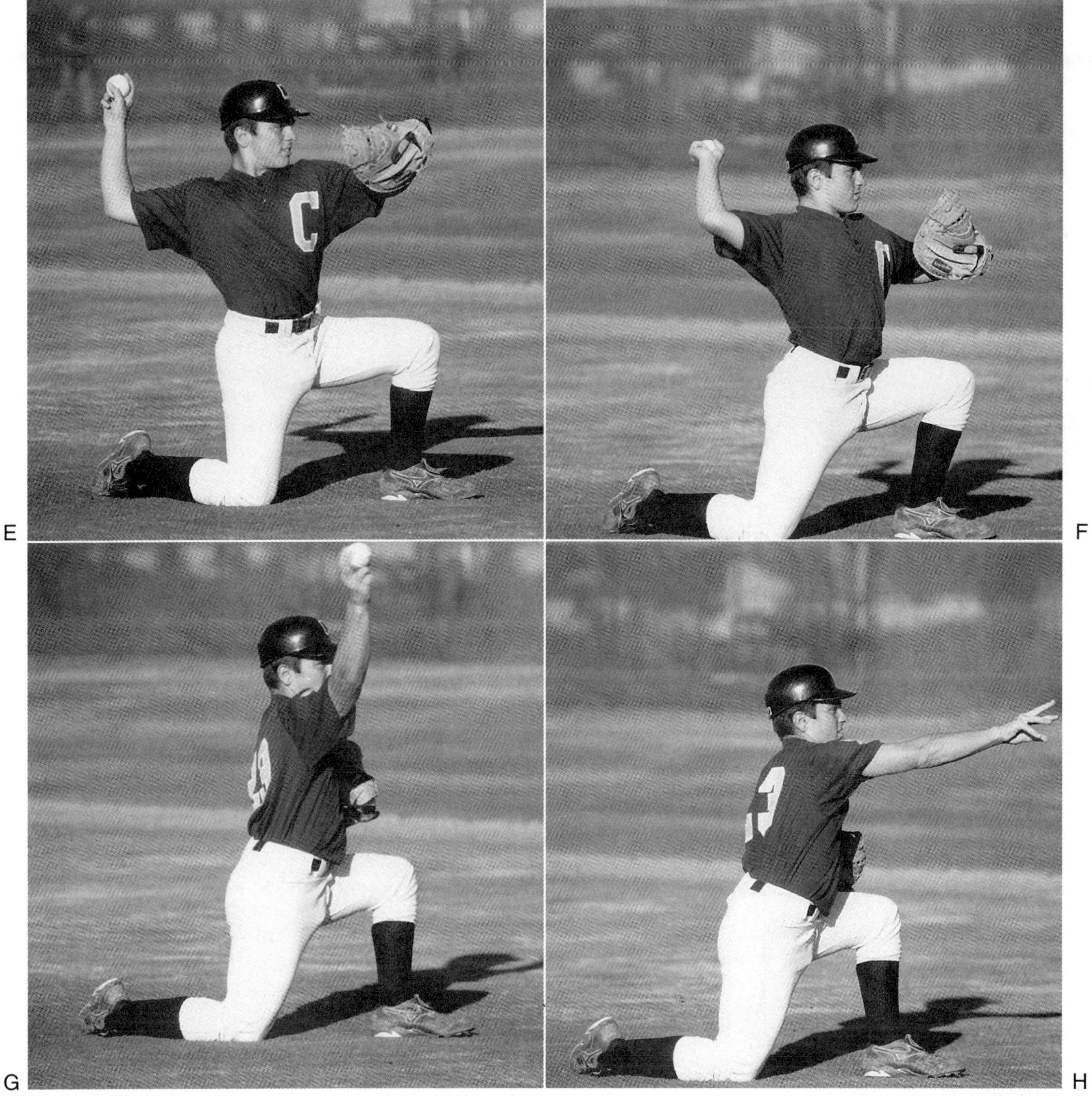

Fig. A-13, cont'd E to H, Pattern throwing from the kneeling position. Emphasis is placed on proper positioning of the hand, elbow, shoulder, and trunk throughout the entire throwing motion.

Continued

(Photos by Marsha Gorman, Camarillo, CA.)

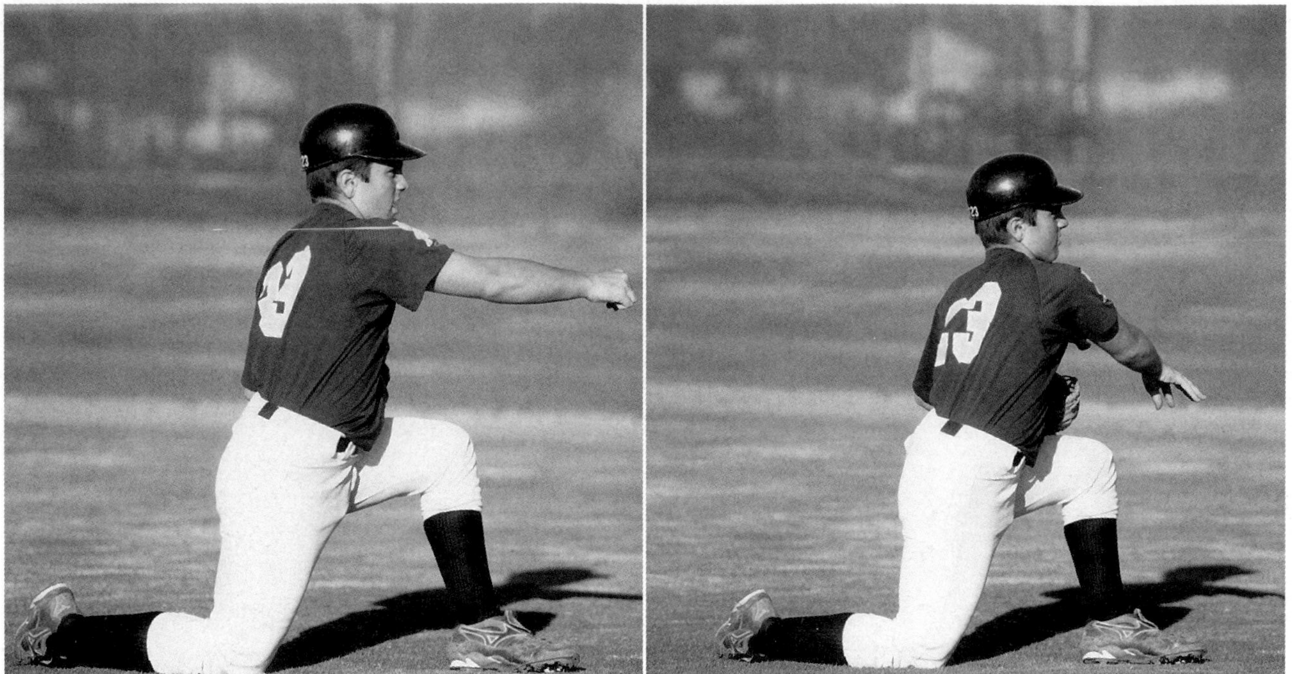

Fig. A-13, cont'd **I** to **J**, Pattern throwing from the kneeling position. Emphasis is placed on proper positioning of the hand, elbow, shoulder, and trunk throughout the entire throwing motion.
(Photos by Marsha Gorman, Camarillo, CA.)

References

1. Adams T: An investigation of selected plyometric training exercises on muscle leg strength and power, *Track Field Q Rev* 84:36, 1984.
2. Astrand P, Rodahl K: *Textbook of work physiology,* New York, 1970, McGraw-Hill.
3. Atwater AE: Biomechanics of overarm throwing movements and of throwing injuries, *Exerc Sport Sci Rev* 7:43, 1979.
4. Broer MR: *Efficiency of human movement,* Philadelphia, 1969, WB Saunders.
5. Browne AO et al: Glenohumeral elevation studied in three dimensions, *J Bone Joint Surg* 72B:843, 1990.
6. Cain PR, Mutschler TA, Fu FH: Anterior instability of the glenohumeral joint: a dynamic model, *Am J Sports Med* 15:144, 1987.
7. Cavagna G, Disman B, Margari R: Positive work done by a previously stretched muscle, *J Appl Physiol* 24:21, 1968.
8. Chu D: Plyometric exercise, *Nat Strength Cond Assoc J* 6:56, 1984.
9. Dickoff-Hoffman SA: Neuromuscular control exercises for shoulder instability. In Andrews JR, Wilk KE, editors: *The athlete's shoulder,* New York, 1994, Churchill Livingstone.
10. DiGiovine N et al: An electromyographic analysis of the upper extremity in pitching, *J Shoulder Elbow Surg* 1(1):15, 1992.
11. Feltner M, Dapena J: Dynamics of the shoulder and elbow joints of the throwing arm during a baseball pitch, *Int J Sports Biomech* 2:235, 1986.
12. DeVries HA: *Physiology of exercise for physical education and athletics,* Dubuque, IA, 1974, WC Brown.
13. Ferrari D: Capsular ligaments of the shoulder anatomical and functional study to the anterior superior capsule, *Am J Sports Med* 18(1):20, 1990.
14. Fleisig GS, Dillman CJ, Andrews JR: *A biomechanical description of the shoulder joint during pitching,* symposium on clinical biomechanics of the shoulder, ACSM Annual Meeting, Dallas, May 1992.
15. Fleisig GS et al: Kinematic and kinetic comparison between baseball pitching and football passing, *J Appl Biomech* 12:207, 1993.
16. Franks BD: Physical warm up. In Morgan WP, editor: *Ergogenic aids and muscular performance,* Orlando, FL, 1972, Academic Press.
17. Gainor BJ et al: The throw: biomechanics and acute injury, *Am J Sports Med* 8:114, 1980.
18. Gambetta V: Conditioning of the shoulder complex. In Andrews JR, Wilk KE, editors: *The athlete's shoulder,* New York, 1994, Churchill Livingstone.
19. Jobe FW et al: *Shoulder and arm exercises for the athlete who throws,* Inglewood, CA, 1996, Champion Press.
20. Lundin PE: A review of plyometrics, *Nat Strength Cond Assoc J* 7:65, 1985.
21. McArdle WD, Katch FL, Katch VL: *Exercise physiology: energy, nutrition, and human performance,* Philadelphia, 1981, Lea & Febiger.
22. Newton R: Joint receptor contributions to reflexive and kinesthetic responses, *Phys Ther* 62:22, 1982.
23. Pappas AM, Zawaki RM, Sullivan TJ: Biomechanics of baseball pitching, a preliminary report, *Am J Sports Med* 13:216, 1985.

24. Payton OD, Hirt S, Newton RA: *Scientific bases for neurophysiologic approaches to therapeutic exercise,* Philadelphia, 1972, FA Davis.
25. Perry J: Anatomy & biomechanics of the shoulder in throwing, swimming, gymnastics, and tennis, *Clin Sports Med* 2:247, 1973.
26. Scoles G: Depth jumping-does it really work? *Athletic J* 58:48, 1978.
27. Siewert MW et al: Isokinetic torque changes based on lever arm placement, *Phys Ther* 65:715, 1985.
28. Smith RL, Brunolli J: Shoulder kinesthesia after anterior glenohumeral dislocation, *Phys Ther* 69:106, 1989.
29. Toyoshima S et al: The contribution of the body parts to throwers performance. In Nelson R, Morehouse C, editors: *Biomechanics IV,* Baltimore, 1974, University Press.
30. Verkhoshanski Y: Perspectives in the improvement of speed-strength preparation of jumpers, *Yessis Rev Soviet Phys Educ Sports* 4:28, 1969.
31. Wilk KE, Arrigo CA: Interval sport programs for the shoulder. In Andrews JR, Wilk KE, editors: *The athlete's shoulder,* New York, 1994, Churchill Livingstone.
32. Wilk KE, Voight ML: Plyometrics for the shoulder complex. In Andrews JR, Wilk KE, editors: *The athlete's shoulder,* New York, 1994, Churchill Livingstone.
33. Wilt F: Plyometrics what it is and how it works, *Athletic J* 55:76, 1995.

APPENDIX B

Transitioning the Jumping Athlete Back to the Court

Christine M. Prelaz

INTRODUCTION

Lower extremity (LE) injuries are prevalent in athletics. These injuries can range from minor sprains or strains to those that result in significant functional limitation and loss of time from work, sport, or both.[28] An estimated 3 to 5 million injuries occur each year among recreational and competitive athletes in the United States.[28] The worldwide annual cost of sports injuries has been estimated at one billion dollars.[31] The National Collegiate Athletic Association (NCAA) reported that the ankle, knee, and lower leg were the most common injury sites among collegiate soccer, field hockey, basketball, and lacrosse athletes in 2000 to 2001.[31] Research studies indicate that both intrinsic and extrinsic factors play a role.[2,31] Recent attention in the literature has focused on the higher incidence of anterior cruciate ligament (ACL) tears in females than in males. Many factors have been suggested, such as ACL thickness, a narrower notch width, hormonal influences, differences in quadriceps and hamstring firing patterns, and landing kinematics. Given the frequency and cost of these injuries, the clinician is challenged to restore the function of these individuals as expediently and as safely as possible.

PROGRAM

Numerous protocols exist for both conservative management and surgical procedures. Each clinician has his or her unique approach to the rehabilitation and surgical management of each specific athletic injury. A survey of current practices in ACL reconstruction by the American Orthopedic Society for Sports Medicine showed that rehabilitation protocols were the most variable factor among other factors that were surveyed.[18] These other factors included weight bearing, immobilization, bracing, length of physical therapy, and when to return to sport. Whatever the injury, a team approach consisting of close communication between the physician, physical therapist (PT), athletic trainer, and other medical specialists should provide the best environment for returning the athlete to sport. The clinician must keep in mind the structures involved, surgical procedures, surgeon's preferences, and healing constraints. It is beyond the scope of this appendix to outline a program for each specific sport or injury. It is the author's goal to provide guidelines, ideas, and resources for returning the jumping athlete back to his or her respective sport successfully and safely.

Readiness to Prepare for Return

Regardless of the injury or surgical procedure, it is the clinician's responsibility to determine the athlete's level of readiness to progress to each phase of rehabilitation. Factors to consider are type and extent of injury, surgical procedure, pain levels, swelling, range of motion (ROM), strength, endurance, flexibility, patient goals, and psychologic readiness. The length of time to return is dependent on these factors. For example, average return to sport after ACL reconstruction is 6 months; a grade II ankle sprain should be able to move through the rehabilitation phase much more quickly; an Achilles tendon repair may be longer.

Goals of the Training Program

Individual goals must be set for each athlete, depending on his or her current functional level, the level of competition he or she is returning to, and the type of sport. In general, the goals of the training program are to restore or improve flexibility, endurance, strength, balance, and agility. A needs analysis of the demands of the sport and an evaluation of the current level of the athlete can assist in establishing specific goals.

Sport-specific training is fundamental in returning the athlete back to his or her respective sport. The same program may also improve sports performance in those without injury. The rehabilitation program should incorporate a whole-body approach, including core strengthening and exercises for the noninjured extremity.

Flexibility

Controversy exists in the literature regarding static stretching.[15] Little evidence indicates that static stretching prevents injury; in fact, pre-exercise static stretching may actually negatively affect performance.[40] Some researchers found decreases in muscle strength[23] and decreases in jumping ability after passive stretching.[14] Shrier[40] contends that regular stretching as part of a comprehensive program (and not before) exercise can increase force, jump height, and speed. The athlete can also perform dynamic stretching by using sport-specific movements. **Ballistic stretching involves bouncing types of movement and is not typically recommended, especially for those who have had prior injury. Despite some of the controversy, most still advocate stretching as part of a comprehensive program (Box B-1).**

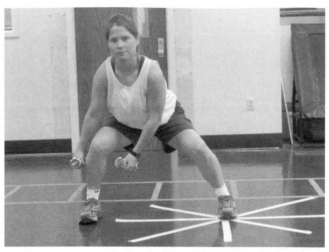

Fig. B-1 Example of closed-chain strengthening (multiangle lunges).

Strength and Endurance

Muscle strength is defined as "the greatest force that can be put forth by a muscle; it is measured with isometric, isokinetic, or isotonic exercises."[19] Before starting any training program, it is important to have a full understanding of the demands of the sport (as well as the individual athlete) to develop a needs analysis. A needs analysis will enable the clinician to design a comprehensive specific program to develop strength, endurance, power, speed, agility, and balance.

Special considerations must be given to an injured athlete with regards to strengthening. Rehabilitation of knee injuries in particular, has presented the clinician with a challenge. For example, one of the main goals of rehabilitation after ACL reconstruction is to restore LE strength while protecting the reconstructed graft and the patellofemoral (PF) joint from excessive stresses. Selective quadriceps muscle atrophy occurs after injury, immobilization, or both. Shelbourne, Whitaker, and McCarrol[39] reported strength deficits in the quadriceps of up to 10% at an average follow-up of 4 years after ACL surgery. Debate exists regarding the use of open kinetic chain versus closed kinetic chain exercises to build quadriceps strength. Several authors have advocated the use of both after ACL reconstruction.[17,30] *A literature review by Ross, Denegar, and Winzenried*[37] *on open kinetic chain versus closed kinetic chain exercises after ACL reconstruction indicates that the greatest amount of ACL strain and PF joint stress occurs at approximately 40 degrees of knee flexion to full extension.*[5,41] It was therefore recommended that open kinetic chain exercises for quadriceps strengthening be performed with knee angles greater than 40 degrees to avoid excessive stress on these structures.[41] The clinician must be aware of the physician's philosophy before implementing the use of open-chain exercises. Closed-chain activities beyond 60 degrees were to be avoided because maximum stress on the PF joint occurs between 60 and 90 degrees of flexion (Fig. B-1).

Because of the predominant atrophy of type I (slow twitch) muscle fibers after injury or immobilization, high repetitions (6 to 10 sets, 12 to 15 repetitions) with low resistance is recommended early in the rehabilitation program.[37] Establishing normal muscle balance for both involved and uninvolved limbs is one of the primary goals. A comprehensive strength-training program should address core, hip, calf, and ankle musculature, as well as establish appropriate quadriceps-to-hamstring ratios.

Box B-1 Flexibility

General Guidelines for Static Stretching
- Initial warm-up
- Stretch slowly, no bouncing
- Stretch until mild tension is felt, not painful
- Hold each stretch 20-30 seconds
- Repeat 2-3 times for each muscle group

Major Muscle Groups to Stretch
- Hamstrings
- Iliotibial band (ITB)
- Gastrocnemius and soleus complex
- Quadriceps
- Low back
- Hip flexors
- Deltoid
- Pectorals/biceps
- Latissimus/triceps

Box B-2 Strengthening

Guidelines: High repetitions, low resistance (4-6 sets of 12-15 repetitions for lower extremity [LE] exercises in early rehabilitation phases). Upper extremity (UE) and core strengthening can follow standard strengthening guidelines. Combinations of traditional and functional training techniques should be used.

- Open kinetic chain knee extension 90-45 degrees (as per physician and clinician philosophy)
- Closed kinetic chain exercises 0-60 degrees
  - Total gym squats (double leg, single leg)
  - Leg press (double leg, single leg)
  - Mini-squats (double leg, single leg) with proper form and control
  - Lunges (multidirectional [weights, sport cord, cable column resistance])
  - Forward/backward/lateral step
- Hamstrings
- Hip abductors/adductors
- Calf raises (bent and straight knee)
- Core strengthening (abdominals, hip musculature, low back)
- Upper body
  - Chest
  - Deltoids
  - Latissimus/posterior shoulder
  - Biceps/triceps

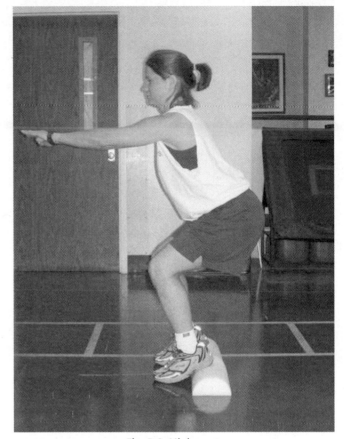

Fig. B-2 Mini-squat.

Strengthening of the hamstrings using both closed- and open-chain methods is important because of their role in assisting in the control of anterior tibial translation. Traditional and functional techniques can be incorporated for both variety and effectiveness (Box B-2 and Figs. B-2 and B-3).

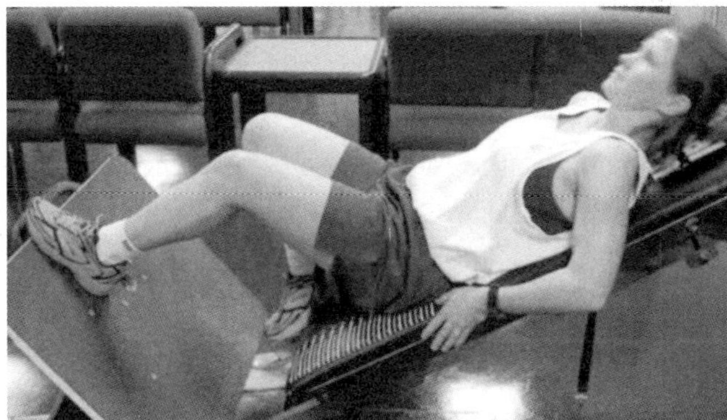

Fig. B-3 Single-leg squat on the Total Gym.

Plyometrics

General Principles

Plyometric exercises use the stretch-shortening cycle (SSC) to store potential energy. The SSC consists of the eccentric phase where preloading occurs as the muscle is placed on stretch, thus storing potential energy. The amortization phase refers to the time period between the eccentric and concentric contraction. The amortization phase must be kept short. The longer it is, the greater the loss of stored energy. The final phase is the concentric phase, in which the stored energy is used in an opposite reaction (i.e., the muscle contracts concentrically to provide the force necessary for the required movement).[29]

When designing a plyometric training program, consideration must be given to age, body weight, current strength and conditioning level, experience, previous injury, and demands of the sport (Box B-3).[29,12]

Warm-Up and Cooldown

Warm-up exercises can consist of a combination of general and specific skill enhancement drills such as marching, skipping, shuffling, and footwork drills.[12] Static and dynamic stretching should also be performed.

Proper Technique

Proper instruction and monitoring of technique is critical not only for proper neuromuscular retraining but also to avoid injury. Verbal, visual, and manual cues may be used

Box B-3 **Plyometrics**

Plyometrics guidelines:

- Proper footwear
- Resilient surface
- Sturdy, safe equipment
- Sufficient and safe training area
- Proper control and technique for all drills before progressing!
- Warm-up: Static and dynamic stretching; skipping, marching, bounding
- Frequency: 2-3 times a week, depending on intensity and other program components
- Volume:
  - Beginner—60-100 foot contacts
  - Intermediate—100-150 foot contacts
  - Advanced—120-200 foot contacts
  - Elite—200-400
- Intensity: Low, medium, high (decrease volume as intensity increases)
- Recovery: 30 seconds to 3 minutes between repetitions (depending on intensity level) Allow 48-72 hours between training sessions.
- Direction: Choose drills that are sport specific for enhancing vertical, horizontal, lateral, or combinations or directions

Progression:

Basic Guidelines	Level of Difficulty Progression
◆ Start simple, progress to complex	◆ Jumps in place
◆ Low volume to higher volume	◆ Standing jumps
◆ General drills progressing to sport-specific exercises	◆ Multiple hops/jumps
◆ Bilateral to unilateral exercises	◆ Bounding/cone drills
◆ Stable to unstable surfaces	◆ Box/depth jumps
Slow speed to faster speeds	

(From Nutting M: Practical progressions for upper body plyometric training, *NSCA Performance Training Journal* 3(2):14-19, 2004.)

to teach the athlete proper control. If the athlete fails to demonstrate proper control during any part of the exercise, then he or she should be stopped and given a brief rest period before continuing. If improper technique is still present, then the exercise should be discontinued for that session. Explaining and reinforcing the importance of proper technique to the athlete will help to prevent overuse and injury during the training program.

Frequency

One to three sessions per week are adequate. Two sessions is the norm for most off-season sports programs.[1] Frequency should be determined by the intensity of the sessions and the phase of rehabilitation or cycle in the sport season.

Volume

Volume is expressed in number of foot contacts per workout. Volume should be 60 to 100 foot contacts for beginners, 100 to 150 for intermediate-level workouts, and 120 to 200 for advanced off-season workouts.[12] If intensity is high, then volume should be low to medium. Volume may also be expressed as a specific distance.[1] The number of contacts should be adjusted down for younger, inexperienced, or postinjury individuals. Elite athletes may perform 200 to 400 foot contacts.[29]

Intensity

Intensity refers to the amount of stress on the tissues during the plyometric activity (Box B-4). It can be classified as low (Figs. B-4 and B-5), medium, or high (Fig. B-6). **In general, as intensity increases, volume should decrease. Athletes weighing more than 220 lb should not perform depth jumps from heights greater than 18 inches.**[29]

Progression

Adequate strength and conditioning levels should be present before the athlete can progress. It is recommended that the athlete be able to squat 1.5 times body weight before starting shock types of plyometric training such as depth jumps.[10] Progression should be based on a current evaluation of the athlete, the establishment of sport-specific goals, attainment of proper technique and control, and the absence of any signs or symptoms of overuse. In general, the following progression guidelines are suggested to avoid overtraining and to prevent injury during the plyometric program:[33]

- Start with simple drills and progress to complex
- Low volume progressing to high volume
- General to specific drills and exercises
- Bilateral to unilateral exercises
- Use of stable before unstable surfaces

Box B-4 Plyometric Exercise Examples

Low Intensity	Medium Intensity	High Intensity
◆ Prancing, galloping, skipping, marching ◆ Skipping rope ◆ Wall jumps ◆ Squat jump ◆ Two-foot ankle hop ◆ Side, forward/backward hops ◆ Dot drill (double leg) ◆ Broad jump	◆ Tuck jump ◆ Split-squat jump ◆ Scissor jump ◆ Barrier jumps (forward/backward, lateral) ◆ Single-leg hop ◆ Dot drill (single leg) ◆ Bounding ◆ Double-leg diagonal barrier jumps ◆ Single-leg dot drills ◆ Hip-twist ankle hops ◆ 180-degree twist	◆ Single-leg triple jump and stick ◆ Single-leg diagonal jumps ◆ Single-leg vertical power jump ◆ Single-leg tuck jump **Shock** ◆ Depth jumps ◆ Box jumps

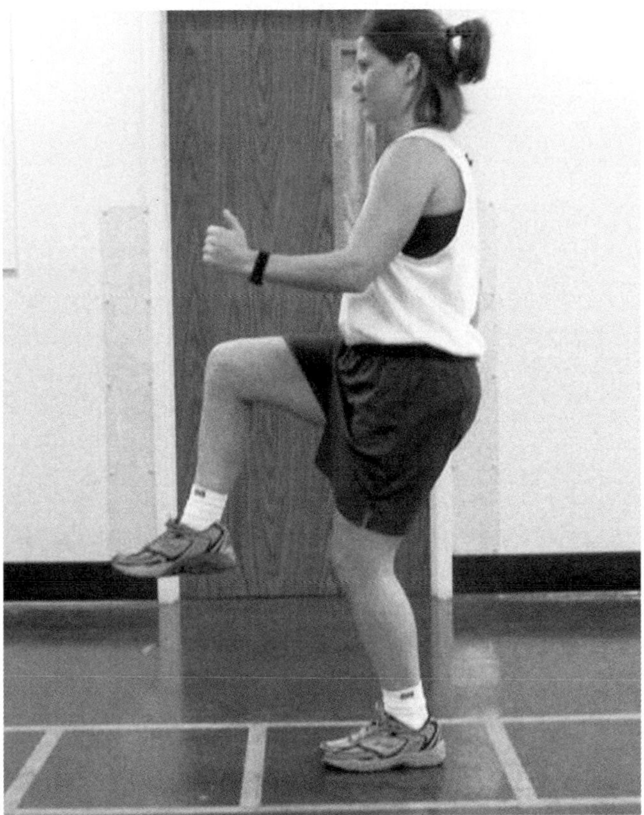

Fig. B-4 Marching (low-intensity plyometric exercise).

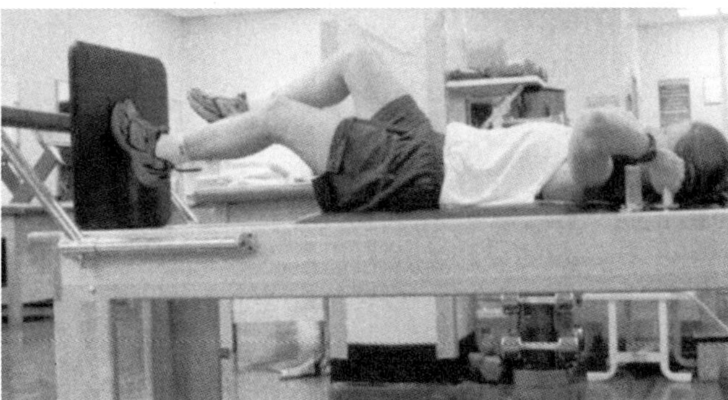

Fig. B-5 Simulated jumping on the Pilates Reformer (low-intensity plyometric exercise).

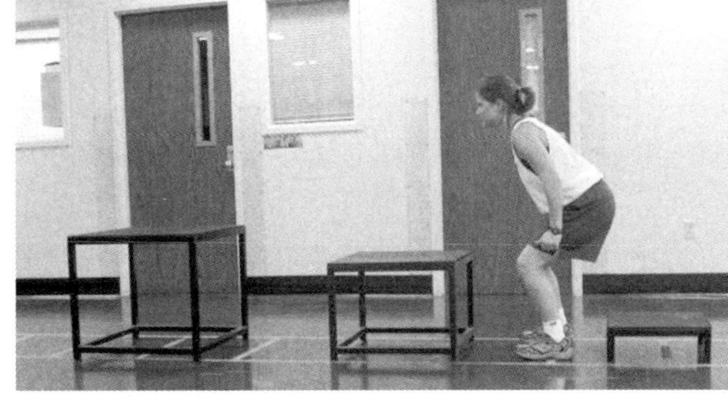

Fig. B-6 Box jumps (high-intensity plyometric drill).

- Slow speed to faster speeds
- Low height to higher height

Recovery

Adequate recovery time must be given between repetitions and sets, as well between workout sessions. Plyometrics are not intended to be an aerobic conditioning workout. Rest time between repetitions and sets is dependent on the intensity of the exercise and the individual. Allow 30 seconds up to 3 minutes for recovery.[29] Plyometric sessions should not be performed on consecutive days. In general, plyometric workouts should allow 48 to 72 hours between sessions.[13]

Direction of Motion

A needs analysis should determine if the sport requires speed and power in a vertical plane, horizontal plane, lateral or diagonal directions, or a combination. Most sports require a combination of directions. Drills that specifically enhance the required components of the sport should be chosen for the program. Proper technique and control is crucial before progressing to the next level!

Speed and Agility

Agility is the ability to rapidly change body direction, to accelerate, or to decelerate. It is influenced by balance, strength, coordination, and skill level. The athlete can improve agility by first developing an adequate base of strength and conditioning that is appropriate for his or her difficulty level. After this is achieved, drills designed to enhance reactive and explosive motor skills can be progressively incorporated (Figs. B-7 and B-8).

Guidelines for speed and agility training are as follows:

- Allow adequate warm-up.
- The athlete should have an appropriate strength and conditioning base for the selected drills.
- Speed and agility should be performed early in the training session or preferably on separate days to maximize training effect, avoid fatigue, and prevent overuse.
- Allow adequate rest between sets and repetitions. Heart rate and respiration should return to almost normal levels after the drill. A 1:4-6 work-to-rest ratio is recommended.[10]
- The number of sessions per week may vary, depending on the sport, the individual's current level, history of injury, intensity of the drill, and period of the mesocycle. Two times a week can be used as a general rule.
- Exercise volume is two to five sets of each exercise.
- The therapist should stress quality not quantity.

Box B-5 lists various speed and agility drills. This list provides examples only; the reader may wish to refer to specific resources on speed, agility, and plyometric training

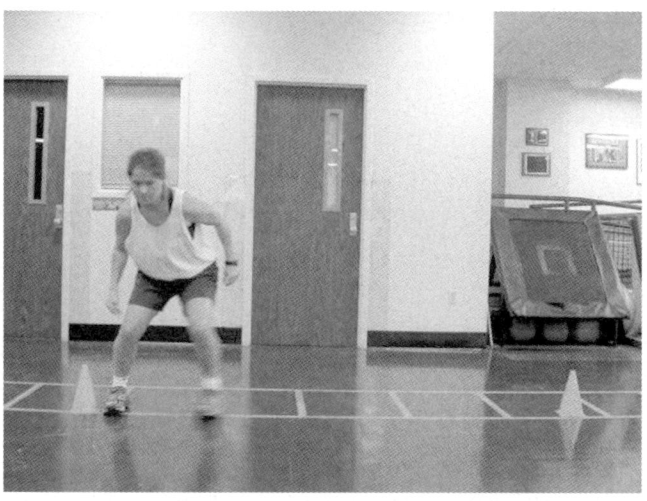

Fig. B-7 Lateral shuffles (agility drill).

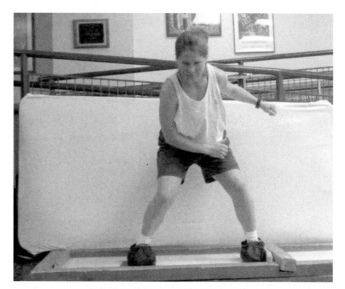

Fig. B-8 Slide board (agility drill).

Box B-5 Speed and Agility

Speed and Agility Guidelines	Speed and Agility Exercise Examples
◆ Adequate strength/conditioning base	◆ High knees
◆ Warm-up	◆ Glut kickers
◆ Perform early in training session, preferably on separate days	◆ Resisted running drills
◆ Allow adequate rest between sets and repetitions (1:4-6 work-to-rest ratio is recommended)	◆ Step hurdles
◆ Number of sessions per week may vary; two times per week can be used as a general rule	◆ Foot tapping
◆ Volume: 2-5 sets of 3-5 exercises (15 seconds progressing to 30 seconds or measured in distance)	◆ Shuttle run
◆ Emphasize quality not quantity	◆ Ladder drills
	◆ Carioca
	◆ Lateral shuffle
	◆ Side-to-side box shuffle
	◆ Directional mirror drills
	◆ *T* drill
	◆ 5 Dot drill (double leg, single leg)
	◆ Figure eights with cones

for a more comprehensive list and description of drills.[8,10,12,35]

Balance and Proprioception

Balance is accomplished by the regulation of three systems: (1) the somatosensory (proprioceptive) system, (2) the visual system, and (3) the vestibular system. Stability is achieved by continuous feedback to the central nervous system from the integration of input from these three systems. The somatosensory system uses several different types of sensory input from proprioceptors and the sensory nerve terminals found in muscles, tendons, and joint capsules. Proprioceptors relay information relating to movement and position sense. The muscle spindle and Golgi tendon organs detect stretch or tension. Information supplied from these receptors is relayed to the cerebellum and cortex via the somatosensory system.

The vestibular system is an intricate system that monitors changes in head position. It detects linear acceleration and angular movement of the head. Vestibular input occurs through the semicircular canals, otoliths, and hair cells located in the inner ear. This sensory information is relayed to the vestibular nuclei and to the cerebellum to help regulate balance.

Visual input received in the cortex and vestibular nuclei provides information for the vestibular and somatosensory systems to make adjustments to maintain stability and balance. Neuromuscular control is the ability to produce controlled movement through coordinated muscle activity.[45] Dynamic joint stability is the ability of the joint to remain stable under the rapidly changing loads during activity.[45] After injury, neuromuscular control, proprioception, and joint position sense can be damaged. Neuromuscular training programs aimed at enhancing or restoring neuromuscular control and proprioception after injury can be found in the literature.* These programs typically incorporate a multilevel approach, which includes combinations of strength training, flexibility, balance, and plyometric exercises. To enhance both static and dynamic balance, training should include stationary and dynamic surfaces such as wobble boards, balance beams, and foam pads. Functional training such as jumping and landing, agility, and perturbation training are also used. Figures B-9 to B-12 illustrate a few examples of balance exercises.

Returning to Sport

As previously stated, the goal of the rehabilitation program is to return the athlete to the highest functional level. Rehabilitation programs are based on current scientific principles that include knowledge of the healing

*References 11, 20, 24, 25, 36.

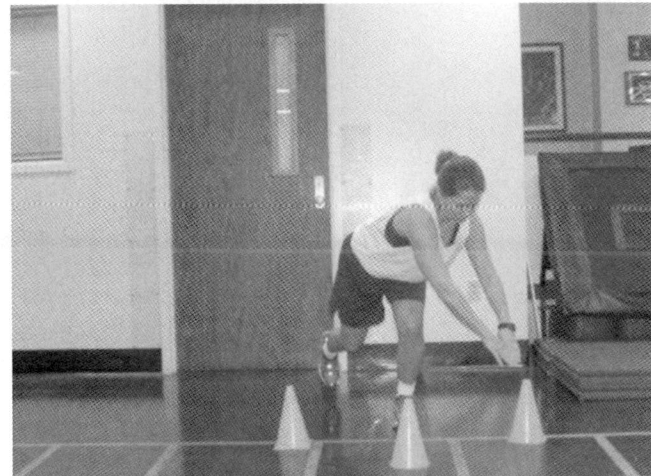

Fig. B-9 Cone reaches (balance exercise).

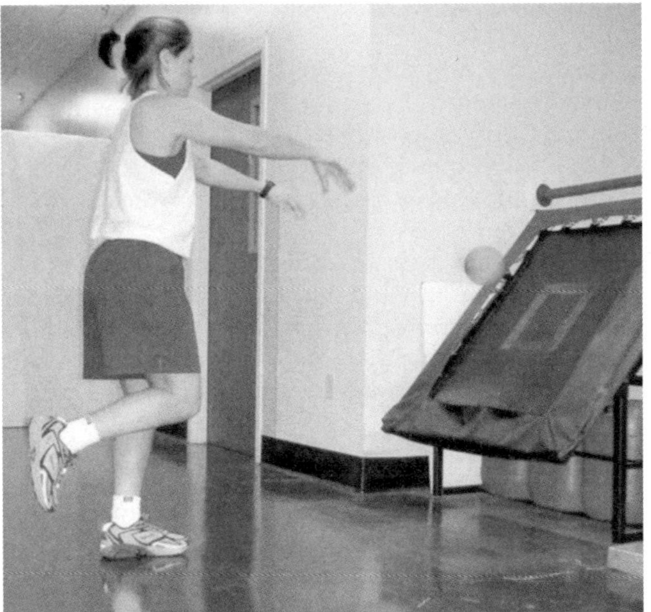

Fig. B-10 Plyotoss (balance and proprioception drill).

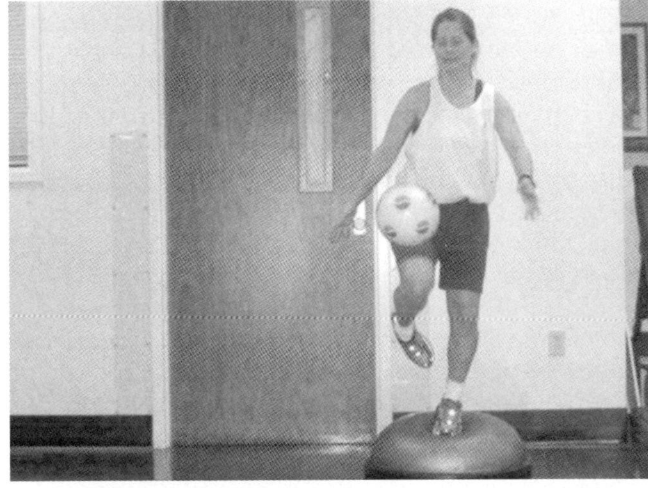

Fig. B-11 Functional activity incorporated with balance (on a BOSU balance trainer).

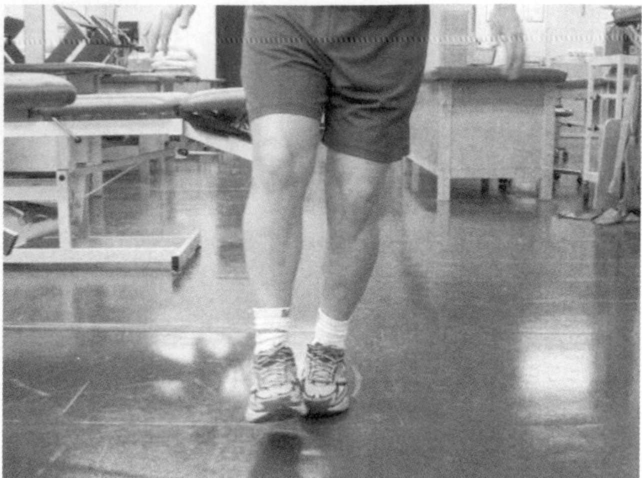

Fig. B-12 Four-way leg kicks (balance and proprioception).

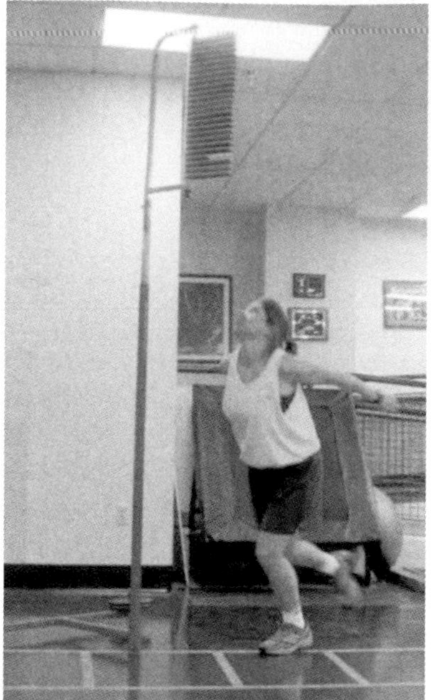

Fig. B-13 Vertical jump test.

process, anatomy, physiology, biomechanics, and kinematics. Typically, return to sport is based on various subjective and objective criteria. Many clinicians have either developed their own compilation of tests or have adopted those used by others to determine when an athlete is ready to return to sport.

Single-leg hop tests are commonly used to determine an athlete's progress in his or her rehabilitation program and determine the readiness to return to sport. Various single-leg hop tests either used alone or in combination have been described in the literature.* These tests include single-leg hop and stop tests,[27] single-leg hop for distance and time, triple hop, and the triple crossover hop.† Several studies have shown these tests to be reliable with intraclass coefficients between 0.66 to 0.97.[3,7,9] Barber and colleagues[22] recommended using at least two hop tests and achieving a limb symmetry score of 85%.

Other test measures have been used to determine return to sport as well. Vertical jump height and isokinetic testing have been used to assess function and strength (Fig. B-13).[6,34] A one repetition maximum (RM) leg press test or squat can also be used to assess strength. The shuttle run and figure-eight run have been used to test the ability to run, cut, and pivot.[4,42,43] The *t*-test and the Edgren Side Step Test are two tests that can be used to assess agility and body control (Fig. B-14).[38] These tests can also be used in the rehabilitation program as functional drills. Speed is typically assessed with a sprint test of a designated distance, which may depend on the specific sport. Speed tests measure the body's displacement per unit of time. Testing speed for clinical purposes is usually limited because of lack of appropriate space. Standard health and fitness tests for flexibility, local endurance, aerobic power, and agility and speed, such as those described in *The Essentials of Strength and Conditioning*,[38] may also be incorporated into the testing protocol and compared with available normative data.

Davies[16] has developed a functional testing algorithm that uses a systematic functional progression of testing and exercise. It is designed to progressively increase stresses on the patient while gradually lessening clinical control. The algorithm includes the following: subjective information, basic measurements, KT 1000 test, balance testing, closed- and open-chain strength testing, two-leg jump test, unilateral hop test, lower extremity functional test (LEFT), and sports-specific testing.[16] Very specific criterion must be met before the athlete is allowed to progress to the next level. Frequent testing and monitoring of the patient allows the clinician to always know the status of that patient. A specific rehabilitation program can then be designed to address individual deficits instead of following a preset clinical protocol.

Recent research by Hewett and associates[26] has focused on biomechanical loading measurements in female athletes in an attempt to predict those who are at risk for ACL injury. They concluded that increased valgus motion and valgus movements at the knee were key predictors for potential ACL injury. If predictive factors associated with LE injuries can be identified, then specific screening programs and training programs could potentially be designed to reduce the risk for injury.

In general, no standard accepted series of tests is available to determine when an athlete is ready to return safely to sport. The decision should be based on ROM, strength, symptomatology, and functional testing. Box B-6 provides

*References 4, 21, 27, 32, 44.

†References 4, 21, 22, 27, 32, 44.

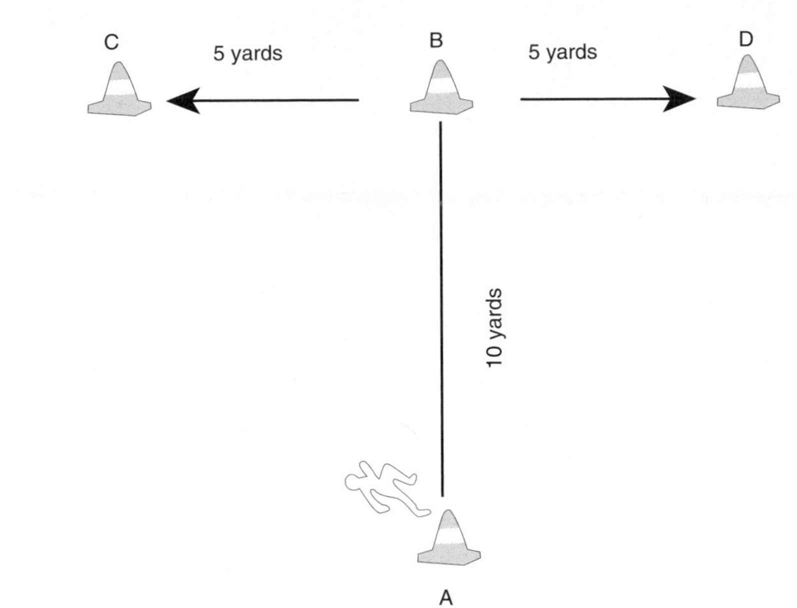

Equipment: four cones, stopwatch, adequate space

Testing Procedure:

- Arrange the four cones in a "T" formation as seen in the figure above
- Athlete should perform adequate warm-up and stretching prior to testing
- The athlete starts at point A
- On "GO," the athlete sprints to point B, touches the base of the cone with the right hand → shuffles to the left 5 yards and touches the base of the cone at point C with the left hand → shuffles to the right 10 yards and touches the base of the cone at point D with the right hand → shuffles to the left, touches the base of the cone at point B with the left hand → then runs backward past point A. The timer stops the watch as the athlete passes point A
- Complete 2 trials, recording the best trial time
  shufflin, fails to face front at all times, or demonstrates poor control
- Disqualification occurs if the athlete does not touch the base of the cone, crosses the feet when shuffling, fails to face front at all times, or demonstrates poor control.

Resource: Semenick[43]

Fig. B-14 *T*-test.

Box B-6 Return to Sport

Assessment	Criterion for Return to Sport

◆ Range of motion (ROM)
◆ Self-report scores (optional): Lysholm, Knee Outcome Survey, International Knee Documentation Committee, Cincinnati Knee Rating Scale
◆ Strength: 1 RM leg press, squat test, isokinetics
◆ Stability: Manual tests, KT-1000
◆ Functional tests:
  ◆ Vertical jump
  ◆ Hop tests (single-leg hop for distance, triple hop for distance, single-leg hop for time over 6 m, crossover hop)
  ◆ Agility/body control: *t*-test, Edgren Side Step Test, shuttle run
	◆ No complaints of pain
	◆ No effusion
	◆ Full and pain-free ROM
	◆ Strength deficit ≥10% compared with uninvolved side
	◆ Functional test score ≥10% deficit compared with uninvolved side (must demonstrate good technique and control)

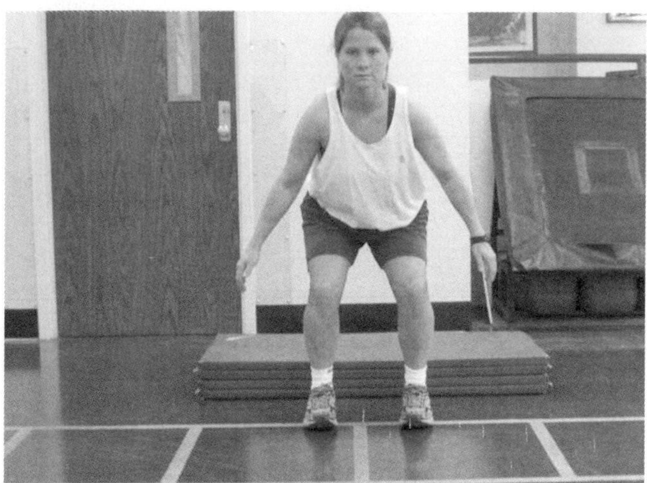

Fig. B-15 Proper landing form.

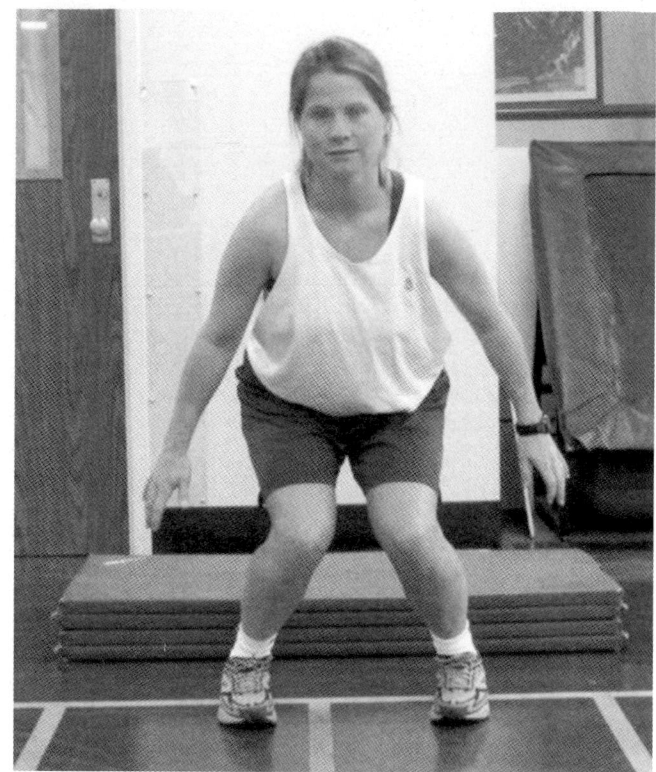

Fig. B-16 Improper landing form.

a list of tests that the clinician may select to assist in the decision. It is recommended that a minimum of two hop tests,[4] a strength assessment, and an agility and body control test be used. The athlete must demonstrate proper form and technique throughout the test procedures (Figs. B-15 and B-16). A deficit of 10% or less with good control is currently used in many facilities to allow return to sport. The tests have obvious limitations; however, they appear to be the most commonly used in various combinations. Further research is needed not only to determine risk factors but also to determine what testing procedures would be best to predict safe return to sport.

SUMMARY

Returning the jumping athlete back to sport as safely and efficiently as possible is the primary goal of the rehabilitation program. The length of time to return depends on many factors. It is the clinician's responsibility to have the scientific knowledge base and clinical skills to determine when and how the athlete is to progress through the program. Current testing procedures have their limitations; however, they provide some objective data to assist the clinician in deciding when the athlete may resume sport activities. It is impossible to design one rehabilitation protocol for all athletes lest it be a "cookbook" approach. Because it was the author's intention to provide guidelines, ideas, and resources for returning the jumping athlete back to sport in this appendix, Box B-7 details only one example of how the various training components can be combined.

Box B-7 **Example Program**

	Weeks 1-3	Weeks 4-6	Weeks 5-8
Monday	◆ Strengthening ◆ Upper-body plyometrics ◆ Core strength ◆ Cardio	◆ Strengthening ◆ Upper-body plyometrics ◆ Core strength ◆ Cardio	◆ Strengthening ◆ Upper-body plyometrics ◆ Core strength ◆ Cardio
Tuesday	◆ Low-intensity plyometrics (4 drills) ◆ Agility ◆ Cardio	◆ 2 low-intensity, 2 medium-intensity plyometric drills ◆ Progress to 4 medium-intensity plyometric drills ◆ Agility ◆ Sport-specific drills ◆ Cardio	◆ 2 medium-intensity plyometric drills, 2 high-intensity plyometric drills ◆ Progress to 4 high-intensity drills ◆ Agility ◆ Sport-specific drills ◆ Cardio
Wednesday	◆ Strength training ◆ Upper-body plyometrics ◆ Core strength	◆ Strength training ◆ Upper-body plyometrics ◆ Core strength	◆ Strength training ◆ Upper-body plyometrics ◆ Core strength
Thursday	◆ Low-intensity plyometrics (4 drills) ◆ Agility ◆ Cardio	◆ 2 low-intensity, 2 medium-intensity plyometric drills ◆ Progress to 4 medium-intensity plyometric drills ◆ Agility ◆ Sport-specific drills	◆ 2 medium- intensity plyometric drills, 2 high-intensity plyometric drills ◆ Progress to 4 high-intensity drills ◆ Agility ◆ Sport-specific drills ◆ Cardio
Friday	◆ Strength training ◆ Core strength ◆ Cardio	◆ Strength training ◆ Core strength ◆ Cardio	◆ Strength training ◆ Core strength ◆ Cardio

References

1. Allerheiligen WB: Speed development and plyometric training. In Baechle TR, editor: *The essentials of strength training and conditioning,* Champaign, IL, 1994, Human Kinetics.
2. Bahr R, Holme I: Risk factors for sports injuries: a methodological approach, *Br J Sports Med* 37(5):384, 2003.
3. Bandy WD, Rusche KR, Tekulve FY: Reliability and symmetry for five unilateral functional tests of the lower extremity, *Isokinet Exerc Sci* 4:108, 1994.
4. Barber SD et al: Quantitative assessment of functional limitations in normal and anterior cruciate ligament-deficient knees, *Clin Orthop* 255:204, 1990.
5. Beynnon BD et al: The strain of the anterior cruciate ligament squatting and active flexion-extension: a comparison of an open and closed kinetic chain exercise, *Am J Sports Med* 25:823, 1997.
6. Blackburn JR, Morrissey MC: The relationship between open and closed chain strength of the lower limb and jumping performance, *J Orthop Sports Phys Ther* 27:430, 1998.
7. Bolgla LA, Keskula DR: Reliability of lower extremity functional performance tests, *J Orthop Sports Phys Ther,* 26:138, 1997.
8. Boyle M: *Functional training for sports,* Champaign, IL, 2004, Human Kinetics.
9. Brosky JA et al: Intrarater reliability of selected clinical outcome measures following anterior cruciate ligament reconstruction, *J Orthop Sports Phys Ther* 29:39, 1999.
10. Brown LE, Ferrigno VA, Santana JC: *Training for speed, agility, and quickness,* Champaign, IL, 2000, Human Kinetics.
11. Caraffa A et al: Prevention of anterior cruciate ligament injuries in soccer: a prospective controlled study of proprioceptive training, *Knee Surg Sports Traumatol Arthrosc* 4:19, 1996.
12. Chu DA: *Jumping into plyometrics,* Champaign, IL, 1998, Human Kinetics.
13. Cissik JM: Plyometric fundamentals, *NSCA Performance Training Journal* 3(2):9, 2004.
14. Cornwell AG et al: Acute effects of passive muscle stretching on vertical jump performance, *J Hum Mov Stud* 40:307, 2000.
15. Croner C: Stretching out, *Biomechanics* 10:1, 2004.
16. Davies GJ, Zillmer DA: Functional Progression of exercise during rehabilitation. In Ellenbecker TS, editor: *Knee ligament rehabilitation,* New York, 2000, Churchill Livingstone.
17. DeCarlo M, Klootwyk TE, Shelbourne KD: ACL surgery and accelerated rehabilitation: revisited, *J Sport Rehabil* 6:144, 1997.
18. Delay BS et al: Current practices and opinions in ACL reconstruction and rehabilitation: results of a survey of the American Orthopedic Society for Sports Medicine, *Am J Knee Surg* 14(2):85, 2001.
19. *Dorland's illustrated medical dictionary,* ed 30, Philadelphia, 2003, Saunders.

20. Fitzgerald GK, Axe MJ, Snyder-Mackler L: The efficacy of perturbation training in nonoperative anterior cruciate ligament rehabilitation programs for physically active individuals, *Phys Ther* 80:128, 2000.
21. Fitzgerald GK et al: A decision-making scheme for returning patients to high-level activity with nonoperative treatment after anterior cruciate ligament rupture, *Knee Surg Sports Traumatol Arthrosc* 8:76, 2000.
22. Fitzgerald GK et al: Hop test as predictors of dynamic knee, stability, J *Orthop Sports Phys Ther* 31(10):588, 2001.
23. Fowles JR, Sale DG, MacDougall JD: Reduced strength after passive stretch of the human plantar flexors, *J Appl Physiol* 89:1179, 2000.
24. Hewett TE et al: The effect of neuromuscular training on the incidence of knee injury in female athletes. A prospective study, *Am J Sports Med* 27:699, 1999.
25. Hewett TE et al: Plyometric training in female athletes. Decreased impact forces and increased hamstring torques, *Am J Sports Med* 24:765, 1996.
26. Hewett TE et al: Biomechanical measures of neuromuscular control and valgus loading of the knee predict anterior cruciate ligament injury risk in female athletes, *Am J Sports Med* 33:492, 2005.
27. Juris PM et al: A dynamic test of lower extremity function following anterior cruciate ligament reconstruction and rehabilitation, *J Orthop Sports Phys Ther* 26:184, 1997.
28. Kraus JF, Conroy C: Mortality and morbidity from injuries in sport and recreation, *Ann Rev Public Health* 5:163, 1984.
29. Kutz MR: Theoretical and practical issues for plyometric training, *NSCA Performance Training Journal* 2(2):10, 2002.
30. Mangine RE, Kremchek TE: Evaluation-based protocol of the anterior cruciate ligament, *J Sport Rehabil* 6:157, 1997.
31. Murphy DF, Connolly DA, Beynnon BD: Risk factors for lower extremity injury: a review of the literature, *Br J Sports Med* 37:13, 2003.
32. Noyes FR et al: Abnormal lower limb symmetry determined by function hop tests after anterior cruciate ligament rupture, *Am J Sports Med* 19:513, 1991.
33. Nutting M: Practical progressions for upper body plyometric training, *NSCA Performance Training Journal* 3(2):14, 2004.
34. Petschnig R, Baron R, Albrecht M: The relationship between isokinetic quadriceps strength and hop tests for distance and one-legged vertical jump test following anterior cruciate ligament reconstruction, *J Orthop Sports Phys Ther* 28:23, 1998.
35. Radcliffe JC, Farentinos RC: *High-powered plyometrics,* Champaign, IL, 1999.
36. Risberg MA et al: Design and implementation of a neuromuscular training program following anterior cruciate ligament reconstruction, *J Orthop Sports Phys Ther* 31(11):620, 2001.
37. Ross MD, Denegar CR, Winzenried JA: Implementation of open and closed kinetic chain quadriceps strengthening exercises after anterior cruciate ligament reconstruction, *J Strength Cond Res* 15(4):466, 2001.
38. Semenick DM: Testing protocols and procedures. In Baechle TR, editor: *The essentials of strength training and conditioning,* Champaign, IL, 1994, Human Kinetics.
39. Shelbourne KD, Whitaker HJ, McCarroll JR: Anterior cruciate ligament injury: evaluation intraarticular reconstruction of acute tears without repair: two to seven year follow-up of one hundred and fifty five athletes, *Am J Sports Med* 18:484, 1990.
40. Shrier I: Stretching out before exercise does not reduce the risk of local muscle injury: a critical review of the clinical and basic science literature, *Clin J Sport Med* 9:221, 1999.
41. Steinkamp LA et al: Biomechanical considerations patellofemoral joint rehabilitation, *Am J Sports Med* 21:438, 1993.
42. Tegner Y, Lysholm J: Derotation brace and knee function in patients with anterior cruciate ligament tears, *Arthroscopy* 4:264, 1985.
43. Tegner Y et al: A performance test to monitor rehabilitation and for re-evaluation of anterior cruciate ligament injuries, *Am J Sports Med* 17:156, 1986.
44. Wilk, KE et al: The relationship between subjective knee scores, isokinetic testing, and functional testing in the ACL-reconstructed knee, *J Orthop Sports Phys Ther* 20:60, 1994.
45. Williams GN et al: Dynamic knee stability: current theory and implications for clinicians and scientists, *J Orthop Sports Phys Ther 31*(10):546, 2001.

APPENDIX

C

New Approaches in Total Hip Replacement: The Anterior Approach for Mini-Invasive Total Hip Arthroplasty

Joel M. Matta

SURGICAL TECHNIQUE

After administration of general or regional anesthesia, both feet are placed in the boots. The patient is placed in the supine position on the PROfx or HANA table, a perineal post is placed and the boots attached to the table (Fig. C-1). The hip that will not be operated on is placed in neutral or mild internal rotation (IR) (to maximize offset), neutral extension, and slight abduction and will serve as a radiographic reference for the operated side. Avoiding external rotation (ER) of the hip to be operated on will make the external landmarks of the hip more reliable and enhance the landmark of the natural bulge of the tensor fascia lata muscle.

The typical team consists of the surgeon, an assistant, an anesthesiologist, a scrub nurse, a circulating nurse-table operator, and a radiograph technician. Although the incision is normally small (8 to 10 cm), the author prefers to drape a relatively wide area. The normal incision starts 2 to 3 cm posterior and 1 to 2 cm distal to the anterio-superior iliac spine (ASIS). This straight incision extends in a distal and slightly posterior direction to a point 1 to 3 cm anterior to the greater trochanter. On thinner people the bulge of the tensor fascia lata muscle marks the center of the line of the incision. After incision of the skin and subcutaneous tissue, the tensor can be seen through the translucent fascia lata. The author places a vinyl circumferential skin retractor (Protractor) undermining slightly the fat layer off the underlying fascia. The fascial lata should be incised in line with the skin incision over the tensor where the fascia lata is translucent and anterior to the denser tissue of the iliotibial tract. The fascial incision should be continued slightly distal and proximal beyond the ends of the skin incision (Fig. C-2).

The surgeon should lift the fascia lata off the medial portion of the tensor and follow the interval medial to the tensor in a posterior and proximal direction. Dissection by feel is most efficient at this point, and the lateral hip capsule can be easily palpated just distal to the anterio-inferior iliac spine (AIIS). A cobra retractor should be placed along the lateral hip capsule to retract the tensor and gluteus minimus laterally, and the sartorius and rectus femorus muscles should be retracted medially with a Hibbs retractor. The reflected head of the rectus that follows the lateral acetabular rim will be visible. A small periosteal elevator placed just distal to the reflected head and directed medial and distal elevates the iliopsoas and rectus femorus muscles from the anterior capsule. The elevator opens the path for a second cobra retractor placed on the medial hip capsule. Using this technique, a view of 180 degrees of the circumference of the hip capsule is obtained within a few minutes (Fig. C-3).

The medial and lateral retraction of the cobras brings the lateral femoral circumflex vessels into view as they cross the distal portion of the wound. These vessels are clamped, cauterized, and transected. Further distal splitting of the aponeurosis that overlies the anterior capsule and vastus lateralis muscle (and at times excision of a fat pad) enhances exposure of the capsule and the origin of the vastus lateralis. The anterior capsule may be either excised or opened as flaps and repaired as part of the closure. (The author prefers to retain the capsule in most cases.) The surgeon should open the capsule with an incision that parallels the anterolateral femoral neck. The

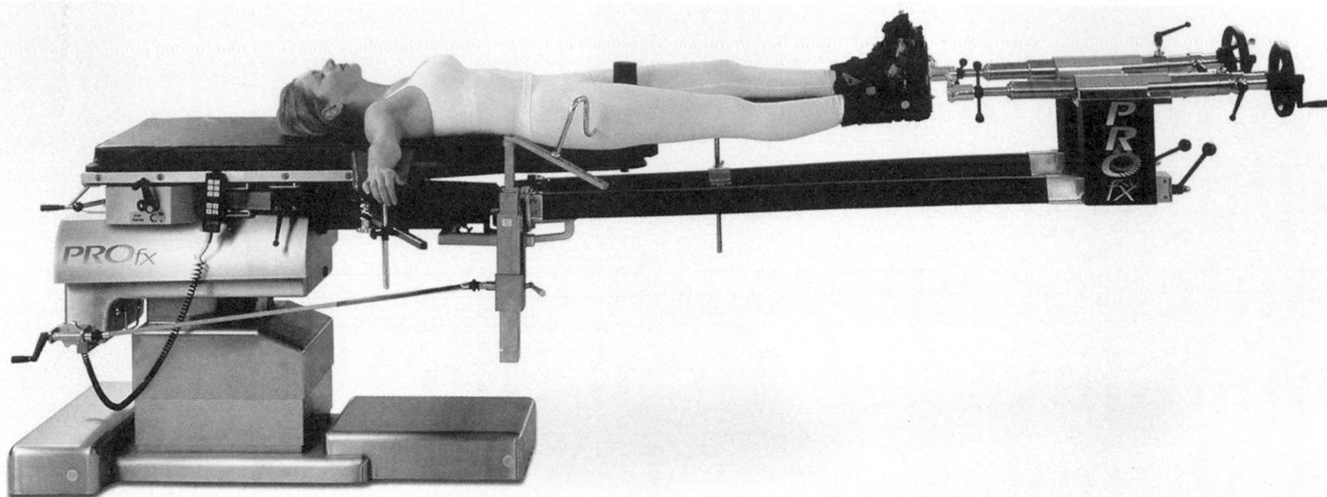

Fig. C-1 Patient positioned supine on PROfx table.

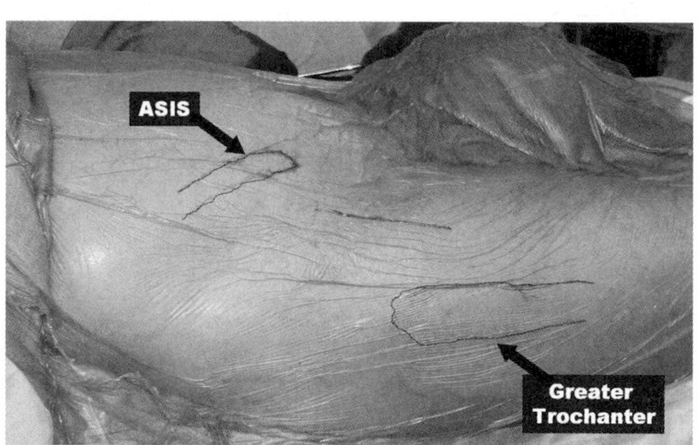

Fig. C-2 8-cm incision.

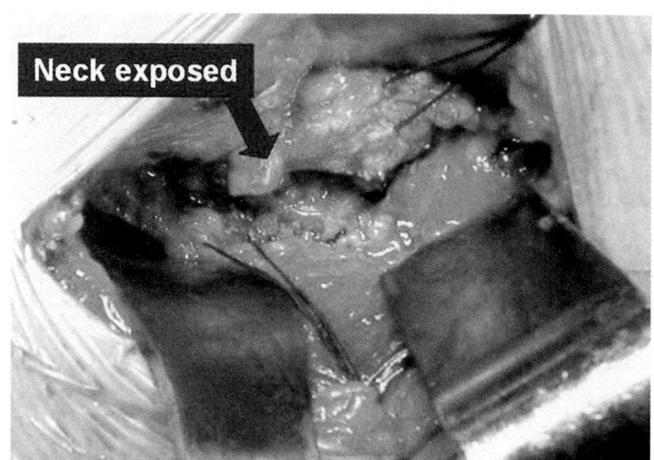

Fig. C-3 Incision of antero-lateral capsule.

proximal portion of this incision crosses the anterior rim of the acetabulum and the reflected capsular origin of the rectus femoris. The distal portion exposes the lateral shoulder of the femoral neck at its junction with the anterior greater trochanter. The junction of the capsule and the origin of the vastus lateralis muscle identify the intertrochanteric line. The distal anterior capsule should be detached from the femur at the anterior intertrochanteric line and suture tags placed on the anterior and lateral capsule at the distal portion of the incision that separates them. The cobra retractors should be placed intracapsular medial and lateral to the neck. Exposure of the base of the neck is facilitated by a Hibbs retractor that retracts the vastus and distal tensor.

A narrow Hohman retractor is now placed on the anterolateral acetabular rim. With this exposure, the anterolateral labrum (and often associated osteophytes) is excised. Distal traction on the extremity will create a small gap between the femoral head and the roof of the acetabulum. A femoral head skid is placed into this gap and then placed in a more medial position. The traction is partially released. The patient's hip should be externally rotated about 20 degrees, and a femoral head corkscrew should be inserted into the head in a vertical direction. As the extremity and hip are externally rotated and leverage is applied to the skid and corkscrew, the hip should be dislocated anteriorly and the femur externally rotated 90 degrees (Fig. C-4).

After dislocation, the surgeon should place the tip of a narrow Hohman retractor distal to the lesser trochanter and beneath the vastus lateralis origin. The capsule should be detached from the medial neck and the lesser trochanter, and the medial posterior neck exposed. The patient's hip is then internally rotated and reduced, the cobra retractors are replaced around the medial and lateral neck, and the vastus origin and distal tensor are retracted with a Hibbs. The surgeon cuts the femoral neck with a reciprocating saw at the desired level and angle as indicated by the preoperative plan (Fig. C-5). The neck cut is completed with an osteotome that divides the

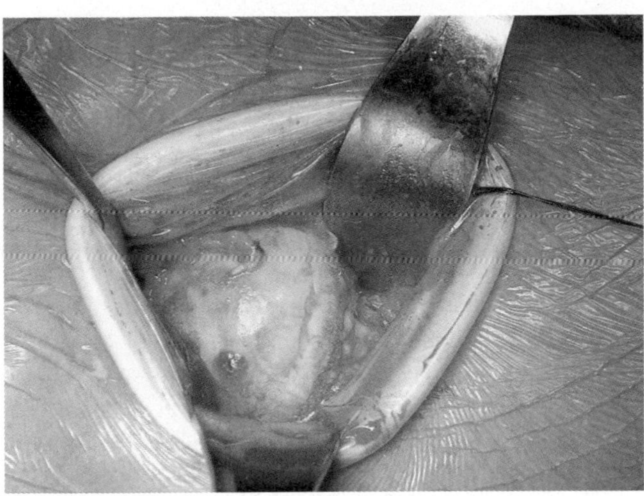

Fig. C-4 90° external rotation allows femoral head dislocation for further exposure.

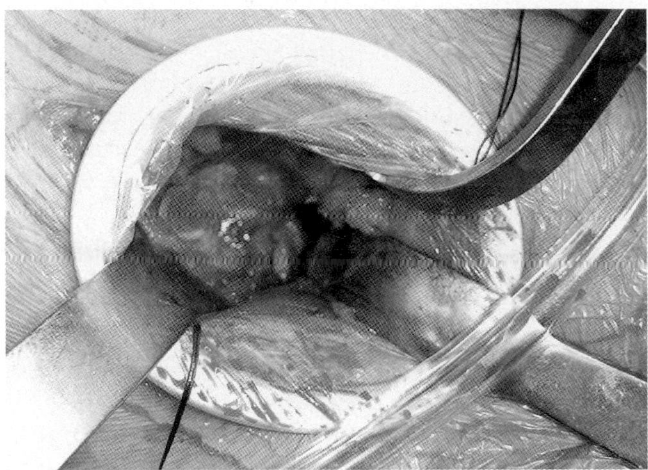

Fig. C-6 Excellent acetabular exposure is achieved.

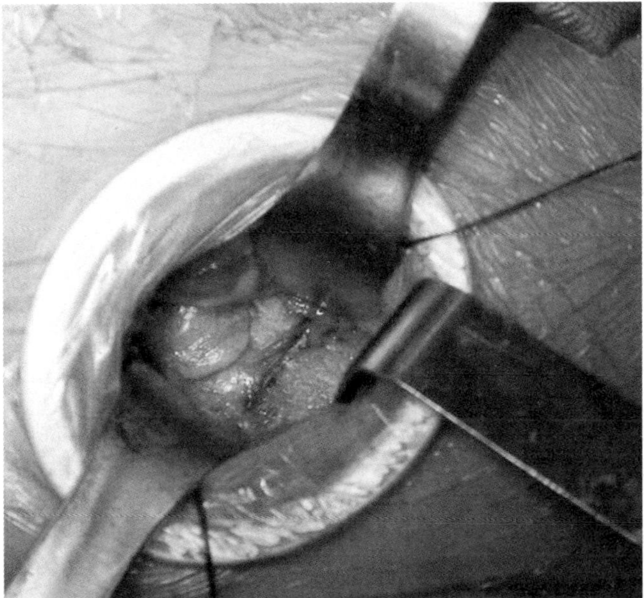

Fig. C-5 Lateral neck cut finalized with osteotome. Head removed.

lateral neck from the medial greater trochanter and is directed posterior and slightly medial to avoid the posterior greater trochanter. The head is extracted with the corkscrew. Light traction will distract the neck osteotomy and facilitate this extraction.

Throughout the procedure the surgeon will find that the tensor fascia lata muscle is potentially vulnerable to injury. If an initial injury to the muscle fibers is avoided, then the muscle seems to hold up well through the procedure. On the other hand, an early laceration to the surface of the tensor seems to hurt its capability of resisting further damage.

The acetabulum is now visualized and prepared. ER of the femur of about 45 degrees usually facilitates acetabular exposure (Fig. C-6). Light traction also limits femoral interference. The author prefers to use a bent Homan retractor above the distal anterior rim of the acetabulum to retract the anterior muscles. The surgeon should take care to place the tip of this retractor on bone and not into the anterior soft tissues. The author places a cobra retractor with the tip on the midposterior rim. The labrum is then excised circumferentially. A transverse release of a prominent band of inferior capsule will facilitate later placement of the acetabular liner. The author usually begins reaming under direct vision and later checks with the image intensifier to confirm depth of reaming and adequate circumference. The indicators of torque and acetabular appearance are also used. The author then inserts the acetabular prosthesis. Most experienced surgeons can easily recognize a properly positioned cup on a radiograph (40 to 45° abduction and 15 to 25° anteversion), and good position can be achieved consistently with the image technique. The liner is inserted in the normal fashion (prior excision of labrum and the inferior capsule release will facilitate this). An osteotome or rongeur should be used to excise projecting osteophytes. The radiograph is the final judge as to whether computer guidance led to the correct result.

After acetabular insertion the gross traction control on the leg spar is released and the femur internally rotated to neutral. The vastus ridge is palpated, and the femoral hook placed just distal to this and around the posterior femur. The femur is then externally rotated 90 degrees and the hip hyperextended and adducted.

For proximal femoral exposure, the author uses a long-handled cobra with the tip on the posterior femoral neck and places the tip of a trochanteric retractor over the tip of the trochanter. The femoral hook now raises the proximal femur until the tissues come under moderate tension.

After this initial maneuver the posterior ridge of the greater trochanter may lie posterior to the posterior rim of the acetabulum. The femur needs to be mobile enough so that lateral and anterior displacement brings the posterior edge of the trochanter lateral and anterior to the posterior rim of the acetabulum. The lateral capsular flap and its tag suture will be clearly visible distal to the trochanteric retractor and attaching to the remnant of the lateral neck. Detachment of this flap from the base of the neck in an anterior to posterior direction facilitates visualization of the medial greater trochanter and enhances femoral mobility (Fig. C-7). The surgeon should use a rongeur to excise the remnant of the lateral neck.

It should be remembered that the obturator internus and piriformis tendons insert on the anterior superior greater trochanter. After release of the lateral capsule, the surgeon should place the tip of the trochanteric retractor closer to the upper border of the trochanter to retract the gluteus minimus muscle and piriformis and obturator internus tendons. Depending on the requirements for femoral mobility, the surgeon may choose to release one or more of the short external rotator tendons and release of the obturator internus tendon particularly when it cannot be flipped over the posterior tip of the trochanter. However, the author prefers to preserve all tendon attachments and strives in particular to preserve the attachment of the obturator externus tendon, because its medial pull on the proximal femur is an important active restraint against dislocation.

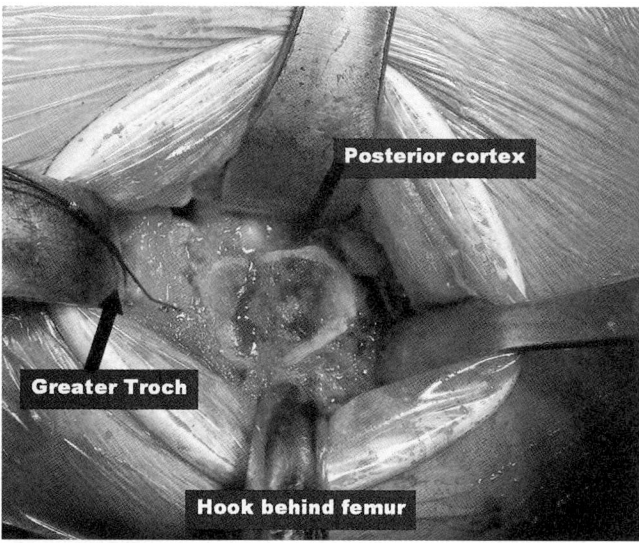

Fig. C-7 Hip hyperextended and adduction with external rotation allows delivery of proximal femur for femoral broaching.

In general, prostheses with less prominence in the proximal lateral area will be easier to insert, will allow preservation of the rotator attachments, and will present a lower risk of trochanteric fracture. However, the instrumentation required most determines the applicability of a stem to the anterior approach. The tip of the first broach enters the neck near the posterior medial cortex (Fig. C-8). When the broaching is complete, a trial reduction is made, with the neck length estimated from the preoperative template.

During trial phase I, the surgeon should check for hip stability in extension and ER with the traction released. He or she should also check for impingement with osteophytes and excise appropriately. The author feels that it is best to rely on the radiograph for length and offset decisions rather than soft tissue tension and intraoperative stability.

After the decision is made for the femoral prosthesis, the femoral hook is replaced behind the proximal femur, traction applied to distract the head, and the hip is dislocated with ER. The femur is then placed into the preparation position (i.e., 90-degree ER, hyperextension, adduction, proximal elevation). The femoral prosthesis is then inserted in the normal fashion. The appropriate-length permanent head can be placed at this time (Figs. C-9 and C-10). With the hip flexed to neutral, the acetabulum is visualized before reduction to ensure that it is clear of bone or cement fragments. Another transparency printed with the image intensifier confirms leg length and offset and serves as the immediate postoperative radiograph.

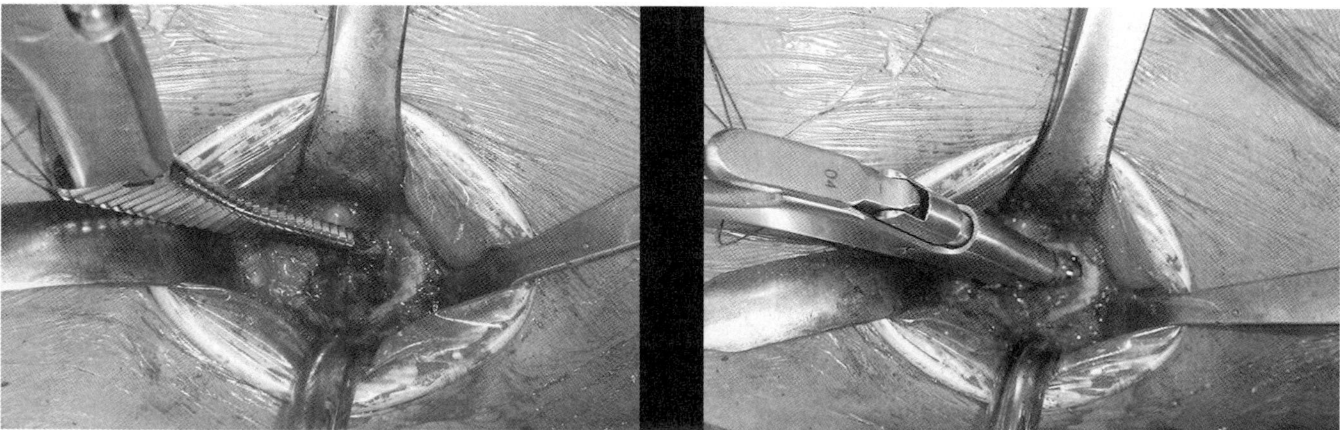

Fig. C-8 Broach insertion easily accomplished through anterior incision.

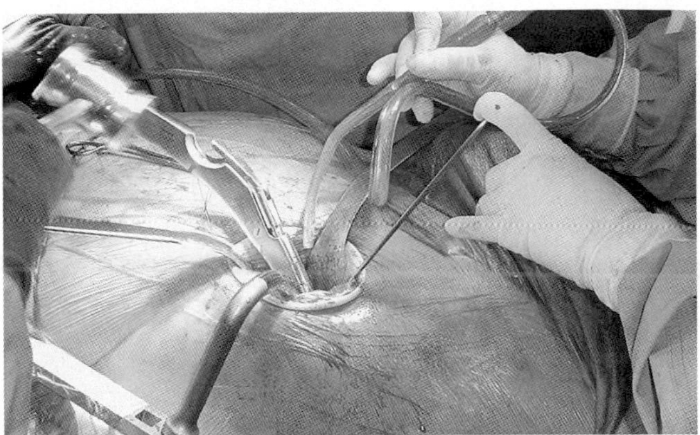

Fig. C-9 Broaching easily accomplished through anterior incision.

Before discharge, radiographs are obtained in the radiology department (Fig. C-11).

A check is made for bleeding and the wound is irrigated. The closure is simple. The anterior and lateral capsular tag sutures are tied together, and further capsular closure is performed if desired. The fascia lata is closed with a running suture, followed by subcutaneous tissue and skin.

After surgery the patient does not follow antidislocation precautions. The patient is encouraged to weight bear immediately, use the hip, and discard external support as symptoms permit.

From November 1996 to April 2005, the author performed 657 primary anterior total hip arthroplasties (THAs), including 67 bilateral THAs. This series of 657 anterior approaches is unselected and consecutive. The surgeries were performed on a Judet or Tasserit table until 2003. Beginning in 2003 the PROfx table became available and is now preferred. The average patient age is 66 and ranges from 29 to 91. The average operative time is 1.2 hours. Average blood loss is 345 mL. The median hospital time is 4 days, and the mode is 3 days. Two early anterior dislocations and one posterior dislocation occurred that were reduced closed and did not recur or require revision. The median time to doing some ambulation without external support is 8 days. The median time for doing all ambulation without external support is 15 days. It is the author's impression that pain is reduced and the recovery rate greatly enhanced. (See the THA slide show at www.hipandpelvis.com for more detailed statistics.)

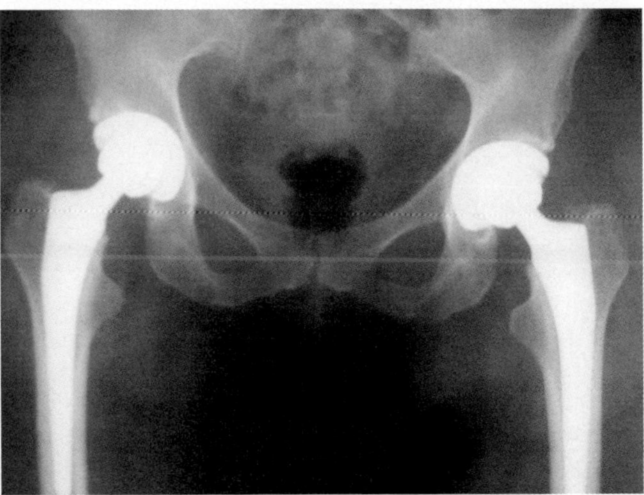

Fig. C-11 Intra-operative imaging ensures length and cup position.

REHABILITATION AFTER ANTERIOR TOTAL HIP ARTHROPLASTY

With this procedure, tendon attachments such as the obturator externus, rotator attachments, and gluteus medius have been preserved. In fact, all the muscle attachments are preserved. The obturator externus has a medial pull on the proximal femur and is an important active

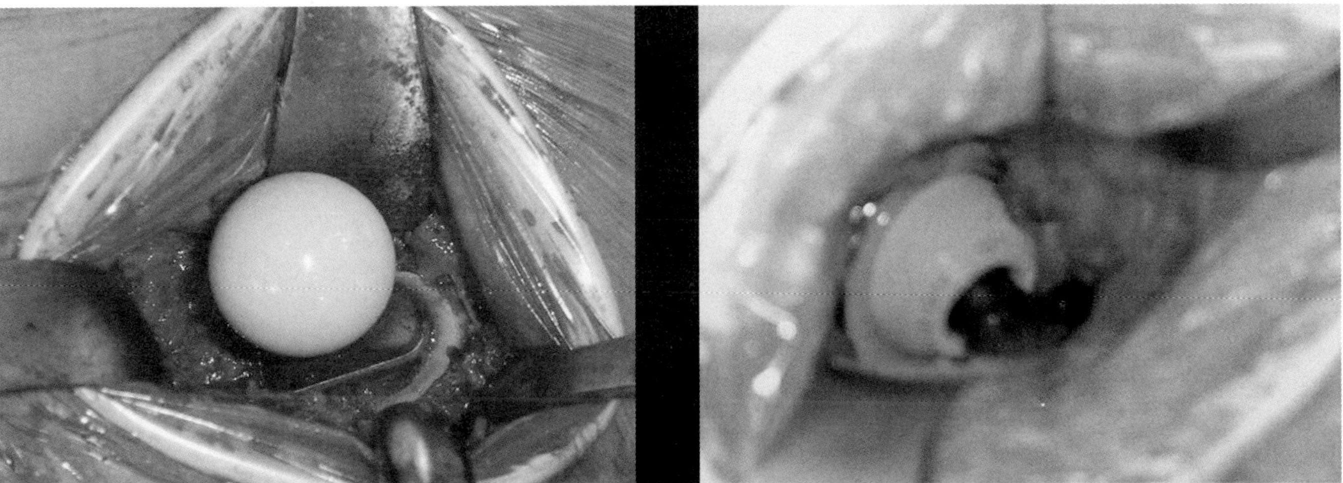

Fig. C-10 *Delta* ceramic head placed and reduced.

contractor against hip dislocation. With the preservation of these muscle attachments and other soft tissues, total hip precautions are not required. Pain is reduced and the recovery rate is enhanced. Weight bearing is immediately encouraged, and assistive devices are discarded when possible.

The rehabilitation process is similar to most total hip replacement (THR) regimens. However, the patient will progress through the process more quickly and with a lower risk of hip dislocation.

In the hospital bed, mobility, transfer training, and gait training are done during the initial treatments. The patient is instructed in ankle pumps. Isometrics such as hip abduction, hip adduction, quadriceps sets, and gluteus sets can also be started immediately. In addition, heel slides are encouraged with assistance, then without any assistance. The patient then progresses to active range of motion (AROM) for hip abduction, adduction, and straight leg raises (SLRs). Patients can be taught pelvic tilts and knee to chest (using the unaffected lower extremity [LE]) for low back discomfort. Heel cord stretches can be done carefully with the leg slightly back and a wedge under the forefoot. Closed-chain exercises like mini-squats, step-ups, and heel raises are begun when the patient can safely perform them.

GENERAL COMMENTS REGARDING HIP REPLACEMENT

The first very successful hip prosthesis was designed and implanted in the 1960s by John Charnley of England. Charnley's design used a one-piece metal stem with a 22 mm diameter head that was cemented into the proximal femur. The acetabular component was made entirely of polyethylene and cemented into the acetabulum. Follow-up studies of the Charnley prosthesis and other similar cemented designs have shown sufficient longevity that the majority of prostheses in surviving patients are still functioning 20 years after implantation. Despite the great success of these hip prostheses, it is recognized that the failure rate increases over time. The mode of failure is typically loosening of the secure bond between the prosthesis and the bone and bone loss associated with this process.

Because of the recognized limits to longevity of these early designs, continued work to improve the design has been conducted, and thereby longevity of hip prostheses has been achieved. Currently the Food and Drug Administration (FDA) (the federal agency regulating hip prostheses) has over 750 approved designs for hip prostheses on file. The majority of new designs, however, have proven to be not as good as Charnley's hip. In addition, some new designs have been shown to equal the longevity of the Charnley hip but have not proven superior to it.

What is the significance of this history for today's hip replacement patient? Just because a hip prosthesis is the latest design does not mean it is better; in fact, it could be worse. Time gives us the answers. We need to continue to look for prostheses with improved longevity; however, a quantum improvement may not be just around the corner, and the current expected longevity may be with us for some time to come.

What has changed? The acetabulum is now almost always implanted without cement. The results of the uncemented acetabulum appear equal to cement, and clinicians hope that the longevity will prove better over time. Some designs of uncemented femoral stems have also shown good longevity comparable to the best-proven cemented stems. It is widely felt that the bearing surfaces have been improved, which means that this surface wears at a slower rate. Although metal against extremely high-density polyethylene is the best-proven bearing, evidence also supports the use of metal-on-metal and ceramic bearings.

Today, development of hip replacement surgery is not limited to efforts to improve the prostheses. Improvements also include surgical approaches that limit the surgical trauma to the soft tissue, thereby accelerating recovery and limiting the possibility of dislocation. The author applauds this trend because it is the basis of the anterior approach for hip replacement described herein.

Possible complications of hip replacement surgery include infection, injury to nerves and blood vessels, fracture of the femur or acetabulum, hip dislocation, and need for revision surgery. Patients should remember that recovery means not only recovery from the surgical procedure but also time to recover from the condition they were in before surgery.

References

1. Matta JM, Ferguson TA: The anterior approach for hip replacement, *Orthopedics* 28(9):927, 2005.
2. Matta JM, Shahrdar C, Ferguson T: Single-incision anterior approach for total hip arthroplasty on an orthopaedic table, *Clin Orthop Rel Res* 441:115, 2005.
3. Yerasimides JG, Matta JM: Primary total hip arthroplasty with a minimally invasive anterior approach, *Semin Arthroplasty* 16(3):186, 2005.
4. Matta JM, Klenck RE. Hipandpelvis.com. Available at: http://www.hipandpelvis.com/

Index

S

T